*F*undamentals of Nursing

Caring and Clinical Judgment

Guidelines for Nursing Procedures

As you provide nursing care you want to communicate through your actions that you are a competent and caring nurse. Through developing systematic work habits you can communicate organization and efficiency that will not only save you time but will give you the appearance of competency and help you focus on the client rather than the procedure. Plan your activities to include CDC Standard Precautions.

As you practice the procedures in this book, include the following activities in each procedure.

Before You Perform a Procedure, Always:

Confirm physician's order. When a nursing procedure is part of medical therapy or the implementation of medical therapy you need to confirm that a physician's order is written and that you are familiar with any guidelines the physician has provided.

Gather equipment. Planning the procedure and gathering the equipment will allow you to work efficiently. You want to gather all the supplies you will need to avoid repeated trips for supplies. However, chose the items wisely. In the hospital setting you cannot replace supplies to a clean storage area after you have taken them to a client's room.

Confirm client's identity. Clients in an inpatient setting are identified with an armband. Check the client's armband against the chart. This check is especially important when the client's level of consciousness is altered or when you are working from a work station where items (especially medications) for multiple clients are stored. Asking the client to state his/her name is considered more reliable identification than asking, "Are you John Smith?"

Explain procedure to client. Form the habit of introducing yourself to the client and explaining what you are going to do. Explain in terms the client can understand. Avoid using medical or nursing jargon.

Arrange the work area. This activity may include raising the bed to a comfortable working height, clearing the over-the-bed table to provide a work surface, and placing the trash can in a convenient place.

Perform hand hygiene. You should perform hand hygiene before every procedure. Washing your hands in the client's presence adds to the client's confidence that you are providing for safety.

Provide for privacy. In a health care setting the client has the right to privacy. Close the door, pull a curtain around the bed, and drape the client if needed to avoid exposing usually private body parts.

After You Finish a Procedure, Always:

Make the client comfortable. Straighten the bed linens, adjust the pillow, and assist the client to a position of comfort. Lower the bed, raise the side rails, position call light. Place water and personal items within easy reach.

Perform hand hygiene. You should perform hand hygiene after every procedure.

Document the care. Document the time of the procedure, the indication for the procedure, what was done, how it was done, supplies used, and pertinent observations made during the procedure.

Other Considerations. If you are unfamiliar with the agency policies and procedures, you should access the policy and procedure manual for guidelines specific to the agency. If you are assisting with an invasive procedure confirm the agency's requirement for written informed consent.

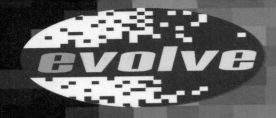

The Latest *Evolution* in Learning.

Evolve provides online access to free learning resources and activities designed specifically for the textbook you are using in your class. The resources will provide you with information that enhances the material covered in the book and much more.

Visit the Web address listed below to start your learning evolution today!

▶▶ *LOGIN: http://evolve.elsevier.com/Harkreader/*

Evolve Learning Resources for Harkreader and Hogan's *Fundamentals of Nursing,* second edition offers the following features:

- **Study Questions**
  Over 600 multiple-choice questions to help test your comprehension

- **Case Studies**
  Real-life examples go beyond the textbook and cover five key content areas: Wound care, Fluid and electrolytes, IV therapy, Enteral tube feedings, and Medication administration

- **WebLinks**
  Links to places of interest on the web specific to each text chapter. Website information is annotated and updated quarterly.

- **Links to Related Products**
  See what Elsevier has to offer in a specific field of interest.

Think outside the book... *evolve.*

Second Edition

*F*undamentals of Nursing

Caring and Clinical Judgment

HELEN HARKREADER, PhD, RN
Professor
Austin Community College
Austin, Texas

MARY ANN HOGAN, RN, CS, MSN
Clinical Assistant Professor
University of Massachusetts–Amherst
Amherst, Massachusetts

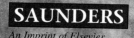
SAUNDERS
An Imprint of Elsevier

SAUNDERS
An Imprint of Elsevier

11830 Westline Industrial Drive
St. Louis, Missouri 63146

Fundamentals of Nursing: Caring and Clinical Judgment

NOTICE

Previous edition copyrighted 2000.

ISBN-13: 978-0-7216-9141-1
ISBN-10: 0-7216-9141-2

Executive Editor: Susan R. Epstein
Developmental Editor: Linda Stagg
Developmental Editor: Robyn L. Brinks
Publishing Services Manager: John Rogers
Senior Project Manager: Beth Hayes
Senior Designer: Kathi Gosche
Cover Art: Kathi Gosche

Printed in China

Last digit is the print number: 9   8   7   6   5   4   3

To the nurses who have served our country in military service,
especially those who served in Operation Enduring Freedom.
To the faculty and students at Austin Community College
who have strongly influenced my teaching style and nursing practice.
Helen Harkreader

To my children,
Michael Jr., Kathryn, Kristen, William, and Donna,
who are sources of unending joy in life.
To my husband,
Michael,
whose kind words of encouragement mean so much.
To the memory of my parents
Joseph and Marian,
who taught me to pursue my dreams.
To all of my past and present students,
who will help shape the future of nursing.
Mary Ann Hogan

About the Authors

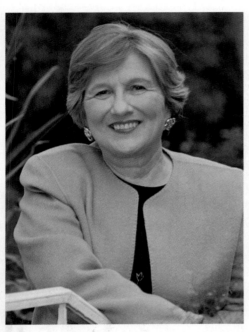

Helen Harkreader, PhD, RN, has practiced as an acute care adult health nurse in general medicine, intensive care, oncology, gastrointestinal, and surgical nursing units. Having begun her teaching career in 1971, she has taught nursing in both baccalaureate and associate-degree nursing programs. While she has taught at all levels of undergraduate programs in Texas, Arkansas, and Iowa, her primary interest is teaching beginning nursing students. Dr. Harkreader believes that her role as a teacher is to foster the individual growth of nursing students and uses the Myers-Briggs Type Indicator as a tool to help students bring their individual strengths to nursing practice. The greatest compliment students can give her is that she has made them think. Dr. Harkreader has conducted research on the effects of positioning on ventilation-perfusion ratios, caregiver burden as a factor in nursing home placement, and the utilization of vocational nurses. Dr. Harkreader received her undergraduate degree from Texas Christian University, her master's degree as a Clinical Specialist in Medical-Surgical Nursing from the University of Iowa, and her PhD in adult health nursing from the University of Texas at Austin. She is a member of the American Nurses Association. She serves as Professor of Nursing at Austin Community College in Austin, Texas.

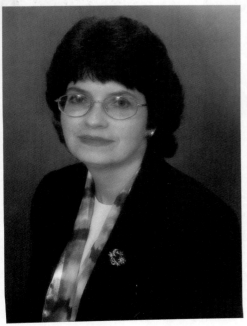

Mary Ann Hogan, RN, CS, MSN has practiced nursing in critical care and adult acute care units in Massachusetts and Connecticut. She began teaching in 1981 and has taught in diploma, associate-degree, and baccalaureate nursing programs. Ms. Hogan has taught fundamentals of nursing, medical-surgical nursing, and leadership and management in various nursing programs. Her ongoing interest in beginning nursing students stems from the belief that early learning has a tremendous impact on subsequent development as a nurse. Ms. Hogan's area of research interest is health-related behavior changes in older adults. She has an ongoing interest in assisting nursing students to prepare for the NCLEX-RN licensing examination and is a former NCLEX item writer. Ms. Hogan received her Bachelor of Science degree from the University of Massachusetts–Amherst and her Master of Science Degree in Nursing from Anna Maria College in Paxton, Massachusetts. Ms. Hogan is certified by the American Nurses Credentialing Center as a Clinical Specialist in Medical-Surgical Nursing and is a member of the American Nurses Association. She is a Clinical Assistant Professor at the University of Massachusetts–Amherst.

Contributors to the Second Edition

Elizabeth B. Abrahams, RN, MSN, ONC
Clinical Nurse Specialist
Materials Management
Inova Health System
Falls Church, Virginia

Dee Baldwin, PhD, RN
Women's Health
Georgia State University
Atlanta, Georgia

Kathleen Barta, EdD, RN
Associate Professor
University of Arkansas
Eleanor Mann School of Nursing
Fayetteville, Arkansas

Lenore L. Boris, JD, MS, BSN, RN
Labor Representative
New York State Nurses Association
Latham, New York

Joan Engebretson, DrPH, RN HNC
Associate Professor
University of Texas Health Science Center at Houston
Houston, Texas

Janet S. Hickman, EdD, RN
Professor and Graduate Program Coordinator
West Chester University
West Chester, Pennsylvania

Karen Y. Hill, PhD, RN
Associate Professor of Nursing
Southeastern Louisiana University
School of Nursing
Hammond, Louisiana

Doris S. Holeman, PhD, RN
Associate Dean and Director
School of Nursing and Allied Health
Tuskegee University
Tuskegee, Alabama

Janene Council Jeffery, RN, MSN, CDE
Professor, Associate Degree Nursing Program
Austin Community College
Austin, Texas

Lorraine E. Kenny, MS, RN
Special Project Manager–Nursing
Governors State University
University Park, Illinois

Eileen Klein, EdD, RN
Austin Community College
Austin, Texas

Kathryn Lauchner, PhD, RN
Professor of Nursing
Austin Community College
Austin, Texas

Janna Lesser, PhD, RN
Assistant Professor
Florida State University School of Nursing
Tallahassee, Florida

Susan J. Lewis, PhD, ARNP, CS
Advance Practice Nurse
Adult Psychiatric Mental Health Nursing
Department of Veterans Affairs Medical Center
Louisville, Kentucky

Nancy J. MacMullen, PhD, APN/CCNS
University Professor
Governors State University
University Park, Illinois

Kristen L. Mauk, PhD, RN, CRRN-A, APRN, BC
Associate Professor of Nursing
Valparaiso University
College of Nursing
Valparaiso, Indiana

Martha Meraviglia, RN, CNS, PhD
Assistant Professor in Clinical Nursing
University of Texas at Austin
School of Nursing
Austin, Texas

Barbara S. Moffett, PhD, RN
Professor of Nursing
Southeastern Louisiana University
Hammond, Louisiana

Janet B. Moore, MS, RN, CS
Director
Robin Read Adult Day Health
West Springfield, Massachusetts
Part-time Faculty
Elms College
Chicopee, Massachusetts

Hilario A. Pascua, MSN, CS, ARNP
Veterans Administration Medical Center
Mental Health and Behavioral Science Services
Louisville, Kentucky

Cecilia Prado, MSN, RN
Professor, Associate Degree Nursing
Austin Community College
Austin, Texas

Joyce Z. Thielen, MS, RN, CS
Assistant Professor of Nursing
Elms College
Chicopee, Massachusetts

Marshelle Thobaben, RNC, MS, PMHNP, PHN, FNP
Chair, Department of Nursing
Professor
Humboldt State University
Arcata, California

V. Doreen Wagner, RN, MSN, CNOR
Assistant Professor of Clinical Nursing
North Georgia College and State University
Dahlonega, Georgia

Reviewers to the Second Edition

Marianne Adam, MSN, RN, CRNP
Assistant Professor
St. Luke's School of Nursing at Moravian College
Bethlehem, Pennsylvania

Tracy C. Babcock, MSN, BSN
Adjunct Assistant Professor
Montana State University College of Nursing
Bozeman, Montana

Sylvia Baird, RN, BSN, MM
Manager Patient Safety
Spectrum Health
Grand Rapids, Michigan

Martha Baker, PhD, RN, CS, CCRN
Associate Professor of Nursing
Missouri Southern State College
Joplin, Missouri

Doris Bartlett, RN, BSN, MS
Lecturer
Bethel College
Mishawaka, Indiana

Julie K. Baylor, MSN, RN
Assistant Professor
Bradley University
Peoria, Illinois

Jan Boundy, RN, PhD
Professor, Director of Graduate Program
Saint Francis College of Nursing
Peoria, Illinois

Therese M. Bower, EdD, RN, CNS
Nursing Instructor
Firelands Regional Medical Center School of Nursing
Sandusky, Ohio

Anna M. Brock, PhD
Professor
University of Southern Mississippi
Hattiesburg, Mississippi

Gayle K. Campbell, RN, BSN, BAHS, BBA, MBA
Health Science Coordinator
Georgian College Midland Ontario
Ontario, Canada
Community Clinical Director
Laurentian University
Sudbury, Ontario, Canada

Darlene Nebel Cantu, RNC, MSN
Director
Baptist Health System
School of Professional Nursing
San Antonio, Texas
Faculty at San Antonio College in Nursing
San Antonio, Texas

Barbara Caton, RN, MSN
Assistant Professor
Southwest Missouri State University–West Plains
West Plains, Missouri

Ellen K. Cervellon, RNC, MSN, CRNI
Interim Director of Emergency Services
San Leandro Hospital
San Leandro, California

Laura H. Clayton, RN, MSN
Assistant Professor
Shepherd College
Shepherdstown, West Virginia

Carol deBlois, BSN, MA, CNOR
Director
Bridgeport Hospital School of Nursing
Bridgeport, Connecticut

Karen Delrue, RN, MSN, CEN
Clinical Nurse Specialist
Emergency Services
Spectrum Health
Grand Rapids, Michigan

Janice H. DeMots, BSN, MSN
Instructor
Milwaukee Area Technical College
Milwaukee, Wisconsin

H. Michael Dreher, DNSc, RN
Assistant Professor and Associate Director
Undergraduate Nursing Programs
College of Nursing and Health Professions
Drexel University
Philadelphia, Pennsylvania

Ellen K. Duvall, BSN, MAEd, MS(N), RN
Assistant Professor
Cox College of Nursing and Health Sciences
Springfield, Missouri

Katherine Federer, RN, AA
Director of Training
Westchester House
Chesterfield, Missouri

Elizabeth Follis, RN, MS
Nursing Faculty
Northeastern Oklahoma A&M College
Miami, Oklahoma

Henry B. Geiter, Jr., RN, CCRN
Adjunct Instructor
St. Petersburg College
St. Petersburg, Florida
Critical Care Nurse
Bayfront Hospital
St. Petersburg, Florida
Critical Care Transport Nurse
Sunstar–AMR
Largo, Florida

Carrol Gold, PhD, RN
Dean and Professor
West Suburban College of Nursing
Oak Park, Illinois

John P. Harper, MSN, BC, RN
Nurse Educator, Critical Care
Delaware County Memorial Hospital
Drexel Hill, Pennsylvania

Linda C. Haynes, PhD
Assistant Professor
Louise Herrington School of Nursing
Baylor University
Dallas, Texas

Dorothy G. Herron, PhD, RN, CS
Assistant Professor
School of Nursing
University of Maryland
Baltimore, Maryland

Janice J. Hoffman, RN, MSN, CCRN
SPRING Program Director
The Johns Hopkins Hospital
Baltimore, Maryland

Glenda C. Johnson, RN, BSN, MSA
Nurse Educator
Louise Obici School of Professional Nursing
Suffolk, Virginia

Stephen P. Kilkus, RN, MSN
Health Educator and Coach
Heartspace Coaching, LLP
Madison, Wisconsin

Maryanne F. Lachat, RNC, PhD
Associate Professor
School of Nursing and Health Studies
Georgetown University
Washington, DC

**Erica Lambert, DipTeach, BNSg, Grad Cert
    Health Administation**
NIL
MRCNA, AARN
Brisbane, Queensland,
Australia

Virginia D. Lester, RN, BSN, MSN
Clinical Nurse Specialist (inactive status)
Assistant Professor in Nursing
Angelo State University
San Angelo, Texas

Suzy Lockwood-Rayermann, RN, PhD
Assistant Professor
Texas Christian University
Harris School of Nursing
Fort Worth, Texas

Rosemary Macy, RN, MSN
Assistant Professor
Boise State University
Boise, Idaho

Peggy Matteson, RNC, PhD
Faculty and Director of Program
Congregational Health and Parish Nursing
Andover Newton Theological School
Newton Centre, Massachussetts

Mary Jo Mattocks, RN, MN, PhD
Nurse Clinician
Benefits Healthcare
Great Falls, Montana

Sharon A. McGahan, EdS, RN, MSN
Assistant Professor, Nursing
Truman State University
Kirksville, Missouri

Ruth Novitt-Schumacher, RN, MSN
Instructor
University of Illinois at Chicago
College of Nursing
Chicago, Illinois

Patricia K. O'Brien, RN, BSN, MSN
Instructor
Penn Valley Community College
Kansas City, Missouri

Brenda Condusta Pavill, PhD, RN
Professor
College Misericordia
Dallas, Pennsylvania

Melissa Powell, RN, MSN
Assistant Professor
Eastern Kentucky University
Richmond, Kentucky

Marisue Rayno, MSN
Clinical Educator
Good Shepherd
Allentown, Pennsylvania

Christine M. Rosner, RN, PhD
Lecturer
School of Nursing
Holy Family College
Philadelphia, Pennsylvania

Alwilda Scholler-Jaquish, PhD, APRN, BC
Assistant Professor
School of Nursing
Texas Tech University Health Sciences Center
Lubbock, Texas

April Sieh, RN, MSN
Associate Professor of Nursing
Delta College
University Center, Michigan

Mary E. Stassi, RN, C
Coordinator Health Occupations
St. Charles Community College
St. Peters, Missouri

Denise M. Tate, MSN, RN, C, CTN
Nursing Instructor/BSN Program Coordinator
St. Peter's College
Englewood Cliffs, New Jersey

Marilyn M. Teeter, MSN, RN
Associate Professor/Coordinator
Nursing Program
Gettysburg Campus of the Harrisburg Area
    Community College
Gettysburg, Pennsylvania

Paige Thompson, RN, DNSc(c)
Associate Professor
St. Luke's School of Nursing
Moravian College
Bethlehem, Pennsylvania

Kathleen L. Upham, MSN, ONC
Assistant Professor of Nursing
Coastal Georgia Community College
Brunswick, Georgia

Lois L. VonCannon, MSN, APRN, BC
Clinical Assistant Professor
University of North Carolina–Greensboro
Greensboro, North Carolina

Melinda A. Warfield, MSM, BSN, RN, BCNA
Health Unit Manager
Michigan Department of Corrections
Ionia, Michigan

Jennifer H. Whitley, RN, MSN, CNOR
Instructor
Associate Degree Nursing Program
Calhoun Community College
Decatur, Alabama

Melissa T. Williams, MSN, BSN, CNS, PALS
Assistant Professor
Augusta State University
Augusta, Georgia

Rosemary H. Wittstadt, EdD, RN
Assistant Professor
Towson University
Department of Nursing
Towson, Maryland

Contributors to Previous Edition

Kay C. Avant, PhD, RN, FAAN
Associate Professor and Chairperson
Family Health Nursing Division
School of Nursing
The University of Texas at Austin
Austin, Texas

Margaret L. Bell, PhD, RN
Assistant Professor
Department of Chronic Nursing Care
The University of Texas Health Science Center
San Antonio School of Nursing
San Antonio, Texas

Laura Bradford, PhD, RNC
Unit Director
Special Care Nursery
Rush–Presbyterian–St. Luke's Medical Center
Chicago, Illinois

Chyi-Kong Karen Chang, MSN, RN
Teaching Assistant
University of Illinois at Chicago
Chicago, Illinois
Formerly Visiting Assistant Professor and Assistant Professor
Purdue University
West Lafayette, Indiana

Carolyn Chambers Clark, EdD, ARNP, FAAN, HNC, DBFN
Adjunct Professor
Graduate Program in Nursing
Schiller International University
Dunedin, Florida
Faculty Mentor
Doctoral Program in Health Services
Walden University
Minneapolis, Minnesota

Jeannette Marie Daly, PhD, RN
Geriatric Nurse Researcher
Department of Family Medicine
University of Iowa
Iowa City, Iowa

Laura Dulski, MSN, RN
Staff Nurse
New Life Family-Centered Care Unit
Rush–Presbyterian–St. Luke's Medical Center
Chicago, Illinois

Carson A. Easley, MS, RN
Instructor of Nursing
Associate Degree Nursing Program
Antelope Valley College
Lancaster, California

Shirley Eden-Kilgour, MSN, RN, FNP
Assistant Professor of Nursing
College of Nursing and Health Professions
Arkansas State University
Jonesboro, Arkansas
Retired Professor of Nursing
Loewenberg School of Nursing
University of Memphis
Memphis, Tennessee
Family Nurse Practitioner
Charter Lakeside Behavioral Health Systems
Memphis, Tennessee

Kathleen A. Ennen, MS, RN
Doctoral Student
University of Illinois at Chicago
Chicago, Illinois
Part-Time Faculty
Parkland College,
Champaign, Illinois

Sally Evankoe, BSN, MS, RN
Instructor
Maternal Child Nursing
College of Nursing, Rush University
Chicago, Illinois

Nancy Evans, BS
Health Science Writer/Editor
San Francisco, California

Joanne H. Frey, PhD, RN
Assistant Professor
University of Massachusetts at Boston
Boston, Massachusetts

Richard Henker, PhD, RN
Assistant Professor
University of Pittsburgh
Pittsburgh, Pennsylvania

Donna D. Ignatavicius, MS, RN, Cm
Clinical Nurse Specialist
Medical-Surgical/Gerontology Nursing
Calvert Memorial Hospital
Prince Frederick, Maryland

Susan M. Irvin, MSN, RN
Clinical Coordinator
Ambulatory Surgery Unit
Memphis Veterans Administration Medical Center
Memphis, Tennessee

Konnie Sue Kyle, MSN, RN, CNRN
Director
Orthopedics, General Surgery, and Neurosurgery
St. Francis Hospital and Medical Center
Topeka, Kansas

Delois Laverentz, MN, RN, CCRN
Formerly Assistant Professor
Fort Hays State University
Hays, Kansas

Jeanne Lawler-Slack, DnSc, RN
Associate Professor and Practitioner-Teacher
College of Nursing
Rush University
Chicago, Illinois

Marilyn S. Leasia, MSN, RN, FNP
Nurse Practitioner
Department of Medicine
Montefiore Medical Center
New York, New York

James Higgy Lerner, RN, LAc
Private Practice
Acupuncture and Oriental Medicine
Chico, California

Gwyneth Lymberis, MS, RN, ANP
Assistant Professor
Borough of Manhattan Community College
The City University of New York
New York, New York

Donna W. Markey, MSN, RN, ACNP-CS
Clinician IV, Surgical Services
University of Virginia Health System
Charlottesville, Virginia

Barbara McKinney, MSN, RN
Formerly Clinical Instructor
Ashland Community College School of Nursing
Ashland, Kentucky

Beverly M. Miller, MSN, RN
Geriatric Nurse Practitioner
Memphis Veterans Administration Medical Center
Memphis, Tennessee

Frances Donovan Monahan, PhD, RN
Professor and Director
Department of Nursing, SUNY Rockland
Suffern, New York
Nursing Faculty
Regents College
Albany, New York

Virginia Nehring, PhD, RN
Associate Professor
College of Nursing and Health
Wright State University
Dayton, Ohio

Beatriz Nieto, MSN, RN, CNS
Assistant Professor
Department of Nursing
The University of Texas–Pan American
Edinburg, Texas

Laura Roddy Redic, MA, MSN, RNC
Formerly Assistant Professor of Nursing
University of Arkansas at Pine Bluff
Pine Bluff, Arkansas

Betty Kehl Richardson, PhD, RN, CS, AANC
Professor, retired
Austin Community College
Austin, Texas
Private Practice
Marriage and Family Counseling
Austin, Texas

Carol F. Roye, EdD, RN, CPNP
Associate Professor
Hunter-Bellevue School of Nursing
New York, New York

Barbara C. Rynerson, MS, RN, CS
Associate Professor Emerita
The University of North Carolina School of Nursing
Chapel Hill, North Carolina

Betty Samford, MSN, RN
School of Nursing
University of Texas at Austin
Austin, Texas

Katherine S. Schulz, RD, MS, LDN
Dietetic Consultant
State of Tennessee
Jackson, Tennessee

Brenda Leigh Yolles Smith, EdD, RN, CNM, ICCE
Associate Professor
College of Nursing
University of Tennessee at Memphis
Memphis, Tennessee

Carol E. Smith, PhD, RN
Professor, School of Nursing
University of Kansas
Kansas City, Kansas

Nancy Spector, DNFc, RN
Assistant Professor
Loyola University
Chicago, Illinois

Karen Stanley, MSN, RN, AOCN
Clinical Nurse Specialist
Pain and Symptom Management
Kaiser Permanente Fontana Medical Center
Fontana, California

Judy Sweeney, MSN, RN
Assistant Professor
School of Nursing
Vanderbilt University
Nashville, Tennessee

Rachel A. Taylor, PhD, RN
Former Assistant Professor
Department of Health Care Systems
College of Nursing
University of Tennessee at Memphis
Memphis, Tennessee

Daria Virvan, MSN, RN, CS
Nurse Psychotherapist
Town Center Psychiatric Associates
Rockville, Maryland

Phyllis Russo Wells, MSN, MEd, MPH, RNC
Women's Health Nurse Practitioner
New Horizons OB-GYN, PC
Stockbridge, Georgia

Bernie White, MSN, RN
Assistant Professor
Creighton School of Nursing
Creighton University
Omaha, Nebraska

Suzanne S. Yarbrough, PhD, RN
Assistant Professor
School of Nursing
University of Texas Health Science Center at San Antonio
San Antonio, Texas

Charlotte F. Young, PhD, RN
Retired Associate Professor
Department of Nursing
College of Nursing and Health Professions
Arkansas State University
Jonesboro, Arkansas

Deborah K. Zastocki, BSN, MA, EdM
Nursing Faculty
William Paterson University
Wayne, New Jersey
Senior Vice President
Clinical Services and Operations
Chilton Memorial Hospital
Pompton Plains, New Jersey

Sheila Rankin Zerr, BSc, MEd, RN, PHN
Visiting Faculty
School of Nursing
University of Victoria
Victoria, British Columbia
Visiting Faculty
School of Nursing
University of British Columbia
Vancouver, British Columbia

Acknowledgments

The preparation of a fundamentals textbook is truly a team effort. We wish to thank all the people on the team for their contribution.

Susan Epstein, Executive Editor, contributed keen insight in textbook development and gave her own unique flair to the project. Linda Stagg as Developmental Editor worked tirelessly to manage the details and keep the project on track from start to finish. With an ever watchful eye she helped develop the ideas for revision into reality. The production team of John Rogers, Publishing Services Manager, and Beth Hayes, Senior Project Manager, ensured a well-coordinated and smooth production process. Beth oversaw the editing and production process, bringing greater clarity and consistency to the text, while working closely with the development team, the typesetter, and the printer to transform the manuscript into a book. Kathi Gosche as Senior Designer oversaw the layout and design to give the book a fresh and sparkling new look yet in keeping with the theme of the first edition.

We thank Mike DeFilippo for his photographic expertise and St. Luke's Hospital for the generous use of their facility for our photo shoot.

We do not want to forget those who contributed to and reviewed the first edition, because we relied heavily on their work for the second edition. We received many helpful suggestions from students and faculty who used the book and feel the book is stronger for their input. Thanks to the contributors and reviewers of the second edition. We hope all of you are as proud of the product as we are.

Preface

Welcome to the profession of nursing. *Fundamentals of Nursing: Caring and Clinical Judgment,* second edition will serve as a guide as you begin the process of developing your practice of nursing. It will give you information about the context of nursing practice, how nurses think, and the people who are recipients of nursing care, as well as the needs and problems that nurses can help people manage. The ideas and techniques in this book should not be taken as the only way to practice nursing but should serve as a beginning to stimulate your creativity to develop a nursing practice that is truly your own.

The first edition of this book was well received by nursing students and faculty across the United States and is being used abroad. We are grateful for the feedback we received from the users of the book and those who reviewed for the second edition that enabled us to refine many areas of the book and better assist your study of nursing.

Changes in the second edition were made with you, the student, in mind. The second edition retains and builds upon the strengths of the first edition, adding content and features to enhance learning and address current practice. While we have reduced the number of chapters by combining and reorganizing content, we were able to retain key content and features from the first edition, including the content on home health and community care.

We are especially pleased that we have included new guidelines from the CDC for hand hygiene, the latest in immunization recommendations, the HIPAA regulations and their impact on nursing, input for our wound care recommendations from a leading expert, and a new series of photographs for inserting an intravenous catheter. The content on rehabilitation in the Managing Functional Limitations chapter has been thoroughly updated. Managing Client Care has been revised to focus more on the organization of the health care environment and on leadership/management concepts. The nursing care plans now incorporate NOC and NIC. A new procedure on Assisting the Adult Client With Feeding has been added.

HOW THE BOOK IS STRUCTURED

Unit I is designed to help you understand the context of nursing practice as a profession, as a service to a multicultural society, and as part of the health care team. As with any profession, the *profession* of nursing controls the *practice* of nursing. Chapters in this unit also discuss legal and ethical parameters of nursing practice, cultural considerations in client care, and the health care delivery system as a context for nursing practice.

Unit II is designed to help you develop a pattern of thinking that will give structure to your practice of nursing. Additionally, you will be introduced to the concepts of caring, critical thinking, and clinical judgment, skills that are growing in importance as health care grows in complexity. The nursing process is the method of studying how nurses think. Although the nursing process is divided into five phases that involve five types of thinking (assessment, diagnosis, planning, intervention, and evaluation), this unit shows the interrelationships among the five types of thinking. This unit concludes with content on documentation of the care that you have provided.

Unit III discusses some key "tools" used in nursing practice. While the use of technology is paramount in health care, these "tools" of nursing are more closely related to the mental processes and human relationships nurses use in practice than to the technology of health care. Independent nursing practice often primarily uses the tool of a therapeutic relationship with the client, in which the client makes decisions about health management and learns effective methods of health care. Additionally you will learn to use the tools of teaching, managing care, and research in your practice.

Unit IV describes the well client across the life span and examines some of the client's needs to maintain health. You will be introduced to growth and development and factors affecting health at each stage of life.

Units IV through XV present common client problems organized around Marjory Gordon's Functional Health Patterns. These patterns focus your assessment on the client problems that are amenable to nursing care. You can use the Functional Health Patterns to systematically assess your clients, thus ensuring comprehensive assessment for any presenting problem. At the start of each chapter in these units, you will find a *Key Nursing Diagnoses* box to help serve as a focus for the chapter content, as well as a *chapter-opening case study* to enable you to study the content in the context of a real-life person. The case study is continued throughout the chapter in brief vignettes with critical thinking questions to help you reflect on the client's problems and explore solutions. A *Nursing Care Plan* and *Sample Documentation Note* for the case study client is also provided.

Unit XVI will help you integrate the information from Units V through XV to plan care for surgical clients. The client who needs surgical intervention has needs in each Functional Health Pattern.

Special Features

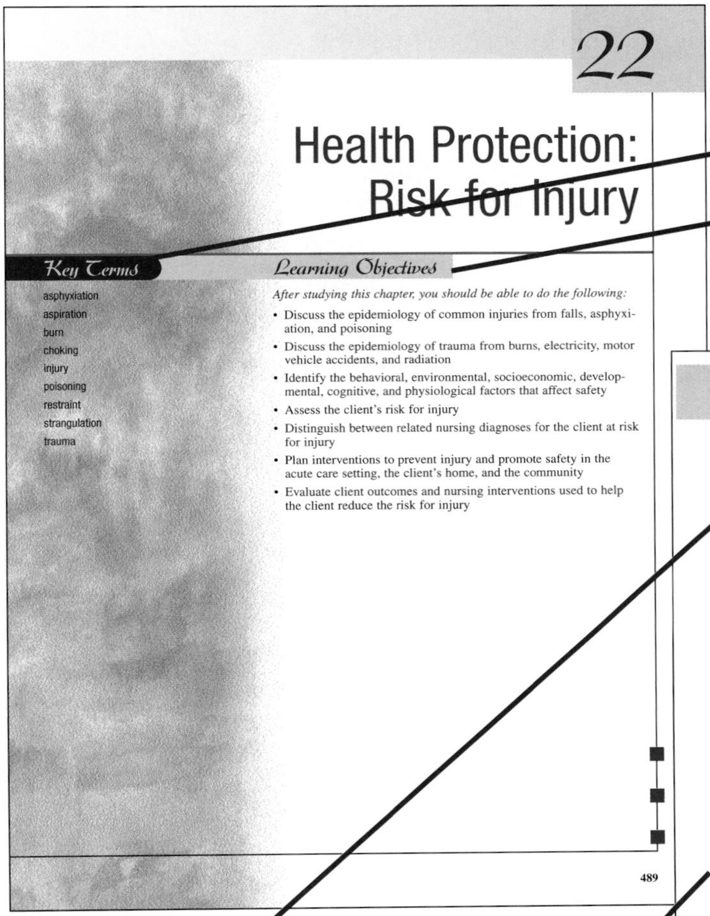

Key Terms and **Learning Objectives** at the beginning of each chapter place focus on key information.

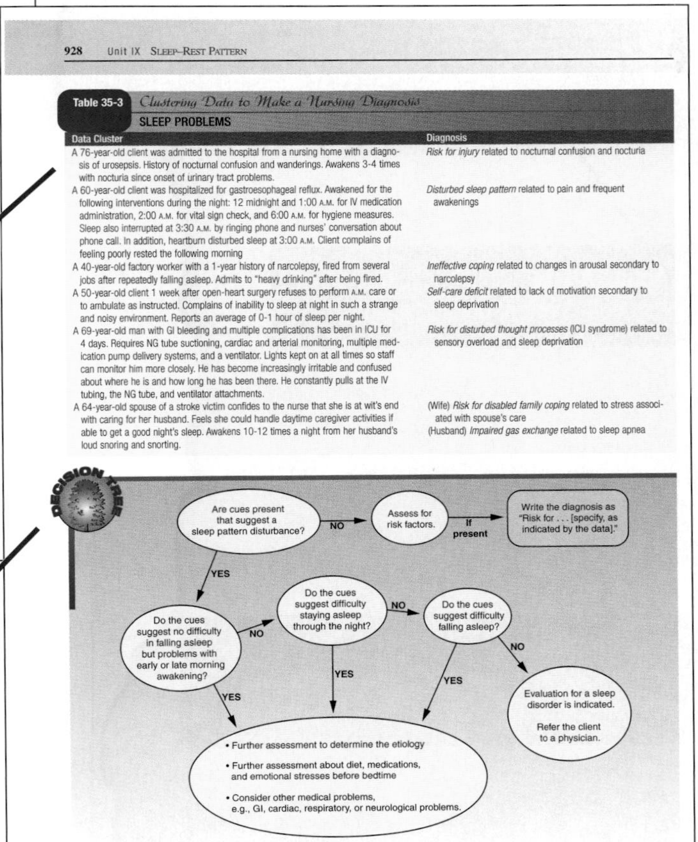

Cluster Data Tables and **Decision Trees** help accurately formulate nursing diagnoses by applying the diagnoses to different client scenarios and showing how to differentiate between closely related diagnoses.

22

Health Protection: Risk for Injury

Key Terms

asphyxiation
aspiration
burn
choking
injury
poisoning
restraint
strangulation
trauma

Learning Objectives

After studying this chapter, you should be able to do the following:

- Discuss the epidemiology of common injuries from falls, asphyxiation, and poisoning
- Discuss the epidemiology of trauma from burns, electricity, motor vehicle accidents, and radiation
- Identify the behavioral, environmental, socioeconomic, developmental, cognitive, and physiological factors that affect safety
- Assess the client's risk for injury
- Distinguish between related nursing diagnoses for the client at risk for injury
- Plan interventions to prevent injury and promote safety in the acute care setting, the client's home, and the community
- Evaluate client outcomes and nursing interventions used to help the client reduce the risk for injury

489

---

928   Unit IX SLEEP–REST PATTERN

Table 35-3 Clustering Data to Make a Nursing Diagnosis

SLEEP PROBLEMS

Data Cluster	Diagnosis
A 76-year-old client was admitted to the hospital from a nursing home with a diagnosis of urosepsis. History of nocturnal confusion and wanderings. Awakens 3-4 times with nocturia since onset of urinary tract problems.	Risk for injury related to nocturnal confusion and nocturia
A 60-year-old client was hospitalized for gastroesophageal reflux. Awakened for the following interventions during the night: 12 midnight and 1:00 A.M. for IV medication administration, 2:00 A.M. for vital sign check, and 6:00 A.M. for hygiene measures. Sleep also interrupted at 3:30 A.M. by ringing phone and nurses' conversation about phone call. In addition, heartburn disturbed sleep at 3:00 A.M. Client complains of feeling poorly rested the following morning	Disturbed sleep pattern related to pain and frequent awakenings
A 40-year-old factory worker with a 1-year history of narcolepsy, fired from several jobs after repeatedly falling asleep. Admits to "heavy drinking" after being fired.	Ineffective coping related to changes in arousal secondary to narcolepsy
A 50-year-old client 1 week after open-heart surgery refuses to perform A.M. care or to ambulate as instructed. Complains of inability to sleep at night in such a strange and noisy environment. Reports an average of 0-1 hour of sleep per night.	Self-care deficit related to lack of motivation secondary to sleep deprivation
A 69-year-old man with GI bleeding and multiple complications has been in ICU for 4 days. Requires NG tube suctioning, cardiac and arterial monitoring, multiple medication pump delivery systems, and a ventilator. Lights kept on at all times so staff can monitor him more closely. He has become increasingly irritable and confused about where he is and how long he has been there. He constantly pulls at the IV tubing, the NG tube, and ventilator attachments.	Risk for disturbed thought processes (ICU syndrome) related to sensory overload and sleep deprivation
A 64-year-old spouse of a stroke victim confides to the nurse that she is at wit's end with caring for her husband. Feels she could handle daytime caregiver activities if able to get a good night's sleep. Awakens 10-12 times a night from her husband's loud snoring and snorting.	(Wife) Risk for disabled family coping related to stress associated with spouse's care
(Husband) Impaired gas exchange related to sleep apnea

DECISION TREE

Figure 35-5. Decision tree for *Disturbed sleep pattern.* Diagnoses are shown in rectangles. Within these rectangles, diagnoses shown in **bold** type are NANDA-approved nursing diagnoses; diagnoses shown in regular type are not NANDA-approved nursing diagnoses.

Case Studies open each clinical chapter and continue with vignettes throughout.

Key Nursing Diagnoses at the beginning of each chapter serve as the focus for assessment, planning, expected outcomes, and interventions.

Action Alerts highlight situations that require important nursing actions.

Cross-Cultural Care boxes focus on the client in the case and highlight considerations for his/her cultural group.

CHAPTER 22 Health Protection: Risk for Injury   1

Juanita Soto is a 75-year-old widow who lives alone in a two-story house. Her sons and daughters live in distant cities and visit her whenever they can. She relies primarily on her neighbors and friends for help. Juanita has been relatively healthy most of her life and has been able to keep up her home despite the fact that 5 years ago she was diagnosed with rheumatoid arthritis. During the last 4 months, however, her condition has worsened. She now uses her wheelchair to get around the house, although she sometimes uses a cane to navigate the flight of stairs that leads downstairs to the washer and drier. She complains of pain and weakness in her hands and

legs. At her last physician visit, she was referred to a local home health agency for evaluation of her condition and her needs.

During the initial assessment visit, the home health nurse notes that, in addition to having limited hand and leg movement, Juanita is partially blind in one eye. The nurse also notes that Juanita's home needs some repairs—especially the stairs, which are old and have no railing for support. Because of the many physical and environmental factors identified, the nurse considers the diagnosis of *Risk for injury.* The nurse also considers related nursing diagnoses for clients with safety needs (see below).

KEY NURSING DIAGNOSES FOR   Health and Safety

Risk for injury: At risk for injury as a result of environmental conditions interacting with the individual's adaptive and defensive resources
Risk for trauma: Accentuated risk for accidental tissue injury (e.g., wound, burn, fracture)
Risk for poisoning: Accentuated risk for accidental exposure to, or ingestion of, drugs or dangerous products in doses sufficient to cause poisoning

Risk for asphyxiation: Accentuated risk for accidental asphyxiation (inadequate air available for inhalation)
Risk for aspiration: At risk for entry of gastrointestinal secretions, oropharyngeal secretions, or solids or fluids into tracheobronchial passages

---

CONCEPTS OF SAFETY

Every person has an inherent need to be and feel safe. Feeling safe allows us to think and act with confidence. Although at birth we depend on someone else for our safety, as we mature we become responsible for our own safety, and eventually we may become responsible for the safety of others. Thus safety is a need that remains with us throughout our lifetime.

Client safety is a major issue in all health care settings. Injuries affect people of all ages, developmental stages, and socioeconomic groups. Injuries can result from behavioral, environmental, or physiological hazards. No matter the cause, they can have devastating effects on both the client and the family when they result in pain, emotional distress, financial hardship, permanent disability, and even death.

Epidemiology of Injury
An *injury* is trauma or damage to some part of the body. According to the National Center for Health Statistics (Anderson, 1999), accidental injuries are the fourth leading cause of death in the United States. Injury can result from physical, mechanical, biological, or chemical agents. Accidents that result most commonly in death include motor vehicle accidents and falls.

Falls. Older people form the group affected most often by falls, both at home and in institutional settings. Falls are the leading cause of injury-related deaths among people age 65 and older, with 82% of the deaths occurring in persons age 75 and older (CDC, 2000a). When a fall occurs, morbidity, immobility, early nursing home placement, or death may result (Fuller, 2002). Because they occur frequently and have serious consequences, falls are one of the most serious problems that acute and long-term care facilities must manage.

Falls occurring in the home are a major concern and account for most reported home accidents in people age 75 and older. The pathophysiological changes that occur with aging—such as an altered gait, decreased mobility, incontinence, and confusion—place many older adults at increased risk for falling (Fuller, 2002).

Action Alert! Assess older clients for unsteady gait, impaired memory or judgment, weakness, and a history of falls.

When older clients fall, the biggest concern is the threat of hip fracture. Hip fracture is the primary cause of approximately 300,000 hospital admissions each year. In most cases, the affected person is age 65 or older and is more likely to be female (CDC, 2000a).

Falls tend to occur in the home when mobility and coordination are limited, when the person is in a hurry, or when the person is stressed or faced with obstacles. Stairways are commonly involved in falls at home. Factors that contribute to these falls include poor lighting, obstacles on the stairs, and poorly repaired steps. Falls that occur in the bathroom commonly involve a slippery tub or shower.

One day when the home care nurse comes to visit with Mrs. Soto, her daughter is there. The daughter is telling Mrs. Soto that she should sell her home and come to stay with the daughter's family. Can you list the possible concerns that prompted Mrs. Soto's daughter to make this suggestion?

Asphyxiation. *Asphyxiation* refers to an interruption in breathing that results from a severe lack of oxygen because there is either no source of air, an inadequate amount of oxygen in the air, or a condition where the air

---

2   Unit 5   HEALTH PERCEPTION–HEALTH MANAGEMENT PATTERN

FOCUSED ASSESSMENT FOR RISK FOR INJURY
To assess the general category of *Risk for injury,* you need to observe the client's physical and psychological status and elements of the environment that are unsafe. Often, a combination of factors from the internal and external environments defines the client's risk.

Defining Characteristics. Internal risk factors for injury are classified as biochemical, physical, and psychological (NANDA, 2000). Biochemical factors of the neurological system include sensory, integrative, and motor dysfunction. Additionally, hypoxia affects the ability to form reasoned judgments. Immune/autoimmune dysfunction, malnutrition, and an abnormal blood profile can make even minor injuries serious. Physical factors include altered mobility and the client's developmental status, with the very young and very old being the most vulnerable. Depression and anxiety are psychological factors that affect a person's ability to reason or to be alert to environmental hazards.

DIAGNOSIS

The main nursing diagnosis used to describe alterations in safety is *Risk for injury.* (The term *alteration in safety,* when used in nursing, implies a modification in behavior, ability, or the environment that increases risk.) This diagnosis can be used for clients in the home setting, in long-term care facilities, and in the hospital or acute care setting. Depending on the safety issue involved, a diagnosis can be written to address the specific risk for an individual client. Examples include *Risk for trauma, Risk for poisoning, Risk for asphyxiation,* and *Risk for aspiration.*

Risk for trauma and *Risk for injury* are closely related concepts. *Risk for injury* is useful in an institutional setting, where you can protect clients from a broad array of risk.

PLANNING

Planning involves identifying appropriate nursing interventions for clients who have actual or potential safety risks, as outlined in the Nursing Care Plan chart (p. •••). Nursing interventions are individualized for each client and take into consideration the severity of the risk and the client's developmental stage, level of health, and lifestyle. The main goal for the diagnoses of *Risk for injury* and *Risk for trauma* is that the client will remain free from injury.

When planning care for a client with an increased *Risk for injury,* focus mainly on prevention. You can prevent injuries by helping the client identify potential hazards and measures needed to address them. Therefore, depending on the nursing diagnosis for a particular client, specific outcomes must be identified and included in the plan of care.

Expected Outcomes for Risk for Injury
The client will be able to do the following:

- Identify safety measures to prevent falls, such as removing safety hazards in the home, using assistive devices correctly, installing ramps or safety bars as needed in the home
- Use medical equipment correctly, employing recommended safety precautions
- Not fall while performing usual activities of daily living
- Not be injured by medical or other hospital equipment, therapeutic interventions, or other hazards in the environment during hospitalization
- Understand and utilize methods of calling for assistance in the hospital
- Recognize internal risk factors that increase vulnerability to injury
- Be protected from risk for fire, electrical hazards, and other environmental hazards in a health care facility

INTERVENTION

When a client is at risk for an alteration in safety status, nursing interventions can be instituted to help prevent hazards, trauma, or disease. Nursing interventions should be individualized for each client. They should be holistic in nature and should take into consideration all the factors that are unique to the client, including age, developmental level, health care needs, abilities, support systems, strengths, and weaknesses.

Prevention is a major category of nursing interventions that you should incorporate into the client's plan of care. Preventing hazards, trauma, and illness can be done by focusing on providing or promoting a safe environment, preventing falls, enhancing safety efforts, arranging ongoing surveillance measures to identify risk factors, and providing instruction to increase awareness, knowledge, and a sense of physical and psychological safety and well-being.

Cross-Cultural Care   CARING FOR AN OLDER MEXICAN-AMERICAN CLIENT   Box 22-6

Mrs. Soto, the client described in this chapter's case study, lives in a city on the border of Texas and Mexico. She was born in Mexico and maintains close ties with family in Mexico. The following are some key facts to keep in mind when caring for Mexican-American clients:
- Mexican Americans are the most successful of all ethnic groups at retaining their culture and language.
- In southwestern cities, Mexican Americans often live in *barrios* (Hispanic ethnic neighborhoods), where their primary interactions are with members of their own ethnic group.
- More than half (51%) of older Mexican Americans were born in Mexico.
- Older adults constitute less than 4% of the population of Mexican Americans.

Holmes, E. R., & Holmes L. D. (1995). *Other cultures, elder years.* Thousand Oaks, CA: Sage.

Procedure 22-1 USING PROTECTIVE RESTRAINTS

TIME TO ALLOW
Novice: 10 min.
Expert: 5 min.

Restraints are any device or method used to restrict or control a client's behavior for the purpose of protecting the client from harm or from causing injury to others. A person can be restrained by confinement to a room or a bed or restrained by the use of drugs that decrease angry or aggressive behavior. The term *restraints* most often refers to restraining devices used to prevent the person from moving the arms or legs.

DELEGATION GUIDELINES
The decision to restrain a client may not be delegated to a nursing assistant. Physical restraint requires a physician's order. As a registered nurse, you will be able to determine whether to restrain a client when the client is deemed to be in immediate danger of causing harm to self or others and no other more appropriate means of managing the behavior exist. However, you must inform the physician and provide direction to continue the restraints. You may delegate observation of the restrained client to a nursing assistant. You may elect to delegate supervision or assistance with eating, toileting, and repositioning to a nursing assistant, and the reapplication of restraints in these circumstances may be delegated to a nursing assistant. However, you must provide specific criteria for observation and supervision.

EQUIPMENT NEEDED
- Restraints: jacket, vest, waist, wrist, or ankle restraint
- Padding as needed

1. Follow preliminary guidelines for nursing procedures (see inside back cover).

2. Assess the need for restraints. *The client's behavior could cause self-harm (risk for fall, risk for suicide, risk for wandering into unsafe areas) or injury to others. Alternatively, it could interrupt medical therapy, thus increasing the risk for complications, delaying the healing process, or causing an early death.*

3. Consider alternatives to restraints. *Discuss with the physician and with the client's family.*

4. Choose the least restrictive type of restraint.
   a. A *jacket restraint* allows the client to turn from side to side in the bed but prevents getting out of bed or a chair. It secures both the shoulders and the waist.
   b. A *belt restraint* secures the person at the waist only. Less restrictive than a jacket, it is also not as protective. It also allows the client to turn from side to side in bed.
   c. A *wrist restraint* secures one or both of the client's hands. By positioning the client's hand or hands away from tubes and dressings, the wrist restraint prevents the client from removing an intravenous line, a nasogastric tube, an indwelling urinary catheter, or a wound dressing. It also can prevent infiltration of an intravenous drug by immobilizing the client's arm. And it can prevent the client from striking people standing nearby.
   d. An *ankle restraint* secures one or both ankles and prevents injury caused by thrashing about in bed. It also prevents the client from dislodging a femoral arterial line.
   e. A *mitten restraint* prevents use of the hands while allowing free arm movements. It is useful for a client who is disturbed by wrist restraints but needs to be prevented from dislodging an intravenous line, an indwelling urinary catheter, a nasogastric tube, or a wound dressing.

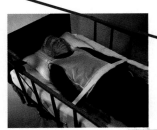

Step 4a Jacket restraint. (Courtesy Medline Industries, Mundelein, IL.)

Procedures include Time to Allow, Delegation Guidelines, Equipment Needed, and Rationales.

Streamlined procedures include only key steps needed to grasp essential information

Procedures include **Age-Related** and **Home Care Considerations.**

Sample Documentation Notes show students how to effectively document care.

Procedure 22-1 USING PROTECTIVE RESTRAINTS—CONT'D

h. Tie the restraint to the bed frame rather than a side rail (see illustration). *The side rail can be moved, which may make the restraint too tight (and harmful to the client) or too loose (ineffective).*
i. Tie the restraint in a location where the client cannot reach it but where an attendant can quickly and easily release it in an emergency.
j. Use a slipknot, and never tape a restraint knot.

6. Monitor the client and intervene to prevent complications.
   a. Observe the client every 30 minutes.
   b. Check the client's skin and circulation every 30 minutes.
   c. Provide a regular schedule of toileting.
   d. Turn the client at least every 2 hours; position for comfort.
   e. Orient the client to the environment every time you check.
   f. Assess the client's respirations, cough, and deep breathing every 2 hours.
   g. Reassess the need for restraints every 2 hours.
   h. Help the client with food and fluid intake as needed.

7. Document the following properly:
   a. Rationale or behavior that led to restraint
   b. Type of restraint and time it was applied
   c. Ongoing assessment and interventions to prevent complications
   d. Time restraints are discontinued and client's response

PEDIATRIC CONSIDERATIONS
Restraints for children depend on the age of the child. Employ the principle of least restrictive environment, but maintain safety. For some procedures the infant may be held in the mothers arms. For the infant or toddler, a mummy or papoose style of restraint is used for short procedures when it is important that the child be still (e.g., when passing a nasogastric tube, inserting an intravenous catheter, or suturing a laceration).

GERIATRIC CONSIDERATIONS
The older client should receive care in the least restrictive environment possible. Also exercise caution to avoid injury to delicate skin.

HOME CARE CONSIDERATIONS
When the client's behavior in the home requires protection to prevent falls or other self-harm, you should work with the family to provide the protection in the least restrictive manner. If the client needs frequent personal care, a hospital bed may be helpful to family caregivers because of the ease of raising the bed to a working height and of lowering the bed to transfer the client to a chair. If the side rails are sufficient restraint, a hospital bed is a good solution. Otherwise, placing the mattress on the floor may give freedom from restraints and afford protection from falling when trying to get out of bed. Also talk to the family about supervision, and help them work out a schedule to ensure that the client is attended closely.

EVALUATION

The effectiveness of nursing interventions used to promote safety and prevent injury is evaluated by comparing the expected outcomes to the goals devised during the planning phase. Nursing interventions are considered effective if the client remains free from injury.

Evaluation of safety is an ongoing process throughout the client's illness or hospital stay. You should continuously reevaluate the client's situation and determine whether new threats to safety have developed or previous ones remain. Additionally, continuous reevaluation will help you make good judgments about discontinuing unnecessary restrictions, especially the use of restraints. The evaluation phase requires frequent assessment of the client's situation to identify specific needs for support services, such as home health care, nursing home placement, or physical and occupational therapy. A care plan for Mrs. Soto can be found in Box 22-11.

SAMPLE DOCUMENTATION NOTE FOR MRS. SOTO
Discharge per wheelchair to son's automobile. Alert and oriented, able to walk the length of the hall without dizziness. Son has acquired a walker for his mother's use. Referred to Spring Valley Home Health for evaluation of home setting for safety needs, ability to perform activities of daily living, correct use of walker, need for meals on wheel, and physical therapy services. Will see primary physician on Friday for follow-up.

appropriate for the child's age and weight. Sharp objects, such as knives and other kitchen utensils, matches, and toxic substances should be kept out of children's reach.

As can be seen from these examples, many safety measures can be emphasized to children's parents, caregivers, or family to help them promote safety and avoid accidents. Community resources are also available and can be accessed through referrals. An important aspect of promoting safety lies in getting clients and their families involved in planning and implementing the safety measures needed to decrease the risk for injury. Solicit involvement of clients and their families through family conferences in which you help them define their mutual goals. This involvement enhances their motivation and increases the likelihood of positive outcomes and the long-term lifestyle changes required.

Most accidents are preventable. By educating yourself, your clients, and their families, you can help reduce the risk for injury, trauma, asphyxiation, poisoning, and aspiration in their homes.

Providing Safety in Institutions

CREATING A SAFE INSTITUTIONAL ENVIRONMENT. In a health care institution, the client, especially one who is incapacitated by illness or disability, depends on the staff to provide a safe environment. This requires a team effort by nursing services, housekeeping, maintenance—indeed, every employee of the institution. Safety issues are similar to those in the home, but a hospital has more equipment, hazardous chemicals, and a large number of people using the facility. Every employee should be trained in electrical safety and fire safety as well as in safe interactions with clients.

Stay aware of the risk for electrical injury, especially in situations that combine moisture with electrical equipment. These situations may involve spills on the floor, a leaking or disconnected intravenous line, or a client with moist skin caused by diaphoresis.

You can help prevent electrical injuries by making sure that electrical equipment stays in good working order and by using devices equipped with three-pronged grounded plugs (Figure 22-8). The third prong of the plug is called the *ground*

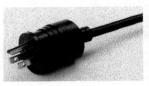

Figure 22-8. A three-pronged grounded plug, used to prevent electrical injuries. (Courtesy Lion Electric, South Norwalk, CT.)

because it is specifically designed to carry any stray electrical current into the earth. The two regular prongs carry power to the equipment being used. However, simply having a three-pronged plug does not ensure that the plug is grounded. The maintenance department should check the grounding periodically. Box 22-7 includes additional ideas to reduce the risk for electrical injury. Identifying and correcting potential sources of danger can prevent electrical shock.

Action Alert! Prevent electrical shocks by using grounded equipment. Teach others to avoid the use of faulty equipment and to never overload electrical outlets or extension cords.

Although fires are uncommon in modern buildings when safety precautions are followed, fire safety programs increase the readiness to respond correctly to a fire. Any fire that arises in a health care setting requires quick actions in response. A common response plan incorporates the acronym RACE to help prioritize those actions. It stands for *rescue, alarm, confine,* and *extinguish.*

The first priority in case of fire is to rescue or remove all clients from immediate danger. The second priority is to call for help. Activate the nearest fire alarm, or report the fire to the switchboard operator, whichever is faster. The switchboard operator will page the code for a fire and its location.

Teaching for Self-Care
Preventing Electrical Shocks   Box 22-7

Purpose: To provide information about electrical safety.

Expected Outcome: The client will demonstrate electrical safety practices.

Client Instructions

Equipment
- Make sure that equipment is grounded; the use of a three-prong outlet does not ensure that the outlet is grounded.
- Do not use electrical cords that are frayed or that have visible damage.
- Repair or replace all malfunctioning equipment. If you drop a piece of electrical equipment, have it tested before reusing it.
- Experiencing shocks while using equipment means that it is not safe; have it tested before continuing to use it.
- Learn about all electrical equipment that you intend to use before attempting to use it.

Electrical outlets
- Do not overload.
- Cover outlets not currently in use, especially if small children are present.
- Install outlets with ground fault circuit interrupters near sources of water, such as bathroom and kitchen sinks.
- Never pull a plug from the socket by the cord. Grip the plug firmly and pull it straight out of the socket.

Extension cords
- Avoid using extension cords when possible.
- Anchor extension cords to the floor using specially... prevent tripping over the cord.

Nursing Care Plan **AN ELDERLY CLIENT WITH A HEAD INJURY**   Box 22-11

ADMISSION DATA

Mrs. Juanita Soto is a 75-year-old Hispanic woman who will be discharged from the hospital in a few days and needs reevaluation by her home health nurse. Mrs. Soto had been admitted through the emergency room to the general medical nursing unit after sustaining a head contusion when she fell trying to get out of the shower. Mrs. Soto informed the nurse, "I never have hurt myself this much before. Usually, I catch myself before I fall all the way, but this time I could not. I guess I'm not as strong as I used to be. Since my husband died, I have lived by myself. My sons and daughters live far away, and I don't want to be a burden on anyone." Mrs. Soto lives alone in a two-story woodframe home.

NURSING REPORT TO HOME HEALTH AGENCY

Client was admitted because of a head contusion sustained while trying to get out of the shower. Her son is present and staying with her while she is in the hospital. Client stated that this has happened before but not to this extent. States that she had been feeling weaker. Has limited movement in hands and legs and is partially blind in one eye.

Mrs. Soto is referred back to the home health agency by her physician. Her daughter had expressed concern about her mother living alone safely and being able to manage her arthritis. Because Mrs. Soto refused to leave her home, the physician requested an evaluation by the home health nurse.

PHYSICIAN'S REFERRAL REQUEST

Evaluate client's ability to perform activities of daily living and instrumental activities of daily living. Arrange for home health aide and Meals on Wheels if needed. Monitor compliance with arthritis medication and assess for side effects. Assist client to plan for two 30-minute to 60-minute rest periods during the day. Arrange for physical therapy to teach isometric and range-of-motion exercises. Home paraffin therapy before exercise, BID.

HOME NURSING ASSESSMENT

The home assessment revealed an older, two-story home with no safety equipment in the bathroom, some throw rugs, inadequate lighting at night, cluttered hallways, and broken stairs with no railing.

NANDA Nursing Diagnosis	NOC Expected Outcomes With Indicators	NIC Interventions With Selected Activities	Evaluation Data
RISK FOR INJURY: FALL	**SAFETY STATUS: FALL OCCURRENCE**	**FALL PREVENTION SURVEILLANCE: SAFETY**	**FIRST HOME VISIT**
Related Factors:			
• Fall related to limited movement	• Number of falls:	• Identify cognitive or physical deficits that may increase potential of falling at home.	• Mrs. Soto maintains order in her home and is familiar with environment.
• Partially blind in one eye	• While standing		• Basement stairs are a hazard; son will repair stairs to basement.
• Lives alone	• While walking	• Monitor gait, balance, and fatigue level with ambulation.	• Not safe to cook hot meals; will arrange Meals on Wheels with provider who caters to Hispanic food preferences.
• Age 75	• While sitting		
	• From bed	• Provide assistive devices.	• Living in her familiar community is an important value to Mrs. Soto.
	• While transferring	• Remove hazards from home (e.g., throw rugs).	• She has neighbors who are willing to visit frequently and perform small tasks.
	• Climbing steps	• Provide grab bars for bathtub, shower chair, nonslip floor.	• She has limited range of motion in lower extremities and sometimes uses a cane to get around; also uses a wheelchair.
	• Descending steps	• Increase lighting in home.	• She has shoes with nonskid soles.
			• She stated that the stairs were going to be fixed by her son while he was there.
			• Her home is about 50 years old; it has four bedrooms and two baths. The bathroom floor has tile, and she usually has throw rugs on the floor because it tends to be cold. She expressed concern over the cost of grab bars.

CRITICAL THINKING QUESTIONS

1. How would you handle the subject of using a copper bracelet rather than the medication the physician has ordered?

2. How would you approach the subject of having a caretaker live with Mrs. Soto?

3. Would adult day care be helpful in this situation?

Nursing outcome and intervention labels from Johnson, M., Bulechek, G., McCloskey Dochterman, J., Maas, M., & Moorhead, S. (2001). *Nursing diagnoses, outcomes, and interventions: NANDA, NOC, and NIC linkages.* St Louis, MO: Mosby.

Teaching for Wellness and **Teaching for Self-Care boxes** focus on sharpening teaching skills, health promotion and illness prevention, and restoration of health after illness.

Nursing Care Plans now incorporate NIC and NOC.

Critical Thinking Questions help explore alternate solutions to client problems.

Contents in Detail

The Nursing Profession

Learning Objectives

After studying this chapter, you should be able to do the following:

- Describe the evolution of nursing from ancient civilizations to the present, including the influence of religious, scientific, and political developments

- Compare the different educational programs in nursing

- Describe the influence on professional nursing practice contributed by standards of professional nursing, professional organizations, and professional nursing roles

- Describe the relationship of the evolution of nursing to changes in the health care delivery system, current social issues, and the profession's political agenda as health care moves into the 21st century

Through the years, the definition of nursing evolved, yet the focus of providing humanistic and holistic care has always been preserved. **Nursing** is an accountable discipline guided by science, theory, a code of ethics, and the art of care and comfort to treat human responses to health and illness. Nursing practice puts the science and art of nursing into action.

The American Nurses' Association (ANA) represents professional nurses in the United States. As a means of defining nursing, the ANA document *Nursing's Social Policy Statement* recognizes the contribution of the science of caring in four essential realms of contemporary nursing practice (ANA, 1995):

1. Attention to the full range of human experiences and responses to health and illness without restriction to a problem-focused orientation
2. Integration of objective data with knowledge gained from an understanding of the client's or the group's subjective experience
3. Application of scientific knowledge to the processes of diagnosis and treatment
4. Provision of a caring relationship that facilitates health and healing

These definitions of nursing and nursing practice emphasize human responses to health and health problems instead of the disease processes. Disease is the domain of physicians or the practice of medicine. Nursing and medicine complement one another in working toward optimal health for humankind.

EVOLUTION OF THE NURSING PROFESSION

Contemporary nursing practice requires a combination of intellectual achievement, ethical standards, scientific knowledge, technological skills, and personal compassion. Gradually, over centuries, these elements have evolved and blended together. During this evolutionary process nursing practice has been influenced by external factors such as economics, religion, politics, scientific advancements, wars, and changing lifestyles.

This chapter begins with a brief journey into the evolution of nursing as a profession. An awareness of this history enhances our collective understanding of the intellectual and societal roots or origins of nursing.

Ancient Civilizations Through the Renaissance

Anthropologists speculate that in most ancient civilizations, women were responsible for nurturing, nourishing, and providing care to children and ill family members. In essence, nursing in its early history was a community service that preserved and protected the family (Donahue, 1996).

In many cultures, illness was believed to be directly related to religious beliefs, mythical magic, and evil spirits that took control of the body. Medicine men, healers, or shamans exorcised these evil spirits from the sick using incantations, vile odors, massage, charms, and even sacrifices. Women delivered custodial care and seldom assisted the medicine men, who were aided by men (Hamilton, 1996).

Some ancient peoples, such as the Aztecs, Mayans, and Toltecs, recognized that illness was at least partly caused by physical factors. Illness was treated with massage, bloodletting, minerals and herbs, suturing of wounds, amputation of limbs, extraction of teeth, and even trephining, the drilling of holes in the skull (Hamilton, 1996).

Under the influence of Christianity, educated and wealthy women dedicated themselves to caring for the sick and poverty stricken (Donahue, 1996). One of the earliest records of nursing influenced by Christianity was the formation of the Order of the Deaconesses. In A.D. 60, Phoebe, a Roman matron, had the distinction of being named "the first deaconess," a church official ordained to meet the needs of women converts. A secondary function of the deaconess was visiting the sick (Jamieson, Sewall, & Gjertson, 1959). From this role Phoebe became known as the "first visiting nurse" (Deloughery, 1998).

The Middle Ages (from AD 476 to 1453) separated ancient from modern times. The first 500 years of this period are often called the Dark Ages because all but the nobles and the clergy were largely uneducated and because these years were marked by war, poverty, social injustices, illness, and general misery among the people. The bubonic plague killed about a third to half of Europe's population during this period. This widespread disease stimulated hospital construction, although early hospitals had no ventilation, heat, plumbing, or lighting and hardly any sanitation services.

The plague also contributed to the founding of many nursing orders, such as the Augustinian Sisters, the first nursing order to provide only nursing services. Gradually, the number of deaconesses diminished as monks and nuns took over the operation of hospitals.

The Crusades also stimulated expanded nursing and health care. Nurses were also knights and were employed in battle as well as in hospital settings (Doheny, Cook, & Stopper, 1987). Groups of knights, such as the Knights Hospitallier of St. John of Jerusalem, cared for the wounded and ill along the crusade routes (Figure 1-1). As the number of all-male military nursing orders increased, all-female religious orders were nearly destroyed. A number of other religious orders also evolved, such as the Franciscans and Dominicans.

The Renaissance was a period of renewed interest in philosophy, science, and the arts. Learning flourished, and by 1500, a trend toward nursing education had developed. Universities were constructed throughout Europe, but even as medicine moved into the university setting, nursing remained behind.

Slowly, monasteries and religious orders declined because of increased Protestantism, and male nurses vanished from the nursing profession (Doheny, Cook, & Stopper, 1987). The home became the main locality for nursing care. The only sick who were hospitalized were poor, and care was delivered by recruited prostitutes and female criminals. This era in Europe has been described as the darkest age of nursing because there was little to no organization, education, or social standing left in nursing.

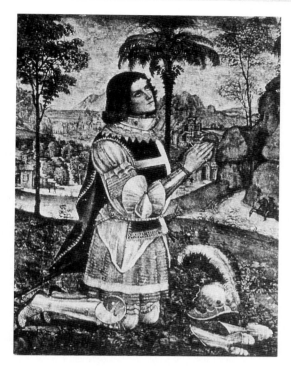

Figure 1-1. A Knight Hospitallier of St. John of Jerusalem. (Courtesy the National Library of Medicine.)

Colonialism and Revolution

Beginning in the last decade of the 15th century, many European powers sought to expand their territories in the New World by founding colonies in North, Central, and South America and in Africa. Early colonists experienced some of the same health care problems seen in Europe. Infectious diseases, nutritional disorders, starvation, and complications of pregnancy were common. Nursing and medical care consisted of folk remedies (Hamilton, 1996).

By the mid-17th century, health care delivery started to improve as medical knowledge began to be developed in the British colonies. The first colonial hospital was established in what later became New York in 1658 (Selevan, 1984). However, the nurses in colonial hospitals were typically untrained men.

Despite these advances, health care was poor. Physicians were not required to have a license to practice medicine, and charlatans were common. Hospital care was available only in the largest colonial cities, and rural colonists relied on visiting physicians and home remedies. The mentally ill went without treatment or were warehoused in hospitals where they were shackled and confined together in filthy, dungeonlike rooms (Hamilton, 1996).

When the 13 American colonies declared independence from England in 1776, their soldiers were poorly dressed, inadequately armed, hungry, and ill. Soldiers were exposed to impure water, dirty camps, and unsanitary hospitals, and scarlet fever, smallpox, and dysentery devastated their ranks. It has been speculated that more soldiers of the American Revolution died from disease or complications of care than

from wounds (Selevan, 1984). The newly formed United States recognized the need for clean hospitals and trained nurses to supervise soldiers' care while in combat (Chitty, 2001). Nurses played a role in the war by directly caring for soldiers at the battlefront and in hospitals.

Industrialization

The Industrial Revolution, which began in England and France during the mid-18th century and in Germany and the United States in the 19th century. A population explosion following migration from rural to urban areas, and changing work modes led to undesirable work conditions, negative attitudes toward the working class, and a much lower standard of living. Families often lived in overcrowded conditions with poor ventilation, heating, and cooling. In urban areas, water supplies, sanitation, garbage collection, and plumbing were poor. In addition, techniques for preserving foods and for basic hygiene were not yet developed. Factories paid starvation wages for long hours of dangerous work. Child labor was common. All of these negative factors increased the incidence of illness, injury, and early mortality.

As consciousness of these barbarous methods slowly began to heighten, society's attitude toward health care became more compassionate. Caring for the sick became socially acceptable, even praiseworthy. Hospitals opened to care for those with work-related illnesses and injuries, and physicians recognized the need for competent hospital nurses. Nursing textbooks on management and techniques were written.

Several groups sought to care for the sick, injured, and poor, such as the Sisters of Charity, who developed a nurse training program. The Kaiserwerth School of Nursing was established in Germany in 1836. Students from many countries were taught practice, theory, and codes of conduct related to nursing (Doheny, et al., 1987).

In the United States, an attempt to organize a school of nursing was made in 1839 by Dr. Joseph Warrington of the Nurse Society of Philadelphia. The classes, which were taught to nurses and medical students together, gave women minimal instruction in obstetrics to enable them to provide maternity nursing services in the home setting (Jensen, Spaulding, & Cody, 1955).

The Influence of War

Advances in military technology in the early 19th century ushered in an age of modern warfare characterized by a tremendous escalation in the rates of crippling injuries, loss of limbs, and mortality. This led to an increased demand for trained military nurses.

Crimean War. The Crimean War was fought in what is now part of the Ukraine, between 1854 and 1856. Great Britain, France, Turkey, and Sardinia united as allies to defeat Russia. This war is important to the history of nursing because of the role played by Florence Nightingale, considered to be the founder of modern nursing (Figure 1-2, p. 4).

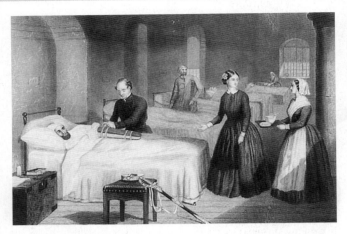

Figure 1-2. Florence Nightingale (1820-1910). (Courtesy the National Library of Medicine.)

Florence Nightingale was born in 1820 into an upper-class English family. As a child, she enjoyed wealth, education, and extensive travel. While accompanying her mother to visit the sick, she became aware of the inadequate care of hospitalized patients, and at age 31 she entered nursing training at Deaconess Institute in Kaiserwerth. In 1853, she completed additional training with the Sisters of Charity in Paris, and shortly thereafter she became administrator of a charity hospital for governesses.

In 1854, as the Crimean War began, Nightingale prepared and led a group of 38 nurses to British military hospitals in Turkey to care for the wounded and to institute reform. Smith (1984) states that once in Turkey, Nightingale found a hospital so crowded that patients lay on the floor still in bloody uniforms. Bath equipment, sheets, cutlery, and laundry facilities were practically nonexistent.

With much compassion, Nightingale established sanitary conditions. Hospital units were cleaned and clothing was washed regularly. The soldiers received nursing care both day and night. Nightingale's reforms reduced the mortality rate of the soldiers from 42.7% to 2.2% in 6 short months (Cohen, 1984; Donahue, 1996; Woodham-Smith, 1951).

Because Nightingale and her nurses made their rounds carrying oil lamps, she became known as "the Lady with the lamp." This remains the symbol of the nursing profession.

After the Crimean War, Nightingale served on several commissions and wrote about health, sanitation, hospitals, and nursing education (Hamilton, 1996). Her most distinguished books are *Notes on Hospitals* (1858) and *Notes on Nursing: What It Is and What It Is Not* (1860).

In 1860, the Nightingale Training School for nurses opened at St. Thomas' Hospital in London. The 1-year course offered classroom and clinical experience, later known as the Nightingale Plan. This plan became the model for nursing education and was used in the United States and Canada. Three schools of nursing based on her training school model opened in Boston, Connecticut, and New York. The women who graduated from these first schools led nursing into the twentieth century.

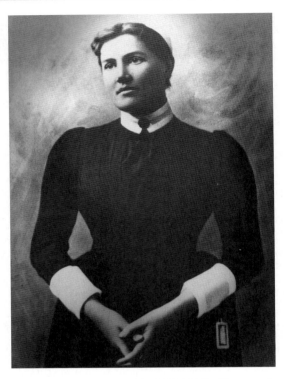

Figure 1-3. Isabel Hampton Robb (1860-1910). (Courtesy the Alan Mason Chesney Medical Archives of the Johns Hopkins Medical Institutions.)

American Civil War. With the American Civil War (1861-1865), early nursing leaders began to emerge. Table 1-1 summarizes the primary contributions of selected early nursing leaders. These women were willing to take risks when human rights were put in jeopardy or threatened. Women volunteered to care for soldiers on both the Confederate and the Union sides of the war. Their contributions included the implementation of sanitary conditions in field hospitals.

It was also during the Civil War that the value of primary prevention became understood in the United States. Clean surroundings, good nutrition, and nurses in control of the environment were recognized as positive factors for healing. It was clear that training nurses would be beneficial.

Isabel Hampton Robb was a graduate of the Bellevue Hospital Training School in New York (Figure 1-3). She became the first principal of the Johns Hopkins School of Nursing. In 1894, she wrote a standardized nursing text to be used in the United States: *Nursing: Its Principles and Practice for Hospital and Private Use* (Donahue, 1996). In 1896, Robb helped found the Nurses Associated Alumnae of the United States and Canada. The Canadian affiliation was removed in 1899, and in 1911 the group became known as the American Nurses' Association. Robb was instrumental in establishing the National League of Nursing Education that is now known as the National League for Nursing.

Mary Adelaide Nutting, also from Canada, was in the first graduating class at Johns Hopkins School of Nursing. She actively worked for nurses to be educated in the university setting. Nutting was the first nurse to be appointed to a

Nursing Leader	Key Date	Contribution
		Table 1-1 Primary Contributions of Selected Early Nursing Leaders
Sojourner Truth	1827	Abolitionist, lecturer, women's rights worker. A Black nurse who made enormous contributions during the American Civil War. Worked as a nurse/counselor for the Freedman's Association after the war.
Harriet Ross Tubman	1840	A Black nurse who led more than 300 slaves to freedom during the American Civil War. Recognized for her kindness and attention to the sick and suffering.
Florence Nightingale	1854	A war nurse and founder of modern nursing education. A publisher and nurse theorist.
Mary Ann Ball	1861	Appointed Superintendent of the Women Nurses of the Army. Devoted herself to the care of the mentally ill and to improvement of jail conditions.
Dorothea Dix	1861	"Mother Beckerdyke" was one of the greatest heroines of the American Civil War. Searched for survivors on the battlefield and organized diet kitchens and ambulance services.
Linda Richards	1872	A graduate of New England Hospital for Women and Children. The first trained nurse in the United States. Later, developed and established the first nursing school in Japan.
Lavinia Lloyd Dock	1873	A well-known nurse who was actively involved in early 20th-century women's rights issues and the suffragette movement.
Mary Eliza Mahoney	1879	Completed the 16-month training course at the New England Hospital for Women and Children to become America's first Black "trained nurse."
Clara Barton	1881	Famous American Civil War nurse who used her work and ideas from the battlefield to develop the American Red Cross.
Mary Agnes Snively	1884	Responsible for the direction of Canadian nursing education. Director of the Toronto General Hospital Canadian Nurses Association.
Isabel Hampton Robb	1886	An outstanding nurse who was first president of the Nurses Associated Alumnae of the United States and Canada. Was first principal of Johns Hopkins School of Nursing, cofounder of the *American Journal of Nursing.*
Betty Moulder and Ada Stewart	1888	First nurses employed as occupational health nurses.
Annie Goodrich	1893	Head of the United States Army School of Nursing in 1918. Was Assistant Professor of Nursing at Columbia Teachers College and Dean of Nursing at Yale University. Served as president of the American Nurses Association (ANA).
Lillian Wald	1893	Founded the Henry Street Settlement service, providing health care for the poor on New York's Lower East Side. Formed the National Organization of Public Health Nursing (the first specialization in nursing) in 1912.
Mary Adelaide Nutting	1894	An early nurse activist at Columbia Teachers College. Known as "the first nursing professor in the world." Influential in raising educational standards for nurses working toward undergraduate and graduate nursing degrees.
Namahyoke Curtis	1898	The first trained Black nurse employed as a contract nurse by the United States War Department during the Spanish-American War.
Clara Maas	1898	A nurse volunteer who participated in the yellow fever research experiment in Havana, Cuba, and died from yellow fever after the Spanish-American War.
Jessie Sleet (Scales)	1900	The first Black public health nurse.
Martha Franklin	1916	Founded the National Association of Colored Graduate Nurses (NACGN).
Margaret Sanger	1916	Founded the first birth control clinic in America, the forerunner of Planned Parenthood.
Francis Reed Elliott	1918	The first Black nurse accepted by the American Red Cross Nursing Service.
Frances Payne Bolton	1923	Provided financial support that was instrumental in the development of the nursing school at Case Western Reserve University.
Mary Breckinridge	1925	Conducted research to differentiate between nursing and nonnursing tasks. Successful in influencing upgraded nursing education.
Isabel Maitland Stewart	1925	Founded the Frontier Nursing Service, which provided the first organized midwifery service in the United States.
Lucille Petry	1949	The first woman appointed to the position of Assistant Surgeon General of the United States Public Health Service.
Mildred Montag	1952	Conducted research; was instrumental in the development of the first Associate Degree nursing program.

university professorship at Columbia University Teachers College, and she directed the newly established department of nursing and health (Donahue, 1996).

In 1879 Mary Mahoney became the first professional Black nurse in the United States. She campaigned for respect for cultural differences. Today, the ANA bestows the Mary Mahoney Award in recognition of individuals who make sig-

nificant contributions toward improving relationships among diverse cultural groups.

In 1893 Lillian Wald founded public health nursing when she opened the Henry Street Settlement Service in New York City. Wald, the first community health nurse, recognized the importance of teaching people about health promotion practices and the means to prevent illness. Programs aimed at tuberculosis control and infant welfare were started. The institutional base later shifted to the government, and public health services were offered through local health departments.

Spanish-American War. The Spanish-American War (1898) offered trained nurses an opportunity for employment in military hospitals. The war revealed American deficiencies, especially the lack of emergency nursing reserves. Although the American army casualties were small, their military camps were shattered by epidemic diseases such as typhoid fever, malaria, dysentery, and food poisoning. The Nurses' Associated Alumnae of the United States and Canada offered to help the government to secure skilled nurses. However, the Daughters of the American Revolution had already volunteered their untrained services for nursing care of the troops.

Clara Louise Maas volunteered to serve in the Spanish-American War as a contract nurse. She became actively involved in yellow fever research experimentation, and in 1901, after being bitten by a mosquito, she died. She was the only American and the only woman to die during the experiments.

During this time Anita Newcomb McGee, a physician, was appointed to be in charge of the Army Nursing Service as acting assistant surgeon in the United States Army. Dr. McGee preferred to enroll nurses who had a certificate of graduation from a training school for nurses. These nurses were then placed under the direction of the Red Cross, which assisted with their expenses while in service (Jamieson, Sewall, & Gjertson, 1959). Through Congress, the nurses worked on a contract basis, receiving $30 per month plus room and meals. Approximately 8000 volunteer nurses were placed under contract and began what is now the Army Nursing Corps. Dita H. Kinney, head nurse of the United States Army Hospital at Fort Baynard, eventually replaced Dr. McGee.

World War I. In 1917, the United States entered World War I. The number of nurses available could not meet both civilian and military needs. Once again, an untrained volunteer system provided military nursing care. Concerned nursing leaders established the Army School of Nursing in 1918 to train volunteers. The school was headed by Annie Goodrich, an assistant professor of nursing at Teachers College.

After the war, the Rockefeller Foundation established a committee to study nursing education. Findings from this study, called the Goldmark Report, revealed the faults associated with hospital nursing programs and identified lack of funding as the obstacle to higher educational standards in nursing (Kalisch & Kalisch, 1986). At this time, the Rockefeller Foundation funded the expansion of nursing programs at Vanderbilt University, Yale University, and the University of Toronto.

During the 1920s, hospitals and nursing schools began to expand. Nursing schools depended on hospitals for support, and the hospitals depended on the students to carry the nursing workload. Eventually, this apprenticeship method of educating nurses became increasingly criticized. More and more, male hospital administrators and physicians governed the almost exclusively female student population. This type of paternalism slowed nursing's progress toward professionalism for several decades (Kalisch & Kalisch, 1986).

Many trained nurses became involved in the women's suffrage movement. Women were not considered equals of men, society did not value education for women, and women did not have the right to vote. Lavinia Dock, a well-known, early 20th-century nurse, was instrumental in furthering women's issues and the suffrage movement. By the mid-1900s, more women were going to college even though only limited numbers of nursing programs were available in the university setting.

The Great Depression and the drought of the 1930s brought financial destruction to a country already exhausted by war. As prosperity diminished, so did the use of private-duty nurses. There was a shortage of funds for visiting nursing services and too many trained nurses on hand. Gradually, hospitals became the primary setting for care for the sick. The decline in home-based nursing care would last until the late 1980s (Chitty, 2001).

World War II. World War II (1939-1945) had an enormous effect on nursing. Qualified nurses were in demand. Training for nurses became associated with classrooms and organized curricula (Figure 1-4). In 1941, the U.S. Congress passed the Lanham Act to fund nursing education and improve existing educational facilities (Donahue, 1996). Federally subsidized nursing programs were developed to offer women and men a career in nursing while serving their country.

After the war, a small number of nurse officers entered undergraduate and graduate nursing programs. The GI bill of rights assisted them in accessing further education. However, many chose to return to traditional homemaking roles. The "baby boom" and economic burst after the war stimulated the construction of hospitals. Within a few years, a shortage of registered nurses created unfavorable working conditions for hospital-based nurses (Chitty, 2001).

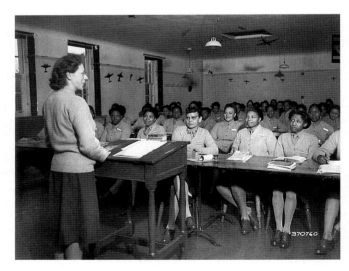

Figure 1-4. During World War II, training for nurses became associated with classrooms and organized curricula. (Courtesy the National Archives at College Park.)

As dissatisfaction grew, the ANA sanctioned state units to form collective bargaining units. This move created an ethical dilemma for many nurses. Now they would have to decide between their duty to care for clients or their duty to themselves and their families.

In the late 1940s, nursing as a profession sought to meet the needs of society and to organize the profession to meet those needs. The war years had underlined the requisite for nurses to speak with professional unity. Work began on the professional issues of education and organizational unity.

Korean War. During the Korean War (1950-1953), the nurses of the U.S. armed forces (Army, Navy, and the new Air Force Nursing Corps) were called on to serve their country. The army instituted combat emergency teams or units called the Mobile Army Surgical Hospital (MASH). The MASH could be moved at a moment's notice and was usually staffed by 10 physicians, 12 nurses, and 90 corpsmen. It could and did set up anywhere. Within a few hours, 200 to 300 wounded soldiers could be treated. Hamilton (1996) reports that the success of these units revealed the tremendous contribution of nurses in demanding circumstances. This experience paved the way for development of intensive care units and better emergency or trauma medical treatment.

Fear of a severe nursing shortage was instrumental in increasing recruitment of students to nursing schools to offset the depleted numbers of professional nurses in civilian hospitals. A significant change in nursing education that affected the profession also occurred at this time: the development of associate degree programs in community colleges.

Mildred Montag of Teachers College developed a new model of nursing education as a result of research she had conducted (Montag, 1951). She began the piloting of the new model of associate degree nursing programs in 1952, and by 1957 a rapid proliferation of community college nursing programs had begun. The nurse of this new program was to be a nurse technician, operating below the level of the professional nurse but above that of the practical nurse (Donahue, 1996). Because of major nursing shortages and to meet societal needs, however, the nurse with an associate degree became the third level of entry into nursing practice.

Vietnam War. From 1957 to 1975, nursing was kept busy with the Vietnam War. The appointment of male nurses to the armed forces nursing corps was made possible by a congressional bill passed in 1966. As a result of the bill, the number of male nurses increased and some all-male nursing units were even established for short periods. Hospitals were fixed facilities during this conflict, and helicopters became the means of evacuation and immediate care by medics and flight nurses.

During this time, civilian hospitals expanded rapidly and installed intensive care units and recovery rooms, creating the need for more advanced technical nursing skills. Specialization advanced at a rapid rate as a consequence of technological changes and new knowledge. This increased specialization introduced constraints in staffing within hospitals. No longer was the nurse able to move freely from one unit to another unless clients in those units had similar health problems and could be treated by the same general modes of therapy.

This was a time of professional awakening for nursing. The concept of nursing diagnosis, introduced in the 1950s, contributed to the development of nursing as a science. Master's degrees in nursing clinical specialties and doctoral degrees in nursing were being offered in major universities. Nurse practitioner programs opened, associate degree nursing programs proliferated, and financial support from the federal government for nursing education was reaching an all-time high.

Many nurses became employed outside the hospital, and this quickly became the age of nurse entrepreneurship. As nurse-owned businesses grew, the number of certified practitioners working individually and in joint practice with physicians also grew (Hamilton, 1996).

Contemporary Developments

The 1980s witnessed changes in the medical, technical, and organizational domains of American society, and these changes had major effects on who received services, who provided them, and what types of services were available. The introduction of diagnosis-related groups (DRGs) for Medicare by the federal government in 1983 was an effort to contain the rapidly rising cost of health care. DRGs, health maintenance organizations (HMOs), and emergency care centers have all been reflections of the financially driven health care system of the 1980s.

The 1990s were also a decade of profound change in health care delivery and health care settings. This era is characterized by efforts toward cost containment and heightened efficiency in health care, which eliminated some nursing positions within hospitals. At the same time, the need for nurses in outpatient and home health agencies grew. The aging of the nursing workforce and increased numbers of nurse retirees have helped to shape the current nursing shortage.

While advanced practice nursing specialties grew, a new trend, *managed care,* emerged in an effort to maintain quality health care at the lowest cost. A large number of registered nurses were employed in the role of case manager to review clients' cases and coordinate care in various health settings. Advanced practice nurses, such as the clinical nurse practitioner and the clinical nurse specialist, were employed in the traditional and nontraditional health care settings. Third-party payment for these nursing services by insurers was secured as a result of the health care dollar crisis of the 1990s. Home nursing care delivery expanded as a major cost-effective measure during this era.

In 1993, President Clinton focused attention on the need for preventive services in the proposed Health Security Act of 1993. Primary prevention was not a new idea for nurses. In an attempt to represent the interests and the role of nursing, representatives of more than 60 nursing organizations developed their own reform plan, called *Nursing's Agenda for Health Care Reform.* The reform focused on primary care, prevention, and community outreach.

PROFESSIONAL NURSING EDUCATION

Since the first schools of nursing opened their doors in the 18th century, nursing education has expanded in response to ongoing changes and advances in health care. Today's nursing roles are more complex and require additional knowledge in the physical, biological, and social sciences, along with nursing practice and theory.

Entry-Level Education

Currently, four types of state-approved educational programs prepare students for entry into professional nursing practice as a **registered nurse (RN).** They are diploma programs, associate degree programs, baccalaureate degree programs, and graduate degree entry programs. Graduates are eligible for licensure as an RN in a particular state after successfully passing the National Council Licensure Examination for Registered Nurses (NCLEX-RN). Thereafter, nurses can become licensed in other states using a process called licensure by endorsement.

Diploma Programs. In the United States, the diploma nursing program is a 2- or 3-year program frequently affiliated with a hospital. However, some diploma programs are associated with a college or university and students receive college credit for all nonnursing classes. The programs retain some of the apprenticeship traditions of the past and prepare nurses for a high technical level of practice. The number of diploma programs has drastically declined over the past few decades as the programs either close or become associate degree–granting programs.

Associate Degree Programs. Associate degree programs are 2-year programs offered by community colleges as well as by other colleges and universities. The program focus is on scientific and practical courses in nursing. Upon graduation, students receive an associate degree in nursing (ADN).

Baccalaureate Degree Programs. The basic baccalaureate nursing program is located within a university or college and requires 4 years of study, including general education courses. The focus is on achieving a level of critical inquiry, clinical judgment, decision-making ability, and clinical knowledge imperative for professional nursing practice.

Many baccalaureate programs admit RNs with previously earned diplomas or associate degrees. Some universities offer an independent study program (external degree) without class structure. Most baccalaureate nursing programs accept student transfer credits from accredited universities and colleges. Additionally, transferring students can take challenge examinations for college credit.

Graduate Degree Entry Programs. Master's and doctoral entry-level programs are offered by only a few universities. These programs prepare college graduates who have degrees in disciplines other than nursing to be entry-level nurse generalists with advanced knowledge and skill levels. These programs may offer tracks of specialization, such as for nurse practitioners, nurse administrators, and nurse midwives.

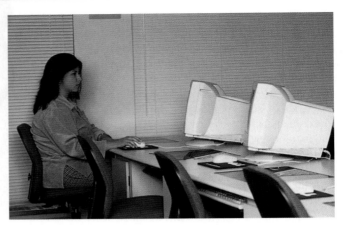

Figure 1-5. A graduate nurse taking the NCLEX-RN examination.

Regardless of their level of entry into the profession, graduates take the same NCLEX-RN (Figure 1-5).

Advanced Practice Education

Today, more nurses are earning master's and doctoral degrees to increase their nursing knowledge and expertise. These advanced degrees are also useful for those who wish to provide leadership in the policy-making arena of health care, in clinical practice and administration.

Master's Degree Programs. Master's degree programs in nursing, which usually take about 2 years to complete, prepare advanced practice nurses, such as nurse practitioners or clinical nurse specialists, nurse educators, and nurse administrators. Special emphasis is given to advanced scientific concepts and clinical practice. Theory and research in nursing form the foundation of the curriculum. As advanced practice roles evolve both in the United States and in the international nursing community, additional research will be needed to document the effectiveness of these roles (Ketefian, Redman, Hanucharurnkul, Masterson, & Neves, 2001).

Doctoral Degree Programs. A nurse doctorate requires in-depth inquiry and scientific research into a specific field of learning. Doctoral programs produce nurse philosophers, ethicists, theorists, and researchers. Many universities now require that nursing faculty members hold doctoral degrees. Clinical agencies are beginning to ask for nurses with doctorates to serve as nurse executives or directors of education and research. Professional organizations are also looking to nurses with doctoral degrees to represent them to those who make decisions about health policy and even to consumers.

Continuing Education

Continuing education (CE) is a term used to describe programs or courses that assist professional nurses in developing and maintaining the clinical expertise that promotes quality nursing care. CE is designed to enhance knowledge and skills in practice, administration, research, and education. CE for nurses is offered in workshops, institutes, short courses, conferences, telecourses, evening courses, and even supplements in professional nursing journals. The use of computers as resources for CE is growing rapidly. It is mandatory in many states to obtain a certain number of contact hours or continuing education units (CEUs) within each year or registration cycle to maintain professional licensure. A CE program may be approved to grant contact hours or CEUs if it meets certain criteria set by an approving authority.

CE should not be confused with **in-service programs,** which are designed to increase knowledge and skills needed for nursing practice in a particular agency. Topics for in-service programs often relate to new policies, procedures, or equipment.

PROFESSIONAL NURSING PRACTICE

Standards of Professional Nursing

Professionalism is behavior that upholds the status, methods, character, and standards of a given profession. But what is a profession? According to Kelly (1981), a profession has the following eight characteristics:

- The services provided are vital to human beings and the welfare of society.
- There exists a special body of knowledge that undergoes continual growth through research.
- The services provided involve intellectual activities and individual responsibility or accountability.
- Practitioners receive education in institutions of higher learning.
- Practitioners have autonomy and control their own policies and activities.
- Practitioners are motivated by the service they provide and consider their work important to their lives (altruism).
- Practitioners' decisions and conduct are guided by a code of ethics.
- High standards of practice are encouraged and supported by an organization.

These characteristics distinguish professions from some other careers or occupations.

States and provinces regulate the professional practice of nursing through nurse practice acts, which legally define the scope of nursing practice in a given state. Even though nurse practice acts differ somewhat from state to state, they are similar in that they serve to protect the public by regulating and monitoring standards of practice and by ensuring that minimum standards for entry into the nursing profession are met. These same activities help meet the needs of the nursing profession as well.

Standards of nursing practice are a set of nursing actions that are generally agreed on by nurses as constituting safe and effective client care. They establish the foundation for the professional practice of RNs. The development and implementation of these standards are major functions of nursing's professional organizations. Chapter 10 further discusses standards of clinical nursing practice. Appendix A provides the American Nurses' Association Standards of Clinical Nursing Practice.

Professional Nursing Organizations

According to Merton (1958), "A professional organization is an organization of practitioners who judge one another as professionally competent and who have banded together to perform social functions which they cannot perform in their separate capacities as individuals." Thus the professional organization deals with events of concern to the profession.

Nursing organizations set standards for nursing practice and education. Active involvement in nursing organizations enhances a sense of professional commitment. Clearly, these organizations empower nurses through educational programs and professional publications. The functions of a nursing professional organization include the following:

- To establish, maintain, and improve nursing standards
- To hold all members accountable for using nursing standards
- To educate the public to appreciate the nursing standards
- To protect the public from individuals who have not attained or who willfully do not follow the standards of nursing practice
- To protect individual members of the profession from one another

Once standards of nursing practice are put into effect, they are used to monitor licensure, accreditation, certification, quality assurance, peer review, and public policy as these factors relate to the profession of nursing (Phaneuf & Lang, 1985).

In North America, there are two similar professional organizations for registered nurses. One is the American Nurses' Association. Its members are state nurses' associations and individual nurses belonging to the state organization. The ANA sponsors workshops for nurses and publishes the *American Journal of Nursing.* The ANA also offers specialty certification (Box 1-1, p. 10).

The ANA is part of the International Council of Nurses (ICN), which promotes international associations of nurses and improves nursing practice standards while seeking higher status for nurses. The council provides nurses with an international power base.

The National League for Nursing (NLN) is a nonprofessional nursing organization. Nurses on any level, and even nonnurses, can join this organization, as can nursing agencies. The organization's main function is to promote increased development of nursing services and education in nursing.

The National Student Nurses Association (NSNA) is the pre-professional organization for student nurses in the United States. A requirement for membership in this organization is enrollment in a state-approved nursing education program.

Other organizations include the American Academy of Nurses (AAN), whose purpose is to recognize nurses who have made major contributions to the profession of nursing. The international honor society for nursing, Sigma Theta Tau, is a member of the Association of College Honor Societies. Students in baccalaureate, master's, doctoral, and postdoctoral programs are eligible to be inducted as members.

Specialty nursing organizations support specialty practice and often provide certification in their areas (Box 1-2, p. 11). These organizations focus on specific areas of nursing practice such as oncology nursing. They strive to improve the standards of practice and welfare of nurses in that specialty.

Box 1-1   American Nurses' Association Certifications

ADVANCED PRACTICE CERTIFICATION

APRN, BC (Advanced Practice Registered Nurse, Board Certified)   A current registered nurse license from the U.S. or its territories and a master's or higher degree in nursing for the specialty is required. Educational program must include a minimum of 500 hours of supervised clinical practice. Criteria for specific specialties are presented in application catalogs.

Nurse Practitioners

- Acute Care Nurse Practitioner
- Adult Nurse Practitioner
- Family Nurse Practitioner
- Gerontological Nurse Practitioner
- Pediatric Nurse Practitioner
- Adult Psychiatric and Mental Health Nurse Practitioner
- Family Psychiatric and Mental Health Nurse Practitioner

Clinical Nurse Specialists

- Clinical Nurse Specialist in Community Health Nursing
- Clinical Nurse Specialist in Gerontological Nursing
- Clinical Nurse Specialist in Home Health Nursing
- Clinical Nurse Specialist in Medical-Surgical Nursing
- Clinical Nurse Specialist in Pediatric Nursing
- Clinical Nurse Specialist in Adult Psychiatric and Mental Health Nursing
- Clinical Nurse Specialist in Child/Adolescent Psychiatric and Mental Health Nursing

NURSING ADMINISTRATION, ADVANCED

RN, CNAA, BC (Register Nurse, Certified in Nursing Administration, Advanced, Board Certified)   A master's degree is required. You must complete the equivalent of 24 months of full-time practice and 30 contact hours in the specialty.

Advanced Diabetes Management for Nurses, Dietitians, and Pharmacists   A current professional license and master's degree is required. You must complete at least 800 hours of direct clinical diabetes management; however, exceptions (refer to catalog) apply depending on licensure.

- RN, BC-ADM (Masters prepared nurses who are not Nurse Practitioners or Clinical Nurse Specialists)
- APRN, BC-ADM (Clinical Nurse Specialist and Nurse Practitioner)
- RD, BC-ADM (Registered Dietitian)
- RPh, BC-ADM (Pharmacist)

DIPLOMA AND ASSOCIATE DEGREE CERTIFICATION

RN, C (Registered Nurse, Certified)   A current registered nurse license from the U.S. or its territories and a diploma or associate degree in nursing is required. You must have practiced the equivalent of 2 years full time as a nurse with a minimum of 2000 practice hours and 30 contact hours in the last 3 years.

- Cardiac/Vascular Nurse
- Gerontological Nurse
- Medical-Surgical Nurse
- Pediatric Nurse
- Perinatal Nurse
- Psychiatric and Mental Health Nurse

BACCALAUREATE AND HIGHER LEVEL CERTIFICATION

RN, BC (Registered Nurse, Board Certified)   A current registered nurse license from the U.S. or its territories and bachelor's degree in nursing is required. You must have practiced a minimum of 2 years with at least 2000 hours of practice in the specialty and 30 contact hours in the 3 years proceeding application.

- Cardiac/Vascular Nurse
- College Health Nurse
- Community Health Nurse
- General Nursing Practice
- Gerontological Nurse
- Home Health Nurse
- Medical-Surgical Nurse
- Nursing Professional Development
- Pediatric Nurse
- Perinatal Nurse
- Psychiatric and Mental Health Nurse

INFORMATICS

RN, C or RN, BC (Registered Nurse, Certified or Board Certified) Credential depends on whether baccalaureate degree is in nursing. A bachelor's degree in nursing or relevant discipline is required. You must complete at least 2000 hours of practice within the last 3 years.

NURSING ADMINISTRATION

RN, CNA, BC (Registered Nurse, Certified in Nursing Administration, Board Certified)   A bachelor's degree in nursing is required. You must complete the equivalent of 24 months of full-time practice and 30 contact hours in the specialty within the 5-year period of application.

MODULAR CERTIFICATION

RN, C (Registered Nurse, Certified)

*Eligibility **with** Core Nursing Certification*—A current registered nurse license from the U.S. or its territories and proof of a current, nationally recognized, core nursing specialty certification is required. You must complete at least 2,000 hours of practice in the specialty within the last 2 years.

*Eligibility **without** Core Nursing Certification*—A current registered nurse license from the U.S. or its territories. You must complete at least 2,000 hours of practice in the specialty within the last 2 years.

- Ambulatory Care Nursing
- Nursing Case Management

From **American Nurses Credentialing Center.** (January 2003). Certification brochure. Washington, DC: Author. www.nursecredentialing.org

---

The National Federation for Specialty Nursing Organizations (NFSNO) represents the largest number of registered nurses practicing in the United States. The organization's goal is to promote excellence in specialty nursing practice. Approximately 39 organizations are members. Membership consists of two representatives from each organization plus representatives from the ANA and the NLN.

Professional Nursing Roles

In the past, a nurse's role consisted of providing care and comfort to clients and performing specific nursing functions. The role of modern nursing has expanded to include a heightened emphasis on illness prevention, health promotion, and concern for the client's holism. Today's nurse engages in approximately eight interrelated roles: caregiver, advocate, crit-

Box 1-2 Examples of Specialty Organization Certifications*

American Association of Critical Care Nurses (AACN)
  Certified Critical Care Registered Nurse (CCRN)
American Association of Occupational Health Nurses (AAOHN)
  Certified Occupational Health Nurse (COHN)
American Association of Nurse Anesthetists (AANA)
  Certified Registered Nurse Anesthetist (CRNA)
American College of Nurse Midwives (ACNM)
  Certified Nurse Midwife (CNM)
American Society of PeriAnesthesia Nurses (ASPAN)
  Certified Post-Anesthesia Nurse (CPAN)
Association of Operating Room Nurses (AORN)
  Certified Nurse Operating Room (CNOR)
Association for Practitioners in Infection Control (APIC)
  Certified in Infection Control (CIC)
Association of Rehabilitation Nurses (ARN)
  Certified Rehabilitation Registered Nurse (CRRN)
Emergency Nurses' Association (ENA)
  Certified Emergency Nurse (CEN)
International Association for Enterostomal Therapy (AET)
  Certified Enterostomal Therapy Nurse (CETN)

National Association of Pediatric Nurse Associates/Practitioners (NAPNAP)
  Certified Pediatric Nurse Practitioner (CPNP)
National Association of School Nurses (NASN)
  Certified School Nurse (CSN)
Oncology Nursing Society (ONS)
  Oncology Certified Nurse (OCN)
The Organization for Obstetric, Gynecologic, and Neonatal Nurses (NAACOG)
  Reproductive Nurse Certified (RNC)
    Ambulatory Women's Health Care
    High-Risk Obstetric Nurse
    Inpatient Obstetric Nurse
    Low-Risk Neonatal Nurse
    Maternal Newborn Nurse
    Neonatal Intensive Care Nurse
    Reproductive Endocrinology/Infertility Nurse
  Neonatal Nurse Practitioner (NP)
  Ob/Gyn Nurse Practitioner (NP)
  Women's Health Care Nurse Practitioner (NP)

*Certificates may be awarded by closely related, but separate and independent, organizations.

ical thinker, teacher, communicator, manager, researcher, and rehabilitator.

CAREGIVER. The nurse addresses the client's holistic health care needs to promote health and the healing process. In the role of caregiver, the nurse provides treatment for specific disease processes and applies measures to restore the emotional and social well-being of the client.

ADVOCATE. The nurse protects the client by preventing physical and/or chemical injury. In the role of **client advocate,** the nurse assists clients in expressing their rights whenever necessary. The nurse also works to preserve clients' legal and human rights in times of health and illness, and during the process of dying. Chapter 2 discusses the legal and ethical contexts of nursing practice.

CRITICAL THINKER. Nurses use decision-making and critical thinking skills in conjunction with the nursing process. Before actually delivering nursing care, the nurse plans the best method of care delivery for each client. Refer to Chapter 5 for additional information on critical thinking and clinical judgment.

TEACHER. The nurse provides clients and family members with information about health, treatment or therapy, and lifestyle changes. As a teacher, the nurse determines if the client understands the information presented and reinforces the learning as necessary. The nurse then evaluates the client's progress toward health-related goals. The nurse uses teaching methods that are compatible with the client's knowledge, education, and literacy levels. For more in-depth information, refer to Chapter 13.

COMMUNICATOR. Open and consistent communication is vital for effective nursing practice. The nurse must possess excellent communication skills to provide care, rehabilitation, teaching, comfort, and protection to clients.

MANAGER. Nurses are responsible for the management and coordination of client care. All nurses need good man-

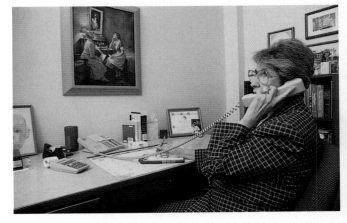

Figure 1-6. Whether a nurse serves as a nurse–manager or as a manager of assistive personnel, management skills are essential.

agement skills, whether they supervise others in the provision of nursing care or whether they provide direct care themselves (Figure 1-6). Chapter 14 will further describe the role of the nurse as manager.

RESEARCHER. Nursing research provides the evolving body of knowledge and theory for our profession. Research nurses may be employed in an academic area, a community agency, or an independent professional agency. The nurse researcher usually conducts studies and investigates problems to improve client health and nursing care. A graduate degree in nursing is usually the minimal educational requirement, although many nurse generalists participate in research. Chapter 15 discusses nursing research as a tool for professional practice.

REHABILITATOR. Ensuring that a client returns to a maximal state of functioning requires rehabilitative activities administered by nurses along with members of other disciplines, such as physical therapy. When clients experience alterations in health, the nurse's role is to promote client adaptation and coping.

CONTINUING EVOLUTION

Now is an exciting time to enter the profession of nursing. Nursing will continue to evolve into the 21st century as the health care delivery system develops in response to social and political pressure.

Nursing's political agenda is a critical element in maintaining nursing's mission of high quality health care.

Nursing and the Health Care Delivery System

In the United States, health care is one of the largest industries. The health care delivery system is a complicated social organization, a unique and interdependent system that provides health care for individuals, families, and groups. Health care providers in this system are professionals or paraprofessionals with special education in health care delivery.

The most common setting for nurses in health care delivery continues to be the acute care hospital, although many sources have predicted that, over time, the number of nurses employed in hospitals will continue to decline. Approximately 59% of RNs employed in nursing in the year 2000 were working in hospitals (Health Resources and Service Administration, 2002).

Nonetheless, the health care delivery system comprises many other entities such as clinics, practice associations, schools, industries, long-term care facilities, military facilities, independent practitioners' offices, and home health agencies. Noninstitutional settings had the largest percentage gain in RN employment from 1980 to 2000. The number of RNs employed in public health and community settings increased by 155% between 1980 and 2000, and the number employed in ambulatory care increased by 127% (Health Resources and Service Administration, 2002). These trends are expected to continue as health care delivery continues to shift into community-based settings.

Individuals who receive nursing care are often referred to as consumers, patients, or clients. The term is largely determined by the health care setting. A consumer is an individual, group, or community that uses a service. Thus anyone using health care services or products becomes a health care consumer. A patient is an individual who is waiting to receive, or is undergoing, care and medical treatment. A client is an individual who employs the services of another who is qualified to provide the desired service. More information on health care delivery systems is in Chapter 4.

Social Issues Affecting Nursing

Technological advances, demographic changes, and various social movements are current challenges facing nursing in the 21st century. Since World War II, technological advances in equipment, drugs, testing procedures, and treatment modalities have increasingly affected health care delivery. Nursing has integrated these technological advances while still focusing on client needs. Nursing has also assisted clients to adapt to the use of technology in their care.

Demographic changes, such as the population's increasing life span and the growing incidence of chronic long-term illness, have affected health care delivery. In the United States in 1998, approximately 7% of the population were between the ages of 65 and 74, 4.4% were between the ages of 75 and 84, and 1.5% were age 85 and older (U.S. Census Bureau, 1999). This increasingly older population is mainly a result of effective health promotion and disease prevention techniques. However, although elderly people are living longer, many over 65 have multiple-system medical problems and one or more chronic illnesses. Therefore geriatric nursing and home health care have become increasingly important nursing specialties.

Beginning in the 1960s, society has increasingly scrutinized health care services. The initial consumer movement in health care sought to address the dehumanization of health care services. Over the last few decades, consumer groups have demanded controls on spiraling health care costs. This has prompted diversification in the financing of health care, such as HMOs and new types of health insurance. Additionally, health care consumers are now more aware of "client rights," such as the right to information. Nurses also continue to support clients' rights by acting as client advocates. Finally, consumers are focusing increasingly on health promotion and illness prevention. The nursing community has responded by developing nursing curricula, community programs, specialized health promotion, and preventive teaching for clients in these two areas.

The women's movement in this century has greatly influenced society. Female clients have assumed more responsibility for their own care. Also, women's health issues are receiving more attention and more research than even a decade ago. The movement has also influenced nursing by inspiring nurses to pursue more autonomy and accountability in their clients' care.

The human rights movement in the last half of the 20th century is changing society's attitude toward people who are not representative of the dominant culture or who have special health care needs. Nurses recognize and respond to these clients' special needs by providing holistic care. In addition, advocates lobby for legislation to ensure that all clients receive quality care without sacrificing autonomy, dignity, or other basic human rights. Many schools of nursing have included the study of cultural diversity as a component of the curriculum to enable nurses to provide care that takes into account client needs and preferences based on culture.

Nursing's Political Agenda

Politics have always permeated the health care delivery system and the profession of nursing. Today nurses are involved in politics within the work environment, professional nursing organizations, and the community, and at the level of government.

In the 1960s, women involved in the feminist movement believed that anyone could utilize personal experience to understand and become involved in the bigger political picture and issues. The personalization of the political process has become a fundamental principle of professional nursing.

Before the 1970s, nurses were not organized. Therefore they had very little influence on legislation involving health care (Doheny, et al., 1987). The development of nursing's formalized political action and the establishment of the Nurses Coalition for Action in Politics (N-CAP) in 1974 as a political arm of the ANA changed that. The ANA now has a political action committee, ANA-PAC, which endorses candidates who have exhibited voting records and demonstrated leadership consistent with ANA's political agenda. Endorsement by a group that represents 1.7 million potential voters is important to any candidate; however, nursing's political message is not always heard as one voice. The major nursing associations have formed a special tri-council to present a united front so that nursing will carry more political weight and have a louder voice.

Until recent years, nurses lacked the political education needed to advance in politics (Mason & Talbott, 1985). Nursing curricula now support nurses' involvement in politics. Professional nursing organizations are also encouraging political involvement. Lobbyists have been employed by many professional nursing organizations to persuade Congress and state legislatures to increase the quality of health care and to address state and federal nursing issues. Nurses are increasingly being elected into political offices.

Nursing in the 21st Century

For the nursing graduate, the future holds numerous social, technological, and political changes. The coming changes will shape nursing into a stronger and more efficacious profession if nursing prepares itself for predicted future trends.

Technology will continue to develop rapidly. Nursing informatics will revolutionize nursing (Figure 1-7). The frontline clinician will be required to access new information systems and store, retrieve, and interpret client care data. The Internet will increasingly allow nurses to be part of a global network of people (researchers, families, nurses, and people with disease) all sharing new health information. Nurses will also help consumers to access the information they need and will provide them with the knowledge to use it.

Other technological advances, such as genetic engineering, implanted ambulatory monitoring devices, new imaging devices, medical artificial intelligence techniques (such as computer-assisted surgery), and more precise techniques for electrocardiographic and fetal monitoring, will have a large impact on nursing. Nursing has already evolved to a point where many nurses are comfortable utilizing sophisticated technology while focusing on meeting the human needs of clients.

During the 21st century, societies will continue to move toward globalization, with an increased sharing of products, attitudes, and financial investments. Third-world countries will develop and contribute enormously to the global market (Chitty, 2001). There will be a blending of many cultural lifestyles. Social changes throughout the world and the global response to terrorism are likely to modify the profession of nursing.

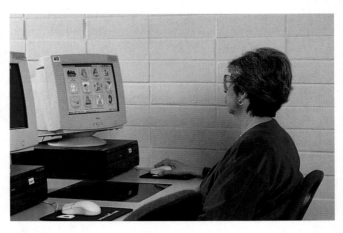

Figure 1-7. In the 21st century, nursing informatics will revolutionize nursing, and computer skills will be essential to nurses at every level of practice.

Clients will continue to make increasingly independent choices about their health care services and settings. They may be more likely to combine conventional therapies with complementary healing techniques, such as homeopathy, neuropathy, therapeutic touch, reflexology, Qigong, acupressure, aromatherapy, kinesiology, and nutritional therapy. Sibbald (1995) and other experts on nursing and health care also predict the following:

- Neighborhoods will employ nurses who will work in 24-hour nurse-managed clinics.
- Nurse practitioners will cross medical thresholds to provide services usually provided by physicians.
- Nurse therapists and nurse entrepreneurs will provide numerous services for clients and their families.
- Rather than working for one hospital, nurses will be employed by a "service" made up of several institutions.
- Hospital stays will be exceedingly short, and early discharge will become even more important.
- Nurses will be strong and autonomous practitioners whose practice and care delivery focuses much more on health than on illness.

Of course, all of these predictions will greatly influence nursing education and care delivery. It will be important for you as a new nurse to use your knowledge, your skills, and the results of ongoing nursing research to provide the best care possible to clients. It will also be important to become involved in professional organizations and communicate with legislators to help shape the future of the nursing profession.

Key Principles

- Nursing is an accountable profession guided by science, theory, a code of ethics, and the art of care and comfort to treat human responses to health and illness. Nursing practice puts the science and art of nursing into action.
- The early history of nursing was heavily influenced by religion and by war.

- Florence Nightingale is considered the founder of modern nursing. Because Nightingale made rounds carrying an oil lamp, she became known as "the Lady with the lamp." This became her trademark and remains the symbol of the nursing profession worldwide.
- There are currently four types of educational programs that prepare students for entry into practice of professional registered nursing: the diploma program, the associate degree program, the baccalaureate degree program, and graduate degree entry programs.
- A registered nurse license is granted after the candidate completes an accredited program of nursing and satisfactorily completes the National Council Licensing Examination for Registered Nurses (NCLEX-RN).
- Graduate nursing programs improve nursing through advancement of theory and science by preparing nurses, clinicians, practitioners, educators, researchers, and administrators.
- Continuing professional education promotes continued quality and competency in nurses as they provide health care services to the public.
- Nurses function in a variety of roles that are not mutually exclusive but often occur together. Understanding the roles helps to clarify the nurse's responsibilities.
- Professional and nonprofessional nursing organizations and associations fulfill essential functions for the profession as well as for the individual nurse.
- Developments such as alternative methods of health care delivery, the continuing impact of health care costs, and efforts toward health care reform have led to nurses being more politically active and aware.
- An awareness of nursing history provides a context for understanding important nursing concerns such as autonomy, professional unity, education, and current practice, which can in turn promote further growth of the profession.

Bibliography

*American Nurses' Association. (1987). *The scope of nursing practice*. Kansas City, MO: Author.

*American Nurses' Association. (1995). *Nursing's social policy statement*. Washington, DC: Author.

American Nurses' Association. (1998). *Standards of clinical nursing practice* (2nd ed.). Washington, DC: Author.

American Nurses' Association. (2003) *Standards of clinical nursing practice*. (3rd ed.). Washington, DC: Author.

American Nurses' Credentialing Center. (2001). *Certification catalog*. Washington, DC: Author.

*Carnegie, M. E. (1986). *The path we tread: Blacks in nursing, 1854-1984*. Philadelphia: Lippincott.

Chitty, K. K. (2001). *Professional nursing: Concepts and challenges* (3rd ed.). Philadelphia: Saunders.

*Cohen, L. B. (1984). Florence Nightingale. *Scientific American 250*(128), 137.

*Conway-Welch, C. (1996). Who is tomorrow's nurse and where will tomorrow's nurse be educated? *Nursing and Health Care: Perspectives on Community 17*, 286-290.

Deloughery, G. (1998). *Issues and trends in nursing* (3rd ed.). St Louis, MO: Mosby.

*Dock, H. K., & Stewart, I. M. (1925). *A short history of nursing* (3rd ed.). New York: Putnam.

*Doheny, M., Cook, C., & Stopper, C. (1987). *The discipline of nursing: An introduction* (2nd ed.). Norwalk, CT: Appleton & Lange.

*Donahue, M. P. (1996). *Nursing: The finest art—an illustrated history* (2nd ed.). St Louis, MO: Mosby.

*Hamilton, P. M. (1996). *Realities of contemporary nursing* (2nd ed.). Menlo Park, CA: Addison-Wesley.

Health Resources and Service Administration. (2002). *Seventh National Sample Survey of Registered Nurses*. Retrieved July 27, 2002, from http://bhpr.hrsa.gov/healthworkforce/rnsurvey/.

Humphrey, C. J. (2001). Nursing rated most ethical profession. *Home Healthcare Nurse 19*(2), 63.

*Jamieson, E. M., Sewall, M. F., & Gjertson, L. S. (1959). *Trends in nursing history* (5th ed.). Philadelphia: Saunders.

*Jensen, D., Spaulding, J., & Cody, E. (1955). *History and trends of professional nursing* (4th ed.). St Louis, MO: Mosby.

*Kalisch, P., & Kalisch, B. J. (1986). *The advance of American nursing* (2nd ed.). Boston: Little, Brown.

*Kelly, L. (1981). *Dimensions of professional nursing* (4th ed.). New York: Macmillan.

Kenner, C. (2001). Nursing: One strong voice? *Nursing Outlook, 49*(6), 283.

Ketefian, S., Redman, R. W., Hanucharurnkul, S., Masterson, A., & Neves, E. P. (2001). The development of advanced practice roles: Implications in the international nursing community. *International Nursing Review, 48*, 152-163.

*Mason, D. J., & Talbott, S. W. (1985). *Political action handbook for nurses*. Menlo Park, CA: Addison-Wesley.

*Merton, R. K. (1958). The function of the professional organization. *American Journal of Nursing, 58*, 50-54.

*Miraldo, P. S. (1991). The nineties: A decade in search of meaning. *Nursing and Health Care, 11*(1), 221.

*Montag, M. (1951). *The education of nursing technicians*. New York: Putnam.

Murphy, M. C., & Gosselin, T. (2001). A vision of unity: Nurses must seek professional unity and respect through education. *American Journal of Nursing,* April (Suppl), 44-46, 49-50, inside back cover.

*National League for Nursing. (1990). *Nursing in America: A history of social reform* [videotape]. New York: Author.

*Nightingale, F. (1860). *Notes on nursing: What it is, and what it is not*. London: Harrison. (Reprinted in F. L. A. Bishop & S. Goldie. [1962]. *A bio-bibliography of Florence Nightingale*. London: Dawsons of Pall Mall.)

*Phaneuf, M. C., & Lang, M. (1985). *Issues in professional nursing practice: Standards of nursing practice*. Kansas City, MO: Author.

Salmon, M. E. (1999). Thoughts on nursing: Where it has been and where it is going. *Nursing and Health Care Perspectives, 20*(1), 20-25.

*Schraeder, B. D. (1988). Entry-level graduate education in nursing: Master of Science programs. In *Perspectives in nursing, 1987-1989*. New York: Author.

*Selevan, L. C. (1984). Nurses in American history: The revolution. In *Pages from nursing history: A collection of original articles from the pages of Nursing Outlook, the American Journal of Nursing and Nursing Research*. New York: American Journal of Nursing.

*Sibbald, B. (1995). 2020 vision of nursing. *Canadian Nurse, 91*(3), 33-36.

*Smith, F. T. (1984). Florence Nightingale: Early feminist. In *Pages from nursing history: A collection of original articles from the pages of Nursing Outlook, the American Journal of Nursing and Nursing Research*. New York: American Journal of Nursing.

U.S. Bureau of the Census. (1999). *Statistical abstract of the United States, 1999* (119th ed.). Washington, DC: Author.

*Woodham-Smith, C. (1951). *Florence Nightingale*. New York: McGraw-Hill.

*Asterisk indicates a classic or definitive work on this subject.

2

Legal and Ethical Context of Practice

Key Terms

accreditation
administrative law
advance directive
assault
autonomy
battery
beneficence
certification
civil law
common law
confidentiality
contract
credentialing
criminal law
defamation
defendant
durable power
  of attorney
  for health care
ethics
false imprisonment
fidelity
fraud

informed consent
invasion of privacy
justice
law
liability
license
living will
malpractice
morals
negligence
nonmaleficence
plaintiff
procedural law
professional
  misconduct
public law
registration
statutory law
substantive law
tort
values
values clarification
veracity

Learning Objectives

After studying this chapter, you should be able to do the following:

- Describe examples of the sources and types of law in nursing practice
- Describe the professional sources of regulation of nursing practice
- Describe the legal sources of regulation of nursing practice
- Apply ethical principles to clarify values and make decisions in nursing
- Discuss selected client rights and their influence on nursing practice
- Describe two initiatives to improve the quality of nursing care delivered to clients
- Summarize actions that can be taken to safeguard one's own nursing practice

Decision making in nursing practice involves the interplay of multiple systems of ethics and legal issues. Ethics is the system of beliefs about what is right or wrong in human conduct; it involves moral conduct and moral judgment. Law is the system of man-made rules and regulations by which a society is governed and through which people can live together. Our actions are at times determined primarily by laws, at times by ethics, and at times by a combination of the two.

Ethical decision making involves the nurse's personal value system, the client's value system, and a professional code of ethics. Personal values may conflict when the client's life choices contributed to a chronic illness, an unmarried teenage girl gives birth to a baby, or an emergency room client refuses a life-saving transfusion of blood. Resolving ethical or moral dilemmas in nursing practice requires an understanding of ethical principles and decision making. Further assistance is found in the well-established concepts of informed consent, advanced directives, a nursing code of ethics, and other professional guidelines.

In some cases, consensus on a moral or ethical dilemma has been reached by a majority in our society, and the consensus has been written into law. Abortion, though considered morally wrong by some, is nevertheless legal. Assisted suicide, viewed by some as morally right, remains illegal. The development of a law lags behind discussion about the best course of action, as illustrated by national debates on euthanasia, the medical use of marijuana, stem cell research, and other issues posing medical–ethical dilemmas. Doing what is ethically right and acting within the law requires continual re-examination of our practice.

A clear understanding of the responsibilities and obligations imposed by law is essential to the safe, effective practice of professional nursing. As you begin your pursuit of a career in nursing, legal directives dictate the educational and entry requirements that you must fulfill before you can practice. Likewise, laws define various roles within nursing, including those of the licensed practical nurse, the registered professional nurse, the nurse anesthetist, the nurse midwife, and the nurse practitioner. Laws also regulate reimbursement by third-party payers for these services.

Also found within the law are guidelines for the practice of professional nursing and sanctions that can be imposed when nursing practice fails to meet minimum standards. Finally, the basis for lawsuits involving your professional practice is found in the law. Understanding the legal and ethical context of your practice of professional nursing is essential to providing safe, efficient, and comprehensive care to your clients. This chapter is a broad overview of the legal and professional guidelines and the ethical considerations that will influence your practice of nursing.

CONCEPTS OF LAW

Law is a body of rules of action or conduct prescribed by a "controlling authority," in this case the government. The Constitution of the United States created three branches of government and granted them the power to create "rules of action or conduct" governing many of the interactions between individual persons, between people and government, between people and businesses, between one business and another, and between one government and another.

A prescribed hierarchy of power exists within the levels of government, with the federal government having the highest authority. Thus local law cannot contradict or be inconsistent with state law, and state law must be congruent with federal law.

Sources of Law

Four sources of law exist at both the state and the federal level. They are the constitutions and the three branches of government (Figure 2-1). Laws arising from each of these sources come into being, and are modified or eliminated, through a process unique to the source. You need to understand the source of laws if you want to become involved in creating, modifying, or eliminating a law that regulates nursing practice.

The federal and state constitutions establish and outline the limits of power at different levels of government. Additionally, the constitutions grant broad individual rights and responsibilities. Some of the rights particularly pertinent to nursing practice are the rights of privacy, freedom of speech, and due process. The right of privacy is embodied in your obligation to maintain client confidentiality. Freedom of speech relates to a professional registered nurse's right and obligation to share information with clients. Due process gives protection to individuals and guides execution of disciplinary proceedings.

The legislative branch of government is an elected body of people who are chosen to represent the interests of their constituents. The federal and state legislatures write laws, or statutes, known as **statutory law.** Examples of these laws that affect health care and nursing include nurse practice acts and the laws that created Medicare and Medicaid.

The executive branch of government has the dual responsibility of establishing the details of laws enacted by state or federal legislatures and ensuring the enforcement of laws. The executive branch works through various administrative agencies, such as the departments of health, housing, and education.

Administrative agencies, whether state or federal, are empowered to establish administrative rules and regulations through specific hearings and rule-making procedures. The resulting rules and regulations, known as **administrative law,** conform to enacted law (i.e., statutory law) and provide the detail necessary to implement them. For example, statutory laws establish the profession of nursing and the authority for administrative functions of the state boards of nursing. State boards of nursing provide the rules and regulations detailing how the profession of nursing will be practiced in each state. These rules and regulations are enforceable as law.

The judicial branch of government is responsible for resolving disputes and interpreting all types of laws. The accumulated judicial decisions have created a body of law known as *judicial, case, decisional,* or *common law.*

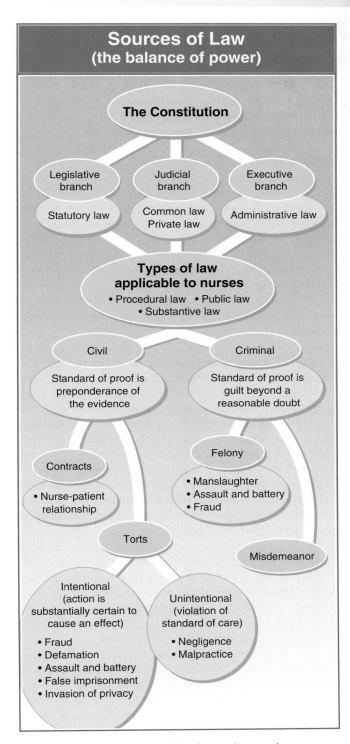

Sources of Law
(the balance of power)

The Constitution

Legislative branch

Judicial branch

Executive branch

Statutory law

Common law
Private law

Administrative law

Types of law
applicable to nurses
• Procedural law • Public law
• Substantive law

Civil

Criminal

Standard of proof is preponderance of the evidence

Standard of proof is guilt beyond a reasonable doubt

Felony

Contracts

• Manslaughter
• Assault and battery
• Fraud

• Nurse-patient relationship

Torts

Misdemeanor

Intentional (action is substantially certain to cause an effect)

Unintentional (violation of standard of care)

• Fraud
• Defamation
• Assault and battery
• False imprisonment
• Invasion of privacy

• Negligence
• Malpractice

Figure 2-1. Sources of law for nursing practice.

Types of Law

Laws differ in the topics they address, the procedures used to resolve disputes, and the remedies that are available. The types of law include administrative law, civil law, criminal law, common law, procedural law, public law, statutory law, and substantive law. These categories are not mutually exclusive, nor is this listing the only way that various types of laws can be categorized. The practice of pro-

fessional nursing is touched by all types of laws in some way.

Civil Law. **Civil law** regulates disputes between individuals and between individuals and groups. The source of much of it is judicial or common law. Civil law includes laws relating to contracts and ownership of property. A common feature is that a monetary award is provided for damages or as compensation when another person causes injury.

Torts. A **tort** is a civil wrong committed by one person against another person or that person's property. It may be intentional or unintentional. When the tort is intentional, the injury suffered by the victim was intended by the wrongdoer. Intentional torts include fraud, defamation, false imprisonment, assault and battery, and invasion of privacy. Unintentional torts include negligence and professional malpractice.

INTENTIONAL TORTS

FRAUD. **Fraud** is the false representation of some fact with the intention that it will be acted upon by another person. It would be fraud for you as a nurse to falsely represent yourself to a client as being certified in a specialty area of nursing. It is fraud to include false statements about past employment on an employment application, or about academic credentials or professional activities on a resumé, for the purpose of deceiving the potential employer.

DEFAMATION. **Defamation** is either a false communication or a careless disregard for the truth that results in damage to someone's reputation. Defamation can take two forms: libel and slander. *Libel* is defamation that occurs through printing, writing, or the use of pictures. A nurse who makes false statements about a client or co-worker in the client's record or the local newspaper could be guilty of libel. *Slander* is spoken defamation either by making a false statement or by making a legally unprotected statement that damages a reputation. An example of slander is telling a client that another nurse is incompetent.

ASSAULT AND BATTERY. **Assault** is an attempt or a threat to touch another person unjustly. **Battery** is the actual willful touching of another person that may or may not cause harm. The terms assault and battery are distinct but are often heard together because an assault precedes a battery. A nurse who threatens a client with an injection or urinary catheterization could be found guilty of an assault. For a nurse to be guilty of battery, the touching must be wrong in some way, such as being done without permission, or done in a way that causes harm or embarrassment. The nurse who proceeds with an injection despite a client's objection could be guilty of battery.

FALSE IMPRISONMENT. **False imprisonment** involves restraining a person, with or without force, against that person's wishes. Detaining clients against their wishes, such as preventing a client from leaving a health care facility, could be false imprisonment. However, a different analysis may be applied to clients suffering from diseases that affect judgment, such as Alzheimer's disease, before determining that a nurse's action constituted false imprisonment.

A less obvious example of false imprisonment is the use of restraints in managing clients. The use of restraints relates not only to false imprisonment but also to the issue of maintaining client rights and dignity. Concerns about the inappropriate use of restraints have been great enough that some states have issued guidelines for their use. These guidelines require a thorough assessment of the client to determine the least restrictive measures to safely accomplish the goal for which restraints are being considered.

If a client or legal representative gives permission for the restraint, there is no liability for false imprisonment. You should carefully document in the client's record the circumstances resulting in permission to restrain, and undertake an ongoing assessment of the necessity for continued restraint.

Invasion of Privacy. Invasion of privacy can occur when the nurse unreasonably intrudes on the client's private affairs. Soliciting information not required for the client's care and discussing client information with persons not entitled to that information (such as employers or estranged spouses) are two examples of nursing actions that could be interpreted as invasion of privacy. Much information is acquired about a client in the course of providing nursing care. You must exercise prudence in using and sharing this information to protect the client's right to privacy.

Other acts could constitute invasion of privacy and expose you to liability as well. They include unnecessarily exposing a client during transportation between departments in a health facility, failing to ensure the anonymity of clients involved in research projects, or sharing information about social or rehabilitative services that your client is receiving.

In the course of providing care to clients, photographs are sometimes obtained. At a professional meeting you may be eager to share photographs of an interesting wound or other medical condition. Photographs with clients prominently featured may be used to advertise the opening of a new health care facility. Without permission from the client, such photographs can be deemed an invasion of privacy. Similarly, observing a procedure done to a client is an invasion of privacy if consent has not been obtained.

UNINTENTIONAL TORTS

Negligence. Negligence occurs when harm or injury is caused by an act of either omission or commission by a layperson. Negligence can also result from failure to use the kind of care a reasonably prudent layperson would use in a similar situation. Examples include carelessly failing to lock the brakes on a wheelchair before transferring a client, leaving an infant on an examining table without taking steps to prevent falling, and failing to take the temperature of a client who complains of feeling warm and lethargic.

Malpractice. Malpractice describes acts of negligence by a professional person as compared to the actions of another professional person in similar circumstances. The difference between negligence and malpractice is significant. Remember that, with negligence, the nurse is judged against what an ordinary, reasonable layperson would do or not do in similar circumstances.

Nurses can be held liable for negligence or malpractice. **Liability** implies a legal obligation for which the nurse can be held responsible and accountable. To prove liability for negligence or malpractice, each of four elements must be proven: duty, breach of duty, causation, and damages. *Duty* involves the obligation of the nurse to use due care; that is, to exercise the kind of care a reasonably prudent nurse would use. The kind of care appropriate for a particular client is defined by standards of care. *Breach of duty* is the failure to meet the standard of care. *Causation* is demonstrated when the failure to meet the standard of care results in harm to the client. Finally, for liability to be established, the client must have suffered an actual harm or injury, called *damages*. Table 2-1 provides examples of the elements of liability for malpractice.

The standard of care is derived from professional standards, legal regulation of nursing practice, and the employer's expectations for nursing practice. Together, these sources outline the kind of care a reasonably prudent nurse would provide for a particular type of client in a particular setting. Compare the following two nurses:

- Nurse A works in a high school. This nurse's practice is guided by, among other things, a nurse practice act, standards developed by the National Association of School Nurses, and the school nurse job description. When a high school student sustains a serious injury during football practice, the position requires giving first aid, calling an ambulance, and sending the client to the nearest emergency room.
- Nurse B works in an emergency room. The nurse practice act and the employer's job description also guide this nurse's practice. However, the teenager brought from the high school now needs definitive care. Nurse B will provide that care in accordance with standards established by the Emergency Nurses Association.

Liability can ensue for almost any activity involved in the practice of nursing. Further, no practice setting is exempt from potential malpractice litigation. However, there are areas in which allegations of malpractice against nurses occur more frequently. Some of the common areas of concern are outlined in Table 2-2.

When clients believe they have been injured as a result of a nurse's negligence or malpractice, they may start legal proceedings. The **plaintiff,** who is the party bringing a lawsuit, alleges certain facts and outcomes. The **defendant** is the person against whom a lawsuit is filed. The nurse, as defendant,

Table 2-1	Elements of Liability for Malpractice
Element	**Example**
Duty	The nurse is responsible for accurate assessment and timely reporting of changes in a client's condition.
Breach of duty	The nurse fails to note that a client's thumb is warm to touch, red, swollen, and painful.
Causation	Failure to note the signs and symptoms of an infection leads to amputation of the thumb.
Damage	Loss of the thumb seriously limits the client's use of the hand.

Table 2-2	Areas of Potential Liability for Nurses
Area	**Examples**
Failure to monitor and assess	• Failure to recognize significant changes in a client's condition • Failure to report significant changes in a client's condition. • Failure to obtain a complete database • Failure to monitor a client as indicated by the client's condition
Failure to ensure safety	• Inadequate monitoring of a client • Improper use of restrictive devices • Failure to identify a client's risk for injury • Inappropriate use of equipment
Medication errors	• Failure to question medication orders that are unclear • Failure to adhere to established procedures in medication administration • Failure to recognize adverse drug reactions • Lack of familiarity with medication • Lack of communication in verbal or written medication orders
Improper implementation of skills or procedures	• Failure to maintain currency in clinical skills • Failure to adhere to proper techniques • Failure to follow agency policy • Performance of unfamiliar skills • Failure to initiate appropriate actions based on assessment
Documentation errors	• Failure to document nursing actions • Failure to document information relevant to a client's condition • Failure to document in accordance with agency policies

must show that the plaintiff is unable to prove the four elements of negligence or malpractice liability. The procedures for malpractice litigation are complex. Nurses named in a lawsuit are always advised to seek their own legal representation even if their employer is also named as a defendant.

Settlement of the legal action can occur in one of three ways. The parties may negotiate a settlement out of court. A negotiated settlement does not necessarily mean the nurse is guilty of negligence or malpractice. However, the cost of litigation and the potential liability may suggest settlement as the best option. If there is no settlement, the case goes to court. Both plaintiff and defendant attempt to persuade the court to rule in their favor. After hearing all the facts and arguments, a decision regarding liability is made. A third possible method of settling a lawsuit in some states is to present the case to a malpractice arbitration panel.

If you are named in a lawsuit, obtain legal counsel and work closely with your attorney, who probably will want to be present at all discussions of the case, including those with representatives of your health care agency. If the agency requests information, review the request with your attorney before supplying information. Avoid discussion with the plaintiff, the plaintiff's attorney, and witnesses for the plaintiff. Do not attempt to alter or enhance the client's medical record. Rather, try to put in writing everything that you can remem-

ber about the case. Your attorney will advise you of your options in each phase of the litigation.

Contracts. A **contract** is an agreement between two or more individuals that creates certain rights and obligations in exchange for goods or services. Contracts can cover many of the services a nurse offers, either as an employee or as an independent provider of services. Nurse entrepreneurs provide many services, including writing books, providing health teaching, consulting on breastfeeding and infant care, and monitoring high-tech venous access devices. A portion of contract law specifically addresses contracts concerning the sale of goods, which is relevant when a nurse is purchasing goods or products for a business.

Contracts come in many forms; they can be oral or written, implied or express. Several elements must be met for a valid contract to exist. All parties must be capable of entering into a contract. Examples of people who lack capacity include minors and persons declared incompetent by a court. The legal term *mutual assent* is used to describe another element. It refers to the idea that the terms of the contract must be clearly communicated and accepted. *Consideration,* a legal term for giving something of value, is also a required element. Finally, offenses that could void the agreement, such as fraud, illegality, and misrepresentation, must be absent.

Whatever the form of a contract, questions can and often do arise concerning whether the parties entered into a legally enforceable contract. The obligations incurred under a contract have value for each party. Hence, if the question arises as to whether there actually was a contract, the answer has serious consequences for both parties.

Additional questions can arise even if there is a valid and enforceable contract in place. *Can the contract be assigned?* Assignment means that one of the parties gives his or her rights under a contract to another party. For example, instead of receiving payment for services, the nurse could request that the money be donated to a charity. *Can the contract be delegated?* Delegation transfers the duty or obligation under the contract to another person. For example, the nurse may agree to teach a cardiopulmonary resuscitation class but, in the event of illness, can delegate the responsibility to another nurse. Assignment or delegation can be limited by the terms of the contract.

Finally, legal disputes can occur when one party or the other fails to perform his or her obligations under the contract. A breach of contract results from a partial or total failure to fulfill one's obligations. When a breach occurs, the non-breaching party is entitled to damages. Remedies for a breach can include monetary payment or specific performance, which is a court-imposed requirement to perform as originally agreed.

Contract law directly or indirectly influences your practice of nursing. As nurses create new businesses, they are increasingly involved in situations that are governed by contract law. Contract law (and employment law) also governs the relationship between a nurse and an employer. A nurse who breaches contractual obligations faces monetary penalties or loss of employment but is usually not at risk of losing the license to practice nursing.

Criminal Law. **Criminal law** defines specific behaviors determined to be inappropriate in the orderly functioning of society. A crime is an act that violates the duties we owe to the community. Generally, statutory law creates our duties. Examples of criminal acts include larceny, homicide, manslaughter, rape, burglary, kidnapping, and arson.

Punishment for a criminal offense varies with the severity of the crime. Punishment may consist of a fine, probation, imprisonment, or death. A felony is a crime of a serious nature and is likely to be punished by imprisonment or death. A misdemeanor is a crime of a minor nature; it may be punished by a fine, a short prison term, or both.

Some actions that a nurse may take are clearly criminal matters. One example is failure to comply with the mandates of the Controlled Substance Act by engaging in activities such as diverting narcotics for personal use or selling narcotics diverted from clients. Other nursing actions that are potentially criminal in nature include participating in active euthanasia, bombing an abortion clinic, or disconnecting a life-support system. There has even been a case of alleged nursing malpractice involving a fatal overdose of medication that was considered so grievous as to warrant criminal charges.

The number of criminal actions that nurses have been involved in is quite small. When they do occur, these cases are monitored closely to determine their impact on the practice of nursing. More frequently, nurses are involved in civil lawsuits.

Common Law. **Common law** includes standards and rules applicable to our interactions with one another that are recognized, affirmed, and enforced through judicial decisions. This court-made law is based on the principle of *stare decisis,* or "let the decision stand." The court's decision becomes the rule (the law) to follow for subsequent cases involving similar facts. The prior court decision will be applied less rigorously or even not at all if it can be shown that the subsequent case is dissimilar and therefore that the law should not apply. With regard to nursing practice, most laws in the areas of negligence and malpractice are judicial.

Procedural Law. **Procedural law** establishes the manner of the proceeding used to enforce a specific legal right or obtain redress. A nurse who is threatened with the potential loss of a nursing license for professional misconduct relies on procedural law to ensure a fair hearing. The procedural laws related to civil, criminal, and administrative actions vary in detail and can be quite complex. A nurse facing any kind of legal action finds that procedural laws direct the course of the legal action. However, a nurse who relies on procedural law without the benefit of legal representation is at a disadvantage in any legal action.

Public Law. **Public law** regulates the relationship of individuals to government agencies and may be administrative, constitutional, or statutory. The defining characteristic is that the law is applicable to a whole group of people. An example of a public law is the requirement that everyone working in a health care setting, including nurses, be tested annually for tuberculosis.

Statutory Law. **Statutory law** is law enacted by the state or federal legislative branch of government. An example of a federal statutory law relevant to nursing practice is the Americans with Disabilities Act (ADA). To illustrate, a nurse who is permanently disabled is protected by the ADA from employer discrimination. Examples of relevant statutory laws at the state level include nurse practice acts and child- or elder-abuse reporting laws.

Substantive Law. **Substantive law** is the part of law that actually stipulates one's rights and duties, in contrast to procedural law, which guides the enforcement of rights. Substantive law includes the laws of contracts, real estate, torts, and inheritance. Substantive law creates your obligations as a professional nurse. To illustrate, your obligation to assess clients and report changes in their status is a matter of substantive law.

Understanding the Law

All levels of government work together to provide the legal framework for the safe practice of professional nursing. However, laws related to the practice of nursing are not permanently fixed. Changes affecting the profession of nursing and its practitioners can and do occur. As a prudent nurse, you must familiarize yourself on an ongoing basis with the legal changes that affect your practice.

As our health care system and medical technology undergo dramatic changes, questions arise in the practice of nursing about whether specific situations or tasks are safe and "legal." *Is it legal to staff a 40-bed unit with only one registered nurse (RN) or to have a staffing ratio of one RN per four intensive-care-unit clients? Is it legal for an RN to insert fetal scalp electrodes or to discontinue central lines?* Many people believe that the law provides specific answers to these and hundreds of other questions, but in many instances, the law is subject to interpretation. It is uncomfortable and potentially illegal to practice in the "gray areas" of nursing (Figure 2-2).

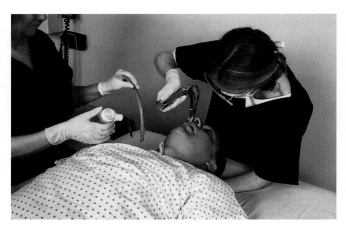

Figure 2-2. As professional practice changes, questions arise about the legal guidelines for practice.

Be aware that administrative agencies offer opinions about the intent and interpretation of rules and regulations, and professional nursing organizations often attempt to clarify practice issues. Ultimately, the courts may provide an interpretation when a specific question is litigated. Understanding your legal obligations and staying abreast of legal changes is the best way to safeguard your professional nursing practice.

Understanding Your Legal and Professional Obligations

Failure to understand your legal and professional obligations as a nurse could jeopardize your livelihood and your ability to practice as a professional nurse. Illegal or incompetent practice could result in professional discipline, a civil lawsuit, a criminal lawsuit, or disciplinary action by your employer. It is important to note that these actions are independent; therefore, more than one can be brought against you at the same time for the same incident.

Furthermore, a determination of "no wrongdoing" in one action does not mean that you will be cleared of wrongdoing in the other potential actions. The procedure used to execute each legal action, the possible outcomes, and the law on which the action is based is different.

PROFESSIONAL REGULATION OF NURSING PRACTICE

To practice nursing in a safe, efficient, competent manner, you must understand both the legal regulation of nursing practice and the voluntary professional regulation of nursing practice. There are several types of laws that direct nursing practice. However, even strict adherence to laws governing nursing practice may be insufficient to guide you in daily efforts to provide quality nursing care. Supplemental voluntary guidelines are provided by professional nursing organizations, the Centers for Disease Control and Prevention (CDC), employer directives, and educational programs. These guidelines do not carry the force of law, but they provide direction for your day-to-day efforts to give competent and legal nursing care.

Professional Nursing Organizations

The American Nurses' Association (ANA) is a professional organization for registered nurses. RNs can also join any of the professional nursing organizations that represent their area of specialization. Most of these organizations have established standards of practice that provide more specific guidance to the professional nurse than might be found in the law. Although the recommendations contained in the standards are not law, they are used to evaluate the quality of care provided by the nurse.

Standards of Practice

Standards of practice provide direction for the provision of nursing care, including your role in professional activities. They reflect the nursing profession's autonomy in establishing standards of professional practice. Standards are written statements that define the acceptable level of performance in the profession. Standards also provide a set of expectations that can be consistently applied to evaluate nursing performance. Values of the profession are reflected in practice standards, including the definition of professional nursing (McCloskey Dochterman & Grace, 2002).

Standards also sometimes address educational qualifications. For example, the law may not specify that a nurse working in labor and delivery must take a fetal monitoring course. The standard of practice, however, as outlined by the Association of Women's Health, Obstetric, and Neonatal Nurses, recommends that these nurses take such a course.

Burkhardt and Nathaniel (1998) note that standards may provide a detailed description of specific acts you must perform in care delivery, or they may outline the process to be followed. For example, the ANA's *Standards of Clinical Nursing Practice* (1998) delineates the steps of nursing care. Each step of the nursing process is identified, including descriptive behaviors. The standards can be used as guides to determine if the care you provided was in keeping with acceptable practice within the profession.

Centers for Disease Control and Prevention

The CDC is a federal agency of the U.S. Public Health Service. The CDC focuses on epidemiology, prevention, control, and treatment of communicable diseases. It offers guidance to nurses about reporting, treating, and managing communicable diseases—such as sexually transmitted diseases, tuberculosis, and acquired immunodeficiency syndrome (AIDS). Isolation procedures and other infection-control recommendations come from the CDC as well.

Employer Policies and Procedures

Employers should not ask nursing employees to function outside the scope of nursing practice as defined by law. However, employers can and do develop guidelines for the practice of nursing in a specific employment setting. Ideally, these guidelines are within the law and are consistent with established standards of practice.

An employer uses at least two methods to convey its expectations of nurses. First, the employer provides a job description to each new employee. It is important to read and understand what your employer expects of you. Although you may have expertise in starting intravenous (IV) therapy, your new community health employer may not want you to restart an IV line on your home care client. It may seem to you to be a waste of resources to ask the client to leave the home and go elsewhere to have an IV line restarted. Nevertheless, the employer is within its rights to ask you not to perform that task. If you fail to adhere to the job expectation, you may not only lose your job but also be exposed to legal liability.

Employers also use written policies and procedures to convey their expectations about the way you will practice nursing. Occasionally, there is more than one safe and efficient way to perform a specific nursing task. Cost factors, staffing limitations, liability considerations, or other factors may direct an employer to require a specific method for performing

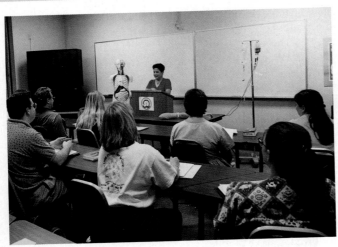

Figure 2-3. Continuing education promotes continued competence in nursing practice.

a nursing procedure. To minimize your legal liability, it is absolutely essential to be familiar with your employer's policies and procedures, to function within your job description, and to practice consistently within established standards.

Educational Programs

Continuing education promotes competence in nursing practice (Figure 2-3). Some states mandate continuing education; however, even without this legal requirement, you have a professional obligation to maintain currency in your nursing practice.

You can obtain the newest information to keep your practice current by attending educational programs, reading professional publications, and maintaining membership in professional nursing organizations. These resources may also provide you with information about legislation that could affect your practice. Evidence of your efforts or lack thereof to keep your practice current may affect the determination of your liability in a legal action.

LEGAL REGULATION OF NURSING PRACTICE

Nurse Practice Acts

Among the powers granted to states is the ability to regulate the practice of health care providers, including RNs. Regulation of the health care professions protects the public by excluding uneducated or unlicensed persons from practicing in a health care profession and by defining the nature and scope of professional practice.

Physicians were the first health care providers to lobby for state regulation of the health care professions through licensure. The broad definition of medicine contained in legislation had a significant impact on licensure of the other health care professions. The nursing profession and others had to carefully construct practice acts that excluded responsibilities addressed in the previously adopted, well-accepted definition of medical practice. The historic dominance of medicine in defining the health care professions continues to challenge the

nursing profession as nurses move into more advanced-practice roles such as nurse anesthetist, nurse midwife, and nurse practitioner.

Common Features of Nurse Practice Acts. A nurse practice act is the most important law affecting your nursing practice. However, each state has its own, and the definitions and descriptions of nursing sometimes differ from state to state. This has created problems for the nursing profession, particularly with regard to reimbursement for services. If the nursing profession cannot reach consensus on a definition of nursing, how can reimbursement be regulated? What services does nursing provide that should be reimbursable?

Despite the differences in the nurse practice acts of the states, they share some common topics. Nurse practice acts usually define terms found within the law, such as "treating" and "diagnosing." A nurse practice act defines the practice of nursing, both registered professional nursing and licensed practical nursing. Historically, some states attempted to list all the tasks registered nurses were legally allowed to perform. Such listings became very restrictive because of technical advances in the practice of nursing and the shifting of responsibilities from physicians to nurses. Subsequent revisions to nurse practice acts allowed flexibility by defining nursing in terms of broad categories of the services provided. These services may include assessing health responses, treating health problems, teaching on health-related topics, and providing supportive care. A nurse practice act also delineates the rules and regulations that govern nursing practice for the licensed practical nurse, the nurse practitioner, the nurse anesthetist, and the nurse midwife.

Often the relationship of the professional nurse to other health care providers is outlined in a nurse practice act. Nurses typically are obligated to implement medical regimens prescribed by physicians and dentists. The care nurses provide to clients independent of a physician's order must be consistent with the treatments ordered by the physician. There is variation from state to state about whether nurses can or must execute the orders of physician assistants, nurse practitioners, respiratory therapists, physical therapists, or other health professionals.

A nurse practice act establishes the requirements for obtaining a license to practice nursing. Completion of a basic accredited nursing educational program is a necessity. A passing score on the National Council Licensure Examination (NCLEX) is also required. Sometimes additional requirements, such as good moral character or a minimum age, must be met for licensure in a particular state.

Another common feature of a nurse practice act is the creation of a state board for nursing. The state board is created to assist in matters related to professional licensing and conduct. The specific functions and composition of a state board of nursing vary somewhat from state to state, but a board must comply with the provisions of the nurse practice act that created it. A board does have the power to create rules and regulations (administrative law) to execute its responsibilities. It can also modify these rules as the need arises.

Professional Misconduct. Finally, a nurse practice act defines **professional misconduct,** which is a violation of the act that can result in disciplinary action against a nurse. In some states, the actual language for professional misconduct, disciplinary proceedings, curricula, and other topics pertaining to the profession of nursing are not found specifically in the practice act but may be found in education law or health law. These other laws may be referenced in the nurse practice act and always work in concert to create the legal context for professional practice. Unprofessional conduct in the practice of nursing covers a wide area. Some actions viewed as professional misconduct are outlined in Box 2-1. Many states provide a nursing handbook to applicants for nursing licensure that contains the nurse practice act and other relevant law.

Disciplinary Actions. Disciplinary actions for professional misconduct are part of administrative procedure. A specific state agency, such as the Board of Nursing, the Office of Professional Discipline, or the Office of Regulation of the Professions is designated to review and manage allegations of professional misconduct. The state agency investigates the allegation, prosecutes or settles a disciplinary proceeding, and enforces the penalty imposed. The disciplinary proceeding may involve a hearing before an administrative officer if a settlement cannot be reached.

Penalties that a state agency can impose range from relatively mild to quite severe, and they may be temporary or permanent. The state agency may find that allegations are unfounded and take no action. An administrative warning may be issued to resolve a violation involving a minor or technical matter. The most serious penalty is revocation of the nursing license.

Other possible penalties include censure and reprimand, a fine (not to exceed a specified dollar amount), a requirement to perform community service, a requirement to complete a specified course of education or training, and an annulment of registration or license. Suspension of license is another penalty that can be imposed. A total suspension may be given for a specified period of time or until a course of therapy or

treatment is completed. A partial suspension, which allows you to work in nursing but not in the area or task (e.g., giving medications) to which the suspension applies, is also possible. The suspension could last until successful completion of a course of retraining.

Penalties for professional misconduct can have a significant impact on your ability to practice nursing. However, because this type of action is an administrative proceeding and not a lawsuit, nurses sometimes fail to recognize the seriousness of the proceeding and therefore do not seek legal representation. Any potential disciplinary action must be viewed very seriously. At the first notice that you are under investigation, you should seek legal representation.

Control of the Profession of Nursing

Credentialing refers to the methods by which the nursing profession attempts to ensure and maintain the competency of its practitioners. The nursing profession uses several methods of credentialing, including accreditation, licensure, and certification. These efforts are designed to assure the public that only those persons who have met specified requirements provide nursing care.

Accreditation. **Accreditation** is a process that monitors an educational program's ability to meet predetermined standards for students' outcomes. The accreditation process examines program length, teaching methods, course objectives, clinical sites, and numerous other factors related to the structure, functioning, and stated outcomes of the educational program. A determination is then made as to whether the educational program meets the minimal standards for basic nursing education. The goals of accreditation include maintaining minimal educational standards and fostering the continuous improvement of nursing education programs.

Accreditation can be granted by a governmental agency, such as a state board of nursing, or by a voluntary organization, such as the National League for Nursing Accrediting Commission (NLNAC) or the Commission on Collegiate Nursing Education (CCNE). As a legal requirement, all nursing education programs must be accredited by the state. Accreditation by a voluntary organization is often truly voluntary, but it may be required by a state for the school to maintain state accreditation.

The NLNAC has been the major nursing education program–accrediting body for all levels of nursing education. The CCNE, an autonomous arm of the American Association of Colleges of Nursing (AACN), is another voluntary organization that accredits nursing education programs. The AACN recognizes the bachelor of science in nursing (BSN) as the minimal educational requirement for what the organization holds to be professional-level nursing practice. The AACN does not seek to deny entry of associate degree graduates into nursing. The AACN supports articulation models that move nurses with an associate degree in nursing (ADN) into higher degree programs. However, the accreditation activities of the CCNE are restricted to ensuring quality and integrity in

---

Box 2-1 Examples of Professional Misconduct

- Exercising undue influence on the client
- Moral unfitness
- Revealing personal information without the client's prior consent
- Practicing beyond the scope permitted by law
- Delegating professional responsibilities to a person not qualified to perform them
- Abandoning or neglecting a client
- Harassing, abusing, or intimidating a client physically or verbally
- Failing to maintain a record reflecting evaluation and treatment of a client
- Failing to exercise appropriate supervision over persons who can practice only under supervision of a licensed professional
- Guaranteeing satisfaction or cure from the performance of professional services
- Failing to wear an identification badge
- Failing to use scientifically accepted infection control techniques

baccalaureate and higher degree nursing programs. Associate degree programs are free to pursue accreditation through the NLNAC.

Licensure. A **license** grants its owner formal permission from a constituted authority to practice a particular profession. The power to grant licenses to professional health care providers is reserved for the state. The state requires the applicant to meet certain criteria to be granted a license, which indicates to the public that this person has met minimal competency standards, thus protecting the public's health and safety. All states now have mandatory licensing acts, which define the practice of nursing and the requirements for licensure.

A major exception to the requirement that you must have a license to practice nursing exists for nursing students. Students enrolled in a recognized, accredited educational program do not need to be licensed to practice nursing, provided such practice is part of the clinical and academic requirements of the educational program and occurs under the supervision and guidance of nursing faculty. Nursing students employed in health care settings in unlicensed roles as aides, client care technicians, and other positions must be cautioned to avoid applying newly acquired skills belonging solely to the domain of licensed professionals. Legal protection is not available to nursing students practicing nursing outside of their educational programs.

States require licensed professional nurses to register. **Registration** is a process by which an applicant provides specific information to the state agency administering the nursing registration process. Information may include current address and telephone number, proof of continuing education, testimonies that no legal actions have been taken against the nurse, and other information. After the initial licensing and registration of the professional nurse, registration renewal may be required every 2 to 4 years. In addition to paying a registration fee, you may need to prove that you have completed specific coursework (e.g., an infection-control update) for a particular type of registration.

In some jurisdictions, the terms *licensure* and *registration* are synonymous. Technically, however, the terms have different meanings. Licensure is a grant to an individual to practice the profession of nursing. Registration is a method of making sure that the state agency has the most current information about a person to whom they have granted a license. Even in a state that recognizes the distinction between licensure and registration, nurses cannot practice without both a license and a current registration.

The recent dramatic changes in the health care delivery system have resulted in rising concerns about nursing licensure. Although these issues may seem theoretical and outside the experience of the beginning practitioner, potential changes in nursing licensure may at some point affect your nursing career. You have a professional obligation to be aware of issues involving your nursing license, and thus your livelihood.

Reciprocity of RN licensing between states is an issue undergoing change. A registered nurse licensed in one state who wants to practice in another state can apply for reciprocity of license. Generally this involves completion of an application and payment of a licensing fee. A nurse can hold licenses from different states but cannot practice in a given state without holding its license.

License reciprocity has limitations. Time delays, differing licensing requirements, tracking of disciplinary actions, telemedicine, and other factors have led to calls for reform of licensing regulations. One suggestion is multistate licensure—a system in which a single license allows a nurse to practice in more than one state.

Some states have adopted a version of multistate licensing called mutual recognition. This model allows a nurse to have one license (in his or her state of residency) and to practice in other states, subject to each state's nurse practice law and regulation. To achieve mutual recognition, each state must enact legislation authorizing the Nurse Licensure Compact and adopt administrative rules and regulations for implementation of the compact.

State boards of nursing have not reached consensus on multistate licensure. The concept would seem to facilitate physical mobility and telehealth practices. However, the impacts have not been fully explored. What would be the impact on the disciplinary processes of state boards? Would a nurse be subject to discipline in several jurisdictions? How would differences in practice (e.g., delegation to unlicensed personnel) be handled? How are data shared between states? These and other questions have yet to be adequately addressed.

An ongoing concern within professional nursing is the concept of institutional licensure for nursing. Currently, the state issues a license to practice nursing to an individual. The boundaries of your professional practice are determined by the state. In effect, you agree to practice nursing according to the rules set forth by the state. As an outcome of this arrangement, you have flexibility to change employers with only minor variations in your professional obligations as a nurse.

In an effort to control the cost, quality, and productivity of the workforce, health care institutions have proposed changes in nurse practice acts that would give them control of nurse licensure. The health care institution would be the gatekeeper, deciding who is qualified to practice nursing within that institution. The institution would review the credentials of the applicant for a nursing position and determine suitability to practice "nursing." Or the institution could provide the education, thus creating a "nurse" tailor-made to the practice setting of the institution. However, under this system, the individual nurse could lose employment mobility, leverage for pay and benefits, and control over individual practice. By decentralizing the practice of nursing, institutional licensure would seriously undermine the collective action of professional nurses to control the defining standards for the professional practice of nursing.

Another ongoing issue in professional nursing is the legal protection of the term *nurse*. Licensure of professional RNs originally came about to protect the public from uneducated persons seeking employment as nurses. The terms *licensed* and *registered* are used to notify the public that these nurses have met minimal educational and licensing requirements. In some states, however, the term *nurse* is not restricted to persons who have met the educational and licensing requirements of nursing. Thus one could advertise and gain employment as a nurse without the appropriate education and credentials. Although employers would recognize the distinction between a nurse, a licensed practical nurse, and a registered professional nurse, families seeking a nurse to provide home care to an ailing relative might not have a sophisticated understanding of the terms. They might thus hire someone ill equipped to provide safe and competent nursing care.

A third licensing issue within the profession of nursing is agreement on the requirements for licensure of persons functioning as nurse practitioners. Nurse practitioners work mainly in primary care settings, providing assessment, teaching, and care to a given client population. It can be argued that nurse practitioners are not performing any functions that fall outside the scope of practice of a registered professional nurse and, therefore, do not need a separate license. Yet many nurse practitioners believe that a separate license is needed, particularly if they are prescribing medications. States have approached the licensing of nurse practitioners differently. Educational requirements, licensing, and scope of practice vary among the states. Future efforts may focus on bringing uniformity to these issues.

The dramatic changes in the health care delivery system and the creation of new roles for nurses have created a new licensing concern. Many managed care organizations operate in more than one state. As a case manager or telephone "telehealth advisor" for such an organization, you could find yourself working with clients in states other than the one in which you are licensed. If you are providing professional services to clients in other states, the potential exists for you to be charged with practicing in that state without a license.

Certification. Although not required by law, nurses often seek certification to receive recognition for their expertise in a particular area of nursing. **Certification** is a voluntary process by which a nurse can be granted recognition for meeting certain criteria established by a nongovernmental association. A nurse can become certified in many areas of nursing, including geriatrics, pediatrics, emergency nursing, community health nursing, school nursing, maternal–child health, and even such newly identified specialty areas as forensic nursing. Certification is offered through the ANA and many specialty-nursing organizations. Requirements vary but typically include specific educational preparation, experience in the specialty area, evidence of continuing education, and successful completion of a certification examination.

In some states, certification can have a second meaning. In New York, for example, certificates are issued to registered professional nurses to reflect their academic preparation as a nurse practitioner. The specific requirements for education and experience for certification as a nurse practitioner are outlined in the law. This legal requirement for certification is entirely different from the certification offered by the professional nursing organizations.

There is a lack of agreement within the nursing profession about the benefits of either voluntary or legal certification. Proponents of certification believe it identifies nursing expertise and is analogous to board certification of physicians. They suggest that this formalized recognition of nursing expertise could be used to leverage higher salaries. Nurses who question the benefits of certification point out the lack of agreement on what certification means in nursing and suggest that certification may be splintering the profession without creating the anticipated economic advantage.

Other Laws Affecting Nursing Practice

Several laws not directly focused on the practice of nursing have a significant impact on the way you must practice nursing. These laws, which apply not only to nurses but to all health care providers regardless of setting, include the Occupational Safety and Health Act, the Controlled Substance Acts, the Health Care Quality Improvement Act, the Americans with Disabilities Act, and Good Samaritan Laws.

Occupational Safety and Health Act. The Occupational Safety and Health Act of 1970, known as OSHA, established legal standards that define safe and healthful working conditions. OSHA is periodically updated and expanded, and it affects you as a nurse in two ways. First, it sets standards for your working conditions. For example, OSHA directs the manner in which potentially toxic or flammable chemicals are handled. The use and care of electrical equipment is another area OSHA regulates.

Second, some of the requirements of the law dictate how you manage clients. For example, OSHA provides standards for the management of contaminated equipment and supplies and the types of isolation techniques used for infectious clients. Promoting health and safety is both your professional obligation and your legal mandate.

Controlled Substance Acts. Several laws have been enacted that address standards for drug development and marketing. These laws affect the process by which new drugs become available to clients. Most significant for you is the Comprehensive Drug Abuse Prevention and Control Act of 1970. This law was enacted to regulate the distribution and use of drugs with the potential for abuse. These drugs include narcotics, depressants, stimulants, and hallucinogens. Your nursing obligations under this law include proper storage and documentation of controlled substances. Failure to meet the requirements of this law is grounds for charges of professional misconduct and potential criminal action against you.

Health Care Quality Improvement Act. One of the difficult issues in attempting to protect the public from unsafe and incompetent health care providers has been the tracking of information related to adverse licensure actions, malpractice payments, and adverse professional actions. The Health Care Quality Improvement Act of 1986 was created to collect data about unsafe and incompetent practitioners. The law, which does apply to nurses, has limited the ability of health care practitioners who had adverse action taken against them in one state from moving to another state without disclosing their previous performance.

Americans With Disabilities Act. The ADA, passed in 1990, was enacted to protect persons with disabilities from discrimination in such areas as housing, employment, education, and health services. The act uses a broad definition of disability that includes persons with AIDS or infected with the human immunodeficiency virus (HIV) and persons recovering from drug or alcohol addiction. Many of your clients may be disabled. As a result, you may be assisting your clients to assert their rights under this law, particularly if you work in an outpatient or community health setting.

Good Samaritan Laws. Because of your education and experience as a nurse, you may feel a special obligation to provide aid to people in emergency situations. In most states, there is no legal requirement for any person, including a health care provider, to provide assistance at the scene of an emergency. You (just as any other person) could choose to help or to leave the scene. However, a few states have enacted legislation requiring a person trained in health care to stop and aid the injured, and it is important that you know whether your state is one of these. Even without a legal obligation, you may feel an ethical obligation to assist in such circumstances (Figure 2-4).

Inevitably, the question arises as to your potential exposure for legal liability if you render care at the scene of an accident. To encourage health care providers to assist in emergency situations and to protect providers who do offer care in these circumstances from legal liability, most states have passed Good Samaritan laws. These laws differ among states but all offer some protection from the fear of a lawsuit when giving emergency care.

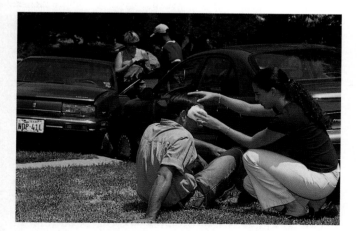

Figure 2-4. Good Samaritan laws offer some protection from legal liability for health care workers who stop to offer assistance at the scene of an accident.

The accident victim may not be able to consent to care, which is a requirement in nonemergency situations. Without such consent, and with the limitations of the situation at hand, you are expected to give the kind of help a reasonably prudent person with your background would give in a similar circumstance. Good Samaritan laws do not provide you with absolute immunity from legal liability. If the care you provide can be shown to be grossly negligent, you could still face liability.

Employment Law

Employment law governs employment practices and encompasses such areas as at-will employment, personal employment contracts, and collective bargaining. It also influences when and how employment may be terminated.

Most nurses work as employees rather than as independent contractors or nurse entrepreneurs. An employee is a person who works for someone else in return for a salary or wages. The agreement to work with the promise of being paid is a contract for hire and can be express or implied, oral or written. The employer has the power to control the details of the work. The employer's expectations as to the work to be done and the manner in which it is to be done are usually found in the job description and the employer's policies and procedures.

In contrast, an independent contractor agrees to provide a specific service for a fee. The independent contractor has control over the details of providing the service. The employer's control is limited to establishing the end product of the contractor's work. For example, a home care agency can hire a nurse as an independent contractor to monitor its clients who have total parenteral nutrition. The independent contractor decides in what order to visit clients, what time of day to see them, and other particular details of monitoring this group of clients. The services provided must be consistent with standards of practice and with the agreement reached with the employer. The contract with the employer may specify details of providing the service (e.g., clients must be seen no less than once a day). However, the independent contractor can decide that the employer's conditions are not acceptable and refuse to provide services for that particular home care agency.

Nurses who establish a health-related business may find themselves in the position of employer. If you are the sole employee of your business, your activities will be covered by the contracts you develop with your clients. However, if you employ other people in your business, your concerns about employment law will be from the perspective of an employer. Your rights and obligations as an employer are covered in a variety of employment-related laws, including the Fair Labor Standards Act, Workers' Compensation laws, and the National Labor Relations Act.

At-Will Employment. Although most nurses still work as employees of hospitals, an increasing number work in community health, ambulatory care, long-term care, and other health care delivery settings. Regardless of the setting, the employee is usually either an at-will employee or an employee covered by a collective bargaining agreement. The at-will employment doctrine allows both the employer and the employee to terminate the employment relationship at any time and for any reason. Several exceptions to the at-will doctrine exist. Some states have modified the at-will doctrine to permit termination only for "just cause." Most nurses are at-will employees.

Collective Bargaining. About 17% of registered professional nurses are covered by *collective bargaining agreements,* which are contracts between an employer and a labor organization that represents the nurses. The labor organization may be a professional nursing association that engages in collective bargaining, or a union. In an employment setting covered by a collective bargaining agreement, the labor organization represents the interests of the bargaining unit. The bargaining unit may include only registered nurses or it may include other health care workers (e.g., licensed practical nurses, nurse's aides, physical therapists, and other workers in the facility). Excluded from the bargaining unit are persons in management positions within the agency.

The employer and the labor organization are obligated to negotiate and reach agreement on the terms and conditions of employment for the members of the bargaining unit. The terms and conditions include pay and benefits, such as vacations, holidays, health insurance, sick leave, personal leave, and rules pertaining to such issues as lunch breaks, coffee breaks, absenteeism, tardiness, dress codes, overtime work, and safety.

Personal Employment Contracts. As an employee, you can theoretically have a personal employment contract with an employer, but the number of nurses who do is low. Typically, nurse executives, nursing faculty, nurse anesthetists, nurse midwives, and nurse practitioners have individual employment contracts. The contract is between the nurse and the employer and describes position responsibilities, terms and conditions of employment, fringe benefits, and other aspects of the employment relationship.

Employer Actions. As a registered nurse, you face three kinds of threats to your livelihood and continued practice of nursing. The first threat involves the employer's right to discipline you through a verbal or written warning, suspension, or termination of your employment. The second threat involves obligations your employer may have for reporting you to the state agency that handles allegations of professional misconduct or substance abuse. Finally, your employer may be required to provide information damaging to your career during litigation of a lawsuit brought against you. It is important to note that these actions are independent, and therefore more than one can be brought against you at the same time for the same incident.

An employer can discipline you for reasons unrelated to your professional practice of nursing. Employment issues common to any employee also affect nurses. Excessive absences or tardiness, failure to notify your employer when you will be absent, poor customer service skills, and poor personal hygiene are the types of issues employers regard as legitimate

grounds for discipline. You may even be terminated for these reasons despite your flawless practice of nursing.

Employers also discipline nurses for reasons more closely related to the practice of nursing. A nurse who is unable to perform to the employer's expectations as outlined in the job description can face discipline. Frequent client complaints, questionable clinical skills, substandard documentation, and failure to master skills needed for the particular clinical area are examples of grounds for discipline. These deficiencies can also be justifiable causes for termination of employment even if they have not resulted in any client harm.

Usually, an employer does not terminate employment without first going through a process of notifying and advising the employee of action required to continue employment. The process of progressive discipline is addressed in a collective bargaining agreement if a union represents the employee. Even without a collective bargaining obligation, most employers have a policy of progressive discipline as a means of avoiding a wrongful discharge lawsuit brought by a disgruntled former employee.

In some instances, nursing practice that is so substandard or that results in client harm obligates an employer to report the nurse to the state agency that investigates allegations of professional misconduct or drug violations. The state agency may impose various forms of discipline if allegations prove to be true. Types of discipline include reprimand, fines, temporary suspension, and permanent license revocation. Criminal prosecution is also a possibility if the alleged misconduct involves violation of criminal statutes. Specific state statutes vary, but allegations of client abuse, substance abuse, illegal activity, or the death of a client under certain conditions are all examples of situations that may obligate an employer to generate a report. This reporting is independent of a disciplinary action the employer may initiate.

Similarly, you may be involved in litigation arising from your employment. The employer is also usually sued. Although the situation that caused a lawsuit occurred in the place of employment, the employer will not necessarily seek to terminate the employment relationship. However, during the course of the lawsuit, the employer may provide evidence damaging to your continuing practice as a nurse.

A determination of "no wrongdoing" in one action does not mean that you will be cleared of wrongdoing in the other potential actions. Suppose a postpartum client complains to your employer that you did not provide all the care she believed she should have received. The client is angry enough that she decides to report you to the state agency that addresses allegations of professional misconduct. The state agency determines that your practice met the standard of care and declines to take any disciplinary action against you. Meanwhile, your employer, concerned that this is the second time it has received complaints about your nursing care, suspends you from work for 2 days.

All potential legal actions determine the extent to which you meet or fail to meet your legal and professional nursing responsibilities. However, the procedures used to execute each legal action, the law on which the action is based, and the possible outcomes vary. You should be aware that professional discipline, civil or criminal lawsuits, and employer sanctions all represent threats to your license and must be addressed appropriately.

THE ETHICAL CONTEXT OF PRACTICE

In nursing, as in life, it is not always easy to determine the best course of action in a given situation. You are dedicated to meeting the needs of your clients, yet institutional policies must be followed, physicians' directives implemented, professional standards upheld, and legal requirements met. You also must have a willingness to listen to your own inner wisdom. When two or more of these domains are in conflict, you may face a dilemma of ethics.

In today's health care arena, ethical issues abound. As technological advances extend life for clients with chronic illnesses, practitioners grapple with the issue of quality of life versus sanctity of life. At the same time, the shrinking health care dollar has led to shorter hospital stays and insurance company restrictions on reimbursement for various tests, equipment, supplies, medications, and procedures. As resources dwindle, the baby boom generation is aging. Should care and services be rationed? And if so, how will such decisions be made, and by whom?

Organ transplantation, in vitro fertilization, genetic engineering, assisted suicide, care of clients with communicable illnesses, umbilical cord blood storage, and allocation of resources are some of the high-profile issues currently being addressed by practitioners. In addition, within your daily practice, you will also confront issues of informed consent, confidentiality (especially with data stored on computer), client advocacy, the competency of caregivers, withholding of food and fluids, and refusal of treatment.

Technical skills and a familiarity with your professional and legal obligations are essential for safe and effective nursing care. However, beyond that you must also develop skills in ethical decision making. Ethical decision-making skills are needed to deal with those situations that have not yet been addressed in law or professional practice standards. You must be able to identify and discuss ethical dilemmas in nursing practice, apply ethical standards to resolve those dilemmas, and provide the rationale for ethical decisions to clients, families, and other health care professionals. Thus you must be equipped to make decisions about ethical issues in a consistent and objective manner in a rapidly changing and constantly demanding health care delivery system (Federwisch, 1997).

Morals, Values, and Ethics

The words *ethics, morals,* and *values* are often used interchangeably to indicate behaviors or ideas that the speaker feels are right, good, just, or proper. Some might say, for example, that it is unethical or immoral to smoke cigarettes in front of children, or that anyone who does so lacks values. However, within the domains of philosophy, sociology, and law, these three terms have separate and unique definitions (Table 2-3).

Morals. **Morals** are standards of conduct that represent the ideal in human behavior, to which society expects its members to adhere. Moral development is the imprinting of the moral standards put forth by society as the norm for human conduct. Imprinting of moral conduct begins in early childhood. It is seen, for example, when parents teach their children to tell the truth. External forces, such as fear of consequences, may govern adherence to such standards. As we mature, it is expected that moral conduct becomes part of our nature rather than an avenue to avoid unpleasant consequences.

As a nurse, you are expected to be a moral agent. That is, you are expected to perform the duties and functions of nursing within established standards of conduct. You are also expected to possess and use moral standards in making decisions. Therefore you must first possess the knowledge to recognize a moral conflict. Jameton (1984) identifies three components of a moral conflict:
- Moral uncertainty, when a person is unsure what values and principles are applicable or if an ethical problem really exists
- Moral dilemma, when moral principles are in conflict
- Moral distress, when the person understands what ought to be done but no supportive systems are available to help in reaching a decision or implementing an action

Table 2-3	Terms in Ethics	
Term	**Definition**	**Example**
Ethics	• Promotes ideal human behavior • Examines what ought to be done • Seeks to provide guidelines or principles to direct human action	• Exploration of ethical principles and moral standards of conduct. • Having a high regard for the uniqueness of the human experience
Morals	• Standards of conduct that represent "ideal" human behavior • Standards identified by society as the norm of conduct • Conduct that is expected regardless of consequences to the individual	• The expectation that members of society will be honest and tell the truth in all situations, even if they experience negative consequences • Behaviors that are judged as the "right" thing to do, such as demonstrating respect for clients
Values	• Ideals, beliefs, and patterns of behavior that are prized and chosen by individuals • Learned behavior acquired from cultural, family, and community life experiences	• Personal values, such as belief in strong family connections and the desire to be accepted by others • Professional values, such as dedication, integrity, and competence

Once you recognize moral conflict, you must then be able to implement moral reasoning. Deloughery (1998) cites research by Rest (1986) that describes moral reasoning in four stages:

- Recognition of a conflict of values or principles
- Selection of an action
- Intention to implement morally correct behavior
- Performance of a selected behavior that resolves the dilemma

Values. **Values** are ideals, beliefs, and patterns of behavior that are prized and chosen by a person, group, or society. Like morals, values provide a foundation for principled behavior. Values shape decisions in everyday life, from the clothes we wear to the movies we prefer to the food we eat and the cars we buy. Therefore it is not unusual to expect that our values will be evident in our behaviors.

TYPES OF VALUES. Values that people hold as important in their private lives are called personal values. They are learned from various experiences in the family and community and are seen as compatible with lifestyle choices. Having strong family connections, having good health, being accepted by others, and being honest are all examples of personal values.

Professional values are qualities that are identified as the acceptable standard of conduct for members of a profession or group. Examples of professional values include integrity, dedication, and fairness. In your position as a health care professional, you are expected to demonstrate personal and professional values that reflect a respect for human dignity, that honor client rights, that demonstrate care and concern, that support equity, and that honor truth.

DEVELOPMENT OF VALUES. Values are learned behaviors that are influenced by culture, ethnicity, education, and life experiences. Values are acquired through structured and unstructured learning, experiences in our homes and communities, and interactions with family, teachers, clergy, and social organizations. As children we are exposed to the values of adults who have influence over our lives. As we mature, we begin to develop our own values, sometimes through trial and error. In childhood a toy may be the most valued object of our young lives. In adolescence, peer opinions begin to be more important than adult and even parent opinions. In adulthood, our behaviors reflect the values we have acquired and use in daily decision making (Burkhardt & Nathaniel, 1998).

Our values reflect what we hold important and what we believe when we act on them in various situations in daily life. When values are freely chosen, they are demonstrated by our behavior through word and deed. For example, if a physician believes that everyone should have access to quality health care regardless of ability to pay, the physician's medical practice demonstrates that belief by providing quality health services to anyone in need.

You will be exposed to many situations in health care that may produce value conflicts. As noted earlier, moral reasoning requires that you recognize conflicts in values or principles. It is important for you to understand your feelings and be able to identify your values about health, illness, aging, access to care, quality of life, dying, and death. If you understand your values and can express them clearly, you will be better prepared to handle difficult situations and make informed decisions.

VALUES CLARIFICATION. An understanding of personal values forms the basis for ethical decision making. The process of **values clarification** allows you to identify your personal values and develop self-awareness. This process is essential in nursing because your values provide the platform on which you will make decisions and take action. A three-step model for values clarification is described in Table 2-4. Using the model, consider the following situation:

Mary is a 22-year-old college student who is concerned about the weight she has gained during her last semester. Some of her friends have decided to start smoking to control their appetite. Mary is considering this option but finally decides that she values her health and will look for a more healthy way to lose weight.

Step 1. *Making a choice.* Mary decided to research the issue. After deciding that overall good health is more important to her than a solution that could lead to nicotine addiction and chronic health problems, Mary decides not to smoke. This choice was based on her valuing good health and finding the possible benefit of smoking not substantial enough compared with the overall risk factors.

Step 2. *Valuing the choice.* Mary is proud of her choice. She affirms it by refusing cigarettes when offered. She readily tells her friends of her decision.

Step 3. *Behavior affirmation.* Mary's makes it clear that she has chosen not to smoke. Her apartment and car have "No smoking" signs. She asks to sit in the nonsmoking sections of restaurants. And when friends ask, "Do you mind if I smoke?" she answers, "Yes."

Ethics. **Ethics** is the branch of philosophy that attempts to determine what constitutes good, bad, right, and wrong in human behavior (Stewart & Blocker, 2000). The study of ethics entails the examination of human behavior in terms of what ought to be done in the course of human interactions, and it seeks to provide guidelines or principles as a way to direct human action (Pojman, 1990). *Bioethics* is a specialized area of

Table 2-4	Levels of Values Clarification	
Level	Implication	
1. Making a choice	• Freedom to choose	
	• Knowledge of other possible choices	
	• Knowledge of consequences	
2. Valuing our choice or intrapersonal affirmation	• Owning the choice as ours	
	• Feeling positive about making the choice	
	• Sharing our choice with others	
3. Behavior affirmation	• Using behavior consistent with choice	
	• Acting on choice when it is not convenient or comfortable	

ethics that is concerned with human conduct in health care (Deloughery, 1998).

Ethical Principles

Principles are basic truths or laws that guide conduct and behavior. Ethical principles, also called standards, provide the framework for the practice of professional nursing. Such principles guide actions by providing the basis for rule development within the profession (Yoder-Wise, 2003). The following seven principles are considered essential to the delivery of ethical nursing care.

Autonomy. **Autonomy** refers to a person's right to make individual choices—that is, to self-determine. It is essential that you respect your clients' rights to make their own health care choices. To support autonomy, you provide detailed and realistic information to clients, who then freely choose from the available options. You support clients' decisions even when they are different from your preferences.

Beneficence. **Beneficence** is the promotion of good. It requires the performance of actions that are of benefit to others. The good of actions must be weighed against any possible harm. For example, failing to turn a bedridden client who complains of pain during the turning may produce the short-term good of reduced discomfort, but it may also cause the harm of impaired skin integrity and musculoskeletal deformities.

Confidentiality. As a nurse, you will hear, see, and gather data about clients that is confidential in nature. **Confidentiality** is the client's right to privacy in the health care delivery system. Confidentiality means maintaining another's privacy by safeguarding information that is entrusted to you. Through the assessment process, you are privy to intimate details about a client's health history. Before you collect data, it is important that clients understand that such information will be documented in the medical record and therefore will be available to other health care providers. This fact may influence the type and amount of information that a client shares.

It is your responsibility to assure clients that information is held in confidence and used as a means of meeting their health care needs. Because clients have to depend on strangers when they are most vulnerable, you are in a position to protect them from indiscriminate disclosure of health care information that may cause harm. For example, the disclosure of a client's HIV-positive status could cause the loss of his job and exposure to social isolation and discrimination.

Maintaining confidentiality demonstrates the kind of respect that is the cornerstone of the nurse–client relationship (Burkhardt & Nathaniel, 1998). A further discussion of confidentiality can be found under Client Rights, later in this chapter.

Nonmaleficence. The word *maleficence* means evil or harm. Thus **nonmaleficence** requires the practitioner to do no harm. Nonmaleficence is the complement of beneficence. It says that your actions should not cause undo harm to clients. Provision of safe and effective nursing care may require you to perform acts that cause fear, discomfort, or pain—inserting a feeding tube, for example, or giving an injection. The good of these acts (beneficence) is weighed against both the temporary pain and the potential for serious harm if the interventions are withheld. Nonmaleficence also requires that your actions be performed according to acceptable standards of practice because failure to follow such standards could result in client injury.

Fidelity. **Fidelity** means honoring agreements and keeping promises. When you say, "I'll give you your pain medication at 9 o'clock" or "I'll be sure to speak with your doctor about your concern," your clients hear this as a promise or commitment to their welfare. Keeping such promises is your responsibility. When you cannot honor a promise at the specified time, you must either inform the client and perform the action as soon as possible, or have another caregiver complete the task.

Justice. **Justice** is moral rightness, fairness, or equity. It is therefore concerned with fair and equal treatment of all clients. In applying the principle of justice, you must consider whether it requires that everyone be treated the same or that the same principles and standards be applied to all. For example, equal treatment of two cancer clients may not be possible if one has a strong financial and emotional support system and the other is homeless and mentally ill.

The issue of justice arises in attempts to allocate health care resources and ensure equal access to health care for all. With the aging of the baby boom generation, the need for health care may become greater than available resources. You will have an integral role in promoting equal or fair access to health care. You must therefore be politically astute regarding issues related to resource allocation, and vocal in advocating for equality of access (Fowler & Levine-Ariff, 1987).

Veracity. **Veracity** means adhering to the truth. It therefore requires truth-telling consistently and continually. In applying the principle of veracity, you tell the complete truth and not an altered version assumed to be in the client's best interest. Veracity also relates to the principle of autonomy because clients can make the best decisions for themselves only when given complete facts. This issue is most crucial when dealing with terminally ill clients and their right to know their prognosis. Often it is you who must answer clients' questions regarding death and dying.

It is important to remember that respect for others guides the implementation of all ethical principles. When you respect others, you spontaneously ensure freedom of choice, promote good, prevent harm, keep promises, act fairly, and remain truthful (Yoder-Wise, 2003).

Common Ethical Problems

Nursing care is often provided to clients who are at risk for ethical dilemmas, such as geriatric clients, terminally ill clients, or clients involved in research studies. Although you will have a certain degree of autonomy in care delivery, it is important to remember that nursing is not practiced in a vacuum. By its very nature, it is provided in collaboration with clients, families, physicians, and other health care practitioners in various practice arenas (Figure 2-5).

You may find yourself in conflict with clients—for example, the client with diabetes who refuses to follow the dietary regimen and is frequently readmitted for out-of-control blood glucose levels. You may experience frustration and even anger because of the client's seeming unwillingness to implement self-care measures. If you place a high value on maintaining good health, you may find it difficult to interact with a client who refuses to follow a regimen that manages a chronic illness. Yet you must also respect the client's autonomy. The needs of the client are paramount, and you must put aside feelings of anger and frustration and deliver the care that meets the client's needs. Nursing with care and concern is important to the profession and must be demonstrated in spite of personal feelings.

Ethical problems may also stem from your interactions with physicians, such as when physician's orders are contra-

dictory to client wishes or when the physician has not informed a terminally ill client of the diagnosis and the client repeatedly questions you. This leaves you feeling caught in the middle, and it can make you want to avoid the client because of the uncomfortable feelings generated by the questions. To whom do you owe loyalty? Is it your responsibility to inform the client of the medical diagnosis? What do you think? In the day-to-day activities of nursing care, ethical problems may also revolve around the following:

- Failure of a co-worker to provide adequate care to a client
- Unit staffing patterns that negatively influence the provision of safe nursing care
- Insurers that limit the type of care a client may receive or that require discharge when a client would benefit from additional hospital days

As you can see, issues of ethics may be unavoidable in the day-to-day delivery of nursing care. Developing skills to identify when there is conflict of values or ethical principles increases your ability to be effective in care delivery. Also, being knowledgeable of the steps in the ethical decision-making process provides you with the tools to ensure that client needs are being served.

Ethics in Nursing

As a profession, nursing has established standards of behaviors that govern the practice. These standards are called codes of ethics. In the United States, the ANA *Code for Nurses* (2001) is the document governing ethical nursing practice (Box 2-2). The ANA *Code for Nurses* identifies the goals and values of the profession and sets forth the philosophy of the profession. It includes interpretive statements that explain how each goal is realized in nursing practice. Not surprisingly, the code focuses on the protection of the client and the identification of standards for a nurse's interactions with clients. Because it identifies the behaviors required for ethical practice, the code can be used as a guide for evaluating nursing actions. It may also be used as a guide to ethical decision making. Although the code is not law, it is the standard by which nursing actions are judged throughout the profession.

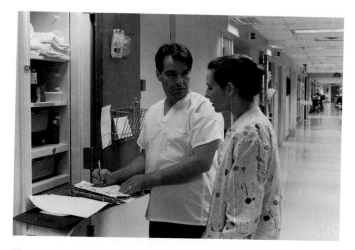

Figure 2-5. Nursing is not practiced in a vacuum but in collaboration with others.

Box 2-2 American Nurses' Association *Code for Nurses*

1. The nurse, in all professional relationships, practices with compassion and respect for the inherent dignity, worth, and uniqueness of every individual, unrestricted by considerations of social or economic status, personal attributes, or the nature of health problems.
2. The nurse's primary commitment is to the patient, whether an individual, family, group, or community.
3. The nurse promotes, advocates for, and strives to protect the health, safety, and rights of the patient.
4. The nurse is responsible and accountable for individual nursing practice and determines the appropriate delegation of tasks consistent with the nurse's obligation to provide optimum patient care.
5. The nurse owes the same duties to self as to others, including the responsibility to preserve integrity and safety, to maintain competence, and to continue personal and professional growth.

6. The nurse participates in establishing, maintaining, and improving health care environments and conditions of employment conducive to the provision of quality health care and consistent with the values of the profession through individual and collective action.
7. The nurse participates in the advancement of the profession through contributions to practice, education, administration, and knowledge development.
8. The nurse collaborates with other health professionals and the public in promoting community, national, and international efforts to meet health needs.
9. The profession of nursing, as represented by associations and their members, is responsible for articulating nursing values, for maintaining the integrity of the profession and its practice, and for shaping social policy.

Sanctions can be imposed against a nurse who is found to be practicing outside the framework of the code.

Another code for professional nursing is the *Code for Nurses: Ethical Concepts Applied to Nursing*, by the International Council of Nurses (2000) (Box 2-3). As you review, note the similarities. For example, both codes address respect for human dignity, rights, and confidentiality, and competence and responsibilities of the nurse in the delivery of health care. Additionally, the codes provide a framework for ethical practice in professional nursing and can be used as a standard in legal proceedings.

Accountability and Responsibility. As a nurse, you are responsible and accountable for your actions. That is, you are *responsible* for providing care within established standards of the profession. For example, you are responsible for implementing care using the nursing process. This means you assess client needs, identify nursing diagnoses, identify outcomes, formulate a plan of care, implement actions, and evaluate the effectiveness of nursing care provided (ANA, 1998). As a nursing student, you are responsible for acquiring the knowledge and skills necessary to become a safe practi-

tioner. Included in this knowledge and skill development are the awareness of ethical principles and the process of ethical decision making. Once you have attained licensure to practice as an RN, you are responsible for maintaining competency in nursing knowledge and skills and demonstrating ethical principles in care delivery.

Being *accountable* means that you are answerable for the outcomes of actions taken. You are answerable to clients, institutions, the profession, peers, and society. In addition, you are answerable to yourself in terms of ensuring that your conduct reflects ethical behavior. If you assess that a client has a high risk of injury from falls and you do not develop and implement a plan of care to protect the client from injury, you are accountable if the client is injured. You are accountable to the client, the family, the nursing service area, and the institution. In this instance, you are also answerable to yourself and the profession because the nursing care provided did not demonstrate implementation of the nursing process or provision of care within ethical principles (nonmaleficence). You are accountable for the outcomes of your nursing judgment, and this accountability cannot be alleviated by physicians' orders or institutional policies (ANA, 2001).

Box 2-3 The ICN Code of Ethics for Nurses

An international code of ethics for nurses was first adopted by the International Council of Nurses (ICN) in 1953. It has been revised and reaffirmed at various times since, most recently with the review and revision completed in 2000. The ICN Code of Ethics is also available in French, Spanish, and German.

PREAMBLE

- Nurses have four fundamental responsibilities: to promote health, to prevent illness, to restore health and to alleviate suffering. The need for nursing is universal.
- Inherent in nursing is respect for human rights, including the right to life, to dignity, and to be treated with respect. Nursing care is unrestricted by considerations of age, color, creed, culture, disability or illness, gender, nationality, politics, race, or social status.
- Nurses render health services to the individual, the family, and the community and coordinate their services with those of related groups.

THE CODE

The *ICN Code of Ethics for Nurses* has four principal elements that outline the standards of ethical conduct.

ELEMENTS OF THE CODE

1. Nurses and People

- The nurse's primary professional responsibility is to people requiring nursing care.
- In providing care, the nurse promotes an environment in which the human rights, values, customs, and spiritual beliefs of the individual, family, and community are respected.
- The nurse ensures that the individual receives sufficient information on which to base consent for care and related treatment.
- The nurse holds in confidence personal information and uses judgment in sharing this information.

- The nurse shares with society the responsibility for initiating and supporting action to meet the health and social needs of the public, in particular those of vulnerable populations.
- The nurse also shares responsibility to sustain and protect the natural environment from depletion, pollution, degradation, and destruction.

2. Nurses and Practice

- The nurse carries personal responsibility and accountability for nursing practice, and for maintaining competence by continual learning.
- The nurse maintains a standard of personal health such that the ability to provide care is not compromised.
- The nurse uses judgment regarding individual competence when accepting and delegating responsibility.
- The nurse at all times maintains standards of personal conduct that reflect well on the profession and enhance public confidence.
- The nurse, in providing care, ensures that use of technology and scientific advances are compatible with the safety, dignity, and rights of people.

3. Nurses and the Profession

- The nurse assumes the major role in determining and implementing acceptable standards of clinical nursing practice, management, research, and education.
- The nurse is active in developing a core of research-based professional knowledge.
- The nurse, acting through the professional organization, participates in creating and maintaining equitable social and economic working conditions in nursing.

4. Nurses and Co-workers

- The nurse sustains a cooperative relationship with co-workers in nursing and other fields.
- The nurse takes appropriate action to safeguard individuals when their care is endangered by a co-worker or any other person.

Advocacy. To advocate for someone means to speak for that person when the person is unable to speak for himself or herself. You will often find yourself in the role of advocate for clients when they are incapacitated or diminished by illness. Thus you may be called upon to assert the client's wishes or desires regarding health care choices. You must be prepared to advocate for clients and families and to provide channels for effective communication of client and family wishes.

You must actively advocate for clients when they are vulnerable and unable to promote their own needs. It is important for you to have knowledge of the clients' values so you can assist in decision making that is consistent with their lifestyle choices. This may be accomplished by providing necessary information, by helping clients explore options, or by doing both. The overall goal of advocacy is to ensure that clients receive the best possible care and to support their right to have health care that is consistent with their values and beliefs (Fowler & Levine-Ariff, 1987).

Making an Ethical Decision. Some decisions in our lives have choices with clearly distinct advantages. For example, choosing to pursue higher education, although it may not be easy, provides a great deal of satisfaction—personally, professionally, and, one hopes, financially—upon completion. Many decisions are routine and require little deliberation, such as clothing choices, what to eat for breakfast, and when to retire for the evening. You are often called upon to make decisions that are not as easy, and the choices may conflict (Box 2-4).

When two or more principles are in conflict or when the choices are unfavorable (i.e., no available solution is satisfactory), you have an ethical dilemma. For example, a geriatric male client is restrained because of his unsteady gait. You are concerned about his risk of injury from falling. The client is oriented and says repeatedly that he does not want to be restrained. In this situation, the principles in conflict are autonomy versus beneficence. You respect the client's right to be autonomous and make his own decisions, yet you are also bound to protect him from injury and prevent unnecessary harm.

You will face situations like this one daily. You are expected to implement actions that result in good outcomes for the client yet remain in keeping with the client's wishes and desires. Following is a discussion of a six-step ethical decision-making process that will help you identify ethical dilemmas, implement solutions, and evaluate outcomes. It will help you move beyond feelings of uncertainty and helplessness to naming and clarifying the problem and implementing solutions. Review of work by Jameton (1984) provides the basis for the following steps in the ethical decision-making process.

Identify the ethical dilemma. Is the situation truly an ethical dilemma, with conflicting principles or values, or is it a legal issue or a problem of faulty communication? Legal and communication issues may be present in any ethical dilemma, but in the absence of conflicting principles, legal counsel or clarification of communication may be appropriate rather than ethical analysis.

Gather pertinent data. Everyone involved in the case is a source of potentially significant data. Documents such as

---

> **Box 2-4   Ethics Discussion Scenario**
>
> John and Mary both have the chance to obtain the answers to the next exam and secure an A in a very difficult course required for completing their degree. John rejects the offer outright. He never considers it an option because he views it as morally wrong and dishonest.
>
> Mary considers the offer and weighs her options. She has been struggling with work and school and "acing" the next exam would greatly relieve some of the pressure. She knows she is smart enough but has not had enough time to study. She is sorely tempted but finally rejects the offer because she does not want to take the chance of getting caught and being expelled from school.
>
> - Is either of these students more moral than the other?
> - If so, who?
> - What is the rationale for your choice?
> - What values are evident in this scenario?

the health history, nurses' notes, and consent forms are also important to research. Questions to ask include the following: What are the relevant facts at issue in the dilemma? Who are the principal people involved? Are values in conflict with expected outcomes? Is there a clear therapeutic regimen for the client? Do cultural or spiritual factors need to be considered in the decision? Do institutional values and systems support the nursing decisions made? Is there a mechanism for implementing actions? Have policies, procedures, protocols, and economic factors been considered?

Examine the dilemma for the ethical principles involved. At this point it is important to have a clear understanding of the principles that are key to making an ethical decision in each case. Questions to ask include the following: With whom must the final decision be made, and is that person competent or empowered to make decisions? *(autonomy)* What is the overall good to be accomplished? *(beneficence and nonmaleficence)* Have the principal decision makers been given all necessary information? *(veracity)* Whose interests are being served? *(justice)* Have there been promises made or are there expectations of behaviors from caregivers? *(fidelity)* Determine which principles are applicable and which are in conflict. Does honoring one over another oppose legal requirements or institutional policies?

Examine all possible solutions. Explore all possible, reasonable actions in terms of ethical principles. In considering solutions, it is important to evaluate realistically which options you can implement within legal guidelines and agency policy. Activities such as facilitating communication, providing facts, and ensuring that participants are aware of all reasonable options are always within the purview of nursing. Additionally, you must be aware of the likely outcomes of the various possible solutions. Will the consequences of actions taken be those that are intended? Will the intended good be served?

Choose solutions. After careful deliberation, choose a solution (or solutions) and take action. The chosen solutions must be consistent with ethical principles and be based on ethical analysis.

Box 2-5 Case Study Using the Six-Step Ethical Decision-Making Process

Michael R. is a 25-year-old African-American client diagnosed with sickle cell disease who has undergone multiple hospital admissions in the last 2 years. He is admitted to Catherine's med-surg unit for the sixth time in the last 5 months. Catherine has cared for him on his last two admissions. She is again assigned to his care. She is aware that an ongoing issue with Michael is pain management. She is concerned when she reads the prescribed pain-management regimen.

His physician prescribed the same regimen during his last two admissions and the client frequently complained of inadequate pain relief, asking for more medication before it was time for his next dose. Because of constant pain and inadequate relief, Michael was often angry and frustrated. The nurses have labeled him hostile and difficult to work with. They expressed relief that Catherine would provide his care.

Catherine notes that the physician prescribed Demerol, 50 to 100 mg, and Vistaril, 50 mg IM every 4 to 6 hours. She knows that the nurses have a tendency to give the lower medication dose and closer to the 6-hour mark rather than the 4-hour mark. She has read recent research suggesting that morphine is a better medication for pain relief in sickle cell clients than Demerol.

Catherine also believes that patient-controlled analgesia (PCA) would probably be best for Michael. However, he is uninsured and she is afraid that the hospital would not assume the cost of PCA. She is unsure whether the physician would be willing to change the orders or listen to her ideas.

Catherine feels that Michael will have the same issues of pain management arise during this hospitalization. She is concerned that he is not getting the best possible care for his condition because of the prescribed pain management, his financial status, and nursing attitudes. She is unsure of what steps to take or what she should do. What follows is a six-step ethical decision-making process using this situation as the example.

STEP 1: IDENTIFY THE ETHICAL DILEMMA

What is the situation that raises ethical problems? Is it a matter of ethics, a legal issue, or a question of communication? Are there ethical principles in conflict?

The client is not a private paying client. Some nurses have said that when he rates his pain at 10+ he doesn't appear to be in a great deal of pain. The physician in question is not noted for listening to nurses' opinions sabout issues that he considers to be medical practice.

Catherine has been feeling dissatisfied with the care that Michael received in the past. She is concerned that she is not protecting his rights or advocating for him. She has voiced her concern to a couple of co-workers, who did not validate her feelings. No formal action has been taken.

STEP 2: GATHER PERTINENT DATA

Review all significant data. Identify the relevant facts. Who are the people involved? Is there a conflict of values? Are there cultural influences? What are the economic and financial implications?

Is the prescribed regimen consistently implemented? Is there a mechanism for implementing action? Are there supportive nursing policies?

Catherine feels that the nursing staff is not showing care and concern. She wonders if the nurses are sensitive to cultural variations in expressing pain. She feels that adequate pain management is possible for Michael, but that the current regimen is neither effective nor implemented appropriately. She thinks that Michael should have more involvement in decision making about his pain management. Nursing policies document standards of nursing practice and nursing care that are helpful guidelines.

STEP 3: EXAMINE THE DILEMMA FOR ETHICAL PRINCIPLES

What principles are key to making a decision here? What is the overall good to be accomplished (beneficence)? Have the principal decision makers been given all the necessary information? Whose interests are being served (justice)? What are the expectations from caregivers (fidelity)?

Catherine feels that Michael can expect pain relief. The good of the client should be the primary concern. She also feels that he can expect to be treated with respect and have his dignity maintained.

She remains unsure of the physician's response but thinks he should be approached. She feels that the nursing staff needs more information regarding pain management for clients with sickle cell disease.

STEP 4: EXAMINE ALL SOLUTIONS

What are all the possible and reasonable actions? What options open to Catherine are legal and within agency policy? What are the possible outcomes and consequences of actions taken? Will the intended good be served?

Catherine considers the options open to her:
- She can voice her concern to the physician and discuss nursing concerns with the unit staff.
- She can consult with the charge nurse and unit director.
- She can involve the client in decision making.
- She can consult with the unit's clinical nurse specialist and nursing education department.
- She can plan a client care conference.
- She can develop a collaborative plan of care using the nursing process.
- She can say nothing and not make waves while trying to give Michael the best care possible when she is on duty.

STEP 5: CHOOSE SOLUTIONS

After deliberation, choose solutions and act on them. Are solutions chosen consistent with ethical principles?

Catherine chooses to speak with the charge nurse and share her concerns. She shares the research information and asks for a client care conference. She involves the clinical nurse specialist in the conference. The client is involved in the decision-making process and included in the care conference. From the conference, a plan of care is developed that includes recommendation for a referral to a pain-management specialist.

Catherine approaches the physician and discusses her concern. He was aware of the conference but did not choose to participate. He does not change his orders but does make a request for the pain-management specialist to see the client.

STEP 6: EVALUATE SOLUTIONS CHOSEN

Was the solution effective and the expected outcome achieved? Was the ethical problem resolved or were additional problems identified?

Consultation with the pain-management specialist resulted in a change in the client's pain-management regimen and client education regarding self-care. He was put in a pain-management protocol study and was able to receive a PCA pump.

Catherine observed that Michael experienced effective pain relief. Other nurses said that they found him pleasant and approachable when his pain was managed. Some of the staff voiced that Catherine had gone overboard for one client.

The unit director recommended that nursing forums should be instituted on a quarterly basis to provide information on ethical principles and identify ethical issues. The nurse educator is planning seminars on the topics of pain management and cultural sensitivity.

Evaluate solutions chosen. Examine solutions chosen for effectiveness. Reflect on whether expected outcomes were reached. Questions to ask include the following: Did solutions chosen resolve the ethical dilemma? What was the effect on those involved? Were additional ethical issues identified? Was the chosen solution the best one in light of the outcomes generated?

Often there is more than one possible solution. The ethical decision-making process assists you in reaching the best solution for a particular situation. The process may also help you to overcome the initial feelings of helplessness that you may experience when facing an ethical dilemma (Box 2-5). Keep in mind that a single perfect answer may not result from this process. Instead, you will search for the answer closest to the intended good for the primary parties involved in the dilemma.

Guides to Ethical Decisions in Nursing

INSTITUTIONAL ETHICS COMMITTEES. Institutional ethics committees are multidisciplinary committees of health care professionals within a facility that perform a variety of tasks related to ethical issues within that facility. Nursing is represented on such committees, but it is usually not in the majority and may be represented only at the administrative level. Ethics committees provide consultation, education, case review, decision making, and mediation when conflicts arise between health care professionals in the identification and resolution of ethical dilemmas (Figure 2-6). They are integral to the development of facility policies and procedures regarding ethics and to the implementation of such policies and procedures (Fowler & Levine-Ariff, 1987).

NURSING ETHICS FORUMS. Heitman and Robinson (1997) describe a nursing ethics forum that can provide a mechanism for nurses to identify and address ethical issues that affect delivery of nursing care. These forums are separate from institutional ethics committees and may be hospital-wide or unit based, involving nursing rounds or case review. Nursing ethics forums focus on assisting you in developing skills in ethical analysis and decision making. They may begin informally as discussions of issues that you have identified as ethical dilemmas.

Nursing forums can provide education in ethical theories, principles, and decision-making models. They can help you

develop skills in ethical analysis and decision making by doing the following (Heitman & Robinson, 1997):

- Providing education in ethical theories, principles, and decision making
- Providing a format for nurses to exchange ideas and talk about ethical issues
- Providing a mechanism for early detection of ethical dilemmas
- Creating a format for recommendations to the institutional ethics committee

It is important that you be knowledgeable about concepts of ethical decision making and able to articulate and apply such concepts in ethical dilemmas. The services of a clinician who has expertise in ethics should be obtained to provide the needed information and instruction.

In many health care settings, you are the primary practitioner with whom clients and families interact. As such, you may be the first to obtain information regarding clients' health care choices. Your nursing skills must include the ability to recognize potential and actual ethical dilemmas. However, you do not solve ethical problems in isolation. Within a health care institution, a nursing practice committee and an institutional ethics committee are forums for resolving ethical problems. A nurse can also look outside the facility to religious leaders or medical–ethical experts to obtain support and guidance in dealing with ethical problems.

Providing nursing care within an ethical framework is the cornerstone of professional nursing practice. To practice within such a framework, you must incorporate ethical principles and standards into your nursing behaviors.

CLIENT RIGHTS

Self-determination has long been valued in Western society, especially regarding health care choices. The American Hospital Association's Patient Care Partnership: Understanding Expectations, Rights, and Responsibilities supports this value:

Self-determination has long been valued in Western society especially regarding health care choices. The American Hospital Association supports this value through the Patient's Bill of Rights in 1975 and the Patient Care Partnership: Understanding Expectations, Rights, and Responsibilities in 2003. Both these documents describe the rights of patients to have informed consent and to refuse treatment. The more recent Patient Care Partnership clearly outlines the elements of informed consent. The American Hospital Association clearly supports the idea that patients should be involved in their treatment and asking questions about their care.

The ethical principle of autonomy, discussed earlier, is clearly reflected in this passage. Although autonomy calls on you to respect client health care decisions, this is possible only when the client's choices are made known.

The health care client has specific rights that affect the relationship between the client and the health care provider and between the client and the health care delivery system. These rights protect each client's ability to determine the level and type of care received. Several of these rights interface with your practice of nursing. Informed consent

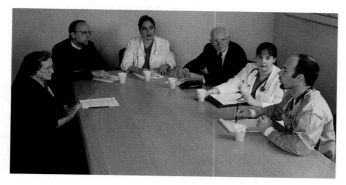

Figure 2-6. An ethics committee at work.

advance directives, do-not-resuscitate orders, organ transplant preferences, and client confidentiality are among the client's rights that direct, in certain instances, how you must practice nursing.

Informed Consent

Informed consent involves the legal right of clients to receive adequate and accurate information about their medical condition and treatment. Such information is necessary for clients to exercise their right to select and consent to particular treatments. The presumption of the law is that all adult clients possess the decision-making capacity to make informed decisions regarding their treatment choices.

If a health care provider believes an adult client is incapable of making informed decisions, an evaluation by a specialist must take place and an opinion rendered before the client is denied the right of informed consent. When the court determines that a client is incapable of making decisions, it may appoint a personal guardian to make decisions on the client's behalf. In some states, statutes have been enacted that identify a ranked listing of who should be consulted to make decisions. The list may begin with a spouse and continue to adult children, parents, and then a sibling.

Minor children are viewed under the law as lacking decision-making capacity. Therefore the parent or legal guardian provides informed consent after receiving all the required information. In some cases, minors are able to provide their own consent for treatment, such as for a sexually transmitted disease or when the minor is married or otherwise emancipated.

Courts have established the information to be shared with a client to obtain informed consent (Box 2-6). A physician is responsible for conveying information and obtaining informed consent for medical procedures. If you are involved in obtaining informed consent for a medical procedure, in most states you are only witnessing the signature of the client on the informed consent form. You may be the person who actually ensures that the client signs the informed consent form. However, you should ask the client to sign a consent form only if the physician has instructed the client and you have determined that the client has reasonably understood the information. You should obtain informed consent for nursing care and procedures.

Advance Directives

An **advance directive** is a written document that provides direction for health care in the future, when clients may be unable to make personal treatment choices. It allows clients to express their preferences for health care prior to an event that renders them incapable of indicating their treatment choices. Individual state laws provide for specific kinds of advance directives, including living wills and the durable power of attorney for health care.

A **living will** is a document that provides written instructions about when life-sustaining treatment should be terminated. Additionally, it may indicate when and if a person may be hospitalized and what types of treatment may be implemented. Ideally, these preferences are discussed in advance with family and friends who may become involved in decision making, so the person's wishes are clearly understood by all. Some living wills may contain general statements requesting that no extraordinary means be used to extend life. The more general the statements, the more open they are to interpretation. California was the first state to recognize living wills with the passage of its Natural Death Act in 1976.

A **durable power of attorney for health care,** also called a proxy directive, is a document that designates a person to make decisions about the client's medical treatment in the event that the client becomes unable to do so. The designated person may be a family member, an attorney, or a friend who is aware of the client's wishes. Like the living will, the durable power of attorney for health care is most effective when the client has written specific instructions. Again, ideally, the client will have discussed his preferences with the person he appoints as his agent.

Often, a nurse is the first health care provider to become aware that a client has executed an advance directive. Thus it may be up to you to make sure that a copy of the advance directive becomes part of the client's record. It may also be up to you to inform the physician about the client's advance directive. In any event, you should ensure that both requirements are met.

When working with a client's significant others, it is especially important to ensure that the decision maker is the person *legally* authorized to make the decisions. Several different family members or significant others may voice conflicting opinions about the client's care. Your obligation is to consult with the person legally authorized to make treatment decisions, even when this person is not clearly identifiable.

State laws and statutes about advance directives may vary. It is important for hospital policies and procedures to be developed and implemented in line with regulatory requirements, and for you to become familiar with such policies and procedures.

Box 2-6   Informed Consent Checklist

The client has received the following information:
- ❏ Diagnosis
- ❏ Name of procedure, test, or medication
- ❏ Explanation of procedure, test, or medication
- ❏ Reasons for recommending the procedure, test, or medication
- ❏ Anticipated benefits
- ❏ Major risks of the procedure, test, or medication
- ❏ Alternative treatments
- ❏ Prognosis if treatment is refused

The nurse has performed the following duties:
- ❏ Assessed barriers, such as hearing impediments, transcultural factors, pain, anxiety, and other factors that could influence the client's understanding of the information
- ❏ Assessed the influence of education, age, developmental level, and emotional status on the client's ability to understand the information
- ❏ Ensured that information was provided in a manner that facilitated understanding
- ❏ Determined that the client is voluntarily giving informed consent

Organ Transplants. As is the case for other treatments, clients have the right to decline organ transplant as a treatment option. Clients also have the right to determine whether they want to donate their organs and tissues for someone else's benefit at the time of death. The desire to donate organs can be expressed through a written document executed before death. In the absence of an express written directive providing an informed consent for donation, the Uniform Anatomical Gift Act would control the donation of any organ.

The Uniform Anatomical Gift Act is law in all states and provides a list of individuals who can provide informed consent for the donation of the deceased individual's organs. The persons on the list must be contacted in order, usually a spouse first, followed by adult children and parents of the deceased.

Do-Not-Resuscitate Orders. Implicit in the client's right to informed consent is a client's right to refuse treatment. In fact, clients have a right to refuse treatment even if that treatment is needed to sustain life.

Cardiopulmonary resuscitation (CPR) is one type of treatment refused by clients. Most health care agencies have developed policies to guide health care providers when clients choose not to be resuscitated. These policies should include a written order for a do-not-resuscitate (DNR) status, review of the order on a regular basis, and evidence of informed consent by the client or legal representative in requesting a DNR. Additionally, DNR and CPR must be specifically defined, so that the client continues to receive any desired treatment.

Confidentiality

Confidentiality is the client's right to privacy in the health care delivery system, as discussed under Ethical Principles earlier in this chapter. As a nurse, you have an ethical obligation to maintain client confidentiality. You are party to much sensitive and private information about clients and must exercise discretion in sharing that information. Sharing information about a client with people who are not involved in the client's care, such as disclosing information about one client to another client, is a violation of client confidentiality. Talking about a client in the hallways, cafeteria, grocery store, social club, or anywhere else with people who are not involved in the client's care is also a violation of client confidentiality. Additionally, disclosure of confidential information could expose you to liability for invasion of your client's privacy.

Even if your conversation partner is involved in caring for the client, in public places you must guard against disclosing information within earshot of others. Some nurses mistakenly think that they have not breached client confidentiality if they talk about the client without using a specific name. If sufficient information is conveyed for another person to identify the person under discussion, however, client confidentiality has indeed been violated and charges of invasion of privacy could be forthcoming.

Increasingly, clients are enrolled in health care networks that offer a range of services, including ambulatory care, hospitalization, rehabilitation services, home care services, and other health-related benefits. Ensuring the provision of care falls to case managers, discharge planners, and other care coordinators. Such planning requires access to confidential information. Additionally, third-party payers and utilization review departments access confidential information to address payment issues. This information is often transmitted by electronic means to the agencies within the network. The difficulty in maintaining client confidentiality is thus compounded by a greater number of persons accessing sensitive client information and the means by which the information is shared.

Any request for client information you receive should be evaluated very carefully. Address two questions. First, does the person requesting client information have a need to know the information requested? Suppose you work in a home care agency. Client information might be shared with the agency's social worker for the purpose of helping the client receive social services, but the social worker may not need to know all the details of the client's medical care. Furthermore, the office administrative assistant may recognize your client as a neighbor and ask you probing questions about your client's condition. The state nurse practice act, ethical considerations, and nursing standards of care require you to protect client confidentiality.

The second question to ask yourself is whether the client has authorized the release of information. When clients consent to receive services from a particular health care agency, they usually sign a consent form for treatment that includes an authorization for information to be shared with people in the agency involved in the client's treatment. Beyond this, requests for information come from concerned family, friends, or employers. Requests also come from other health care providers, lawyers, insurance companies, and public news sources. Carefully consider whether the client has authorized release of information to these persons. When in doubt, consult with your supervisor.

Specific federal or state statutes protect the confidentiality of some client groups. Persons receiving treatment for drug and alcohol abuse, mental health care, sexual assault, HIV infection, and AIDS are among the groups whose confidentiality receives additional protection under the law. If you work with clients in these categories, you should familiarize yourself with the particulars of confidentiality requirements.

QUALITY IMPROVEMENT INITIATIVES

Quality improvement initiatives are activities that health care agencies undertake to contain costs, improve quality, and increase competitiveness. Some of the costs an agency seeks to reduce are those related to legal liability arising from adverse occurrences. *Adverse occurrence* is a term sometimes used to describe errors in practice or the injury or death of a client. Health care agencies have used several methods to manage adverse occurrences. These include incident reports, risk management committees, quality assurance committees, safety programs, and quality improvement programs.

Risk management programs and quality improvement programs are somewhat different in focus, but both can potentially reduce legal liability. Continuous quality improvement, total quality management, and quality initiatives are programs that have proliferated in recent years in health care facilities. These programs focus on improving the quality of client care or the efficient operation of the business by examining the processes used to deliver health care services. For example, a quality improvement initiative might examine how waiting time in an outpatient clinic can be reduced.

In contrast, incident reports and risk management programs identify and analyze risks with the objective of taking corrective action and thus reducing legal liability. A risk management program might examine the excessive number of client falls at the entrance to a long-term health care facility. You may become involved in both types of programs.

Incident or Adverse Occurrence Reports

An incident or adverse occurrence report is a tool used by health care facilities to document situations that have caused harm or have the potential to cause harm to clients, employees, or visitors. Medication errors, client falls, and accidental needlesticks are common situations documented on an incident report. The report is not part of the client's medical record and should not be referenced in the client's record. These reports are used to identify patterns of risk so that a corrective plan can be developed. The report also serves as a record of the facts surrounding the event should litigation arise at some point in the future.

The nurse who identified the potential or actual harm or who created the situation leading to actual or potential harm initiates the incident report. The incident report identifies the people involved in the event (including witnesses), describes the event, and records the date, time, location, actions taken, and other relevant information. A physician completes the report after examining the client, employee, or visitor if actual or potential injury occurred. Often, suggestions are solicited for how this event can be avoided in the future.

In some instances, incident reports can be used in a court of law. Documentation should be as factual as possible and avoid accusations. Questions of liability are for the court to decide and therefore conclusions about who is responsible for the event should be avoided in the incident report.

Risk Management Programs

Risk management programs have several components. An ongoing safety program is essential to ensure the safety of clients, employees, and visitors. Periodic inspections of electrical equipment, monthly fire drills, and monitoring of the disposal of hazardous wastes, are often included in safety programs. Educational programs about potential risks help reduce accidents and injuries. Identifying known risks (e.g., by putting up warning signs for construction or ice on the walkway) are also activities of a risk management program.

A health agency may have a designated risk manager. This person can be an invaluable resource to answer questions regarding potential risks and liabilities.

SAFEGUARDING YOUR PRACTICE

The legal threats to your continuing practice as a professional nurse are very real. Clients deserve and demand that only those persons who are able to provide safe, competent quality care should practice nursing. Administrative procedures, lawsuits, and disciplinary practices by employers help ensure that unsafe and incompetent nurses are removed from the practice of nursing. Despite the demands and complexity of nursing, you can take steps to safeguard your nursing practice and avoid having legal action taken against you.

Know Your Obligations and Responsibilities

The first step in safeguarding your practice is to thoroughly understand your professional, legal, and ethical obligations and responsibilities. It is as important to be competent in the professional and legal aspects of your practice as it is to be technically competent. Read your state's nurse practice act. Read your job description and your employer's policies and procedures. Follow legislative bills that may affect your practice. Track court decisions that clarify the specifics of your practice and identify your potential legal exposure (the Internet can help you find them). Read the standards of practice that apply to your area of nursing and comply with the guidance provided. These actions are important steps in making sure that your practice conforms to the expectations inherent in your license to practice nursing.

Practice Competently

The competent practice of nursing requires that, as your professional practice develops, you expand on the skills and knowledge you acquired as a nursing student. You are expected to maintain competency in three domains:

- *Technical competency:* You perform skills accurately, safely, and in a manner consistent with established procedures.
- *Cognitive competency:* Having acquired knowledge and information, you understand the needs of your clients and implement appropriate nursing care.
- *Interpersonal competency:* You further develop effective communication techniques for working with professional colleagues and maintaining therapeutic relationships with clients.

Keep in mind that clients who believe their nurse is caring and respectful are less likely to sue. The combination of technical, cognitive, and interpersonal competencies applied within the legal limits of nursing practice is an effective safeguard for your nursing practice.

Know Your Strengths and Limitations

The nursing profession is characterized by endless opportunities. The number of work settings, types of clients, specific expectations of a nursing position, conditions of employment, work hours, and any number of other factors combine to create a vast array of nursing opportunities, some of which will match your temperament, skills, knowledge, and interests. The key to finding an appropriate nursing position is an accurate assessment of your professional and personal strengths and weaknesses.

No nurse can function equally effectively in all settings. A nurse accustomed to the collegiality of an institutional setting may find the independence of community health nursing unnerving. An experienced intensive care nurse may feel that work in a physician's office is not challenging enough and may overlook critical elements of practice. A nurse who is mismatched with or overwhelmed by the demands of a particular position or type of client is inviting disciplinary or legal action.

Keep Current

A license to practice nursing signifies that you have met the minimum standards for a beginning practitioner. The expectation is that you will ultimately become a master practitioner of your chosen profession. This can occur only if you acknowledge your role as lifelong learner. Action follows acknowledgment. Attending in-service programs, pursuing continuing education courses, reading professional publications, and attending professional meetings are evidence of your commitment to continued professional growth.

Projections made about the relevancy of the nursing information you master today suggest that much of what you know will be obsolete in 3 years. Indeed, 25 years ago, standard precautions were unheard of and gloves were worn only to keep your hands clean. At that time, AIDS, Ebola, hepatitis C, and other very serious illnesses had not yet been identified. Nursing is an evolving profession. It is incumbent upon you to keep your practice current. An outdated practice is a practice ripe for a lawsuit.

Document Your Care

Documentation of your activities while practicing nursing will not compensate for failing to render nursing care that is consistent with established standards of practice. However, timely, accurate, complete, and appropriate documentation of the care you give can provide evidence that you executed your professional responsibilities in accordance with your legal and professional obligations. Client records are legal documents that may be entered as evidence in a lawsuit. In either a lawsuit or an insurance claim, documentation may be the factor upon which liability determinations are made.

There are many types of documentation formats. In all cases, the content of the documentation requires that you make decisions about the words you use, the relevance of the information you provide, the completeness of your notations, and the inclusion of certain information. Information conveyed should be an accurate, complete, objective, and relevant assessment of your client and the nursing care you provided. As in other forms of communication, however, excellent documentation takes practice.

The client record is a legal document that should provide a complete and accurate picture of the client's condition and the nursing care provided. Nurses are sometimes reluctant to document adverse events that happen to clients. But falls, medication errors, and other adverse incidents must be documented as completely and accurately as any other information pertinent to the client's care. Document the event in a straightforward manner, including all the steps you took to respond appropriately to the situation.

Purchase Professional Liability Insurance

Despite competent or even expert nursing care, clients are not always satisfied with the outcomes of their health care experiences. Also, the responsibilities and complexities of practice in today's rapidly changing health care environment can create situations that expose you to greater legal risk. Although it is virtually impossible to practice flawless nursing, the cost of an error in your practice could be a lawsuit. Increasingly, nurses are being named with the agency and the physician in a lawsuit. Insurance coverage will not reduce the risk of being sued, but at least the financial impact of a lawsuit can be minimized.

In the past, plaintiffs have named in a lawsuit those persons or institutions believed to have the most money. Thus the hospital and physicians were typically sued, whereas nurses were overlooked because they lacked "deep pockets." Yet with the rise in nurses' salaries, the protection against being sued attributed to the deep-pockets theory is becoming increasingly suspect. Indeed, some people believe that a nurse who has individual liability insurance is more likely to be sued.

In a variety of employment settings, you may be told that you are covered by your employer's liability insurance and do not need to purchase individual liability insurance. Your employer's lawyers also may have an excellent record of representing their nurse employees. If you have individual insurance coverage, the approach of your insurance company to the management of a lawsuit may differ from the approach of your employer's lawyers. The resulting adversarial relationship between you and your employer could be detrimental to a mutually agreeable resolution of the lawsuit.

Despite these risks, however, there are several sound reasons why you should purchase your own professional liability insurance even if you are covered under an employer's insurance plan. One is to ensure that, if you are named as a defendant in a lawsuit, your best interests will be represented. An employer's first obligation is to reduce or eliminate its own liability. One way of doing that may be to shift responsibility for the incident to you by trying to demonstrate that you practiced incompetently, that you exceeded the limits of your job description, or that you did not follow agency policies and procedures. These would represent attempts to prove that you, and not the agency, should be held liable.

A second reason you should have your own professional liability insurance is to protect you when you are providing care or giving advice outside of work. An employer's insurance will cover only your professional activities while working for the employer. You may want to believe you are a nurse only while at work, but family, friends, and neighbors know otherwise. The first aid you provide at your daughter's soccer game, the health education and screening done during a health fair at the local retirement community, the advice you are asked to give to the neighbor's ailing father you meet at the grocery store, and countless other occasions may expose you to liability. You must protect yourself whether or not you are providing professional services during your employment hours.

Key Principles

- Laws are rules or standards of conduct. Laws are developed by the different branches of government and are statutory, administrative, or judicial, or they arise from constitutions. Governments enact and enforce laws.
- Many different types of law affect the practice of nursing. These include civil, criminal, common, private, procedural, public, statutory, and substantive law.
- Specific laws that secondarily affect the practice of nursing include the Occupational Health and Safety Act, Controlled Substance Act, Americans with Disabilities Act, and Health Care Quality Improvement Act.
- Legal liability may result from intentional torts involving assault and battery, defamation, fraud, false imprisonment, or invasion of privacy.
- Negligence and malpractice are unintentional torts. Liability is determined by proving duty, breach of duty, causation, and damages.
- Voluntary professional standards also regulate nursing practice. Standards of care and practice are developed by professional nursing organizations and organizations that accredit educational programs or institutions.
- Failure to adhere to legal and professional directives regarding the practice of nursing can result in professional discipline, legal liability, or employer disciplinary actions. A nurse may simultaneously be involved in two or more of these actions.
- Employer job descriptions, policies, and procedures direct the practice of nursing in a specific employment setting. These directives should conform to professional and legal practice guidelines.
- Nurse practice acts regulate nursing practice in a specific state and provide mechanisms for disciplinary action against nurses practicing in that state.
- The nursing profession attempts to ensure the competency of its practitioners through individual licensure and certification methods and through educational program accreditation.
- Clients have specific rights, including confidentiality, informed consent, use of advance directives, and control over decisions about organ transplant and life-sustaining measures.
- Health care agencies undertake quality improvement initiatives to contain costs, improve quality, and increase competitiveness. They try to reduce potential legal liability through the use of risk management programs and incident or adverse occurrence reporting mechanisms.
- Members of the nursing profession ensure competent and safe professional practice by reading professional publications and attending continuing education programs, professional meetings, and in-service programs.
- Legal safeguards for nurses begin with competent practice. Additional safeguards include understanding professional responsibilities and obligations, recognizing individual strengths and limitations, keeping knowledge and skills current and accurate, documenting care appropriately, and purchasing individual professional liability insurance.
- Ethical principles in conjunction with professional and legal obligations provide the framework for professional nursing and guide nursing actions during care delivery. The principles of autonomy, beneficence, confidentiality, nonmaleficence, fidelity, justice, and veracity are considered essential to nursing.
- In the United States, the American Nurses' Association *Code for Nurses* governs ethical nursing practice. The code sets forth the philosophy of the profession and identifies the goals and values of nursing. The code also provides a guide to ethical nursing practice and can be used to evaluate nursing actions.
- Ethics is the branch of philosophy that attempts to determine what constitutes good, bad, right, and wrong in terms of human behavior. The study of ethics helps you determine the correctness of actions in situations that have ethical implications.
- The term *moral* is often used to describe ethical behavior. Morals are standards of behavior to which society expects members to adhere. Nurses are expected to be moral agents who perform duties within established standards of moral conduct.
- Values are ideals and beliefs that are chosen and prized by an individual, group, or society. Values form the basis for ethical decision making. Thus it is important for nurses to clarify values because they provide the platform from which decisions are made and actions are taken.
- In the delivery of health care, nurses are often required to make decisions that affect clients; therefore, it is important for nurses to recognize ethical dilemmas and apply ethical standards in resolving those dilemmas.
- Models for ethical decision making provide systematic and thoughtful mechanisms to examine issues and determine if ethical dilemmas exist. This systematic analysis helps you in clarifying a problem, identifying possible solutions and actions, and evaluating actions taken.
- Advance directives provide a guide to ethical decisions that identify client wishes about health care. They support client self-determination (autonomy), which is a key ethical principle. Other guides to ethical decisions in nursing include informed consent, a client's written instructions, institutional ethics committees, and nursing ethics forums.

Bibliography

*American Hospital Association. (1992). *Patient's bill of rights.* Washington, DC: Author.

*American Nurses' Association. (2003). *Standards of clinical nursing practice.* Washington, DC: Author.

*Asterisk indicates a classic or definitive work on this subject.

American Nurses Association. (2002). *Code of ethics for nurses.* Geneva, Switzerland: Author.

American Nurses' Association. (2001). *Code of ethics for nurses with interpretive statements.* Washington, DC: Author.

*American Nurses' Association. (2001). *Code for nurses.* Washington, DC: Author.

Anderson, E. R., & Gold, J. (1996). Medical malpractice insurance: Nurses take on bigger health care role and bigger legal risks. *Journal of Nursing Law, 3,* 27-33.

Association of Women's Health, Obstetric and Neonatal Nurses. (1997). *Fetal Monitoring Principles and Practices.* Washington, DC: Author.

Ballard, D., & Cohen, J. (1995). Confidentiality of patient records in the computer age. *Journal of Nursing Law, 2,* 49-61.

Beauchamp, T., & Childress, J. (2001). *Principles of biomedical ethics* (5th ed.). London: Oxford University Press.

Bernzweig, E. P. (1996). *The nurse's liability for malpractice: A programmed course* (6th ed.). St Louis, MO: Mosby.

*Black, H. C. (1999). *Black's law dictionary* (7th ed.). St Paul, MN: West.

Brent, N. J. (2000). *Nurses and the law: A guide to principles and applications* (2nd ed.). Philadelphia: Saunders.

Brown, S. M. (1999). Good Samaritan laws: Protection and limits. *RN, 62*(11), 65-68.

Burkhardt, M., & Nathaniel, A. (1998). *Ethics and issues in contemporary nursing.* Albany, NY: Delmar.

Calfee, B. E. (1996). Labor laws: Working to protect you. *Nursing, 26*(2), 34-40.

Cameron, M. E. (2000). An ethical perspective: Value, be, do—Guidelines for resolving ethical conflict. *Journal of Nursing Law, 6*(4), 15-24.

Chally, P. S. (1998). Ethics in the trenches: Decision making in practice. *American Journal of Nursing, 90*(6), 17-20.

Deloughery, G. (1998). *Issues and trends in nursing* (3rd ed.). St Louis, MO: Mosby.

DeMarco, R. (1998). Caring to confront in the workplace: An ethical perspective for nurses. *Nursing Outlook, 46,* 27-32.

Fade, A. E. (1995). Advance directives: An overview of changing right to die laws. *Journal of Nursing Law, 2,* 27-38.

Federwisch, A. (1997). Making difficult daily choices: Ethics are everywhere. *Nurseweek, 10*(2), 1, 6.

*Fowler, M., & Levine-Ariff, J. (1987). *Ethics at the bedside: A source book for the critical care nurse.* American Association of Critical Care Nurses. Philadelphia: Lippincott.

Goldsborough, R. (1999). Doing the right thing: Computers and ethics. *RN, 62*(12), 19-20.

Gordon, S., & Fagan, C. M. (1998). Commentary: Preserving the moral high ground. *American Journal of Nursing, 98*(6), 31-32.

*Gosfield, A. (Ed.). (1993). *1993 Health law handbook.* Deerfield, IL: Clark Boardman Callaghan.

Hall, J. (1996). *Nursing ethics and law.* Philadelphia: Saunders.

Haynor, P. (1998). Meeting the challenge of advance directives. *American Journal of Nursing, 98*(3), 27-32.

Heitman, L., & Robinson, B. (1997). Developing a nursing ethics roundtable. *American Journal of Nursing, 97*(1), 36-38.

Helm, A., & Kihm, N. C. (2001). Is professional liability insurance for you? Before you say no, weigh these considerations. *Nursing, 31*(1), 48-49.

Hendin, H. (1999). Suicide, assisted suicide, and medical illness. *Journal of Clinical Psychiatry, 60*(Suppl. 2), 46-50; discussion, 51-52, 113-116.

Infante, M. (1996). The legal risks of managed care. *RN, 59,* 57-59.

*International Council of Nurses. (2000). *Code for nurses: Ethical concepts applied to nursing.* Geneva, Switzerland: Author.

*Jameton, A. (1984). *Nursing practice: The ethical issues.* Englewood Cliffs, NJ: Prentice-Hall.

Johnston, L. (1999). The advanced practice nurse: Changing the practice law—What did we learn? *Clinical Nurse Specialist, 13*(5), 243-247.

LaDuke, S. (2000). The effects of professional discipline on nurses. *American Journal of Nursing, 100*(6), 26-33.

Mathes, M. (2000). Ethics, law, and policy: Ethical challenges and nursing. *Medical-Surgical Nursing, 9*(1), 44-45.

McCloskey-Dochterman, J. C., & Grace, H. K. (2002). *Current issues in nursing* (6th ed.). St Louis, MO: Mosby.

New York Regulations of the Commissioner. Part 64: *Nursing.* Albany, NY: The State Education Department.

New York Rules of the Board of Regents. Part 29: *Unprofessional Conduct.* Albany, NY: The State Education Department.

New York Title VIII Education Law. Article 130: *General Provisions.* Subarticle 3: *Professional Misconduct.* Albany, NY: The State Education Department.

New York Title VIII Education Law. Article 139: *Nursing.* Albany, NY: The State Education Department.

Parks, B. (1998). Advanced directives: Do they really mean what they mean? *Journal of Emergency Nursing, 24*(5), 382-383.

Paul, S. (1999). Developing practice protocols for advanced practice nursing. *AACN Clinical Issues, 13*(5), 243-247.

Pinch, W. (1996). Is caring a moral trap? *Nursing Outlook, 46,* 130-135.

*Pojman, L. (1990). *Ethics: Discovery of right and wrong.* Belmont, CA: Wadsworth.

*Raths, L.E., Hormin, M., & Simon, S.B. (1978). *Values and teaching: Working with values in the classroom.* Columbus, OH: Charles E. Merrill Books.

*Rest, J. R. (1986). *Moral development: Advances in research and theory.* New York: Praeger.

Rice, V., Beck, C., & Stevenson, J. (1997). Ethical issues relative to autonomy and personal control in independent and cognitively impaired elders. *Nursing Outlook, 45,* 27-34.

Sheehan, J. (1996). Safeguard your license: Avoid these pitfalls. *RN, 59,* 59-62.

Sheehy, S. B. (1999). Understanding the legal process: Your best defense. *Journal of Emergency Nursing, 25*(6), 492-495.

Smith, R., Hiatt, H., & Berwick, D. (1999). Shared ethical principles for everybody in health care. *Nursing Standards, 13*(19), 32-33.

*Stewart, D., & Blocker, G. (2000). *Fundamentals of philosophy* (5th ed.). New York: Prentice-Hall.

Ulrich, C. M. (2001). Need for knowledge of ethics. *Journal of Nursing Scholarship, 33*(4), 306.

Wilkinson, A. (1998). Nursing malpractice. *Nursing, 28*(6), 34-40.

Yoder-Wise, P. (2003). *Leading and managing in nursing* (3rd ed.). St Louis, MO: Mosby.

Zimmermann, P. G. (2000). The use of unlicensed assistive personnel: An update and skeptical look at role that may present more problems than solutions. *Journal of Emergency Nursing, 26*(4), 312-317.

3

Cultural Context of Practice

Key Terms

cultural competence

culture

diversity

ethnic

ethnicity

ethnocentrism

humanistic care

multicultural society

stereotyping

transcultural nursing

universality

Learning Objectives

After studying this chapter, you should be able to do the following:

- Discuss culture and ethnicity as they relate to the delivery of nursing care
- Define humanistic care
- Outline the elements and objectives of transcultural nursing
- Describe the dangers of stereotyping
- List and explain the six concepts included in transcultural assessment
- Understand basic aspects of the Irish-American, African-American, Mexican-American, Chinese-American, and Navajo cultures
- Anticipate the effects of cultural characteristics on the successful delivery of health care

CONCEPTS OF CULTURE

Simple observation leads to the conclusion that, although people are all equal, they are not all alike. At least some of the differences among people stem from the behaviors, beliefs, and values learned from their families and other members of the society around them. Indeed, these cultural and ethnic influences can make people seem very different from one another.

As a nurse, you must be able to transcend the differences among people. You must seek to understand clients of all cultural backgrounds and to provide them with care that enhances their individual health and well-being. To do so, you will need a sound understanding of the effects of culture and ethnicity. And you will need to be able to work comfortably with clients who hold different beliefs and values from your own.

Culture and Ethnicity

Culture can be defined as a patterned behavioral response that develops over time as a consequence of imprinting the mind through social and religious structures and intellectual and artistic manifestations (Giger & Davidhizar, 1999). Culture is shaped by the values, beliefs, norms, and practices held in common by members of the cultural group. It guides a person's thinking, acting, and being, and it becomes a patterned expression for that person (Giger & Davidhizar, 1999).

Madeleine Leininger, a nurse anthropologist, defines culture as the learned, shared, and transmitted values, beliefs, norms, and lifeways of a particular group that guide thinking, decisions, and actions in a patterned way (Leininger, 1991). Most definitions of culture imply a dynamic, ever-changing process through which a group defines itself through art, music, stories, and lifestyles.

For most people, cultural background and ethnic background are intimately related (Spector, 1999). The term **ethnic** refers to groups of people of the same race or national origin (within a larger cultural system) that are distinctive based on traditions of religion, language, or appearance. A person's **ethnicity** reflects the characteristics a group may share in some combination (Box 3-1).

Multicultural Societies

The United States and Canada are examples of multicultural societies. A **multicultural society** is a society composed of more than one culture or subculture. It includes many groups that participate in and enjoy the larger culture. In such a society, the larger culture provides common interests and values. These shared interests and values help to create a social order that provides benefits to the society at large. In the United States, shared values include a democratic structure, equality among peoples, freedom of speech, and the right to the pursuit of happiness.

The United States contains many distinct ethnic groups that maintain some characteristics of their origins. This is largely because the United States is home to immigrants from every country in the world. Some nations—such as Germany,

---

Box 3-1 Characteristics of Ethnic Groups

PRIMARY CHARACTERISTICS

An ethnic group shares one or more of the following:
- Race
- Color
- National or geographic origin
- Religious beliefs
- Cultural origin

SECONDARY CHARACTERISTICS

Group identity is evident in one or more of the following:
- A sense of identity as a group
- Distinctive customs, art, music, literature
- Elements of lifestyles
- Language, accent, or dialect
- Style or manner of dress
- Food preferences, spices, methods of cooking
- Attitudes derived from group identity
- Moral values
- Economic or political beliefs
- Special political interests as a group
- Health care practices

England, Wales, and Ireland—are well represented. Others—such as Japan, the Philippines, and Greece—have smaller populations in the United States. People from around the world continue to enter the United States, particularly from Vietnam, Laos, Cambodia, Cuba, Haiti, and Mexico, and South and Central American countries (Spector, 1999).

In the United States, although cultures have blended to some degree, many cultural groups have remained visible and intact and function as a social force within the larger society. The social emphasis before the 1960s was on creating a "melting pot" society in which all members would blend together and create a common culture. Various cultures have blended together through marriage, membership in social organizations, and assimilation. However, a homogenized society runs the risk of losing distinctive contributions from cultural subgroups.

The multicultural societies of the United States and Canada represent all of the cultural and racial groups of the world (Figure 3-1, p. 44). However, the mix of cultural and ethnic populations is shifting. Experts project that by the year 2021 the number of Asian Americans and Hispanic Americans in the United States will triple, and the number of African Americans will double (U.S. Department of Commerce, Bureau of the Census, 1992, a,b).

These projections have important implications for society as a whole, and nursing in particular well into this new millenium. Recognizing the multicultural nature of society may be helpful in improving communication between groups and increasing the likelihood that individuals will work together through common concerns and create ways to solve societal problems. Understanding the cultural context of care for multiple cultural groups will increase your ability to provide individualized care and to influence health care institutions to

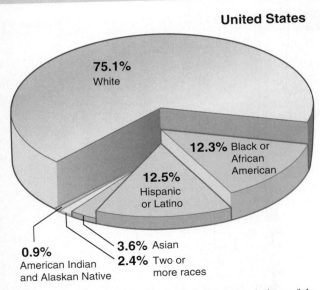

United States

75.1% White

12.3% Black or African American

12.5% Hispanic or Latino

0.9% American Indian and Alaskan Native

3.6% Asian

2.4% Two or more races

Figure 3-1. Racial and ethnic distribution of the populations of the United States. (Data from the United States Census. Bureau of the Census 2000 Redistricting [Public law 94-171], Summary file, Table PL1.)

meet the needs of diverse groups. The challenge will be to provide culturally appropriate care to clients with widely diverse backgrounds.

Transcultural Nursing

Nurses attempt to understand health problems from the client's unique perspective, and knowledge of the client's culture becomes a key to optimal client care. **Transcultural nursing** is culturally competent nursing care focused on differences and similarities among cultures, with respect to caring, health, and illness, based on the client's cultural values, beliefs, and practices (Leininger, 1991). To administer culturally appropriate care, you must avoid projecting onto the client your own cultural uniqueness and worldview. You must remember that each person is a product of past experiences, beliefs, and values that have been learned and passed down from one generation to the next (Giger & Davidhizar, 1999).

Providing care within the framework of the client's culture can yield a number of benefits:

- Increased understanding of health care behavior that can be used as a basis for practice
- Improved health resulting from internally consistent health practices
- Improved compliance with the health regimen
- Increased satisfaction with services
- Creation of methods or techniques that may be useful cross-culturally

Central to the concept of transcultural nursing is the concept of care as the essence of nursing. Cultural care has many meanings, expressions, and forms. To care for another person is to take the person under your protection, using the culture's own "forms, patterns, expressions, and structures of care to

know, explain, and predict well-being, health, or illness status" (Leininger, 1991, p. 23).

Transcultural nursing offers a way to provide humanistic care. **Humanistic care** includes understanding and knowing a client in as natural or human a way as possible while helping or guiding the client to achieve certain goals, make improvements, reduce discomforts, or face disability or death. The goal of humanistic care is to gain full understanding of human beings and their humanity (Leininger, 1991). Three elements important to recognize when seeking to provide humanistic care are ethnocentricity, stereotyping, and cultural competence.

Ethnocentricity. Self-esteem means to hold oneself in high regard. Part of the self is produced by the cultural group with which a person identifies and from which the person has learned how to behave and what to value. **Ethnocentrism** is the belief that one's own ethnic beliefs, customs, and attitudes are correct and thus superior. Ethnocentrism includes positive regard for that part of oneself that is culturally based. However, ethnocentric behaviors in a multicultural society produce conflict between cultural groups. One way to overcome the conflict is to identify beliefs and values that are common across all cultures, even those expressed through different behaviors and customs.

All cultures have strengths and weaknesses. Strengths of a culture are those elements that enhance the life and well-being of the members of the group. For example, children who have pride in their cultural heritage have a good foundation for healthy self-esteem in adulthood (Figure 3-2). Weaknesses (such as alcohol dependency) are elements that can have detrimental effects on the group as a whole or on a significant number of people in the group. Most human characteristics can be strengths or weaknesses, depending on the circumstances and the behaviors that result.

Stereotyping. The danger of having a little knowledge about a culture is the belief that it is enough to provide culturally competent care. Instead, it may lead to stereotyping. **Stereotyping** is the assumption that an attribute present in some members of a group is present in all its members. A stereotype may be associated with a negative attribute, but not always. For example, knowing that the Chinese use acupuncture to treat many ailments might lead you to assume that a Chinese-American client would be interested in or would even prefer acupuncture as anesthesia for a minor surgical procedure. In reality, both traditional and Western medicine are taught in Chinese medical schools, and many Chinese physicians do not use acupuncture.

If you assume that you know something about a person just because that person is Appalachian, Bostonian, Canadian, or Mexican American, you are stereotyping. This is a dangerous way of characterizing other people, even when the assumption may have some elements of truth. In trying to establish rapport, the *process* of getting to know the person may be more important than knowledge of the person.

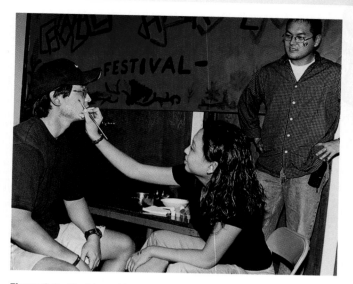

Figure 3-2. Healthy self-esteem in young adulthood is tied to appreciation of one's cultural heritage. These Korean Americans demonstrate pride in their cultural heritage through participation in a cultural celebration.

Cultural Competence. Cultural competence can be described as having enough knowledge of cultural groups that are different from your own to be able to interact with a member of a group in a manner that makes the person feel respected and understood. However, knowledge alone is not enough. You will need an attitude that appreciates differences before you can see the strengths of a client whose values, beliefs, and behaviors differ from yours. In addition, it is important to clarify your own values as a prerequisite to caring for clients of differing cultures (Table 3-1, p. 46).

Because it is difficult to acquire enough knowledge of multiple cultures to fully understand the cultural perspective of every client you will encounter as a nurse, it is important to develop positive attitudes that are helpful to working with different peoples. Culturally competent practitioners have five attributes: awareness, sensitivity, recognition, respect, and the ability to compromise.

AWARENESS. Awareness includes recognizing the values and beliefs of both your client and yourself. It therefore requires you to clarify your own values, as suggested earlier, and to actively seek to understand and appreciate the values of others. Thus becoming aware requires an attitude of discovery, active listening, and the desire to learn.

It is normal to filter observed behaviors through your own values and beliefs. This filtering produces bias or preconceived beliefs about the meaning of behavior or about the beliefs of another person. Bias can be favorable or unfavorable, and it is not necessarily correct.

SENSITIVITY. Sensitivity means recognizing the possibility of different meanings of behavior and looking objectively for cues that suggest the meaning. It also requires you to validate your interpretation with the client.

RECOGNITION. Recognizing the customs and behaviors of clients from different cultures requires knowledge.

Obtaining that knowledge requires curiosity. You must have the desire to explain why you are seeing, hearing, or experiencing something about a client.

Although you can gain a certain amount of knowledge from books, understanding will be enhanced when you live among and interact with persons of different cultures. Naturally, you will not be able to live among people from all the cultures that you will encounter in nursing practice. However, learning to recognize and value the differences of even one or two other cultures will heighten your observations of all cultures.

RESPECT. Respect may be the most important attitude to convey when working with persons of a different culture. When you respect others, you recognize and acknowledge their worth and uniqueness. You also recognize and honor their rights and privileges.

Respect dictates that you refrain from interfering with the beliefs and values of another. To develop respect, you must believe that there is value in diversity and then actively look for the value in lifeways that are different from your own.

COMPROMISE. You may need a willingness to compromise when a client's values and beliefs about health care, life, family, responsibility, or medical treatment differ from yours. An attitude of compromise implies that there is more than one right way to do anything.

DIVERSITY AND UNIVERSALITY. Another framework for developing cultural competence is Leininger's theory of diversity and universality. It postulates that "care or caring patterns include assistive, supportive, facilitative, and enabling acts or attitudes that influence the well-being or the health status of individuals, families, groups, and institutions as well as general human conditions" (Leininger, 1991). Caring acts and attitudes can be classified into those that are universal across cultures and those that are diverse. The term **universality** describes a common mode or value of caring or a prevailing pattern of care across cultures. **Diversity** refers to the differences in modes or patterns of care between cultures and includes specific patterns of care within cultural groups.

This model assigns three major modalities to guide culturally sensitive nursing care. *Cultural care preservation/ maintenance* includes helping clients to continue cultural practices that have importance to them. This may include using folk medicine, practicing religious rites, eating traditional cultural foods, or providing interpreters when the client's primary language is not the dominant language.

Cultural care accommodation/negotiation includes changing your behaviors or actions to be more fully understood and accepted by the client. This may include, for example, modifying your manner of addressing the client, extending visiting hours, or ensuring that the client is not interrupted during prayers or meditation.

Cultural care repatterning/restructuring includes helping the client change patterns of living that are not beneficial to healthy life patterns. An example is teaching the client different methods of food preparation, such as steaming or baking instead of frying with saturated fats.

Table 3-1	Values Clarification: Providing Culturally Competent Care	
Value	**Related Actions**
Make a commitment to providing culturally competent care.	• Make a commitment to providing the best nursing care possible in a manner that respects the values, beliefs, and lifeways of the person for whom you are caring.
	• Learn about other cultures so you can take a positive approach to their health practices and use group characteristics to improve health. You will see in other cultures what you expect to see; look for strengths. Health teaching is more successful when it builds on strengths.
	• Examine your own culture—not only the larger common culture but also specific subgroups to which you belong. Review your attitudes and beliefs about health and objectively assess their origin and logic.
	• Examine biases, prejudices, and stereotypes that could contribute to ineffective nursing care. Plan ways to avoid the pitfalls that could harm the nurse–client relationship and lead to ineffective care.
	• Analyze your own communication (including facial expressions and body language) and how it may be interpreted.
Act in concert with the value of culturally competent care.	• Convey respect for the individual and respect for the individual's values, beliefs, and cultural practices.
	• Recognize that almost any human characteristic can be both a strength and a weakness, depending on the circumstances.
	• Recognize that cultural symbols and practices can bring comfort.
	• Support the client's practices, and incorporate them into nursing practice whenever possible.
Honor the value in differences.	• When you encounter different beliefs and values, reserve judgment until you can better understand the source of the beliefs and their meaning in the person's daily life. Do not assume that beliefs and values are wrong simply because they differ from yours.
	• Recognize differences in the ways clients communicate, and do not assume the meaning of a specific behavior (such as lack of eye contact) without considering the client's cultural background.
	• Relate your client's differing cultural beliefs to your own. In this way, you convey interest and respect for the client's beliefs.
Validate your perceptions of each client.	• Ask if a cultural practice is acceptable, desirable, or important.
	• Recognize individual differences. People vary within cultural groups and may make individual choices rather than follow traditional ways.
	• Learn how each client views health, illness, grieving, and the health care system.
	• Remember that clients may return to preferred cultural practices during illness; for example, the client who has learned English as a second language may revert to the primary language.

TRANSCULTURAL ASSESSMENT MODEL

The Giger and Davidhizar (1999) transcultural assessment model considers six cultural phenomena that may vary with application, yet are present in all cultural groups. These phenomena are communication, space, social organization, time, environmental control, and biological variation (Table 3-2).

Communication

Communication difficulties between people of different cultures involve more than speaking a different language. Misunderstanding also arises in the use of idiomatic language (language that is peculiar to a dialect, region, or social group). For example, the word *croaked* may be slang for "died," but it does not have the same meaning when translated to another language. Nor is it understood by people who have no experience in the social context in which the phrase is commonly understood.

Even nonverbal communication can lead to misunderstandings. Gestures, facial expressions, and body language may carry certain meanings commonly understood in one culture, but they would be misunderstood in another. Also, clients from different cultures may misinterpret gestures that Western nurses use to convey empathy and caring. For example, actions such as gentle touch on the hand, maintaining eye contact, or smiling and nodding may seem intrusive, disrespectful, or dismissive to clients of certain cultures.

Space

Personal space includes a person's body and the space around it. The level of discomfort generated when personal space is invaded is highly personal and is also related to culture. U.S. citizens, Canadians, and Britons require considerable personal space. Latin Americans, Japanese, and Arabs need a smaller amount of personal space (Watson, 1980). In the United States, close personal space is generally reserved for intimate friends or family and is related to the amount of trust one has in another person. Personal space can be used to meet the needs of security, privacy, autonomy, and self-identity.

In the United States, three categories of personal space describe our physical distance from others. The intimate zone is within 18 inches of the body. The intimate zone is used when comforting, protecting, or counseling, and it is reserved for people who have a close personal bond. The personal zone is 18 inches to 3 feet from the body and is maintained with friends and some counseling sessions. The social zone is 3 to 6 feet from the body and is used for impersonal business being conducted with people who are working together.

You have probably noticed that you usually begin a nurse-client relationship in the social zone and then move to the

Table 3-2 Elements of Transcultural Assessment

Element	Definition
Communication	A continuous process by which one person may affect another through written or oral language, gestures, facial expressions, body language, space, or other symbols
Space	The area around a person's body that includes the individual body, surrounding environment, and objects within that environment
Social organization	The aggregate of family and other groups within a society that dictates culturally accepted role behaviors and rules of behavior. Behaviors are prescribed for such significant life events as birth, death, childbearing, and illness.
Time orientation	A person's focus on the past, the present, or the future. Most cultures include all three time orientations, but one orientation is more likely to dominate the cultural perspective.
Environmental control	The perceived ability of an individual or persons from a particular cultural group to plan activities that control nature, such as illness causation and treatment
Biological variation	Biological differences among racial and ethnic groups may include physical characteristics, such as skin color, and physiological variations, such as lactose intolerance.

From Giger, J., & Davidhizar, R. E. (1999). *Transcultural nursing: Assessment and intervention* (2nd ed.). St Louis, MO: Mosby.

Table 3-3 Selected Consequences of Time Orientation

Orientation	Possible Consequences
To past	• When traditions conflict with a prescribed treatment regimen, the person may have trouble accepting or maintaining the plan of care. • In contrast, a strong connection with the past may ground the person with others in the same culture and provide a sense of self that encourages positive health practices.
To the present	• A present-oriented person may have little concern for long-term preventive health practices and may respond better to short-term goals. • In contrast, a present-oriented person may be most able to enjoy the here-and-now and may engage fully in exercise, enjoy nutritious food, and appreciate the company of others—all attributes associated with good health.
To the future	• This person has little focus on the difficulties and inconvenience of the present, focusing instead on the future goals. • The present is important only if what is happening now will help the person realize long-term goals. • This person may have little trouble following a treatment plan as long as its benefits are clear. • However, the person may have great difficulty dealing with chronic illnesses for which no complete cure is known. • A future-oriented person naturally tends to become more of a present-oriented person with age because, as the future life becomes shorter, the present becomes more important.

personal zone as the relationship is established. Of necessity, you enter the intimate zone when you are providing personal care and therapeutic treatments. Most clients intuitively understand and accept this level of personal space in a health care environment. However, you cannot assume that all clients will feel this way. Space varies among cultural groups.

Social Organization

Social organization refers to family structure and organization, religious beliefs, and the group's participation in social activities. Among most cultural groups in the United States, the family is the basic unit of organization. However, there is a great deal of variety in the nature and structure of family relationships. For example, many Hispanic families have grandparents, aunts, uncles, and cousins in important roles. Similarly, Native Americans have a tribal organization of which the nuclear family is a subunit.

Time

Time can mean many things. It typically is measured, as in the period between one sunrise and the next, or the passage of years or decades. Time can refer to a duration, such as how long a person has to complete a task or how long a movie lasts. It can also refer to specific appointments, such as the time for a meeting or the time to take a medication.

Cultures vary in their awareness of time and how they use this awareness in managing their lives. Some people are more likely to focus on the task at hand as though there is nothing else to do, giving it their full attention for as long as it takes to complete. Other individuals compartmentalize time. They are more likely to set a specific amount of time for a task and work to get it done in that amount of time.

Additionally, individuals may be described as oriented toward the past, present, or future (Table 3-3). Culture is only one of many factors that influence time orientation. For example, parents who have lost a child may focus on the life of the child and be unable to engage in the present or plan for the future. Poverty focuses a person's attention on the immediate. People involved in social, political, or educational activities may be focused almost exclusively on the future, neglecting their health in order to achieve a long-term goal.

Environmental Control

Environmental control refers both to the perception of control over the environment and to methods used to control the environment. Environmental control can be seen in a culture's attitude toward nature and in its commitment to preserving the natural environment. But the environment can also include health care, religion, work, and governmental organizations.

Your perception of being able to control your environment depends on whether you operate primarily from an internal locus of control or from an external locus of control. Persons with an internal locus of control feel empowered to influence their environment. Persons with an external locus of control are more likely to believe that events are primarily caused by chance, fate, or luck. They may feel helpless to change their environment or circumstances. These individuals may readily relinquish control to others, allowing others to make decisions for them.

Biological Variations

Biologically, humans of all races are the same, with minor variations in skin color, facial features, and body size. When a variation is shared by enough people, a group is formed. Genetic variations that produce different health problems in different races are uncommon but do exist. For example, Tay-Sachs disease is more common in people of Jewish ancestry. Thalassemia is more common among people of Mediterranean descent. Sickle cell disease is more common among African Americans.

Most illnesses that are more common in particular groups can be traced to environmental and lifestyle factors. Nevertheless, knowledge of culture is sometimes useful in identifying the lifestyle variables that contribute to disease. It is also useful to direct screening programs to groups that have a high incidence of a particular illness.

UNDERSTANDING SPECIFIC CULTURES

For the most part, a person is born into a cultural group and stays in that group. However, culture is partly a matter of choice. You may choose to continue to closely identify with the group to which your parents belonged, or you may adopt the ways of the larger culture around you. This second choice may have benefits but also carries the risk of inducing a feeling of alienation from the part of you that came from cultural teachings and lifeways. This may require you to know not only which group you belong to but also the degree to which you identify with that group.

The following descriptions provide highly generalized information about certain subgroups of larger cultural groups. They do not apply to each person who belongs to a subgroup. Brief descriptions cannot capture the rich cultural heritage and subtle patterns of behavior that are commonly understood in a given culture. Nevertheless, these descriptions may provide the first step in your goal of providing culturally competent care.

Irish Americans are a subset of white-skinned people of European descent. African Americans are a subset of black-skinned people. Mexican Americans are a subset of the rapidly growing Hispanic culture. Chinese Americans are a subset of the Asian culture, and Navajos are a subset of the Native American culture.

European Americans

Members of the European-American cultural group have roots in a combination of European countries—Germany, England, Italy, Ireland, and others—and therefore cannot be entirely understood through a study of the whole. Although many have integrated into the larger society and are less aware of the influence of their roots, their responses to illness and health care continue to reflect the origins of their ancestors. Additionally, some pockets of European groups have retained a specific cultural identity.

Irish Americans are an example of a group for whom assimilation has been more the norm than maintaining cultural identity. In 1960, more than half of Irish-American men married outside their cultural group. Today, some descendants of the original Irish immigrants identify themselves as Irish Americans, but others see themselves as members of other cultural groups or claim no specific cultural identity. With assimilation into the cultural mainstream of U.S. society, Irish Americans have gained economic and educational mobility. They are more likely to be professionals or managers.

Irish immigrants include two distinct groups. The Scotch Irish arrived during the colonial period. They were predominately Protestant and were culturally distinct from the Celtics, who immigrated in the later nineteenth and early twentieth century. When we talk about Irish Americans today, we are more likely to be describing the Irish Catholics of Celtic origin. Westward migration was associated with jobs building canals and railroads. Irish immigrant laborers were often in conflict with other immigrant labor groups, especially the Chinese.

By the early twentieth century, the second- and third-generation Irish Americans had moved into white collar jobs. Women were secretaries, nurses, and teachers. Men were skilled laborers, policemen, and firemen. The high percentage of Irish policemen and firemen resulted from political favors granted by officials elected through block voting in the Irish community. Although the Irish had not been well known for an interest in education, higher education became a means of upward mobility for many Irish Americans. The history of the Irish in America resulted in a belief that assimilation was the route to success in America.

Communication. Although the official language of Ireland is Irish (Gaelic), the British domination of Ireland required the people to speak English. English is recognized as the second official language and is universally spoken throughout Ireland. About 27% of the population knows both Irish and English (Giger & Davidhizar, 1999). Historically, the Irish had an advantage over other immigrants because of the high percentage who spoke English. Among more recent immigrants, Gaelic may be the spoken language.

Craic is an Irish expression for good, fun conversation among equals. Irish Americans are good company because they are often warm, sociable people, with family and friends being an important part of their lives. Wit and humor are a prominent part of communication that adds to their sociability. The "gift of gab" or "blarney" includes storytelling, laughter, and conversation. Weaving the truth into mythical stories is considered an Irish art form (Sullivan, 1997).

Family/Social Structure. A repeated theme among Irish Americans is the significance of family and family structure with close family bonds. Some Irish Americans tend to delineate roles and behaviors within the family according to gender. Irish-American women may view their role as primary caretaker of the family. Intermarriage between Irish-American families in the United States is one of the clearest distinctions of social acceptance and social equality in the community. There are few bachelors and spinsters in the Irish-American community.

Irish Americans have enjoyed a significant rise in the political arena in the United States. This resulted primarily from their strong sense of group solidarity, their fluency with the spoken word, and their personal charm. Religion and religious views are of paramount importance to some Irish Americans in maintaining the social integrity of the individual. The lack of recognition of the significance of religious beliefs may serve to augment problems and difficulties encountered with illness (Giger & Davidhizar, 1999).

Health/Health Practices. Irish Americans are perceived as having an external locus of control. They tend to cling to a past-oriented value orientation regarding the family and family relationships, and they tend to consider past values and traditions to be of paramount importance to future growth and development.

Ignoring bodily complaints appears to be a culturally prescribed and supported defense mechanism for some Irish Americans. The use of the defense mechanisms of ignoring and denying seems to be the typical way to cope with psychological and physiological needs (Giger & Davidhizar, 1999).

Some Irish Americans may subscribe to folk medicine beliefs that can be perceived as neutral health practices (neither having benefit nor producing harm). Examples are "blessing of the throat" and the wearing of religious medals to prevent illnesses. For some Irish Americans, the first level of intervention for illness is often home treatment. They may believe that a physician should be seen only in an emergency. Some folk practices may be viewed as beneficial, such as getting plenty of rest and going to bed early, enjoying fresh air and sunshine, and exercising.

Irish Americans have been ranked the highest or near the highest in terms of heavy alcohol intake. The use of alcohol is influenced by a variety of factors, including patterns and characteristics of the family and social and economic conditions. Some Irish Americans drink for reassurance and to escape what is viewed as an intolerable burden (Giger & Davidhizar, 1999).

African Americans

The term *African American* is a descriptor that suggests pride in a cultural heritage that is a combination of African and American. It can mean the descendants of people who were brought to America as slaves or more recent immigrants from Africa. The term Black suggests group pride and is used by some African Americans to describe their cultural group. The term African American places the emphasis on cultural heritage, whereas the term Black emphasizes biological racial identity. *African American* will be used in this chapter as a means of emphasizing the cultural characteristics.

African Americans include immigrants from African countries, the West Indian Islands, the Dominican Republic, Haiti, and Jamaica. The largest importation of slaves to America from the west coast of Africa occurred during the seventeenth century, and not all African Americans are the descendants of these slaves. The first English settlers brought African slaves and servants with them. Over time other Africans immigrated to America as free persons. The history of African Americans in the northern states differs from that in the southern states. In the North, African Americans who were slaves were freed by their owners and allowed to live their own lives. In the South, most slaves were prohibited from learning to read or write and were denied access to medical care and education.

Communication. The African-American dialect may be a product of the English learned by different tribes or of different languages intermingled. The syntax and grammar reflect in part the English dialect of southern white Americans. Patterns of speech have developed that are somewhat unique to African Americans. The dialect (or variation within a language) spoken by African Americans may differ from Standard English in pronunciation, grammar, and syntax. It is helpful for nurses to learn strategies for communicating (Box 3-2, p. 50).

Family/Social Structure. Historically, because of prejudice and legalized segregation, African Americans were isolated from the mainstream of society. Assimilation into mainstream society has been slow because of continued racial prejudice and a desire to build the solidarity of a strong African-American community in predominantly African-American neighborhoods, churches, and schools.

The African-American community has maintained a core of strength through its churches and schools that can be expected to continue as a force in solving the problems of the community. Religion is taken very seriously, and many African Americans actively participate in church-related activities and believe strongly in the power of prayer.

The family structures of African Americans in the United States include the male-headed (patriarchal) family structure and the female-headed (matriarchal) family structure. More than half of African-American families have a female head of household. African-American women are responsible for maintaining and protecting the health of family members, and they are assuming significant leadership roles in the community as professionals and businesswomen. Large family

---

Box 3-2 **Strategies for Communicating With Clients From Different Cultures**

- Take a little extra time to establish a level of comfort between yourself and the client.
- Ask questions in an unhurried manner. Rephrase a question and ask it again if the answer seems inconsistent with other information the client has provided.
- Observe for cultural differences in communication, and honor those differences. Use eye contact, touch, and seating arrangements that are comfortable for the client.
- Ask the client about the personal meaning of health and illness, and understanding of treatments and planned care. Investigate how his illness is likely to affect his life, relationships, and self-concept. Find out what he considers to be the cause of his illness. Ask how he prefers to manage his illness.
- To establish a therapeutic relationship, listen to the client's perception of her needs, and respect her perspective.
- Listen actively and attentively; try not to anticipate the client's response.
- Talk to the client in an unhurried manner that considers social and cultural amenities.
- Give the client time to answer.
- Use validation techniques to verify that the client understands. Remember that smiles and head nodding may indicate that the client is trying to please you, not necessarily that you are understood.
- Sexual concerns may be difficult for clients to discuss. Having a nurse of the same sex may facilitate communication.
- Use alternative methods of communication, such as a foreign language phrase book, an interpreter, gestures, or pictures, for clients who do not speak English.
- Learn key phrases in languages that are commonly spoken in your community.

---

networks or community groups, such as churches, provide support during times of crisis and illness.

Grandmothers tend to play an active role in the lives of the African-American family. In fact, children may be raised by grandmothers. Grandmothers may assist with financial support. And they may be actively involved in the care of an ill child. Including a grandmother in the plan of care, therefore, can be of vital importance.

Health/Health Practices. The definition of health for many African Americans stems from African beliefs about life and the nature of being. Some Africans believe that life is a process rather than a state (Spector, 1999). The nature of a person is viewed in terms of energy force rather than matter. When one possesses health, one is in harmony. Many African Americans believe in the power of some people to heal and help others (McQuay, 1995).

Traditional healers are usually women who use herbs and roots to treat illness. The reliance on healers reflects the deep religious faith of African Americans. Some belief in voodoo or hoodoo is still present. Health is maintained with proper rest, diet, and a clean environment. Treating illness through prayer and laying on of hands is practiced in some religious groups. Home remedies and folk medicine are used by some African Americans, and local hospitals are avoided except in extreme emergencies. Fear of hospitals has grown out of lack of access to health care facilities and a continued concern that equal treatment will not be offered.

Lack of access to health care services, low income, and the tendency to self-treat and wait until symptoms become severe tend to increase the morbidity rate among African Americans (McQuay, 1995). An African American may perceive receiving health care as degrading or humiliating. Some fear or resent health care centers; they may tend to feel alienated by the system and experience a sense of powerlessness. Some clients believe they are being talked down to by the health care providers and that providers fail to listen to them. Consequently, they choose to suffer in silence. Therefore you should actively ensure that a prescribed treatment or special diet is consistent with the client's needs, cultural background, income, and religious practices. The treatment plan and rationale must be shared with the client, and it is important that the client understand what is being prescribed.

Among African Americans, skin color may vary from a light, almost white color to a very dark brown. Melanin provides protection from the effects of the sun. African Americans and other dark-skinned people have a lower incidence of skin cancer than light-skinned people.

Hypertension is common among African Americans; they have a higher hypertension-related mortality rate than other groups. Sickle cell disease and lactose intolerance are genetic disorders prevalent in African Americans; other diseases and disorders common to this culture include cancer, cardiovascular disease, cirrhosis, and diabetes. African-American children have a tendency to weigh less at birth.

Hispanic Americans

Members of the Hispanic-American community have origins in Spain, Cuba, Central and South America, Mexico, Puerto Rico, and other Spanish-speaking countries. This ethnic community is very diverse. It includes people with black skin and people with white skin. The Mexican-American subgroup is one of the most prominent.

Most Mexican Americans reside in Texas, the Southwest, and California. In early U.S. history, Mexican Americans helped build many southwestern cities. Settlers learned skills such as mining, farming, and ranching. Most Mexican Americans have remained close to the region of the country that was settled by their ancestors (Giger & Davidhizar, 1999). As new immigrants arrive, they have tended to gather in these areas as well. However, they have also migrated as farm workers to other areas of the country.

Many Mexican Americans can trace their ancestry back to Indian groups such as the Incas and Mayas, who developed complex Mexican civilizations before the arrival of the Spanish explorers. Many Mexican Americans are a blend of both Indian and Spanish European cultures (Giger & Davidhizar, 1999).

Mexican Americans have been successful at retaining a unique cultural identity within the dominant culture, unlike early European immigrants, who assimilated into the overall U.S. culture. Traditional gender and family roles continue to be part of the heritage that separates Mexican Americans from other cultural groups. Some are well educated, and others are migrant workers who move around the country seeking work harvesting seasonal crops.

Communication. For many Mexican Americans, Spanish is the primary language, spoken in many dialects and differing widely between Hispanic groups. Some Mexican Americans place a high value on diplomacy and tactfulness and communicate in a manner that avoids direct confrontation and arguments, which are considered rude and disrespectful. Through the use of elaborate, often indirect communication, the Mexican American tries to accomplish the goal of communication while maintaining politeness and respect. Self-disclosure is avoided with strangers, including health care professionals. In communicating, Mexican Americans may incorporate the use of senses as well as words, and they are characterized as tactile in their relationships.

Most Mexican Americans can speak at least some English, but they may use it selectively. It is not uncommon to use English in the workplace and Spanish at home or with friends. Children of newer immigrants who have not yet mastered English may have a hard time in school. In general, Mexican-American children are more likely to grow up bilingual than European-American children in the same regions. In health care situations, you may observe a client speak to his family in Spanish, to you in English, and, when very stressed, to both his family and you in a mix of both English and Spanish.

Family/Social Structure. The strength of the nuclear family (parents and children) is the foundation of the Mexican-American community. For most Mexican Americans, extended family relationships have special significance, and the family may be the most significant social organization (Murillo, 1978). The Mexican-American family takes pride in family accomplishments and usually does not seek help from outsiders to meet needs or resolve problems. Men may assume the dominant role of breadwinner and decision maker. Women often work at jobs outside the home, and they are taking significant leadership roles in the community as educators, attorneys, and businesswomen.

Health/Health Practices. Mexican Americans are more likely to perceive an external locus of control. They may perceive life as being under the influence of a divine will. They may also have a fatalistic belief that they are at the mercy of the environment and have little control over what happens (Giger & Davidhizar, 1999).

Some Mexican Americans may view health as purely the result of good luck or a reward from God for good behavior. Individuals are expected to maintain their equilibrium in the universe by conducting themselves in the proper way, eating the proper foods, and working the proper amount of time. The prevention of illness is an accepted practice that is accomplished with prayer, by wearing religious medals or amulets, and by keeping relics in the home. Illness may be viewed as

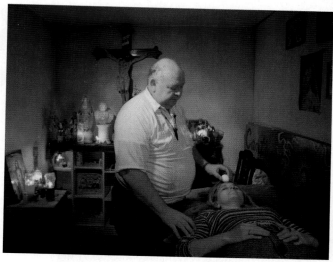

Figure 3-3. Within the Mexican-American folk medicine system, the curandero is the folk healer.

an imbalance in the individual's body or as a punishment for wrongdoing.

Some Mexican Americans believe that an imbalance may exist between hot and cold or wet and dry. These forces are embodied in four body fluids (or humors): blood, which is hot and wet; yellow bile, which is hot and dry; phlegm, which is cold and wet; and black bile, which is cold and dry. When all four humors are balanced, the body is healthy. When an imbalance occurs, an illness is present. If an illness is categorized as hot, it is treated with a cold substance. A cold disease, in turn, must be treated with a hot substance. The classification of what is a hot disease or a cold disease varies from person to person.

Within the Mexican-American folk medicine system, the *curandero* is the folk healer (Figure 3-3). The *curandero* views illness from a religious and social context rather than the scientific perspective that dominates Western society (Giger & Davidhizar, 1999). The *curandero* is a holistic healer and can be either female or male.

In the folk medicine system, illness may be caused by *susto* (fright), *mal ojo* (evil eye), *envidia* (envy), or *empacho* (gastrointestinal ailment). The most popular form of treatment by folk healers involves herbs, especially when used as teas. Treatments may also include massage, cleanings *(limpias),* diet, rest, prayers, and supernatural rituals. Rituals include elements of both Catholic and Pentecostal rituals and artifacts: money offerings, confession, candle lighting, wooden or metal offerings in the shape of anatomic parts *(milagros),* and laying on of hands. The *herbero* is a folk healer who specializes in the use of herbs and spices for preventive and curative purposes. *Brujos* (male witches) and *brujas* (female witches) are another level of healers. They practice black magic and may not be sought until other forms of healing have been tried.

Roman Catholicism is the predominant religion practiced by Mexican Americans. During times of crises, Mexican Americans may rely on a priest or prayers. Rituals, such as making promises, lighting candles, or visiting shrines may be practiced when a family member is ill.

The incidence of diabetes among Mexican Americans is five times the national average, and complications are more frequent. The client with multiple health problems is a special concern in this population. Hypertension is a significant health problem. Urban, elderly Mexican Americans are at risk for many age-related chronic health conditions associated with migrant status, lower levels of education, nutrition, and poverty. Alcoholism is also a crucial health problem among Mexican Americans (Giger & Davidhizar, 1999). Men are most often affected, because the male role may be correlated with the ability to ingest large amounts of alcohol.

Asian Americans

Asian Americans numbered 7.3 million in 1990, and estimates put the population at about 20 million by the year 2020 (Russell, 1996). In 1990, 24% of the Asian-American population was Chinese American. Chinese Americans are immigrants and their descendants, mainly from Taiwan, Hong Kong, and mainland China.

Chinese Americans have various degrees of acculturation. Some adhere to Chinese culture, some adopt both cultures, and some adapt entirely to American culture (Chang, 1999). To assess the effect of Chinese culture on the health status and health care behaviors of Chinese Americans, you should study communication styles, English proficiency, interpersonal interactions, social support systems, health care practices, the use of Chinese medicines, and biological variations pertinent to Chinese Americans (Chang, 1999; Grossman, 1996).

Many religions exist among Chinese Americans, such as Buddhism, Taoism, Christianity, Islam, beliefs in myths and fortunes, and worship of ancestors and deified heroes. When they are ill, Chinese Americans may practice one or more religions to help themselves get well. Respect these practices as long as the client's faith does no harm to health.

The teachings of Confucius form a primary force in Chinese culture. Confucius was a Chinese sage who established rules and codes of ethics for personal and interpersonal behaviors to maintain order and harmony in society. Lao Zi, another Chinese sage, greatly influenced Chinese medicine (Boxes 3-3 and 3-4). Confucius encouraged people to pursue the virtues of loyalty to family, friends, and the government. He also encouraged filial piety to parents, love, faithfulness, righteousness, and peacefulness. Confucius emphasized harmonious relationships with nature and each other. He suggested accommodating rather than confronting and seeking group consensus rather than advocating individual concerns. A person is expected to demonstrate these virtues, to exert self-control, to be self-reliant, and to behave modestly. Otherwise, one brings shame to oneself, family members, and society. (Chinese call this losing face.) Consequently, Chinese Americans may be group oriented (Hall, 1976), tending to conform to the group and avoiding conflicts or being different. Chinese Americans may seem quiet, unassertive, agreeable, and pleasant. They may suppress the exhibition of neg-

---

Box 3-3	**Principles of Chinese Medicine**

A Chinese sage named Lao Zi developed a religion called Taoism and influenced the fundamental principles and practices of Chinese medicine (Reid, 1993). Taoism hypothesizes that two opposing and interacting forces—yin and yang—exist in the universe and in the body. Yin is a negative, recessive, female force. Yang is a positive, dominant, male force. In Chinese medicine, a balance between yin and yang yields optimal health. Imbalance between these two forces results in disease (Chang, 1999; Reid, 1993).

The underlying principle of Chinese medicine is to maintain and restore the balance between yin and yang forces in the body. Food, symptoms, diseases, and medicine are classified into yin and yang groups. Yang symptoms or diseases are treated with yin foods and medicines. Yin symptoms or diseases are treated with yang foods and medicines. For example, yang symptoms include a red complexion, restlessness, thirst, constipation, dark urine, and nervousness. They are treated with foods that have yin qualities, such as oranges, limes, watermelon, and cucumber. Yin symptoms include coldness, loose stools, clear urine, a poor appetite, pallor, and fatigue. They are treated with foods that have yang qualities, such as lamb, beef, chicken, ginger, chili, and peanuts (Chang, 1999; Reid, 1993).

Chinese medicine is also based on an invisible life force or energy, called qi (pronounced chee), that moves around the universe and within the body. The circulation of qi and the quality and quantity of qi determine the yin–yang balance. Many forms of exercise, external therapies, and herbal medicines are used to promote the circulation of qi, maintain the yin–yang balance, and restore health (Reid, 1993).

---

ative emotions, such as anger, sadness, worry, and depression (Chang, 1999).

Communication. English proficiency and communication styles affect the interactions of Chinese Americans with health care providers and the health care delivery system. Once Chinese Americans are in the health care delivery system, they may experience an undue amount of stress. They may not understand their health condition and may be unable to express their concerns or needs. Even when able to express concerns, they may be misunderstood.

To reduce your Chinese-American clients' stress, you may help them in the following ways:

- Find a translator who can speak their dialect, or use family members who are fluent in English to help them understand their health status and care.
- Use plain and simple English to explain things; avoid jargon or medical terms.
- Provide written materials in addition to verbal information to clients and to family members to facilitate understanding.
- Find resources that are written in Chinese.

During the process of acculturation, some Chinese Americans may feel shame and develop low self-esteem and feel helpless, powerless, and depressed because of their limitations in English and reduced social support. Because the Chinese culture emphasizes self-control and self-reliance, a Chinese American may feel shame in verbalizing emotional and social problems. The person may verbalize only physical symptoms. You can help by using therapeutic communication

Box 3-4 *Considering the Alternatives*
Traditional Chinese Medicine

Description and History: Chinese medicine has a rich scholarly heritage of healing that goes back more than 5000 years. One of the earliest recorded compilations of Asian medicine, the *Emperor's Classic of Internal Medicine,* describes Chinese medicine from the third century BC. Chinese medicine is based on Asian philosophy, which is different from Western philosophy. Asian philosophy is circular, rather than linear, and includes opposites in a single unit, as seen in the familiar yin/yang symbol. New ideas are added and cumulate, rather than replacing old ideas and practices.

Important Concepts:
Tao: The goal of life is to flow or be in harmony with the Tao, which is the way life unfolds, the way of nature, life, and death.
Yin/yang: These polar opposites represent the fundamental dualities of the universe; they are united through the Tao.
Chi: The universal force or subtle material or vital life force that maintains health and vitality. Chi is carried through the body via pathways or *meridians.* Specific points located along these meridians are stimulated through acupuncture or acupressure to balance and improve the flow of Chi. Chi is combined with *essence* (a gift of one's parents) and *spirit* (a gift of heaven) to describe the human condition.
Five phases: Earth (nourishment), *metal* (strength), *water* (change), *wood* (growth), and *fire* (love) describe not only human experience but all dynamic relationships in nature. Health and illness are conceptualized and described through this framework. All healing is focused on the restoration of balance within the person and restoring harmony with the environment.

Therapeutic Techniques: The practice of traditional Chinese medicine (TCM) in Asian countries includes moxibustion, herbalism, cupping, ChiGong, massage, and acupuncture. In Western countries, the most common practices are acupuncture and acupressure. Although Chinese herbal treatments are available in some areas with Asian populations, their use is not widespread in the West. A thorough history of the client's complaint, examination of the tongue, and a thorough analysis of the pulse are used to make a diagnosis in TCM.

Treatment is often acupuncture, the strategic placement and manipulation of fine needles along the meridians, corresponding to various organs and the flow and balance of Chi. Moxibustion involves heating herbs to stimulate acupuncture points. Cupping is placing a heated cup on the skin to stimulate circulation and extraction of toxins. Herbal preparations constitute a dominant aspect of TCM. ChiGong is an ancient form of exercise integrating breathing, movement, and meditation to restore balance to Chi. Massage may also be used to stimulate the Chi along the meridians or to stimulate acupuncture points.

Practitioners: Acupuncture has gained much popularity in the West. Most states now license acupuncturists, and many schools of acupuncture have been established. Many health care providers, physicians, nurses, and other professionals are now certified to perform acupuncture. Some controversy exists related to differing lengths of programs. All licensed acupuncturists must ensure proper hygiene and use disposable needles.

Potential Benefits of Acupuncture: Acupuncture has been accepted clinically and supported by research for use in chronic and acute pain. Evidence of its efficacy, especially for musculoskeletal pain, is excellent. Research has also demonstrated its effectiveness in treating nausea related to pregnancy, surgery, and chemotherapy. Research into its use in addictive disorders also appears promising. The National Institutes of Health Consensus Committee reported in 1997 that acupuncture "is an effective treatment for nausea caused by cancer chemotherapy drugs, surgical anesthesia and pregnancy; and for pain resulting from surgery and a variety of musculoskeletal conditions" (NIH, 1997).

Concerns About TCM: If acupuncture is given by a licensed professional, concern over unclean needles is diminished. Most TCM methods, like Western treatments, are more successful when used early in disease trajectories; it is important that biomedical treatment not be delayed by using TCM alone in the early stages. The use of Chinese herbs is completely unregulated in the United States; often these biological agents are imported from Asia and are contaminated with other substances. Little research has been conducted regarding their efficacy, side effects, contraindications, or safety.

Resources
Books
Beinfeld, H. Y., & Korngold, E. (1991). *Between heaven and earth: A guide to Chinese medicine.* New York: Ballantine Books.
Ergil, K. (2001). Chinese medicine. In Micozzi, M. (Ed.), *Fundamentals of complementary and alternative medicine* (2nd ed.). New York: Churchill Livingstone.
Kaptchuk, T. (1983). *The web that has no weaver.* New York: Congdon & Weed.
Sheikh, A. A. & Sheikh, K. S. (1989). *Eastern and Western approaches to healing: Ancient wisdom and modern knowledge.* New York: Wiley.

Websites
Acupuncture, www.acupuncture.com.
National Institutes of Health Consensus Reports, http://consensus.nih.gov/cons/107/107_statement.htm.
Office of Complementary and Alternative Medicine, www.nccam.nih.gov.
Foundation for Traditional Chinese Medicine, www.ftcm.org.uk.

From National Institutes of Health. (Nov. 3-5, 1997). Acupuncture. NIH Consensus Statement Online. 15(5):1-34. Available from http://consensus.nih.gov/cons/107/107_statement.ntm.

skills to identify psychosocial problems underlying physical symptoms (Chang, 1999).

Chinese communication styles tend to be covert and highly contextual (Hall, 1976). Chinese Americans use implicit, subtle, and indirect communication styles. During communication, they perceive not only explicit information but also implicit clues, such as facial expression, body movements, the use of physical space, gestures, and tone of voice. Because Confucius teachings emphasize harmonious relationships and respect for elders and authoritative figures, and discourage individual opinions, Chinese Americans may avoid direct conflicts. They may consider it shameful to express their disagreement: they would lose face. Instead, Chinese Americans may express disagreement in a nonverbal way. They may lose eye contact, change the subject, or appear reluctant (Chang, 1999; Grossman, 1996). When they dislike or disagree with a health care provider, they may switch to another health care provider rather than confront the original one. When communicating with

Chinese Americans, assess their communication style, be sensitive to nonverbal communication clues, and encourage them to verbalize any questions, concerns, or disagreements.

Family/Social Structure. Chinese Americans tend to have a hierarchy in the social and family structure. Husbands and elders have authority over wives and children. Elders and people in authoritative positions are highly respected. Chinese culture expects children to take care of their parents when they grow up. If children do not take care of their parents, the parents may feel shame and consider the children disloyal to their family.

Under the influence of democracy and American culture, Chinese Americans may challenge traditional social structure and values. They may come to value the individual more than the group. They may alter the line of authority in the family. The conflicts between traditional values and American culture may create stress. Some stress may cause physical symptoms and psychological problems. For example, elder immigrants may feel some loss of self-respect because they depend on their children for financial, physical, and psychosocial support. As a result of this dependence, the elder immigrants may experience loneliness and emotional isolation. However, they may complain only about problems with sleep or appetite because they are ashamed to admit emotional problems (Mackinnon, Gien, & Durst, 1996). Some may develop further mental illnesses and commit suicide (Tien-Hyatt, 1987).

When caring for Chinese Americans, assess their family structure, the line of authority, and their social support. You may include family members in the plan of care. You may also involve the person who is authoritative to the client to help the client reach therapeutic goals. To identify psychosocial problems, encourage the client to express thoughts and feelings without feeling shame. For a client with limited social support, help identify available community resources to increase the client's sense of self-reliance and self-esteem (Chang, 1999).

Health/Health Practices. Chinese culture does not emphasize control of the environment but rather maintenance of a harmonious relationship with nature and balance in life. To maintain health, some Chinese Americans may perform traditional Chinese exercises, such as tai chi or qi-kung, to facilitate the flow of qi and the yin-yang balance within the body. They believe that fresh air is important for quality qi. They usually exercise early in the morning in the park while the air is fresh. They may also prefer to keep windows open to allow the flow of fresh air instead of using air-conditioning (Chang, 1999; Chen, 1996).

When Chinese Americans are ill, several types of problems may occur. One is that the person may take Western medicines together with Chinese herbal medicines, and both may have similar effects. Caution the client about overmedication and suggest not taking both types of medicines together.

Some Chinese Americans may save prescribed medications for later use. They may be afraid of drug side effects or of overdose. They may not see the need to continue taking medication when they do not feel ill anymore. This practice may be detrimental to their health, especially when the medicine is insulin, an antihypertensive drug, a corticosteroid, and so on. Teach clients about medications, and emphasize the importance of taking them as prescribed, without stopping or self-regulating. Encourage the client to work with health care providers for any problems related to medicines.

Some Chinese Americans may observe the yin-yang quality of foods and eat only foods that can balance the yin-yang quality of their diseases. For example, after giving birth (yin quality), some Chinese Americans drink only warm milk or hot water (yang quality) and will not drink or eat anything cold (yin quality). Respect this belief, and help the client obtain the preferred foods and drinks.

Some Chinese may use external Chinese medicine, such as acupuncture, moxibustion, skin-scraping, or suction-cupping, to promote the circulation of qi and to restore health. Acupuncture uses hair-thin needles inserted at special sites. This procedure may leave no marks and has been reported to control pain effectively (*Compton's Interactive Encyclopedia*, 1996).

Some of these procedures can produce skin lesions. For example, moxibustion involves placement of a burning moxa (an herb) over vital points. A crater about 1 cm in diameter on the skin may develop. Skin-scraping involves scraping skin firmly at selected points with a blunt spoon or coin until bright red stripes appear. Multiple linear bruises over the neck, the bridge of the nose, along the spine, or over the chest may be observed. Suction-cupping involves the use of an ignited cotton swab inside a glass cup that is quickly placed on a treatment site to create suction. The suction cup is left on the skin 15 to 20 minutes. Circular lesions about 2 inches in diameter may be observed as a result (Boyle & Andrews, 1999; Louie, 1985; Reid, 1993; Spector, 1999). When these lesions are present, do not mistake them for physical abuse. Provide care as needed to prevent infection.

Several symptoms or diseases are genetically linked to Chinese Americans. Mongolian spots (bluish pigmentation, usually at the coccygeal area) are often observed on Chinese infants. They should not be mistaken for bruises.

More than half of Chinese babies develop neonatal jaundice. The bilirubin level usually peaks at 5 or 6 days (Boyle & Andrews, 1999). Prepare Chinese-American mothers before discharge to be aware of jaundice, and teach them ways to reduce or treat it.

Chinese Americans typically weigh less than whites. Their drug metabolism may also be different from that of whites. Therefore they may develop side effects or toxic effects when they take the dosages usually prescribed for whites. You need to observe if lower dosages are needed to reduce side effects (Chang, 1999; Louie, 1995).

High incidences of lactose deficiency, thalassemia deficiency, and glucose-6-phosphate dehydrogenase (G6PD) deficiency have also been reported among the Chinese (Chang, 1999). After drinking milk, some Chinese Americans may experience abdominal cramps, diarrhea, or flatus. Thus they may avoid drinking milk. Thalassemia deficiency causes rapid destruction of red blood cells. Clients require monthly blood transfusions for life. If both parents are thalassemia carriers, infants or mothers may develop complications, such as stillbirth or preeclampsia (Anionwu, 1996). G6PD deficiency may result in anemia because of rapid destruction of red blood cells when some Chinese Americans take certain drugs (Chang, 1999). Screening for these deficiencies and providing information and genetic counseling are the best preventive care.

Chinese Americans are at high risk of developing hepatitis B, tuberculosis, nasopharyngeal cancer, esophageal cancer, stomach cancer, and liver cancer (Chang, 1999; Louie, 1995). The consumption of fermented, moldy, and pickled foods may contribute to the development of esophageal and liver cancers (Chang, 1999). Crowded living arrangements may be one of the contributing factors for tuberculosis. To help Chinese Americans, you may provide them information about these diseases to reduce their risk and to help them identify these diseases at an early stage.

In summary, when caring for Chinese Americans, you need to assess the impact of Chinese culture and beliefs on their health status and health care behaviors to help them deal with physical and psychosocial problems, to screen for genetic disorders, and to reduce high-risk diseases.

Native Americans

There are about 200 Native American tribes in the United States, and they are concentrated primarily in western states as the result of forced westward migration. Oklahoma, Arizona, California, New Mexico, and Alaska have the largest numbers of Native Americans (Spector, 1999). Although many live on reservations and in rural areas, just as many live in cities, especially those on the West Coast. The term *Native American* implies tribes residing in the continental United States. One of the largest tribes is the Navajo, and elements of that culture are discussed here.

Communication.
Many Navajo use English as their primary language, but many are fluent both in the Navajo language and in English. Naturally, those who do not speak English will require the assistance of an interpreter when seeking or receiving health care.

Rather than shaking hands, as is common among many Americans, Navajos tend to extend a hand and lightly touch the hand of the person being greeted. The Navajo culture holds a taboo against touching a dead person or an animal killed by lightning. Consequently, a Navajo client or family member may prefer not to touch articles associated with a dead person or animal.

The Navajo people may appear silent and reserved when first meeting strangers. Warm behavior may be demonstrated once the Navajo individual becomes familiar with you (Giger & Davidhizar, 1999). In the Navajo culture, eye contact is considered a sign of disrespect.

Family/Social Structure.
The Navajo culture is very family oriented, and the definition of family may have no limits on

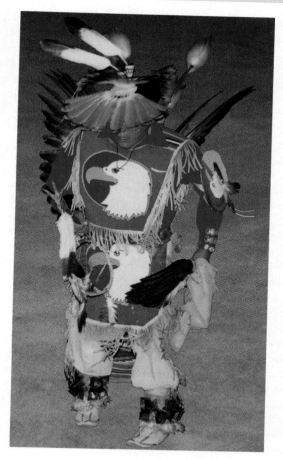

Figure 3-4. Dancers have always been a very important part of the life of the Native American.

number or on relationship. Navajo people believe that family members are responsible for each other. Therefore it is not unusual for many relatives to come to the hospital to care for a Navajo client. Decision making is mutual. The goal of the family is to help its members grow, share resources, and participate in daily activities and significant life events, such as birth, death, marriage, and sickness.

The Navajo culture is neither dead nor static but instead is a living culture, retaining its heritage and advancing with the times. Navajo members may join with other tribes and share their songs and dances to remind the people of their old ways and rich heritage. Dancers have always been a very important part of the life of the Native American (Figure 3-4). Although dance styles and content have changed, their meaning and importance have not.

Health/Health Practices.
The traditional Navajo belief about health is that it reflects living in total harmony with nature and having the ability to survive under exceedingly difficult circumstances. Illness is viewed as a price being paid for something that happened in the past or for something that will happen in the future. Everything is the result of something else.

Native Americans do not subscribe to the germ theory of medicine. Illness is something that must be. The cause of disease or injury to a person or property, or of continued misfortune of any kind, must be traced back to an action that should not have been taken. Examples of such infractions are breaking a taboo or contacting a ghost or witch. To the Navajo, the treatment of an illness must be concerned with the external causative factors and not with the disease or injury itself (Spector, 1999).

The traditional healer of the Navajo is the medicine man. He is a person wise in the ways of land and nature. He knows the interrelationships of humans, the Earth, and the universe. He knows the ways of the plants and animals, the moon, and the stars. The medicine man takes his time to determine first the cause of the illness, and then the proper treatment. To determine the cause and treatment of an illness, he performs special ceremonies that may take several days. Navajos may rely on traditional tribal medicine, the "white man's medicine," or a combination of both. Conflicts can occur in families when there are different degrees of acceptance of scientific medical treatments.

Navajos may be suspicious of people of European descent. Initial reluctance may dissipate when a health professional respects the client's opinion and demonstrates sensitivity to the client's point of view. Nurses and caregivers must avoid "interviewing" Navajos to gain information. Often, simply listening helps the person overcome concerns about interacting with health care providers of a different culture.

Today, Navajos are faced with a number of health problems. Health care skills inherent in the Navajo traditional ways of diagnosing and treating illness have not fully survived their migration and changing ways of life. Because of the loss of these skills and because modern health care centers are not always available, Navajos are frequently in limbo when it comes to obtaining appropriate health care. Additionally, at least a third of Navajos live in poverty. With poverty come poor living conditions, malnutrition, tuberculosis, and high maternal and infant death rates. In 1996, the leading causes of hospitalization for Navajo clients were obstetrical deliveries, accidents (including motor vehicle accidents), respiratory diseases, diseases of the genitourinary system, mental disorders, diseases of the circulatory system, skin diseases, and diseases of the endocrine system (U.S. Department of Health and Human Services, 1997).

Type II diabetes mellitus is a major health problem for Navajos. It tends to occur early, in the teens or early twenties. As a result, complications also occur early, leading to excessive mortality in the early and middle adult years. According to the U.S. Department of Health and Human Services (1997), the age-adjusted death rate is on the rise. It is not known why diabetes is prevalent among Navajos.

Key Principles

- In a multicultural society, distinct cultural groups retain cultural identity and contribute to the overall society the strengths and lifeways of the group.
- Stereotyping is a counterproductive tendency to assume that an attribute present in some members of a group must be present in all members of the group.
- Culture includes the values, beliefs, norms, and practices shared by a particular group that guide thinking, decisions, and actions in a patterned way.
- Six elements by which to describe cultural diversity are communication, space, social organization, time, environmental control, and biological variation.
- To communicate with persons of other cultures, you should respect each individual's values, beliefs, and cultural practices.
- Communication requires validation that all parties in the communication have been understood.
- There is perhaps as much variation within cultures as between cultures.
- Culturally competent nursing care requires understanding the health care setting from the client's point of view.

Bibliography

*Alba, R. D. (1990). *Ethnic identity: The transformation of White America.* New Haven, CT: Yale University Press.

Anionwu, E. N. (1996). Sickle cell and thalassaemia: Some priorities for nursing research. *Journal of Advanced Nursing, 23,* 853-856.

*Blessing, P. (1980). Irish. In S. Thernstrom (Ed.), *Harvard encyclopedia of American ethnic groups.* Cambridge, MA: Belknap Press.

*Boyle, J. S., & Andrews, M. M. (1999). *Transcultural concepts in nursing care.* Philadelphia: Lippincott.

Chang, K. (1999). Chinese Americans. In J. N. Giger & R. E. Davidhizar (Eds.), *Transcultural nursing: Assessment and intervention.* St Louis, MO: Mosby.

Chen, Y. D. (1996). Conformity with nature: A theory of Chinese American elders' health promotion and illness prevention processes. *Advanced Nursing Science, 19*(2), 17-26.

*Chen, C. L., & Yang, D. C. V. (1986). The self-image of Chinese-American adolescents: A cross-cultural comparison. *International Journal of Social Psychiatry, 32*(4), 19-26.

Compton's interactive encyclopedia [CD-ROM]. (1996). Carlsbad, CA: Compton's New Media.

*Fallows, M. (1979). *Irish Americans.* Englewood Cliffs, NJ: Prentice-Hall.

Giger, J. N., & Davidhizar, R.E. (1999). *Transcultural nursing: Assessment and intervention* (2nd ed.). St Louis, MO: Mosby.

Grossman, D. (1996). Cultural dimensions in home health nursing. *American Journal of Nursing, 96*(7), 33-36.

*Hall, E. T. (1976). *Beyond culture.* New York: Anchor Press/Doubleday.

Leininger, M. (1991). *Culture care diversity and universality: A theory of nursing* (Publication No. 15-2402). New York: National League for Nursing Press.

*Louie, K. B. (1985). Providing health care to Chinese clients. *Topics in Clinical Nursing, 7*(3), 18-25.

Louie, K. B. (1995). Cultural considerations: Asian-Americans and Pacific Islanders. *Imprint, 42*(5), 41-44, 46.

Mackinnon, M. E., Gien, L., & Durst, D. (1996). Chinese elders speak out. *Clinical Nursing Research, 5*(3), 326-342.

---

*Asterisk indicates a classic or definitive work on this subject.

McQuay, J. E. (1995). Cross-cultural customs and beliefs related to health crisis. *Critical Care Nursing Clinics of North America, 7,* 581-594.

*Murillo, N. (1978). The Mexican American family. In C. A. Hernandez, M. J. Haug & N. N. Wagner (Eds.), *Ethnic nursing care: A multicultural approach* (pp 115-148). St Louis, MO: Mosby.

*Murillo-Rohde, I. (1977). Care for all colors. *Imprint, 24*(4), 29-32, 50.

*Primeaux, M. (1977). Caring for the American Indian patient. *American Journal of Nursing, 77,* 91-94.

Purnell, L. D., & Paulauka, B. J. (Eds.). (1998). *Transcultural health care: A culturally competent approach.* Philadelphia: Davis.

Reid, D. P. (1993). *Chinese herbal medicine.* Boston: Shambhala.

Russell, C. (1996). *The official guide to racial and ethnic diversity.* Ithaca, NY: New Strategist.

*Sowell, T. (1981). *Ethnic America: A history.* New York, NY: Basic Books.

Spector, R. E. (1999). *Cultural diversity in health and illness.* (5th ed.). Upper Saddle River, NJ: Pearson Education.

Stokes, L. G. (1977). Delivering health services in a Black community. In A. M. Reinhardt & M. B. Quinn (Eds.), *Current practice in family-centered community nursing* (pp 51-65). St Louis, MO: Mosby.

Sullivan, M. (1997) *The hidden people.* Retrieved from http://home.earthlink.net/~_maireidsullivan/craig.html.

*Takaki, R. (1993). *A different mirror: A history of multicultural America.* Boston: Little, Brown.

*Tien-Hyatt, J. L. (1987). Self-perceptions of aging across cultures: Myth or reality? *International Journal of Aging and Human Development, 24*(2), 129-148.

U.S. Department of Commerce, Bureau of the Census. (1992a). *Population estimates and projections* (Publication No. 25-1024). Washington, DC: U.S. Government Printing Office.

U.S. Department of Commerce, Bureau of the Census. (1992b). *Population projections of the United States by age, race, and Hispanic origin: 1990 to 2050* (Publication No. 25-1095). Washington, DC: U.S. Government Printing Office.

U.S. Department of Commerce, Bureau of the Census. (June 12, 1993a). *News release, Commerce News.* Washington, DC: U.S. Government Printing Office.

U.S. Department of Commerce, Bureau of the Census. (1993b). *We, the American Asians.* Washington, DC: U.S. Government Printing Office.

U.S. Department of Commerce, Bureau of the Census. (2000). Retrieved from http://www.census.gov.

U.S. Department of Health and Human Services, Indian Health Service. (1997). *Trends in Indian health.* Retrieved from www.ihs.gov/PublicInfo/Publications/trends97/trends97.asp.

U.S. Department of Health and Human Services, Public Health Service, National Institutes of Health. (1982). *Diabetes in the 80s: Report of the National Diabetes Advisory Board.* Washington, DC: U.S. Government Printing Office.

Walch, T. (1994). *Immigrant America: European ethnicity in the United States.* New York: Garland.

*Watson, O. M. (1980). *Proxemics behavior: A cross cultural study.* The Hague, Netherlands: Mouton.

4

The Health Care Delivery System

Learning Objectives

After studying this chapter, you should be able to do the following:

- Compare the four types of health care services
- Identify health care personnel and describe their training, roles, and responsibilities
- Discuss inpatient, outpatient, and community settings for the delivery of health care
- Compare the types of health care financing
- Discuss current issues and opportunities in health care delivery

The health care delivery system in the United States is a complex array of services working together as independent units with an interdependent relationship based on government regulation and systems for payment of services. The goal of these services is to provide accessible, available, affordable, quality health care. It is not truly a system in the sense of being a well-ordered, coordinated body of connected parts, but it is a system in the sense that the parts are interdependent with each affecting the work of the others.

Each person or group concerned with the system has a unique perspective on the meaning and relationship of the parts of the whole. Clients and their families, such as the parents of a child with a serious illness, seek the health care delivery system as a beneficent domain—that is, a source of nurturance and healing with solutions to their health problems. Health care providers view the system as a means to provide care to their clients. Economists on the other hand see it as a huge service industry consisting of public and private businesses providing health care services to consumers. Legislators may see it as a political agenda driven by demand from their constituents. Social theorists may claim that the system is the property of all citizens, who should be granted universal availability and coverage.

Understanding the strengths and weakness of the health care delivery system begins with knowledge of the nature of comprehensive health care services and the people and institutions that provide those services. However, full understanding takes into account the methods of health care financing, the social and economic factors affecting health care, and the framework for redesigning the system to better meet the goal of a healthy society. Indeed, these are the forces that have created the health care delivery system over the last century and that have created the opportunities and issues in health care for the twenty-first century.

SCOPE OF HEALTH CARE SERVICES

Over the last century, identification and treatment of an illness or disease has largely governed the direction of health care delivery. However, four types of services have evolved as a means to provide comprehensive health care: health promotion and illness prevention, diagnosis and treatment, rehabilitation, and supportive care. These components produce a system to provide health care services for the individual, family, aggregates, and communities.

Health Promotion and Illness Prevention

Health promotion is a means to modify a client's knowledge, attitudes, and skills to adopt behaviors leading to a healthier lifestyle thus achieving a higher level of wellness from any point on a continuum from health to illness. **Illness prevention** involves the use of immunizations and medications that avert disease or detect disease in its earliest, most treatable stages.

Although the treatment of illness has made tremendous advances in the last century, the overall improvement in general health and longevity of the past few decades owes less to medical care and more to healthy behaviors and improved environmental quality. If this continues to be true for the next decades, the health care delivery system should emphasize health promotion and illness prevention.

Diagnosis and Treatment

The diagnosis and treatment of illness will continue to be a major component of the health care system. Technological advances have allowed physicians to diagnose illnesses far sooner and treat them more effectively than in the past. However, the emphasis on high technology may cause clients to feel that the providers' focus is on the machine or procedure rather than the person's health needs. The client needs to understand the medical diagnosis and treatment and assume responsibility for managing the treatment plan at home.

Rehabilitation

Rehabilitation has the goals of restoration of function, maintenance of the remaining levels of physical and mental function, and prevention of further deterioration. Rehabilitation activities are applied to a wide range of health problems, such as stroke, joint replacement, burns, or spinal cord injury, which can occur on an acute, chronic, or time-limited basis. Rehabilitation services are required by clients whose past illnesses or injuries have left them with residual physical or mental impairments that affect their ability to function normally. In addition, people are living longer with chronic illness and often need rehabilitation services.

Supportive Care

Supportive care includes medical, nursing, psychological, and social services aimed at helping the client manage a chronic illness, disability, or terminal illness when rehabilitation or restoration is not a realistic goal. This care can be provided in a hospital, a nursing home, a hospice, or in the client's home setting and aims to meet the physical, emotional, and spiritual needs of the client and the family. The objective is to help clients achieve or maintain the highest level of functioning possible, thus permitting the greatest degree of independence and participation in their community.

HEALTH CARE PERSONNEL

The accelerating employment growth in health services during the 1980s and early 1990s has slowed in recent years, but the industry continues to be a major source of new jobs in the United States (Engel, 1999). Health care jobs are expected to be among the most rapidly growing fields over the next 10 years (Hecker, 2001). Although physicians remain the most prominent members of the health care system, many other specialties have evolved to participate in today's multidisciplinary team approach to care.

Registered Nurses

A registered nurse is a graduate of a state-approved school of nursing and licensed by the state to practice nursing as defined by the nurse practice act in that state. Nurses are the largest single group of health care professionals in this country. Although most nurses work in hospitals, they also work in long-term care facilities, rehabilitation centers, public and private agencies, schools, ambulatory care centers, and nursing education. There are 2,696,540 (Division of Nursing, 2001) registered nurses, or 828.4 per 100,000 people in the United States (National Center for Health Statistics, 1998). Registered nurses focus on health promotion and disease prevention and are major care providers for sick and injured clients. The evolving health care system has created the need for nurses trained in many specialties.

Advanced Practice Nurses

Advanced nurse practitioners include clinical nurse specialists and nurse practitioners. Advanced nurse practitioners have a master's degree that includes academic work in a clinical specialty or in nurse practitioner skills. Nurse practitioner programs require a designated amount of clinical practice. Advanced practice nursing is regulated by the various state boards of nursing, and the states vary with regard to the authority to write prescriptions and the nature of required supervision by a physician.

Physicians

A physician is a graduate of a college of medicine or osteopathy and licensed under the medical practice act by the state to diagnosis and treat disease. Physicians practice in a variety of settings and practice arrangements. Some are employed by hospitals as staff physicians, in federal or state government agencies, public health clinics, community health centers, and prisons. However, most physicians are in private practice as solo or group practitioners. The number of physicians has steadily increased from 14.1 per 10,000 of the population in 1950 to 27.8 per 10,000 in 1999 (American Medical Association, 2000/2001).

Increasingly, physicians are specializing. Physicians trained in family medicine, general internal medicine, and general pediatrics are considered primary care providers or generalists. Board certification in a specialty requires additional years of training and a specialty board examination. Common medical specialties include cardiology, dermatology, family medicine, neurology, obstetrics and gynecology, ophthalmology, pediatrics, psychology, radiology, and surgery. Primary care physicians may refer clients to specialists on the basis of evaluation of the client's medical needs.

Physician Assistants

The American Academy of Physician Assistants (2001) defines physician assistants (PAs) as "health care professionals licensed to practice medicine with physician supervision." As part of their comprehensive responsibilities, PAs conduct physical exams, diagnose and treat illnesses, order and interpret tests, counsel on preventive health care, assist in surgery, and, in most states, write prescriptions. Thus physician assistants practice only under the supervision of a physician and are not meant to be a separate profession such as nursing. Physician assistants practice in a variety of settings including physicians' offices, hospitals, ambulatory care centers, nurs-

ing homes, government agencies, and community health centers. According to the American Academy of Physician Assistants (2001), there were 52,716 physician assistants as of December, 2000.

Most of the programs that train physician assistants grant a baccalaureate degree upon graduation. The National Commission on Certification of Physician Assistants provides PAs with their certification after completion of education and clinical experience requirements.

Allied Health Practitioners

Allied health workers can be divided into two broad categories: therapists and technologists, and technicians and assistants in fields such as physical therapy, respiratory therapy, surgery, radiology, laboratory analysis, and sonography. Generally, *technicians and assistants* are prepared in 2 years or less and require supervision from therapists or technologists to evaluate the treatment process. *Therapists and technologists* receive more advanced training to evaluate clients, diagnose problems, and develop treatment plans (Jonas, 1998). Additionally, the terms *technician* and *assistant* are being used as job titles for personnel with only on-the-job training.

Pharmacists

A pharmacist is a graduate of an accredited program of study in pharmacology and licensed to prepare, compound, and dispense drugs when presented with a prescription from a physician, dentist, or some other licensed practitioners with prescriptive authority. A pharmacist takes an active role on behalf of clients by interpreting, evaluating, and implementing medical orders, assisting providers in making appropriate drug choices, counseling clients, and assuming direct responsibilities collaboratively with other health care professionals and with clients to achieve the desired therapeutic outcome.

Social Workers

Social workers help clients and families cope with problems resulting from long-term illness, injury, and rehabilitation. They also often work in clinical settings as case managers to facilitate appropriate client discharge and follow-up care and to ensure proper use of community services. Social workers may have a bachelor's, master's, or doctoral degree in social work; a graduate degree is often required for those engaged in clinical practice. Social workers' licensure and scope of practice are regulated in all 50 states.

Spiritual and Religious Personnel

Pastoral care workers provide spiritual care, which is an integral part of holistic health care. Clients and their families come from diverse religious backgrounds, ranging from Christianity to Taoism, and others practice no formal religion at all. The health care team must be comfortable with and receptive to clients' spiritual needs (Sumner, 1998). Many hospitals have a department of full-time pastoral care employees to minister to their clients, families, and staff (Jonas, 1998).

Alternative Practitioners

Complementary and alternative medicine practitioners use many healing methods, from ancient arts such as traditional Chinese medicine and acupuncture to recently discovered food supplements (Box 4-1). Viewed by many with skepticism and sometimes even labeled as quackery, the use of alternative therapies is growing in typical health care settings. Some think these methods could reduce the need for physicians and therefore the cost of health care. Proponents believe that some forms of alternative medicine may prove to be superior to traditional Western medicine. Nontraditional or alternative thera-

pies include homeopathy, herbal formulas, acupuncture, therapeutic touch, and biofeedback. Even meditation imagery, massage, spiritual guidance, and prayer are often included in discussions of nonconventional and alternative therapy options. Dietary changes and vitamin supplements have become popular for preventing or treating health problems for several reasons: dissatisfaction with traditional medicine, a desire to manage symptoms not well understood by traditional medicine, and the expectation that we can live longer and better. The lack of definitive research does not seem to deter the marketing of these therapies.

Box 4-1 *Considering the Alternatives*
Complementary and Alternative Therapies in Health Care

Description and History: Complementary and Alternative Medicine (CAM) is one of the fastest-growing health-related industries in the United States, Europe, and other English speaking countries. CAM incorporates a wide range of therapies and health-related activities that are not traditionally taught in medical schools. Many of these therapies originated in healing systems from historically or geographically different cultures. Surveys suggest a continuing trend of increased use, representing a significant shift in the public orientation to health care.

The majority of users are well educated and combine CAM activities with biomedical treatment. They use CAM for promoting optimal health, treating symptoms of chronic conditions, treating side effects of biomedical treatments, and treatment of a disorder.

Both the nursing and the medical professions have organizations related to holistic health: the American Holistic Nurses Association (AHNA) and the American Holistic Medical Association (AHMA). This shift in health care on the part of professionals and the lay public coincides with the increasing emphasis on health and with the expansion of health care to include concerns about quality of life and prevention of diseases and disability. Over two thirds of the medical schools in the United States now have courses on CAM.

The National Institutes of Health (NIH), following a mandate by congress, established the Office of Alternative and Complementary Medicine in the early 1990s. This was upgraded to the National Center for Complementary and Alternative Medicine (NCCAM) in 1998 with the mission of supporting research and disseminating knowledge to the public. In 2002, the White House Commission presented its report recommending continued research, education, and dissemination of information as well as an office to address concerns related to regulating safety, efficacy, and preparation of providers. Some health care organizations are offering CAM to their clients and some insurance companies now cover select modalities.

Important Points: The term *alternative therapy* refers to therapies that are used in place of biomedical treatment or physically or chemically invasive treatments. It is important to differentiate these from the more gentle complementary therapies. The term *complementary therapy* is more appropriate for most of the currently popular modalities, as they are generally used in combination with biomedicine, most are oriented toward health, and they are not performed by physicians. The current trend is to combine the best of both biomedicine and complementary medicine in integrated health care. Many complementary therapies are intended to act gently to stimulate the natural healing potential of the individual. NCCAM classifies CAM into the following domains:
1. *Alternative medical systems* are scholarly systems of healing, such as traditional Chinese medicine (TCM) and Ayurvedic medicine homeopathy.

2. *Mind-body interventions* facilitate relaxation and other modalities that might enhance health through the psychoneuroimmunologic framework.
3. *Biologically based therapies* include diet modifications, diet supplements, and other biologically based modalities.
4. *Manipulative and body-based methods* include bodywork, massage, and other structural manipulations.
5. *Energy therapies* include magnets, touch therapies, and other modalities known as biofield therapies.

Practice of Complementary and Alternative Therapies: Although the therapies practiced under the CAM umbrella have not traditionally been taught in medical schools, some have been taught in schools of nursing, are described in the nursing literature, and are listed in the Nursing Interventions Classification (NIC). Many nurses incorporate complementary modalities into their practice, using, for example, active listening, touch therapy, nutritional counseling, exercise and physical movement, and psychological support. An additional certificate is required for some complementary modalities, such as massage therapy, therapeutic touch, healing touch, and visualization. A number of healers operate as independent practitioners of various methods. The NIH is supporting research to determine the safety and efficacy of these modalities, but it is yet in the early stages.

Practitioners of Complementary and Alternative Therapies: Although many of these modalities are incorporated into the professional practice of a nurse, physician, or other health care provider, many practitioners have no health care background. There is no standard regulation or licensure for CAM practitioners. For some, a certificate process is in place, but further regulation has not been established. Some groups are organizing to develop some professional status; they are seeking licensure status and positioning themselves to receive third-party reimbursement. Others operate on a more individual intuitive basis. This is often confusing for the consumer.

Potential Benefits of Complementary and Alternative Therapies: As many complementary therapies act to bolster the body's natural health-promoting capacity, their beneficial effects may be more generalized and more effective. Some may be effective in the very early stages of a disease. Others have efficacy in symptom control, such as in reducing pain or side effects of treatments. Many have demonstrated efficacy in reducing anxiety and stress. There is some speculation that the relationship between a CAM provider and the client is more engaging, which may explain some of the positive benefits of CAM modalities. NCCAM is currently studying the placebo effect.

Continued

Box 4-1 *Considering the Alternatives*
Complementary and Alternative Therapies in Health Care—cont'd

Concerns About the Practice of Complementary and Alternative Therapies: The first area of concern relates to the lack of regulation. As many of these therapies have not been subjected to research, and the practitioners and many of the products are underregulated, there is a potential for harm. Some CAM practitioners may exploit or actually harm clients. Others, although well intentioned, do not have any medical knowledge and may inadvertently harm vulnerable clients by giving inappropriate advice. Additionally, many practitioners do not have a background in health care ethics and may violate confidentiality, they may not provide informed consent, and they may not have professional accountability.

A second major concern is that of replacing or delaying effective biomedical treatment. Some providers are highly critical of CAM because they fear that clients will spend valuable time and resources pursuing CAM treatments and thus fail to get an effective biomedical treatment.

A third area of concern is about the interaction of a CAM therapy with biomedical treatments. Dietary supplements, herbs, and other substances may have a synergistic, cumulative, or counteractive effect with medications. Nurses should always ask clients about herbs, diet supplements, or over-the-counter medications in their assessments.

The fourth concern is about the interaction of the CAM treatment and the disease process. For example, using very vigorous bodywork with a client with a clotting disorder could lead to injury.

Resources
Books
Dossey, B., Keegan, L., & Guzzetta, C. (Eds.). (2000). *Holistic nursing: A handbook for practice* (3rd ed.). Gaithersburg, MD: Aspen.
Micozzi, M. (Ed.). (2001). *Fundamentals of complementary and alternative medicine* (2nd ed.). New York: Churchill Livingstone.
Synder, M., & Lindquist, R. (Eds.). (1998). *Complementary/alternative therapies in nursing* (3rd ed.). New York: Springer.

Journals
Advances in Mind Body Medicine
Alternative and Complementary Therapies
Alternative Therapies in Health and Medicine
HerbalGram
Holistic Nursing Practice
Journal of Holistic Nursing

Websites
Center for Mind Body Medicine, http://www.cmbm.org/.
Commonweal, http://www.commonweal.org/.
Fetzer Foundation, www.fetzer.org.
Integrative Medicine, http://www.integrativemedicine.com.
National Center for Complementary and Alternative Medicine (NCCAM), www.nccam.nih.gov.

HEALTH CARE SETTINGS

Health care delivery occurs within a continuum of health care settings and services from outpatient to inpatient, and from acute care to long-term care. *Inpatient* denotes care given in the context of an overnight stay in a hospital or other facility. Inpatient treatment is provided in long-term care facilities such as nursing homes, psychiatric hospitals, and rehabilitation centers. *Outpatient* services do not require an overnight inpatient stay in a hospital or long-term care facility. Outpatient services, also called ambulatory care, include a wide range of services, from routine tests and treatments to complex procedures and therapies. The managed care environment has made outpatient settings increasingly important in the delivery of health care services.

Services based in the community are provided through voluntary, public, or proprietary organizations and include adult day care, respite care, congregate meals, transportation, and case management programs. A variety of funding sources include Medicare, Medicaid, Title II of the Older Americans Act established in 1965, and other federal, state, and local social services programs. The extent of services provided and the eligibility requirements vary by service, funding source, and locality.

Hospitals

A hospital is an institution for the medical and nursing care of ill and injured persons needing complex services with a high risk of complications. Hospital services are appropriate when intensive monitoring is required for the early detection or prevention of complications or deterioration of the client's condition. Hospitals offer a variety of inpatient and outpatient services for management of acute and subacute conditions. Services may also include emergency, rehabilitative, and skilled nursing care.

Although some hospitals serve multiple purposes in a community, in general there are three levels of hospitals. The first tier of the hospital system includes the general hospital, the community hospital, and the rural community hospital. The general hospital offers a range of medical, surgical, obstetrical, pediatric, and emergency services. A community hospital serves a specific location (an area of a city, a rural community) or population (women, children, heart patients). Rural hospitals are often more limited in the scope of their services than urban hospitals. Poor economic conditions, isolated rural areas, weather conditions, limited availability of transportation, and long distances affect rural residents' access to health care. Rural hospitals also have difficulty recruiting health care providers such as pediatricians, obstetricians, internists, dentists, and nurses.

The second tier is a larger, usually urban, general hospital with a full range of services including up-to-date, high-technical-level care by specialists. The third tier or tertiary care hospitals are large medical centers that provide highly sophisticated, cutting-edge care and maintain extensive research and teaching programs. Tertiary care centers draw clients from a larger geographical region.

Hospitals are also classified as public or private. Public hospitals are owned by agencies of federal, state, or local government. Federal hospitals are maintained for special groups of federal beneficiaries, such as military and governmental personnel, veterans, and Native Americans. State governments generally limit themselves to operating hospitals intended to safeguard public health by treating mental illness and contagious diseases such as tuberculosis.

Private hospitals are owned and operated by corporations or charitable organizations. As health care grew to be one of the largest industries in the United States, multihospital chains developed in response. The change in reimbursement methods and a need to constrain costs while still providing a variety of health care services forced cost constraints that allowed large corporations to have an advantage over smaller, single-hospital systems.

Emergency and Rescue Care

Ambulance service and first aid treatment to victims of acute illness, accidents, and disasters by trained emergency medical technicians (EMTs) are the most common mobile medical services. EMTs are trained to provide critical early treatment, on site and in transit, that is often life saving. Most urban centers have developed formal emergency medical systems to provide a quick response to emergencies. Rural areas access medical centers through ambulance services and helicopter medical transport units. Specialized ambulance services, such as cardiac care units and shock/trauma units initiate complex care at the scene and during transport.

Most hospitals provide some level of emergency services. The hospital emergency department provides services around the clock for clients with emergent problems, as well as services after office hours for other clients. A trauma center has a full range of services for complex trauma victims.

Psychiatric Care

In both public and private psychiatric facilities, the number of beds devoted to inpatient psychiatric services has decreased over the past two decades. New treatment techniques, consumer protection laws, and issues of cost are responsible for the shift from inpatient care to community care. However, the result of the shift to community care and the client's right to refuse treatment has been an increased number of homeless people who are not managing their mental illness well.

Rehabilitative Care

Rehabilitation hospitals specialize in providing restorative services to rehabilitate chronically ill and disabled clients (Figure 4-1). Clients who are discharged from a short-term inpatient stay may transfer to a freestanding rehabilitation hospital, a rehabilitation unit in a general hospital, or an outpatient rehabilitation service. Most rehabilitation hospitals offer nursing, physical therapy, psychological services, social services, and vocational services.

Long-Term Care

Long-term care describes a range of health and housing services provided to people unable to care for themselves independently or in need of assistance to maintain their independence. In addition to traditional nursing home care, options include assisted living facilities, residential care facilities, and retirement centers. Assisted living provides services associated with a resident's activities of daily living. Residential care, also known as sheltered care or board and care, offers some services, such as meals and assistance with taking medicine. Retirement centers offer residents the opportunity to

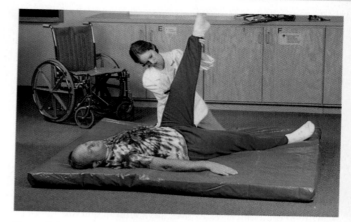

Figure 4-1. Rehabilitation hospitals specialize in providing restorative services to rehabilitate chronically ill and disabled people.

maintain their own lifestyle while having some services available for those who need them.

More than half of the financial support for long-term care comes from public funds such as Medicaid and Medicare. Long-term care is heavily regulated through licensure and certification requirements.

After a hospital stay, Medicare will pay for care for a short period of time when the care can be expected to assist the client to return to independent living. The care has to include medically necessary services requiring professional skills. Skilled care, as a Medicare level of care, is offered on special hospital units, in nursing homes, and in subacute care hospitals. Subacute care addresses the needs of clients who have recovered from the acute phase of an illness or injury but still require ongoing nursing and medical monitoring and treatment.

For clients who are unable to care for themselves and have no expectation of improvement, the only source of public funding for long-term care is Medicaid. To receive Medicaid funding for long-term care, they have to demonstrate financial need. As a result, clients must spend almost all of their resources before qualifying for Medicaid.

Hospice

Hospice is a cluster of special services that address the special needs of dying people and their families. It blends medical, spiritual, legal, financial, and family-support services. Hospice is a model of care that regards the client together with the family as the unit of care. It is a concept, not a location. The venue of care can vary from a specialized facility to a nursing home to the client's own home. Services can be organized out of a hospital, a nursing home, a freestanding hospice facility, or a home health agency.

Physicians' Offices

Private physicians working solo, in partnerships, or in private group practices are the dominant providers of outpatient care. The physician's office is the usual setting for most basic outpatient services, such as physical examinations, diagnostic and screening services, minor illness care, medication administration, counseling and advice, and routine treatment follow-up. Today this office is most likely to be part of a group practice or medical clinic complex.

Ambulatory Care Centers

The ambulatory care center provides health services on an outpatient basis to those who visit a hospital or other health care facility and depart after treatment on the same day. This category covers managed care programs and hospital-based ambulatory services, including clinics, walk-in and emergency services, mobile units, and health promotion centers. Freestanding "surgi-centers" and "urgi- or emergi-centers," health department clinics, neighborhood and community health centers, organized home care, community mental health centers, school and workplace health services, and prison health services are additional examples of ambulatory care settings.

Mobile medical services take advanced diagnostic services to clients in rural communities in a convenient and cost-effective manner. For example, mobile eye care and dental care units can be brought to a nursing home site or to a workplace, where they can efficiently serve a large number of clients. Mobile diagnostic services include mammography, magnetic resonance imaging, and cardiac assessment and health screening services such as blood sugar, blood pressure, and cholesterol checks.

Adult Day Care Centers

Adult day care (ADC) is a daytime program offered in an institutional setting that provides a wide range of health, social, and recreational services to frail (usually older) adults who require supervision and care while members of the family or other informal care givers are away at work (Shi & Singh, 1998). ADC is generally a structured, comprehensive weekday program that provides personal care, midday meals, social services, and transportation in a protective setting. It complements informal care given in the home by family members and helps delay or prevent institutionalization. ADC may also work as respite to help reduce caregiver stress. Many ADC programs provide a mix of medical, maintenance, and social-psychological services. Group socialization and recreational activities are important as well.

Respite Care Services

Respite care is defined as a service that provides temporary relief to informal caregivers such as family members. Respite care is the most frequently suggested intervention to address family caregivers' feelings of stress and burden. ADC, home health care, and temporary stays in nursing homes, hospitals, group homes, or foster care homes are examples of respite care services or programs. In-home respite care provides temporary homemaker, chore, or home health services. The focus of respite care, regardless of how it is provided, is to give the client's informal caregivers time off while meeting the needs for assistance of frail, older, or disabled chronically ill clients.

School Health Clinics

Almost all educational institutions provide some form of ambulatory health services to students. Services are provided by local health departments or by school boards in conjunction with the local health department.

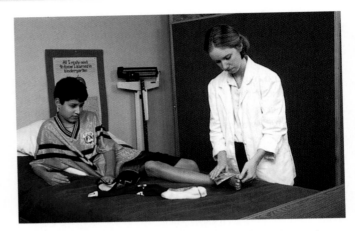

Figure 4-2. The work of most school-based health programs is carried out by a registered nurse and is confined to basic first aid, case finding, and prevention of certain chronic or epidemic diseases.

The work of most school-based health programs is supervised by a registered nurse and confined to basic first aid, case finding, and prevention of certain chronic or epidemic diseases (Figure 4-2). Very little disease treatment is done in the health program of a public school (kindergarten to 12th grade). Vision and hearing screenings and various immunizations are commonly offered. When indicated, referrals for diagnosis and treatment are made to the student's parents and physician. Colleges and universities provide a broader set of services, including many basic diagnostic and treatment services. In some school settings there are programs to help students deal with mental, physical, and substance abuse problems (Jonas, 1998).

Occupational Health Services

Industrial or occupational health services are provided in most large businesses and factories. The actual number of these "in-plant" health units in the United States is unknown. In smaller firms it may be simply a first-aid box; larger firms may provide systematic health services staffed by industrial nurses and part-time physicians. In a few firms the health services are comprehensive, with complete care for all health disorders, whether or not the disorders are work related (Jonas, 1998).

Optimal health accomplished through changes in lifestyle improves the overall health of America's workforce. Work-site health promotion or wellness programs create awareness of health factors, help employees make lifestyle changes, and develop workplace environments that are conducive to health.

Home Health Care Services

Home health care services, such as nursing, therapy, and health-related homemaker or social services, are brought to clients in their own homes because these clients are unable to leave their homes safely to get the care they need. Home health care is provided to clients and their families at their place of residence to promote, maintain, or restore health and minimize effects of disability and illness. Home health care services are provided mainly to older adult clients. Seventy-five percent of home health care clients are age 65 or over.

Community Health Centers

Community health centers concentrate on the delivery of primary health care services to the community as a whole and to individuals. They serve as a primary care safety net for our nation's poor and underserved in both inner-city and rural areas. Community health centers have become expert in managing the health care needs of these special populations. Long-standing outreach programs, case management, transportation, translation services, alcohol and drug abuse screening and treatment, mental health services, health education, and social services are provided to roughly 30% of the country's indigent population served by these centers nationwide (Shi & Singh, 1998).

HEALTH CARE FINANCING

Over the past few decades a complex blend of private and public mechanisms has arisen to affect how Americans pay for health care. Since the early 1980s, the basic approach for reimbursing hospitals, physicians, and long-term providers of services has been restructured.

After Medicare, private health insurance has been the most prevalent source of financing for the United States health care system. Insurance is a mechanism created to help protect against risk, and it protects against potential substantial financial loss from a low-probability event. A person protected by insurance against a specific risk is called the insured, and the insuring agency that assumes the risk is the insurer.

However, the term *health insurance* is often used to mean a wide array of health care financing mechanisms, including the "social insurance" of Medicare and the public assistance of Medicaid, the self-insurance plans used by employers, and the managed care programs of health maintenance organizations (HMOs) and preferred provider organizations (PPOs). Clients pay for some of their health care themselves. Persons not covered by either private or government-sponsored health financing programs are called uninsured. Medicare and private health insurance plays an important role in influencing the direction and structure of our nation's health care system.

The American health care system is the most expensive and unique system in the developed world. In 1997 about $4,000 per person was spent on health care as compared with the next most expensive country, Switzerland, which spent $2,500 (Organization for Economic Cooperation and Development, 1998). However, over the years public outlays for health care financing have increased and private financing has shrunk proportionately. In 1997, the number of people without health insurance increased to 43.4 million, or 16% of the population (U.S. Bureau of the Census, 1997, 1998). Although this figure declined in 2000 (U.S. Bureau of the Census, 2000a) to 14% of the population (38.7 million people), it will rise again as unemployment and poverty rates grow. The figures for children show that 21.5% had no health insurance in 2000 (U.S. Bureau of the Census, 2000b). There has been a decline in the growth of private health care expenditures since the early 1990s, whereas the government's share of the nation's health care bill in 1997 rose to $507 billion, or 46% of the total, an increase from 40% in 1990. Private resources financed 54% of personal health services, $585 billion in 1997, down from 60% in 1990 (Levit et al., 1998). All of the money to pay for health care services ultimately comes from the American people.

Private Health Insurance

Private health insurance may be purchased by an individual or a group. Group insurance measures the risk for the insured group, resulting in lower premiums for each member. Indemnity (commercial) health insurance reimburses health care providers on the basis of a fee for each health service provided to the insured person. The traditional method of reimbursement was **retrospective**—that is, the amount of insurance paid was based on the service received. This type of insurance was considered to be catastrophic coverage, thus paying only for major medical events like an automobile accident or major surgery.

Managed Care Organizations

Currently, health care coverage is more likely to be administered by a managed care organization (MCO). MCOs were the most significant development in America's system of health care delivery in the twentieth century. **Managed care** is a system that combines the functions of health insurance and the actual delivery of care in a way that controls utilization and costs of services by limiting unnecessary treatment (Shi & Singh, 1998).

Health care delivery under MCOs is designed to affect the operation and structure of the health care system and thus to affect the use of services by the consumer. Managed care attempts to control cost by controlling access to unnecessary care. The opponents of managed care say it limits consumer choice and access, and it involves insurers in the client-provider relationship.

The primary care physician is the "gatekeeper" in the managed care systems. This provider has the coordinating role for the client's health care needs through being responsible for all primary care for the client and determining when referral to specialists is necessary (Figure 4-3, p. 66). The gatekeeper concept manages the client's use of resources, reduces the self-initiated use of specialty services, and ensures overall coordination without duplication of care.

A **health maintenance organization** is a prepaid health plan that delivers comprehensive health care to members through designated providers, has a fixed monthly payment for health care services, and requires members to be in a plan for a specified period of time (usually 1 year). HMOs are a type of group health care practice that provides basic and supplemental health maintenance and treatment services to voluntary enrollees who prepay a fixed periodic fee that is set without regard to the amount or kind of services received. HMOs are the most common type of MCO. All health care is obtained from hospitals, physicians, and other providers participating in the HMO. The HMO is responsible for establishing standards for the quality of services provided.

The **preferred provider organization,** the most common type of MCO after the HMO, is an organization of physicians,

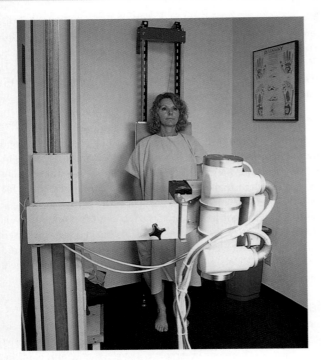

Figure 4-3. Under managed care, the primary care physician serves as a "gatekeeper" for referral for diagnostic procedures and specialty care.

hospitals, and pharmacists whose members discount their health care services to subscribers (clients). A PPO may be organized by a group of physicians, an outside entrepreneur, an insurance company, or a company with a self-insurance plan. The PPO is the insurance industry's response to the growth of HMOs. PPOs negotiate contracts with companies to lock in the business of treating their employees. The PPO makes contractual arrangements with providers for the delivery of health care services on a discounted fee schedule (Shi & Singh, 1998).

An **exclusive provider organization** (EPO) is similar to a PPO in its organization and purpose, but enrollees are restricted to the EPO's list of providers of health care, called exclusive providers. Like HMOs, EPOs use a gatekeeping approach to health care service delivery as a means of decreasing cost.

Government Insurance Plans

Public financing of health care services accounts for roughly 46% of the total expenditures on health care in the United States. Governmental spending supports *categorical programs* designed to provide benefits to certain groups of people. The most well-known examples are Medicare and Medicaid. Like Social Security, Medicare is an *entitlement program.* Because people have contributed toward Medicare through taxes, they are "entitled" to the benefits regardless of their income and assets. In contrast, Medicaid is a welfare program, in which the level of benefits depends on a person's income and assets. Medicare and Medicaid purchase government-funded services from the private sector (Shi & Singh, 1998).

Medicare is a federally funded national health insurance program in the United States for people over 65 years of age and for some chronically ill persons. Medicare is the first na-

medical care. Medicare was enacted in 1965 as Title XVIII of the Social Security Act. Health care services are provided for those disabled persons who are eligible for Social Security benefits and for those who have end-stage renal disease. Although there is no monthly fee for Medicare Part A, which pays for hospitalization and some skilled care afterward, the recipient must pay the first $764, and the number of days is limited. For part B coverage, there is a monthly premium and Medicare pays only 80% of the allowable charges. Most people need supplemental insurance. Medicare recipients can participate in a managed care organization.

Medicaid is the largest health insurer in the United States, covering medical services and long-term care for nearly 40 million people (Centers for Medicare and Medicaid Services [CMS], 2002). It was established along with Medicare in 1965 under Title XIX of the Social Security Act. **Medicaid** is a grant program providing partial health care services for indigent people. Federal and state governments support it jointly. The federal government provides matching funds to the states on the basis of the per-capita income in each state. By law the federal matching dollars cannot be less than 50%, or more than 83%, of the total state Medicaid program costs.

A **prospective payment system** (PPS) is a payment system in which the amount paid for a specific service is predetermined. This system was implemented for short-stay inpatient hospitalizations (Medicare Part A) in the mid 1980s under the Social Security Act of 1983. The predetermined reimbursement amount is set according to **diagnosis-related groups** (DRGs), a system of classification or grouping of clients according to medical diagnosis for purposes of paying hospitalization costs. Payment is based on diagnosis and date of discharge rather than length of stay (per diem). Payment is at a rate set for "bundled services." It involves approximately 500 DRGs corresponding to the most prevalent diagnoses found in clients using inpatient services (Jonas, 1998). The PPS has helped Medicare to control the per-case rate of increase for Part A hospital expenditure reimbursement.

Another form of payment is a **capitation payment system.** In this system, payment for health care services is an arrangement between the purchaser of care and the provider, and the provider receives a flat fee to provide a defined level of care. The enrollee (insured person) may or may not need the services being covered. Thus the provider theoretically has an investment in keeping the enrollee healthy.

In the United States, health care is not administered or controlled by a central department or agency of the government. However, many other industrialized countries maintain central control of health care delivery. Three basic types of basic systems are in use.

In the Canadian system, the government finances health care through general taxes, but private providers deliver health care services. Canada's system demonstrates that the use of a national health care budget can be effective in controlling the growth of health care expenditures.

In Great Britain the government's National Health Service not only finances the program but also manages the infrastructure for the delivery of medical care. Under this system the government operates most of the medical institutions, and physi-

In Germany's system of socialized health insurance, employers and employees finance health care through government-mandated contributions. Private providers deliver health care. Private, not-for-profit insurance companies, called sickness funds, are responsible for collecting the contributions and paying physicians and hospitals.

Generally, the three national health care systems described have common features: (1) every citizen is entitled to a defined set of health care services, (2) national budgets determine total health care expenditures and allocate resources, and (3) the budget limits determine the availability of services and the payments to providers. The governments control the proliferation of health care services, especially those that involve high technology. Resource allocation determines the extent to which the governments can offer citizens health care services (Shi & Singh, 1998).

The United States has long resisted the idea of moving from a private practice model for delivery of health care to a national health plan. However, the issue continues to be discussed. Oregon has led the way in developing a model for a state-administered health care system that guarantees certain basic services to all its citizens. In 1989, the Oregon state legislature passed the Basic Health Services Act, creating the Oregon Health Services Commission (OHSC) (1991). The OHSC defined basic health care as a bottom-line standard for the services to be available to all people. The OHSC created three levels of health care benefits: "essential," "very important," and "valuable to certain individuals." It also developed a priority list of 709 health services (Hadorn, 1991).

Oregon's health plan was originally seen as extreme, but rationing of health care is no longer seen as radical. Every state is struggling to keep Medicaid costs under control. So far, the Medicaid portion of the Oregon plan has been successful, signing up about 126,000 new members since 1994 (Bodenheimer, 1997; Montague, 1997).

While many people resist the idea of rationing health care, the current system of delivery does in essence ration health care. Instead of being rationed by the state, it is rationed by the HMOs.

ISSUES AND OPPORTUNITIES IN HEALTH CARE DELIVERY

In the last few decades, the United States has experienced great changes in its demographics, family structures, communities, and lifestyles. Unemployment and poverty clash with rising health care costs, and this has raised many legal and ethical issues related to the distribution and availability of health care services. Fortunately, opportunities to influence the future quality and financing of health care services exist.

Issues Affecting Health Care Delivery

Changes in the composition of a population are important for the planning of health care services. The age of the population, the contribution of family support systems, and health problems of specific groups affect the need for specific services.

Age of the Population. The health care system can expect an

of the Census (2000b) estimates that people age 65 and over represented 12.1% of the population in 2000. In the year 2010, it is predicted that approximately 40 million, or 14% of Americans, will be age 65 years or older, with about 4.3 million age 85 years and older. People in the 85 or older category are the fastest-growing group of the U.S. population. Older adults consume more health care services than the younger population. A growing older adult population will have a serious impact on health care expenditures in the future. By 2010, it is estimated that the proportion of children (age 14 and under) in the population will be only 20% (U.S. Bureau of the Census, 2000).

The median age of the population in the year 2000 is 35 years (U.S. Bureau of the Census, 2000b). However, subgroups such as Hispanics have a lower median age than the general population.

Characteristics of the Family. Family support systems have declined as America has evolved from a rural economy with large families to a nation of city dwellers with small families often a long distance from their family of origin. The last U.S. census showed a trend toward increasing urbanization and persistent rural losses. In 1990, 79% of the population lived in urban areas, up from 63% in 1960.

Additionally, the size of the average American family had declined to 2.62 people in 1992. One-parent families continue to increase, contributing to the small average family size. Only 26% of American households with children under the age of 18 years include a married couple. Women living alone head 11.7% of all households in the United States and are likely to be part of the 89% of all households receiving at least one noncash benefit such as Medicaid or food stamps (World Almanac, 1995).

At the same time, there are 25.8 million family caregivers providing $200 billion worth of health care services per year, almost double the annual amount the United States spends on nursing home and home health care. Cutting costs in the health care delivery system will shift the burden of caregiving to an already strained family system (Gordon, 2001).

Cultural Diversity. The changing ethnic composition of the United States is creating a demand for a health care system more responsive to minority population needs. Hispanics, Asians, and Muslims are among the minority groups whose presence is visibly increasing in the United States. There will be a growing demand for health providers who speak languages other than English and understand the health needs of a multiethnic society.

Lifestyle. The nature of common health problems has changed from primarily acute disease to chronic or "lifestyle" diseases. The major causes of death in the United States are from chronic diseases such as heart disease, stroke, cancer, and chronic obstructive pulmonary disease. One in six deaths in this country is attributable to smoking. Dietary practices have a direct role in five of the top ten causes of death and contribute to three more through alcohol abuse. Lifestyle diseases are the result of human behaviors.

Additionally, Americans are more vulnerable to health problems from our interactions with other countries. Diseases distant lands. Through global telecommunications and expanding travel, we live in a world of people who continuously exchange ideas and influence each other's national cultures, languages, and lifestyles.

Affluence and Poverty. For people who live in the right geographic region of the United States, have the right health care coverage, and have a disease on which the health care professionals have chosen to focus, the American health care system is the best in the world. However, the distribution of and access to health care services for the American people is significantly uneven.

The uneven distribution of wealth is a contributing factor to the uneven distribution of health care. American workers' wages have stagnated or declined in recent decades. Additionally, the wealth and income in the United States are becoming increasingly concentrated in the hands of just a few people, producing a large gap between those who have and those who do not. One in seven Americans lives below the poverty level. One in five children under 18 years and one in four children under 3 years are living in poverty. Two of every five Hispanic children and one of every two black children are poor (World Almanac, 1995).

Many Americans living in poverty are the victims of social and environmental ills such as drug addiction, acquired immunodeficiency syndrome (AIDS), crime, and prostitution. Their children likewise suffer from addiction, low birth weight, and resultant mental and physical problems. Women, Blacks, and Hispanics experience poverty at a higher rate than other Americans. Although the socioeconomic status of our nation's older adults (older than 65 years) varies dramatically on the basis of their sources of income and assets, over one fifth of the older adult population is considered poor or near-poor.

The need for health services for vulnerable populations is closely tied to the economic conditions often produced by their health conditions. Homelessness may result from health problems or staggering medical bills. The treatment of AIDS is an economic hardship even with health insurance. Substance and alcohol abuse are costly experiences crossing all economic and social levels in our country. Women, children, and older adults who are chronically ill, disabled, mentally ill, cognitively impaired, neglected, or abused make up the high-risk categories of vulnerable populations that make increasing demands on society as a whole and on the health care system in particular.

Opportunity for Redesigning the System

The American health care system will continue to face the challenge of balancing three competing goals—containing costs, improving access to health care services, and enhancing the quality of care. The dehumanization of the reformed and reengineered health care system of the 1990s led to consumer activism in the political areas of clients' rights and client safety. Tumultuous change in the health care delivery system requires health care providers, including nurses, to be vigilant to ensure that the level of quality achieved not be left to chance. For their part, consumers must insist that an adequate

mechanism for assessing value and effectiveness of care and services be in place to monitor and report to federal, state, and private sector providers. Consumers must be willing to respond to lack of satisfaction in their health care and health services in the same way they would any other product or service, if necessary by lobbying for legislation, by legal action, and with media campaigns. Today's consumers are better educated, more aggressive, and not limited to thinking that "the doctor knows best" or that illness prevention is the only way to improve their health and overall quality of life (Box 4-2).

Cost of Care

The most significant problem in the health care delivery system is how to pay for the increasingly staggering cost of services. Spending for health care topped $1.1 trillion in 1998—13.5% of the gross domestic product. The Centers for Medicare and Medicaid (CMS) predict that this figure could rise to 16.2% by 2008 (Alliance for Health Reform, 2000). Although managed care has been effective in decreasing the cost of care, it may have reached the limits of cost savings that can be accomplished with reduction in hospitalization days. A major area of growth in cost is in the area of prescription drugs, because of both high drug use in older adults and the high cost of newer prescription drugs.

Savings could possibly come through better coordination of care (especially for clients with complex, expensive, or chronic conditions), the use of advanced practice nurses as providers, controlling the cost of prescription drugs, controlling the profits of MCOs, controlling expensive litigation, giving individuals and families more power in the system, decreasing the amount of time spent complying with regulations, reducing overhead cost, and reducing the incidence of errors. Because many of these issues affect their profession, nurses must understand how economic forces drive change and how the system must continue to evolve to meet the needs of society, and how it must respond to fulfill the profession's responsibility to meet the health care needs of society.

Economic constraints and cost-cutting measures exacerbate ethical problems in the delivery of health care. The ever-increasing availability of technology is creating situations that require decision making about who receives what services. These decisions must be made under complex and stressful circumstances (Figure 4-4). Competition pushes health care executives to walk a fine line between what is good for the business and what is ethical.

Access to Health Care. Health care in this country is neither universally available nor universally accessible. There are wide variations depending on residence (urban or rural), health care insurance, economic status, and skill in negotiating the system. **Access** to health care is a complex construct representing the personal use of health care services and the structures or processes that facilitate or impede that use. *Realized access* is the actual use of health care providers and services. Whether access is equitable or inequitable depends on what determines realized access. For example, to the extent that they are precursors of need,

A PATIENT'S PERSPECTIVE
"Sad to Say, This May Be as Good as It Gets in Today's Health Care System."

Box 4-2

If every pregnancy and childbirth were like my first experience, people would never have big families. As a health science editor, I considered myself well prepared to deal with the health care system, especially during what should be a normal physiological process. Never in my worst nightmares had I imagined what actually happened.

Five months into my pregnancy, I realized I was in the wrong place to get the right kind of care. There was little or no personal interaction or education. If I had a problem or a question, I had to tell it to an answering machine. I decided it was time to take charge and make a change.

On the basis of advice from three different people, I went to a practice associated with the university medical center. They made me feel better instantly. There were five physicians, two nurse midwives, four nurse practitioners, and one maternity triage nurse—what I now know was an ideal situation. Whenever I called with a question or a problem, I talked with a person, not a machine. The triage nurse was always available, either immediately or through her beeper.

At 27 weeks, after being really sick all week, I became dehydrated and went into preterm labor. I was hospitalized and spent 2 days in labor and delivery, terrified that I would lose the baby. At 31 and 32 weeks, it happened again—2 more days in labor and delivery.

When I began having preterm labor every week, my doctor intervened and advised my employer that I needed some flexibility in my work life. Easing my schedule helped a lot; the last month was much easier. In my 40th week, I went into labor on my way to the office.

During the next 38 hours, I saw every doctor in the practice but only two nurses. One of them stayed with me for the entire last day; she was a saint. I was given epidural anesthesia twice—the first one wore off, and the second was given too close to the time when I needed to push, so I felt like I had no legs; I couldn't push. The baby was stuck and they had to use forceps. Then whoosh—there she was—the beautiful, perfect baby we had hoped for.

In the first hour after delivery, things began to get confusing. I got very brief instruction in breastfeeding and then they had to take the baby away because I was in an older, unsecured section of the hospital. Next morning, two different nurses gave me two different sets of instructions for breastfeeding. Finally, the discharge nurse gave me yet another set of instructions about breastfeeding. Baby and I went home Christmas day, a Thursday, and had no success with breastfeeding because all the various recommendations were so conflicting. I was exhausted, confused, and frustrated. The baby was hungry. My breasts were engorged and a terrible pain was beginning to build in my abdomen.

By Monday the abdominal pain was excruciating, so I went to the clinic and was examined by my least-favorite physician, who diagnosed the problem as constipation or gas and recommended milk of magnesia. Two days later, on New Year's Eve, my temperature was 102.5° F and I was immobilized by the pain. This time the doctor told me to drink plenty of fluids. Finally, on Friday, I was doubled over in pain, ghostly white, feverish, too weak even to hold my daughter. The doctor said to meet him in the emergency department, which I did at 2 PM. After poking and prodding my tender abdomen, he did an ultrasound but was still baffled. Around midnight he concluded that it might be appendicitis and decided to operate.

Surgery solved the mystery. A fibroid tumor on my uterus had caused the preterm labor; fueled by the pregnancy hormones, my uterus began shrinking, causing the tumor to pull at the appendix until it burst.

I was in the hospital for 5 days after the appendectomy. The surgeon thought it was too soon after delivery to remove the tumor. Each doctor from the obstetric clinic came in to apologize for not diagnosing my problem sooner. During those 5 days, I tried valiantly to maintain my milk supply by using a breast pump (the one they brought in was industrial size!), and it was a real disaster. Not a single medical-surgical nurse could remember how to operate the pump.

Later I made two more trips to the emergency department because the pain just wouldn't stop. The surgeon said the fibroid would have to come out, but I disagreed. Enough was enough. It took a month just to be able to walk again, and 9 months later I still don't have any feeling in my abdomen.

I did go back to breastfeeding for a time, but it was a struggle. After 4 months, I gave up.

I'm an educated health care consumer. I was in one of the best medical centers in the country—certainly the best in the region—but my care left a lot to be desired. Yet I would recommend that hospital and that ob-gyn group because I believe, sad to say, this may be as good as it gets in today's health care system.

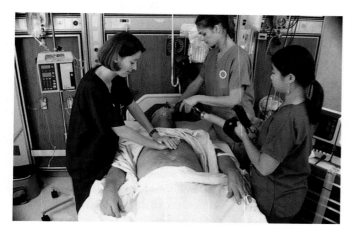

Figure 4-4. Modern technology leads daily to situations that require decision making under complex and stressful circumstances.

age, gender, and ethnicity are indicators of equitable access or inequitable access when they determine who obtains access to health care.

Effective access is the link between utilization of health care services (realized access) and health outcomes that include enhanced health status and consumer satisfaction. Evaluating the effectiveness of access involves assessment of health care utilization within the context of predisposing, enabling, need, and health behavior variables. Predisposing variables are factors (such as age, gender, and social support) that could influence a person's health status after treatment. The presence of enabling resources such as health insurance and income can lead to expeditious medical treatment that takes advantage of state-of-the-art technology. Its absence can lead to delays in seeking medical care and result in episodic, fragmented treatment with the potential for a negative impact on outcomes and on satisfaction with the care received.

To help formulate public policy that works to enhance access to health services, consumers need to get involved in the political process. For example, older adults have had a major impact in influencing the political process in our country. As a group they are better educated than ever; organizations such as the American Association of Retired Persons (AARP) have a legislative agenda and their own lobbyists in Washington, D.C. to advance their causes. Their ability to influence legislation and policy relating to specific issues of concern lies in numbers—their voting power. In contrast, the change in work patterns from a blue-collar manufacturing workforce with dwindling union membership to a white-collar, services-based workforce has affected organized labor's ability to influence politicians and has allowed businesses to receive more support for their issues.

Quality of Care. The U.S. health care system is a patchwork of many subsystems loosely connected to provide medical care rather than health care to those who are insured. Although the system is undergoing major changes, most of these are focused on improving delivery of and payment for illness care rather than providing better health care. Reform should look to systems that would integrate services and activities to minimize risks and provide early detection and treatment of emerging diseases. These systems must also place a greater emphasis on wellness and public health for the health care system reform to eventually affect the overall health of the American population.

Technological Progress. The technological advances of recent decades have significantly affected the delivery of health care and its outcomes. Selected developments include computerized clinical laboratory and diagnostic equipment, multiple organ transplants, improved invasive and noninvasive surgical techniques, genetic engineering, and the use of lasers. These advances have allowed the health professions to treat certain conditions more quickly, more safely, and more effectively, with less pain and fewer complications.

In spite of their benefits, many fear that "high-tech" equipment and procedures will increase the use of machines and decrease human interaction. It is this fear of depersonalization of health care that is fueling the demand for more humane or "high-touch" care systems, such as hospice care, birthing rooms, and neighborhood clinics. Some high-tech equipment, notably computers, can also be used to increase human contact. For example, electronic mail and internet services can be used to help people communicate and share information with each other. The use of computers in health care institutions and agencies is likely to intensify. They have become critical to various functions within a health care organization, such as client records, billing and accounting, information processing and retrieval, hiring and staffing, and ordering and tracking supplies.

Unquestionably, computers have helped to improve the delivery of health care services in our country. Integrated computerized systems within health care agencies link a client's care with every department within the facility. Outside the hospital, computer-assisted communication techniques are making speedy transmission of health information

and new knowledge a powerful influence in molding public opinion.

Environmental Health Challenges. In addition to the behavioral and biological factors that determine health, a complex array of environmental influences must also be considered. Environmental determinants of health can be divided into three components: physical, social, and psychological. In a health context, the physical environment includes hazards such as air, noise, and water pollution, with the potential consequences of hearing loss, infectious diseases, gastroenteritis, cancer, emphysema, and bronchitis. The social environment produces child abuse, homelessness, and drug abuse. The psychological environment produces diseases related to stress.

Social and psychological components of environmental health can be combined to address the major issues of behavior modification, perceptual problems, and interpersonal relationships. Crowded living spaces, physical or social isolation, rapid and persistent change, and increased social interchange may all contribute to homicide, suicide, stress, and environmental overstimulation, which negatively affect the overall health of the individual and the community. Professional nursing must be involved in policy-making decisions that set standards for and controls on responsible agencies and industries. These decisions should be directed toward the control of potential threats to health and safety in our physical environment.

Quality Improvement. The growth of managed care with its emphasis on cost containment has prompted the concern that containing costs will diminish and disrupt quality. Differing definitions of quality by clients, providers, and payers translates into different expectations of the health care delivery system and evaluations of its quality. Quality can mean improved health in populations, client satisfaction with the level of care received, reduction in complications that result from errors, reduced death rates, prolonged life, or access to multiple options in care.

The basic goal of the health care system in the United States is to provide those services that will optimize the overall health of the resident population. The key to achieving this goal is the commitment to quality—its assurance, monitoring, evaluation, and improvement. The Joint Commission on Accreditation of Healthcare Organizations (JCAHO) has published standards to help health care organizations continuously improve and meet this basic goal.

The future of our health care delivery system and the quality of its services will depend on the ability of health care professionals to work with consumers, policy makers, and payers. The ethical dilemmas of access, impact of technology, cost versus quality versus amount of service, business orientation of the delivery system, provider turf battles, and availability of alternative health and illness care treatments will challenge everyone to be partners. Professionals, policy makers, providers, payers, and consumers must act in concert with each other to ensure that basic health care services are delivered by a system that acknowledges the ties between quality and the caring interaction.

Key Principles

- The diagnosis and treatment of identifiable disease or illness has largely governed health care delivery in the United States.
- *Health promotion,* aimed at modifying a client's knowledge, attitudes, and skills to adopt behaviors leading to healthier lifestyles, may contribute more to longevity than medical care.
- *Illness prevention* that relies on strategies described as primary prevention, such as immunizations, health screenings, and medications that avert disease, may be more cost effective than treatment of illness.
- Registered nurses focus on health promotion and disease prevention and are also the major care providers of sick and injured clients.
- Physicians, the major providers of health services, play a central role in the diagnosis and treatment of diseases, illnesses, and injuries.
- The American Academy of Physician Assistants (1996) defines a *physician assistant* as "a member of the health care team who works in a dependent relationship with a supervising physician to provide comprehensive care."
- Allied health workers can be divided into two broad categories: therapists and technologists, and technicians and assistants.
- The role of the pharmacist includes instructing clients about medications as well as advising physicians and other health care providers about new and complex pharmaceutical management regimens.
- Social workers help clients and families cope with the problems resulting from long-term illness, injury, and rehabilitation. They often work in clinical settings as case managers to facilitate appropriate client discharge and follow-up care, and to ensure proper use of community services.
- The term *inpatient* is used in conjunction with an overnight stay in a hospital or other facility. Inpatient treatment is provided in long-term care facilities such as nursing homes, psychiatric hospitals, and rehabilitation centers.
- Outpatient services do not require an overnight inpatient stay in a hospital or long-term care facility, although these institutions may offer these services.
- Managed care is a system that combines the functions of health insurance and the actual delivery of care, where costs and utilization of services are controlled.
- Changes in the composition of a population are important for the planning of health care services.
- Economic markets exist for allocating scarce resources to pay for the provisions of goods and services.
- The U.S. health care system will continue to face the challenge of balancing three competing goals—containing costs, improving access to health care services, and enhancing the quality of the delivered health care services.

Bibliography

Alliance for health reform: Source book for journalists. (2000). Health care costs (Chapter 6). Retrieved from http://www.allhealth.org/sourcebook/chp_06/ch06_main.htm.

American Academy of Physician Assistants. (2001). *PA fact sheet.* Arlington, VA: Author. Retrieved from http://www.aapa.org/.

American Medical Association. (2000/2001). *Physician characteristics and distribution in the U.S.* Chicago: Author.

American Nurses' Association. (2001). *Nursing's agenda for health care reform.* Washington, DC: Author. Retrieved from http://www.nursingworld.org/readroom/rnagenda.htm.

Bodenheimer, T. (1997). The Oregon health plan: Lessons for the nation. *New England Journal of Medicine, 337*(9), 651-655.

Carville, J. (1996). *We're right, they're wrong.* New York: Random House.

Centers for Medicare and Medicaid Services. (2002). Retrieved from http://www.medicare.gov/basics/overview.asp.

Division of Nursing. (2001). *Preliminary findings from the national sample survey of registered nurses 2000.* Washington, DC: Health Resources and Services Administration, Department of Health and Human Services. Retrieved from ftp://ftp.hrsa.gov/bhpr/nursing/samp-survpre.htm.

Engel, C. (1999). Health services industry: Still a job machine? *Monthly Labor Review.* Washington, DC: Bureau of Labor Statistics. Retrieved from http://stats.bls.gov/opub/mlr/1999/03/contents.htm.

Gordon, S. (2001). Families on call. *The American Prospect, 12*(1). Retrieved from http://www.prospect.org/print/V12/1/gordon-s.html.

Hadorn, D. C. (1991). The Oregon priority-setting exercise: Quality of life and public policy. *Hastings Center Report, 21*(3), 11-16.

Hecker, D. C. (2001). *Monthly labor review.* Washington, DC: Bureau of Labor Statistics. Retrieved from http://stats.bls.gov/opub/mlr/2001/11/art4full.pdf.

Jonas, S. (1998). *An introduction to the U.S. health care system* (4th ed.). New York: Springer.

Leininger, M. M. (1991). *Culture care diversity and universality: A theory of nursing* (Publication No. 15-2402). New York: National League for Nursing Press.

Levit, K., Cowan, C., Braden, D., Stiller, J., Sensenig, A., & Lazenby, H. (1998). National health expenditures in 1997: More slow growth. *Health Affairs, 17*(6), 99-110.

Montague, J. (1997). Why rationing was right for Oregon. *Hospitals & Health Networks, 71*(3), 64-65.

National Center for Health Statistics. (1998). *Health United States, 1995* (Public Health Service Publication No. 96-1236). Hyattsville, MD: Department of Health and Human Services.

*Oregon Health Services Commission. (1991). *Prioritization of health services: A report to the governor and legislature.* Salem, OR: Author.

Organization for Economic Cooperation and Development. (1998). *OECD health data 1998: A comparative analysis of 29 counties.* Paris: Author.

Shi, L., & Singh, D. A. (1998). *Delivering healthcare in America: A systems approach.* Gaithersburg, MD: Aspen.

*Steinbrook, R., & Lo, B. (1992). The Oregon Medicaid demonstration project: Will it provide adequate medical care? *New England Journal of Medicine, 326*, 340-344.

Sumner, C. H. (1998). Recognizing and responding to spiritual distress. *American Journal of Nursing, 98*(1), 26-31.

The World Almanac and Book of Facts 1995. (1994). Mahwah, NJ: Funk and Wagnall.

U.S. Bureau of the Census. (1997, 1998). *Current population reports: Health insurance coverage, 1997 and 1998.* Washington, DC: U.S. Government Printing Office.

U.S. Bureau of the Census. (2000a). *Current population reports: Health insurance coverage, 2000.* Washington, DC: U.S. Government Printing Office. Retrieved from http://www.census.gov/hhes/www/hlthins.html.

U.S. Bureau of the Census. (2000b). *Fact finder: Profile of general demographic characteristics: 2000.* Washington, DC: U.S. Government Printing Office. Retrieved from http://factfinder.census.gov/.

U.S. Bureau of the Census. (2002). *National Population Projections,* Summary files. Retrieved from http://www.census.gov/population/

*Asterisk indicates a classic or definitive work on this subject.

Caring and Clinical Judgment

Learning Objectives

After studying this chapter, you should be able to do the following:

- Discuss the importance of theory in nursing practice
- Compare and contrast nursing theories about caring
- Differentiate between critical thinking, problem solving, decision making, diagnostic reasoning, and clinical judgment
- Describe the elements of the T.H.I.N.K. model of critical thinking
- Discuss Benner's stages of skill proficiency in nursing practice
- Recognize obstacles to critical thinking
- Describe the five interwoven phases of the nursing process
- Apply the T.H.I.N.K. model to the nursing process

THINKING ABOUT NURSING

When we think about the profession of nursing, a set of words and images come to mind: caring, tender loving care, compassion, and an expectation of clinical competence. We might have a mental picture of a female nurse dressed in white, wearing a white cap and a flowing navy blue cape with a red cross on it. Although starched white uniforms and caps are no longer worn, the mental image of the qualities of the nurse represented by these symbols continues. To understand the source of this mental image, we can try to understand what has guided the development of today's practice of nursing.

In 1859, Florence Nightingale published *Notes on Nursing, What It Is and What It Is Not.* This small but incredibly important volume established nursing as a profession, a profession that provides a kind of caring often equated with motherhood but in fact more than and different from that kind of nurturing. Furthermore, nursing has developed as both an art and a science. To explain the relationship between the art and the science of nursing, Parse (1992) defines nursing as a basic science, the practice of which is a performing art. She states that the knowledge base of the discipline is the science of the art, and the performance is the art creatively lived. When you think about how you apply theory—what you have learned in the laboratory and classroom—to a real clinical situation, you as the nurse *perform* the practice of nursing. You do this *creatively,* using both your assessment data and your knowledge base to individualize care for each of your clients and their families.

The science of nursing continues to be a topic of significant debate in the current nursing literature. Simply stated, nursing science focuses on *phenomena* related to human health, such as facts, behaviors, problems, and events that describe a reality. From the description of the phenomena, the concepts present in nursing practice can be named and their relationships described.

A **concept** is an idea, thought, or notion conceived in the mind. It may be *empirical* or *abstract.* **Empirical** concepts can be observed or experienced through the senses. A stethoscope is an example of an empirical concept; it can be seen and touched. **Abstract** concepts are those that are not observable, such as caring and hope. All concepts become abstract in the absence of the object. For example, once you have become familiar with a stethoscope, you are able to see the concept of a stethoscope in your mind without having one physically present. Abstractions such as hope or caring are more difficult to mentally visualize.

Chinn and Kramer (1999) define a **theory** as "a creative and rigorous structuring of ideas that project a tentative, purposeful, and systematic view of phenomena" (p. 51). From their view, theories are *tentative,* and therefore open to revision as new information emerges. More simply stated, theories suggest a direction or structure of how to view facts and events. Think about how your view changes when you put on a pair of sunglasses. Nursing theories can be thought of as different colored lenses, each color both affecting and structuring how you perceive your professional practice.

Theories cannot be equated with scientific laws, which predict a given outcome every single time. Laws compose the basis of the natural sciences such as chemistry. However, as nursing is a human science, the rigor and objectivity of the chemistry laboratory are both inappropriate and impossible to duplicate in nursing practice. As the research base from which nursing theories are developed is tested, the predictability of nursing theories will become more reliable.

Theories are composed of concepts and their definitions, and of prepositions that explain the relationships between the concepts. For example, when Nightingale proposed a beneficial relationship between sunlight and health, she had the beginning of a nursing theory. A complete theory is one that contains context, content, process, and goal (Barnum, 1998). Context is the environment in which the nursing act takes place, content is the subject matter of a theory, process is the method the nurse uses to apply the theory, and the goal is the intended aim of the theory—what the nurse hopes to achieve.

Two major and opposing schools of thought exist in nursing science today. The *received view* is the scientific position, which requires that all truths be confirmed by sensory experiences. It is objective and value free and requires study of the smallest parts of phenomena using the scientific method. In this view, the whole is equal to the sum of its parts. Nursing theories that view human beings as biopsychosocial–spiritual entities are reflective of the *received view* and are considered to be the majority view in nursing practice today.

The *perceived view,* on the other hand, views human beings as irreducible wholes in constant interrelationship with the universe. Nursing theorists of the received view define health as a state of well-being as measured against norms, whereas perceived view theorists view health as something that the client determines it to be. This perceived view is currently considered the minority view in nursing practice.

Nursing theories interpret and explain the reality of nursing, thus guiding practice, education, and research activities for nursing as a profession. When nurses have a theoretical base of knowledge, they have professional autonomy. That is, nurses make decisions on the basis of nursing theory as opposed to always taking direction from another profession. Theory is useful for demonstrating that although nursing is a practice discipline, it is also a profession with a unique body of knowledge, needed and trusted by society to (1) help individuals, families, groups, and communities retain and promote health and (2) intervene when there is illness and disease. Thus theory underlies both the science and art of nursing.

The concepts of person, environment, health, and nursing are the most recognized organizing realities of nursing theory. These concepts have provided the boundaries and the shared viewpoint that have helped nurses focus their practice over the last half century. Recently, nurse scientists have added caring to this group of concepts. Clarification of caring may broaden the boundaries of nursing and reaffirm our long-standing social directive. **Caring** is to be attentive to or watch over the needs of another person, thus implying responsibility in the context of a human relationship (Figure 5-1, p. 74).

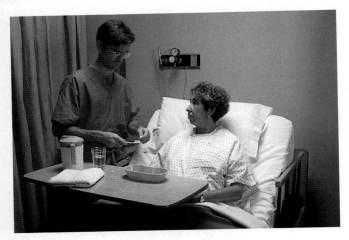

Figure 5-1. In entering into relationships with clients, nurses use the self to establish a caring relationship.

Nursing theory and research can be viewed as interdependent components of the scientific process. When constructing a theory, the theorist must be knowledgeable about the empirical findings and formalize the available knowledge by validating or verifying knowledge through research activities. A theory is accepted when the consensus of the nursing profession is that the theory provides an adequate description of reality. In the broadest sense, nursing research and theory development are necessary for the continued evolution of nursing as a science.

Historical Perspective

The following historical perspective gives an overview of the nursing theorists. Although no one of these theorists is recognized as having provided a complete theoretical basis for nursing practice, each has added to our understanding of nursing through explanations of the phenomena of nursing practice. The bibliography at the end of this chapter includes references to original theoretical works and texts that focus on nursing theory to give you depth and breadth of understanding about each theory.

Nightingale. *Florence Nightingale* wrote extensively on what she and other nurses were attempting to do during the Crimean War. She gathered statistics on the death rate in the hospital before and after nurses intervened. She was our first researcher, using statistics to show the effect of nursing care. She was our first theorist, recognizing the importance of the environment and basing her theory of nursing on it. She believed environment included all external conditions and influences that affect life including ventilation, food, warmth, odors, noise, and light (Nightingale, 1859). Through being supportive and physically present, nurses also enhanced a sense of well-being in suffering clients.

To teach new recruits to nursing how to give nursing care, curricula were created to help teach students about nursing using Nightingale's approach. Students were taught how to manipulate the environment and support the client as the client sought health.

The 1950s. During the 1950s, nursing education was in the early stages of moving into college and university settings, and the scientific basis for nursing practice was developing. There was a need to prepare nurses at the graduate level for positions in nursing administration and education. Columbia University's Teachers College developed graduate education programs to meet these needs, and the first wave of nursing theorists were graduates of these programs. These theorists include Peplau (1988), Henderson, (1966), Hall (1959), and Abdellah (Abdellah, Beland, Martin, & Matheney, 1960).

The nurse theorists of this era operated from a biomedical model and nursing research. This model focused primarily on what nurses do—that is, their functional roles, and most theorists considered client problems and needs to be the focus of nursing practice.

However, *Hildegarde E. Peplau* focused on the nurse-patient relationship. She introduced her interpersonal concepts in 1952 and departed from the biomedical model by basing them on several psychosocial theories. Peplau is known as the first to borrow from other scientific fields and to relate the data to nursing theory. Her ideas and theory development are the basis for psychiatric nursing practice and have contributed to all nursing practice. Peplau believed that in the nurse-client relationship, the nurse assumes many roles: stranger, teacher, resource person, surrogate, leader, and counselor. She also identified four phases of the nurse-client relationship: orientation, identification, exploration, and resolution.

Virginia Henderson (1966) defined nursing as doing for clients what they would do for themselves if they had the necessary knowledge, will, or strength. Her definition of nursing was adopted by The International Council of Nursing and later by the World Health Organization. Henderson also identified 14 basic client needs that define the components of nursing care. From Henderson's perspective, nursing has the basis for a comprehensive and systematic approach to care. Henderson's basic needs have evolved into nursing diagnoses as we use them today.

However, Henderson's model did not seem to adequately include the "caring" component of nursing. *Lydia E. Hall* (1959) presented her theory of nursing by drawing three interlocking circles, each circle representing a distinct aspect of nursing: care, core, and cure. This is the first theoretical model that speaks specifically to the concept of caring. Hall defined the care circle as representing the nurturing component of nursing. She further defined nurturing as the care and comfort of the person and the provision of the person's teaching and learning activities.

Faye G. Abdellah and her colleagues (1960) laid the foundation for a process of critical thinking in nursing practice when they developed a problem-solving approach to deal with the 21 nursing problems they had identified in clinical practice. Nursing practice changed when her book *Patient Centered Approaches to Nursing* was published in 1960. Its list of nursing problems outlined everything nurses did, from improving nutrition to increasing comfort. This approach built on Henderson's model and formed the basis for the nursing process as a way of approaching nursing care problems.

The 1960s. In the 1960s, theories of nursing roles moved from a focus on problems (or needs) and function, to a focus on the relationship between the nurse and the client. In these theories, the process (between nurse and client) of nursing is as important as the procedures and practices. Here the interest is not only how nurses practice but also how clients perceive their situation, and the effects of nursing on that perception. Theorists representative of this era include Henderson (1960, 1966), Orlando (1961/1990), and Levine (1967, 1996).

In 1961, *Ida Jean Orlando* suggested that all nurses use interpersonal relationships to meet the needs of the client as defined by that client, not as defined by the nurse. Orlando also introduced the nursing process as a tool for nursing practice. She delineated automatic actions and deliberate actions from the three elements of a nursing situation: client behavior, nurse reaction, and nursing actions. The client became more important as a member of the health care team.

Building on work of earlier theorists, *Myra E. Levine* (1967) further developed the idea of a comprehensive approach to client care and hypothesized the mechanism of the relationship of nursing actions to improved client health. She suggested that the focus of all nursing actions is to conserve the client's energy, structural or physiological integrity, personal integrity, and social integrity. Based on Levine's nursing activity analysis, these four components became *four conservation principles* used by nurses to help clients adapt to the environment. She presented the client holistically and as the center of nursing activities.

The 1970s. In the 1970s, new theories were developed to explain the unique nature of nursing and to provide holistic caring for clients of all backgrounds. These theories elaborated on previous ones to provide increasingly complex explanations of the practice of nursing. Theorists included Rogers (1970), King (1971), Orem (1971), Neuman (1974), Roy (1976), Paterson and Zderad (1976), Newman (1979), and Watson (1989).

The theories presented in this decade were diverse. One group furthered the holistic approach to nursing practice. Rogers and Newman introduced the concept of human beings as irreducible energy fields, the first of the perceived-view theorists. King, Roy, and Neuman based their theories on general systems theory.

Other groups expanded on the importance of the nurse-client relationship. Paterson and Zderad based their theory on existential philosophy, and Watson addressed the nurse's role of caring and healing as it pertains to sustaining humanity and wholeness.

Martha E. Rogers (1970) saw human beings as dynamic energy fields integral to or interwoven with environmental fields, both identified and recognized by their pattern, existing in a multidimensional universe. Rogers's theory of unitary human beings focuses on integration of humans with environment and the interrelationships of energy fields. Her theory is well known for capturing the complexities of interactions between nurse, client, and environment. She emphasized that

nursing was not something a person does but a body of abstract knowledge, a learned profession that is both science and art. Rogers's theory was revolutionary and provided the foundation for a large body of research.

Betty Neuman (1974) introduced a comprehensive conceptual model for nursing that is based on a "systems" point of view to evaluate nursing problems. She views the client as a system functioning harmoniously in relation to environmental influences. The focus of this model is the stability of the client system as it encounters stressors in the environment. The goal of keeping the client system stable is achieved through nursing actions derived from prevention measures.

The work of *Imogene M. King* (1971) can be categorized as a systems model derived from three dynamic interacting systems: personal systems or individuals, interpersonal systems or groups, and social systems or society. King defines nursing as a human interaction process between nurse and client, who communicate to set goals, explore actions for reaching the goals, and then agree on which actions are to be used. Her theory of goal attainment highlights the importance of the decision-making process and the outcomes of nursing care.

Dorothea E. Orem (1971) defines nursing as a human service and theorizes that the special concern of nursing is assisting people to achieve self-care. Orem's focus is primarily on the needs of the client and the actions of nursing to meet those needs. Her theory of self-care maintains that nursing care is needed when people are affected by limitations that do not allow them to meet their self-care needs. According to Orem, the need for nursing care stems from a client's self-care deficit.

The adaptation model of *Sister Callista Roy* (1976) views humans as biopsychosocial beings who exist through adaptation within an environment. Her model combines divergent thinking, such as systems, stress, and adaptation, into a convergent view of a client interacting with the environment. Roy's model differentiates nursing from medicine by focusing its activity on client adaptation as opposed to health or illness alone.

Josephine G. Paterson and *Loretta T. Zderad* (1976) introduced the theory of humanistic nursing. This theory relates to nursing practice that is developed from the lived experiences of the nurse and the person receiving care. It is based on existential thought.

Margaret Newman (1979) describes health as expanding consciousness. She views health as a fusion of disease and nondisease. She defines nursing as caring in the human health experience and believes that caring is a moral imperative for nursing.

Jean Watson (1989), in her philosophy and science of caring, wrote that caring must be central to nursing practice to preserve human dignity and humanity. As a moral ideal, nursing practice is based on humanistic or altruistic values in the development of a helping-trust relationship between the nurse and the client. Watson's theory includes 10 *carative factors* that represent both feelings and actions pertaining to the nurse and the client and that include elements to be felt, experienced, expressed, and promoted by every nurse. Examples of carative factors include developing a helping-trusting, human caring relationship with the client and the instillation of faith-hope. Her theory contributes to nursing by sensitizing nurses to humanistic aspects and caring.

The 1980s. As it now had a solid theoretical base, nursing knowledge was able to grow rapidly in the 1980s. Many nursing theories were revised on the basis of research findings that refined and expanded them, and new theories were developed. The works of Johnson (1980), Leininger (1980), Parse (1981), Erickson, Tomlin, and Swain (1983), Benner (1984), and Eriksson (1987) developed from the perspective of previous nursing theory and began the process of connecting theory to practice.

In fact, by 1988, the theory of nursing was sufficiently advanced to warrant it own scientific publication, and *Nursing Science Quarterly* debuted. This journal, edited by Rosemarie Rizzo Parse, is devoted exclusively to the presentation of nursing theory and research based on nursing theory.

Building on the systems theory approach, *Dorothy E. Johnson* (1980) presented a behavioral system model in which the various parts of the system strive to achieve balance. She believes that each individual has patterned, purposeful, repetitive ways of acting that compose that person's behavioral system. She identified seven subsystems. The role of the nurse in this model is to foster balance, or equilibrium, in the individual.

Madeleine M. Leininger (1980) expanded on the theme of the importance of care in the nurse-client relationship. She believes that caring is the central theme in nursing knowledge and practice. Educated in cultural and social anthropology, Leininger states that caring varies among cultures in its processes and patterns, is largely culturally derived, and is culturally expressed. Her theory of transcultural care focuses on culture-specific and culture-universal nursing practices. She identifies culture as the broadest and most holistic way to view, understand, and be effective with people.

In 1981, *Rosemarie Rizzo Parse* connected several themes in her theory of man-living-health. This theory is based on existential-phenomenological philosophy and the work of Rogers (1970). Parse's theory is an example of the perceived view, in which the whole person is in constant and dynamic interaction with the universe. The goal of nursing is quality of life from the client's perspective. In 1992, Parse changed the title of her theory to the "human becoming" (Parse, 1992).

Helen C. Erickson, Evelyn M. Tomlin, and *Mary Ann P. Swain* (1983) explained the role of the nurse. Their theory of modeling and role modeling requires the nurse to assess (model), plan (role model), and intervene on the basis of the client's perspective of the world. At all times the nurse respects the client's self-care knowledge and assists the client to access and use self-care resources.

The phenomenological theory of *Patricia Benner* describes caring as a common bond between people situated in a meaningful relationship. This situation is essential to nursing. Skill and skilled practice, as defined by Benner (1984), refer to skilled nursing interventions and clinical judgment skills in actual clinical situations. She sees clinical nursing practice in terms of nurses making a positive difference by be-

ing in the situation in a caring way. Further development of this research led to an interpretive theory of nursing practice that she (together with Wrubel) explained in *The Primacy of Caring: Stress and Coping in Health and Illness* (1989). The primacy of caring is concerned with helping clients cope with the stress of illness. Benner is credited with helping us understand the decision-making process in nursing.

Katie Eriksson is the author of the theory of caring science. Eriksson is a Finnish nurse-educator and clinician who continues to develop caring science (1987). The emphasis of caring science is the phenomenon of caring, and the aim has been to create a humanistically oriented caring science.

The leading idea of caring science is to alleviate human suffering and to preserve and safeguard life and health. Eriksson clearly states, however, that the core of caring is not primarily tied to specific discipline (2002).

The 1990s. In the 1990s research studies that tested and expanded nursing theory were numerous. Eleven nurse-theorists refined and published their theories.

Ann Boykin and *Savina Schoenhofer* (1993) proposed their theory in their book *Nursing as Caring*. They view caring as a process of daily becoming, not a goal to be attained. The basic premise of this theory is that all persons are caring. Caring is living in the context of relational responsibilities—for self and others. At the heart of the caring relationship is the importance of the person-to-person connection. The focus of nursing is "nurturing persons living in caring and growing in caring" (1993, p. 21). Nursing is the response to the human need to be recognized as a caring person.

ADVANTAGES OF MULTIPLE THEORIES

There were alternative viewpoints as nursing evolved as a profession. Some believed that nursing used only borrowed theory—that is, borrowed from other disciplines. Other nurses demanded that nursing create its own research methods and knowledge so that nursing concepts would be unique. Today we recognize that no discipline owns knowledge. Therefore nursing uses knowledge from other fields and shares knowledge with other disciplines.

What you as a nurse observe, document, choose as an intervention, and evaluate depends on the theoretical perspective that guides your nursing practice. Having more than one theoretical perspective increases your options and choices. The more ways you can analyze the needs of a particular client, the more potential there is for seeing different needs.

Table 5-1 summarizes the work of selected nurse theorists. Table 5-2 summarizes the work of those theorists who focus specifically on caring.

CRITICAL THINKING AND CLINICAL JUDGMENT

The theoretical basis of nursing practice affects how we think about nursing situations. The extent to which your critical thinking and clinical judgment is derived from nursing theories determines the unique contribution you make to health

Table 5-1	Overview of Selected Nursing Theorists	
Theorist	**Key Date**	**Conceptual Focus of Theory**
†Nightingale	1859	Environmental manipulation crucial to health and the client's ability to regain health
†Peplau	1952	Nurse-client therapeutic relationship; the basis for interpersonal psychiatric nursing
†Henderson	1955	Known for her definition of nursing and for the identification of 14 basic needs of clients
†Hall	1959	Nursing represented as core, care, and cure
Orlando	1961	Emphasizes the reciprocal relationship between client and nurse using nursing process
†Rogers	1970	First perceived-view theorist; the science of unitary humans continuously exchanging energy with the universe
King	1971	Nursing as a system; decision-making process and outcomes of mutual goal attainment are specified for nurse-client interactions
Orem	1971	Delineation of the need for nursing care that comes from a client's self-care deficit
Neuman	1970	Nursing as a system, with the client seen as a system functioning in relation to environmental influences
Roy	1976	Clients exist through adaptation to a changing environment, with the nurse as a regulatory mechanism in situations of health and illness.
Parse	1981	Man-living-health theory, perceived-view theory that became the theory of human becoming in 1992

†Deceased

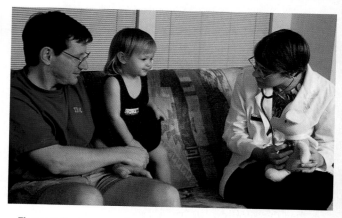

Figure 5-2. A nurse adept at critical thinking uses creativity to overcome barriers to quality nursing care.

Table 5-2	Caring-in-Nursing Theorists
Theorist	**Description of Theory**
Nightingale, 1859	Caring provided by trained nurses is more than and different from the nurturing provided by mothering. Nursing care involves the environment to the benefit of the client's health.
Leininger, 1978-present	Caring is the central theme in nursing knowledge and in culture-specific and culture-universal nursing practice (now known as the theory of culture care diversity and universality).
Watson, 1979-present	Theory of transpersonal caring seeks to connect with and embrace the spirit of the client through processes of caring and healing. From the original 10 carative factors have emerged 10 caritas processes that guide nursing practice. Watson ties the future of nursing to Nightingale's sense of "calling," a sense of deep commitment to human service (Watson, 2001).
Benner, 1984-present	Phenomenologically describes caring as a common bond between people in a meaningful situation, which is essential to nursing.
Eriksson, 1987-present	Caring science focuses on the phenomenon of caring, not on the profession. Caring implies alleviating suffering in charity, love, faith, and hope. Natural, basic caring is expressed through tending, plying, and teaching in a caring relationship (Eriksson, 2002).
Boykin & Schoenhofer, 1993-present	Caring nursing is living in caring and growing in caring. "The intention of nursing as a practice discipline is nurturing persons living in caring and growing in caring" (Boykin & Schoenhofer, 2001, p. 393).

care. As health care becomes more complex, nurses must exercise increasingly complex thinking skills. Indeed, the body of knowledge that nurses need is increasing at such a rate that it is impossible to succeed in nursing simply by applying standardized responses. Even clients who have common needs express those needs in highly individualized ways. Consequently, critical thinking is an important and integral part of nursing practice.

Because critical thinking is an abstract concept rather than something you can observe and measure, defining it can be somewhat difficult. In fact, a number of respected scholars have created different definitions of the critical thinking process. However, all of these definitions include thinking skills that you can learn, practice, and integrate into your nursing care. Using these critical thinking skills will result in sound decisions, safe practice, and creativity in addition to promoting the well-being of your clients.

THE LANGUAGE OF CRITICAL THINKING

Critical thinking is defined as purposeful, self-regulatory judgment that gives reasoned and reflective consideration to evidence, contexts, conceptualizations, methods, and criteria (Facione, 1990).

Critical thinkers examine all elements of a situation and think through alternative strategies to achieve an end. The goal of critical thinking is not to devise a single solution but rather to envision a number of scenarios that could occur depending on actions taken or not taken. Rather than one right answer, critical thinkers determine a number of possible outcomes. They use creativity to overcome barriers (Figure 5-2). Built on the nurse's knowledge, clinical experience, and intuition, critical thinking takes a holistic approach to the client.

Embedded in the broad concept of critical thinking are several more specific thinking skills, including problem solving, decision making, diagnostic reasoning, and clinical judgment. Typically, all of these processes take place within the framework of the nursing process.

Problem solving is defining a problem, selecting information pertinent to its conclusion (recognizing stated and unstated assumptions), formulating alternative solutions, drawing a conclusion, and judging the validity of the conclusion (Watson & Glaser, 1964). Problem solving is a process used to arrive at an answer or a solution. There is an implied gap of information or action that must be bridged to arrive at the solution. There is also the expectation that the solution be "right" according to a particular standard of measure.

Decision making involves choosing between two or more options as a means to achieve a desired result. Typically, the decision is goal directed, in which case the goal or goals direct the outcome. For example, if you were to plan a dinner party, your menu (goal) would direct your decisions in grocery shopping and food preparation. Decision making in the clinical setting yields approaches for nursing care selected from a variety of possible nursing interventions. You must decide which intervention(s) will be most likely to achieve the desired client outcomes.

Diagnostic reasoning is the process of clustering assessment data into meaningful sets and generating hypotheses about the client's human responses. Diagnostic reasoning can be carried out as a deliberate, conscious activity, or it may occur intuitively with little conscious awareness.

Clinical judgment is a conclusion or an opinion that a problem or situation requires nursing care. It includes determining the cause of the problem, distinguishing between similar problems, and discriminating between two or more courses of action.

The **nursing process** is a critical-thinking framework in which you will exercise decision making, diagnostic reasoning, problem solving, and clinical judgment. It is composed of five interwoven phases: assessment, diagnosis, planning, intervention, and evaluation. Although the nursing process is sometimes criticized as being linear or unidirectional, it is more appropriately thought of as a dynamic, constantly interactive process, where new client data and feedback continuously affect each phase. The nursing process provides a framework to guide you to think critically in the clinical setting.

THINKING ABOUT THINKING

To improve your ability to think critically, you need to examine how you think. Thinking about thinking means bringing your mental activities to conscious awareness. It means recognizing the thinking patterns that you use in different situations and evaluating the effectiveness of those patterns in achieving desired results. It means understanding yourself and the elements included in your thinking.

Thinking involves multiple mental functions grouped into two broad categories:
- Taking in information
- Using information to make decisions

Information is perceived through the five senses and stored in the brain. Storing information requires that the information be processed into meaningful patterns so that it can be retrieved or used in some way. The ways in which you process and understand information form your basic functions of thinking.

People have different preferences for processing information, and they seem to create meaning from information more efficiently when they receive it in the manner that most closely matches their preference. For example, some people process information best when they see it (visual learners), whereas others process information best when they hear it (auditory learners). Think about how you learn best. You may find that you learn better if you have both visual and auditory cues.

Thinking is ever changing. Before beginning to read this chapter you may have *thought* about the other choices you have for this period of time. You also may have *thought* about whether you would sit at your desk to read or sit in a comfortable chair. You might have *recalled* that a study-skills teacher told you that concentration improves when you study in one place consistently. Making a decision about each of the options requires thinking. Likewise, every action you will take in nursing practice requires thinking. Clearly, understanding your thinking process will enhance that thinking.

Thinking occurs on more than one level of awareness. Sometimes we consciously think by saying to ourselves that a problem must be solved, a decision must be made, or simply that we will pay attention to a symphony. In any event, cognitive activity is occurring in the brain. Appreciating a symphony is a more passive activity than decision making. However, even when you are making a decision consciously, more-passive activity is also going on in your brain to influence the decision.

The T.H.I.N.K. Model

Nursing educators Rubenfeld and Scheffer (1999) propose a critical thinking model that incorporates five modes or processes of thinking that occur in combination or simultaneously. Whereas some situations may seem to require only one mode of thinking, the authors emphasize the importance of effectively using all of the thinking modes. Together, the five modes constitute a broad definition of critical thinking. You can use the mnemonic device T.H.I.N.K. to help remember them (Box 5-1).

Box 5-1	The T.H.I.N.K. Model

T = Total Recall
H = Habits
I = Inquiry
N = New Ideas and Creativity
K = Knowing How You Think

Rubenfeld, M. G., & Scheffer, B. K. (1999). *Critical thinking in nursing: An interactive approach* (2nd ed.). Philadelphia: Lippincott.

Total Recall. Total recall involves remembering facts, such as names, dates, normal values, and telephone numbers. Thinking based on total recall is useful when you want to dial a phone number, drive to work, perform a nursing procedure, or obtain complete information during a client interview.

How total your recall is depends on your memory and how you process information into memory. One way to increase recall is to put information into patterns of similar or related items. Telephone numbers in the United States—a three-digit area code, a three-digit prefix, and a four-digit number—use a pattern that is easier to remember than a string of 10 numbers. Similarly, grouping clinical data into patterns can help you remember the data.

Another way to aid total recall is to attach significance to a fact by relating that fact to an experience (Rubenfeld & Scheffer, 1999). You may remember how to give an injection to a client at your clinical setting because you practiced injection techniques in the learning laboratory. One of the most important aspects of nursing education occurs in the clinical setting where students actualize what they have read in texts and heard in lectures. It is much easier to recall how a client looked and behaved while in respiratory distress than it is to memorize the signs and symptoms of pulmonary edema. Putting real people's faces into one's memory in the context of the clinical learning setting helps you learn about clinical practice.

Having total recall of essential facts is crucial to thinking. It allows you to sort information in different ways to solve problems, make decisions, or create scenarios. (Remember, however, that the way you sort or cluster information affects the way you interpret that information.) Ready recall of information also frees your mind to engage in other modes of thinking.

Habits. Habits are accepted ways of doing things that work, save time, or are necessary. Habits are behaviors that have been repeated so many times that they become second nature. When a behavior is habitual, you need not think through the individual steps involved. Knowing how to drive a car and knowing how to swim are examples of habitual activities. Most of the activities that you learn in the nursing skills laboratory will become professional habits as you gain experience in nursing practice.

Forming habits allows you to do one thing while thinking about another. Much as you can drive a car while having a conversation, you can change a dressing while considering whether the wound has become infected. Naturally, habitual behaviors can be unsafe if unsafe steps become incorporated into the pattern.

Inquiry. Inquiry means examining issues in depth and questioning things that may seem obvious on the surface. It is the primary kind of thinking by which you reach conclusions. Inquiry involves analyzing information to confirm your hunch about a situation. Through feedback and further analysis, you can validate a conclusion. Nurses use this process to verify that the best interpretation is made of the client's clinical situation. Typically, the client provides the main source of information as well as validation for your perception of reality.

Inquiry also includes the quality of being curious or wondering about the meaning of information. It is a spirit of wanting to know more, to understand, or to be able to explain facts that arise. Having a spirit of inquiry means never being satisfied with an interpretation of facts until you are sure that it is complete and accurate.

New Ideas and Creativity. New ideas and creativity occupy the opposite end of the spectrum from total recall and habit. They emphasize new and different ways of looking at information, and they form the basis for individualized client care. No two clients have identical values, life situations, preferences, and concerns. If you need to teach a person to care for a wound after discharge from the hospital, you need to consider how the client learns, whether the level of anxiety will permit learning to occur at this time, what supplies are available in the home, and the complexity of terminology the client can understand. A creative plan considers all of these variables.

Knowing How You Think. Knowing how you think is called metacognition, which literally means "in the midst of knowing." Knowing how you think means that you recognize when you are using logical reasoning to reach a conclusion. It leads you to ask yourself questions about how you think. Did I get all the facts before making a decision? Am I making assumptions that may not be true? In the example of teaching a client to manage a wound, you recognize that you have made an assumption that all clients want to learn wound care, so you seek validation that the assumption is true. Another question might be, "Do I spend so much time making sure I have all the facts that I am blocked from making a decision?" Box 5-2 lists strategies you can use to gain understanding about how you think.

Critical Thinking as Clinical Judgment

In making a clinical judgment, you form an opinion using critical thinking to identify problems, solve problems, or make decisions. Sound clinical judgments stem from knowledge, clinical experience, and a holistic approach to the

---

Box 5-2   Strategies for Gaining Understanding About How You Think

- Keep a journal of how you use thinking skills. If you find a principle that works for you, jot it down! If something helps to make a thinking connection for you, jot it down!
- Share your journal with classmates in clinical conference. Compare how different thinking styles work for each of you.
- Discuss with classmates the thinking connections that you find difficult. Share problems and solutions.
- Always consider multiple solutions to any problem.
- Keep at it! Remember that critical thinking is the key to good nursing care and the foundation of accountability.

client's needs. As you learn to recognize patterns of behavior, the process also begins to include your powers of intuition.

Kataoka-Yahiro and Saylor (1994) have proposed a model of critical thinking that helps nurses make the clinical judgments needed for effective nursing care. The first component of the model is a *specific knowledge base.* Thinking depends on the knowledge base that each individual brings to the thinking process. The nurse's knowledge base includes sciences, liberal arts, and the nursing content needed to provide nursing care. Physical sciences help you understand the functions of the body and how humans think and respond to health care situations. The liberal arts provide a basis for understanding human values and cultural variations. Nursing knowledge incorporates these elements, contributes understanding of what it means to be ill, and provides methods of increasing the client's level of wellness.

The second component of the model is *experience.* As a nursing student, you bring a unique set of individual experiences to the nursing education. Material presented as part of that education will be understood and applied within your experience. During nursing education, you gain additional experiences through the practice of nursing in the clinical setting. Classmates share clinical experiences in formal clinical conferences. Each of these experiences adds to your knowledge. As your clinical experience increases, so does your ability to think critically in the setting.

The third component of the model is called *competencies* and refers to the cognitive processes used to make clinical judgments. Competencies that you need as a nurse include the following:

- The ability to identify problems caused by illness
- The ability to recognize health needs
- The ability to make decisions about how to improve a client's health
- The ability to recognize when and why nursing care has improved the client's condition

The fourth and fifth components of the model are *attitudes* and *standards* of critical thinking. Attitudes associated with critical thinking include a spirit of inquiry, the desire to understand a situation from more than one perspective, and valuing or seeking the truth. Paul's (1993) work, discussed shortly, expands on the attitudes and standards of critical thinking.

Characteristics of Critical Thinking

In critical thinking, the most fundamental concern is excellence of thought. The idea that the study of critical thinking is important is based on two assumptions: first, that the quality of our thinking affects the quality of our lives, and second, that all of us can learn how to continually improve the quality of our thinking. The idea is to systematically form and shape our thinking to function purposefully to exacting standards. Critical thinking is disciplined, comprehensive, and based on intellectual ideals. As a result of the process of examining critical thinking, well-reasoned thinking develops (Paul, 1993).

Comprehensive critical thinking has the following characteristics (Paul, 1993, pp. 20-23):

- It is thinking that is responsive to and guided by such intellectual standards as relevance, accuracy, precision, clarity, depth, and breadth. Without standards to guide it, thinking cannot achieve excellence.
- It is thinking that deliberately supports the development of intellectual traits in the thinker, such as humility, integrity, perseverance, empathy, and self-discipline.
- It is in thinking that the thinker can identify the elements of thought present in the process. For example, the thinker can make logical connections between the elements and the problem at hand. Paul states that the critical thinker will routinely ask probing questions such as these: What is the purpose of my thinking? What question am I trying to answer? What information am I using? How am I interpreting it? What conclusions am I coming to? What assumptions am I making? If I accept the conclusion, what are the implications and the consequences? Table 5-3 applies these elements to nursing.

Table 5-3	Paul's Elements of Critical Thinking Applied to Nursing
Element	**Application Examples**
Assumptions	• The nurse-client relationship is a helping relationship. • Clients have a right to make decisions about their health care.
Information	• Data, facts, and observations about the client • Knowledge about the pathophysiology and etiology of disease • Knowledge about human behavior
Concepts	• Theories, definitions, principles, and laws that give meaning to information and that are used to interpret clinical data and make decisions about effective management of the client's problems
Purpose of thinking	• To make decisions about data to be collected • To diagnose problems and make clinical judgments • To determine client goals or outcomes
Question of an issue	• To determine the nature of the client's presenting problem • To identify ethical and legal issues in practice
Points of view	• The nurse's and client's perception of the clinical situation • Perspective of health team members
Interpretation and inference	• Diagnostic reasoning that results in nursing diagnoses, plans, and interventions
Implications and consequences	• Client outcomes and modifications of care

- It is thinking that is routinely self-assessing, self-examining, and self-improving. Paul stresses that if students are not assessing their own thinking, they are not thinking critically.
- It is thinking in which there is integrity to the whole system.
- It is thinking that yields a predictable, well-reasoned answer from the comprehensive and demanding process that the thinker pursues.
- It is thinking that is responsive to the social and moral imperative to argue from alternative and opposing points of view and to seek and identify the weaknesses and limitations of one's own position.

Critical Thinking and Nursing. Scheffer and Rubenfeld (2000) conducted a Delphi study to arrive at a consensus statement on the definition of critical thinking in nursing. Fifty-one nurses representing practice, education, and research served on the international panel of experts. After five rounds of data analysis, the following consensus statement was reached:

> Critical thinking in nursing is an essential component of professional accountability and quality nursing care. Critical thinkers in nursing exhibit these habits of the mind: confidence, contextual perspective, creativity, flexibility, inquisitiveness, intellectual integrity, intuition, open-mindedness, perseverance, and reflection. Critical thinkers in nursing practice the cognitive skills of analyzing, applying standards, discriminating, information seeking, logical reasoning, predicting, and transforming knowledge. (p. 357)

Box 5-3 provides descriptions of the habits of the mind and the cognitive skills that nurse-critical thinkers exhibit.

DEVELOPMENT OF CRITICAL THINKING

Critical thinking is a skill that develops over time and with conscious application of total recall, habits, inquiry, new ideas and creativity, and knowing how you think. As you gain more experience in nursing, your thinking will evolve and advance.

Stages of Skill Acquisition

In *From Novice to Expert,* Patricia Benner (1984) applies the Dreyfus model of skill acquisition to nursing practice. The Dreyfus model suggests that a person passes through five levels of proficiency in acquiring and developing a skill. Applying this model to professional nursing practice, Benner identifies these stages as novice, advanced beginner, competent, proficient, and expert (Figure 5-3, p. 82). Each of these stages requires that the nurse be able to think critically; however, the depth and breadth of the nurse's ability to think critically evolves with each stage.

Benner's stages of skill acquisition in professional nursing practice reflect changes in three general aspects. The first change is from reliance on abstract principles stored in memory to the use of past concrete experiences to guide actions. The second change is the individual's perception of the situation; it is seen as a whole in which only certain elements are relevant. The third change is from being a detached observer to being an involved performer.

Novice. Benner describes the behavior of the *novice* nurse as being rule-governed, limited, and inflexible. Critical thinking operates in the total recall mode. Because the novice has no experience of the situation at hand, rules are used to guide performance. The student nurse follows rules because they are "correct." But, Benner cautions, rules legislate against ultimately successful performance because rules do not specify the most relevant tasks in actual situations.

Box 5-3 **Definitions of Habits of the Mind and Skills of Critical Thinking**

HABITS OF THE MIND

- **Confidence:** Assurance of one's reasoning abilities
- **Contextual perspective:** Considering everything relevant to the whole situation, including relationships, background, and environment
- **Creativity:** Intellectual inventiveness, used to generate, discover, or restructure ideas; imaging alternatives
- **Flexibility:** Capacity to adapt, accommodate, modify, or change thoughts, ideas, and behaviors
- **Inquisitiveness:** Eagerness to know by seeking knowledge and understanding through observation and thoughtful questioning to explore possibilities and alternatives
- **Intellectual integrity:** Seeking the truth through science and honest processes, even if the results are contrary to prior assumptions and beliefs
- **Intuition:** Insightful sense of knowing without conscious use of reason
- **Perseverance:** Pursuit of a course with determination to overcome obstacles
- **Reflection:** Contemplation on a subject, especially assumptions and thought processes, for the purposes of deeper understanding and self-evaluation

SKILLS

- **Analyzing:** Separating or breaking a whole into parts to discover their nature, function, and relationships
- **Applying standards:** Judging according to established personal, professional, or social rules or criteria
- **Discriminating:** Recognizing differences and similarities among things or situations and distinguishing carefully as to category or rank
- **Information seeking:** Searching for evidence, facts, or knowledge by identifying relevant sources and gathering objective, subjective, historical, and current data from those sources
- **Logical reasoning:** Drawing inferences or conclusions that are supported or justified by evidence
- **Predicting:** Envisioning a plan and its consequences
- **Transforming knowledge:** Changing or converting the condition, nature, form, or function of concepts among contexts

Scheffer, B. K., & Rubenfeld, M. G. (2000). A consensus statement on critical thinking in nursing. *Journal of Nursing Education 39,* 358.

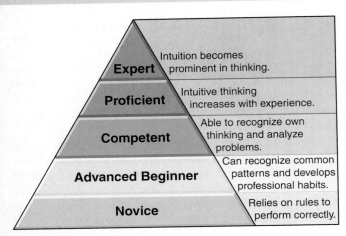

Figure 5-3. Growth in critical thinking from novice to expert. Advancing to expert is not automatic. It requires commitment to continued growth.

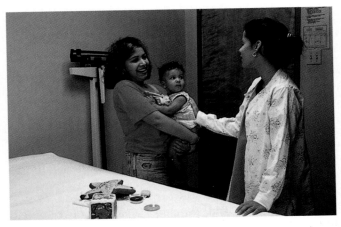

Figure 5-4. An expert nurse uses intuition to ascertain that this mother is happy and the baby is healthy.

Advanced Beginner. According to Benner, the *advanced beginner* (or new graduate) has experienced enough real situations to note the recurring meaningful aspects and attributes in a situation. The advanced beginner can formulate guidelines on the basis of experience but may miss their differential importance, thereby treating them equally. Benner states that the advanced beginner benefits from assistance, given by an instructor or a preceptor, in setting priorities. This stage demonstrates the very beginning of the development of professional habits, part of the T.H.I.N.K. process.

Competent. Benner reports that the third stage of proficiency—*competence*—is typified by the nurse who has been in the same or a similar position for 2 to 3 years. In this setting, the nurse begins to interpret actions in light of long-range goals or plans with conscious awareness. The plan dictates which aspects of the current and future situation are most important and which can be ignored. Therefore the competent nurse can develop a plan on the basis of considerable conscious, abstract, and analytical contemplation of the problem. The competent nurse lacks the speed and flexibility of the proficient nurse but does have a feeling of mastery and the ability to manage the required nursing care. In this stage, the nurse relies on all modes of the critical thinking process.

Proficient. Benner describes the *proficient* nurse as one who perceives each situation as a whole, rather than its individual aspects. She states that the nurse's perception is the key element in this stage. The perspective is not consciously thought out; instead, it "presents itself" on the basis of experience and recent events. Proficient nurses understand a situation as a whole because they perceive its meaning in terms of long-term goals. They operate in a holistic mode where, on the basis of their clinical experience, they can clearly understand nuances in clinical situations. It typically takes 3 to 5 years in one setting to become proficient. This is an advanced level of critical thinking, possibly involving highly complex clinical situations.

Expert. Benner states that the *expert* nurse no longer relies on an analytical principle to connect the understanding of a situation with an appropriate action. The expert nurse has an intuitive grasp of each situation and zeroes in on the accurate region of the problem without wasteful consideration of alternative actions (Figure 5-4). It takes 5 to 15 years in a setting for a nurse to become expert. Practice at this stage demonstrates the highest level of critical thinking in that the expert nurse knows holistically what to do without consciously thinking through all the data.

Advanced Clinical Judgment. Benner, Hooper-Kyriakidis, and Stannard (1999) studied the nursing practice of critical care nurses. They identified two pervasive habits of thought and action that provide a rich description of clinical judgment—*clinical grasp* and *clinical forethought*. Clinical grasp describes clinical inquiry in action and includes problem identification and clinical judgment across time. It has four components: making qualitative or subjective distinctions, engaging in detective work, recognizing changing clinical relevance, and developing clinical knowledge in specific client situations.

Clinical forethought structures the practical logic of clinicians. It refers to at least four habits of thought and action: future-think, clinical forethought and specific diagnosis, anticipation of risks for a specific client, and seeing the unexpected. These aspects of clinical judgment are advanced nursing practice skills that the novice nurse can watch for and observe in experienced nurses.

Obstacles to Critical Thinking. A number of obstacles impede the developing and exercising of your critical thinking skills. By being aware of them, you can ensure that your thinking remains sound.

One of the most common obstacles involves overuse of the habit mode. Nurses tend to develop routines and habits to make sure that work gets done efficiently. However, habits can narrow the focus of your thinking. Unquestioned habits may cause you to miss important cues and could be dangerous to your clients. Every person for whom you provide care is unique. By assuming that habitual behaviors will be correct for all clients, you leave yourself open to mistakes.

Another obstacle to good thinking is anxiety, especially severe anxiety, which can render even the most prepared person unable to perform. Dealing with anxiety requires you to focus on yourself, thus reducing the focus and energy available to your clients.

Working under deadlines may affect your ability to think critically because you simply may not have enough time to think through all available information before arriving at a solution. You may make decisions prematurely, without all the facts or before the client is ready. Clearly, clinical practice often takes place under real time pressures, depending on the setting. One way to overcome this obstacle is to prepare as thoroughly as possible for the clinical experience at hand. Also, make good use of your clinical instructor.

Another obstacle to developing critical thinking skills is an overcommitment to ideological, religious, or political principles—to the extent that your mind is closed to other ideas. It is important that you understand your own biases as well as those that your client might have.

Finally, lack of confidence in your thinking can be an obstacle to critical thinking. Nursing students sometimes lack the confidence to stand up for what they believe; it may feel safer to back away from an authority figure (staff nurse, instructor, or physician) than to defend your position. However, if you think clearly, logically, and with consideration for the values of others, then you can always have confidence in your thinking.

CRITICAL THINKING AND THE NURSING PROCESS

In clinical practice, the nursing process provides the structure in which critical thinking, diagnostic reasoning, and clinical judgment take place. It is composed of five interrelated phases: assessment, nursing diagnosis, planning, intervention, and evaluation (Figure 5-5, p. 84).

Assessment

In the first phase of the process, *assessment,* you collect data that you then can use to identify client needs that can be managed or treated with nursing care. The focus of your assessment may be narrow or broad and may generate a large amount or a relatively small amount of data, depending on the setting and the client's condition. A specific nursing theory may be chosen to direct the structure of your assessment.

A comprehensive assessment is holistic and includes a physical examination, a health history, and a psychosocial-cultural assessment. Client-centered data are usually collected to understand the client's history in the areas of health needs. This health history is organized in a framework that is most pertinent to identifying the care needs of the client. Most health care agencies have a form for collecting a health history. Proceeding though scripted questions, you listen for cues

that suggest a problem or a need. These cues direct you to explore those areas of concern in more depth. Critical thinking directs this exploration.

The nursing assessment is performed in all nursing specialties and settings. You may encounter clients in the hospital setting where a presenting problem or illness becomes the starting point of the assessment. In contrast, in a community setting, you may screen healthy clients for risk factors for a particular disease.

As you collect assessment data, you will engage in critical thinking, mentally grouping data into clusters for specific meaning related to the client's situation. You will listen actively and make observations about the client. As the pieces of data form meaningful patterns or information clusters, you will critically analyze them. This is the process of diagnostic reasoning. Diagnostic reasoning is not innate; it is a skill that you can learn and improve with practice, experience, and an ever-increasing knowledge base.

As a result of your assessment, you will arrive at one of the following outcomes:

• You will identify no problem.
• You will identify a potential problem.
• You will identify an actual problem that needs further assessment.

The process of taking a health history is addressed in detail in Chapter 6.

Nursing Diagnosis

Once you have clustered the data pieces obtained through assessment, you will assign specific diagnostic labels to those clusters. The North American Nursing Diagnosis Association (NANDA) has adopted a *nursing diagnosis* classification system to promote the standardization of diagnostic labels used by nurses and, consequently, the quality of care delivered by nurses. NANDA defines a nursing diagnosis as a clinical judgment about individual, family, or community responses to actual and potential health problems or life processes. These responses include physiological, cognitive, emotional, and social changes that influence how an individual functions.

Each nursing diagnosis has five components: a label, a definition, a set of defining characteristics (signs and symptoms), a group of related factors, and risk factors. The nursing diagnoses you choose for each client will be based on assessment data for that client; their accuracy depends on the quality and completeness of the data collected. The data on which you base your nursing diagnoses should be the best and most reliable available to you.

As specified by NANDA, nursing diagnoses provide the basis for selecting nursing interventions to achieve the outcomes for which you are responsible. Your clinical judgment determines which diagnosis you will attend to first.

Planning

The third phase of the nursing process is *planning.* In this step, you set goals and plan nursing care. Collaboration with the client is essential to successful planning. If a goal that you create on your own holds no importance for the

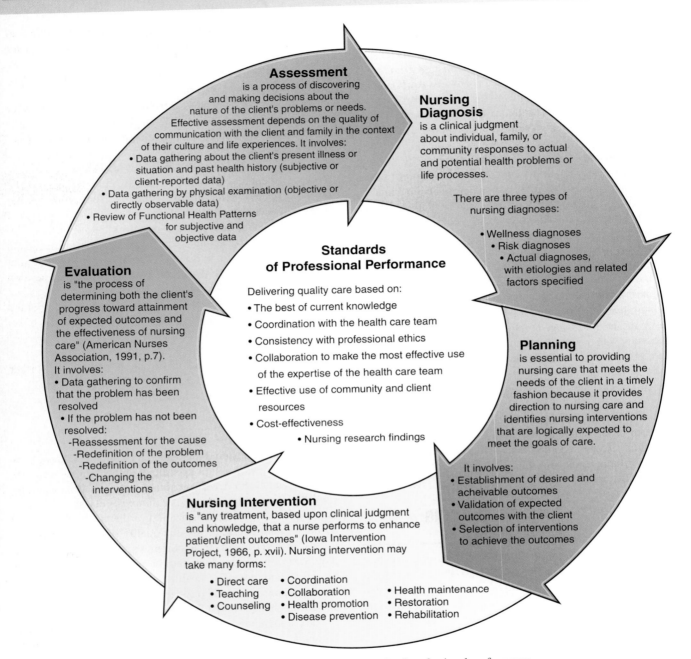

Figure 5-5. The nursing process and standards of professional performance.

client, the client will have little interest in pursuing the goal and no incentive to become interested (Figure 5-6). This is why the goals (or outcomes) of the planning process must be client oriented. The goals you establish should state, in measurable terms, what the client will be doing and how the client will be doing it after nursing care has been delivered. Determining realistic and achievable outcomes means that you can be held accountable for the results of your nursing care.

Planning nursing care involves setting priorities. This can be done by ranking the goals, or by identifying goals as having high, medium, and low priority. High-priority goals should be attended to first or are the focus of your nursing

care. Setting priorities involves critical thinking, clinical judgment, and a good knowledge base.

Document your plan of care in the client record and also on the nursing care plan so that all nursing personnel can work from the same plan. Because the nursing process is dynamic, information obtained during the planning stage is added to the assessment data, and it may alter the nursing diagnoses and goals.

Intervention

The fourth phase of the nursing process is the *intervention* phase, in which you execute the care plan. *Independent* interventions are those that the nurse is licensed to carry out inde-

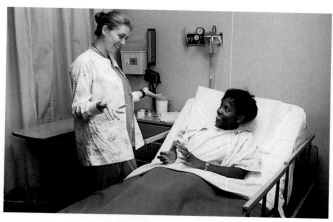

Figure 5-6. Planning for interventions that are acceptable to the client requires the nurse to use creativity to engage the client in the process.

pendently. They include counseling, providing comfort measures, teaching, offering emotional support, managing the environment, and assessing. *Dependent* interventions are those activities carried out under a physician's order. An example is administration of an intravenous infusion.

Evaluation

The final phase of the nursing process is *evaluation*. In this phase, the planned outcomes of nursing care are measured against the actual outcomes. Outcomes can be met, unmet, or partially met and are recorded as such. When outcomes are unmet or partially met, reassessment is necessary to determine why this result occurred. The care plan is then revised accordingly.

Clinical pathways and case maps are evaluation tools that can help nurses monitor client progress. They show the average path that a client with a certain diagnosis is likely to take. These evaluation tools provide you with a daily measure of the client's progress on the clinical path. They are examples of building quality assurance measures into nursing care.

APPLYING T.H.I.N.K. TO THE NURSING PROCESS

You will use each of the five modes of critical thinking outlined in the T.H.I.N.K. model while carrying out the nursing process. Doing so will help you to more accurately and completely provide for each client's needs.

Using T.H.I.N.K. in Assessment

Total recall is used in assessment when you follow a specific list of questions, or a guide, to collect assessment data. An assessment guide ensures that your assessment covers all essential elements of data collection. *Habits* come into play when you develop consistent patterns of behavior that you use in the assessment process. You use *inquiry* when you explore abnormal findings and form additional questions to obtain more information that may improve your understanding of the problem—and perhaps reveal the cause of the problem. You use *new ideas and creativity* by listening to what is not said as well as to what is said and by formulating questions that help

the client express sensitive feelings or describe embarrassing symptoms. You use *knowing how you think* by asking yourself such questions as Have I been thorough? Have I identified all the necessary cues? Is there sufficient evidence to support my conclusions?

Using T.H.I.N.K. in Diagnosis

You use *total recall* and *habits* to cluster assessment data into meaningful patterns. *Inquiry* is used as you ask yourself how the data patterns affect the client's health. *New ideas and creativity* are used in the process of diagnostic reasoning to arrive at nursing diagnoses. *Knowing how you think* assists you in the analytical process of diagnosing.

Using T.H.I.N.K. in Planning

You use *total recall* to remember the usual goal for the problems that you have identified. *Habits* help you to develop goals and outcomes that are measurable and achievable. *Inquiry* is used to validate goals with the client, thus making sure that you and the client agree. *New ideas and creativity* may be needed when the client denies that a problem exists or is unwilling to engage in behaviors that improve health. *Knowing how you think* leads to questions about the logic used in connecting the expected outcomes to solving the problems that have been identified.

Using T.H.I.N.K. in Intervention

Total recall is used to remember the steps of a procedure and the principles or elements that are critical to safe and effective intervention. You rely on *habits* to achieve a well-organized, smooth procedure. *Inquiry* helps you to determine if the methods of intervention are the best for the particular client situation. *New ideas and creativity* modify the intervention for client preferences or situational variables. *Knowing how you think* helps you to evaluate the methods of intervention by asking such questions as Was the client comfortable? Was the intervention successful?

Using T.H.I.N.K. in Evaluation

Total recall and *habits* are used to compare the goals of care with the outcomes of care. *Inquiry* helps you to determine client satisfaction (or dissatisfaction) with the achieved outcomes. *New ideas and creativity* may be necessary to modify the plan of care. *Knowing how you think* helps you to assess an outcome objectively.

Key Principles

- The basis of any discipline is theoretical. Theories identify important concepts and the relationships between them.
- Theories help the nurse learn, organize knowledge, apply knowledge, seek new knowledge, and communicate quickly and effectively with other nurses.
- Nursing theory provides a basis for clinical practice.
- More than any other single component, nursing theory helps the nurse to engage in thoughtful, experienced, skillful care of clients, whether that client is an individual, family, or community.

- T.H.I.N.K. is a mnemonic device for a model that reflects the key elements of critical thinking: total recall, habits, inquiry, new ideas and creativity, and knowing how you think.
- Nurses typically develop skill proficiency in the following order: novice, advanced beginner, competent, proficient, and expert.
- Obstacles to critical thinking include an inadequate knowledge base, an overreliance on habits, anxiety, too little time to make reasoned decisions, zealous adherence to circumscribed sets of beliefs, and lack of confidence in thinking ability.
- The nursing process is composed of five interrelated phases: assessment, diagnosis, planning, intervention, and evaluation. It provides a framework in which to exercise critical thinking.

Bibliography

*Abdellah, F., Beland, I. L., Martin, A., & Matheney, R. V. (1960). *Patient centered approaches to nursing.* New York: Macmillan.

*Adams, B. L. (1999). Nursing education for critical thinking: An integrative review. *Journal of Nursing Education, 38,* 111-119.

Alligood, M. R., & Marriner-Tomey, A. (2002). *Nursing theory: Utilization and application.* St Louis: MO: Mosby.

Barnum, B. S. (1998). *Nursing theory: Analysis, application, and evaluation* (5th ed.). Philadelphia: Lippincott.

*Benner, P. (1984). *From novice to expert: Excellence and power in clinical nursing practice.* Menlo Park, CA: Addison-Wesley.

Benner, P., Hooper-Kyriakidis, P., & Stannard, D. (1999). *Clinical wisdom and interventions in critical care: A thinking-in-action approach.* Philadelphia: Saunders.

*Benner, P., & Wrubel, J. (1989). *The primacy of caring.* Menlo Park: CA: Addison-Wesley.

Boykin, A., & Schoenhofer, S. O. (1993). *Nursing as caring: A model for transforming practice.* New York: NLN Press.

Boykin, A., & Schoenhofer, S. O. (2001). Nursing as caring. In M. Parker (Ed.), *Nursing theory and nursing practice* (pp. 391-402). Philadelphia: Davis.

Chinn, P., & Kramer, M. K. (1999). *Theory and nursing: A systematic approach* (5th ed.). St Louis, MO: Mosby.

Erickson, H. C., Tomlin, E. M., & Swain, M. A. P. (1983). *Modeling and role modeling.* Lexington, KY: Pine Press.

Eriksson, K. (1987). *Pausen: En beskrivning av vardvetenskapens kunskapsobjekt* [The pause: A description of the knowledge of caring science]. Stockholm, Sweden: Almqvist & Wiksell.

Eriksson, K. (2002). Caring science in a new key. *Nursing Science Quarterly, 15,* 61-65.

*Facione, P. A. (1990). *Executive summary-Critical thinking: A statement of expert consensus for purposes of educational assessment and instruction.* Millbrae, CA: California Academic Press.

George, J. B. (Ed.) (2002). *Nursing theories: The base for professional practice* (5th ed.). Upper Saddle River, NJ: Prentice Hall.

*Hall, L. E. (1959). *Nursing: What is it?* Publication of the Virginia State Nurses Association.

*Hammers, J., Abu-Saad, H., & Halfens, R. (1994). Diagnostic process and decision-making in nursing: A literature review. *Journal of Professional Nursing, 10*(3), 154-163.

*Harmer, B., & Henderson, V. (1955). *Textbook of the principles and practice of nursing.* New York: Macmillan.

Henderson, V. (1960). *Basic principles of nursing care.* Geneva: International Council of Nurses.

Henderson, V. (1966). *The nature of nursing.* New York: Macmillan.

*Hickman, J. S. (1993). A critical assessment of critical thinking in nursing education. *Holistic Nursing Practice, 7*(3), 36-47.

Hicks, F. D. (2001). Critical thinking: Toward a nursing science perspective. *Nursing Science Quarterly, 14,* 14-21.

*Johnson, D. E. (1980). The behavioral system model for nursing. In J. P. Riehl & C. Roy (Eds.), *Conceptual models for nursing practice* (2nd ed.) (pp. 207-216). New York: Appleton-Century-Crofts.

*Kataoka-Yahiro, M., & Saylor, C. (1994). A critical thinking model for nursing judgment. *Journal of Nursing Education, 33,* 351-355.

*King, I. (1971). *Toward a theory for nursing: General concepts of human behavior.* New York: Wiley.

Krichbaum, K., Lewis, M., & Duckett, L. (1997). Critical thinking: What is it and how do we teach it? In J. C. McCloskey & H. K. Grace (Eds.), *Current issues in nursing* (5th ed.). St Louis, MO: Mosby.

Leininger, M. M. (1978). *Transcultural nursing: Concepts, theories, and practice.* New York: Wiley.

Leininger, M. M. (1980). Caring: A central focus of nursing and health care services. *Nursing and Health Care, 6,* 209-212.

Leininger, M. M. (1991). *Cultural care diversity and universality: A theory of nursing.* New York: National League for Nursing.

*Leininger, M. M. (2001). Theory of culture care diversity and universality. In M. Parker (Ed.), *Nursing theories and nursing practice* (pp. 361-376). Philadelphia: Davis.

Levine, M. (1967). The four conservation principles of nursing. *Nursing Forum, 69*(10), 93-98.

*Levine, M. (1996). The conservation principles: A retrospective. *Nursing Science Quarterly, 9,* 38-41.

Marriner-Tomey, A., & Alligood, M. R. (2002). *Nursing theorists and their work* (5th ed.). St Louis, MO: Mosby.

Meleis, A. I. (1997). *Theoretical nursing: Development & progress* (3rd ed.). Philadelphia: Lippincott.

*Neuman, B. (1974). The Betty Neuman health care systems model: A total person approach to patient problems. In J. P. Riehl & C. Roy (Eds.), *Conceptual models for nursing practice* (pp. 99-114). New York: Appleton-Century-Crofts.

*Neuman, B. (1995). *The Newman systems model.* Norwalk, CT: Appleton & Lange.

*Newman, M. A. (1994). *Health as expanding consciousness* (2nd ed.) (Publication No. 14-2626). New York: NLN Press.

Newman, M. A. (1979). *Theory development in nursing.* Philadelphia: Davis.

*Nightingale, F. (1859, 1992). *Notes on nursing* (Com ed.). Philadelphia: Lippincott.

North American Nursing Diagnosis Association. (1999). *Nursing diagnoses: Definitions and classification, 1999-2000.* Philadelphia: Author.

Orem, D. E. (1971). *Nursing: Concepts of practice.* New York: McGraw-Hill.

*Orem, D. E. (2001). *Nursing: Concepts of practice* (6th ed.). St Louis, MO: Mosby.

*Orlando, I. J. (1990). *The dynamic nurse-patient relationship.* New York: Putnam. (Original work published 1961.)

Parker, M. (2001). *Nursing theories and nursing practice.* Philadelphia: Davis.

Parse, R. R. (1981). *Man-living-health: A theory of nursing.* New York: Wiley.

Parse, R. R. (1992). The performing art of nursing [Editorial]. *Nursing Science Quarterly, 5,* 147.

---

*Asterisk indicates a classic or definitive work on this subject.

*Parse, R. R. (1998). *The human becoming school of thought.* Thousand Oaks, CA: Sage.

Paterson, J. G. & Zderad, L. T. (1976). *Humanistic nursing,* New York: Wiley.

*Paul, R. W. (1993). *Critical thinking: What every person needs to know in a rapidly changing world* (3rd ed.). Rohnert Park, CA: Center for Critical Thinking.

*Paul, R. W. (1995). *Critical thinking: How to prepare students for a rapidly changing world.* Santa Rosa, CA: Foundation for Critical Thinking.

*Peplau, H. E. (1988). *Interpersonal relations in nursing.* New York: Putnam. (Original work published 1952.)

*Rogers, M. E. (1970). *An introduction to the theoretical basis of nursing.* Philadelphia: Davis.

Rossignol, M. (1997). Relationship between selected discourse strategies and student critical thinking. *Journal of Nursing Education, 36*(10), 467-475.

*Roy, C. (1976). *Introduction to nursing: An adaptation model.* Englewood Cliffs, NJ: Prentice-Hall.

*Roy, C., & Andrews, H. A. (1991). *The Roy adaptation model: The definitive statement.* Norwalk, CT: Appleton & Lange.

*Rubenfeld, M. G., & Scheffer, B. K. (1999). *Critical thinking in nursing: An interactive approach* (2nd ed.). Philadelphia: Lippincott.

*Scheffer, B. K. & Rubenfeld, M. G. (2000). A consensus statement on critical thinking in nursing. *Journal of Nursing Education, 39,* 352-359.

Vaughn-Wrobel, B. C., O'Sullivan, P., & Smith, L. (1997). Evaluating critical thinking skills of baccalaureate nursing students. *Journal of Nursing Education, 36*(10), 485-488.

Watson, G., & Glaser, E. M. (1964). *Watson-Glaser critical thinking appraisal.* New York: Harcourt, Brace World.

Watson, J. (1989). *Nursing: Human science, human care.* New York: National League for Nursing.

Watson, J. (1999). *Postmodern nursing and beyond.* Edinburgh, UK: Churchill Livingstone.

*Watson, J. (2001). Theory of human caring. In M. Parker (Ed.), *Nursing theory and nursing practice* (pp. 343-354). Philadelphia: Davis.

Wilkerson, J. M. (2001). *Nursing process and critical thinking* (3rd ed.). Upper Saddle River, NJ: Prentice Hall.

Client Assessment: Nursing History

Learning Objectives

After studying this chapter, you should be able to do the following:

- Make preliminary decisions in preparation for data collection
- Understand data collection as a critical thinking process
- Employ interviewing techniques in taking a health history
- Develop a systematic framework for organizing data
- Document the assessment in the client's health record

Assessment is the process of gathering information about a client's health status to identify concerns and needs that can be treated or managed by nursing care (Figure 6-1). The **data** gathered consist of subjective and objective information about the client, such as signs and symptoms of disease, results of diagnostic tests, and the client's health practices. Data collection marks the beginning of the nursing process and continues throughout the process. As you gather data you organize the information into groups or meaningful clusters that describe the problems to be treated. Thus assessment also involves analyzing data to identify a client's problems and arrive at appropriate nursing diagnoses.

Assessment begins before the actual collection of data; that is, assessment begins with thinking about the data you will need and the best method of obtaining the data (Figure 6-2). Assessment is an active mental process requiring critical thinking about the data to be collected rather than merely obtaining answers to a specific list of questions. To gather information wisely, you need well-developed skills in observing and listening. At the same time, the mental skills of translating, reasoning, intuiting, and validating will make the data meaningful.

Data are more useful when the assessment process is organized in a framework that helps you to identify the nature of data to be collected and classify them into common problem areas. As you collect data in each category prescribed by the framework, you will produce an initial clustering of information about the client. The framework for data collection affects which problems are distinguished or emphasized. For example, if you studied colors by examining red, blue, and yellow, all colors could be put into one of those categories. However, you would not be able to identify or classify the uniqueness of purple, green, and orange, much less the millions of subtle shades in between. In the same fashion, data about a client can be classified by physiological systems, but you might fail to identify social, psychological, and spiritual problems that influence the client's health. In this chapter you will learn to organize data using functional health patterns.

Rarely will you perform assessment as a single isolated step in the nursing process. Rather, as you elicit information about a client, you will begin to consider nursing diagnoses and formulate plans. In some cases, during the assessment you will include interventions such as giving information to the client. In other words, assessment is often combined with teaching. In other cases, assessment and implementation take place almost simultaneously, as when the person has a compromised airway or needs emergency surgery. In all cases, assessment serves to establish priorities for care.

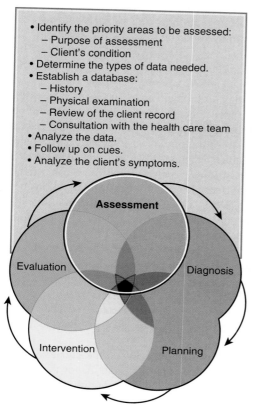

Figure 6-1. Assessment is the process of gathering information about a client's health status to identify concerns and needs that can be treated or managed by nursing care.

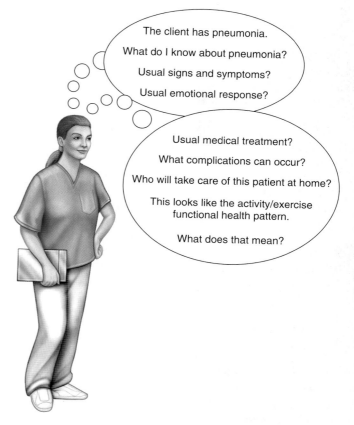

Figure 6-2. Assessment begins with thinking.

PRELIMINARY DECISION MAKING

Any time you interact with a client, for virtually any reason, you will assess the person's problems, needs, and concerns. To efficiently and correctly collect data, you must make decisions about the type of assessment required, the sources of data to be consulted, how to structure and focus the assessment, and how much information to collect before developing a plan of action.

Purpose of Assessment

An assessment may have a comprehensive focus or a specific, narrow focus. Depending on the purpose, assessment may involve asking two or three specific questions, or it may involve spending an hour in an in-depth conversation with the client. The purpose of the assessment may be to do any of the following:

- Establish a database with which to plan and evaluate comprehensive care
- Identify actual and potential problems to make nursing diagnoses
- Focus on a specific problem
- Determine immediate needs to establish priorities
- Determine the cause (etiology) of a problem
- Determine related or contributing factors
- Identify strengths as a basis for changing behavior
- Identify the risk for complications
- Recognize complications

Types of Assessment

To help you begin to identify the purpose of your assessment, consider four major types of assessment: initial, focused, emergency, and ongoing. The initial assessment is made at the first contact with the client. A focused assessment is a detailed examination of a specific problem. An emergency assessment identifies or rules out life-threatening problems and those problems that need immediate treatment to prevent complications. Ongoing assessment refers to the data collection that takes place during every contact with the client throughout the client's association with the health care agency.

Initial Assessment. Assessment on initial contact with the client is typically more comprehensive than subsequent assessments. It begins with the problems that prompted the client to seek nursing services, and it obtains a holistic overview of the client's level of functioning. The nature of the client's problems—and therefore of the services to be provided—dictate the course and depth of the assessment. The objective is to rule out as well as to identify problems.

The initial encounter with a client commonly occurs when the client has sought services for a specific problem, desires a general health status evaluation, or seeks wellness care. The client entering the hospital for surgery or for treatment of a medical condition has a specific problem and needs nursing care aimed at managing the treatment for the problem. The client entering a long-term care facility needs a general evaluation of health status to ensure that medical problems are stabilized and to identify the scope of anticipated nursing care. Wellness services typically take place in community settings, such as schools or clinics, where the nurse may screen for health problems in addition to helping clients manage specific concerns. In any setting, the focus of the nursing assessment is to identify how the nurse can help the client.

The focus of the initial assessment relates directly to the goals of prevention, maintenance, restoration, or rehabilitation. As a screening procedure, assessment is an overview designed to detect risk factors and evidence of certain problems. When prevention is the focus, assessment examines risk and lifestyle factors. A health maintenance assessment examines health and health behaviors. When the goal is restoration, assessment focuses on the need for support of body functions and the detection and prevention of complications. Rehabilitation considers the potential for restoring function and the resources needed to modify the lifestyle. Over the course of an illness, assessment will focus on different goals. For example, for a client recovering from open-heart surgery, restoration of health is the immediate goal. As the client recovers, the goal shifts to rehabilitation.

Not every assessment is comprehensive. In general, the thoroughness of an assessment is directly proportional to the length of expected care. If the client has an acute, short-term problem, such as a need for sutures in an accidentally inflicted minor wound, you will gather only minimal lifestyle information. However, when caring for clients with serious injuries resulting in admission to a rehabilitation unit, you are able to provide better long-term care by knowing the client's complete health history.

Focused Assessment. Once the client's general problems have been identified, you may perform a focused assessment on each problem or problem area. The focused assessment examines the evidence in detail, considers possible etiologies, looks for contributing factors, and considers client characteristics that will help solve the problems. Imagine, for example, that you have identified a diagnosis of *Ineffective individual coping (use of alcohol as primary coping mechanism)* for a client. You then can focus on this diagnosis to gather information about the person's pattern of drinking, defense mechanisms that maintain the behavior, effects on the family, and other information helpful in developing an appropriate plan of care.

Focused assessment also takes place when the client has a complaint or describes a new problem. Common complaints include pain, shortness of breath, difficulty urinating, and visual changes. You must be prepared to assess the severity of the problem, determine a possible cause, evaluate effects on the client's health, and decide on an appropriate course of action.

Emergency Assessment. When the client's situation is life threatening or time is an important factor in preventing complications, assessment will include only key data directly related to the immediate problem. The initial information you collect will vary, depending on the urgency of the situation. Additional data can be collected after the client's condition is stable. As always, emergency assessment follows the ABCs, which means airway, breathing, and circulation. Naturally, the client needs an open airway to take in oxygen-laden air, be able to make a respiratory effort, and circulate blood to transport oxygen to the person's tissues. When you observe an emergency team in action, it may seem that many activities are taking place all at the same time, but the procedure is actually orderly and based on the ABCs.

Ongoing Assessment. Assessment continues throughout the client's health care experience. Reassessment may occur monthly, weekly, daily, or hourly, depending on the client's condition and the nature of the services being offered. For the critical care client, assessment takes place continually via electronic monitoring equipment. Assessment also takes place continually while a client is receiving anesthesia and afterward until its effects have worn off. A client taking a new once-daily medication may need daily assessment until the medication's effects are clear. Weekly assessment may be appropriate for a client on a weight-loss program. Clients in a nursing home may have a formal assessment only once a month.

Nurses routinely make decisions about the frequency, the depth, and the breadth of client assessment. To make these decisions effectively, you must anticipate the potential for a client's condition to change, the speed at which it could change, and the evidence that would indicate a change. For example, when a client takes a new medication, assessment decisions are based on the expected effects of the medication, how rapidly those effects occur, and potential adverse effects.

Types of Data

As you listen to and interact with a client, you will gather some information that is directly observable and some that is not. Information not directly observable typically comes from the client's description of a problem. Either type of information can provide a **cue,** an indicator of the presence or existence of a problem or condition that represents a client's underlying health status. The data of greatest significance in diagnosing a particular illness, disease, or health problem are called **cardinal signs and symptoms.**

Subjective Data. Information that is provided by the client and that you cannot observe directly is called **subjective data.** When subjective data supplied by the client describe characteristics of disease or dysfunction, those characteristics are known as **symptoms.** Pain, nausea, cramps, dizziness, and ringing in the ears are examples of symptoms because you cannot observe them directly. The client must inform you of their presence.

You may be able to directly observe evidence related to the client's symptom. For example, you may notice grimacing, an increased heart rate, and a doubled-over posture in a client who complains of pain. However, these observations could apply to pain, nausea, or cramps and can be confirmed only by asking the client to name the complaint. You may help the client describe or quantify subjective findings, but you should not make judgments about whether or not the symptom exists. The client is the best—indeed, the only—source of information about subjective findings.

Objective Data. Characteristics about the client that you can observe directly are called **objective data.** When these data indicate characteristics of disease or dysfunction, they are known as **signs.** Objective data can be observed through your senses of sight, hearing, taste, touch, and smell. These data can be measured (or quantified) and they can be reliably replicated from one examiner to the next, a concept called *inter-rater reliability.*

For example, you can measure the size of a wound and the amount of drainage it produces. The number of red blood cells in a sample of blood can be counted. Because they are factual, objective data have a high degree of certainty. However, objective information is not necessarily superior to subjective information.

Sources of Data

When assessing a client, you will need to make decisions about the most effective use of multiple sources of data, possibly including the client, the client's significant others, your colleagues, and the client's records. You will need to confirm that each data source is appropriate, reliable, and valid for each assessment. *Appropriate* means that the source is suitable for a particular purpose, person, or occasion. *Reliable* means that you can trust the information to be accurate and honestly reported. *Valid* means that the information can be substantiated or confirmed.

Client. Usually, the client is in the best position to provide accurate, reliable, and valid information about subjective data that describe health problems. In fact, some symptoms can be validated and accurately described *only* by the client. Always start by considering the client as the primary source of assessment data. However, sometimes a client may be too ill to provide information, may be confused, or may suffer from memory loss or otherwise not be able to provide accurate information.

Significant Others. You may ask the family for information when the client is unable to give reliable information or simply prefers to have a family member help describe events. Family members may be able to contribute significant details, provide a different perspective, or clarify the information. Additionally, it is often important to help the family feel included in the process.

Before discussing the client's problems with family members or significant others, however, you must consider the client's right to confidentiality. Although many times an ill person relies on a family member to help remember details and ask important questions, that client may prefer to maintain some privacy from the family. Making an accurate determination of the client's wishes requires you to respond sensitively to subtle cues that may suggest the client's willingness, even preference, to have a family member remain in the room while you conduct the interview. Remember that you are in a position to ask family members to leave during the interview unless the client expresses the desire to have them stay.

Colleagues. All members of the health care team who have worked with the client can be important sources of data. Each team member will have a unique perspective on the client's problems, and therefore team members may make different observations. For example, the physical therapist may recognize that pain is preventing the client from walking or getting adequate exercise; the dietitian may suggest that pain is interfering with the client's ability to learn important information about a newly prescribed diet.

In contrast to nurses in hospitals, nurses who work in the home setting may have fewer opportunities to confer face-to-face with other members of the health care team. Consequently, other forms of communication may become more important in ensuring complete assessment and continuity of care. Usually, the client's record provides the primary method of communication to ensure continuity of care among various health care team members.

Client Records. The client has a right to expect members of the health care team to communicate adequately with each other. Likewise, the client has a right to expect you to be informed about the reason for admission or care. If the client has a medical or nursing record in the agency, you will usually begin by reviewing that record.

For the admission assessment of a hospitalized client, the record will indicate the reason for admission and the physician's admitting orders. In a home health agency, the initial record may show the reason for the referral and a brief history of the current problem. At a follow-up visit in a clinic setting, reviewing the record will help you detect any ongoing problems as well as any new problems. Naturally, clients will feel more confidence in the health care team if you and other members take time to review the record before beginning an assessment, and if you can avoid collecting data that are already in the record.

Standards of Practice for Assessment

One characteristic of a profession is that it has the means to regulate and control its practice. As the official voice of nurses in the United States, the American Nurses' Association (ANA) develops and disseminates Standards for Clinical Practice (ANA, 1998) (see Appendix A). These standards are broad guidelines that require clinical judgment. They may be used in a court of law when determining what a reasonable and prudent nurse would do in a similar situation.

COLLECTING THE DATA

Assessment requires more than obtaining the answers to an established list of questions; it is a process of discovery, of gathering information in a manner that reveals the client's needs. The health assessment forms used by many health care facilities provide plausible and reasonable guides to data collection; however, forms are not a substitute for critical thinking skills (ANA, 2001). Whether or not you use a health assessment form, you will gather data using active listening and active processing.

Active Listening and Active Processing

When assessing a client, you will be (1) observing and listening to the client and (2) processing information through translating, reasoning, intuiting, and validating. To accomplish these goals effectively, you will use **active listening.** In other words, you will attend to what the client says and help the client clarify and elaborate and give additional pertinent information.

Additionally, you will use **active processing,** which involves a systematic series of mental actions to analyze and interpret the information about the client. When you process information actively, you help yourself form mental impressions by thinking through such questions as "How does this information fit with what I know about a certain disease or health problem?" and "What questions do I need to ask to see how well it fits the pattern?"

Active listening and active processing are closely related concepts that occur simultaneously. Together they require you to use all your senses, to make judgments about the meaning of information, and to validate that meaning. For example, you may see that a client is exhibiting a particular symptom, hear the client describe an alteration in health, and then make a judgment about the meaning of these cues for this client. Finally, you may think about other experiences involving these cues and ask further questions.

As you assess a client, your mind continually shifts back and forth from general or global scanning to focusing on a specific problem. An initial assessment often follows a standardized format that directs your mental activity toward the global scan. Proceeding through specified questions, you listen for cues that suggest a problem or a need, or for other cues relevant to the present circumstances. Then you ask questions to follow up any cues that arise so you can determine whether a problem exists.

After categorizing this specific information in the context of the global assessment, you continue scanning for problems. Assessment of a specific cue may lead to one of the following three conclusions:
• No problem exists.
• A potential problem exists.
• An actual problem exists and needs further assessment.
Some potential problems may need further assessment; others may need to be noted only for future reference. Box 6-1 illustrates a conversation with a client in which the nurse is actively processing information to guide continued assessment questions.

Observing. Assessment involves using all of your senses to observe the client. You will observe the client's physical condition for cues that need to be followed up with appropriate questions. Observations of difficult breathing, pale skin, or other physical signs help you know how to proceed with the assessment.

Additionally, you will observe the client's behavioral responses. For example, watch for consistency or discrepancy between nonverbal and verbal responses. Interpret eye con-

Box 6-1 Active Processing

The line on the simple assessment checklist reads *Recent weight gain/loss?* Rather than simply placing a check mark on the form to confirm that the client has lost weight recently, the nurse follows up with the following conversation:

Nurse: How much weight have you lost?

Client: About 30 pounds in the past 2 months.

Nurse: How do you account for losing so much weight?

(The nurse knows weight loss can be associated with cancer. This question is looking for any other possible cause.)

Client: I don't know. I guess I just haven't had much appetite.

Nurse: Have you had any nausea or vomiting?

(The nurse is still exploring for other possible causes.)

Client: No.

Nurse: Have you had any blood in your stool? Or had black, tarry stools?

(Not finding any explanation for the weight loss, the nurse moves to other warning signs of cancer.)

Client: I haven't seen any blood, but I have sometimes had really dark, sticky bowel movements. Does that mean something?

Nurse: Well, it could be blood. I don't really know what it means. Have you discussed it with your doctor?

(The nurse has begun to explore a plan with the client.)

Client: I know I need to. I guess I don't want to know. My father died of cancer.

(The client has revealed a need for teaching.)

Nurse: Blood can mean several things, only one of which is cancer. How long ago did your father die?

(The nurse is looking for further information before being satisfied with the teaching.)

Client: Oh, it's been 30 years. They didn't know how to treat cancer then. I guess I really should see about it.

Nurse: We can do a screening test for blood in your stool. However, even if it is negative at this time, I want you to make an appointment with your doctor. If there was blood in your stool, it would be best to make sure it is not from cancer. Will you do it?

Client: Yes.

Nurse: Remember that cancer is only one of the possibilities. If it turns out to be cancer, you know that there are many new treatments that were not available when your father died. However, whatever the cause, you need to see the doctor.

(The nurse then gives the client a Hemoccult test slide and instructions to collect the specimen.)

---

tact, body language, and facial expressions in the context of what the client says in response to your questions.

Listening. Listening is an active process that involves hearing what the client says as well as the meaning behind it. This type of listening requires practice. When you listen actively, you can immediately formulate questions that help the client describe a problem completely by providing all pertinent information. For example, if the client has difficulty describing the intensity of nausea, you may suggest using a scale from 0 to 10, with 10 being the worst nausea imaginable. And it may be helpful to know if eating makes the nausea better or worse.

Failing to listen attentively to both what a client says and does not say can keep you from identifying a problem or understanding it completely. Denying the possible seriousness of a problem can cause the client to withhold information. The client may leave out important details, believing that the problem is not important or that certain symptoms are not relevant and that seeking help was not appropriate.

Naturally, most clients describe their problems from a layman's point of view. Consequently, they often include extraneous information. You must decide how long to listen before refocusing the client to more pertinent data. If you interrupt the client too soon or too abruptly, the client may feel misunderstood and will probably feel that you have little interest in helping to identify the problem.

Translating. Assessment further involves translating information into clear, succinct, meaningful statements that will be understood by other health care personnel. The client may express concerns in slang terms or lengthy descriptions. You will then translate and document these descriptions in medical terminology, which has the advantage of abbreviating the description and conveying meanings that are commonly understood by other health care team professionals. However, if you feel that a medical term or interpretation could be misinterpreted, choose instead to document the client's own words.

Grouping data into meaningful patterns is also part of translation. For example, you would group cyanotic skin color, restlessness, and rapid respirations together because they all relate to tissue oxygenation.

Reasoning. Assessment includes actively processing information to make mental connections of the data to diseases, health patterns, or the current situation. Nurses who have a wide knowledge base are more likely to make appropriate mental connections. For example, the nurse who understands pathophysiology can determine whether the client's signs and symptoms are consistent with normal progression of an illness or whether a complication may be developing. Knowing the problems or complications that can occur with an illness, medical treatment, or surgical procedure can help you determine the meaning of the data you collect.

Reasoning also includes recognizing and understanding psychological and social responses to a health problem. These responses must be distinguished from the signs and symptoms of the illness itself.

Reasoning includes making **inferences** from the data, which means that you attach meaning to the data or reach a conclusion about the data. Inferential reasoning is based on a premise or proposition that supports or helps to support a conclusion. Correct inferential reasoning is based on knowing that the facts are correct, that the premise is correct, and that the known information is sufficient to reach the conclusion.

Box 6-2   Understanding Inferential Reasoning

CORRECT INFERENTIAL REASONING

Fact: *Mr. Smith has a bowel movement every 3 days, and the stool is soft and easily passed.*
Premise: *Constipation is the presence of hard, dry stool that is difficult to pass.*
Conclusion: *Mr. Smith is not constipated.*
Explanation: *Asking whether information included in the premise is sufficient to establish the presence of constipation can corroborate this correct conclusion. Because the premise includes a standard definition of constipation, the conclusion is based on sufficient evidence.*

INCORRECT INFERENTIAL REASONING

Fact: *Mr. Smith has swelling in his ankles and feet.*
Premise: *Persons with right-sided heart failure have swelling in their ankles and feet.*
Conclusion: *Mr. Smith has congestive heart failure.*
Explanation: *Although the premise is correct, the information in both the fact and the premise are insufficient to support the conclusion. Because ankle swelling can result from other problems besides heart failure, more evidence is needed to determine that heart failure has caused Mr. Smith's swollen ankles.*

Box 6-2 illustrates examples of correct and incorrect inferential reasoning.

You will routinely make inferences about the meaning of information as you collect it. However, reaching a conclusion too rapidly can result in errors. Always validate the data and explore the problem further. Look for evidence that you can use to judge the extent of the problem, and look for logical relationships between the data and the probable causes.

Using Intuition. Intuition is an ability to understand the whole without having to systematically examine the parts. It is knowing without always knowing why you know. The knowing comes in a flash of understanding, or a gestalt, without being aware of the thinking that has preceded the understanding. This kind of thinking starts with the whole and then examines the parts to validate that the thinking is correct.

Some people appear to be naturally intuitive thinkers, having developed a preference for intuitive reasoning from early childhood. However, poorly developed or untrained intuition skills can lead to faulty reasoning, and an excessive reliance on intuitive reasoning raises the danger of accepting a conclusion without verifying that the facts support the conclusion. A novice should never rely on intuition alone.

Intuition can be developed through repeated systematic examination of data to arrive at an appropriate conclusion. After multiple experiences with similar situations and similar correct conclusions, you will begin to develop intuitive reasoning as a valid basis for nursing actions.

Well-developed intuitive reasoning distinguishes the expert nurse from the novice (Figure 6-3). With intuition, the nurse acts correctly, seemingly without thinking, and cannot always explain the basis for the action. Intuition is efficient reasoning that allows the nurse to act quickly to save a life or prevent a complication. It allows the nurse to recognize a client's feelings or sense a level of understanding and respond appropriately (Benner, 1999; Benner, Tanner, & Chesla, 1996).

Validating. Validation means substantiating or confirming the accuracy of information using another source or another method. Cross-validation of both objective and subjective data increases the accuracy of all the data. For example, you can validate your interpretation of nonverbal behavior by ask-

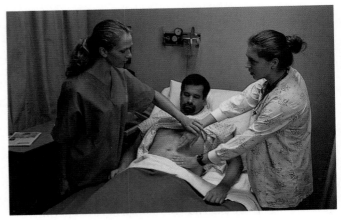

Figure 6-3. Well-developed intuitive reasoning distinguishes the expert nurse from the novice. Here, an expert nurse guides a novice nurse through a systematic physical examination guided by intuitive reasoning.

ing the client about it. When the client reports symptoms (subjective data), you can try to validate them with objective findings. Imagine that a client has reported being constipated; you can look for such objective evidence as lack of a bowel movement, a hard and dry stool, or a distended abdomen.

Sometimes family members or significant others can be used to validate information given by the client. The family can be especially helpful when the client has developed symptoms too gradually to be aware of their onset.

When the client and a family member provide conflicting reports, you must make a clinical judgment about which information to accept. Sometimes you can validate the most accurate account by using other sources, such as the medical or health record, objective observations, other family members, or the judgments of other team members. For example, suppose a client reports having an occasional alcoholic beverage, whereas a family member reports that the client is a heavy drinker. You check the medical or health record and find that the client's blood alcohol level on admission indicates heavy drinking. This information does not confirm that the client continually drinks large amounts of alcohol, but it does provide evidence that supports the family member's position.

INTERVIEWING

An **interview** is a planned series of questions designed to elicit information for a particular purpose. Whether you enter a client's room to assess a complication or a complaint, make a phone call to a home health client, or take an initial history, the interview has a definite purpose. You know in advance exactly what information is needed. An interview can be formal or informal; the following principles can be applied to either.

A well-conducted interview helps the client explain his or her own interpretation and understanding of the condition or reason that prompted the visit. The interview usually begins with an open approach that allows the client to talk until you develop an understanding of the client's perspective. Next, you will ask a series of questions while continuing to give the client some control of the interview. The client should feel like your partner in explaining and defining health problems.

The initial assessment interview begins with information about the client's **chief complaint,** which is the problem that caused the client to seek health services, call the doctor, or request a visit with a nurse; it is the client's description of the problem. The initial assessment typically includes both nursing and medical emphases. The **nursing history** is a narrative of the client's past health and health practices that focuses on information needed to plan nursing care. The medical history focuses on illness and the treatment of disease. The medical and nursing histories have some elements in common. Both types are collected through interviewing the client and they use an assessment framework to ensure thoroughness. The physical examination follows the assessment interview.

Phases of the Assessment Interview

A successful interview depends on preparation that anticipates the client's needs and sets the stage for the interview. Additional skills are engaged to ensure that the assessment is comprehensive and that the time with the client is productive. Interviewing skills are engaged in each of four phases of the interview process: preparation, orientation, the working phase, and termination.

Preparation. You need to prepare for each assessment both mentally and physically. Doing so allows you to assess each client systematically and thoroughly. The extent of your preparation depends on the purpose of the assessment. It may be as brief as asking a colleague to provide one or two pertinent pieces of information before entering a room to assess a client's report of pain. A comprehensive health assessment requires more extensive preparation.

As part of your preparation, you will set the stage for the assessment interview. Ideally, a comprehensive health history should take place in a private setting because some of the conversation may be sensitive or embarrassing to the client.

Of course, all client information is confidential. Assure the client that the information you solicit will be shared only with the health care team and only for purposes related to providing care. Do not suggest that any information will be kept confidential from the health care team. In some cases, you may need to inform the client of your obligation to share information with legal authorities; as needed, do so before asking for information that may be incriminating.

Additionally, the client should be comfortable and have any immediate needs met before the interview begins. Immediate needs may be as simple as going to the bathroom, or they may require you to treat pain or reposition the client to ease difficult breathing. The client's condition always determines how much information can be collected in one sitting. Before beginning the interview, assess the client's probable reliability in providing or reporting health information.

Orientation. The **orientation phase** is a brief exchange to establish the interview's purpose, the examination procedures, and the nurse's role in the interview process. The orientation phase in the initial interview is important because it establishes the nurse-client relationship as a legally binding contract. The nurse should be seen as a person who can be trusted with confidential information, trusted to provide competent care, and trusted in some cases with the client's life. The relationship will benefit from establishing an atmosphere that communicates care for the client.

Therefore, the first step in client assessment is establishing a nurse-client relationship based on mutual trust and understanding. In other words, you must build rapport with the client. *Rapport* means that there is a sense of understanding and trust between the nurse and client, suggesting that each of you has a vested interest in the client's well-being. When rapport is present, the client is more likely to reveal personal information.

Your demeanor can help establish rapport and trust to the extent that you portray yourself as a professional, knowledgeable person who is interested in the client. In a social relationship, flirting, giggling, joking, exchanging personal stories, or talking about sports events are expected forms of interchange. In a professional relationship, however, the conversation focuses on the reason for the relationship: the client. The client is the most important person in the relationship. A small amount of social interchange can help some clients be more comfortable with you, but you must avoid using a client relationship to meet your own personal or social needs.

Begin the assessment by identifying the client's immediate concerns and addressing them. A mother admitted to the hospital for elective surgery may need to know how to use the telephone to call her children before she will be interested in talking about the upcoming surgery. One client who is admitted for open-heart surgery may be worried about the surgery itself, whereas another may have questions about the postoperative diet and smoking cessation plan. Allow the client's questions and concerns to shape and focus the assessment, but do not limit the interview to these areas. Box 6-3 (p. 96) lists key points for the orientation phase.

Working Phase. The **working phase** is the phase of the interview process in which the client and nurse work together to review the client's health history and establish potential and actual problems that will be addressed as part of the care plan. The nurse gains insight about the client's concerns and expectations. The client feels assured these concerns will be addressed.

Termination. Skillfully ending the interview leaves both the nurse and the client feeling satisfied that the purpose has been accomplished, the client has been understood, and there is no unfinished business. The nurse prepares the client for **termination** of the interview by announcing in advance the approximate length of time the interview will take. The client will know how much time the nurse expects to devote to the process. As the interview nears an end, it may be helpful to state that you have just a few more questions. The last phase of the interview allows time for the client to ask questions and address any additional concerns that have not been covered in the interview.

Types of Interviews

You will need to choose the method of conducting an interview on the basis of the type of information you need to collect, the purpose of the interview, and the client's skill in describing problems. Interviews can be primarily directed or nondirected. Most interviews will make use of a combination of approaches.

Directed. In a directed interview, you maintain control over the interview by asking a list of questions that call for specific information from the client. The directed interview is used to elicit specific information and to ensure that the interview covers all relevant areas of assessment. One advantage of the directed interview is its ability to focus the client on information that is pertinent to the immediate concern and avoiding extraneous information. The directed interview is an efficient way to collect data in a short time.

The directed interview makes use of **closed questions,** questions that call for a specific, short response from the client. For example, to assess pain the nurse asks, "Do you

have pain? Where is the pain? Describe the pain? How severe is the pain?" The directed interview may also use **leading questions,** questions that suggest a possible appropriate response. An example of a leading question is "Are you frightened that the diagnosis will be cancer?" Using closed questions can help you collect the most pertinent information in the shortest time.

The directed interview has the disadvantage of not providing the opportunity for clients to freely express their concerns, fears, or feelings. You can obtain the most basic and necessary information, but the client may be left feeling that you are not concerned enough. Clients need to express their feelings and describe their symptoms from their own point of view to feel understood.

Nondirected. The nondirected interview gives more control to the client, thus allowing freer expression of concerns and feelings. Many clients try to "make sense" of their symptoms and may have associated meanings and antecedents to events surrounding the onset of symptoms that may or may not be relevant. The nondirected interview offers the client the opportunity to discuss and seek clarification about these meanings and events.

The nondirected interview uses primarily **open-ended questions** that ask for longer, interpretive responses. Open-ended questions do not call for a specific answer and may be phrased as a request rather than a question, such as "Tell me about the events that brought you to the hospital." or "Describe your symptoms." Open-ended questions are more useful for eliciting information from the client's point of view. A disadvantage on the nondirected interview is the client can become involved in discussing tangential information that is not pertinent.

ORGANIZING THE DATA

A **database** is all of the information that has been collected about the client and recorded in the health record as a baseline for the initial plan of care. It typically includes the data from the physician's client history and physical examination, the nurse's assessment, laboratory and diagnostic test results, and input from other members of the health care team. The database is used for comparing the client's response to treatment with the client's baseline condition.

A health care agency establishes a **minimum data set** that specifies information that must be collected from every client entering or being admitted to an institution. There is usually some commonality among clients in a particular setting that directs the decision about what to include in the minimum data set. Many institutions have assessment forms designed to ensure the collection of the minimum data set. Box 6-4 illustrates a typical minimum data set for a hospitalized client.

Beginning the Health History

Health care agencies generally use a standardized assessment tool or form on which to record your health history interview. This tool may vary, depending on the goals for care and the

Box 6-4 Typical Minimum Data Set for Admission of a Hospitalized Client

AT ADMISSION

Admitted from (home, physician's office, emergency medical service, or emergency department)
- Mode of arrival (ambulatory, wheelchair, or stretcher)
- I.D. band on (yes/no)

PRESENT ILLNESS

- Vital signs
- Height and weight
- Time and type of last oral intake
- Chief complaint
- Observations

ALLERGIES

- List drugs, food, other
- Describe reaction
- Allergy band on (yes/no)

PROSTHESES

- Dentures
- Glasses
- Contact lenses
- Hearing aid
- Artificial limb
- Artificial eye
- Other

EQUIPMENT: ADAPTIVE DEVICES USED

- Safety rails
- Pickup extension
- Ramp
- Chairlift

MEDICATION HISTORY

- List dose, frequency, date and time of last dose
- Medications brought to hospital
- Disposition (list medications)
- Valuables (to safe, policy explained, to home [with whom])

MEDICAL HEALTH HISTORY

- Previous illness or hospitalization
- Bleeding tendencies
- Circulatory problems
- Previous transfusion
- Hypertension
- Asthma
- Hay fever
- Arthritis

- Heart problems
- Kidney problems
- Cancer
- Diabetes
- Epilepsy

FUNCTIONAL STATUS (ACTIVITIES OF DAILY LIVING)

- Primary language spoken
- Diet
- Hygiene (bathing, dressing, grooming)
- Sleeping patterns
- Communication/speaking
- Comprehension
- Seeing/hearing

MOBILITY (DESCRIBE LIMITATIONS)

- No limitations
- Unable to sit
- Unable to stand
- Requires walker/cane
- Requires wheelchair
- Requires partial/complete assistance

ADMISSION INSTRUCTIONS GIVEN

- Bathroom emergency light
- Visitor policy
- Meals/guest meals
- Smoking
- Room: Bed control, phone, call light, TV control, side rails
- Electric appliances OK. or Maintenance notified of non-U.L. equipment

SOCIAL ASSESSMENT/DISCHARGE PLANNING

- Religion
- Culture
- Apparent family support system
- Are any persons in your home dependent on you?
- Obvious family conflicts that may impair health care in the future
- Able to administer all medications
- Indications of possible neglect or abuse
- Do you anticipate any problems after discharge?
- Able to return to previous living situation
- Will you need help when you go home?
- Independence in the home setting?
- Are you being seen by any health service/agency?
- Do you have any suggestions that will help us with your care here?
- Identified client/family education needs
- Person to notify in emergency
- Respondent (if other than client)

type of services offered by the agency. Acute care agencies with short-term stays will need only the information necessary to manage the short-term experience. Some information is gathered for the purpose of helping clients plan their care after discharge. If a client appears to need extensive assistance with discharge planning, additional information may be gathered.

Some agencies use a form organized as a review of body systems, whereas functional ability or other nursing assess-

ment schemata organize other forms. In all cases, the goal is to achieve a systematic, comprehensive assessment appropriate to the services of the agency. No matter what organizational framework you use, your assessments will be more efficient when you use a consistent, thorough pattern.

In an effort to reduce the time spent documenting, ensure comprehensive assessment, and meet the legal requirements for documentation, assessment forms have been developed that allow you to complete a checklist and possibly write brief notes. Computerized charting systems take the idea one step further, and you may choose from a list to record your findings. You may need to add a narrative nursing note to be sure you have completely documented the assessment.

Usually, a systematic assessment begins with an exploration of the client's biographical data, expectations and goals, reason for the visit, and medical and family histories. It then can expand into a holistic approach on the basis of an assessment framework (functional health patterns or body systems) that addresses all aspects of the client's health.

Biographical Data.
Biographical data consist of information that identifies and describes the person, such as name, address, age, gender, religious affiliation, race, occupation, other people residing in the household, and the number of dependent children. This kind of information is also referred to as **demographical data** because it is factual information that can be aggregated to describe populations of clients. Biographical information helps the health provider anticipate problems common to a particular group. For example, the probable causes of difficulty in urinating would be different in a 55-year-old man and in a 16-year-old boy. Biographical data may also be collected by having the client complete an admission form or by reviewing the client's record.

Expectations and Goals.
In describing their symptoms or concerns, clients may provide cues to their feelings about their illness, expectations of the health care encounter, or health care goals. You should listen for information that suggests that the client fears a serious or life-threatening problem. Sometimes you can provide information that calms those fears or helps the client gain a realistic perspective.

The client's goals and expectations are affected by the setting. In home health, the client may be seeking information to decide whether to call a physician or information to determine whether the family has the resources to manage a problem. The family may expect you to give them information or help them manage the problem. The hospitalized client may be expecting a short hospital stay, full recovery, and immediate return to usual activities. Other expectations of the hospitalized client include to be free from pain, to be treated with respect, to be safe, and to receive appropriate treatment for the presenting problem. The nurse needs to know if the client's expectations and goals match those of the health care team.

Social and cultural history provides cues to the person's values and experience with health care (Figure 6-4). It may also suggest the need to investigate problems that are more likely to occur within a particular group. Care can be planned that is consistent with the client's values.

Reason for the Visit.
The health care provider usually begins by finding out the reason for the encounter from the client's point of view. The physician often writes only brief descriptions of the client's problems in the medical record; therefore, you may need a more complete description from the client.

Most clients appreciate the opportunity to review the details of the experience that has led them to seek health care.

While listening to the client's account of the reason for the visit, you are gathering information about the client's knowledge level and feelings about the problem and areas for teaching. Using active listening techniques, you may discover that the client has misunderstandings about the medical treatment plan. If you cannot remedy these misunderstandings, you will need to share this information with the physician.

HISTORY OF PRESENT ILLNESS. Information about the history of the present illness helps to anticipate problems the client may have and to understand the illness from the client's point of view. Having described the reason for the visit, the client may have given a complete account of the history of the present illness. If not, you can help the client fill in missing information. It is helpful to know when the symptoms began, the severity of the symptoms, and what actions were taken to control them. The client who enters the hospital may have been managing an illness for a long time through outpatient services, or the symptoms may have had a sudden onset. The following questions may be helpful: Have you been seeing a physician for this problem? What did the doctor tell you about the problem? What medications have you been taking? Did the medication help? Have you received other treatment?

ASSESSING THE CHIEF COMPLAINT. You can encourage the client to describe the chief complaint by asking questions such as these: How can I help you? What brought you to the hospital? or Tell me about your problem. Told in the client's own words, the chief complaint establishes the purpose of the contact, provides direction for the assessment, and establishes the nurse-client relationship.

Then you will gather information to fully describe the client's problem. Ask questions that help the client describe the specific signs and symptoms associated with the problem and provide a history of the present illness. The following seven variables provide a core description of most problems. Although all the variables may not apply to every symptom, using this general pattern of assessment will help you to be thorough.

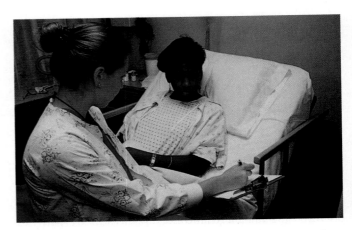

Figure 6-4. The social and cultural history provides important clues to the client's health-related values and to the client's experience with the health care system.

LOCATION. Symptoms are often associated with a particular body part. Ask the client to be specific about the location of pain, numbness, or other sensation. For example, you might ask, "Can you point to the exact location of the pain in your abdomen?" or "Where does it hurt?" The location of a rash or other lesion may help identify the cause.

QUALITY. You are seeking the client's description of how the symptoms feel. Avoid giving the client words to describe the symptom but, if the client cannot find any words, you can offer choices. People will often describe a symptom by using an analogy, such as "pins pricking my skin," "a knife stabbing me," "something very heavy on my chest," or "something tearing." Clients' choices of analogies are fairly consistent for particular diseases and therefore may provide a definitive cue to the medical diagnosis.

QUANTITY. Measuring quantity is an attempt to determine the intensity or severity of the symptom. Quantity can be elicited as frequency, volume, number, effects on activity, and extent. You might ask, "How severe is your symptom?" or "How often does it occur?" To get more objective data about pain, it may be useful to have the client rate the pain or other symptom on a scale of 0 to 10, with 10 being the most severe pain imaginable.

CHRONOLOGY. It may be helpful to know how long the client has had the symptom. Was the onset insidious (slow, gradual) or acute (sudden)? Is the symptom constant or does it come in episodes? Does the intensity vary with time? Does the symptom disturb the client's sleep?

SETTING. Where was the client, and what was happening when the symptoms first occurred? The setting may suggest that stress, activity, or environmental pollution is affecting the symptom. For example, the onset of asthma when the person goes to a park may suggest an environmental trigger for the attack.

AGGRAVATING OR ALLEVIATING FACTORS. Ask what the client has found to be helpful in relieving the symptom. What attempts has the client made to relieve the symptom? Is there any activity that makes it worse? Does eating make it worse or better? Does resting help? Was aspirin used to reduce a fever?

ASSOCIATED FACTORS. Look for anything else that might have been missed. Associated factors will vary according to the nature of the problem. You may ask about common associations. For example, for a client with diarrhea and abdominal cramps, ask if that person has recently traveled to a foreign country or eaten a food that might have produced the problem. The client may have an idea about what brought on the problem.

Medical History. A medical history is a review of problems or diseases that required or continue to require treatment by a physician. You are looking for any past medical problems that might influence the present illness by contributing to the problem or that might require altering the care for the current problem. A medical history may be elicited through a written checklist of common chronic problems, filled out by either the client or the nurse. Specific questions are asked about each ill-

ness in the client's history. By using a checklist, the client is encouraged to be thorough, and the focus of the interview is narrowed to pertinent information.

The medical history also includes a history of allergies to medications, pollutants, foods, and pollens. When the planned treatment includes the administration of medications, it is most important to ask about allergies to medications. If the client reports an allergy, obtain information about the type of reaction and how the reaction has been managed in the past.

Family History. As you ask about the client's medical history, you will also ask about the family history of any illnesses that are genetic or familial. As the name implies, genetic illnesses are passed through genes. Familial illnesses tend to be more prevalent in families, but the cause of the increased incidence in a family may be unknown. Familial illness may have a basis in lifestyle, diet, stress, or environmental factors.

REVIEW OF FUNCTIONAL HEALTH PATTERNS

One method of holistic assessment that provides information from a nursing rather than a medical perspective uses **functional health patterns,** a concept that refers to the positive and negative behaviors a person uses to interact with the environment and maintain health. During assessment, you will examine the client's behaviors to determine whether each pattern is functional or dysfunctional. Assessment includes the usual pattern of behavior, complaints, limitations, problems associated with the pattern of behavior, behaviors used to manage the problem, and the client's coping skills. Each pattern is examined for biological, social, psychological, cultural, developmental, and spiritual factors influencing behavior. Box 6-5 lists categories of information to be assessed in each health pattern.

A few key questions in each category may be sufficient to determine that the person does or does not have a problem (Box 6-6, p. 100). If a problem is suggested, you will ask fur-

Box 6-5	**Assessment of Health Patterns**

For each pattern, assess the following categories:

FUNCTIONAL PATTERN

- Present function
- Personal habits
- Culture and lifestyle factors
- Age-related factors

DYSFUNCTIONAL PATTERN

- History of dysfunction
- Diagnostic tests
- Risk factors associated with medical treatment plan
- Types of adaptations used

WHEN A PROBLEM IS IDENTIFIED IN A FUNCTIONAL PATTERN

- Relationship to other functional patterns

| Box 6-6 | Nursing History Questions Arranged by Functional Health Pattern |

HEALTH PERCEPTION–HEALTH MAINTENANCE PATTERN

- Client's description of general health
- Health practices; may include those related to managing a specific chronic illness
- Use of alcohol, tobacco, and other substances
- Home, school, and occupational safety
- Client's description of the cause of the illness (if present) and actions taken to manage it

NUTRITIONAL–METABOLIC PATTERN

- Does the client seem well nourished and well developed in general appearance?
- Is the client overweight or underweight for the age and height?
- What is the client's usual dietary pattern? Describe typical daily food and fluid intake.
- Does the client adhere to a special diet?
- How does the client's skin look? Are there lesions? Is the skin dry?
- What is the client's body temperature?
- What was the client's recent cholesterol level?
- Does the client have diabetes or a family history of diabetes?
- Does the client have dental problems?
- History of gastrointestinal or endocrine problems?

ELIMINATION PATTERN

- What are your usual bowel and bladder habits?
- What are the frequency, consistency, and color of your stool?
- Do you have difficulty with urination?
- Do you experience incontinence?
- How would you describe your use of laxatives or other aids to elimination?
- Do you have a history of bowel or bladder problems?

ACTIVITY–EXERCISE PATTERN

- What are your usual daily activities?
- What is your general level of physical fitness?
- Do you have a history of cardiac or respiratory problems?
- What activities give you the most pleasure?
- Do you need help with home maintenance?
- What is your activity tolerance?
- What is your usual pattern of exercise?
- Do you lead a sedentary lifestyle?
- Are you satisfied with your level of activity?
- Do you smoke? How many packs per day? For how many years?
- Are you able to feed yourself, bathe, go to the toilet, groom yourself, and move about in bed?
- Can you do the shopping and cooking, maintain your home, and achieve general mobility?
- Do you use a cane or walker or need help for walking?

SLEEP–REST PATTERN

- What is your usual pattern of sleep?
- Do you feel rested in the morning?
- Do you use sleep aids?
- Are you able to sleep through the night?
- Do you have trouble falling asleep?

COGNITIVE–PERCEPTUAL PATTERN

- Do you have any difficulty with vision? Do you need glasses for reading or distance vision?
- Do you have any difficulty with hearing? Do you use a hearing aid?

- What is your name? Where do you live? What brought you to the hospital? What day is it?
- How long have you been here?

SELF-PERCEPTION–SELF-CONCEPT PATTERN

- What can you tell me about yourself?
- How will this hospitalization affect your life?
- How would you describe your support systems?
- Who relies on you?
- Where do you go for moral support?
- What do you do to "take care of yourself?"
- How do you feel about being ill? In the hospital?
- Do you have anxiety? How does it affect you?
- Do you have a history of anxiety disorders? Have you used psychotropic drugs? Alcohol? Street drugs?

ROLE–RELATIONSHIP PATTERN

- Who are the members of your household?
- How would you characterize the strength of your marriage?
- Is your family dependent on you? How are they managing during your hospitalization or illness?
- What are the ages of your children? Where do they live?
- Do close family ties characterize your family?
- When someone is ill, how does your family offer support?
- Do you have trouble sharing your problems and concerns with others?
- Do you have concerns that this illness will affect your ability to perform in your occupation?
- If you are unable to continue in your present occupation, are you in a position to retire?
- Do you have problems with your children that are difficult for you to manage?

SEXUALITY–REPRODUCTION PATTERN

- How would you characterize your satisfaction with your sexual relationship?
- Would disruption of your sexual relationship with your spouse be a factor in making a decision about having this surgery (taking this medication)?
- What was the date of your last menstrual period?
- At what age did you start menstruation? Are your menstrual periods regular?
- Do you use birth control? What method do you use?
- How many times have you been pregnant? How many live births?

COPING–STRESS TOLERANCE

- How are you managing (name the current problem or situation)?
- Have you talked to your (significant other) about (the current situation)?
- Have you informed your family and friends of your (current situation)?
- How would you characterize the level of stress in your life over the past year?
- Do you have someone with whom you are comfortable talking about problems or changes in your life?
- Do you use alcohol or other drugs to relieve stress?

VALUE–BELIEF PATTERN

- Is your life satisfying? Is your life good?
- What are your plans for the future?
- Do you have a religious affiliation?
- Do you actively practice a religion?
- Is spirituality important in your daily life?
- Will this hospitalization interfere with any religious practices?

ther questions. However, assessment of functional patterns includes the client's strengths as well as weaknesses, problems, and limitations. Information about methods of health maintenance can be combined with indicators of physical function to develop possible causal relationships between the two. Additional questions are asked not to identify problems but to elicit the client's usual pattern of function. You need this information to more effectively support the client's usual pattern of functioning while providing care.

Clustering of data by functional health patterns also helps you identify problems that are responsive to nursing intervention and helps you assign appropriate nursing diagnoses to dysfunctional patterns. Nursing care is more concerned with helping the person manage or function with a health problem than with diagnosing and treating illnesses. Therefore the focus of functional health patterns is on nursing diagnoses rather than on medical diagnoses.

Marjorie Gordon (2002) introduced a formal framework for assessing functional health patterns in 1982. She identified patterns of human function in 11 categories that address physical, psychological, spiritual, and social needs. Rather than treating the illness, nursing care is aimed at maintaining or improving the client's functional status in each of the 11 areas.

Health Perception–Health Maintenance Pattern

The health perception–health maintenance pattern describes the client's personal view of health and behaviors associated with the quest to be healthy. The client's risk factors for altered health and altered health maintenance should be explored. Although health maintenance is inherent in the other 10 patterns of functioning, exploring the health perception–health maintenance pattern separately gives you the opportunity to focus on health behaviors and risk factors. Important components of this pattern of behavior include the beliefs held by a person about control over health and the actions taken to change the state of health.

Assessment of the client's lifestyle can reveal areas where health can be improved. Knowledge of the client's health-seeking behaviors will provide you with cues to help the client plan care that will improve health. Assessment would include health-related activities in each of the functional patterns.

Assessment of health perceptions may begin by asking the client to describe any current health problems. Information about health perceptions and beliefs may be inherent in the response.

Another way to elicit information about health perceptions is to ask, "Have you had a similar experience in the past?" You may get information about previous illnesses or hospitalizations, including the client's perceptions of these experiences. In eliciting information about the current illness, ask the client to describe it, including the onset and the cause. Ask about previous treatment, whether the client complied with the treatment regimen, and whether the client anticipates having any problems in self-care as a result of the illness. When assessing health perception–health maintenance, you are looking for evidence of a healthy lifestyle.

Asking about the use of alcohol, illegal drugs, over-the-counter drugs, and tobacco products should be a routine part of a health assessment. A nonjudgmental manner is essential to getting truthful information. Accurate information is particularly important if the hospitalized client is expected to have anesthesia or to be confined long enough for withdrawal symptoms to occur.

You also need to know whether the client has sufficient information to understand and manage the presenting health problems. Allow time to address the client's concerns, and frequently ask whether the client has any questions. By having the client describe problems and review information received from a physician, you can often detect whether the person has any misunderstandings.

Nutritional–Metabolic Pattern

The nutritional–metabolic pattern includes the client's dietary habits in relationship to metabolic need, and indicators of metabolic function, such as the skin, mucous membranes, and body temperature. Nutritional patterns are learned from early childhood; they may be modified by lifestyle changes, new knowledge, economics, or health problems. General health is affected by nutritional intake (Figure 6-5).

You will assess the dietary pattern to ascertain the feasibility of improving the client's general health in relationship to the health problems or potential health problems of obesity, undernourishment, uncontrolled diabetes, or high cholesterol. Metabolism is related to the gastrointestinal system and the endocrine system; therefore gastrointestinal, thyroid, and pancreatic functions are included.

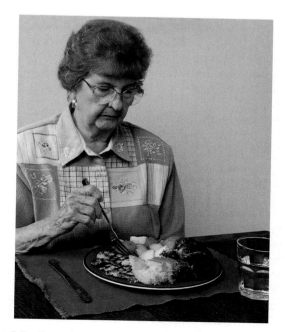

Figure 6-5. General health is affected by nutritional intake. This woman understands the importance of maintaining a well-balanced diet in older adulthood, even though it is difficult on a retiree's fixed income.

Elimination Pattern

The elimination pattern overlaps with the effects of the nutritional pattern. Nutritional intake and fluid intake are important determinants of the pattern by which a person eliminates wastes from the body. This pattern includes bowel and bladder habits, the effect of activity on elimination, and the use of laxatives and other aids to elimination. Fluid loss through the skin must also be considered. The elimination pattern describes the function of the gastrointestinal tract, kidneys, and bladder.

Activity–Exercise Pattern

The activity–exercise pattern includes the person's ability to be active and the level of activity the person chooses. Energy is expended in exercise, daily routines, leisure, and recreation. The person's ability to engage in activity affects both productivity and the quality of life. The activity–exercise pattern includes the person's physical capability for self-care, an attribute that also depends on cognitive function, mobility, resources, knowledge, and motivation.

Assessment includes obtaining information about limitations of mobility, type of exercise, duration of exercise, ability to perform activities of daily living, and satisfaction with level of activity. The person's ability to perform activities is related to the musculoskeletal system, the neurological system, the cardiovascular system, and the respiratory system. You may need to assess each of these areas in depth, or simple observation may be sufficient to recognize, for example, that the client is or is not capable of adequate self-care.

Sleep–Rest Pattern

All persons need sleep and rest, but the amount they need is variable. Assessment of the sleep–rest pattern includes the usual pattern of sleep and rest, aids to sleep, the person's satisfaction or feeling of being rested, and routines associated with sleep and rest. Problems related to the sleep–rest pattern may form the presenting complaint, or they may be secondary to the chief complaint.

Cognitive–Perceptual Pattern

The cognitive–perceptual pattern includes sensation, perception, and cognition. Sensation is the reception of stimulation through receptors of the nervous system. Sensory functions include vision, hearing, touch, taste, smell, and proprioception (the sense of position). Pain is a sensation and therefore included in this functional pattern. Perception is the ability to receive input from the senses, interpret the information in the brain, and interpret it in a meaningful way. The closely related concept of cognition is the act or process of knowing. Cognitive functions include memory, thoughts, language, and reasoning.

Assessment of the cognitive–perceptual pattern includes neurological assessment and the mental status examination. Additionally, you will assess how a cognitive–perceptual problem alters the client's daily life and how the client compensates for the deficit.

Begin your assessment of the cognitive–perceptual pattern by spending a few minutes getting acquainted and conversing with the client. Listen for cues that the client is hearing and understanding you; is oriented to time, place, and person; and has memory of recent and past events. Evaluate the client's language for unusual speech patterns and reasoning. You may perform this assessment without asking any questions specific to the pattern.

Self-Perception–Self-Concept Pattern

The self-perception–self-concept pattern includes how the person views the self. Self-concept is an attitude, a feeling about self, or an evaluation of self; self-esteem is the affective component of self-concept that describes an attitude, feeling, or evaluation of self-worth. To understand a client's self-concept, you will need information about the person's perception of cognitive, affective, and physical abilities as well as the perception of body image and identity, the general sense of worth, and the general emotional pattern.

When assessing this pattern, you would like to know if the client has mental problems or emotional needs that must be addressed to provide the best care. It is particularly important for the home care nurse to recognize depression, because this condition has a high potential for interfering with the client's ability to comply with the therapeutic regimen. The home care client may have anxiety about managing at home and getting help when it is needed. The hospitalized client is at high risk for anxiety because of the potentially serious nature of problems that require hospitalization.

You will assess this pattern through active listening rather than by asking specific questions. Listen for negative self-talk, lack of confidence, and beliefs about how others regard the client. Also consider body posture, eye contact, voice tone, speech patterns, and general appearance.

Role–Relationship Pattern

Roles are the parts one plays in one's own life. Typically, they relate closely to relationships with children, spouse, friends, and co-workers. For example, a person may have the roles of mother, teacher, friend, and colleague. Roles and relationships are the means through which the need for love and belonging is met and self-esteem is developed.

Examining living arrangements, support systems, and family life assesses the role–relationship pattern. Complaints may include isolation, loneliness, abuse, and marital problems.

Sexuality–Reproductive Pattern

Sexuality is present from birth to the end of a person's life. The expression of sexuality varies among individuals by age, culture, beliefs, health, life circumstances, and social norms. Assessment of the sexuality–reproductive pattern must include the person's satisfaction and perceptions of appropriate sexual and reproductive behavior. Many of the external indicators of sexual patterns may be misleading or lead to stereotypical assumptions that may not be valid.

Generally, the sexuality–reproductive pattern is not assessed explicitly unless you have a specific reason to do so.

For example, the client may indicate that a potential problem exists or that a potential problem is secondary to the problem for which the client is seeking treatment. Possible indicators include the strength of the client's relationship with a spouse, flirting behavior, an overtly sexy way of dressing, a single parent, children with different fathers, discomfort with persons of the opposite sex, and adults who remain unmarried beyond the usual age for marriage.

Coping–Stress Tolerance Pattern

Stress is a part of life that results from both positive and negative experiences, from hardships and joys, and from internal and external forces. A person's experience of stress varies with the perception of stress-producing events and the person's skills in managing both the events and the responses to them. During assessment, you would consider the client's evaluation of the current situation and experience with similar situations. In addition, how the client managed stressful situations in the past may provide useful information.

You may not assess this pattern directly, although hospital nurses commonly ask about previous reactions to hospitalization. In the process of describing the previous experience, the client often provides cues to how he or she coped with the experience. One client may say, "I don't know how I could have managed without my wife," whereas another may suggest that a warm, friendly relationship with the nurses helped in managing the experience. The home care nurse may get cues from the home environment. A well-ordered, well-planned living environment may suggest that order and planning are a possible coping strategy.

Value–Belief Pattern

The value–belief pattern describes the philosophical position that guides a person's choices or decisions in life. The spiritual self is a major component of this pattern. It also reflects what the individual perceives as important to quality of life. Often, values and beliefs are derived from a religious or other formal philosophical base. Family strongly influences the formation of values and beliefs as well. Health care that is consistent with and supportive of the person's value system is most likely to result in positive health outcomes. Table 6-1 illustrates assessment data obtained for a client and grouped by functional health patterns.

DOCUMENTING THE DATA

The assessment data that you collect must be documented in the client's medical record so that the entire health care team has access to it. Thus the record serves as a means of communication and sharing information for the health care team. The database includes the information contributed by all members of the health care team.

Clearly, it is crucial that data recorded about the client be accurate, complete, and concise. The data will be used to make treatment decisions not just for nursing care but for medical care, respiratory care, physical therapy, diet therapy, and others. The record should contain all information

Table 6-1 Data Illustrating Functional Health Patterns

A 50-year-old man is admitted to the hospital for abdominal pain. He is being evaluated for a bowel obstruction. Although pain applies specifically to the cognitive/perceptual pattern, it has the potential to affect all other functional patterns as well. Assessing its relationship to other functional patterns might reveal findings such as those listed here.

PATTERN	POSSIBLE FINDINGS
Self-Perception–Self-Concept	Client has never been hospitalized and denies that anything could be seriously wrong. "I must have food poisoning. The doctor will probably give me an antibiotic and send me home. One of the guys at work had the same thing." Well-developed muscles emphasized by tight-fitting shirt with rolled-up short sleeves. Attempts to flirt with the nurses.
Values–Beliefs	Lists *Christian* as religious preference. Wife says she will call the minister if he has to go to surgery, but her husband does not attend church very often.
Roles–Relationships	States he is angry at his wife because she insisted that he come to the hospital. Is employed as a lineman for the city utility company and is concerned because a recent electrical storm has left a number of power lines down. Has a 30-year-old son who is married and works with his father as a lineman. A 33-year-old daughter is unmarried and lives in another city.
Elimination	Usually has a daily bowel movement after breakfast. Has not had a bowel movement in 5 days. Abdomen hard and distended. Bowel sounds absent. Voids without difficulty. Urine dark and concentrated. Results of abdominal CT scan pending. Father and one uncle died of cancer of colon.
Activity–Exercise	Usually engages in daily weight lifting but has not exercised since the onset of pain 3 days ago. No history of cardiovascular problems. Has never had cholesterol checked. Vital signs: blood pressure 100/70, pulse 108, respiration 34, temperature 101.2∞ F. Skin is pale, cool, and clammy. Became dizzy after getting out of bed to go to the bathroom. Hemoglobin and hematocrit levels slightly elevated. Skin turgor sluggish. Eyes sunken. Breath sounds diminished in lung bases.
Cognitive–Perceptual	Complains of severe, diffuse abdominal pain; a 7 on a scale of 0 to 10. Agrees to take pain medication to make his wife happy. Alert and oriented.
Nutritional–Metabolic	Has not eaten much for 3 days and nothing for 24 hours. Last meal caused severe nausea followed by vomiting. Appetite is generally good. Often eats in fast-food places for lunch. Coffee, eggs, and toast for breakfast. Wife prepares a balanced meal for supper. No family history of diabetes. Intravenous infusion of D_5/NS started in left forearm at 125 ml per hour. Nasogastric tube to low intermittent suction. Serum sodium and potassium levels slightly high.
Sexuality–Reproductive	Appears to have a close relationship with wife.

pertinent to the client's condition. Statements should be succinct, using the least number of words needed to convey meaning accurately. Often, potential or actual problems identified on an assessment form will need to be described in more detail in your nurse's notes.

Only factual information should be documented. Clear documentation differentiates between objective and subjective data. When the data come from the client, always indicate that the client has stated the information. Avoid including your opinions. Almost always, it is better to chart the facts that caused you to develop an opinion rather than the opinion itself. More information on documentation appears in Chapter 11.

Key Principles

- Assessment does not exist in isolation from the other steps of the nursing process; making diagnoses, planning, and establishing outcomes take place simultaneously with assessment.
- Critical thinking is a necessary part of assessment to know what questions to ask, what the answers mean, how to follow up, and how to recognize the etiology of the problem.
- The most appropriate format for assessment depends on the purpose and type of the assessment.
- Using multiple sources of data increases the accuracy of the database.
- Prudent health assessment requires that you collect data about sensitive subject matter in a private setting.
- Assessment requires active listening and active mental processing, not merely asking a list of questions.
- During assessment, the client's immediate concerns should occupy your focus of attention.
- Assessment begins with the chief complaint, proceeds to health history, and ends with a physical examination.
- When a symptom is revealed, it should be followed with questions that help the client describe the symptom.
- A systematic method of data collection can help ensure a comprehensive, holistic assessment.
- The collected data are documented in the health record to aid continuity of care and communication with the health care team.

Bibliography

American Nurses Association. (1998). Standards of clinical nursing practice (2nd ed.). Washington, DC: Author.

*American Nurses Association. (2003). *Nursing: Scope and Standards of Practice* (3rd ed.) (Publication No. 9801ST). Washington, DC: Author.

American Nurses Association. (2001). Don't just simply "follow the form." *Same-Day Surgery, 25*(6), 66.

Benner, P. (1999). Nursing leadership for the new millennium: Claiming the wisdom and worth of clinical practice. *Nursing and Health Care Perspectives, 20*(6), 312-319.

*Benner, P. A., Tanner, C. A., & Chesla, C. A. (1996). *Expertise in nursing practice: Caring, clinical judgment, and ethics*. New York: Springer.

Beyea, S. C., & Nicoll, L. H. (1999). Common sense: A key component of decision making. *AORN Journal, 70*(6), 1076-1077.

Bowles, K. (2000). The relationship of critical-thinking skills and the clinical-judgment skills of baccalaureate nursing students. *Journal of Nursing Education, 39*(8), 373-376.

Boychuk-Duchscher, J. E. (1999). Catching the wave: Understanding the concept of critical thinking. *Journal of Advanced Nursing, 29*(3), 577-583.

Camann, M. A., & Chase, L. (2001). Older adults: The case for comprehensive assessment. *Caring, 20*(1), 26-28.

Chien, W. T., Kam, C. W., & Lee, I. F. (2001). An assessment of the patients' needs in mental health education. *Journal of Advanced Nursing, 34*(3), 304-311.

Fitzgerald, M. A. (2000). To the test: Assessment skills. *Advance for Nurse Practitioners, 8*(1), 29.

Frye, B., Alfred, N., & Campbell, M. (1999). Use of the Watson-Glaser Critical Thinking Appraisal with BSN students. *Nursing and Health Care Perspectives, 20*(5), 253-255.

Gordon, M. (2002). *Manual of nursing diagnosis* (10th ed.). St Louis, MO: Mosby.

Hansten, R., & Washburn, M. (2000). Intuition in professional practice: Executive and staff perceptions. *Journal of Nursing Administration, 30*(4):185-189.

Harbison, J. (2001). Clinical decision making in nursing: Theoretical perspectives and their relevance to practice. *Journal of Advanced Nursing, 35*(1), 126-133; discussion 134-137.

Herbig, B., Bussing, A., & Ewert, T. (2001). The role of tacit knowledge in the work context of nursing. *Journal of Advanced Nursing, 34*(5), 687-695.

Jarvis, C. (2001). *Physical examination and health assessment* (3rd ed.). Philadelphia: Saunders.

Keegan, L. (2001). The environment as a healing tool. *Nursing Clinics of North America, 36*(1), 73-82.

Kunkler, C. E. (1999). Neurovascular assessment. *Orthopedic Nursing, 18*(3), 63-71.

Valk, M., Post, M. W., Cools, H. J., & Schrijvers, G. A. (2001). Measuring disability in nursing home residents: Validity and reliability of a newly developed instrument. *The Journals of Gerontology, Series B Psychosocial Sciences and Social Sciences, 56*(3), 187-191.

Ward, D. (2000). Implementing evidence-based practice in infection control. *British Journal of Nursing, 9*(5), 267-271.

*Asterisk indicates a classic or definitive work on this subject.

Assessing Vital Signs

Learning Objectives

After studying this chapter, you should be able to do the following:

- Identify the rationale for the assessment of vital signs
- Interpret deviations from the normal ranges of each vital sign according to the client's age
- Describe the normal physiological features of each vital sign
- List factors that influence temperature, pulse, respirations, and blood pressure
- Safely and accurately measure axillary, oral, rectal, and tympanic temperatures; apical and radial pulses; respirations; and blood pressure
- Measure vital signs in an organized, accurate manner
- Document and report vital sign measurements correctly

Vital signs are a basic component of assessment of the physiological and psychological health of a client. Body temperature, pulse, respiration, and blood pressure are the signs of life, and their assessment allows you to (1) identify specific life-threatening clinical problems and select nursing interventions and (2) detect changes in the client's health status. You may assess vital signs to establish a client's baseline, to detect a change in condition, or to make a nursing diagnosis. There are many situations in which you may assess a client's vital signs:

- As part of a physical examination
- To establish a baseline on admission to a health care facility
- For routine monitoring during the client's stay in a hospital
- To determine the effects of surgery or other invasive procedure
- To determine the effects of medications on temperature or the cardiovascular or respiratory systems
- To evaluate the effectiveness of the medical treatment plan
- To evaluate the effectiveness of nursing interventions, such as ambulation
- To detect improvement or deterioration in the client's condition
- To validate health status on discharge from a nursing unit

As in any scientific measurement, accuracy depends on precision of measurement. A careless assessment can result in inaccurate planning, interventions, and evaluation. Perform the procedures methodically to ensure accurate readings and maintain your client's safety.

INTERPRETING VITAL SIGNS

To form conclusions about the significance of vital sign measurements, you need to analyze the data in relationship to other findings in the assessment. The significance of vital signs does not stem from a single value but from the *relationship* of the vital signs to each other and to other assessment findings. Additionally, the *trend* of changes in vital signs should guide your conclusions about the client's condition.

First, compare the client's readings with the average normal parameters. Normal values are different for children, adults, and older adults (Table 7-1). For example, 30 respirations per minute is normal for an infant but abnormally high for an adult.

Next, compare the data with the client's previous readings to consider normal for the specific client. Have any or all vital signs increased or decreased since the previous measurement? If the previous measurement was recent, is the client's condition changing quickly? If the condition is changing for the worse, how soon will you need to assess the vital signs again to verify the continuing trend? This may be as soon as 5 or 10 minutes. Do you need an emergency plan to prevent serious or fatal consequences?

Next, compare the data you obtained with the client's complete health history and condition. In a client with a history of hypertension, expect a blood pressure that is higher than normal. In a client who just underwent surgery, pain may cause an increased pulse and blood pressure. Perhaps the client is taking a drug that adversely affects the vital signs. For example, some medications, such as digitalis, may slow the heart rate. Others, such as aminophylline, may speed the heart rate. Be sure to review any over-the-counter medications or herbal supplements the client may have taken recently. Overall, the goal is to consider whether the client's vital signs are consistent with the history and current clinical status. If not, measure the vital signs again to make sure your readings are correct. If changes in the client's vital signs stem from a medication, consult the physician, who may change the dose.

Additionally, consider the effects of the environment, level of activity, and mental status on your results. Generally vital signs should be assessed in quiet, comfortable, resting conditions. Is the room hot or cold? Does the client appear anxious, angry, or stressed? Has the client been exercising? Is the client a child who is upset and crying?

Action Alert! Reassess elevated blood pressure and pulse after the client has sat quietly for 10 to 15 minutes.

Through interpretation of vital signs, nurses make decisions about the frequency of vital sign assessment. Although a physician's order or nursing unit policy typically specifies the minimum frequency for measuring vital signs, you are responsible for assessing vital signs any time a need arises. For example, if the client's temperature rises above 100.4° F (38° C), you may decide to measure

Table 7-1	Average Range for Vital Signs According to Age-Group				
Age-Group	Temperature (Oral, in °F)	Pulse per Minute	Respirations per Minute	Blood Pressure (in mm Hg) Systolic	Diastolic
Newborn	N/A	100 to 180 (Mean, 125)	35 to 40	60 to 90	20 to 60
Infant up to age 1	99.4	100 to 160 (Mean, 120)	30 to 40	85 to 105	50 to 65
Toddler ages 1 to 3	99.0 to 99.7	80 to 120 (Mean, 110)	25 to 40	95 to 105	50 to 65
Preschooler ages 3 to 6	98.6	70 to 110 (Mean, 100)	22 to 35	95 to 100	55 to 60
Child ages 6 to 12	98.6	65 to 100 (Mean, 90)	20 to 30	100 to 110	60 to 70
Adolescent ages 12 to 18	97.8 to 98.6	60 to 90 (Mean, 80)	16 to 20	110 to 120	60 to 65
			12 to 16	110 to 130	65 to 80
Adult	98.6 ± 1	60 to 100 (Mean, 75)	12 to 20	100 to 130	60 to 85
Older adult	97.6 ± 1	60 to 100 (Mean, 75)	12 to 20	120 to 140	70 to 85

the temperature again in 60 minutes, even though the physician may have ordered temperature assessment every 4 hours.

> *Action Alert!* Increase the frequency of vital sign assessment if the client is at risk for a complication or a change in condition. Frequent assessment is indicated for fever, infection, recent surgery, chest pain, or shortness of breath.

COMMUNICATING VITAL SIGNS

Whether your client's vital signs are normal or abnormal, you are responsible for communicating your findings to other health care providers. Document the vital signs in the client's nursing record in a manner that is readily available. A typical graphic record is easily read and shows trends in vital signs, and it may be used even where records are computerized. (Figure 7-1)

> *Action Alert!* Verbally report significantly abnormal vital signs or changes to the nurse in charge or to the physician. Changes in vital signs are key parameters for making changes in the treatment plan.

Additionally the client and family may request information about vital signs. Be prepared to provide health teaching about how to measure and interpret vital signs. Many clients must track vital signs as part of their ongoing health maintenance. For example, a client who takes an antihypertensive medication may need to routinely take blood pressure measurements.

TEMPERATURE

Body temperature is measured to monitor for signs of inflammation or infection, but it may also be used to monitor for problems in thermoregulation. It reflects the balance between heat produced in the body and heat lost from the body. In a healthy individual, the body effectively maintains a balance between heat production and heat loss. **Thermogenesis** is the generation of heat from the chemical reactions that take place in cellular activity. In the presence of inflammation or infection, these chemical reactions accelerate, causing a rise in body temperature. Heat is dispersed from the body through radiation, conduction, convection, and evaporation, a process called **thermolysis** (see Chapter 27).

Although the average normal body temperature is 98.6° F (37° C), heat production varies with the **basal metabolic rate,** which represents the amount of energy needed to maintain essential basic body functions, expressed as calories per hour per square meter of body surface. Heat production increases with muscular activity, stimulation of the sympathetic nervous system (which produces epinephrine and norepinephrine), and stimulation of the thyroid gland (which produces thyroxine). Thus normal body temperature varies by approximately plus or minus 1 degree.

Understanding Thermoregulation

Thermoregulation balances heat production and heat loss to maintain a constant body temperature in a range between 96.8° F and 99.4° F (36° C and 37.4° C). The body temperature has a rhythmic biological variation throughout each 24-hour period, which is called circadian rhythm. For most people, temperature is lowest in the morning because the basal metabolic rate slows during the inactivity of sleep. In the afternoon, the increased activity of the day may raise the temperature by about 1° F. Stress, strong emotions, and exercise

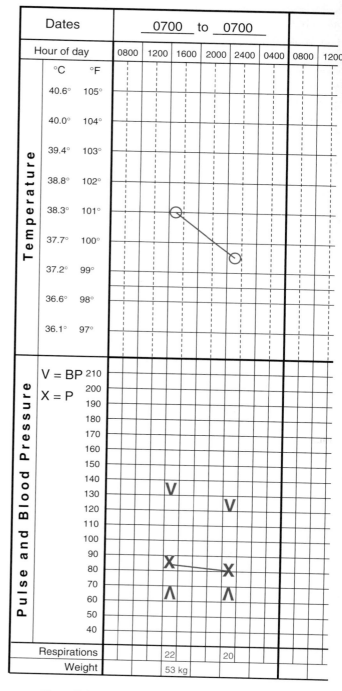

Figure 7-1. An example of how to chart vital signs.

can increase cellular activity and thus also raise temperature within a normal pattern of variation.

Other factors can alter temperature as well. For example, estrogen causes women to have a slightly higher average temperature than men. Newborns, children, and older adults have a reduced capacity for thermoregulation. A cold environment speeds up heat loss, and a warm environment slows heat loss. Internally, infection and inflammation can raise body temperature through their pyogenic influence on the medulla of the brain.

Physiological compensatory mechanisms are involuntary and intended to help maintain a normal core temperature in the body. The autonomic nervous system helps to keep the core body temperature at 98.6° F (37° C) through receptors in the skin, abdomen, and spinal cord. These receptors sense internal and external temperature changes and send this information through the nervous system to the hypothalamic region of the brain. The data are integrated, and the appropriate effector mechanisms (such as blood vessels, sweat glands, and skeletal muscles) are activated.

The cardiovascular system plays an important role in maintaining body temperature through its vast network of blood vessels. An increase in body temperature causes blood vessels near the skin surface to dilate, a process called vasodilation. By bringing an increased volume of warmed blood to the skin surface, vasodilation enhances heat loss. In contrast, a decrease in body temperature causes vasoconstriction, which keeps warmed blood closer to the center of the body, thus maintaining its core temperature. By insulating the body, fat helps to control heat loss as well.

Keep in mind that the body's cells function within a relatively narrow range of normal temperatures (Figure 7-2). However, the cells can tolerate a change in temperature for a short time and may even benefit from it. For example, the increased heat of a fever is thought to benefit the immune system and increase its activity. However, prolonged, extreme temperature elevation (hyperthermia) or reduction (hypothermia) can lead to tissue damage and death. High temperatures damage cells by inactivating proteins and enzymes. Low temperatures damage cells when ice crystals form and puncture the cell membranes.

We assist the body to maintain a normal body temperature by changing our behavior; for example, we may move to the shade, regulate the thermostat, or remove extra clothes. Naturally, if a client cannot alter his temperature, is unconscious, or is unaware of the environment, you may need to intervene and help with temperature regulation. Even when clients can regulate temperature normally, your assessment of their temperature offers vital information about their condition.

Measuring Temperature

Temperature can be measured using either the Fahrenheit or the centigrade (also called Celsius) scale (see Figure 7-2). The Fahrenheit scale has long been the standard in English-speaking countries and continues to be in common use despite the movement of the scientific community to the centigrade scale. A hospital may use the centigrade scale, and you may need to discuss this with clients who are used to the more commonly understood Fahrenheit scale. Any reading can be converted from one scale to the other by completing a simple calculation (Box 7-1). Depending on your client's needs, you may use a

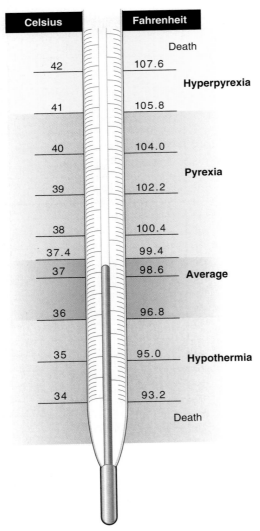

Figure 7-2. Range of normal body temperature and alterations in body temperature on the Celsius and Fahrenheit scales.

Box 7-1 **Conversion Formulas for Fahrenheit and Celsius Scales**

CONVERTING FROM FAHRENHEIT TO CELSIUS

- Subtract 32 from the Fahrenheit reading.
- Multiply the resulting number by 5/9.

For example, the following formula shows the conversion of 98.6° F to Celsius:

$$98.6° F - 32 = 66.6 \times \tfrac{5}{9} = 37° C$$

CONVERTING FROM CELSIUS TO FAHRENHEIT

- Multiply the Celsius reading by 9/5 (or 1.8).
- Add 32 to the resulting number.

For example, the following formula shows the conversion of 37° C to Fahrenheit:

$$37° C \times \tfrac{9}{5} = 66.6 + 32 = 98.6° F$$

glass thermometer, an electronic thermometer, a tympanic thermometer, chemical dots, or an intravenous catheter to measure temperature.

Glass Thermometer.

Most glass thermometers are calibrated hollow cylinders with a liquid-filled bulb at the base. When the liquid is heated, it expands and rises in the hollow tube. Temperature is measured by the height of the column of liquid. The most common liquids are mercury and alcohol.

For infection-control purposes, glass thermometers are color coded to signify rectal or oral use (Figure 7-3, *A*). The rectal thermometer is always red tipped, and it always has a blunt tip to avoid trauma to delicate membranes.

Glass thermometers are no longer commonly used in health care settings. Although they are inexpensive, easy to use, and easily disinfected, and can be used multiple times for the same client, glass thermometers frequently contain mercury, which is poisonous. If the glass breaks, the mercury must be recovered according to strict guidelines established by the Occupational Safety and Health Administration (OSHA). Furthermore, this type of ther-

mometer cannot be shared between clients, its small calibrations can be difficult to read, and it can take 5 to 7 minutes to get an accurate reading. The readings are recorded to the nearest 0.2° F.

The use of medical devices that contain mercury, such as thermometers and sphygmomanometers, is being reduced or eliminated. Mercury-filled thermometers are being removed from retail stores. All forms of mercury are toxic to humans, but organic forms (i.e., methylated mercury) are much more toxic than the inorganic forms used in medical devices. However, if improperly disposed of, the inorganic form changes to an organic form. Disposal of mercury from medical facilities accounts for about 10% of the mercury contamination in our environment. Short-term exposure to high levels of mercury can produce severe respiratory irritation, digestive disturbances, and marked renal damage. With long-term exposure, mercury is a neurotoxin.

Action Alert! Do not attempt to clean up a mercury spill yourself. Call the hazardous waste disposal team at your agency.

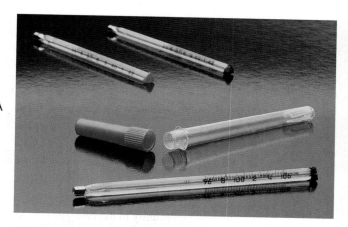

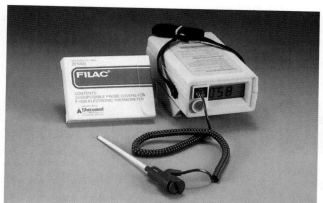

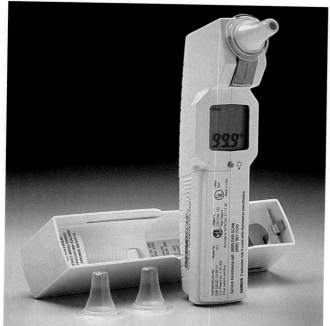

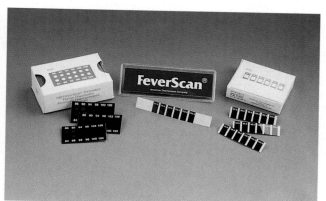

Figure 7-3. Types of thermometers. **A,** Glass thermometers. **B,** Electronic thermometer. **C,** Tympanic thermometer. **D,** Disposable temperature strips. (**A** courtesy American Diagnostic Corporation, Smithtown, NY; **B** through **D** courtesy Medline Industries, Mundelein, IL.)

Electronic Thermometer. You are more likely to use an electronic thermometer that has a heat-sensitive probe attached by a thin wire to a battery-powered control unit (Figure 7-3, *B*). It offers a convenient, safe, accurate, and fast method for measuring temperature. The reading is quickly displayed on the unit and is easy to read. Typically, the unit beeps when the measurement is complete. Readings can be measured to the nearest 0.1°.

An electronic thermometer can be used for oral, axillary, or rectal temperature measurements, and it can be used with multiple clients. The use of disposable probe covers (also called sheaths) avoids the transmission of microorganisms between clients. For visually impaired clients, electronic thermometers are available that give auditory temperature readings. The disadvantages of electronic thermometers are their high cost and the need for regular maintenance.

Tympanic Thermometer. The tympanic thermometer was designed to measure temperature quickly and easily in clients who cannot easily hold a thermometer in their mouth. A heat-sensitive probe is placed into the ear canal to measure the temperature of the blood in the tympanic membrane (Figure 7-3, *C*). Readily visible measurements are displayed on the unit and reflect temperature to the nearest 0.1°. The unit can be used for multiple clients because the disposable probe covers avoid the transmission of microorganisms. Tympanic thermometers are more costly than glass thermometers and must be regularly checked for accuracy.

Temperature Strip and Chemical Dot. A temperature strip or chemical dot is an inexpensive, disposable product for measuring temperature. Although the strip or dot lacks precision, it can ensure infection control for a client in an isolation unit, and it is easy to use at home (Figure 7-3, *D*). As the client's temperature rises or falls, the strip or dot changes color.

The disadvantage of the strip or dot is that it gives less accurate and variable readings. In addition, sweating can alter the contact between the device and the client's skin, and this change may alter the temperature reading.

Core Body Temperature. Core body temperature can be directly measured using a urinary bladder probe or a central intravenous catheter. The central venous catheter uses a thermistor attached to the central line. It is more accurate and reliable for measuring core temperature, but it is used only for clients in intensive care units because of the potential complications of infection and air emboli. Both methods require expertise in using the device.

Routes for Measuring Temperature

The oral, rectal, axillary, and tympanic sites for measuring body temperature have been chosen because these sites approximate the core body temperature (Procedure 7-1) and provide reasonably consistent readings for most clinical purposes. Core body temperature is the temperature at the center

Text continued on p. 113

PROCEDURE 7-1 ASSESSING TEMPERATURE

TIME TO ALLOW
Novice: 2 min.
Expert: 2 min.

We measure body temperature primarily to detect inflammation and infection, and it can be an independent or a dependent nursing action. However, because some disorders and medications can have an effect on body temperature, its measurement can give important information about a client's health.

DELEGATION GUIDELINES
The measurement and recording of body temperature is a simple, low-risk procedure that you may delegate to a nursing assistant. Be sure the assistant indicates the route by which the temperature is to be taken. You remain responsible for your knowledge of the temperature measurement and your assessment of changes in the client's temperature.

EQUIPMENT NEEDED
- Thermometer (oral, rectal, electronic, tympanic)
- Water-soluble lubricant
- Disposable probe covers
- Clean gloves and tissues
- Watch with a sweep second hand

1. Follow preliminary guidelines for nursing procedures (see inside front cover).

2. Select an appropriate route, and obtain a corresponding thermometer. You may choose the oral, rectal, axillary, or tympanic route, whichever is safest and most convenient for the client. For consistency of results, use the same route for succeeding temperature measurements.

3. Prepare the thermometer.

GLASS THERMOMETER
a. Ensure that the glass thermometer (see Fig. 7-3, *A*) is clean and free of defects. Follow agency policy for storage and cleaning. A common practice is to provide each client with an individual thermometer. The thermometer is cleansed with an alcohol wipe between uses, wiping

from the stem to the bulb using a rotating motion. Any disinfectant should be thoroughly rinsed away in cool water before use. *Hot water will expand the liquid and can break the glass. Consider covering the thermometer with a disposable sheath to protect both you and the client, and use a clean sheath for each measurement (see illustration). A well-designed sheath inverts on itself as it is removed, thus preventing you from contact with oral mucus. The sheath also helps contain the glass if the thermometer breaks.*

b. Ensure that the liquid is confined to the bulb (i.e., the thermometer registers $\leq 96°$ F or $\leq 35.6°$ C). Hold the thermometer firmly by the tip. Using a flicking wrist motion, shake the thermometer. This action forces the liquid into the bulb. Check the reading on the thermometer to ensure that it is below body temperature. *Hold the thermometer with the numbers positioned to be read from left to right. Slightly rotate the thermometer toward yourself until the column of liquid is visible. Most thermometers have a white or yellow background to increase visibility of the liquid. You should be viewing the liquid against the background.*

ELECTRONIC OR TYMPANIC THERMOMETER

a. If using an electronic thermometer (see Figure 7-3, *B*), turn on the device by removing the probe. If using a tympanic thermometer (see Figure 7-3, *C*), turn on the unit.

b. Place a disposable sheath or cover over the probe (see illustration). *A probe cover prevents transmission of microorganisms between clients.*

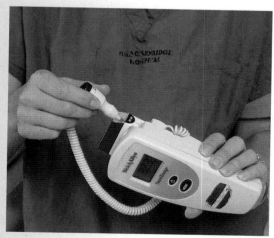

Step 3b. Placing a disposable sheath, or cover, on the probe.

4. Measure the temperature.

ORAL ROUTE

a. Place the thermometer or electronic probe under the client's tongue, in the sublingual pocket next to the frenulum linguae, for 2 to 4 minutes or according to your facil-

ity's policy (glass thermometer) or until unit beeps (electronic thermometer). *Although most glass thermometers are calibrated to register in 1 minute, waiting at least 2 minutes results in 2 more reliable measurement.*

b. Have the client close his or her mouth and hold the thermometer in place with the lips (see illustration). Make sure the bulb remains in direct contact with the sublingual tissue. *Warn the client not to bite on the thermometer, especially a glass one, because the glass could break.*

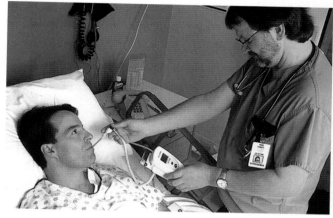

Step 4b. Holding the probe in place for oral temperature assessment.

RECTAL ROUTE

a. Position the client in the side-lying (left Sims') position, and drape for privacy. *The left Sims' position allows easy access to the client's anus. Appropriate draping helps to minimize the client's discomfort.*

b. Put on clean gloves. *Taking a rectal temperature has a higher risk of contact with fluid from mucous membranes.*

c. Lubricate the bulb of the thermometer with water-soluble jelly. *Lubrication prevents rectal trauma.*

d. Gently insert the thermometer about 1.5 inches into the rectum. *Angle the thermometer toward the client's umbilicus during insertion.*

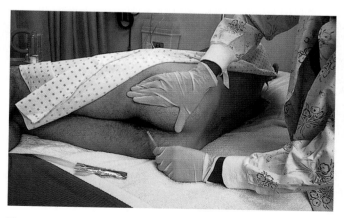

Step 4e. Holding the probe in place for rectal temperature assessment.

PROCEDURE 7-1   ASSESSING TEMPERATURE—CONT'D

e. Hold the thermometer in place for 2 to 4 minutes or according to your facility's policy (see illustration, p. 111).

AXILLARY ROUTE

a. Place the thermometer in the center of the client's axilla, and leave it in place for 8 to 10 minutes or according to your facility's policy (see illustration). *To secure the thermometer and make sure the bulb of the thermometer remains in contact with the axillary skin, have the client cross his or her arm across the chest.*

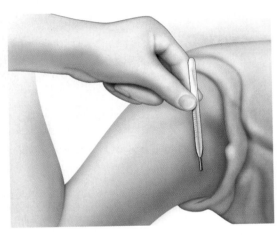

Step 4a. Axillary. Placing the probe for axillary temperature assessment.

TYMPANIC ROUTE

a. Pull the client's auricle back, and then gently obtain the temperature measurement (see illustration). *For a child, pull the auricle down and back. For an adult, pull the auricle up and back. Doing so will straighten the ear canal and help to direct the probe toward the tympanic membrane.*

b. Place the probe into the ear canal, pointing the tip of the probe toward the client's nose. *The probe must be directed toward the tympanic membrane. Errors in measurement occur when it is directed toward the wall of the ear canal.*

c. Holding the probe steady, quickly press the activation button.

d. A buzzer will sound when the temperature has been measured. *A tympanic reading usually takes only 2 or 3 seconds.*

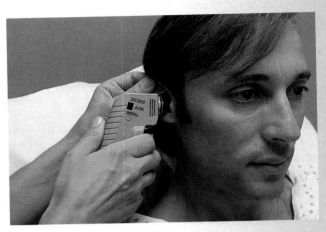

Step 4a. Tympanic. Inserting the tympanic probe into the ear canal.

5. Read the temperature measurement.

a. After an appropriate time or after the electronic thermometer beeps, remove the thermometer from the client's mouth, axilla, ear canal, or anus.

b. After removing a glass rectal thermometer, wipe it with a tissue, using a rotating motion from stem to bulb. Discard the tissue, or remove the disposable sheath. *This cleaning pattern moves from clean to contaminated areas of the thermometer and prevents transmission of microorganisms.*

c. Read the temperature measurement indicated on the thermometer. If using an electronic thermometer, obtain the measurement, and then discard the probe cover directly into the trash by pressing the release button. *This prevents transmission of microorganisms.*

6. Document the client's temperature in his medical record as soon as you obtain the reading. *Note whether the reading was oral, rectal, or axillary by writing oral, R, or Ax next to the measurement. Report an abnormal temperature to a charge nurse or physician. A normal oral temperature is 98.6° F (37° C), a normal rectal temperature is 99.6° F (37.5° C), and a normal axillary temperature is 97.6° F (36.5° C).*

PEDIATRIC CONSIDERATIONS

Rectal temperatures are taken only when there is no other feasible route. Rectal temperatures can cause rectal perforation in young infants and are especially contraindicated in the neonate, the immunosuppressed child, or the child with rectal surgery, diarrhea, or a bleeding disorder. If it is necessary to take a rectal temperature insert a well-lubricated thermometer no more than the length of the bulb.

of the body or in the deep tissues of the body (e.g., in the cranium and thoracic, abdominal, and pelvic cavities). It is more constant than skin temperature. The traditional method for temperature measurement in adults is to place the thermometer (glass or electronic) under the tongue in the pocket created by the frenulum linguae.

To accurately reflect the core body temperature by the oral route, you must consider factors that affect the temperature of the mucous membranes. The client must be able to follow directions and breathe with the mouth closed. Nasal oxygen cannulae and nasogastric tubes do not seem to affect the reading adversely. However, if the client has just eaten, ingested fluids, or smoked a cigarette, wait 15 to 30 minutes before obtaining the temperature reading. Avoid using this method for any client who could be injured by the thermometer, who cannot breathe with a closed mouth, or who cannot follow simple instructions.

The rectal or axillary route is sometimes used for infants and for small children who cannot hold a thermometer safely in their mouths. It is also used for adults who are unconscious or confused, have respiratory difficulty, or have had recent oral surgery. However, this route should be used with caution, especially with uncooperative or combative clients. The rectal route is contraindicated for clients who have had rectal or perineal surgery or injury, and for clients who have severe hemorrhoids. It is also not used with cardiac clients because the thermometer can stimulate the vagus nerve, slowing the heart rate. The axillary route is less invasive than the rectal route but offers less accurate readings because it measures only surface body heat. It is contraindicated if the client is uncooperative or combative.

The tympanic membrane thermometer is a fast, safe, easy, and noninvasive method that can be used for children and adults. It is reliable and accurate when used properly. However, it is contraindicated for clients who have had a recent ear infection or ear surgery.

After obtaining a client's temperature by any route, document your reading in the client's medical record. Temperature readings are usually charted on a graph with connecting lines to illustrate trends over time (see Figure 7-1). Rectal and axillary temperatures are charted with the designations R and Ax, respectively. Document other factors associated with temperature, such as diaphoresis or chills, in your nurse's progress notes.

PULSE

A pulse wave is created throughout the arterial system with each contraction of the ventricle of the heart (systole). It is best felt with the tip of a finger at a point where the artery is close to the surface and rests against a bone. Thus the pulse is a rhythmic fluctuation of fluid pressure against the arterial wall created by the pumping action of the heart muscle. Between contractions, the heart muscle rests (diastole), and the pulse wave disappears.

Understanding Pulse Characteristics

The characteristics of the pulse are described as rate, rhythm, and strength. Examining these characteristics gives you infor-

mation about the strength of the myocardial contraction, its rhythm, the volume of blood in the vascular system, and the patency and resiliency of blood vessels. Abnormal pulse patterns are described on the basis of changes in the client's heart rate, rhythm, and strength (Table 7-2).

Rate. The pulse rate of a normal adult varies from 60 to 90 beats per minute, although the range of normal may extend from 50 to 100. A heart rate less than 60 beats per minute is called **bradycardia.** A heart rate greater than 100 is termed **tachycardia.** Rate cannot be viewed as the sole criterion for normal, however; instead, it must be considered together with any signs and symptoms that might produce, or be produced by, an abnormal rate. The heart rate is primarily controlled by the two opposing parts of the autonomic nervous system. The sympathetic nervous system increases the heart rate, and the parasympathetic system decreases it. Both of these changes stem largely from the body's response to the cells' need for oxygen.

Any psychological stressor (producing anxiety, fear, or anger) or physiological stressor (such as exercise or a loss of blood) causes the body's compensatory mechanisms to launch a fight-or-flight response. Information is relayed to the cardiac center in the medulla, and the sympathetic nervous system is stimulated to produce changes in the pulse.

Other factors can influence the pulse rate as well (Table 7-3, p. 114). For example, infants and children have a higher basal metabolic rate and thus a slightly higher pulse rate than

Table 7-2	Pulse Patterns
Pattern	**Description**
Pulsus paradoxus	A regular rhythm of an increase and then a decrease in the pulse amplitude associated with respirations (may also be heard on the blood pressure measurement). May be a sign of a serious cardiac or respiratory condition.
Pulsus alternans	A regular rhythm with a pattern of a strong normal pulse followed by a weak pulse (every other beat is strong). One of a group of signs that indicate a failing heart.
Pulse bigeminy	Cardiac arrhythmia results in an irregular rhythm with a pattern of a strong normal pulse (beat originating in the sinus node) followed quickly by an early, weak pulse (beat originating elsewhere in the heart). May progress to ventricular fibrillation and death.
Sinus rhythm	The electrical impulse is generated in the normal pacemaker (sinus node). Usually a regular rhythm with a rate between 60 and 100 beats per minute for an adult.
Tachycardia	Regular rhythm with a rate higher than 90 to 100 beats per minute for an adult. Decreases cardiac output by decreasing ventricular filling time. If prolonged, may lead to shock.
Bradycardia	Regular rhythm with a rate less than 50 to 60 beats per minute for an adult. Rate is insufficient to meet the demands for oxygen. May lead to cardiac standstill.
Sinus arrhythmia	Slightly irregular rhythm that speeds up and slows down with respirations. Originates in the sinus node. Does not usually affect cardiac output or vital signs.

Table 7-3	Factors That Influence Pulse Rate
Factor	**Influence**
Age	Infants and children have a slightly higher heart rate than adolescents and adults. As the client ages, the pulse rate gradually decreases.
Emotions and stress	Anxiety, fear, anger, and pain stimulate the sympathetic nervous system and cause the pulse rate to increase. Relaxation stimulates the parasympathetic nervous system and decreases the rate.
Exercise	Exercise increases the oxygen demand, and the rate increases. A conditioned athlete can have a slow but effective resting heart rate.
Rest and sleep	During rest and sleep, oxygen needs decline, and the rate decreases.
Temperature	Hyperthermia and fever increase the heart rate. Hypothermia decreases the heart rate.
Dehydration, shock, and hemorrhage	Decreases in blood volume or cardiac output result in an increased pulse rate because of sympathetic stimulation.
Hypoxia and hypoxemia	When oxygen levels in the blood decrease, the heart rate increases in an attempt to compensate.
Vomiting	Vomiting stimulates the vagus nerve and causes the pulse rate to drop.
Head injury and increased intracranial pressure	Head injuries cause the pulse to decrease.
Electrolyte balance	Changes in potassium and calcium affect the pulse rate and rhythm.
Medications	Certain medications cause the heart rate to increase, such as adrenalin and atropine, and others decrease the pulse, such as digitalis.

adults. Some medications (such as digitalis) slow the heart rate, and others (such as amphetamines) increase it. Low blood pressure, dehydration, fever, and pain can each stimulate the sympathetic nervous system. In contrast, rest and relaxation can stimulate the parasympathetic nervous system.

Rhythm. Normally the myocardial contraction is initiated in the sinus node in the atrium and produces a normal rate and regular rhythm. However, chemical disturbances, such as inadequate oxygen in the heart muscle and electrolyte imbalance, may cause the heart to beat irregularly. Some children, and even some adults, have a variation in rhythm in which the heart rate increases with inhalation and decreases with exhalation. Even though this is normal, all irregular rhythms should be reported to the nurse in charge or to a physician.

Strength. The quality of the pulse reflects the strength of the cardiac contraction and the volume of blood available in the vascular system. A normal contraction of the heart muscle combined with an adequate blood volume will create a strong pulse wave. A weak heart contraction combined with a low blood volume will create a weak, thready pulse wave. An increased heart contraction combined with a large blood volume will create a full, bounding pulse wave.

A number of conditions can alter the strength of a client's pulse. For example, heart failure can cause the

strength of the heart's contraction to vary on alternating beats while the rhythm remains regular, a condition called pulsus alternans.

You also may detect an abnormality (in adults) in which the strength of the client's pulse wave increases during inhalation and decreases back to normal during exhalation, a condition called pulsus paradoxus. This can also be heard when measuring blood pressure. Finally, the nervous system can alter the strength of the client's pulse. Stimulation of the sympathetic nervous system increases the force of myocardial contraction, increasing the amount of blood ejected from the heart with each beat (stroke volume) and creating a large pulse. Stimulation of the parasympathetic nervous system decreases the force of contraction, thus decreasing stroke volume and creating a small pulse.

Measuring Pulse

Significant clinical decisions, such as the administration of medications, are based on pulse values. To facilitate accurate pulse measurement, you should apply light pressure over the client's artery with the pads of one of your two middle fingers. Press firmly enough to detect the pulse wave without occluding the artery. If you use your thumb or index finger, you may feel your own pulse rather than the client's (Procedure 7-2).

Peripheral Pulses. Peripheral pulse sites are located where arteries lie over bony surfaces. Nine sites are available to assess peripheral pulses: the carotid artery in the neck; the brachial, radial, and ulnar arteries in the upper extremities; and the femoral, popliteal, dorsalis pedis, and posterior tibial arteries in the lower extremities (Figure 7-4, p. 116). The temporal artery can also be used, but it is not easily palpated in all people.

The most common site for assessing the quality, rate, and rhythm of the pulse is the radial artery. The radial artery, on the inner surface of the wrist on the thumb side, is easily accessed and palpated. Other sites (e.g., at the cardiac apex and the carotid and femoral arteries) are used for special purposes. In an emergency or during cardiopulmonary resuscitation (CPR), you may assess the client's heart rate using the carotid or femoral pulse in an adult or the brachial pulse in an infant.

Other pulses also have specific uses. The brachial artery, located in the antecubital fossa (the inner aspect of the elbow), is used for blood pressure assessment. The popliteal artery, located behind the knee, can also be used for blood pressure assessment. The dorsalis pedis and posterior tibial arteries are used to assess the status of the peripheral vascular system rather than for counting the rate and assessing the rhythm of the heart.

No matter how you measure a client's pulse, always document your findings immediately in the client's medical record (see Figure 7-1). If you obtained an apical pulse, note it with an A. Place other information about the client's pulse in your nurse's notes or a progress report.

Apical Pulse. The **apical pulse** is the heart rate counted at the apex of the heart on the anterior chest. If a client has weak or ineffective heart contractions, cardiac disease, an irregular heart rhythm, or a history of taking cardiac medications that

PROCEDURE 7-2 ASSESSING RADIAL AND APICAL PULSES

TIME TO ALLOW
Novice: 1 min.
Expert: 1 min.

A person's pulse reflects the function of his heart and the condition of his arterial system. Usually, we measure a client's radial pulse in his wrist. In some cases, however, we need to measure the apical pulse instead of or in addition to the radial pulse.

DELEGATION GUIDELINES

The measurement and recording of the radial and apical pulse rates is a simple procedure that you may delegate to a nursing assistant who has received training in this technique. Training should include careful instructions about specific findings that necessitate your immediate notification. You remain responsible for knowledge of the pulse measurement and your assessment of a client with any reported irregularities.

EQUIPMENT NEEDED

- Stethoscope
- Watch with sweep second hand

1. Follow preliminary guidelines for nursing procedures (see inside front cover).

2. Prepare the client for pulse measurement.
a. Place the client in a comfortable position. Have the client relax. *If the client is not relaxed, wait 10 or 15 minutes before obtaining the pulse reading. This will enhance the accuracy of your reading by preventing false elevations caused by stress or anxiety.*

3. Measure the pulse.

RADIAL PULSE MEASUREMENT

a. Place the client's arm across his or her abdomen or in another relaxed, comfortable position. Locate the client's radial pulse (see illustration).
b. Place the pads of your middle fingers on the inside of the client's wrist. *Do not use your thumb or first finger to palpate the pulse because they have pulses of their own.*
c. Compress the radial artery firmly against the underlying bone.

d. Occlude the pulse, and then gradually release pressure until the pulse becomes palpable. *Occluding and then restoring the pulse verifies its presence.*
e. Assess the quality and rhythm of the client's radial pulse as you count the pulse. *If the radial pulse is irregular or weak, you will need to assess the client's apical pulse. If the radial pulse is regular and of normal strength, count the number of beats for 30 seconds and multiply by 2. If it is irregular, count for a full minute. For rapid approximation, you can count for 6 ($\times$10), 10 ($\times$6) or 15 ($\times$4) seconds. The most accurate count requires counting for a full minute.*

APICAL PULSE MEASUREMENT

a. Place the client in the supine position and locate the apical pulse at the fifth intercostal space to the left of the midclavicular line on the client's anterior thorax (see illustration). *If you have difficulty hearing, a left-lying position or*

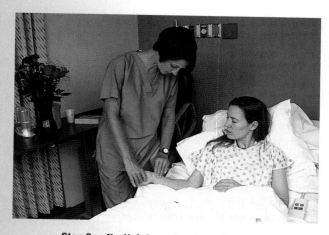

Step 3a. Radial. Locating the radial pulse.

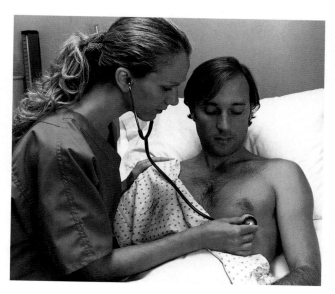

Step 3a. Apical. Locating the apical pulse.

a forward-leaning position (with the client seated) enhances transmission of heart sounds through the chest wall.

b. Keep the client covered appropriately, exposing the chest only as needed.

c. If necessary, lift a female client's breast to find her apical pulse. *Finding the correct anatomic location of the apex increases the accuracy of the apical pulse measurement.*

d. Place the diaphragm of your stethoscope firmly against the client's chest. Avoid rubbing it against clothing or linens. *The diaphragm is used for high-pitched sounds, such as heart tones. Firm skin contact enhances sound transmission. Clothing may cause interfering noises.*

e. Assess the rate and rhythm of the client's apical pulse. *The apical pulse is the most likely to reveal irregularities of heart rhythm. Count the apical pulse for 1 full minute. This will increase the accuracy of your reading.*

4. Document the rate and any abnormality of rhythm or strength as soon as you obtain the reading. Report an abnormal pulse to a charge nurse or physician.

PEDIATRIC CONSIDERATIONS

An apical pulse is recommended for an infant or a child younger than 2 years.

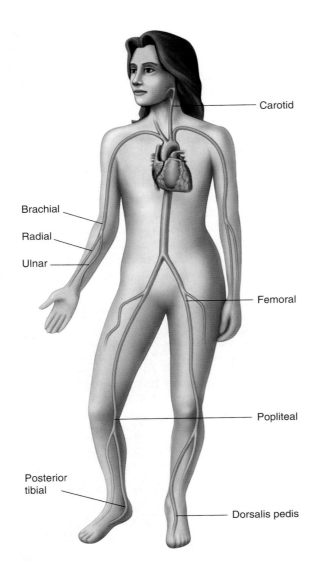

Figure 7-4. The eight sites commonly used to assess peripheral pulses.

Carotid

Brachial

Radial

Ulnar

Femoral

Popliteal

Posterior tibial

Dorsalis pedis

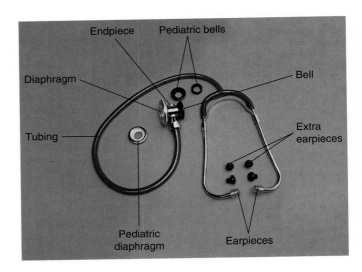

Figure 7-5. Components of a stethoscope.

Endpiece Pediatric bells

Diaphragm

Bell

Tubing

Extra earpieces

Pediatric diaphragm

Earpieces

affect the heart's action, you may not be able to palpate all cardiac contractions at the radial pulse site. For these clients, apical pulse measurement is a more accurate means of assessment. The apical pulse is preferred for infants and children because it can be difficult to palpate their peripheral pulses. You may choose to perform an apical pulse measurement instead of a radial pulse measurement on any client for whom you think it would be helpful.

To take an apical pulse you will need a stethoscope. A stethoscope consists of earpieces connected to two stiff tubes that join with a single flexible tube that ends in a sound-transmitting device that has a diaphragm on one side and a bell on the other (Figure 7-5). Place the earpieces into your ear canals with the ends pointing slightly toward your nose, not the back of your head. Use the bell to assess low-frequency sounds and the diaphragm to assess high-frequency sounds. Remember that a stethoscope does not

Table 7-4	Factors That Influence the Palpation of Pulses
Factor	**Influence**
Heart failure and myocardial infarction	Injury to the heart muscle impairs contractility and decreases the stroke volume. Ineffective contractions may be unable to transmit a palpable fluid wave to the peripheral pulse sites. Pulses may be difficult to palpate, and the client may have an apical-radial pulse deficit.
Artery patency	A clot in an artery causes the pulse to be absent distal to the occlusion.
Arteriosclerosis	Hardening and stiffening of the artery makes palpation more difficult.
Low blood volume	The client will have a weak, thready pulse that may be difficult to palpate.
High blood volume	The client will have an overly strong, bounding pulse.

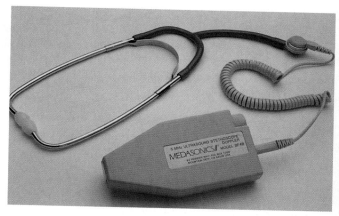

Figure 7-6. A Doppler ultrasound stethoscope. (Courtesy Medasonics, Inc., Newark, CA.)

magnify heart sounds. It simply focuses them into the end piece and eliminates outside sounds. To decrease the transmission of microorganisms, wipe the diaphragm and bell with alcohol between clients.

When you listen to the client's anterior chest, you will hear two sounds produced by a normal heart. The first heart sound, called S_1, results when the mitral and tricuspid valves close during systole. This creates the "lubb" of the "lubb-dupp" heart sound. It can be heard best at the apex of the heart, near the fifth intercostal space, just left of the midclavicular line. The second heart sound, called S_2, results when the aortic and pulmonic valves close during diastole. This creates the "dupp" of the "lubb-dupp" heart sound. It can be heard best at the base of the heart, by the second intercostal space, right or left of the sternal border. When assessing a client's apical pulse rate, count S_1 and S_2 together ("lubb-dupp") as one beat.

Apical-Radial Pulse. To gain further information about the effectiveness of the heart as a pump in the event of dysrhythmias and cardiac disease, take an apical-radial pulse to assess for a pulse deficit. When the apical pulse rate exceeds the radial pulse rate, the difference is described as a **pulse deficit.** To be accurate, both pulses must be counted simultaneously. Because it is difficult to count both pulses at the same time, work together with a colleague to assess apical-radial pulse. One of you auscultates the apical rate while the other palpates the radial pulse. Both of you start counting at the same time, count for a full minute, and compare your findings. The difference is documented as a pulse deficit.

Pulse Quality. Quality refers to the strength or weakness of the pulse. A weak pulse is caused by any condition that slows or restricts the blood flow, such as decreased blood volume, weak heart contractions, or partial obstruction of arteries (Table 7-4). For example, vasoconstriction can cause the artery to become so narrowed that the pulse wave is difficult to feel. Likewise, in shock, the blood volume may be reduced to a point at which you can no longer feel the pulse wave. In

contrast, in vasodilation and overhydration, the extra blood volume can make the pulses pronounced.

Additionally, to produce a palpable pulse, the wall of an artery must have enough elasticity to respond to the pulse wave. The more elastic the walls of the artery, the more easily the wave can distend the artery and create a pulse wave. The harder and stiffer the wall of the artery, the less the pulse wave can distend it. The result is a weak pulse that is difficult to palpate.

When you have trouble palpating a pulse wave, you may need to use a Doppler ultrasound stethoscope to assess the weakened pulse (Figure 7-6). By enhancing pulse sounds, it can also improve the accuracy of your assessment. The Doppler stethoscope can help you detect a pulse when you cannot palpate one. It may be especially helpful for a client who has total occlusion of an artery. To use the device, place the transducer over the artery while listening through the earpieces. A sensor picks up the arterial pulse wave and magnifies the sound, giving it a "whooshing" sound. Like any device used on multiple clients, the transducer should be cleaned between clients, following the manufacturer's directions.

RESPIRATION

To survive, the cells of the body must receive enough oxygen to meet their metabolic needs. They must also release carbon dioxide, the major byproduct of metabolism. As you know, breathing—also known as respiration—accomplishes these purposes.

Understanding Respiration

A person's respiratory rate and depth vary with the cellular demand for oxygen and with levels of carbon dioxide and hydrogen ions (pH) in the blood (see Chapter 33). Receptors throughout the body feed to the brain information about the level of oxygen available to cells. The brain, in turn, regulates the person's respiratory rate. For example, peripheral chemoreceptors located in the aorta and the carotid arteries are especially sensitive to low blood levels of oxygen (hypoxemia). Central chemoreceptors in the medulla are especially sensitive to high levels of carbon dioxide (hypercapnia) and changes in pH.

When these receptors sense a change in oxygen, carbon dioxide, and hydrogen ions, they communicate via the autonomic nervous system to the respiratory center in the medulla for integration. As a result, the rate, depth, rhythm, or effort of respiration may change. During rest and sleep, cells need less oxygen, and respirations become shallow, quiet, and slow.

Measuring Respirations

The act of breathing is primarily involuntary. In fact, people usually are not aware that they are breathing. When you measure respirations, you are assessing this natural, involuntary function. However, breathing can come under voluntary control as well. When a person concentrates on her breathing, the rate may change. Consequently, when you assess a client's respirations, you should do so when the client is not aware of your actions. This ensures that you will be assessing the client's natural respirations. To keep the client unaware of your assessment, try counting respirations just after you take the client's pulse, while still holding the wrist (Procedure 7-3). Count one cycle of inspiration and expiration as one breath. Make sure to assess the client's complete breathing pattern, including rate, rhythm, depth, and effort.

A quiet, easy respiration, with a rate between 12 and 20 breaths per minute in an adult at rest, is known as **eupnea.** A rate of more than 20 breaths per minute is called **tachypnea,** and a rate less than 12 breaths per minute is called **bradypnea.** Children normally have slightly higher respiratory rates than adults.

Normally, breathing has a regular rhythm with periodic sighing. Irregular breathing in an adult is often accompanied by dyspnea and can result from head injury, increased intracranial pressure, or cardiovascular dysfunction (Table 7-5). Report irregular breathing to the nurse in charge or a physician immediately. Infants and children normally have a slightly irregular pattern of breathing.

PROCEDURE 7-3 ASSESSING RESPIRATIONS

TIME TO ALLOW
Expert: 1 min.
Novice: 1 min.

Respiration is a largely involuntary process, but it may come under voluntary control at times. By assessing respirations without the client's knowledge, you can gain important information about the client's respiratory and cardiovascular systems.

DELEGATION GUIDELINES
The measurement and recording of the client's respiratory rate is a simple procedure that you may delegate to a nursing assistant who has received training in this technique. Training should include specific instructions about findings that necessitate your immediate notification. You must complete the full respiratory assessment if one is indicated (Chapter 33).

EQUIPMENT NEEDED
- Watch with a sweep second hand

---

1. Follow preliminary guidelines for nursing procedures (see inside front cover).

2. Make sure the client is relaxed and quiet. Make sure that the client's anterior thorax is easily visible and that the lungs can complete the full excursion of respiratory movement without hindrance. The client may be sitting or lying down. *If necessary, wait 10 or 15 minutes before counting respirations. Anxiety, discomfort, and exercise increase the rate and depth of respirations and may result in a false reading.*

3. Make sure the client does not know you are counting the respirations. *If aware, the client may alter the respirations or concentrate on them, which can alter the natural count. Many nurses simply continue holding a client's wrist after taking a pulse measurement. The client thinks the pulse measurement is still continuing while the nurse has begun counting respirations.*

4. Watch the rise and fall of the client's chest. Count each cycle of inhalation and exhalation as one breath. *If necessary, you may place your hand on the client's lower thorax or abdomen and palpate the movement.*

5. Count the client's respirations. *For an adult with a regular rhythm, count for 30 seconds, and multiply your result by 2. For an infant, a child, or an adult with an irregular rhythm, count for a full minute to obtain the most accurate reading. Infants and children normally have a slightly irregular rhythm.*

6. Document the respirations as soon as you obtain the reading. *Normal respirations are 12 to 20 per minute, regular, of moderate depth, and effortless.*

7. Report abnormal respirations to a charge nurse or physician.

Table 7-5 Breathing Patterns

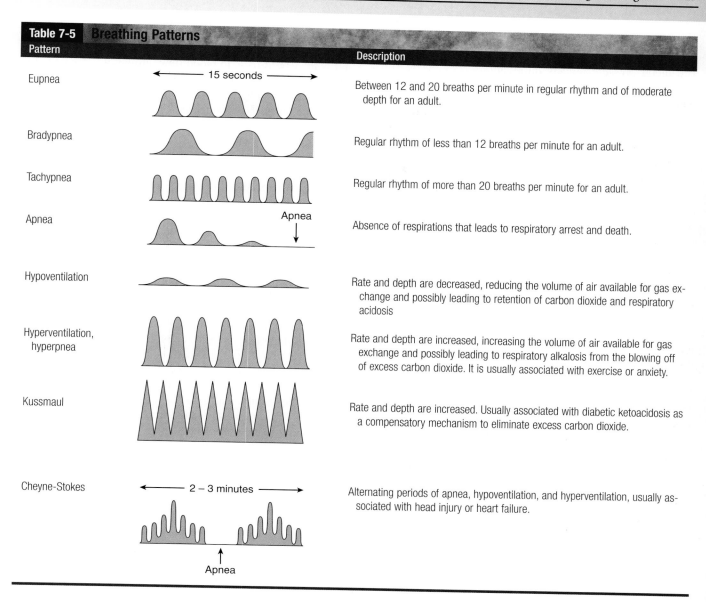

Pattern	Description
Eupnea	Between 12 and 20 breaths per minute in regular rhythm and of moderate depth for an adult.
Bradypnea	Regular rhythm of less than 12 breaths per minute for an adult.
Tachypnea	Regular rhythm of more than 20 breaths per minute for an adult.
Apnea	Absence of respirations that leads to respiratory arrest and death.
Hypoventilation	Rate and depth are decreased, reducing the volume of air available for gas exchange and possibly leading to retention of carbon dioxide and respiratory acidosis
Hyperventilation, hyperpnea	Rate and depth are increased, increasing the volume of air available for gas exchange and possibly leading to respiratory alkalosis from the blowing off of excess carbon dioxide. It is usually associated with exercise or anxiety.
Kussmaul	Rate and depth are increased. Usually associated with diabetic ketoacidosis as a compensatory mechanism to eliminate excess carbon dioxide.
Cheyne-Stokes	Alternating periods of apnea, hypoventilation, and hyperventilation, usually associated with head injury or heart failure.

The normal rhythmic volume of ventilation, called **tidal volume,** indicates the volume of air exchanged with each breath (about 500 cc with each breath). Because you will not be able to measure this volume while taking vital signs, you will need to estimate whether the client is exchanging an adequate volume of air with each breath. With normal depth, you will see a moderate amount of chest movement. With deep breathing, the chest expands fully. With shallow breathing, you may see little chest movement at all. Fast, deep breathing is known as hyperventilation or hyperpnea (see Chapter 39). Slow, shallow breathing is known as hypoventilation (see Chapter 33). Normal respiration includes periodic deep breaths known as sighing. Sighing is a protective mechanism that periodically expands unused alveoli and prevents their collapse.

Normal ventilation is effortless and quiet. It results from movements of the intercostal muscles and diaphragm.

Accessory muscles are not used. Exercise, shortness of breath (dyspnea), or respiratory diseases can lead to an exaggerated respiratory effort to breathe. Infants and children often flare their nostrils if they are having difficulty breathing.

On occasion, you may use a stethoscope to count a client's respirations, especially if they are shallow and slow. You also may use palpation to assess slow, shallow respirations. Place your hand on the client's lower chest or abdomen and feel for a slight rise and fall with each breath. No matter which assessment method you use, document the client's respirations immediately after obtaining the reading (see Figure 7-1). Other information about the client's respirations can be documented in your nurse's notes or a progress report. For example, you would document other indicators of respiratory status, such as pulse oximetry readings, a blue tinge to the client's skin or mucous membranes, or restlessness.

BLOOD PRESSURE

The blood pressure reflects information about the person's cardiovascular system. Blood pressure is the pressure (measured in millimeters of mercury) of the blood against the inner walls of the arteries. The pressure is recorded at the highest point of pressure and at the lowest point of pressure.

During myocardial contraction (systole), when blood is ejected from the heart and into the arteries of the body, blood pressure reaches its height. During diastole, when the heart rests, blood pressure falls to its baseline level. These values are known as **systolic blood pressure** and **diastolic blood pressure.** The difference between the systolic and diastolic blood pressures is the amount of pressure that produces the palpable pulse, and it is known as the **pulse pressure.** For an adult, systolic pressure normally varies from 100 to 130 mm Hg. Diastolic pressure normally varies from 60 to 85 mm Hg. Blood pressure is usually expressed and documented as a ratio of systolic over diastolic. Pulse pressure is normally about 30 to 50 mm Hg. By correlating a client's blood pressure readings with the history and other signs and symptoms, you can draw important conclusions about health changes.

Understanding Blood Pressure

Several factors combine to form the reading that you report as a person's blood pressure (Figure 7-7). One of the most important is the volume of blood in the person's vascular system. Less blood yields a lower blood pressure; more blood yields a higher blood pressure. A second factor is the action of the heart. An increased cardiac output raises blood pressure, and a decreased cardiac output lowers it. A third factor is the impediment to blood flow through the vascular system, known as **peripheral vascular resistance.** The diameter of the vessel and the viscosity of the blood create resistance. When vascular resistance increases, blood pressure rises, and vice versa.

Compensatory mechanisms involving the brain, kidneys, and adrenal glands combine with these factors to help keep blood pressure in the normal range. For example, when nervous system receptors (baroreceptors) in the great vessels sense a drop in blood pressure, they relay that information to the pressure center in the medulla. The sympathetic nervous system is then activated. In response, blood vessels constrict, and blood volume rises in response to sodium retention by the kidney and catecholamine (epinephrine and norepinephrine) production by the adrenal glands. When the parasympathetic nervous system is activated, a series of events occurs to cause the blood pressure to decrease.

Other factors that help to regulate blood pressure to some degree include the viscosity of blood; the velocity of blood flow; levels of oxygen and carbon dioxide in the blood; the client's age, emotions, pain, and exercise; time of day; stressors; and medication use (Table 7-6). Finally, hemorrhage, shock, dehydration, and blood loss reduce blood pressure by lowering the circulating blood volume. Renal failure and other causes of fluid overload can raise blood pressure. Head injuries can raise blood pressure as well, by interfering with regulatory mechanisms in the medulla.

Factors That Increase Blood Pressure

- Increased peripheral vascular resistance
  – Vasoconstriction
  – Increased blood viscosity

- Increased blood flow
  – Increased cardiac output
  – Increased blood volume

Factors That Decrease Blood Pressure

- Decreased peripheral vascular resistance
  – Vasodilation

- Decreased blood flow
  – Decreased cardiac output
  – Decreased blood volume

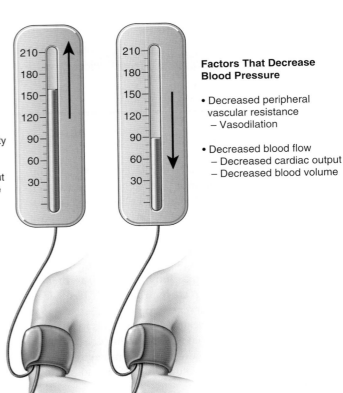

Figure 7-7. Physiological factors affecting blood pressure.

Measuring Blood Pressure

To measure a person's blood pressure, you will use a sphygmomanometer and a stethoscope to listen to a series of sounds, usually in the client's brachial artery. A sphygmomanometer includes a pressure manometer (Figure 7-8, p. 122), an inflatable cuff, and a pressure bulb. The manometer can function either with air (aneroid) or with mercury. Additionally, a variety of automatic blood pressure cuffs are available ranging from inexpensive over-the-counter models to high-tech models that can be programmed to inflate the cuff and check the blood pressure at preset intervals. Mercury-filled manometers are being phased out in many health care settings because of the mercury hazard. All devices record blood pressure standardized to millimeters of mercury (mm Hg). Before taking a person's blood pressure reading, you should calibrate the manometer to zero to avoid a false high reading.

To most accurately detect significant changes, blood pressure should be measured under constant conditions. The site for measurement (usually the upper arm) should be level with the left ventricle. The person should be in a comfortable, relaxed position without crossing the legs or constricting the abdomen. Box 7-2 (p. 122) can help you understand the possible effects of seemingly small variations in posture or body alignment.

You will also need to choose a blood pressure cuff of a size appropriate for your client (Procedure 7-4, p. 123). Cuffs come in newborn, infant, child, and adult sizes for both arm and leg measurements. The inflatable bladder inside the cuff should be long enough to almost encircle the limb. The cuff's width should be about two-thirds the length of the upper arm or thigh. A too-narrow cuff will produce a false high reading. A too-large cuff will produce a false low reading. Place the cuff directly over the client's brachial artery to ensure complete and equal compression.

To hear the sounds on which you will base your blood pressure measurement, you will need to know how to use a stethoscope correctly. Some of the sounds are very faint, and the possibility of error is considerable (Table 7-7, p. 125). To improve the sound, place the diaphragm of the stethoscope directly over the brachial artery. To ensure the accuracy of your measurement, insert the stethoscope earpieces so the tips point toward your nose, not the back of your head. Turn the television or radio down or off and, if necessary, ask people in the room to be quiet. You will need to practice and refine your technique for measuring blood pressure to make sure you can do it accurately.

The five distinct sounds you will listen for when measuring blood pressure are called **Korotkoff's sounds** or Korotkoff's phases. When blood is flowing freely through an artery or the artery is totally obstructed, no sound can be detected even with a stethoscope. However, if you partially constrict the artery, turbulent blood flow vibrates the walls of the artery and produces sound. Thus the blood pressure cuff is used to temporarily obstruct the artery. As you slowly release pressure from the cuff, the obstruction is gradually reduced,

Table 7-6	Factors That Influence Blood Pressure
Factor	**Influence**
Age	Newborns and infants have the lowest blood pressure. Blood pressure increases as age increases. It is highest in older adults because of a decrease in the elasticity of vessels, which causes an increase in resistance to blood flow. However, even in older adults a blood pressure above 130/85 should not be considered normal.
Stress and emotions	Anxiety, pain, tension, worry, and stress raise blood pressure by stimulating the sympathetic nervous system, which causes vasoconstriction and a resulting increased heart rate.
Medication	Medications that lower blood pressure include narcotics, tranquilizers, hypnotics, diuretics, antihypertensives, and certain cardiac medications (particularly vasodilators). Medications that raise blood pressure include antihistamines, estrogen, and corticosteroids (glucocorticoids and mineralocorticoids).
Diurnal variation	Blood pressure is typically lowest in the early morning, with decreased activity, and highest in the afternoon or evening, with increased activity.
Sex	After puberty, males tend to have higher blood pressure than females. After menopause, women tend to have higher blood pressure than men of the same age.
Environment	A hot environment can lower blood pressure by causing vasodilation. A cold environment can raise it by causing vasoconstriction.
Exercise	Blood pressure increases with activity and exercise because the sympathetic nervous system responds to the body's increased need for oxygen.
Body position	Blood pressure is lowest in the recumbent position. It is slightly higher in the standing position because of sympathetic nervous system stimulation.
Right versus left arm	About one fourth of the population has a difference of 10 ($\pm$5) mm Hg between the right and left arms.
Arm versus leg	There is a difference of 10 to 40 mm Hg in systolic blood pressure between measurements taken using the arm and measurements taken using the leg.
Vasodilation	Parasympathetic nervous system stimulation causes blood vessels to increase in lumen diameter, thus lowering blood pressure. This may happen in response to warm temperatures, fever, and relaxation, for example.
Vasoconstriction	Sympathetic nervous system stimulation causes blood vessels to decrease in lumen diameter, thus raising blood pressure. This may happen in response to cold temperatures, for example.
Head injury	Injuries to the head and increased intracranial pressure result in increased blood pressure.
Reduced blood volume	Blood pressure decreases if the circulatory system contains an inadequate volume of blood, as from low cardiac output, hemorrhage, or shock.
Increased blood volume	Too much fluid in the cardiovascular system increases blood pressure.

THE STATE OF NURSING RESEARCH: Blood Pressure Accuracy

Box 7-2

What Are the Issues?

Cardiovascular disease is a major cause of death and disability. Untreated hypertension can lead to vessel damage, stroke, and heart attack. Blood pressure measurements reflect cardiovascular integrity, and blood pressure screening is one way to identify persons with hypertension. It is important that the blood pressure reading be accurate and reliable. Many variables affect the accuracy of the blood pressure measurement, including equipment, experience of the provider, and recent activities of the client. Body posture is one variable that can be controlled prior to the blood pressure assessment.

What Research Has Been Conducted?

One group of researchers (Foster-Fitzpatrick and others, 1999) studied the effects of leg crossing on blood pressure in a sample of adult volunteers. Using a manual cuff, they found that systolic blood pressure was significantly increased when the person's legs were crossed. Keele-Smith and Price-Daniel (2001) studied blood pressure assessment in a sample of 103 senior citizens. They took measurements with the people's legs crossed and uncrossed and found that the systolic blood pressure was almost 6 mm Hg higher when the legs were crossed. Whether the person had hypertension or not, the systolic blood pressure was higher with the legs crossed. Even though the difference was small, the researchers felt it was significant and could alter treatment decisions, especially in people with borderline hypertension.

What Has the Research Concluded?

Researchers found that blood pressure readings are altered when people cross their legs. They recommend that vital sign assessment protocols include a request that clients rest their feet flat on the floor when the blood pressure is assessed in a sitting position. Consistent protocols allow comparisons in blood pressure readings over time.

What Is the Future of Research in This Area?

Because blood pressure is now measured with many types of electronic devices as well as in the traditional way, and the finger, wrist, or upper arm may be used as the site for the measurement, the issue of standardization is more important than ever. New methods of assessing blood pressure must be standardized, and nurses should use these standards to ensure consistency and accuracy.

References

Foster-Fitzpatrick, L., Ortiz, A., Sibilano, H., Marcantonio, R., & Braun, L. T. (1999). The effects of crossed leg on blood pressure measurement. *Nursing Research, 48*(2), 105.

Keele-Smith, R., & Price-Daniel, C. (2001). Effects of crossing legs on blood pressure measurement. *Clinical Nursing Research, 10*(2), 202-213.

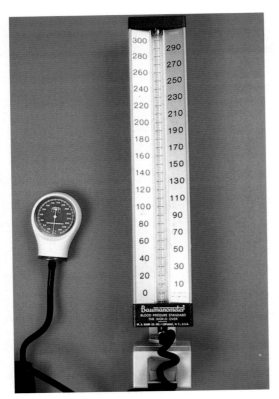

Figure 7-8. Manometers: aneroid *(left)* and mercury *(right).* (From Polaski, A. L., & Warner, J. P. [1994]. *Saunders' fundamentals for nursing assistants: Slide package.* Philadelphia: Saunders.)

and the sounds change. When the blood flows freely again, the sound disappears.

The first sound you will hear as turbulent blood begins flowing through the partially compressed artery is Korotkoff I, a clear tapping sound (Figure 7-9, p. 125). As you continue to release pressure, the other sounds follow. Korotkoff II is a murmur or swishing sound. Korotkoff III is a clear, intense tapping. Korotkoff IV is a distinct change to a muffled sound and indicates the first diastolic blood pressure. Korotkoff V is the disappearance sound caused by freely flowing blood; it indicates the second diastolic blood pressure.

To assess a client's cardiovascular function fully, you may need to check for **orthostatic hypotension,** in which blood pressure drops by 20 mm Hg or more with position changes (see Chapter 32). You will do so by measuring the blood pressure when the client is lying, sitting, and standing. Wait about 2 minutes between position changes to allow the client's compensatory mechanisms to stabilize the blood pressure before you take the next reading. Orthostatic hypotension may result from a reduced blood volume or from certain medications.

Action Alert! Ensure the safety of clients with orthostatic hypotension when they are getting out of bed.

If the client has hypertension, you may not hear Korotkoff II. This absence is called an **auscultatory gap.** You will hear a faint first Korotkoff sound, then silence until the third Korotkoff sound comes in loud and crisp. The cause of this

PROCEDURE 7-4   ASSESSING BLOOD PRESSURE

TIME TO ALLOW
Novice: 2 min.
Expert: 2 min.

Blood pressure is the pressure exerted by blood against the inner walls of the arteries. Measuring a client's blood pressure gives you information about the health of the cardiovascular, circulatory, and renal systems.

DELEGATION GUIDELINES

The measurement and recording of the client's blood pressure is a simple, low-risk procedure that you may delegate to a nursing assistant who has received training in this technique. Training should include specific instructions about findings that necessitate your immediate notification. You remain responsible for assessing any variance or irregularities in the client's blood pressure.

EQUIPMENT NEEDED

- Sphygmomanometer with cuff of correct size
- Stethoscope

1. Follow preliminary guidelines for nursing procedures (see inside front cover).

2. Select a cuff of correct size for the client and the limb you intend to use.
a. Select a bladder that fits almost completely around the client's arm.
b. Select a cuff width that is about two-thirds the length of the client's upper arm. *A cuff that is too wide will result in a false low reading. A cuff that is too narrow will result in a false high reading.*

3. Choose the arm on which you will take the blood pressure reading. *Avoid taking a blood pressure measurement on an arm that is used for hemodialysis or has a shunt, burn, cast, intravenous line, or traumatic injury. Also avoid using an arm contiguous with the site of breast or axillary surgery. If you cannot use one of the client's arms to take a blood pressure reading, use a leg and measure blood pressure at the popliteal artery.*

4. Position the client's arm so it is level with the heart, palm up, in a relaxed and comfortable fashion. If the client is supine, you may place the arm on the bed. If the client is sitting or standing, position the arm on the table over the bed, or hold it with your elbow. *Positioning the arm below heart level will result in a false high reading. Positioning it above heart level will result in a false low reading. Positioning it with palm up exposes the brachial artery.*

5. If the client is changing from a lying to a sitting position, wait at least 2 minutes before taking the blood pressure measurement. *This time allows the body's compensatory mechanisms to stabilize the blood pressure.*

6. Affix the cuff onto the client's arm.
a. Do not place the cuff over the client's clothing.
b. Place the bottom edge of the cuff 1 inch above the client's antecubital fossa (see illustration).
c. Place the center of the cuff directly over the brachial artery.
d. Wrap the cuff snugly around the client's arm while allowing space to place the stethoscope over the brachial artery. *This ensures uniform and complete compression of the brachial artery. A cuff that is too loose will result in a false high reading.*

7. Position the sphygmomanometer at eye level. The liquid in a manometer or the needle of an aneroid gauge should be at zero (see illustration, p. 124). *Positioning the manometer above eye level results in a false high reading. Positioning it below eye level results in a false low reading.*

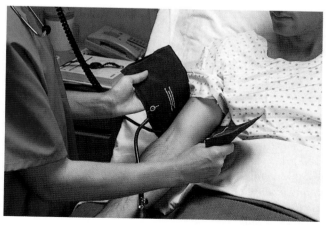

Step 6b. Placing the cuff 1 inch above the antecubital fossa.

PROCEDURE 7-4   ASSESSING BLOOD PRESSURE—Cont'd

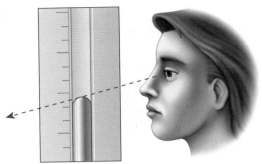

Falsely low reading

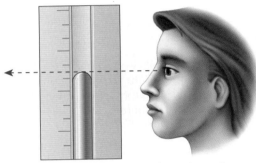

Accurate reading

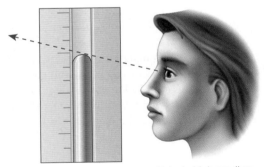

Falsely high reading

Step 7. Effect of viewing the meniscus at different levels. Viewing at eye level gives the most accurate reading.

8. Obtain a palpated systolic blood pressure. *Blood pressure measurement should be performed on each client whose blood pressure is being read for the first time. It ensures that the cuff is sufficiently inflated to give you an accurate systolic reading by auscultation. It also provides information about an auscultatory gap. Failure to identify such a gap results in a false low systolic reading.*

a. Palpate the brachial or radial pulse.
b. Inflate the cuff until the pulse disappears.
c. Release the pressure slowly until the pulse returns, and note this reading.
d. Quickly release the cuff.

9. Obtain the blood pressure reading.

a. Wait 30 to 60 seconds after obtaining the palpatory systolic blood pressure. *If you attempt to obtain the blood pressure reading too soon after obtaining the palpatory systolic blood pressure, you will receive a false high reading.*
b. Place the bell of your stethoscope lightly over the brachial artery (see illustration). *The bell of the stethoscope is used for low-pitched sounds, such as extra heart sounds.*
c. Tighten the screw clamp, and quickly inflate the cuff to 30 mm Hg above the palpatory systolic blood pressure reading. *The auscultatory systolic blood pressure should be slightly higher than the palpatory reading. Slow inflation can result in an inaccurate reading.*

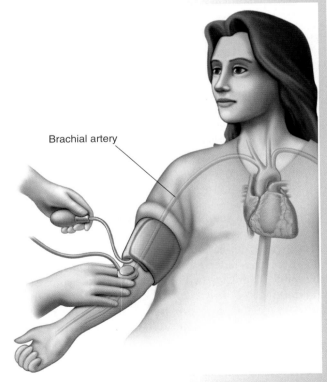

Brachial artery

Step 9b. Positioning the stethoscope over the brachial artery.

d. Deflate the cuff slowly and steadily at 2 to 3 mm Hg per second until you hear a soft, tapping sound. This is the first Korotkoff sound and indicates the client's systolic blood pressure. *Deflating the cuff too rapidly results in a false low systolic reading. Deflating the cuff too slowly results in a false high diastolic reading.*

e. Continue deflating the cuff slowly. Listen for a murmur or swishing sound (Korotkoff II), a clear tapping (Korotkoff III), and a muffling of sound (Korotkoff IV). *Muffling of sound correlates with the beginning of diastole and is the best indicator of diastolic blood pressure in children.*

f. Continue deflating the cuff slowly, listening for the sounds to stop. *Cessation of sounds correlates with the end of diastole (Korotkoff V) and is the best indicator of diastolic blood pressure in adults. In children and athletes, the sounds of phase V may continue all the way to zero.*

10. Deflate the cuff at a moderate rate and completely. If you must take another blood pressure reading, wait 1 to 2 minutes before doing so. *Continued pressure on the blood vessels decreases circulation to the hand, causing the client discomfort. Waiting a minute or two allows normal circulation to return to the hand.*

11. Document the client's blood pressure in the medical record as soon as you obtain the reading. If you identify an auscultatory gap, document the reading (in mm Hg) that corresponds to the length of the silence. *Normal systolic blood pressure is 100 to 140 mm Hg. Normal diastolic blood pressure is 60 to 90 mm Hg. Some facilities require that you document three sounds: systolic blood pressure, muffling, and diastolic blood pressure.*

12. Report an abnormal blood pressure to a charge nurse or physician.

Table 7-7	Blood Pressure Measurement: Sources of Error and the Effect on Results	
Source of Error	**Effect on Blood Pressure Reading**
Cuff size too wide	False low
Cuff size too narrow	False high
Cuff wrapped too loosely	False high
Arm below heart level	False high
Arm above heart level	False low
Manometer below eye level	False low
Manometer above eye level	False high
Cuff deflated too rapidly	False low systolic
Cuff deflated too slowly	False high diastolic
Failure to wait 30 to 60 seconds between successive blood pressure readings	False high
Failure to identify an auscultatory gap with a palpatory systolic blood pressure measurement	False low systolic
Defective equipment, poorly calibrated manometers, hearing impairment, or improper use of stethoscope	Inaccurate readings

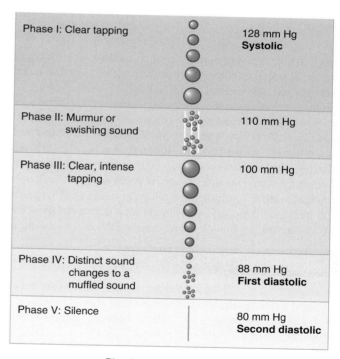

Blood pressure = 128/88/80

Figure 7-9. The Korotkoff sounds (also called phases).

gap is unknown. However, recognizing it is crucial. If you fail to recognize it, you could mistake the third Korotkoff sound (instead of the first) as the client's systolic pressure. Doing so produces a false low systolic reading.

If the normal tapping sounds disappear on inspiration and return on expiration, the client has pulsus paradoxus. Slowly decrease the cuff pressure and listen for the paradoxical pulse to cease. If it is present for more than 10 mm Hg, it may be a sign of serious cardiovascular problems.

If you cannot use the client's arm to measure blood pressure, you may need to use the popliteal artery behind the knee. Use an appropriate thigh-size cuff. Systolic pressures in the leg can differ by 10 to 40 mm Hg from pressures in the

arm. When documenting your findings, make sure to note that your reading is from the client's leg.

Finally, if you have trouble hearing the Korotkoff sounds, you may need to use Doppler ultrasound to measure the client's blood pressure. This problem may result from severe hypotension, shock, or circulatory instability. The Doppler transducer picks up and amplifies blood pressure sounds so you can hear them. However, you will be able to determine only a systolic pressure measurement with this device. If you

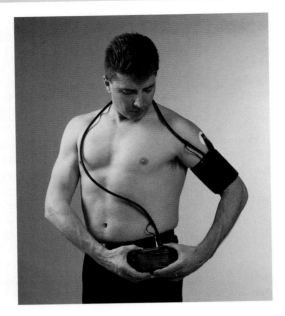

Figure 7-10. An automated blood pressure monitor. (Courtesy Welch Allyn, Inc.)

need to take frequent blood pressure readings, you may want to use an automated blood pressure machine to obtain quick, accurate measurements (Figure 7-10).

In all cases, document your client's blood pressure as soon as you obtain the reading. Make sure you follow your health care facility's policy when documenting pressures. Most continue to use the two-part measurement that lists systolic and diastolic levels. However, a growing number of facilities require a three-part documentation. If yours does, you will need to chart systolic, muffling, and diastolic readings. Along with the numerical readings, you should also document the location from which you took the reading and the client's position.

Key Principles

- Assessment of vital signs provides you with crucial information about a client's psychological and physical state of health.
- The body's temperature is a balance between heat production and heat loss.
- Body temperature is affected by the client's health, age, stress, and time of day.
- Common types of thermometers are glass, electronic, and tympanic.
- Routes for temperature measurement are oral, axillary, rectal, and tympanic.
- The pulse is a wave of blood in the arteries created by the pumping action of the heart.
- Assessment of the radial and apical pulses includes the rate, rhythm, and strength.
- The rate and depth of respirations change according to the body's need for oxygen, the release of carbon dioxide, and the person's emotions.

- Blood pressure is largely a reflection of blood volume, cardiac output, and vascular resistance.
- Blood pressure measurements record the highest pressure (systolic) and the lowest resting pressure (diastolic) of the fluid in the vessels.
- Accurate documentation is essential for communication of vital sign data to other health care providers.

Bibliography

Anonymous. (2001). New products. *Medsurg Nursing, 10*(1), 22.

*Bayne, C. G. (1997). Technology assessment: Vital signs—Are we monitoring the right parameters? *Nursing Management, 28*(5), 74-76.

*Beaudry, M., VandenBosch, T., & Anderson, J. (1996). Research utilization: Once-a-day temperature for afebrile patients. *Clinical Nurse Specialist, 10*(1), 21-24.

Bernardo, L. M, Henker, R., & O'Connor, J. (1999). Temperature measurement in pediatric trauma patients: A comparison of thermometry and measurement routes. *Journal of Emergency Nursing, 25*(4), 327-329.

Braun, S. K., Preston, P., & Smith, R. N. (1998). Getting a better read on thermometry. *RN, 61*(3), 57-60.

*Erickson, R. S., Meyer, L. T., & Woo, T. M. (1996). Accuracy of chemical dot thermometers in critically ill adults and young children. *Image Journal of Nursing Scholarship, 28*(1), 23-28.

Fawcett, J. (2001). The accuracy and reliability of the tympanic membrane thermometer: A literature review. *Emergency Nurse, 8*(9), 13-17.

*Flo, G., & Brown, M. (1995). Comparing three methods of temperature taking. *Nursing Research, 44*(2), 120-122.

Foster-Fitzpatrick, L., Ortiz, A., Sibilano, H., Marcantonio, R., & Braun, L. T. (1999). The effects of crossed leg on blood pressure measurement. *Nursing Research, 48*(2), 105.

*Henker, R., & Coyne, C. (1995). Comparison of peripheral temperature measurements with core temperature. *AACN Clinical Issues, 6*(1), 21-30.

Hirshberg, A. (2001). Accuracy of tympanic thermometers questioned. *Journal of Emergency Medical Services, 26*(6), 17.

Irvin, S. M. (1999). Comparison of the oral thermometer versus the tympanic thermometer. *American Journal of Nursing, 13*(2), 85.

Jevon, P., & Jevon, M. (2001). Practical procedures for nurses: Using a tympanic thermometer. *Nursing Times, 97*(9), 43-44.

Keele-Smith, R., & Price-Daniel, C. (2001). Effects of crossing legs on blood pressure measurement. *Clinical Nursing Research, 10*(2), 202-213.

Kleinpell, R. M. (2001). Danger of mercury lingers in healthcare. *Nursing Spectrum, 13A* (NJ), 6-7.

Lanham, D. M, Walker, B., Klocke, E., & Jennings, M. (1999). Accuracy of tympanic temperature readings in children under 6 years of age. *Pediatric Nursing, 25*(1), 39-42.

McConnell, E. A. (1998). Automated vital sign monitoring devices. *Nursing Management, 29*(2), 49-51.

Molton, A. H., Blacktop, J., & Hall, C. M. (2001). Temperature taking in children. *Journal of Child Health Care, 5*(1), 5-10.

Murphy, L., & Linn, L. (1996). Managing vital signs monitoring problems. *Nursing, 26*(11), 32gg-32jj.

*Asterisk indicates a classic or definitive work on this subject.

Nuckton, T. J., Goldreich, D., Wendt, F. C., Nuckton, J. G., & Claman, D. M. (2001). A comparison of 2 methods of measuring rectal temperatures with digital thermometers. *American Journal of Critical Care, 10*(3), 146-150.

Occupational Safety and Health Administration, U.S. Department of Labor. (Revised February 2000). *Occupational Safety and Health Guideline for Mercury Vapor.* Retrieved from http://www.osha.gov/SLTC/healthguidelines/mercuryvapor/recognition.html.

Powell, K. R., Smith, K., & Eberly, S. W. (2001). Ear temperature measurements in healthy children using the arterial heat balance method. *Clinical Pediatrics, 40*(6), 333-336.

Rhodes, V. A., McDaniel, R. W., Homan, S. S., Johnson, M., & Madsen, R. (2000). An instrument to measure symptom experience: Symptom occurrence and symptom distress. *Cancer Nursing, 23*(1), 49-54.

*Sneed, N. V., & Hollenbach, A. D. (1995). Measurement error in counting heart rate. *Critical Care Nurse, February,* 36-40.

Wilshaw, R., Beckstrand, R., Waid, D., & Schaalje, G. B. (1999). A comparison of the use of tympanic, axillary, and rectal thermometers in infants. *Journal of Pediatric Nursing, 14*(2), 88-93.

*Winslow, E. H. (1995). Research for practice: Are 60-second pulse counts necessary? *American Journal of Nursing, 95*(1), 53.

*Winslow, E. H., Jacobson, A. F., & Beazlie, M. A. (1997). Research for practice: Tympanic thermometers—Accuracy is questionable. *American Journal of Nursing, 97*(5), 71.

Physical Assessment

Key Terms

- accommodation
- auscultation
- bronchial
- bronchovesicular
- ecchymosis
- inspection
- lesion
- ophthalmoscope
- otoscope
- palpation
- percussion
- point of maximal impulse
- precordium
- respiratory excursion
- tactile fremitus
- turgor
- vesicular

Learning Objectives

After studying this chapter, you should be able to do the following:

- Describe the four techniques used in physical examination: inspection, palpation, percussion, and auscultation
- Identify the purpose of the primary instruments used in physical assessment
- Acquire nonthreatening techniques for physical examination to ensure client comfort and prepare the client for each regionally focused area of a complete physical examination
- Perform a complete physical examination on a client using a head-to-toe approach
- Recognize normal physical findings
- Recognize when physical findings deviate from normal

The physical examination is a systematic means of collecting objective assessment data. Objective data may be used to verify findings from the history or to determine the meaning of the findings. Although the history and the physical examination are usually conducted as separate procedures, the information is synthesized to identify and explain the client's problems, which may have psychological, social, or spiritual components.

As you collected the nursing history, you identified problems and possible problems in the client. In doing a physical examination, you are now looking for objective evidence commonly associated with these problems. Your findings may confirm the problems you suspected or at least add evidence to substantiate your hypotheses.

Physical assessments can be either *comprehensive* or *focused*. Ideally, every physical assessment should be comprehensive; that is, it should evaluate every body system and every area of function. However, a comprehensive physical assessment is often limited to the first time that a client sees a specific health care provider or enters a health care agency. Subsequently, assessment is focused on the reason for the visit and the client's current needs. When a client presents in acute distress with need of immediate intervention for a specific problem, assessment is focused on the most important data for the immediate problem.

How quickly you narrow the focus may depend on the client's needs and your knowledge level. A focused assessment assumes you have the knowledge to rule out the need for examination of particular body parts or functions.

Regardless of type, all physical assessment is aimed at detecting problems related to altered function, establishing baseline data against which subsequent data can be compared to judge whether the client's condition is improving or worsening, and identifying factors that place the client at risk for additional health problems. To learn to perform physical assessment, you must first learn to recognize normal findings. As you continue to study each health pattern, you will add knowledge of some common abnormal findings.

PREPARATION FOR PHYSICAL EXAMINATION

Techniques of Physical Examination

The four basic techniques used in physical examination are inspection, palpation, percussion, and auscultation, and they are generally performed in that order. Inspection is always done first. Palpation follows, except during examination of the abdomen, when it is done last so that it does not alter bowel sounds and change the findings on percussion and auscultation.

Inspection. **Inspection** is the systematic visual examination of the client. It involves observation of color, shape, size, symmetry, position, and movement, using the sense of smell to detect odors, and using hearing to detect sounds. For inspection to yield accurate findings, the area to be inspected must be fully exposed and the environmental light must be good. Use natural light when it is important to avoid distortion of color. Use tangential lighting (lighting that shines from one side and casts shadows) to increase your ability to detect variations in body surface such as changes in abdominal contour (Figure 8-1).

Palpation. **Palpation** is examination of the body through the use of touch. It is used to obtain information regarding temperature, moisture, texture, consistency, size, shape, position, and movement. You palpate to assess pulses as well as to check for tenderness, guarding, abdominal distention (enlarged or swollen abdomen), masses, and edema.

When checking temperature, use the back (dorsal surface) of your hand, as it is usually more sensitive than the palm. When assessing factors such as texture, shape, size, muscle tone, movement, or tenderness, use the pads of your fingers.

Palpation may be either light or deep. Use light palpation to examine lesions or masses on the surface of the skin or lying immediately under the skin. A light touch helps you avoid changing the shape of the lesion or mass. For light palpation, place your hand, fingers together, flat on the area to be palpated. Press your finger pads into the area to a depth of 1 to 2 cm (½ to ¾ inch). Repeat this action in ever-widening circles until you have palpated the entire area to be examined. Use light palpation to check muscle tone and to check for tenderness. Light palpation is always done prior to performing deep palpation.

Use deep palpation to identify abdominal organs and abdominal masses. With deep palpation, hold your hand at a 60-degree angle, fingers together, and use your finger pads and fingertips to press inward to a depth of 4 cm (2 inches). For two-handed deep palpation, place one hand on top of the other and palpate as just described. Two-handed palpation may help you keep the lower hand relaxed and thus more sensitive to underlying structures.

Before performing palpation, wash and warm your hands. Make sure your fingernails are short to avoid scratching the client's skin. If the client is ticklish, spread your fingers and add the client's fingers between yours until the hypersensitivity is lessened and the client's hand can be removed. During

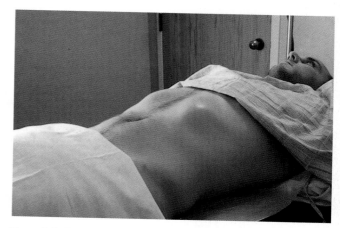

Figure 8-1. Tangential lighting (lighting that shines from one side and casts shadows) increases your ability to detect variations in body surface, such as changes in abdominal contour.

palpation, tell the client to take slow deep breaths through his mouth to decrease muscle tension, which can interfere with palpation. Palpate any tender areas last, and stop palpating if the client has pain at any point during the examination.

Percussion. **Percussion** is the use of short, sharp strikes to the body surface to produce palpable vibrations and characteristic sounds. Percussion is used to determine the size, shape, density, and location of a body organ, and to elicit pain and tenderness. Additionally, it can be used to detect whether tissue or a body cavity is fluid filled, air filled, or solid.

Generally, as the amount of air present in the area being percussed increases, the sounds produced become louder, longer, and deeper. Softer, higher, shorter sounds are produced from more solid areas. The five types of percussion sounds are *resonance* (hollow sound), *hyperresonance* (booming sound), *tympany* (musical or drum sound), *dullness* (thud), and *flatness* (extremely dull sound). Resonance is heard over the normal lung, hyperresonance is heard over an emphysematous lung, tympany is the sound produced by air-filled bowel, dullness is heard over dense structures such as the liver and heart, and flatness is heard over very dense structures such as skeletal muscle and bone.

The two types of percussion are direct and indirect. For direct percussion, you use a sharp, rapid movement of your wrist so that the pad of your middle finger strikes the area of the client's body to be percussed (Figure 8-2, *A*). The striking finger is called the plexor. Direct percussion is used primarily to assess the sinuses in adult clients.

Indirect percussion involves two hands. Place a finger of your nondominant hand in contact with the client's body, then use your plexor to strike your own finger on the client's body (see Figure 8-2, *B*). The finger in contact with the client's body is called the pleximeter and it is struck by the plexor (the middle finger of your dominant hand) just behind the nail bed at the distal interphalangeal joint, which is hyperextended.

Strike the pleximeter with the plexor at a right angle, then withdraw the plexor immediately to avoid damping the resulting vibrations. When performing indirect percussion, strike each area twice and then move to a new area. Keep your other fingers and the palm of your hand off the body part be-

ing percussed, as this will also damp the vibrations. Generally, the thicker the body wall is in the area being percussed, the greater the force of the strike needed to produce a clear tone.

Percussion that uses either the ulnar surface of the hand or the fist to strike the surface to be percussed is called blunt percussion. If the area to be percussed is struck directly, it is direct blunt percussion. It is indirect blunt percussion when the palm of your nondominant hand is placed flat on the area to be percussed and the back of your hand is struck.

Again, make sure your hands are washed and warmed, and that your fingernails are short.

Auscultation. **Auscultation** is the process of listening to sounds generated within the body. Examples of such sounds are those produced by the passage of air in and out of the lungs (breath sounds), those produced by the flow of blood through the heart and blood vessels (heart and vascular sounds), and those produced by the movement of fluid and gases through the intestinal tract (bowel sounds). Each sound is described in terms of loudness, pitch, quality, frequency, and duration. Sounds can be judged abnormal on the basis of where they are located or because changes are noted in one or more of these characteristics.

Auscultation is most often done using a stethoscope, which we will discuss next. However, you may also listen without a stethoscope to detect breath sounds, clicking or popping sounds from joint movements, and other sounds of body functions.

Equipment for Physical Examination

To perform a physical examination, you will rely heavily on the use of your five senses, particularly your ability to observe. Much of the examination is a mental activity rather than something you actually do. However, some equipment is used for specific aspects of the basic physical examination, and additional equipment may be used for special parts of the examination (Figure 8-3).

For most purposes, you will need a stethoscope, sphygmomanometer, and thermometer to take vital signs. A tongue blade and penlight are useful to examine the oral cavity and

Figure 8-2. Techniques for direct percussion (**A**) and indirect percussion (**B**).

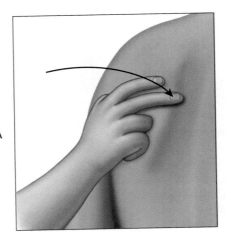
A

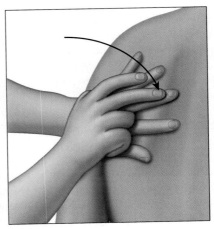
B

throat. The tuning fork, cotton-tipped swabs, and safety pins are needed only for the neurological examination.

For safety and accuracy, conduct the examination in a manner that is both time-efficient and conducive to client comfort and satisfaction. It is essential that all equipment be clean or sterile, accessible, in working order, and warmed if it will touch the client. Most nurses carry a stethoscope and a penlight, as they are most commonly used.

You will need to become proficient in using a stethoscope to detect the sounds created within body cavities and blood vessels. The earpieces should fit snugly to occlude noises other than those transmitted through the tubing, but they should not be uncomfortably tight. An earpiece that is too small may slip into the auditory canal and totally occlude sound. An earpiece that is too large may not occlude outside noises well.

Many stethoscopes have both a bell and a diaphragm. The bell is used to improve detection of relatively soft, lower-pitched sounds such as extra heart sounds or murmurs. The diaphragm improves detection of higher-pitched sounds such as breath sounds, bowel sounds, and normal heart sounds. Thus, the diaphragm is used more often than the bell.

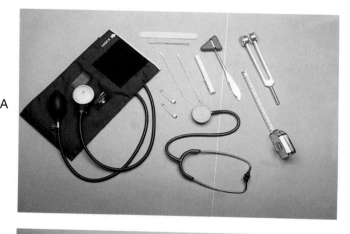

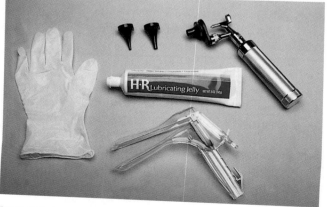

Figure 8-3. A, Equipment used for a basic physical examination: sphygmomanometer, stethoscope, tongue blade, thermometer, safety pins, cotton-tipped applicators, penlight, percussion hammer, tape measure, and tuning fork. **B,** Equipment used for specialized aspects of the physical examination: clean gloves and water-soluble lubricant, otoscope, and vaginal speculum.

The thickness and length of the tubing can affect the quality of sound transmission. The tubing should be thick with an internal diameter of ⅛ inch. Twelve to 14 inches is considered to be the ideal length. You will need to purchase a reasonably good quality stethoscope with interchangeable earpieces to be successful in detecting subtle sounds.

To use a stethoscope you will need to limit extraneous sounds. The room should be quiet. If this involves turning off suction devices that are being used on the client, first ascertain the safety of doing so. Additionally, the room should be warm. Shivering may distort the sound. Listening through clothes can create extraneous noise and damp the sounds. Hair on the chest can mimic abnormal lung sounds.

Practice until you can hear very quiet, soft sounds. Place the stethoscope firmly, but not pressing, on the client's skin and keep the tubing still. As you listen to normal body sounds, imagine the normal function that is occurring and associate the sound with the function. You should mentally "see" what is happening in the body.

CONDUCTING THE PHYSICAL EXAMINATION

It is critical that the physical examination be conducted in a manner that will promote the collection of complete, accurate assessment data. This means that you should follow a regular pattern of examination, position the client for the most accurate collection of data, and describe your findings in a manner that can be understood by other health care providers.

There is no one correct pattern for physical examination; the importance of the pattern is to ensure a comprehensive assessment through systematic data collection. You may choose, for example, a head-to-toe approach, or you may proceed from one body system to the next. (The pattern may be modified as appropriate for the physical condition of the client and the information needed.) The approach you choose should become second nature to you, thus helping to ensure that no aspect of the assessment is overlooked and that the data are organized in a meaningful fashion. The head-to-toe approach helps you proceed from clean to dirty. Thus you are not examining the mouth with a hand that has touched a foot.

To prepare the client, introduce yourself and descri' what the examination will involve. Be sensitive to the clier personal or cultural need for privacy, touch, and commun' tion. Reassure the client about the confidentiality of the amination. Ask the client to immediately report any fa' or discomfort.

Before starting the examination, provide the client w opportunity to use the bathroom and to assume a comf position. Throughout the examination, drape the client vacy. Repositioning will be necessary as the different the body are examined (Table 8-1, p. 132).

For the ambulatory client, the physical examina ally starts with the sitting position. For the hospitali' the examination is often started with the client lyi You need to plan the examination to avoid havin' change positions any more than necessary while s' you to obtain all needed data.

Table 8-1   Client Positions for Physical Examination

Position	Description and Use
Dorsal recumbent	Can be used to examine head and neck, anterior thorax, breasts, abdomen, arms, and legs. Turn the client to examine the back and posterior thorax. With client's knees flexed, can be used to relieve strain on the lower back during the examination. (Perineal and vaginal examination can be done in this position.)
Sitting	Client sits on the end of an examination table or the side of a bed. Better position of anterior and posterior chest than dorsal recumbent position. Client will need to lie down for abdominal examination.
Lithotomy	The feet and legs are put in stirrups. Used for vaginal and rectal examination in a female.
Genupectoral (knee–chest)	Used for a rectal examination.
Prone	Can be used to examine the posterior thorax in this position. Most common use is for range of motion in hip.
Sims'	Can be used to examine the posterior thorax. Used as an alternative position for vaginal and rectal examination when lithotomy position is contraindicated.

To accurately describe the findings of a physical examination, you need to use terms that have a common meaning to other health care providers. To describe the location of the area you are examining, imagine that the body is divided by three planes that divide it into anterior-posterior, inferior-superior, and medial-lateral aspects (Figure 8-4).

The frontal plane divides the body into anterior and posterior surfaces. The anterior surface is called the ventral surface and the posterior surface is the dorsal surface.

The transverse plane divides the body into inferior and superior aspects. The terms *inferior* and *superior* are also used in relation to a point of reference, usually the heart or thorax. For example, the knee is inferior to the thigh and superior to the foot. Similarly, the terms *distal* and *proximal* are used in relation to a reference point. Distal means away from, usually with reference to a point of origin. In other words, the hand is distal to the elbow. Proximal means nearer to a point of origin. The elbow is proximal to the hand.

The sagittal plane divides the body into right and left halves. The sagittal plane is described as the midline. Although medial refers to the center of the body and lateral to the sides, the terms medial and lateral are also used in relation to a point of reference. For example, you might describe a lesion as on the lateral aspect of the right thigh, 2 inches superior to the patella.

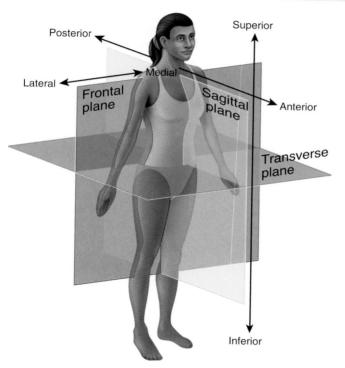

Figure 8-4. The body is divided by three planes. The frontal plane separates the body into anterior and posterior aspects. The transverse plane separates the body into inferior and superior aspects. The sagittal plane runs through the midline and separates the body into left and right halves and lateral and medial aspects.

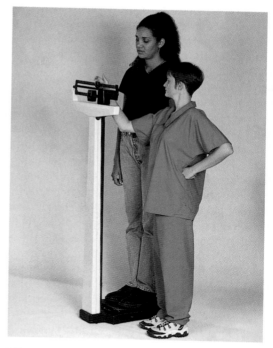

Figure 8-5. For both children and adults, compare height and weight to determine whether the person is overweight or underweight. This is one indicator of general health status and nutrition.

General Survey

The general survey is the first step in physical assessment. It provides information on the overall state of the client. It begins on first meeting the client, continues through the health history interview, and includes the measurement of height, weight, and vital signs. The general survey provides a basic impression of the client derived from overall physical appearance relative to age, body development, height, weight, movement, behavior, and vital signs, and it helps guide both the health history and the detailed physical examination.

Inspection of body posture may reveal significant information about the client's emotional and physical status. Assess it as the client enters the examination room or sits on the examination table, on the bed, or in a chair. Observe posture frontally, laterally, and posteriorly.

Record the client's height and weight as parameters of general health status (Figure 8-5). Measure the height and weight rather than relying on the client's report. However, if it is not possible to weigh and measure the client, record the client's report and note that it is approximate. Medication doses may later be calculated based on the recorded height and weight.

A standardized balance scale is preferable to a spring-loaded scale. This scale can easily be checked for balance at the zero mark each time a client is weighed, and more accurate and consistent weights are obtained. Ideally, in successive assessments, a person is weighed at the same time of the day, wearing the same clothes, on the same scale, and immediately before eating. To measure a client, be sure the client is standing erect and looking straight ahead. No shoes should be worn for the most accurate measurement.

Scales are available to suspend a bedridden client in a sling, to lay an infant on a platform, to roll a wheelchair on a platform, or even as part of high-tech hospital beds. If sheets, clothes, wheelchairs, or items are weighed with the client, weigh the item separately and subtract to obtain the person's total weight.

Height and weight are important measurements in children to determine that growth and development are proceeding at a normal rate. For both children and adults, compare the height and weight to determine if they are overweight or underweight. This is one indicator of general health and nutrition.

Signs of Acute Distress. The general survey begins with observing the client for obvious signs of distress. These include cyanosis, labored breathing, bleeding, diaphoresis, writhing, moaning, or guarding of a body part. If any of these signs is present, determine whether immediate intervention is needed. If no sign of distress requiring immediate intervention is present, the general survey continues.

Age and Developmental and Nutritional Status. Assess the client in terms of apparent age versus reported age. This assessment is based on signs of aging such as skin changes, gait, posture, muscle strength, and mental alertness. It answers the question, "Does the client look older or younger than the actual chronological age?" Obtain height and weight measurements and note general body shape, muscular development, and fat distribution. Draw an impression regarding apparent nutritional status (see Chapter 23). Does the client seem to be well-nourished, malnourished, obese, thin, emaciated?

The general survey includes an assessment of sexual development. Note the client's secondary sexual characteristics, such as facial hair, breast size, and voice quality. Are they appropriate for the client's age and sex?

Observe for normal body proportions, the size and symmetry of facial features, facial mobility, length of limbs, and symmetry of body parts. Also observe the symmetry, smoothness, and coordination of movement, as well as the absence of involuntary movement of the head and limbs; posture, both sitting and standing; balance on standing and walking; speed, smoothness, and style of gait; and use of assistive devices or prosthetic limbs.

Skin color and condition, personal hygiene and dress, and the presence of body and breath odors are all components of the general survey. On encountering a person with a body odor, you must consider cultural variation. Typical values in the United States dictate freedom from body odor as the norm. In many other cultures, however, the presence of normal body odor is the norm. For persons of all cultural groups, however, a fecal, urinary, or other-than-normal body odor is an abnormal finding. Similarly, breath odors, such as a sweet smell, or the smell of alcohol, acetone, or ammonia are abnormal findings. Be alert to the excessive use of perfumes and determine whether they are used to disguise an abnormal odor.

Orientation, Mood, Manner, Affect, and Speech.
Assess the client's level of consciousness (Box 8-1). For example, is the client oriented, alert, aware, and able to respond to questions and instructions quickly and appropriately? This information is obtained by your observation and from the responses to routine questions in the health history.

Observation of the client's mood, manner, affect, and speech is also a part of the general survey. Mild anxiety with a cooperative, attentive attitude, and with mood and affect appropriate to the situation, are normal findings. Abnormal findings include marked nervousness; restlessness; agitation; combative or uncooperative behavior; bizarre mannerisms; apathetic, depressed, or euphoric attitude; and stooped posture. In observing the client's speech, note the speech pattern, pace of speech, use of words, thought pattern, and sentence structure. Also note the tone, clarity, and strength of the voice and whether the client has any speech defects.

Abnormal findings include excessively slow or fast speech; halting, slurred, garbled, or very deliberate speech; an excessively soft or loud voice; or a voice that is weak, hoarse, high-pitched, or monotone. Aphasia, dysphasia, use of inappropriate vocabulary, stuttering, and lisping are also abnormal findings.

Mental Status.
The mental status examination provides a detailed description of the client's cognitive functioning at a given time. You can ascertain whether the client understands what is happening and how well the client can cooperate with the treatment plan. The depth of the mental status examination depends on the reason the client is being

---

Box 8-1 Describing a Client's Level of Consciousness

AWAKE AND ALERT: The client is aware of the surroundings and can respond appropriately to internal and external stimuli. Awake means not asleep and should not be confused with alert.

LETHARGIC OR SOMNOLENT: Easily drifts off to sleep or is not fully alert even though awake. This person may appear to be asleep but can be aroused with difficulty.

OBTUNDED: More difficult to arouse than lethargic. Technically refers to someone who is heavily dosed with narcotics and not only may be difficult to arouse but also may not be breathing adequately.

STUPOR, SEMICOMA, COMATOSE: A state of almost complete unconsciousness. May respond to strong stimuli such as loud noise, shaking, or pain. These terms may represent a continuum, with stupor being the most arousable; however, they are difficult to distinguish. For this reason, record precisely the observations you make, such as spontaneous movement, opening eyes, attempts to speak, or level of pain that elicits a response.

COMA: A state of unconsciousness from which the client cannot be aroused even by painful stimulus. Painful stimulus is applied by rubbing deeply on the chest. If there is no response, the coma is deep. *Caution:* Sternal rubbing can cause bruising and should be used only if absolutely necessary.

ORIENTATION: If the mental status is not certain, ask the client to identify person (state his name), place (where he is), and time (what day it is).

---

seen, the relevant medical problems, and the expected goals for treatment. If mental status is part of the chief complaint or related to the chief complaint, then a thorough mental status examination should be conducted. For example, for the confused client, consider evaluating the elements in the following paragraphs.

General *appearance* may provide a clue to the client's level of functioning. Poor hygiene and grooming can suggest depression, schizophrenia, organic brain disease, or lack of sufficient cognitive functioning for self-care. Bizarre dressing and makeup may be seen in manic-depressive illness.

Assess whether or not the *behavior* is appropriate for the client's reference group, age, and social situation. Unusual, bizarre, or inappropriate behavior may indicate a mental disturbance.

Assess whether or not the client is able and willing to *cooperate with the interviewer.*

Affect refers to the external expression of emotion attached to ideas or mental representation of ideas. Affect is normally an expression of the internal mood of the person. Assess whether the affect is appropriate for the topic of conversation or situation. Inappropriate affect is inconsistent with content of the client's speech or ideas, such as laughing at a sad story. A flat affect is a lack of emotional expression and is associated with depression.

Assess *speech* for clarity, choice of words, rate, and any unusual patterns. Speech may be slowed in depression or rapid in manic-depressive illness. The person with organic brain damage may have difficulty speaking.

Box 8-2	Brief Mental Status Examination

Ask the client to respond to the following instructions and questions:
- State your full name.
- Where are we? Hospital? City? State?
- What is the date today? Month? Year?
- What day of the week is it?
- I am going to name three objects and I want you to repeat them back to me when I ask you.
- Where do you live? Address? City? State?
- How old are you?
- Name the three objects I listed for you.
- Count backward from 100.

Orientation is the most basic assessment. Ask direct questions to determine whether clients knows who they are, where they are, and whether they have some orientation to time (Box 8-2). Orientation to time should take into consideration the normal tendency to lose track of time without the usual cues to the time of day. Most people normally can convey some frame of reference, such as "after lunch" or "nighttime." However, not knowing the day of the week may simply be a function of a lifestyle in which keeping up with the day of the week is not important.

Cognitive functioning refers to the client's patterns of thinking. Assess for logic, relevance, organization, and coherence of the pattern of thinking.

Ask clients if they have any problems with *memory* or concentration, or if they have noticed any changes in memory. Assess recent and remote memory. Assess recent memory by asking about recent events, such as what was eaten for the evening meal or what occurred in today's news. Remote memory is generally considered to deal with events that occurred 6 months or more in the past. The client's birth date, names of children, and names of past presidents may serve as reference points.

Intellectual functioning includes abstract thinking, concentration, content and process of thinking, perceptions, social judgment, and insight.

- *Abstract thinking* is frequently assessed by giving the person a proverb and asking what it means. The client who can think abstractly will give the nonliteral meaning. Useful proverbs include these: a rolling stone gathers no moss, as the twig is bent so grows the tree, a stitch in time saves nine, a penny saved is a penny earned.
- *Concentration* is tested by asking the person to remember a series of numbers or unconnected words and asking him to repeat them later in the examination.
- *Thought* is examined for content and process. Abnormality in content includes looking for delusions. Abnormality of process means that associations between thoughts are vague, or thoughts are loosely connected, poorly organized, or illogical.
- *Perception* is the ability to see the environment as it is; assessment includes asking about illusions and hallucinations. Illusion is misinterpreting external sensory stimuli. Hallucinations are false perceptions of any of the five senses: vision, hearing, taste, touch, or smell.

- *Social judgment* is whether or not the client can compare and evaluate alternatives, make and carry out reasonable decisions, and behave in an appropriate manner for a given social situation.
- *Insight* refers to the client's ability to evaluate and understand the events and behavior that resulted in the present situation.

Vital Signs

The final component of the general survey is vital signs: temperature, pulse, respiratory rate, and blood pressure. Vital signs are an important determinant of the person's overall health. Assessment of vital signs is discussed in Chapter 7.

Assessment of the Skin, Hair, and Nails

Assessment of the skin requires that you be able to recognize a vast array of normal variations in skin color, tone, distribution of pigmentation, effects of the sun, hair growth, and distribution of hair. Physical assessment of the skin, hair, and nails involves the following activities:

- Inspecting the skin for color, cleanliness, hair distribution, and presence of lesions
- Palpating the skin to determine moisture, temperature, texture, mobility, and turgor
- Inspecting the hair for quantity, distribution, color, and cleanliness
- Checking the texture of the hair
- Inspecting the scalp for cleanliness, parasites, and lesions
- Inspecting the fingernails and toenails for color, shape, contour, smoothness, uniformity of thickness, and presence of lesions

Skin

APPEARANCE. To inspect and palpate the skin, expose and cleanse areas as needed. Use good, preferably natural, light to avoid distortion of color. Make the room temperature comfortable to prevent color or other changes that might be caused by excessive heat or cold. In assessing skin color, note general color as well as local or patchy variations.

Normally skin is intact, free of lesions, and pink toned in light-skinned persons and light to dark brown or olive in dark-skinned persons, with an underlying healthy glow. Light-toned lips, palms, nail beds, and soles are common among dark-skinned persons, as are areas of blue-black discoloration over the sacrum and pigmented spots on the nail beds and in the sclera.

Abnormalities of skin color include pallor, cyanosis, flushing, and yellowing. Pallor, which appears as a loss of red tones in dark skin, is best seen in the nail beds, lips, oral mucous membranes, and palpebral conjunctivae. Cyanosis blueness, in light skin is seen as ash gray in dark skin. Ce cyanosis is best seen in lips, buccal mucosa, and the t Peripheral cyanosis is best observed in the nail beds ar skin of the arms and legs. Jaundice (yellow skin f disease) is seen in the bulbar conjunctiva, lips, and l as well as the skin.

LESIONS. Many different types of lesions occur in the skin. A **lesion** is a wound, injury, or pathological change in the body. A thorough description of a lesion is useful in determining whether the lesion is primary or secondary and whether it is benign or malignant. A primary lesion arises from the original source, condition, or set of symptoms in a disease process. A secondary lesion arises as a result of changes or complications from the primary condition.

The characteristics of a lesion may help determine the nature of an injury or of the disease process. Observe characteristics of the lesion. Then palpate to determine whether it is hard, soft, freely mobile with the skin, or attached to underly- ing structures. Also palpate for temperature. Various types of lesions are illustrated in Figure 8-6 and further described in Chapter 26.

Descriptions of skin lesions should include size, color, shape, distribution, and arrangement of the lesions. The size descriptors may include the area of redness, size of a raised area, or depth of the lesion. The color descriptor usually includes redness and blue discoloration. A bruise, or **ecchymosis,** is a hemorrhagic infiltration of the skin producing a bluish discoloration that changes to yellow as the blood cells are broken and reabsorbed. Erythema is redness of the skin caused by congestion of capillaries close to the surface of the skin.

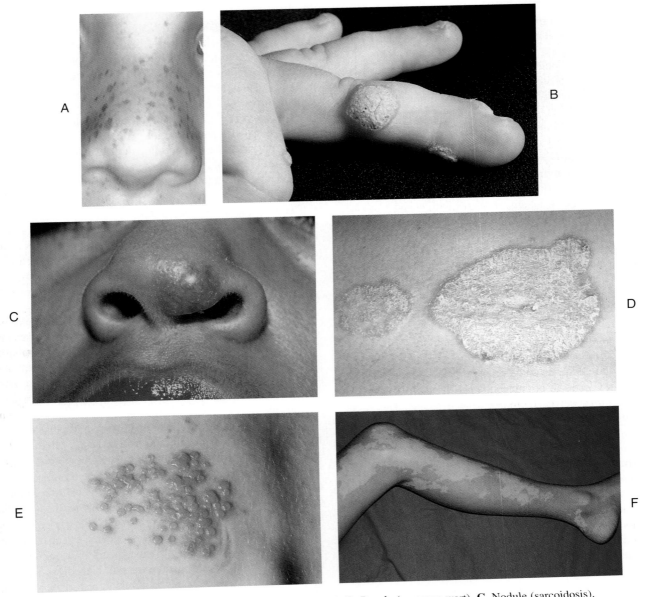

Figure 8-6. Examples of skin lesions. **A,** Macules (freckles). **B,** Papule (common wart). **C,** Nodule (sarcoidosis). **D,** Plaque (psoriasis). **E,** Vesicles and bullae (herpes simplex). **F,** Patches (vitiligo). (**A** from Hurwitz, S. [1993]. *Clinical pediatric dermatology: A textbook of skin disorders of childhood and adolescence* [2nd ed.]. Philadelphia: Saunders; **B, D,** and **E** from Lookingbill, D. P., & Marks, J. G., Jr. [1993]. *Principles of dermatology* [2nd ed.]. Philadelphia: Saunders; **C** and **F** from Callen, J. P., Greer, K. E., Hood, A. F., Paller, A. S., & Swinyer, L. J. [1993]. *Color atlas of dermatology.* Philadelphia: Saunders.)

Continued

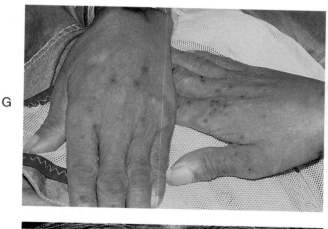

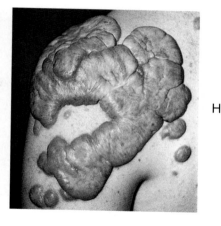

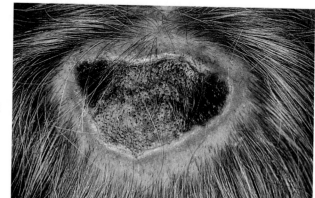

Figure 8-6, cont'd. G, Petechiae. **H,** Keloid. **I,** Necrosis (pressure necrosis after coronary artery bypass). (**G** courtesy Dr. Beverly A. Johnson, Washington, D.C.; **H** from Ignatavicius, D. D., Workman, M. L., & Mishler, M. A. [1999]. *Medical-surgical nursing across the health care continuum* [3rd ed.]. Philadelphia: Saunders; **I** from Callen, J. P., Greer, K. E., Hood, A. F., Paller, A. S., & Swinyer, L. J. [1993]. *Color atlas of dermatology.* Philadelphia: Saunders.)

The shape can be round, oval, irregular, ringlike (or annular), or annular with a center target. The distribution can be regional, generalized, scattered, on exposed body surfaces, at pressure sites, or on intertriginous areas (where skin surfaces touch). The arrangement of skin lesions can be described as linear (in a line), discrete (separate), confluent (running together), arciform (in an arch), or clustered. Additional terms used to describe lesions include the following:

- *Rash:* A skin eruption characterized by macules (flat spots), papules (superficial, circumscribed, solid elevations of the skin less than 0.5 to 1 cm in diameter), vesicles (serous fluid-filled elevations of epidermis—blisters), or erythema
- *Excoriation, abrasion:* Removal of surface skin by scraping or rubbing
- *Fissure:* A thin, linear crack in the epidermis
- *Ulcer:* An open lesion extending deeper than the dermis

MOISTURE, TEXTURE, AND TEMPERATURE. Assess the moistness and texture of the skin using the pads of your fingers. Normally the skin is dry, soft, smooth, and even. Excessively dry, damp, sweaty, oily, rough, thick, or uneven skin is an abnormal finding. Check skin temperature with the back of your hand. It is normally warm or cool, not hot or cold. General skin temperature as well as temperature of any reddened areas should be checked bilaterally. Assess for pus, exudates, or transudate from any lesion. Pus, which contains dead cells and leukocytes, indicates infection. Exudate is fluid with protein and cells that have escaped from blood vessels, usually as the result of inflammation. Transudate is similar but is mostly fluid.

TURGOR AND MOBILITY. Skin **turgor** is a reflection of the skin's elasticity, measured as the time it takes for the skin to return to normal after being pinched lightly between the thumb and forefinger. To check skin turgor and mobility, pinch and lift a fold of skin on the hand or forearm, over the sternum, or over the clavicle. Observe the ease of moving the skin and the speed with which it returns to its original position (Figure 8-7, p. 137). If mobility is normal, the skin moves easily. If turgor is normal, the pinched-up skin fold immediately returns to normal position. Turgor is abnormal if the skin fold remains tented (elevated) for more than 3 seconds. In older adults who have lost subcutaneous adipose tissue and skin elasticity, use the skin over the sternum. In an infant, use the abdomen.

Hair and Scalp. To assess the hair and scalp, ask the client to remove any wig, hairpiece, or other head covering. Observe the quantity, distribution, and color of the hair, then palpate the hair to determine its texture. Abnormal findings include patchy or sudden hair loss, and brittle hair. Next, part the hair in several areas and inspect the scalp. It should be smooth, clean, and intact. Look for discolorations, lumps, scaliness, or open areas. Inspect the base of the hair shaft for nits, which are tiny, white, opaque eggs of head lice found attached to the hair shafts. Palpate the skull for lumps or tender areas.

Nails. Inspect the fingernails and toenails to determine their color, shape, contour, smoothness, thickness, and cleanliness. Abnormal findings are described by comparing the nail to a

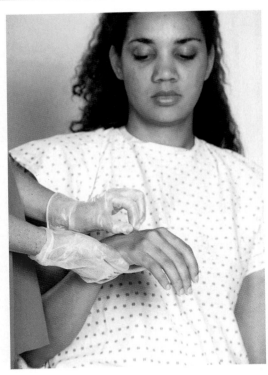

Figure 8-7. Checking skin turgor and mobility in a young person.

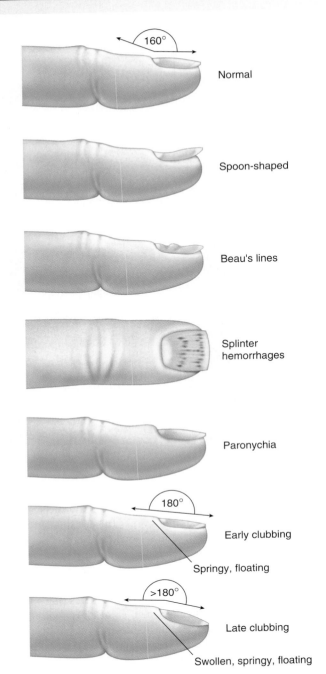

Figure 8-8. Comparing normal and abnormal nails. Examples of abnormal changes in nails include spoon-shaped nails, Beau's lines, splinter hemorrhages, paronychia, and clubbing.

normal nail. Normal nails are clean, curved, and hard, with a pink to light brown nail bed. The angle between the nail and its base is 160 degrees. Abnormal findings include soft or brittle nails, inflammation, and pale or cyanotic nail beds. Cleanliness and grooming of nails are a cue to hygienic practices. Examples of abnormal changes in nails include spoon-shaped nails, Beau's lines, splinter hemorrhages, paronychia, and clubbed nails (Figure 8-8).

Assessment of the Head and Neck

Head and Face. Physical assessment of the head and face involves the following activities:

- Observing the size, symmetry, position, and movement of the head as a whole and of the facial features
- Palpating the skull
- Checking for tenderness of the temporal artery
- Checking the function of the temporomandibular joint
- Checking the function of cranial nerve VII (facial)
- Checking the function of cranial nerve V (trigeminal)

Assessment of the head and face begins with observation of size, position, and symmetry. The head should be normal in size (normocephalic), not abnormally small (microcephalic) or large for the person's age. In older adults, the nose and brows are often prominent and the lower face may appear small, with the mouth shrunken if the person is edentulous (without teeth).

The head should be in a normal upright position, not tilted backward, forward, or to the left or right side. It should also be symmetrical in shape—that is, the same on the right and left sides. The eyebrows, palpebral fissures, and nasolabial folds should be equal (on the right and left) in size, shape, and position. The sides of the mouth should be similar in appearance

and free of any abnormal one-sided droop or sag. Facial movements and expressions should be free, variable, and symmetrical. Distorted, absent, or asymmetrical movement or expression is abnormal. Involuntary movement is also abnormal, although in older adults mild rhythmic tremors are common.

Temporal Artery. Although the temporal artery is not routinely assessed, you may do so by palpating the temporal artery, located superior to the temporalis muscle. The pulsation can be felt in front of the ear. Normally it is nontender, smooth, and pliable. Tenderness or hardness is abnormal. The temporal arteries are often prominent and tortuous in older adults.

Temporomandibular Joint. Examine the temporomandibular joint to determine its range of motion (ROM) and to check for any swelling or tenderness. To do this, place the tips of your index fingers on the sides of the client's face just in front of the tragi of the ears. Ask the client to open the mouth while your fingertips slide into the joint space when the mouth opens.

Normally the mouth will open 3 to 6 cm and the lower jaw can move laterally 1 to 2 cm. Snapping or popping sounds when the mouth is opened are common and not pathological. Restricted motion, deviation of the lower jaw to one side when the mouth is opened, pain, or crepitus (crackling or rubbing sound) are abnormal findings.

Cranial Nerve VII. Cranial nerve VII (the facial nerve) is routinely tested. It is a mixed nerve, which means it has both motor and sensory components, but only the motor component, which innervates the facial muscles and is responsible for closing the eyes and for labial speech, is routinely tested. To test motor function of cranial nerve VII, ask the client to smile, frown, raise his eyebrows, show his upper and lower teeth, and keep his eyes tightly closed while you attempt to open them (Figure 8-9). As the client performs these actions, observe for symmetrical strength and movement. Ask the client to puff out the cheeks. Then use your finger pads to press the puffed cheeks in. Air should escape equally from both cheeks with this maneuver.

Cranial Nerve V. Cranial nerve V (the trigeminal nerve) is also a mixed nerve. Its motor component innervates the muscles of mastication, and its sensory component is responsible for sensation in the face, scalp, cornea, and the mucous membranes of the mouth and nose. Its motor function is tested by asking the client to clench the teeth together while you push down on the chin to try to separate the jaws. Normally the jaw cannot be separated and muscle strength is equal on both sides.

Sensory function of cranial nerve V is tested in two ways. First, ask the client to close the eyes, and then you touch the chin, cheeks, and forehead with a sterile pin or cotton ball. Ask the client to describe what is felt and where it is felt. The client should be able to distinguish sensations of light touch, dullness, and sharpness and identify their location as being on the forehead, cheeks, or chin. Absent, decreased, or unequal sensation is abnormal.

The second test of sensory function involves touching a wisp of cotton to the cornea and observing for the normal blink in response to the touch. For this test, contact lenses must be removed, and the client looks straight ahead while the cotton wisp is brought in from the side to prevent the natural blinking response. This test is often omitted during a normal screening examination.

Eyes. People under age 40 should have their eyes tested every 3 to 5 years. After age 40 the eyes should be examined every 2 years. More frequent examinations are needed if the person

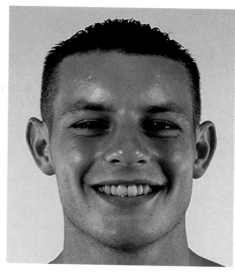

Figure 8-9. Assessing cranial nerve VII function. (From Jarvis, C. [2004]. *Health assessment and physical examination* [4th ed.]. Philadelphia: Saunders.)

has hypertension, diabetes, glaucoma or other eye disease, or bleeding disorders. Physical assessment of the eye involves the following activities:

- Testing visual acuity for distance vision and near vision
- Inspecting the outer eye structures, including lids, lashes, sclera, conjunctiva, cornea, iris, and pupil
- Testing pupillary response to light and accommodation
- Checking extraocular muscular function
- Checking visual fields
- Examining the ocular fundus

DISTANCE VISION. Visual acuity is the clearness of the visual image or the degree of detail the eye can discern in an image, which allows the eye to discriminate between forms. The Snellen chart is used to screen for acuity of distance vision. This chart consists of lines of print that become progressively smaller as one reads from the top to the bottom of the chart. There are three versions of the Snellen chart: one for the preschool child, which has commonly recognized symbols instead of letters; the Snellen E chart, which can be used for the preschool child or others who cannot read; and the standard Snellen chart, which consists of random letters.

The client is positioned 20 feet in front of the chart and is directed to cover one eye with a cover card and read the smallest line of print possible with the other eye. Acuity is recorded as 20 (distance from the chart) over the number printed by the side of the smallest line of print the client can read with at least 50% accuracy. A minus sign and the number of letters of this line that the client read incorrectly follows. An example is 20/80–1, which means that the client was able to read with one error at 20 feet a line of print that a person with normal vision could read at 80 feet.

This procedure is repeated for the other eye. If corrective lenses, glasses, or contacts are worn, distance vision is tested both with and without them and CC (with correction) or SC (without correction) is recorded after the acuity ratio. Normal acuity is 20/20. Legal blindness is defined as 20/200 with correction in either eye. If the client cannot see any print on the Snellen chart, finger counting ability, hand motion, and light perception are tested.

NEAR VISION. Acuity of near vision is tested in adults over age 40 and in those who present with a complaint of difficulty reading. This is done by asking the client to read lines of print of different sizes on a Jaeger chart, which the client holds 14 inches in front of the face. A Jaeger card is similar to a Snellen chart, but the print size is scaled to be equivalent to the print size at 20 feet when read at 14 inches. Results, which indicate the smallest line the client can read, are recorded as J1 (smallest letters) through J12 (largest letters). A person with normal near vision acuity can read J1 with each eye without hesitation and without moving the card. Near vision acuity can also be checked by having the client hold and read any printed materials at a comfortable distance from the face. If this type of test is used, the type of material and the distance it is held from the face is recorded.

OUTER EYE STRUCTURES. To examine the structures of the eye, begin with the outer structures and work your way inward. Begin inspection of the outer eye structures by noting the position of the eyelids in relationship to the globe. Normally no sclera (white) is visible between the upper lid and the iris. The lids are also observed for the presence of abnormalities such as ptosis (drooping of the upper lid), incomplete closure, redness, swelling, and presence of discharge or other lesions. The eyelashes are observed for even distribution and outward curve. Uneven distribution, inward growth touching the globe, crusting, or lesions are abnormal findings.

The globe, conjunctiva, sclera, iris, and pupil are also inspected. The right and left globes should be aligned and neither sunken nor protruding. To inspect the sclera and conjunctiva, separate the lids using your index finger and your thumb and ask the client to look up, down, and to each side. The palpebral (eyelid) conjunctiva is inspected by everting the lower lid with your thumb while asking the client to look up. The sclera should be smooth, moist, and glossy, and the conjunctiva should be clear, pale pink, and glistening, often with small blood vessels visible. The irises should be similar in shape, color, clarity, and markings. The pupils should be 3 to 5 mm in diameter, round, and equal in size in both eyes. Excessively dilated or constricted pupils as well as irregular or unequal pupils are abnormal. Shining a light from the side onto each eye and observing for cloudiness or opacities checks the clarity of the cornea.

PUPILLARY RESPONSE TO LIGHT AND ACCOMMODATION. With the client looking straight ahead into the distance, bring a bright light in from the side (one side at a time) to the front of the pupil to test pupillary response to light. The illuminated pupil should constrict. This is called the direct response. When the other pupil constricts at the same time, the response is called consensual. Bringing the light directly in front of the eye causes both a direct and a consensual response. Bringing the light in from the side elicits only a direct response. Speed and degree of constriction should be equal in both pupils and should be followed by equal dilation. Absence of constriction or an asymmetrical response is abnormal. Degree of constriction is recorded as millimeters before and after exposure to the light, and speed is described as brisk or sluggish.

Accommodation is adjustment of the eye for seeing objects at various distances. To test accommodation, hold a finger or an object such as a pen 10 to 15 cm (4 to 5 inches) in front of the client's nose. Tell the client to look ahead into the distance and then to quickly look at the finger or other object. If accommodation is normal, both eyes converge (move medially) and the pupils constrict. Normal pupillary findings are recorded with the acronym PERRLA, which stands for pupils equal, round, and reactive to light and accommodation.

EXTRAOCULAR MUSCLE FUNCTION. Checking for parallel gaze (corneal light reflex), coordinated eye movement, and convergence tests extraocular muscle function. Shine a light straight into the client's eyes from a distance of 31 cm (12 inches) while the client looks straight ahead to test parallel gaze. Normally the light is reflected on or just medial to the pupil in both eyes. Reflection of the light in a different location in each eye is abnormal.

Coordinated eye movement is checked by holding a finger 31 cm (12 in) in front of the client and moving it from the center to one of the eight locations, holding a moment, and then returning it to center (Figure 8-10, A). This action is repeated for each of the eight locations while the eyes are observed for normal parallel movement. As the gaze moves up and down, the upper lid is observed and should be seen to overlap the iris at all times. Both eyes should remain parallel as the finger is tracked through the eight locations. Weakness of extraocular muscles or cranial nerve dysfunction results in nonparallel tracking. Additionally, you should look for nystagmus, which is involuntary, rapid, rhythmic movement of the eyeball.

Convergence is then tested by asking the client to watch your finger as you move it from out in front of the client's eyes in toward the bridge of his nose. The iris of both eyes should converge or move toward midline as the finger moves toward the nose.

VISUAL FIELDS. The visual field is the entire area seen by the eye in a fixed position. Visual fields are checked using a confrontational test to compare the client's peripheral vision with that of the examiner (Figure 8-10, B). Position yourself in front of the client so that your faces are at the same level. Then direct the client to cover his right eye while looking with his left eye into your right eye. Then cover your left eye and bring a raised finger, pen, or other object held at arm's length between yourself and the client from several points in the right periphery into the visual field. Tell the client to say "Now" when the object comes into view. This should be at the same time the object enters your field of vision. Thus, you can use your visual field to test your client's. This gross check of visual fields is repeated for the other eye. Normal findings are recorded as "Visual fields full to confrontation." Normal results are about 50 degrees upward, 90 degrees to the temporal side, 70 degrees down, and 60 degrees to the nasal side.

OCULAR FUNDUS. You can examine the inner eye by directing a light through the window of the pupil to view the lens, anterior chamber, vitreous, and ocular fundus. Registered

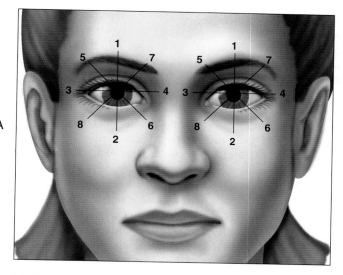

A

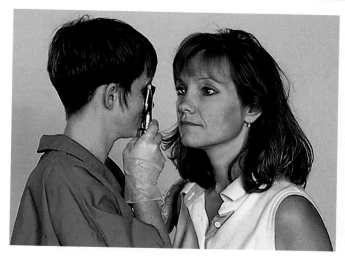

Figure 8-11. Ophthalmoscopic examination.

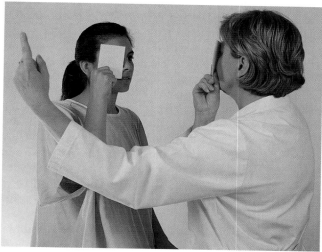

B

Figure 8-10. A, The eight cardinal directions of gaze used in checking for coordinated eye movement. **B,** The visual fields or confrontational test assesses for peripheral vision by comparing the client's peripheral vision to your own.

nurses do not routinely examine the inner eye. However, nurses in some settings or advanced practice nurses may perform this examination, called a funduscopic examination.

The ocular fundus, which is the back portion of the interior of the eyeball, is visible through the pupil by examination with an ophthalmoscope. The **ophthalmoscope** is an instrument used to visualize the retina (including the optic disk, macula, and retinal blood vessels) through the pupil. The examination is done in a darkened room and begins with you about 15 inches away from the client and slightly to the side of the client's line of vision. As the light beam from the ophthalmoscope is shone on the pupil of the eye being examined, an orange-red glow called the red reflex appears in the pupil. This glow should be uninterrupted and fill the pupil. Dark shadows or black dots interrupting the glow are abnormal.

The client must be able to cooperate and hold the eyes still by looking at a distant object that you have identified and that

holds the gaze about 20 degrees upward and to the side. Hold the ophthalmoscope in your right hand and use your right eye to examine the client's right eye (Figure 8-11). The ophthalmoscope is used as an appendage to your own eye. To prevent losing sight of the fundus during the examination, stabilize the ophthalmoscope on your eyebrow or nose and move your head and the instrument as one unit. Rest your index finger on the lens wheel to focus easily during the examination, and rest your thumb on your lower jaw. The light should be adjusted to maximum if tolerated by the client.

The ophthalmoscope contains a set of lenses to control the units of measurement (dioptrics), thus focusing for vision from near to far. The black numbers are positive dioptrics for focusing on nearer objects, and the red numbers are negative dioptrics for focusing on objects farther away.

Start with the lens set at zero and adjust upward for better focus on details found in the examination. Begin about 10 inches from the client at an angle of 15 degrees lateral to the person's line of vision. When you have found the red glow (the reflection of the light off the inner retina), move closer to the client until your heads are almost touching. If you lose the red glow, move back, relocate the glow, and move forward again.

As you advance, adjust the lens to +6 and note any opacity in the lens. These appear as black areas or dark shadows interrupting the red reflex. Continuing to move forward, adjust the lens setting (diopter) to bring the fundus into focus. When both you and the client have normal vision, this should be at 0. Adjust to red dioptrics for nearsighted eyes and to black for farsighted eyes.

Begin the examination of the optic fundus by finding the optic disk (Figure 8-12, p. 142). The optic disk is an area on the nasal side of each retina. The blood vessels of the retina converge at the optic disk. If you do not see the optic disk, track a blood vessel as it grows larger and it will lead you there. Outside the optic disk, the retina is light red to dark brown-red, with the shade varying in accord with skin color.

Assess the structures in the ocular fundus: optic disk, retinal vessels, general background, and macula. The optic disk

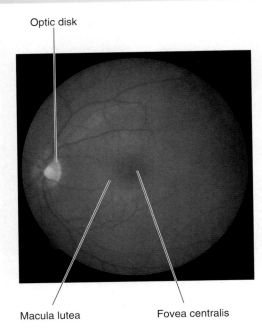

Optic disk

Macula lutea   Fovea centralis

Figure 8-12. Normal ocular fundus, as seen on ophthalmoscopic examination. Note the location of the optic disk. (Courtesy Dr. Harry Kaplan and Dr. Lawrence P. Roach, Philadelphia.)

is normally yellow orange to creamy pink in color, with distinct margins except at the nasal edge. Pallor, hyperemia, irregular shape, or blurred margins are abnormal findings. Visualized retinal vessels should consist of one artery and one vein passing to each quadrant of the retina, with a progressive decrease in the diameter of both veins and arteries as they extend toward the periphery. Arteries are brighter red than veins. Abnormal findings include the absence of major arteries, constricted arteries, dilated veins, and extreme tortuousness. The general background should be free of lesions such as hemorrhage or exudate. The macula lutea is an irregular yellowish depression on the retina, lateral to and slightly below the optic disk. It receives and analyzes light only from the center of the visual field. At the macula, which is about 1 DD (one disk diameter—i.e., the size of the diameter of the optic disk), the color may be darker than that of the rest of the retina, but all areas should be free of clumped pigment, which occurs with aging, trauma, or retinal detachment. Hemorrhage or exudate may represent macular degeneration. For further details on examination of the ocular fundus, a specialty text on physical assessment should be consulted.

Ear. Physical assessment of the ear involves the following activities:
- Inspecting and palpating the external ear
- Inspecting the external auditory meatus
- Using an otoscope to examine the external auditory canal and the tympanic membrane (eardrum)
- Testing the acuity of hearing (cranial nerve VIII)

EXTERNAL EAR. Inspection of the external ears involves noting their placement on the sides of the head, their alignment with each other, and their size, shape, symmetry, and skin color. The top of the pinna (the projecting part of the ear; also called the auricle) is normally level with the outer corner of the eye, and the whole ear is normally angled less than 10 degrees toward the occiput (the back of the head). The skin of the external ear should be the same color as the face and should be intact, smooth, and free of drainage or lesions. In older adults, ear lobes may be pendulous and coarse, and stiff hairs may be present on the external ear.

Next, the external ear is palpated to identify nodules or other irregularities. The pinna is moved up and down, the tragus (the cartilaginous projection anterior to the ear canal) is pressed, and the area behind the ear is pressed, with normal findings being no pain or tenderness on manipulation. The external auditory meatus is inspected for redness, swelling, discharge, and presence of a foreign body; the presence of any of these is an abnormal finding. The size of the opening is noted and should be unobstructed.

EXTERNAL AUDITORY CANAL. The external auditory canal is examined using an otoscope fitted with the largest speculum that can be inserted comfortably into the auditory canal. An **otoscope** is a handheld instrument used to examine the external ear, the eardrum, and, through the eardrum, the ossicles of the middle ear. It consists of a light, a magnifying lens, a speculum, and sometimes a device for insufflation.

With the client in a sitting position, move to the side and slightly to the back of the ear to be examined. Ask the client to tip the head toward the shoulder on the opposite side (Figure 8-13). Grasp the top of the pinna and pull it up and slightly away from the head with your nondominant hand. This pull straightens the ear canal in the adult and is maintained throughout the examination. In the infant, the pinna is pulled downward because the canal is directed downward.

The otoscope is commonly held in an upside down position in your dominant hand, and your hand is kept firmly braced against the side of the client's head so that if the head moves so does the otoscope, thus preventing accidental trauma to the auditory canal. The speculum is slowly inserted at a slightly downward and forward angle approximately ½ inch into the auditory canal. Because of its sensitivity to pain, avoid touching the medial wall of the canal. Watch the insertion and then put your eye to the otoscope.

Once the speculum is inserted, the canal can be observed. If you cannot see anything but the wall of the ear canal, angle the otoscope slightly toward the client's nose. You may need to rotate the otoscope to see the entire eardrum.

Normally the walls are pink and uniform, with small to moderate amounts of cerumen present. Cerumen, or ear wax, is moist and honey colored to dark brown or black in most white or black individuals and dry, gray, and flaky in most Asians and Native Americans. Large amounts of ear wax, swelling, redness, discharge, foreign bodies, or other lesions are abnormal, as are marked pain on insertion of the speculum and foul odor. Sometimes you will have to remove ear wax for good visualization. Ear irrigations are discussed in Chapter 37.

TYMPANIC MEMBRANE. Following inspection of the external auditory canal, the tympanic membrane (eardrum) is

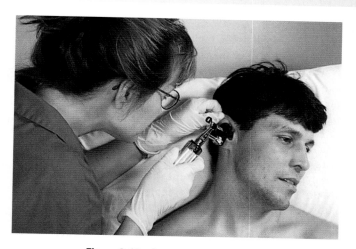

Figure 8-13. Otoscopic examination.

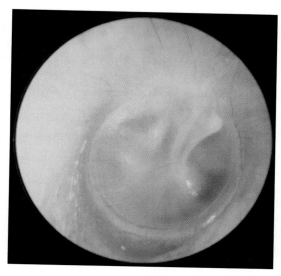

Figure 8-14. Normal tympanic membrane as seen on otoscopic examination. (From Swartz, M. H. [1994]. *Textbook of physical diagnosis: History and examination* [2nd ed.]. Philadelphia: Saunders.)

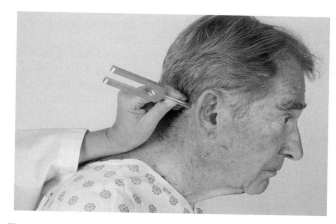

Figure 8-15. Place the stem of the vibrating tuning fork on the mastoid process and ask the client to signal when the sound goes away.

also inspected with the otoscope, and the positions of the handle of the malleus, the umbo, the short process, and the cone of light are noted. The tympanic membrane separates the external and middle ear and is tilted obliquely toward the ear canal. Normally the tympanic membrane is intact, pearly gray, shiny, translucent, and conical, although in older adults it may be whiter, duller, and thicker than in younger adults.

Assess for landmarks. The cone of light seen at the 5 o'clock position in the right ear and at the 7 o'clock position in the left ear is a reflection of the otoscope light. The malleus is the primary landmark. The short process of the malleus stands out as a knob. The manubrium, or the handle of the malleus, extends downward from the short process to the umbo (Figure 8-14). Having the client hold the nose and swallow assesses mobility of the eardrum; the membrane should be seen to flutter. Abnormal findings include perforations, scarring, dullness, blue, red, or amber coloring, retraction with accentuated landmarks, bulging with partially occluded landmarks, and a fluid level in the middle ear.

HEARING ACUITY. Hearing is mediated by the acoustic nerve, which is cranial nerve VIII. Testing of hearing acuity involves checking gross acuity, checking ability to lateralize sound, and comparing air and bone conduction of sound.

Gross hearing is evaluated during the course of normal conversation. The voice test is a more specific measure of gross hearing acuity. For this test, press on the tragus of one of the client's ears with your index finger to occlude the auditory canal. Stand 1 to 2 feet in front of the client. With the client's eyes closed or your mouth covered to prevent lip reading, exhale and whisper words of two equally accented syllables toward the ear being tested. The same procedure is used for the other ear. Normally the client can repeat the whispered words accurately. Repeat with spoken words. Whispered words are higher tones, which are more commonly lost than the lower tones of spoken words.

Lateralization of sound is evaluated by means of the Weber test. For this test, set a 512- or 1024-Hz tuning fork to vibrate lightly by tapping the tines against your hand. The base of the tuning fork is then placed in the middle of the top of the client's head or in the middle of the forehead. Ask whether the client hears the tone only in the right ear, only in the left ear, equally in both, or more in one ear than in the other (specify). Normally the tone is heard equally in both ears. If a *conductive* hearing loss exists, the tone is lateralized to the affected ear because the normal ear is more likely to be distracted by room noises. In the case of *sensorineural* hearing loss, the sound is lateralized to the unaffected ear.

Air and bone conduction are compared by means of the Rinne test. In this test, a lightly vibrating tuning fork is placed on the client's mastoid process and the client is asked to indicate when the tone is no longer heard (Figure 8-15). When the client so indicates, quickly move the tuning fork so that the tines are in front of the auditory meatus. Then ask the client if a tone is heard; if the answer is Yes, have the client indicate when it ends. Then repeat the procedure for the other ear.

Normally, air conduction lasts twice as long as bone conduction, so the client is able to hear the tone when the tines are placed in front of the auditory meatus for as long as the tone was heard when the tuning fork was on the mastoid process. In sensorineural hearing loss, air conduction lasts longer than bone conduction but not twice as long. It is equal to or shorter than bone conduction in conductive hearing loss.

Nose and Sinuses. Physical assessment of the nose and sinuses involves the following activities:
- Checking patency of the nares
- Inspecting the outside and the inside of the nose
- Palpating the sinuses for tenderness
- Testing the function of cranial nerve I

NOSE. Observe the external aspect of the nose for abnormalities such as asymmetry, lesions, or signs of inflammation. Check the patency of the nares by asking the client to close his mouth; then occlude each naris in turn while you feel for exhaled air from the nonoccluded naris. Next, inspect the inside of the nose using an otoscope fitted with a short, wide nasal speculum and magnifying lens. With the client's head tilted back and the handle of the otoscope held to the side, insert the speculum 1 cm into each naris without touching the nasal septum. Direct it back and somewhat upward to allow both the upper and lower nose to be seen.

Normally the mucosal lining of the nose is intact, smooth, and deep pink; the nasal septum is straight, and the turbinates are smooth and of the same color as the rest of the mucosa. The nasal mucosa is redder than the oral mucosa. The septum is somewhat deviated in most adults. The lateral wall of the nose consists of inferior, middle, and superior turbinates. The inferior turbinate is the largest and lies like a finger along the lower lateral wall of the nose.

Pale, bright red, or gray mucosa is abnormal. Bogginess, exudate, swelling, bleeding, ulcers or fissures, polyps, or a perforation or deviation of the septum are other abnormal findings.

SINUSES. The paranasal sinuses are pockets within the cranium that lighten the weight of the skull. They are lined with a ciliated mucous membrane and communicate with the nasal cavity. The frontal and maxillary sinuses are within the frontal and maxillary bones (Figure 8-16). The sphenoid sinuses are deep within the skull in the sphenoid bone, and the ethmoid sinuses are between the orbits of the eyes.

Examination of the sinuses is performed by indirect methods of inspection and palpation of the overlying soft tissues (frontal and maxillary sinuses) and by noting secretions that may drain from the nose. Use the pads of your thumbs to palpate the frontal and maxillary sinuses. Palpate the frontal sinuses by pressing up from under the medial aspect of the brow ridges. Palpate the maxillary sinuses by pressing up and in under the zygomatic arch. Normally the sinuses are nontender on palpation.

CRANIAL NERVE I. To test cranial nerve I, the olfactory nerve, the client closes his eyes while you occlude one naris and hold a substance with a familiar odor under the other. Ask the client if he smells anything and, if so, to identify it. The procedure is then repeated for the other naris. Normally, familiar odors such as coffee or vanilla can be distinguished. The sense of smell is often decreased in older adults.

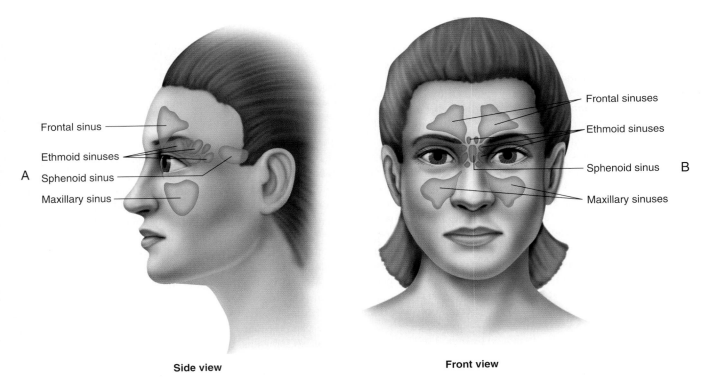

Side view   Front view

Figure 8-16. The paranasal sinuses.

Lips, Mouth, and Throat.

Physical assessment of the mouth and throat involves the following activities:

- Inspecting the lips, gums, teeth, buccal mucosa, roof and floor of the mouth, top, bottom, and sides of the tongue, throat, tonsils, and uvula
- Checking motor function of the palate, pharynx, and larynx (cranial nerve X)
- Testing the client's ability to move the tongue (cranial nerve XII)

LIPS. Observe the color and moistness of the client's lips. Also inspect them for cracking, ulcers, and lumps. Normally the lips are smooth, pink, moist, intact, and free of lesions. A blue tinge to the pink coloration due to the presence of melanin pigment is a normal finding in some dark-skinned people. Abnormal findings include dryness, cracks, fissures, pallor, cyanosis, drooping, and involuntary movements. Inspect the oral mucosa of the lower lip for color and lesions by everting the lip (Figure 8-17, *A*).

MOUTH AND THROAT. Ask the client to remove any dentures and open his mouth. Inspect the buccal mucosa, gums, teeth, roof of the mouth, top, bottom, and sides of the tongue, and floor of the mouth. To allow good visibility of the buccal cavity, good light and a tongue blade are essential (Figure 8-17, *B*). Use the tongue blade to expose the buccal mucosa, which can then be inspected for color, intactness, and presence of lesions.

Like the lips, the buccal mucosa is normally intact, smooth, moist, and pink, with areas of dark pigmentation in dark-skinned clients. The tongue should be shiny, pink, and moist, with an even distribution of papillae arranged in an inverted V.

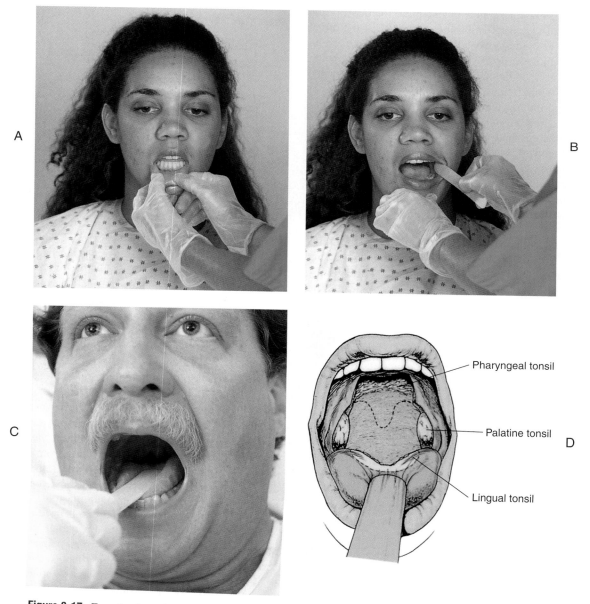

Figure 8-17. Examination of the oral cavity. Inspecting the mucosa of the lower lip (**A**) and the buccal cavity (**B**). Assessing the oropharynx (**C**) and the tonsils (**D**).

Inspect the teeth for dental caries (cavities) and periodontal disease (pyorrhea). The enamel should be smooth, white, and shiny. Brown or black discoloration of the enamel may indicate staining or the presence of caries. Gingivitis (red, swollen gums, bleeding, receding gum lines, and the formation of pockets between the teeth and gums) is characteristic of periodontal disease. In advanced disease, the teeth may be loose and pus may be present.

You should also assess for other inflammatory conditions of the mouth. Glossitis is inflammation of the tongue. Stomatitis is inflammation of the oral mucosa. Fungal infection or oral candidiasis is a common cause of stomatitis. Parotitis is inflammation of the parotid gland (the largest of the salivary glands) and results in obvious swelling of the lower cheek. The most well-known infection of the parotid gland is mumps.

To assess the oropharynx, have the client tilt his head back and open his mouth. Use the tongue blade to depress the tongue about halfway back and shine a penlight on the throat (Figure 8-17, C). Depress one side at a time to avoid eliciting the gag reflex. In the oropharynx, or throat, the uvula should be at the midline. The lingual tonsils lie on either side of the dorsal surface of the tongue. These tonsils normally do not protrude beyond the tonsillar pillar and are of the same color as the rest of the oropharynx. The tonsils may have crypts with exfoliated epithelium that gives a white appearance. Examine the throat for redness, swelling, and the presence of lesions, plaque, or exudate. The tonsils are graded from 1 to 4. Grade 1 is normal. In grade 2, the tonsils are between the pillars and the uvula. In grade 3, the tonsils touch the uvula. In grade 4, one or both tonsils extend to the midline of the oropharynx.

Neck. The neck contains a number of important structures (Figure 8-18). The major blood vessels supplying the head are the carotid artery and jugular vein. The neck is also highly lymphatic, receiving lymph drainage from the head. The esophagus and the trachea course through the neck supported by the cervical spine. Strong muscles support the head and assist with multidirectional ROM. Physical assessment of the neck involves the following activities:

- Observing the shape, symmetry, position, and motion of the neck
- Inspecting the carotid artery and jugular vein
- Inspecting and palpating the trachea
- Inspecting and palpating the thyroid gland
- Palpating cervical lymph nodes

APPEARANCE AND MOTION. With the client in an upright position, begin your assessment of the neck by observing for symmetry and proportion to the head and shoulders. To assess for normal movement, direct the client to put his head back to check extension, put the chin on the chest to check flexion, touch the chin to each shoulder to check rotation, and bend the right ear to the right shoulder and the left ear to the left shoulder without raising the shoulder to test lateral abduction.

Normally the neck flexes 45 degrees, extends 55 degrees, laterally flexes 40 degrees, and rotates 70 degrees (and is free of uncoordinated, uncontrolled movements). This check of

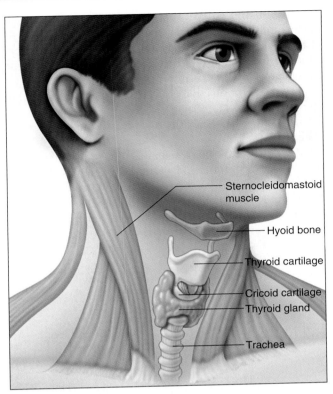

Figure 8-18. Major structures of the neck.

ROM must be performed slowly in geriatric clients, as they may become dizzy with the lateral movements.

Assess for muscle strength by having the client turn his head to one side against the resistance of your hand. Ask the client to shrug his shoulders against the resistance of your hands. The strength should be equal on both sides.

Abnormal findings include unusual shortness of the neck, lack of symmetry, fullness, edema, masses, and scars. In geriatric clients, the neck may appear shortened. This is a normal finding that occurs as a result of muscle atrophy, compression of vertebrae, and loss of fat.

JUGULAR VEIN AND CAROTID ARTERY. Observe the side of the neck over the jugular vein and the carotid artery. Normally the jugular vein is not distended and only a mild pulsation of the carotid artery can be seen. A distended jugular vein or marked pulsations of the carotid are abnormal.

TRACHEA. Observe the middle front of the neck and then palpate for any sign of tracheal deviation from the midline. To palpate for tracheal deviation, place your index finger along one side of the trachea and note the distance between the side of the trachea and the sternocleidomastoid muscle. Repeat this action on the other side and compare the two distances. Normally the distances should be equal, and the trachea should be nontender with distinct rings palpable. Soreness or swelling indicated by nonpalpable rings is abnormal.

THYROID. The thyroid gland has two lobes, one on each side and slightly in front of the trachea. The thin isthmus that connects the lobes lies over the trachea just below the cricoid cartilage.

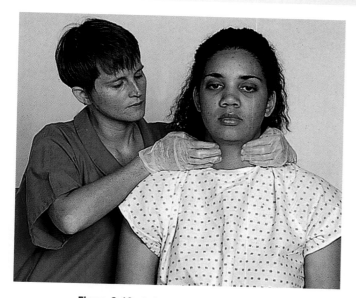

Figure 8-19. Palpating the thyroid gland.

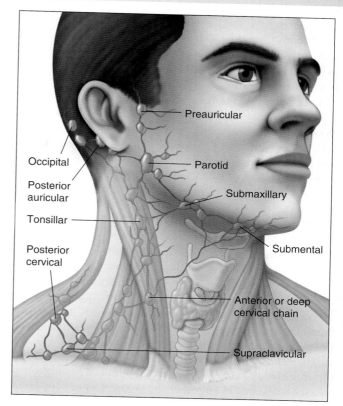

Figure 8-20. The cervical lymph nodes.

To assess the thyroid gland, ask the client to lift his chin so you can observe his neck for a visible thyroid. You may also ask the client to take a sip of water, lift his chin, and then swallow while you watch the movement of the thyroid in the neck. Normally the thyroid is not visible with this inspection.

Next, palpate the size, shape, and consistency of the thyroid. This is done by standing behind the client and asking him to tilt his head back slightly. Place the fingers of both hands on the sides of the client's neck with the index fingers just below the cricoid cartilage (Figure 8-19). Then ask the client to swallow while you feel for the thyroid isthmus to rise. Then move your fingers downward and laterally to identify any palpable parts of the lateral lobes. The normal thyroid feels smooth and rubbery. If palpable, the lobes should be symmetrical and painless.

CERVICAL LYMPH NODES. Lymph nodes in the neck collect lymph from the head and neck (Figure 8-20). There are 10 major groups of superficial cervical lymph nodes:

- Preauricular (in front of the ear)
- Parotid
- Submaxillary
- Submental (midline, beneath the tip of the mandible)
- Anterior or deep cervical chain
- Supraclavicular (between the sternocleidomastoid muscle and the trapezius muscle at the base of the neck)
- Occipital (at the base of the skull)
- Posterior auricular (behind the ear, over the mastoid process)
- Tonsillar
- Posterior cervical (between the sternocleidomastoid muscle and the trapezius muscle in the middle of the neck)

Cervical lymph nodes are assessed by palpating both sides of the neck simultaneously using the pads of your index and middle fingers. Bend the client's head slightly forward or to the side to relax the soft tissues and muscles around the area being examined.

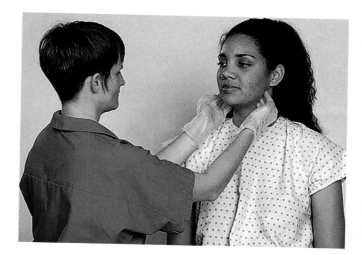

Figure 8-21. Palpating the cervical lymph nodes.

To examine the submental and submandibular nodes, place your fingertips under the mandible and move the skin over the nodes. To assess the supraclavicular nodes, have the client flex his neck forward. Exert light to moderate pressure and move the skin over the underlying tissues beginning in front of the ear and progressing systematically over the areas of the neck where the groups of cervical lymph nodes are located. There is no one right order for palpation of cervical nodes (Figure 8-21). It is simply important that you select an order and use it consistently so that no area is accidentally missed.

Normally, cervical lymph nodes either are not palpable or are smooth, firm, less than 1 cm in diameter (with definite margins), mobile, and nontender. In geriatric clients, submandibular salivary glands commonly prolapse and may be felt as soft masses in the upper neck, below the jaw.

Enlargement of the lymph nodes is called lymphadenopathy. Describe the location, size, presence of tenderness, consistency, inflammation, and whether they are freely moveable. Enlargement can result from infections or neoplasms of the oral pharynx or nasopharynx, from systemic diseases, or from infections such as mononucleosis or measles. Infection of the mouth or oropharynx is the most common cause.

Assessment of the Breasts and Axillae

Breasts. The breasts of both men and women are composed of glandular, fibrous, and adipose tissue. Adult women have more adipose tissue and fully developed (mature) glandular tissue, whereas it is rudimentary in men. However, the breasts in both sexes should be inspected and palpated for malignancy. Breast cancer is rare in men, but one of nine women will acquire breast cancer at some point in life. Therefore, women should be taught breast self-examination (see Chapter 45).

The glandular tissue in the female breast is concentrated in the upper outer quadrant, where a tail of breast tissue projects into the axilla and is known as the tail of Spence. The breast is drained by four groups of axillary lymph nodes: central axillary nodes high in the midaxilla; pectoral nodes, along the outer edge of the pectoral muscle at the anterior axillary line; subscapular nodes, along the posterior axillary line at the lateral edge of the scapula; and lateral nodes, inside the upper arm along the upper humerus.

Physical assessment of the breasts involves the following activities:

- Observing the size, contour, symmetry, skin color and appearance, and vascularity of the breasts
- Observing the areolae for shape, color, and hair
- Observing the size, shape, symmetry, and direction of point of the nipples
- Palpating each breast for consistency, tenderness, and presence of masses or palpable lymph nodes
- Checking for nipple discharge

SIZE, SHAPE, AND SKIN APPEARANCE. To inspect the breasts, begin with the client sitting with her arms at her sides and then ask her to raise her arms over her head, lower them, and press her hands against her hips. If she has pendulous breasts, ask her to lean forward. As the client performs these actions, observe the size, symmetry, contour, vascular pattern, and skin appearance of the breasts.

Normal breasts are symmetrical, although one may be larger than the other. They are conical to pendulous in shape, their contour is even, and the skin is similar to normal skin on the trunk, with a faint, symmetrical vascular pattern evident.

Abnormal findings include asymmetrical breasts; breasts markedly different in size; areas of retraction, dimpling, or flattening; erythematous or peau d'orange (orange peel appearance) skin; and asymmetrical vascular dilation.

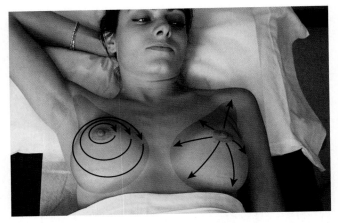

Figure 8-22. Client position and assessment patterns for breast palpation.

PALPATION. First, palpate the breasts with the client sitting with her hands at her sides. Then have her lie on her back with the arm on the side being examined raised and positioned so that its hand is behind her head; place a pillow under the shoulder on the side being examined. This position allows the breast tissue to flatten evenly over the chest wall (Figure 8-22). Palpate in a specific pattern, such as in a spiral working out from the areola, following horizontal or vertical lines up and down the breast, or following spokes of a wheel from the areola to the periphery, to ensure that all four quadrants and the axillary tail of Spence are assessed (Figure 8-23). In palpating the breasts, move the pads of your fingers in a firm circular motion to slide the skin over the breast tissue. In judging the findings, one breast must be compared with the other.

Normally, breast tissue feels uniformly loose or dense, smooth, and either firm or soft. The finding of areas of thickening, palpable masses, or tenderness or pain on palpation (except in the premenstrual female) is abnormal. Following palpation, the nipple of each breast is gently compressed between the thumb and forefinger to check for nipple discharge. With the exception of lactating women, the appearance of discharge with or without nipple compression is abnormal, as is retraction, deviation, or recent inversion of a nipple.

Axillae. Physical assessment of the axillae involves the following activities:

- Inspecting the condition of the axillae
- Palpating the axillae for masses and tenderness

INSPECTION. Inspect each axilla for cleanliness, hair distribution, and skin condition. Axillary hair is a secondary sex characteristic and thus is absent prior to puberty. In older adults, axillary hair is normally sparse and gray. In persons of all ages, the skin of the axilla should be free of redness, crusts, rashes, and other lesions.

PALPATION. Palpate the axillae after inspecting them. Have the client sit with her arms hanging at her sides. Support the client's arm on the side to be examined with one hand and use the fingertips of the other hand to palpate the axilla. With your fingers together, slightly cupped, and as high up in the axilla as

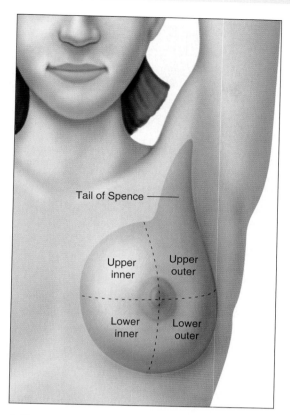

Tail of Spence ————

Upper inner

Upper outer

Lower inner

Lower outer

Figure 8-23. The four breast quadrants and the axillary tail of Spence.

possible, press inward toward the chest wall and move your fingers downward. Repeat this action down the anterior border of the axilla, along the inner aspect of the upper arm and, standing behind the client, down the posterior border of the axilla. Usually no lymph nodes are felt; however, one or more soft, nontender central nodes are an occasional insignificant finding.

Assessment of the Thorax

Assessment of the thorax includes the chest wall, the lungs, the heart, and the great vessels. Begin with either the anterior or posterior chest, using the techniques of inspection, palpation, percussion, and auscultation, and then proceed to the opposite chest wall. In the hospitalized client, it is common to begin with the anterior chest for convenience when the client is lying in bed.

Examining the organs within the chest cavity is an indirect examination that is based on knowledge of the location of the underlying structures. You must become familiar with the landmarks on the chest wall to associate your findings with the underlying structures. Using imaginary reference lines, you will be able to describe the location of your findings in a manner that will have the same meaning to anyone reading your description. Useful landmarks include the ribs, the sternal notch, the angle of Louis, the thyroid process, the vertebra prominens, and the scapula.

As you begin learning to identify key locations on the chest wall, it is useful to count the ribs. Once you are comfortable with

the locations, you will no longer need to count. The first rib is hidden beneath the clavicle; therefore, the first space is the first intercostal space, and the first rib to be felt is the second rib. The angle of Louis separates the manubrium from the body of the sternum. The second intercostal space is at the same level as the angle of Louis. Additionally, the trachea bifurcates at the angle of Louis. All 12 ribs articulate with the thoracic spine.

The right lung has three lobes and the left lung has two lobes. Figure 8-24, *A,* (p. 150) helps you locate the lobes of the lungs using landmarks on the anterior surface of the chest wall. On the right, the horizontal fissure that divides the upper lobe from the middle lobe follows the fourth rib. The fissure between the middle and lower lobes starts at the midclavicular line under the sixth rib and angles diagonally to the midaxillary line in the axilla. On the left, the heart occupies the space that would otherwise be the middle lobe. Only small portions of the lower lobes are accessible anteriorly on either the right or the left side.

Your best access to the lower lobes is posteriorly. With the client's arms raised over the head, the division between the upper and lower lobes starts at the third thoracic vertebra and runs obliquely, following the edges of the scapulae (Figure 8-24, *B*).

On the lateral left side, the upper and lower lobes are divided obliquely from the midclavicular line at the sixth rib to the axilla at the level of the third thoracic vertebra (Figure 8-24, *C*). The same line on the right side divides the upper and middle lobes from the lower lobe. A horizontal line from the fourth or fifth rib at the midclavicular line divides the upper and middle lobes (Figure 8-24, *D*). The right side provides the best access to the right middle lobe.

Chest Wall and Lungs. Physical assessment of the chest wall and lungs should include the following:
- Inspection and palpation of the chest for shape, contour, and symmetry
- Inspection of the pattern of breathing
- Palpation of tactile fremitus
- Palpation of respiratory excursion
- Percussion of the posterior, anterior, and lateral thorax
- Auscultation of the posterior, anterior, and lateral thorax

INSPECTION AND PALPATION. To assess the thorax and lungs, evaluate the anterior, posterior, and lateral areas of the thorax, using the techniques of inspection, palpation, percussion, and auscultation.

ANTERIOR LANDMARKS. The anterior chest is divided into imaginary vertical lines, which serve as anatomic landmarks (Figure 8-25, p. 151):
- The midsternal line, drawn vertically through the center of the sternum
- The left and right midclavicular lines, drawn vertically through the midpoint of the left and right clavicles and running parallel to the midsternal line
- The left and right anterior axillary lines, drawn vertically through the anterior axillary folds and running parallel to the midsternal line

Additional anterior anatomic landmarks include the manubriosternal junction (often called the angle of Louis), the suprasternal notch, the costal angle, the clavicles, and the ribs.

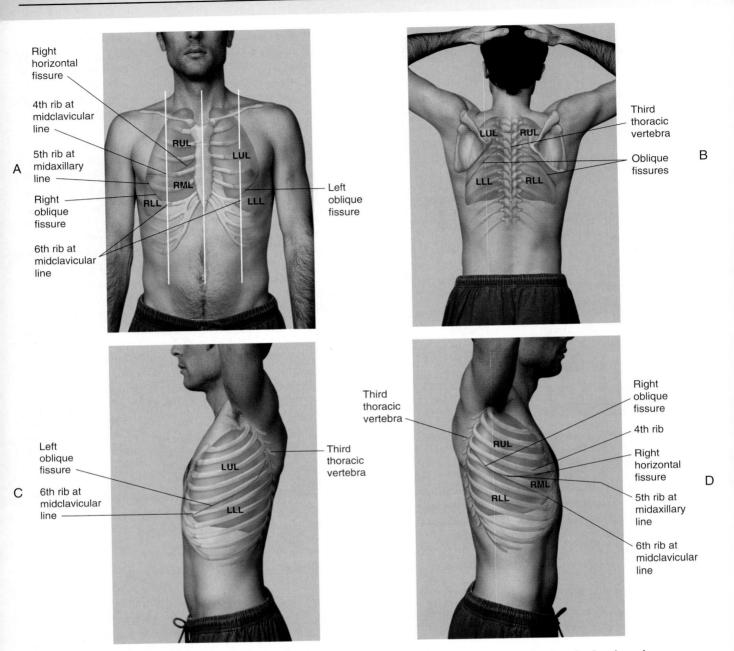

Figure 8-24. Chest landmarks. **A,** Anterior chest landmarks and underlying lungs. **B,** Posterior chest landmarks and underlying lungs. **C,** Left lateral chest landmarks and underlying lungs. **D,** Right lateral chest landmarks and underlying lungs.

Anteriorly, the ribs articulate with the manubrium and the sternum. Posteriorly, they articulate with the vertebral processes. The first seven ribs articulate with the manubrium and the body of the sternum, and the last five ribs are fused into a bony and cartilaginous costal angle anteriorly. This angle should be less than 90 degrees. They are supported and connected by the intercostal muscles and attached to each other by costal cartilage. The exceptions are the 11th and 12th ribs, which remain unattached (or floating) anteriorly. The palpable spaces between the ribs are called intercostal spaces (ICSs) and are numbered in ascending order beginning at the base of the neck and moving downward (i.e., the first left or right ICS, second left or right ICS, etc.). They are used as anatomic landmarks.

POSTERIOR LANDMARKS. The posterior chest is divided similarly into three imaginary vertical and parallel lines that serve as landmarks (Figure 8-26):
- The vertebral or midspinal line, running through the center of the spinous processes
- The left and right midscapular lines, which run vertically through the midpoint of the inferior angle of the scapulae and parallel to the vertebral line

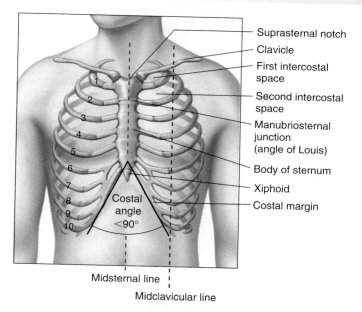

Figure 8-25. Anterior chest landmarks.

Suprasternal notch
Clavicle
First intercostal space
Second intercostal space
Manubriosternal junction (angle of Louis)
Body of sternum
Xiphoid
Costal margin
Costal angle <90°
Midsternal line
Midclavicular line

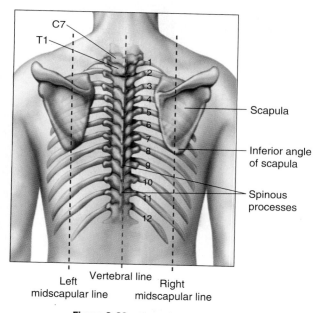

Figure 8-26. Posterior chest landmarks.

C7
T1
Scapula
Inferior angle of scapula
Spinous processes
Left midscapular line
Vertebral line
Right midscapular line

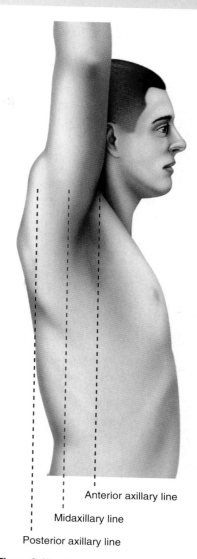

Figure 8-27. Lateral chest landmarks.

Anterior axillary line
Midaxillary line
Posterior axillary line

Additional posterior landmarks include the scapulae, the spinous processes, and the intercostal spaces of the ribs. All 12 of the ribs articulate posteriorly with the thoracic vertebrae.

LATERAL LANDMARKS. The lateral chest is divided similarly into three imaginary lines: the anterior axillary line, the midaxillary line, and the posterior axillary line (Figure 8-27). The midaxillary line is drawn vertically through the midpoint of the left and right axillae. The anterior axillary line is drawn vertically through the anterior axillary folds and parallel to the midaxillary line. Finally, the posterior axillary line is drawn through the posterior axillary folds parallel to the midaxillary line.

SHAPE, CONTOUR, AND SYMMETRY. Begin your assessment of the chest and lungs with the client undressed from the waist up and sitting up on the examining table. Observe the posterior thorax from a midline position behind the client. Observe the anterior thorax with the client lying supine. Note whether the chest is of normal size and contour (Figure 8-28, A and B, p. 152). Does the chest appear asymmetrical? Normally the anteroposterior to lateral ratio should be between 1:2 or 5:7.

Note whether there are congenital anomalies, past traumatic injuries, disfigurements, or surgical alterations. Inspect and palpate the thorax, clavicles, scapulas, ribs, and spine for contour and abnormalities. Note any congenital abnormalities, traumatic injuries, postsurgical alterations, masses, lesions, tenderness, or abnormal slopes or contours. Ask the client to bend over at the waist so that you can further inspect the curvature of the spine.

Figure 8-28, *C* through *F*, illustrates normal variations and abnormalities of chest configuration. Pigeon chest (Figure 8-28, *C*)

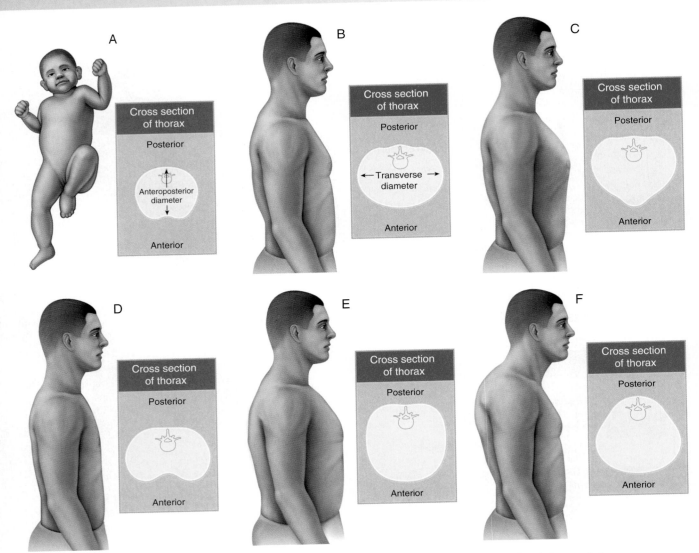

Figure 8-28. Normal configuration of the thorax in an infant (**A**) and an adult (**B**). Normal variations and abnormalities of chest configuration include pigeon chest (**C**), funnel chest (**D**), barrel chest (**E**), and kyphosis (**F**).

and funnel chest (Figure 8-28, *D*) are considered normal congenital variations and are not corrected unless the deformity interferes with cardiopulmonary function or the client desires correction for cosmetic reasons. Barrel chest (Figure 8-28, *E*) is associated with chronic obstructive pulmonary disease. Kyphosis (Figure 8-28, *F*) and scoliosis (see Figure 31-5, p. 772) can be severe enough to interfere with breathing.

PATTERN OF BREATHING. Inspect the client's breathing pattern. Attempt to observe the respirations without making the client aware that you are doing so. A commonly used technique is to pretend you are taking the pulse while you are actually observing the respiratory pattern. Note any abnormalities of breathing rate or rhythm. A rate of 12 to 20 breaths per minute is considered normal for an adult. Inspiration time is slightly shorter than expiration time.

Any variations in rate and rhythm, such as tachypnea (rapid breathing), bradypnea (slow breathing), hyperpnea (sighing), hyperventilation (rapid deep breathing), apnea (periods of cessation of breathing), Cheyne-Stokes respirations (irregular breathing with long pauses), Kussmaul's respirations (rapid, deep breathing seen in diabetic ketoacidosis), wheezing (squeaking or whistling), respiratory lag or pauses, prolonged expiration, bulging of the intercostal spaces, or use of accessory muscles to breathe should be clearly noted.

TACTILE FREMITUS. Palpate for tactile fremitus (also called vocal fremitus). **Tactile fremitus** is a vibration in the chest wall that is felt on the thorax while the client is speaking. It occurs over an abnormal area, such as an area where secretions have collected. Ask the client to repeatedly say "ninety-nine" as you place the ball of your hand (the posterior palm near the proximal finger joints) on each of the target areas diagrammed in Figure 8-29. The pattern shown for palpating for tactile fremitus will later be repeated for percussion and auscultation.

Compare the transmission of the client's voice through the chest wall in opposite symmetrical areas of the chest. The

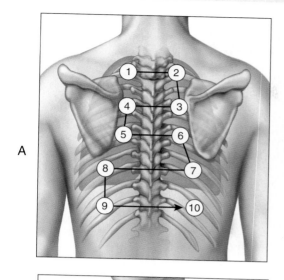

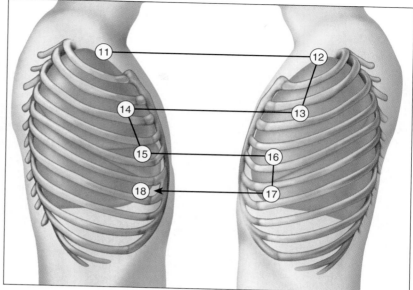

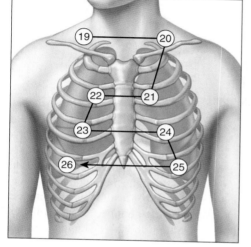

Figure 8-29. Systematic pattern of palpation for tactile fremitus, also used to percuss and auscultate the chest. **A,** Posterior; **B,** lateral; **C,** anterior target areas.

vibratory transmission of the voice should be equivalent in symmetrical areas. Vibratory sensations are decreased in clients with a soft voice, laryngeal disease or obstruction, bronchial obstruction, chronic obstructive pulmonary disease (COPD), effusions (fluid), fibrosis (thickening), pneumothorax (air), or infiltrating tumor. Vibratory sensations are increased with conditions that would increase the transmission of sound, such as a consolidated lung (lobar pneumonia).

RESPIRATORY EXCURSION. Palpate for **respiratory excursion,** which is the ability of the lungs to expand as evidenced by the degree to which the chest wall expands. To do this, stand behind the client with your thumbs placed on the spinous processes at the level of the tenth ribs. Spread your fingers apart over the lateral thorax with your thumbs pointing toward each other and your fingers pointing away from each other (Figure 8-30, p. 154). Press your palms inward toward the spine, moving your thumbs closer together with only a small skin fold between them. Now ask the client to exhale and then to take a deep breath and hold it. Observe the movement

of your thumbs and note the expanded distance between them. Normal respiratory excursion will separate the thumbs by 1¼ to 2 inches. Limited respiratory excursion may occur with chronic fibrotic disease of the lungs, COPD, emphysema, pulmonary tumors, an abdominal mass, or superficial pain.

PERCUSSION. Percuss the posterior and anterior thorax to reveal the nature of underlying tissue. To obtain a percussion "note," press the middle finger of your left hand firmly on the surface. Cock the middle finger of your right hand and strike the middle finger of your left hand between the distal joint and your fingernail. Work your way down the posterior and then the anterior thorax, striking at least twice in each of the percussion target areas in intercostal spaces. Listen for dullness, resonance, or tympany (Figure 8-31, p. 155). Dullness is heard over solid or fluid-filled tissue (e.g., large underlying organs such as the liver or heart). Resonance is heard over air-filled tissue (e.g., most of the lung spaces). Tympany is heard over tissue that is hyperinflated with air or where a large amount of air is common, such as the gastric air bubble.

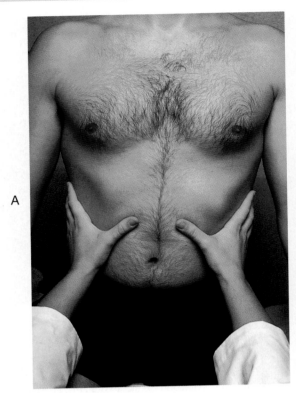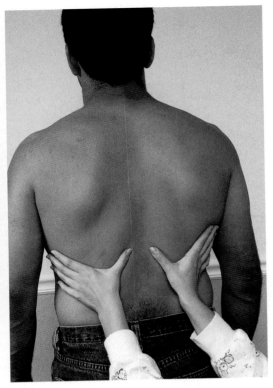

Figure 8-30. Position of the hands for assessing respiratory excursion on the anterior (**A**) and posterior thorax (**B**).

Percuss for diaphragmatic excursion or the ability of the lungs to expand as evidenced by the movement of the diaphragm. Ask the client to exhale and hold it. Percuss downward from a point of resonance toward the diaphragm. Mark the point where dullness is initially heard. Ask the client to then inhale and hold it. Again percuss downward from a point of resonance to the area where diaphragmatic dullness is initially heard. Mark this point and measure the distance between the two points. Normally the diaphragm will descend 3 to 6 cm. Excursion is decreased in COPD.

AUSCULTATION. Auscultate the posterior and then the anterior thorax in the pattern diagrammed for palpation (see Figure 8-29). Have the client (undressed from the waist up) sit up for both posterior and anterior chest auscultations, because abnormal findings may be masked in a supine client. With the diaphragm of the stethoscope on bare skin, listen to the client breathing. Move across and down the posterior and then the anterior chest. Be alert for artifacts and eliminate them before proceeding. Artifacts are sounds made inadvertently from clothing, muscle contractions, paper, scratching, or from your fingers resting on the stethoscope or the client's chest.

Identify the bronchial, bronchovesicular, and vesicular breath sounds (Figure 8-32) and distinguish these sounds from artifactual and abnormal breath sounds. **Bronchial** breath sounds are normal sounds heard with a stethoscope over the main airways, including the trachea and sternum. Inspiration is shorter than expiration. **Bronchovesicular** breath sounds are normal breath sounds that occur between sounds of the bronchial tubes and those of the alveoli, or a combination of the two sounds. Expiration and inspiration are of equal duration and sound like blowing through a hollow tube. **Vesicular** breath sounds are a normal sound of rustling or swishing heard with a stethoscope over the lung periphery, characteristically higher pitched during inspiration and falling rapidly during expiration. Inspiration is longer than expiration.

Adventitious is derived from a Latin word meaning from an outside source. Thus, adventitious breath sounds are produced by a source other than normal lungs. There are basically three types of adventitious breath sounds: discontinuous, or coarse and fine crackles that indicate the presence of fluid in the lung spaces; continuous, including high- and low-pitched wheezes that indicate narrowing or partial obstruction of the airways from inflammation, mucus, edema, a foreign body, or a mass; and rubs, grating sounds heard on both inspiration and expiration and caused by the rubbing together of inflamed pleural surfaces. Note any adventitious sounds, their timing (inspiratory or expiratory), their location, and whether they clear with coughing, deep breathing, or position changes. Adventitious sounds are discussed in Chapter 33.

Heart. Examination of the heart should include the following steps:
- Inspect and palpate the anterior chest, including all six anatomic landmarks.
- Palpate the apical impulse or point of maximal impulse.
- Palpate the carotid pulse.
- Percuss the cardiac border to assess the size of the heart.
- Auscultate the heart for rate and rhythm.

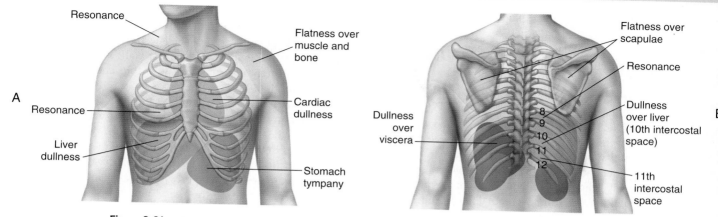

Figure 8-31. Normal percussion notes over the anterior (**A**) and posterior (**B**) chest and upper abdomen.

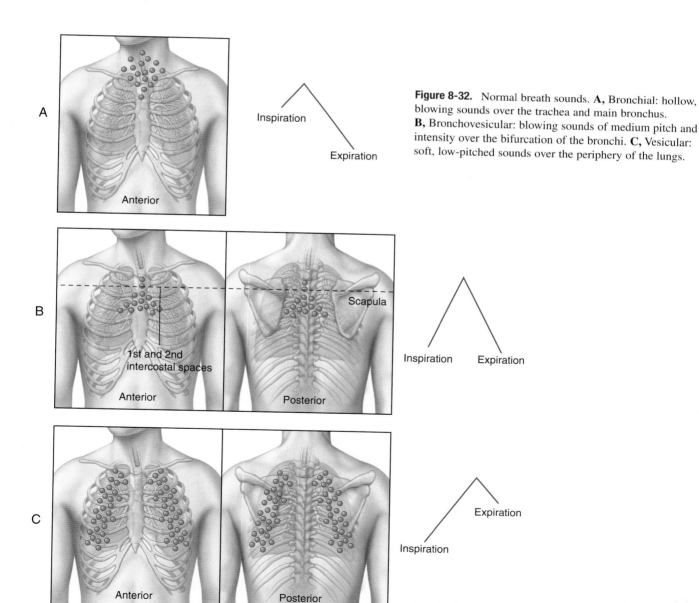

Figure 8-32. Normal breath sounds. **A,** Bronchial: hollow, blowing sounds over the trachea and main bronchus. **B,** Bronchovesicular: blowing sounds of medium pitch and intensity over the bifurcation of the bronchi. **C,** Vesicular: soft, low-pitched sounds over the periphery of the lungs.

- Compare the apical and radial pulses if the rhythm of the heart is found to be irregular.
- Auscultate the heart at each of the six anatomic landmarks.
- Identify and auscultate S_1 and S_2.
- Identify and auscultate systole and diastole.
- Auscultate for extra heart sounds.
- Auscultate and evaluate any heart murmurs.

ANATOMIC LANDMARKS. The location of the heart in the anterior chest begins with identification of the anatomic landmarks that identify the precordium. The **precordium** is the area on the anterior chest overlying the heart and great vessels. The heart extends from the right border of the sternum to the left midclavicular line and from the second intercostal space to the fifth intercostal space. The heart can be thought of as an inverted isosceles triangle in the chest with the base at the top and the apex pointing down and to the left. It is slightly rotated with the right side anterior and the left side posterior.

There are six anatomic landmarks for listening to heart sounds. Four are associated with the heart valves: aortic, pulmonic, mitral, and tricuspid. The areas to listen to for the sounds are not directly over the valves but over the area to which the sound produced by the valve is transmitted (Figure 8-33). Sound is transmitted in the direction of blood flow. Although these areas are depicted as a single spot on the precordium, the valve sounds are heard in a larger area that overlaps with other areas. The area associated with the pulmonic valve is the second intercostal space to the left of the sternum. The area associated with the aortic valve is the second intercostal space to the right of the sternum. The area associated with the tricuspid valve is the fifth intercostal space at the left sternal border. The area associated with the mitral valve is the fifth intercostal space at the left midclavicular line. Erb's point is the fifth area, located in the third intercostal space on the left sternal border, and it is here that some murmurs are best heard. The sixth area is the **point of maximal impulse** (PMI). The PMI is the area of the chest wall where the apex of the heart comes closest to the chest wall; the heart beat is felt there and may even be seen in a thin chest wall. In a healthy adult, the PMI is the mitral area.

EVENTS OF THE CARDIAC CYCLE. The heart is evaluated in relationship to the events of the cardiac cycle. The cardiac cycle is the time from the beginning of the contraction of the ventricles to the beginning of the next contraction. Systole is the contraction phase and diastole is the relaxation phase. When the ventricles contract, pressure immediately increases in the ventricles, causing the mitral and tricuspid valves to close and the aortic and pulmonic valves to open. When the ventricles relax, the pressure drops to below that of the aorta and the pulmonary vein, causing the aortic and pulmonic valves to close. The greater pressure in the atria opens the mitral and tricuspid valves.

Two heart sounds are produced by the events of the cardiac cycle. The first heart sound, S_1, is the heart sound produced by the vibration of the chest wall set in motion by the closure of the mitral and tricuspid valves. S_2, the second heart sound, is produced by the vibration of the chest wall set in motion by the closure of the aortic and pulmonic valves. Thus, S_1 is associated with systole and S_2 is associated with diastole. The heart sounds are often described as a lubb-dupp sound with the lubb being S_1 and the dupp being S_2.

INSPECTION AND PALPATION. Begin the assessment of the heart with inspection and palpation of the anterior thorax. Have the client undress to the waist and examine the client first sitting up, then lying down, under adequate lighting. Be sure to inspect the client from the side and at an angle to take full advantage of lighting.

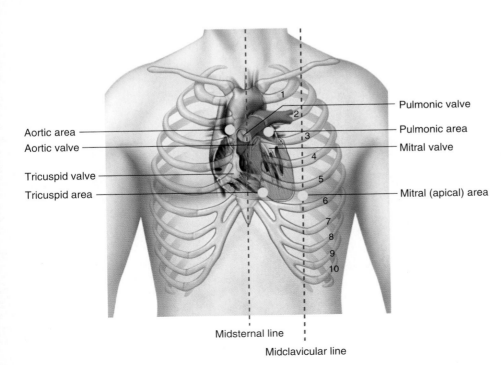

Aortic area
Aortic valve
Tricuspid valve
Tricuspid area

Pulmonic valve
Pulmonic area
Mitral valve
Mitral (apical) area

1
2
3
4
5
6
7
8
9
10

Midsternal line
Midclavicular line

Figure 8-33. Anatomic sites for assessment of the precordium.

Inspect and palpate the aortic area, the pulmonic area, Erb's point, the tricuspid area, the apical area, and the epigastric area just below the tip of the sternum. Palpate the anatomic landmarks of the precordium. Palpate the chest and anatomic landmarks using the ball of the hand and the posterior side of the proximal finger joints placed lightly on the chest surface in each area. Time the occurrence of any perceived pulsations, heaves, or thrills during systole and diastole, and auscultate the heart while palpating the carotid artery simultaneously.

Heaves are forceful pulsations that bound up against your hand. Thrills are vibrations. Normally no lesions, masses, or abnormalities should be noted. There may be a light tapping sensation in the apical landmark (fourth or fifth intercostal space at the midclavicular line); however, any heaves, any thrills anywhere in the precordium, or any pulsations palpable in a location other than the apical landmark should be considered abnormal.

APICAL PULSE. As defined in Chapter 7, the *apical pulse* is the heart rate counted at the apex (the PMI) of the heart on the anterior chest. Palpate and evaluate the apical impulse by placing your hand over the fifth intercostal space at the midclavicular line. Usually you will feel a light tapping sensation occurring in the apical area at the left fifth intercostal space at the midclavicular line. Normally the area of the tapping sensation is limited to 1 to 2 cm in diameter and confined to one intercostal space. Displacement of the apical impulse or an impulse felt in an area that is larger than 2 cm in diameter may be a result of abnormal curvatures of the spine, cardiomegaly, emphysema, obesity, increased musculature, or enlarged breasts. A faint or barely perceptible PMI may also be related to any condition that increases tissue mass or fluid between the heart and the chest wall, such as pericardial effusions (inflammatory fluid in the pericardium), pulmonary effusions (inflammatory fluid in the pleural space), or tumors.

CAROTID PULSE. Palpate and evaluate the carotid pulse. The carotid artery is located in the groove between the trachea and the sternomastoid muscle and can usually be easily felt anywhere along this groove. To locate the most prominent pulse, ask the client to turn his head away from the side chosen for palpation. Observe the neck for pulsations. Figure 8-34 shows the major arteries and veins of the right side of the neck. Place the tips of two fingers held together (usually your index and second finger) lightly over the pulsations. Auscultate the heart simultaneously and determine whether the carotid pulse is regular and synchronous with S_1.

PERCUSSION. Rarely is the technique of percussion employed to determine cardiac size in current practice because chest radiographs now provide a much more reliable assessment of cardiac size and contour. However, when chest radiographs are not readily available, this may be a useful technique to know.

Using the percussion technique described previously, percuss the borders of cardiac dullness and assess the size of the heart. The heart tissue is dull to percussion amid surrounding resonant lung tissue. The left border of cardiac dullness is usually at the fifth intercostal space at the midclavicular line

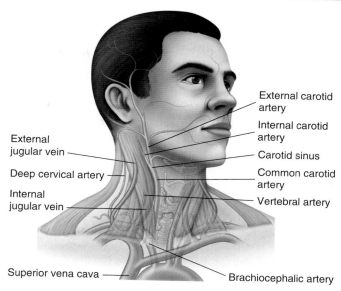

Figure 8-34. Arteries and veins of the right side of the neck.

External jugular vein

Deep cervical artery

Internal jugular vein

Superior vena cava

External carotid artery

Internal carotid artery

Carotid sinus

Common carotid artery

Vertebral artery

Brachiocephalic artery

and at the second intercostal space at the sternum. The right border of cardiac dullness is usually at the sternum.

A number of conditions, such as cardiomegaly (enlarged heart), left ventricular hypertrophy (enlarged left ventricle), pericardial effusions, or a cardiac mass, may account for increased heart size. A small number of clients may have congenital anomalies such as dextrocardia (abnormally rotated or positioned heart) or situs inversus (organs located on the side opposite of normal), which will result in markedly abnormal findings.

AUSCULTATION. Auscultate the heart for rate and rhythm. Using the diaphragm of the stethoscope, auscultate the apical area of the heart for the rate and rhythm, counting the first heart sound (S_1, lubb) and the second heart sound (S_2, dupp) in combination as one beat, lubb-dupp.

Assess the apical heart rate by counting the number of beats in 1 full minute. Assess the cardiac rhythm. Listen to several full cycles, paying particular attention to the length of the systolic pauses between S_1 and S_2. The length of both the systolic and the diastolic pause should be consistent in all cycles. Any variation in length of systolic or diastolic pauses, an abnormally long pause, or a sudden increase in heart rate over 100 cycles constitutes an irregular rhythm.

The average heart rate for adults is between 60 and 100 beats per minute (bpm). The average heart rate for children varies depending on age. Sinus bradycardia, or heart rate less than 60 bpm, may be normal in well-conditioned athletes but is abnormal when associated with hypothermia, hypothyroidism, and drug overdoses (narcotics and digoxin). Sinus tachycardia, or a heart rate greater than 100 bpm, may be normal with increased exercise; however, it is abnormal in association with increased caffeine intake, stimulant overdoses, fever, pain, hyperthyroidism, anxiety, shock, and heart disease. A sinus dysrhythmia, in which the pulse rate changes with respirations, increasing at the peak of inspiration and decreasing with expiration, often occurs in children and young adults as a normal variant. Ventricular premature contractions result in irregular heart rhythms perceived as beats that occur out of sequence and sometimes singularly or in couplets. They may occur frequently or infrequently and are caused by abnormal electrical conduction through the ventricular tissue; they may indicate or be a precursor to a serious arrhythmia.

If the rhythm of the heartbeat is found to be irregular, compare the apical and radial pulses. Compare the rate (per full minute) between the apical and radial pulses. Usually the apical and radial pulses will be equivalent in rhythm. If a pulse deficit occurs, the lost beats were not strong enough to send a pulse wave to the radial artery; the peripheral circulation may be compromised by the deficit.

Auscultate the heart in each of the six anatomic landmarks using first the diaphragm of the stethoscope and then the bell. Apply firm pressure when using the diaphragm and light pressure when using the bell. At each site, listen for the rate and rhythm, S_1, S_2, systole and diastole, extra heart sounds, and murmurs (murmurs will be described shortly).

Since the sounds produced by the closing of heart valves may often be heard throughout the precordium, it is now advised to edge the stethoscope across the base of the heart and down the chest to the apex in a Z-like pattern, which will include the anatomic landmarks while covering more surface area of the heart.

HEART SOUNDS. Identify and carefully auscultate S_1 and S_2. The first heart sound (S_1, or lubb) occurs at the same time as the carotid pulse. It is heard best at the apex of the heart and is louder than the second heart sound (S_2, or dupp) at the apical and tricuspid areas and at Erb's point. It is softer than S_2 at the pulmonic and aortic areas. The second heart sound (S_2, or dupp) is heard best in the aortic area. It is louder than S_1 in the aortic and pulmonic areas and at Erb's point.

As you listen to the heart sounds, listen to S_1 and S_2 carefully and separately. Identify and auscultate systole and diastole. Systole is the shorter pause between S_1 and S_2. Diastole is the longer pause between S_2 and S_1. Usually systole and diastole are silent. Figure 8-35 will help you compare the heart sounds to the events of the cardiac cycle and the electrocardiogram.

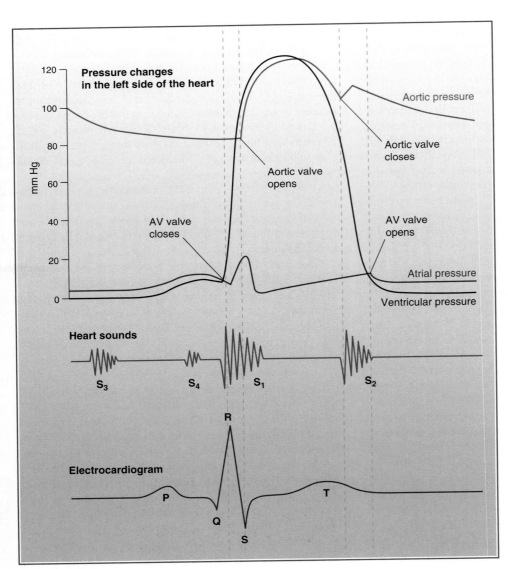

Figure 8-35. Relationship of heart sounds to the events of the cardiac cycle and the electrocardiogram.

Once you have identified S_1 and S_2, note whether the heart sounds are normal, accentuated (loud), or split. A split sound means you can distinguish more than one sound in S_1 or S_2. A physiological split of S_2 can occur with respiration. The change in intrapulmonary pressure causes blood to sequester in the lungs with inspiration, resulting in late closure of the pulmonic valve. Hence, closure of the aortic and closure of the pulmonic valves are heard separately. A physiological split of S_2 is easily identified because it varies with respiration.

EXTRA HEART SOUNDS. Auscultate for extra heart sounds. Note whether there are third (S_3) and fourth (S_4) heart sounds, split sounds, or audible clicks. S_3 and S_4 are sounds produced by rapid ventricular filling. Split sounds are the result of one valve closing before the other. Clicks are the result of diseased valves being forced open or incompletely closing. S_3 and S_4 are a good introduction to extra heart sounds.

The cause of S_3 is vibrations of the ventricle walls when they are suddenly distended by blood from the atria at the end of diastole; S_3 is heard most clearly at the apex of the heart just after S_2. As the atrioventricular valves open, the rush of blood into the ventricles creates vibration that produces sound. It occurs when the ventricles are resistant to filling during the early rapid filling phase of diastole. S_3 is best heard at the apex in the lateral position or lower left sternal border. S_3 is normal in children and in young adults, but after age 40 it is usually taken as a sign of heart failure. The sound of an S_3 can be simulated by rapidly repeating LUBB-dupp-pa.

The cause of S_4 is vibrations created as the atrial contraction forces the last blood into the ventricle just before systole. In Figure 8-35 note the increase in atrial pressure as the atrium contracts in late diastole. S_4 is best heard at the apex of the heart during expiration just before S_1. A physiological S_4 may occur in adults over the age of 40, particularly after exercise, but it usually indicates a pathological condition such as hypertension, fluid overload, or heart failure. An S_4 can be simulated by rapidly repeating deeLUBB-dupp.

S_3 and S_4 are called gallop rhythms because the sound produced resembles the galloping of a horse. S_3 is a ventricular gallop. An atrial gallop is an abnormal cardiac rhythm in which a low-pitched, extra heart sound (S_4) is heard late in diastole, just before the S_1. If both S_3 and S_4 exist, it sounds like deeLUBB-dupp-pa.

MURMURS. Auscultate for heart murmurs. Murmurs are muffled, softened, prolonged heart sounds that occur when there is turbulent blood flow in the heart or great vessels. When auscultated, they are heard as a soft swooshing or blowing sound rather than the clear lubb-dupp of the first and second heart sounds. Three conditions can cause murmurs: increased velocity of the blood, decreased viscosity of the blood, and structural defects in the valves or unusual openings in the heart chambers.

Evaluate all murmurs for intensity, pattern quality, location, radiation, and posture. The intensity (loud or soft) of a murmur may be high, medium, or low, depending on the pressure and rate of blood flow. To more accurately describe their intensity, murmurs can be graded on a scale of 1 to 6 according to the following criteria:

Grade 1: Barely audible
Grade 2: Audible but faint
Grade 3: Moderately loud
Grade 4: Loud and associated with a thrill
Grade 5: Loud and heard with the edge of the stethoscope lifted off the chest wall
Grade 6: Loudest and heard easily without a stethoscope or with a stethoscope held just above the chest wall

Murmurs may also vary in their pattern of intensity (Figure 8-36). They may grow louder in intensity (crescendo), taper off in intensity (decrescendo), or increase in intensity to a peak and then taper off all within one systolic or diastolic pause (a crescendo-decrescendo or diamond-shaped pattern). The murmur may be pansystolic or holosystolic (or pandiastolic or holodiastolic). In other words, it occurs throughout the entire length of the systolic (or diastolic) pause, or it occurs in the early, middle, or late part of systole or diastole. Whatever pattern the murmur exhibits, it should be carefully and accurately described to help differentiate the possible underlying causes. Although some patterns of intensity are in-

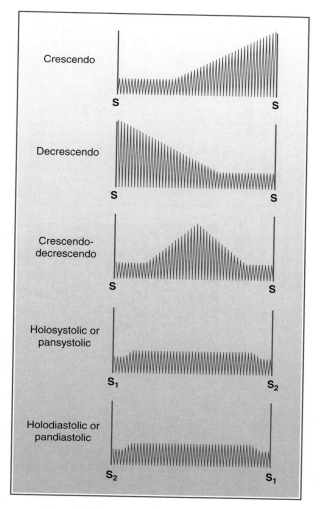

Figure 8-36. Characteristics of heart murmurs.

troduced here, it is beyond the scope of this chapter to provide more detailed explanations of the characteristic murmurs associated with each cardiac abnormality.

The location of a murmur refers to its position within the cardiac cycle. A murmur heard during the lubb, or systolic phase, is a systolic murmur; one heard during the dupp, or diastolic phase, is a diastolic murmur.

A murmur can radiate downstream of the blood flow and be heard in a different area of the precordium. The degree to which a murmur can be heard can vary with posture. Therefore, a thorough examination of the heart includes listening with the client in the supine, forward-sitting, and side-lying positions (Figure 8-37).

Assessment of the Peripheral Vascular System

Include the following in the assessment of the peripheral vascular system:

- Assessment of the client's blood pressure
- Inspection and palpation of the carotid arteries
- Assessment of the jugular venous pulsations
- Assessment of the peripheral venous circulation
- Assessment of the peripheral arterial circulation

Ask the client to undress to underwear and to don an examination gown. The examination of the peripheral vascular system will require that the client sit, stand, or lie down as necessary.

Blood Pressure. Using your stethoscope and sphygmomanometer, assess blood pressure while the client is relaxed and sitting and again just after standing. Blood pressure normally varies in an individual. In general, systolic pressure in the adult varies from 95 to 140 mm Hg, and diastolic pressure varies from 60 to 90 mm Hg. Compare the blood pressures in each arm. A difference of 15 mm Hg or less systolic and 5 mm Hg or less diastolic while the client is standing, and a difference of 5 to 10 mm Hg or less while the client is sitting are considered normal. Assess whether there are orthostatic changes in blood pressure (represented by a difference of greater than 10 mm Hg in diastolic pressures taken from the same arm while the client is sitting and while standing). Orthostatic hypotension is usually defined as a drop in systolic pressure greater than 20 mm Hg. Refer to Chapter 7 for a more thorough discussion of blood pressure and vital signs.

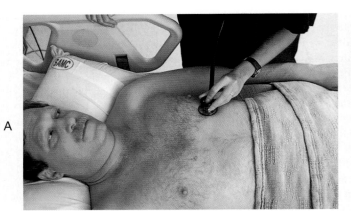

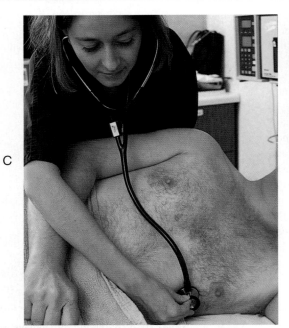

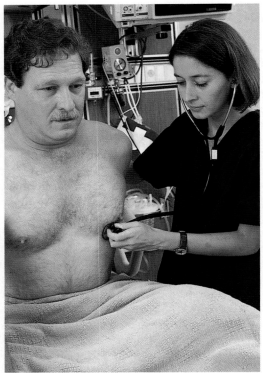

Figure 8-37. Positions for auscultation of the heart. **A,** Supine. **B,** Forward-sitting. **C,** Side-lying.

Carotid Arteries.

Inspect and palpate the carotid arteries. With the client sitting, inspect and palpate the pulsations of the carotid arteries. Use the index and middle fingers together to gently palpate the carotid arteries on either side of the neck near the medial edge of the sternocleidomastoid muscle.

Examine one artery at a time. It may help to turn the client's head slightly away from you for inspection and then back toward you for palpation. Compare and note the rate, rhythm, and strength of pulsations of both carotid arteries. A normal rate varies between 60 and 90 bpm bilaterally. The carotid pulsations should feel strong, elastic, and regular. Note whether the rate is synchronous with the client's heartbeat and whether the rate changes with inspiration or expiration.

Listen for a bruit. A bruit is an abnormal blowing or swishing sound or murmur heard while auscultating a carotid artery, organ, or gland, such as the liver or thyroid. The special character of the bruit, its location, and the time of its occurrence in a cycle of other sounds are all of diagnostic importance. Ask the client to hold his breath (to prevent artifact from the tracheal breath sounds) while you auscultate each carotid artery for bruits using the bell of the stethoscope (Figure 8-38). Assess at the angle of the jaw, middle third of the neck, and just above the clavicle. Use light pressure because compressing the artery can create an artificial bruit.

Normally no bruits should be audible. The presence of bruits indicates thrombosis or severe thickening of the lumen from atherosclerosis.

Neck Veins.

Assess the jugular venous pulsations. A jugular pulsation results from a backward wave associated with events in the cardiac cycle. Next, inspect the jugular veins with the client sitting up at a 90-degree angle and again with the client lying down with the head raised slightly at a 30-degree to 45-degree angle. Assess the level for jugular vein distention on both sides. The pressure in the jugular vein reflects the pressure where the vena cava enters the right side of the heart. Jugular vein distention to more than 3 cm above the sternal angle is associated with increased blood volume or congestive heart failure. Chapter 34 further discusses jugular vein distention.

Peripheral Veins.

Assess the lower extremities for changes in peripheral venous circulation. Inspect and palpate for signs of peripheral venous insufficiency (changes in the skin, changes in temperature, presence of edema, varicosities, phlebitis, and thrombosis). Note signs of pallor, cyanosis, dermatitis, ulcers, necrosis, edema, or cellulitis. Note whether there is clubbing of the client's fingers or toes. Bilateral comparison is useful to distinguish normal from abnormal in one individual.

If edema is present, assess the extent or height of involvement on the leg and whether it is pitting or nonpitting. The edema of peripheral vascular disease is usually ascending. It may begin in the ankles and ascend up the legs, depending on the severity of the vascular compromise. Chapter 34 discusses edema in greater detail.

Inspect and palpate the lower extremities for varicosities. Varicose veins are swollen, distended, and knotted veins resulting from incompetent valves that allow the blood to backflow, thus distending and stretching the veins. They appear as swollen, thick, tortuous veins seen or palpated along the surface of the lower extremities. Inspect and palpate the superficial veins for signs of phlebitis or inflammation. Look for reddened, thickened, or tender veins. If varicosities are present, palpate the vessel with one hand while pressing down on the vessel with your second hand at a point just above the first hand. Palpate for the impulse of blood flow. Normally there should be none. If any varicosities occur in the lower legs, assess for phlebitis (inflammation of a vein).

To check for the presence of phlebitis, *gently* squeeze the calf muscle against the tibia and note the presence of any tenderness. You also can perform a special maneuver to detect deep vein thrombosis (DVT). With the client's knee slightly flexed, dorsiflex the foot. In the presence of DVT, there will be a characteristic, sharp calf pain, which is described as a positive Homan's sign (Figure 8-39). A positive Homan's sign suggests DVT but is not definitive.

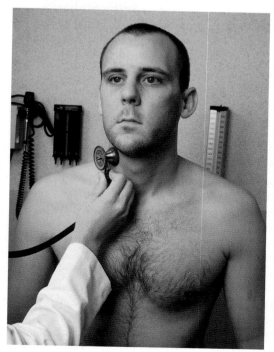

Figure 8-38. Assessing for a carotid bruit.

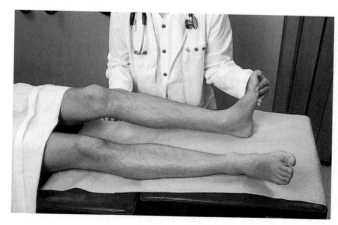

Figure 8-39. Assessing for Homans' sign.

Peripheral Arteries. Assess the peripheral arterial circulation. Inspect and palpate for signs of peripheral arterial insufficiency. Inspect the skin and nails. Note the presence of thin shiny skin, scaly skin, decreased hair growth, or thickened nails. Note whether the extremities are cool to the touch. Note whether the client demonstrates any sensory deficits. Test the client's ability to perceive soft, dull, sharp, and vibratory sensations with the eyes closed.

Check each of the peripheral pulses (radial, ulnar, brachial, femoral, popliteal, dorsalis pedis, and posterior tibial). See Chapter 7 for more information about pulses. Since each person's anatomy varies slightly, pulses are located primarily by touch. Exert light pressure with your index and middle fingertips held together and palpate the arterial pulses. You may need to use deep palpation to locate the temporal artery. Compare all contralateral, or paired, pulses for rhythm, strength, and equality. If the pulse is not palpable, you may need to use a Doppler or ultrasound stethoscope to amplify the sound of the arterial pulsations.

Palpate the radial pulse along the radial groove on the palmar and radial side of the wrist. Palpate the ulnar pulse on the palmar and medial side of the wrist. Palpate the brachial pulse at the antecubital fossa between the biceps and triceps muscles. Palpate the femoral pulse (with the client supine) just below the inguinal ligament and halfway between the symphysis pubis (pubic bone) and the anterior superior iliac spine. Palpate the popliteal pulse (located behind the knee) with the client supine or prone. Ask the client to relax the leg muscles and slightly flex the knee. Palpate the dorsalis pedis pulse with the client supine. It can be found on the anterior or upper aspect of the foot, halfway between the base of the ankle and the second metatarsophalangeal joint. Palpate the posterior tibial pulse just below and behind the medial malleolus with the foot relaxed and slightly extended.

Assessment of the Abdomen

The abdomen is a large oval cavity extending from the diaphragm to the floor of the pelvis. It is lined with the parietal peritoneal membrane that covers the wall of the abdomen and is continuous with the visceral peritoneal membrane that covers the organs of the abdomen. To assess the abdomen, you must know the precise location of the visceral organs underlying the skin and abdominal muscles. A routine nursing examination generally includes inspection, auscultation, and light palpation. Deep palpation and most percussion are more likely to be part of a diagnostic medical examination.

The abdomen can be divided into four or nine sections. Commonly the abdomen is divided into four quadrants by vertical and horizontal lines at the umbilicus (Figure 8-40, *A*). However, the older nine-section method is sometimes useful to describe findings more precisely (Figure 8-40, *B*).

The lower ribs on the right protect the liver and gallbladder, and thus only the lower border of the liver is normally palpable. The lower ribs on the left protect the spleen. The organs of the abdominal cavity are not normally palpable. The lower left colon may be palpable if filled with feces, and the

bladder if filled with urine. The uterus and ovaries are palpable with a bimanual vaginal examination.

The following should be included in assessment of the abdomen:

- Inspection of the abdomen
- Auscultation for bowel sounds and vascular sounds
- Percussion of the abdomen
- Percussion of the size and span of the liver
- Percussion of the gastric air bubble
- Percussion of the kidneys
- Percussion of the spleen
- Palpation of the abdomen in all four quadrants using light and deep palpation techniques
- Palpation of the umbilicus
- Palpation of the liver
- Palpation of the gallbladder
- Palpation of the spleen
- Palpation of the aorta
- Palpation for ascites in the distended abdomen
- Ballottement of a suspected mass

Inspection. To prepare for an examination of the abdomen, ask the client to undress to the waist and don an examination gown. Cover the legs and genitalia with a sheet and have the client lie supine with knees slightly flexed and arms at the side or folded across the chest. You may need to provide pillows for the head and knees to make the client more comfortable. Ask the client to locate any tender areas before proceeding, and examine these areas last. Examine the client with warm hands and a warm stethoscope. Try to distract the client with conversation throughout the examination, and watch facial expressions for any grimaces or confirmations of pain.

Observe the client's posture. Note whether the client is guarding or splinting the abdomen, lying perfectly still, constantly changing positions, frequently leaning forward, or favoring one side or position.

Inspect the skin of the abdomen (refer to Assessment of the Skin, Hair, and Nails, earlier). Note its color, its turgor, and the presence of erythema, ecchymosis, lesions, masses, striae (stretch marks), old scars, or venous abnormalities. Note whether the client has markedly diminished or excessive adipose tissue.

Note the symmetry, the contour (flat, convex, or concave), the presence of surface movements (breathing, peristalsis, aortic pulsations), bulging (hernias, cysts, tumors), obesity, and distention (obstruction, ascites). Asymmetry above the umbilicus may indicate gastric dilation, a pancreatic cyst, or malignancy. Asymmetry below the umbilicus may indicate pregnancy, fibroid uterus, ovarian cancer, bowel or bladder obstruction, hernias, tumors, or cysts. It is normal to see the pulsation of the aorta and waves of peristalsis in thin persons.

Assess for abdominal distention. Inspect the abdomen from all angles while the client is lying supine and again while the client holds a deep breath. Mild distention of the abdomen below the umbilicus may be the normal result of a full bladder or stool in the colon. Abnormal distention of the abdomen occurs with the accumulation of fluid, feces, or gas in

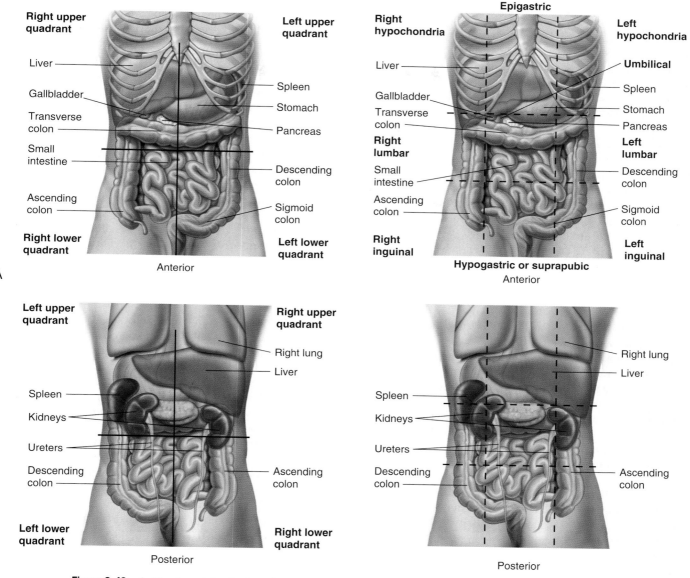

Figure 8-40. **A,** The four abdominal quadrants and their underlying organs. **B,** The nine regions of the abdomen and their underlying organs.

the intestine, often from bowel obstruction or absent peristalsis. It may also be secondary to infection or inflammation, such as in appendicitis or after surgery. The cause might also be inflammation, infection, or free fluid in the peritoneal cavity. If the appendix ruptures, the entire peritoneal cavity becomes inflamed (peritonitis). A glistening, taut abdomen might indicate the presence of ascites, the abnormal accumulation of lymphatic fluid within the peritoneal cavity secondary to liver disease.

Auscultation. Because percussion and palpation can change the bowel sounds, auscultate before you palpate and percuss. Place the diaphragm of the stethoscope lightly on the abdomen to auscultate for bowel sounds. Auscultate the ab-

domen in all four quadrants. Begin in the left lower quadrant (LLQ) and listen for up to 1½ minutes in each quadrant. Usually 10 to 15 seconds provides the information you need.

Bowel sounds are gurgling, high-pitched sounds occurring as peristaltic waves move gas through the intestine. Their occurrence is irregular—there may be anywhere from 5 to 20 or more a minute. After a meal or other stimulus to peristalsis, the bowel is active and produces more frequent sounds.

If bowel sounds are present, note their character and frequency and whether they are normal, hyperactive, or hypoactive. Hypoactive sounds are quiet and infrequent. Hyperactive sounds are loud and frequent. Normal is somewhere in between. The loud, audible sound of the stomach "growling" or the loud, gurgling, tinkling sound of the hyperactive bowel is termed borborygmus. The complete absence of bowel sounds indicates a nonfunctional intestine. You would need to listen for 5 minutes in each quadrant before deciding absolutely that bowel sounds are absent.

If they are absent after 1 to 2 minutes in one quadrant, make note of this and proceed to the other three quadrants. Bowel sounds do not necessarily occur in all four quadrants but should occur in at least one, most frequently the right lower quadrant (RLQ) at the ileocecal valve. However, hyperactive bowel sounds may occur in response to inflammation of the bowel, laxative abuse or overuse, and certain spicy foods. Hypoactive bowel sounds or the complete cessation of bowel sounds may occur in response to conditions that decrease the gastric motility, such as pancreatitis with peritonitis, paralytic ileus (absence of peristalsis), or an intestinal obstruction.

Bowel sounds are described as present, absent, increased, decreased, high pitched, tinkling, gurgling, and rushing. The bowel sounds are higher pitched, with rushing and tinkling sounds, when there is increased tension in the bowel such as occurs in intestinal obstruction.

Auscultate for abdominal bruits. Using the bell of the stethoscope, auscultate for vascular sounds. Listen carefully for bruits, hums, and friction rubs in the epigastric area and in all four quadrants over the aortic, renal, iliac, and femoral arteries. Bruits may occur normally in healthy young adults. However, the presence of bruits, venous hums, or friction rubs may indicate an underlying stricture, thrombosis, or aneurysm. If bruits are present, notify the physician and do not further palpate the abdomen, as this may damage an existing aneurysm.

Percussion. Percuss the abdomen using the percussion techniques previously described. Percuss all four quadrants of the abdomen to determine the nature of underlying tissue. Hollow organs, such as the gastric air bubble in the left upper quadrant (LUQ), produce tympanic sounds, and solid or fluid-filled tissue, such as the liver, kidneys, spleen, pancreas, and distended bladder, produce a dull sound. Percussion for excess flatus may be useful to the nurse in general practice.

If you need to assess for urinary retention, percussion may be a more useful tool than palpation (see later). Percuss the lower abdominal area, just above the symphysis pubis. A distended bladder may sometimes extend almost to the umbilicus and may deviate to one side; however, it is usually just above the symphysis pubis. Percussion of the bladder produces a dull sound when compared to the sound heard in the surrounding gut.

When you have had more experience and training, you may add the technique to percuss the size and span of the liver. The liver is normally dull to percussion. Begin at a point just below the umbilicus on the right midclavicular line and percuss upward to the lower edge of the liver. Mark the area where the dullness of the lower liver border begins. Next, percuss downward from an area of resonant lung to the upper liver edge. Mark the area where the dullness of the upper liver edge begins. Measure between the two marks with a ruler or

tape measure. Record this measure as the liver span. The normal liver span should be from 6 to 12 cm, or 2½ to 5 inches, in width. An enlarged liver (span greater than 12 cm) may indicate cirrhosis, hepatitis, hepatoma, cyst, abscess (localized collection of pus), or other extrinsic mass or malignancy that impinges on the liver.

When you have had more experience and training you may add the technique to percuss the kidneys. Ask the client to sit or stand and percuss the posterior costovertebral angle at the scapular line. The kidneys should be dull and painless to percussion. Tenderness of the costovertebral angle may indicate acute pyelonephritis or glomerulonephritis.

When you have had more experience and training you may add the technique to percuss the spleen in the area of the left tenth rib just posterior to the midaxillary line. Identify the small oval area of splenic dullness. You may also assess for splenic enlargement by percussing the normally tympanic area in the lowest left interspace on the left anterior axillary line. If this area grows dull when the client takes a deep breath, the spleen may be enlarged.

Palpation. Palpate the abdomen in all four quadrants using the technique of light palpation, compressing the skin to a depth of 1 cm (Figure 8-41). Use the finger pads or palmar surface of three or four fingers held together. Move methodically through each quadrant, depressing the abdomen not more than ½ to 1 inch, while using dipping or circular motions. Identify and note the size and location of any abnormalities and areas of increased resistance or tenderness. While distracting the client, return to and further evaluate areas of increased resistance and tenderness to determine whether the resistance is voluntary or involuntary. With the client relaxed, palpate for any abnormal rigidity of the rectus muscles.

Palpate the abdomen in all four quadrants using the technique of deep palpation to a depth of 5 to 8 cm. Use bimanual palpation if necessary to overcome the resistance of a large

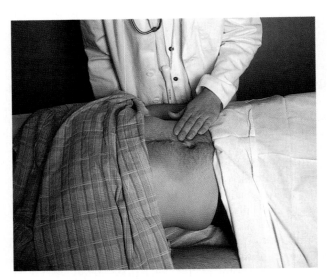

Figure 8-41. Light palpation of the abdomen.

abdomen (Figure 8-42). Using the palmar surface or finger pads of three or four fingers held together, deeply palpate the abdomen, depressing underlying tissue 1 to 3 inches as you move methodically through each quadrant. Move your fingers back and forth over underlying tissue to delineate organs and detect less obvious masses. Deeply palpate for rebound tenderness, which occurs after the sudden release of deep pressure on the abdomen if an acute inflammatory process is present. Proceed cautiously and avoid deeply palpating any areas of known severe tenderness, pulsating masses, or recent surgical incisions.

Palpate the umbilicus for tenderness, masses, bulges, hernias, lesions, and discharge.

Palpate the liver. Place your left hand under the client's right posterior thorax parallel to and at the level of the 11th and 12th ribs. Place your right hand on the client's right upper quadrant (RUQ) over the midclavicular line with fingers pointing toward the head and positioned below the lower edge of liver dullness. Ask the client to take a deep breath while you press inward and upward with the fingers of your right hand. With inspiration, the liver descends lower in the abdomen. Attempt to feel the edge of the liver as it descends (Figure 8-43). The liver edge may normally descend up to 1 inch on deep inspiration, but often it is not palpable, which is also normal. When palpable, the liver edge should feel smooth, firm, and nontender and have a regular contour. If you can feel more than 1 or 2 cm extending from under the ribs, the liver is enlarged. Abnormalities may indicate the presence of cirrhosis, hepatitis, hepatoma, cyst, abscess, malignancy, or other extrinsic mass compromising the integrity of the liver.

Palpation of the gallbladder is usually not performed on routine physical examinations. This technique is usually left to highly experienced practitioners and is performed in the following manner. Ask the client to take a deep breath, and palpate deep below the liver margin for enlargement of the gallbladder. Since the gallbladder is usually not palpable, a palpable gallbladder is more than likely enlarged. An enlarged, palpable, tender gallbladder may indicate cholelithiasis (gallstones), cholecystitis (infection), malignancy, abscess, or obstruction by an extrinsic mass or malignancy. A positive Murphy sign (abrupt cessation of inspiration during deep palpation of the gallbladder) is further indication of an acute process.

Palpate the spleen. Place your left hand under the client's left costovertebral angle and your right hand on the abdomen below the left costal margin. Ask the client to take a deep breath while you press the fingertips of your right hand inward. Palpate the edge of the spleen as it descends with inspiration. The spleen is often not palpable; if it is palpable, it may be enlarged.

Palpate the aorta. Use your thumb and forefinger to palpate the aorta by pressing deeply just to the left of the vertical midline of the abdomen. Unless the client is morbidly obese, the aorta will be palpable with strong and regular pulsations. Faint or irregular pulsations may indicate cardiovascular disease. A distinct pulsating mass indicates an aneurysm and should not be further palpated, to avoid possible inadvertent rupture.

Palpate the bladder. Palpate the area above the pubic symphysis if the client's history indicates possible urinary retention. Use only gentle palpation, as pressing on a full bladder is uncomfortable. It may be sufficient to ask if the client experiences the urge to urinate as you gently press on the lower abdomen. You may be able to feel the top of a full bladder because it rises above the symphysis pubis. Sometimes it will deviate to one side or the other. The alert client will be able to describe the sensation of the urge to urinate when you press on a full bladder.

If the abdomen appears distended, palpate for ascites below the right costal margin. Ask the client to lie supine. Have a colleague assist you by pressing his hand and forearm firmly along the vertical midline of the abdomen. Place your hands on either side of the client's abdomen. Strike one side of the client's abdomen forcefully with your fingertips and, with the other hand, feel for the rebounding impulse of a fluid wave. Another technique for determining the presence of ascites is to percuss for "shifting dullness" in the abdomen. With the

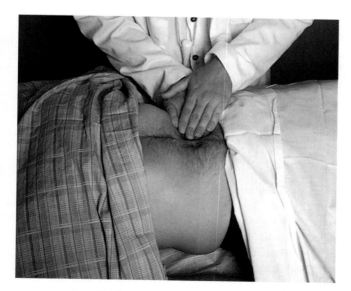

Figure 8-42. Deep palpation of the abdomen.

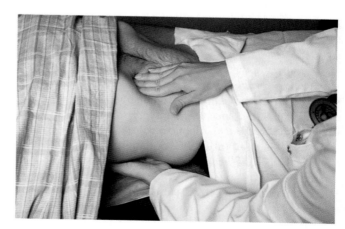

Figure 8-43. Palpating the liver.

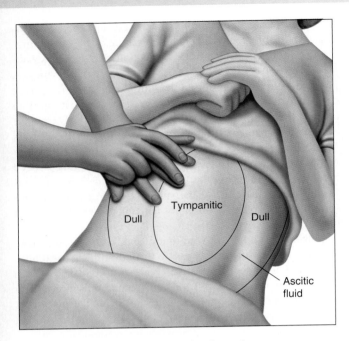

Figure 8-44. Assessing for ascites.

client lying supine, percuss from the midline of the abdomen to the flank. Mark the level of dullness. Ask the client to lie on one side and percuss again over the same area, this time from the flank to the vertical midline of the abdomen (Figure 8-44). Note any change in the level of dullness. If ascites is present, the level of dullness will be slightly higher with the client lying on one side. The presence of ascites may result from a number of medical problems, primarily liver disease, congestive heart failure, or ovarian cancer.

Perform ballottement for any suspected masses. It may be difficult to palpate a suspected mass in a person with marked ascites. In this situation, ballottement may prove helpful in determining the presence of a mass. To perform ballottement for a suspected mass, thrust the fingers of the right hand quickly and firmly into the area of the suspected mass. If the mass is freely mobile, it will initially retreat into the abdomen, and then immediately rebound back against your fingers.

Assessment of the Musculoskeletal System

Include the following in your assessment of the musculoskeletal system:

- Assessment of the client's posture, stance, and gait
- Inspection for gross abnormalities
- Inspection of the skin and surrounding tissues of all the bones, joints, and muscle groups
- Inspection of the temporomandibular joint (TMJ) and jaw and assessment of their range of motion
- Inspection of the neck and spine and assessment of their range of motion
- Inspection of the upper extremities and assessment of their range of motion
- Inspection of the lower extremities and assessment of their range of motion

Posture, Stance, and Gait. Assess the client's posture, stance, and gait by observing inconspicuously as the client enters the examining room. The client should be able to stand erect with head up, face forward, arms hanging straight at the sides, shoulders and hips parallel, and legs straight with both knees and feet side by side and a few inches apart.

The client's paired extremities should appear grossly symmetrical, and equal in size, shape, and length. Note whether the client appears unable to stand erect or exhibits a hunched, bent, or stooped posture. Note any apparent abnormal curvature of the spine as in kyphosis (accentuated lordosis), or scoliosis (a lateral bending of the spine). Also note any contractures or deformities of the extremities. Note whether the client is able to stand on both feet comfortably without assistance or support and without any swaying or loss of balance. Note whether the client is able to stand on one foot at a time without difficulty. Note any evidence of uneven distribution of weight, swaying, stumbling, or loss of balance, favoring one foot, standing on the heels, toes, or edges of the feet, uneven depth of footprints, or toes pointing laterally or medially rather than straight ahead.

Assess gait by asking the client to walk across the room. The client should be able to walk with strides that are equal and symmetrical with respect to timing, weight bearing, and distance. The client's steps should consist of a rhythmic planting of first the heel and then the toe of the foot, and the toes should point forward. While walking, the client may sway slightly as he shifts weight from foot to foot but should not demonstrate an unsteady gait, loss of balance, shuffling, limping, propulsive walking, veering off in one direction, footdrop, foot lag, or any irregularity in the timing of the stride.

Gross Abnormalities. Inspect for any gross or obvious abnormalities that are easily noticed on an initial head-to-toe inspection (such as amputation, congenital deformities, contractures, paralysis, and so on). Inspect and palpate the skin and surrounding tissues of all the bones, joints, and muscle groups (refer to Assessment of the Skin, Hair, and Nails, earlier). Inspect for color, temperature, swelling, edema, skin folds, and lesions. Note any abnormalities.

Muscle Tone and Strength. Assess all muscle groups for bilateral symmetry, tone, and strength. Bilateral muscle groups, or those muscles identically paired, as in the left and right biceps, should be symmetrical in size, shape, contour, position, and alignment of like joints. Note any variances.

Assess all muscle groups for muscle tone. You can assess muscle tone and strength at the same time as ROM by noting the degree of resistance felt on passive ROM (Figure 8-45). Normally a slight resistance is felt.

Assess muscle strength by asking the client to pull away from or push against an opposing force that you impose. Repeat these same maneuvers with the contralateral joint and assess bilateral muscle strength. Usually a particular muscle group has normal tone if slight resistance is demonstrated against passive ROM exercises. A hypertonic muscle exhibits increased resistance to passive ROM exercises. A hypotonic

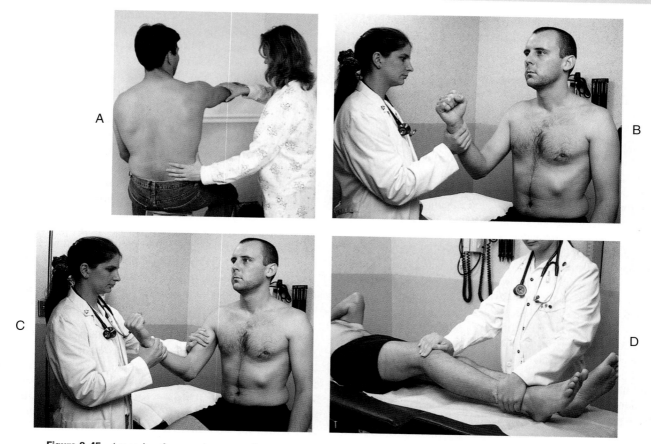

Figure 8-45. Assessing for muscle tone and strength. **A,** Ask the client to flex his shoulder muscle against your hand as you apply resistance. **B,** Ask the client to extend his elbow as you apply resistance. **C,** Ask the client to flex his elbow as you apply resistance. **D,** Ask the client to raise his knee as you apply resistance.

muscle presents as a boggy, flat, flabby, or flaccid muscle that offers little or no resistance against passive ROM exercises.

Assess the strength of all muscle groups. Each muscle group should be relatively equal to the contralateral muscle group. The dominant hand or arm may normally be slightly stronger. Measure (preferably with a tape measure) the size (diameter) of any muscle or muscle group that demonstrates weakness. A smaller size of a particular muscle or muscle group may indicate atrophy, and an unusually large muscle may indicate hypertrophy.

Bilateral Bones and Joints. Assess bones and joints bilaterally for symmetry with respect to size, shape, position, alignment, stability, and ROM. Asymmetry may be the result of congenital anomalies, arthritis, bony tumors, fractures, dislocations, adhesions, or surgery. Malalignment may be secondary to fracture dislocation, congenital anomalies, or surgical procedures. The joints should be able to be moved passively in all directions and degrees expected for the specific groups. There should be no abnormal movements or sounds produced by movement or manipulation of the joints. Any pain or stiffness elicited upon movement of a joint that has no associated fracture or dislocation usually indicates arthritis or damage to a tendon or ligament.

Assess the stability of each joint. To do this, grasp and stabilize the joint on the proximal side with one hand while attempting to move the joint with the other hand from the distal end. Note any abnormal movements, unusual sounds, crepitus, or abnormal ROM or tenderness associated with these movements.

Finally, assess each joint for full passive ROM. Note the angle at which the joint is able to freely bend in each position. A brief overview of ROM as part of a physical examination is presented here. More details are provided in Chapter 32, where ROM is presented as a treatment. When doing a musculoskeletal assessment, it is often easiest to begin with the temporomandibular joint and jaw and then progress from head to toe. For example: assess the neck, then the spine, then the upper extremities, and then the lower extremities.

Jaw and Temporomandibular Joint. Inspect and palpate the jaw and the TMJ. Simultaneously place two or three fingertips of each hand in the depression over the two TMJs. Ask the client to open widely and close his mouth two or three times while your fingertips are in place. Palpate for any unusual clicking sounds, sliding, or "catching" of the joint. With the client's mouth as wide open as possible, the normal distance between the top and bottom front teeth is 3 to 6 cm. Ask the client to slide the lower jaw forward and from side to side. The lower teeth should be able to be moved beyond and overlap the upper teeth. Normal side to side movement is 1 to 2 cm. Note any misalignment of the upper jaw and lower jaw, inability to move the lower jaw sideways or forward (lockjaw), inability to open or close the jaw, or pain on mastication or movement of the jaw.

Neck, Cervical Spine, Thoracic Spine, and Lumbar Spine.

Inspect and palpate the neck, cervical spine, thoracic spine, and lumbar spine, with the client first standing erect and then bending over at the waist. Inspect from directly behind the client and again from the side. Normally the cervical spine is concave, the thoracic spine convex, and the lumbar spine concave. Note any abnormal curvatures, palpable masses, compression fractures, lesions, or pain along the spine. An abnormal curvature of the spine may be a result of kyphosis (an accentuated posterior curvature of the thoracic spine), sway back or lordosis (an accentuated lumbar curvature), scoliosis (a lateral curvature of the spine), ankylosing spondylitis (evidenced by persistence of the lumbar concavity and failure of the spinous processes to separate when the client bends over at the waist), or spondylolisthesis (a forward slipping and fusing of the vertebrae).

Assess the ROM of the neck and spine. Assess flexion by asking the client to touch his chin to his chest. Assess hyperextension by asking the client to bend the head backward with the chin pointing up toward the ceiling. Assess rotation by asking the client to turn the head as far as possible to the left and then to the right with the ears facing the front and back. Assess lateral bending by asking the client to bend the head laterally, attempting to touch the ear to the shoulder. The normal ROM for flexion is 70 to 90 degrees; for hyperextension, 55 degrees; for rotation, 70 degrees; and for lateral bending, 35 degrees.

Assess the ROM of the spine. To assess flexion, ask the client to bend forward at the waist; to assess extension, ask the client to bend backward at the waist. To assess rotation, ask the client to stand with feet planted and toes pointed forward and attempt to rotate the upper torso so that the shoulders attempt to face backward. To assess lateral bending, ask the client to bend laterally at the waist with shoulders pointing toward the floor or feet. Normal ROM for flexion is 75 degrees; for extension, 30 degrees; for rotation, 30 degrees; and for lateral bending, 35 degrees.

Upper and Lower Extremities.

After the assessment of the neck and spine, assess the upper and then the lower extremities. Work your way down from top to bottom, assessing first the right side and then the left side. For example, assess the right and then the left shoulder, then move to the elbows, then the wrists, then the fingers, then the hips, then the knees, then the ankles, and then the toes. After inspection and palpation of each joint and muscle group, assess each for ROM and muscle strength.

Shoulders.

Assess the shoulders for ROM and muscle strength, starting from the anatomic position with the arms at the side. Assess flexion by asking the client to lift the arm forward and above the head until the arm is straight and horizontal to the floor, then move the arm backward toward the spine. Assess extension from the anatomical position by moving the arm backward with the arm straight. Assess horizontal extension by asking the client to abduct the arm to a point horizontal to the floor and then bring the arm back to the anatomic position and across the chest.

To assess abduction, lift the arm away from the body straight up above the head. To assess adduction, adduct the arm toward the midline of the trunk. Note any pain, which may be secondary to arthritis, inflammation, infection, bursitis, tendinitis, bony spurs, calcific deposits, masses, fractures, and dislocations. A frozen shoulder, evidenced by the inability of the client to abduct the arm without characteristic "shrugging" suggests a rupture of the supraspinal tendon or rotator cuff injury. Normal ROM for the shoulders can be expected to be 180 degrees for flexion, 130 degrees for horizontal flexion, 60 degrees for extension, 45 degrees for horizontal extension, 180 degrees for abduction, and 45 degrees for adduction.

Elbows.

Assess the ROM for the elbows. Assess flexion by asking the client to bend the lower arm up toward the biceps. Assess extension by asking the client to open his arm to a fully extended resting position. Assess hyperextension by asking the client to extend his arm beyond the normal resting position. Assess supination by asking the client to turn the lower arm so that the front faces upward. Assess pronation by asking the client to turn the lower arm so that the front faces downward. Normal ROM for the elbows is expected to be 150 degrees for flexion, 150 degrees for extension, 0 to 10 degrees for hyperextension, 90 degrees for supination, and 90 degrees for pronation.

Wrists.

Assess the ROM for the wrists. Assess flexion by asking the client to flex the wrist toward the lower arm. Assess extension by asking the client to extend the wrist backward. Assess radial deviation by asking the client to deviate the wrist toward the radius. Assess ulnar deviation by asking the client to deviate the wrist toward the ulna. Normal ROM for the wrists is expected to be 80 to 90 degrees for flexion, 70 degrees for extension, 20 degrees for radial deviation, and 30 to 50 degrees for ulnar deviation.

Fingers.

Assess the ROM for the fingers. Assess flexion by asking the client to close his fingers into a fist. Assess extension by asking the client to fully open his fingers. Assess abduction by asking the client to spread his fingers apart. Assess adduction by asking the client to cross the fingers together so that they touch and overlap. Assess opposition by asking the client to touch each finger with the thumb of the same hand. Normal ROM for the fingers is expected to be 80 to 100 degrees for flexion, 0 to 45 degrees for extension, and 20 degrees for abduction. Normal adduction is demonstrated if the client is able to cross his fingers. Normal opposition is demonstrated if the client is able to touch each finger to the thumb of the same hand.

Hips. Assess the ROM of the hips. Assess flexion with both a straight knee and a bent knee. Ask the client to first raise his leg straight up without bending the knee and then to raise it again with the knee bent. Assess extension by asking the client to lie prone and then extend the leg backward. Assess abduction by asking the client to abduct a partially flexed leg outward. Assess adduction by asking the client to adduct a partially flexed leg inward. Assess internal rotation by asking the client to flex the knee and swing the foot toward the midline. Assess external rotation by asking the client to flex the knee and swing the foot away from the midline. Normal ROM for the hips is expected to be 90 degrees for straight-knee flexion, 110 to 120 degrees for bent-knee flexion, 30 degrees for extension, 45 to 50 degrees for abduction, 20 to 30 degrees for adduction, 35 to 40 degrees for internal rotation, and 45 degrees for external rotation.

Knees. Assess the ROM of the knees. Assess flexion by asking the client to fully bend the knee so that the posterior calf and posterior thigh are nearly touching. Assess hyperextension by asking the client to extend the knee beyond the normal point of extension. Assess internal rotation by asking the client to rotate the knee and lower leg toward the midline. Assess external rotation by asking the client to rotate the knee and lower leg away from the midline. Normal ROM is expected to be 130 degrees for flexion, 15 degrees for hyperextension, and 10 degrees for internal rotation.

Ankles. Assess the ROM of the ankles. Assess dorsiflexion by asking the client to bend the ankle of the foot so that the toes point toward the head. Assess plantar flexion by asking the client to bend the foot downward with the toes pointing downward. Assess eversion by asking the client to turn the foot away from the midline. Assess inversion by asking the client to turn the foot toward the midline. Normal ROM is expected to be 20 degrees for dorsiflexion, 45 degrees for plantar flexion, 20 degrees for eversion, and 30 degrees for inversion.

Toes. Assess the ROM of the toes. Assess flexion by asking the client to curl his toes under his foot. Assess extension by asking the client to lift the toes to point upward. Assess abduction by asking the client to spread the toes apart. Normal ROM is expected to be 35 to 60 degrees for flexion, 0 to 90 degrees for extension (depending on the specific joint), variable capability for abduction, and inability to adduct the toes.

Reflexes. A muscular reflex is an involuntary response to a stimulus in which the sensory nerve carries the message to the spinal cord and directly back to cause a contraction in a muscle. All muscles contract reflexively when stimulated. However, only a few reflexes are tested clinically as indicators of motor function (Figure 8-46, p. 170).

Reflexes are classified as superficial and deep tendon reflexes. Superficial reflexes are elicited by stroking or stimulating the skin. Deep tendon reflexes are elicited by stretching a tendon by tapping with a percussion hammer. Testing re-

flexes requires sensitivity to slight contractions of muscles. Reflexes are classified as 0, no response; 1+, slightly diminished; 2+, normal; 3+, brisker than normal; and 4+, hyperactive. This scale is subjective and the ratings may vary between examiners and with experience.

The biceps, triceps, and brachioradialis reflexes provide information about the function of the nerves of the cervical spine (C5 to C8). All three are deep tendon reflexes. To test the biceps reflex, have the client partially flex the elbow and rest the arm on his own thigh or on your forearm. Place your thumb in the antecubital space over the biceps tendon. Tap your thumb with the percussion hammer. A positive response is slight movement of the forearm with contraction of the biceps muscle.

To test the triceps reflex, flex the client's arm at the elbow and hold it suspended at a right angle to the shoulder. The arm should be relaxed with the forearm hanging freely. Directly tap the triceps tendon just above the elbow. The forearm should extend slightly. Alternatively, you may have the client hold the forearm across the chest, flexed 90 degrees at the elbow.

To test the brachioradialis reflex, have the client rest the forearm on his thigh. Grasp the thumb to suspend the forearm in a relaxed position. Tap the forearm directly on the lateral aspect of the radial bone 2 to 3 cm above the joint. The forearm should flex slightly, turning toward the supinated position.

In the lower extremity, the knee jerk, Achilles, and plantar reflexes are tested. The knee jerk or patellar reflex tests function of L1, L2, and L3 nerves. The Achilles reflex tests function of S1 and S2 nerves. These are deep tendon reflexes. To test the patellar reflex, have the client sit on a table or bed from which the foot and lower leg can hang freely. Strike the tendon directly below the patella (knee cap). The lower leg should extend.

To test the Achilles reflex, position the person supine with the hip externally rotated and the knee flexed. Hold the foot in a relaxed dorsiflexed position and strike the Achilles tendon with the percussion hammer. You should feel the foot plantar flex against your hand.

The plantar, or Babinski, reflex is a superficial reflex that is present in the first 8 to 10 months of life, then disappears and should be absent in adults. This reflex should be tested with the client in a relaxed supine position. With a blunt instrument, apply firm pressure and draw a line from the heel along the lateral aspect of the sole of the foot and across the footpad under the toes. With a positive response (the Babinski sign), the toes spread outward and the big toe moves upward. This finding in an adult indicates upper motor neuron disease of the pyramidal tract. In a normal adult, the toes curl toward the sole of the feet.

Assessment of the Anus, Rectum, and Prostate
The following should be included in the assessment of the anus, rectum, and prostate:
- Inspection and palpation of perianal tissue and perineu
- Inspection for the appearance of protrusions of masse straining
- Digital examination to palpate the anus, rec prostate

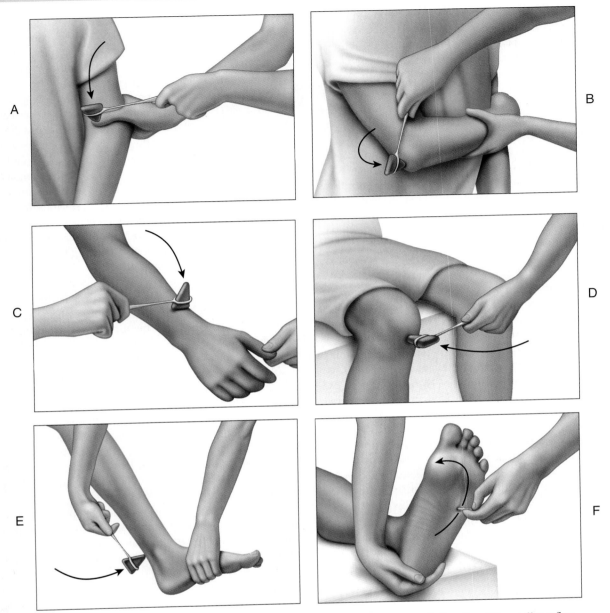

Figure 8-46. Assessing reflexes: biceps reflex (**A**), triceps reflex (**B**), brachioradialis reflex (**C**), patellar reflex (**D**), Achilles reflex (**E**), and plantar (Babinski) reflex (**F**).

- Assessment of the tone and musculature of the anal sphincter
- Palpation of the muscular anal ring and rectum
- Palpation for high masses
- Palpation of the prostate in men
- Palpation of the uterus and cervix in women
- Examination of the fecal material

Perianal Tissue and Perineum. Inspect and palpate the perianal tissue and perineum. Position the client (male or female) on his or her side in the Sims position with knees lightly flexed. Gently retract the buttocks with your gloved hand, and inspect the anal and perianal tissue. Note color, texture, lesions, masses, prolapse, hemorrhoids, erythema, ec-

chymosis, skin breakdown, pressure ulcers, fistulas (an abnormal, tubelike passage between two organs or from an organ to the body surface), sinus tracts (a recess, cavity, or channel), abscesses, masses, lesions, and any evidence of poor hygiene. Perianal tissue may appear slightly darker in pigmentation, and anal tissue is slightly reddened normally.

Ask the client to bear down as though attempting a bowel movement and inspect for the appearance of protrusions, masses, hemorrhoids, prolapse, or polyps.

Digital Rectal Examination. Perform a digital examination to palpate the anus, rectum, and prostate. Press gently against the anal sphincter with your gloved and lubricated index finger pad. Ask the client to bear down and gently press your finger-tip into the opening of the anus. Assess the tone and muscula-ture of the anal sphincter. (Normally the anal sphincter will tighten firmly around the inserted finger and the client may ex-press the urge to defecate.) Palpate the entire surface of the anal sphincter. Ask the client to tighten the buttocks around your fin-ger to allow assessment of tone and strength of the sphincter.

Palpate the musculoanal ring and rectum. Palpate the en-tire surface of the musculoanal ring by turning the finger in a circular motion around its own axis. Then, move further in-ward to the rectum and repeat. Note any palpable lesions, masses, lacerations, or abnormalities or a palpable rectal shelf (often secondary to peritoneal metastatic disease).

Palpate for high masses. With your gloved finger as far into the rectum as possible, ask the client to bear down and palpate for any descending masses. Note the presence of any high mass descending against the inserted fingertip when the client bears down.

Palpate the prostate in men (only after the onset of pu-berty). Turn your finger to palpate the anterior rectal wall. Gently palpate the prostate (Figure 8-47). Try to identify the two lateral lobes and the median sulcus. Normally the prostate feels rubbery and smooth to palpation, and less than 1 cm of the prostate tissue is palpable protruding into the rectal wall. Note any enlargement, irregularity in shape, palpable mass, tenderness, or softening (bogginess).

Palpate the uterus and cervix in women. Turn your finger to palpate the anterior rectal wall. Gently palpate the uterus and cervix. Normally they feel rubbery and smooth. Note any enlargement, irregularity in shape, palpable mass, tenderness, or softening (bogginess).

Withdraw your gloved finger and examine the fecal mate-rial on the glove for color (brown, gray, yellow, black) and consistency (watery, loose, greasy, formed, hard, impacted). Using a Hemoccult card, test the fecal material for occult blood. Normally the stool should appear brown, feel formed, and contain no evidence of frank or occult blood.

Assessment of the Female Genitalia

The following should be included in the assessment of the fe-male genitalia:
- Inspection and palpation of the vulva for lesions, masses, and abnormalities
- Inspection of the pubic hair for infestations, density of growth, and sexual maturity
- Inspection and palpation of the labia majora for lesions, masses, inflammation, swelling, and abnormalities
- Inspection of the labia minora
- Inspection of the clitoris
- Inspection of the urethral meatus and Skene's glands
- Inspection of the hymen and vaginal introitus
- Inspection of Bartholin's glands
- Inspection of the cervix
- Inspection of the vaginal wall
- Palpation of the cervix
- Palpation of the ovaries and adnexa
- Palpation of the uterus

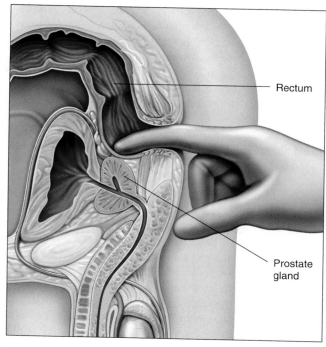

Figure 8-47. Palpating the prostate gland through the anterior wall of the rectum.

External Genitalia. Prepare the client for the examination. Ask the client to urinate and empty her bladder. Have her un-dress from the waist down and assume a semirecumbent posi-tion on the examining table with her knees and thighs draped and her feet in the stirrups. Ask the client to rest her hands on her waist and to relax her knees and let them fall to the side as far as possible.

Wear gloves to inspect and palpate the vulva for lesions, masses, and abnormalities. Touch the client's thigh initially to avoid startling her, then proceed with the examination, parting the pubic hair as necessary to facilitate thorough examination. Palpate any noticeable masses, lesions, swelling, or abnor-malities. Normally the skin is smooth, warm, and pink in light-skinned people and olive to brown in dark-skinned peo-ple, and it may be lighter in color than the rest of the body be-cause of lack of exposure to sun. Note any hematomas, ec-chymosis, irregular pigment, macules, papules, wheals, vesicles, ulcers, or other rashes.

Inspect the pubic hair for density of growth and sexual ma-turity. Part the pubic hair to look for infestations of pubic lice often found at the base or root of the pubic hair. Also inspect for nits (tiny teardrop-shaped white or gray eggs) adhering to the hair stalks. Assess the sexual maturity of the client.

Inspect and palpate the labia majora and labia minora for lesions, masses, inflammation, swelling, and abnormalities. It may be necessary to grasp the labia majora between two fin-gers to accomplish a thorough examination. Part the labia ma-jora with your gloved fingers to inspect the labia minora. Note and thoroughly palpate any observed lesions or abnormalities.

Inspect the clitoris for position, size, lesions, masses, and abnormalities. The clitoris can be found between the anterior junction of the labia majora and the labia minora. Normally the clitoris is a small pink nodular form that does not exceed 0.5 cm in width and 2 cm in length. (In some cultural groups the clitoris may have been ceremonially excised.)

Separate the labia minora and locate the urethral meatus, a small orifice just below the anterior junction of the labia minora. Inspect for lesions, prolapse, polyps, fistulas, edema or tenderness, masses, or discharge. If there is inflammation or if urethritis is suspected, milk the urethra gently by inserting a gloved finger into the vagina and stroking its posterior side in a downward motion toward you. Culture any discharge for gonorrhea, chlamydia, and bacteria. Perform a potassium hydroxide and wet preparation to discern the presence of yeast and *Trichomonas,* respectively.

Inspect the hymen and vaginal introitus. The hymen may be intact in children and virgins; however, usually only remnants of the hymen remain in sexually active women. If the hymen is edematous, torn, or absent in small children, sexual abuse must be considered as a possible cause.

With the labia separated by your gloved finger, inspect the vaginal introitus or vaginal opening. Ask the client to bear down to allow the support of the vaginal outlet to be evaluated. Observe and note any abnormal swelling or bulging. The introitus is usually open and unobstructed, but in older, multiparous women it is not uncommon to observe a cystocele (a bulging mass arising from the anterior wall of the vagina) or a rectocele (a bulging mass arising from the posterior vaginal floor). Cystoceles and rectoceles are caused by inadequate support of the vaginal outlet. A large, smooth, pink, protruding mass may actually be a uterine prolapse with the cervix visible in the vaginal canal. Uterine prolapse can be staged as first degree, second degree, or third degree depending on the severity of drop in the vaginal vault. In first-degree prolapse, the cervix is palpated slightly lower than usual in the vaginal vault; in second-degree prolapse the cervix can be palpated halfway down the vaginal vault; and in third-degree prolapse the cervix is at the introitus or sometimes even visibly protruding from the vaginal opening.

Inspect the Bartholin glands located bilaterally at the base of the vaginal opening. The Bartholin glands are normally not visible other than as a small pinpoint duct opening inside the labia. Palpate the glands between your gloved index finger and thumb by placing one finger inside the vaginal opening and one on the outside of the labia majora. Normally the Bartholin glands are nontender and not palpable. Note any pain, swelling, masses, or discharge. A large nontender unilateral mass may be a Bartholin cyst. A large tender fluctuant unilateral or bilateral mass may be a Bartholin abscess. The abscess may have tracked, spontaneously ruptured, or remained exquisitely tender and fluctuant. Gently compress the glands between two gloved fingers and culture any discharge exuding from the duct openings for gonorrhea, chlamydia, and bacteria.

Internal Genitalia. After you have completed your examination of the external genitalia, prepare to perform the speculum examination of the internal genitalia. Figure 8-48 illustrates a vaginal speculum used to hold the vagina open to visualize the cervix. Lubricate your gloved fingers and speculum with water. Water is used as the lubricant to prevent contamination when a smear for cytology is part of the examination. Insert one or two fingers into the vaginal opening and press downward on the posterior aspect to further open the introitus and facilitate the insertion of the speculum. Insert the closed speculum, holding it so that the blade width is in a vertical position. Gently push in a downward and sloping fashion, while at the same time rotating the blade so that the width is now in a horizontal position. Follow the vaginal canal to the cervix. Open the speculum and manipulate the cervix into position and secure by clamping. Observe the cervix, obtain specimens for cytology, and culture any discharge.

The cervical os appears as a small rounded opening within a central depression on the cervix in nulliparous women. It takes on a more "fish-mouthed" appearance in multiparous women. There are usually no lesions, masses, erythema, or cervical motion tenderness. Usually the cervix appears as a smooth, rounded, pink, moist, sometimes glistening, and firm mass. Although the cervix usually remains about 1 inch in diameter, it enlarges, softens, and becomes bluish-tinged normally in pregnancy and may appear pale during menopause.

The Papanicolaou smear, or Pap smear, is a cytology test to screen for cervical cancer. To obtain a specimen for a Pap smear, use a cytobrush and an Ayre speculum to collect specimens from three sites. Each specimen is placed on a

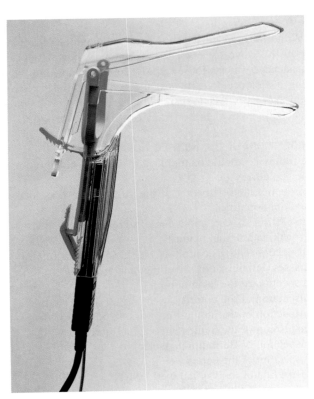

Figure 8-48. A vaginal speculum. (Courtesy Welch Allyn, Inc., Skaneateles Falls, NY.)

separate glass slide, sprayed with fixative within 2 seconds, and labeled with the source. A Pap smear should not be done during the menstrual period or if the client has infectious discharge. Ideally the woman should not have had intercourse, or put douche or anything else in the vagina 24 hours prior to the test.

Unclamp the speculum and hold it open as you withdraw it slowly from the vaginal canal. As you withdraw the speculum, inspect the walls of the vaginal canal. Use a gooseneck lamp or penlight to better illuminate the canal.

Normally you will see rugate homogeneous tissue with thin, clear or cloudy, odorless secretions, which are likely to be more profuse in pregnant women. Note any abnormal findings of masses, lesions, vesicles, papules, warts, or thick, foul-smelling discharge. Palpate the vaginal wall by inserting the lubricated and gloved middle and index finger of the right hand into the vagina (Figure 8-49). Palpate the anterior, posterior, and lateral walls of the vaginal canal.

Palpate the cervix with the tips of your fingers. Note the position, shape, consistency, and mobility of the cervix. Gently move the cervix from side to side and test for cervical motion tenderness, which can be a telltale sign of a pelvic inflammatory disease or other acute pelvic process. Attempt to admit one fingertip into the cervical os to determine its patency. Usually the cervical os remains closed and offers tight resistance. If the os admits one fingertip, or offers no resistance, it is considered open and may indicate a threatened or inevitable abortion or incompetent cervix.

Palpate the ovaries and adnexa. Place your left hand on the client's abdomen about halfway between the umbilicus and the symphysis pubis. Push inward and downward toward the symphysis pubis while at the same time pushing upward on

the vaginal mucosa lateral to the cervix with the fingers of your right hand. Try to palpate the small almond-shaped ovary on either side. Palpate for the adnexa. Normally it is not palpable unless there is an adnexal thickening or mass.

Palpate the uterus with your hands positioned as just described. Push downward toward the symphysis pubis with your left hand while pushing upward on the cervix with the fingers of your right hand. Attempt to grasp the uterus between the fingers of your two hands. Note the position, size, shape, consistency, and mobility of the uterus. Note also whether the uterus is tender. The fundus will not be palpable above the symphysis pubis. If it is enlarged, soft, or tender, it may indicate pregnancy, fibroids, hydatidiform mole, or the presence of a mass.

Assessment of the Male Genitalia
The following should be included in the assessment of male genitalia:
- Assessment of sexual maturity
- Assessment of the prepuce or foreskin
- Assessment of the glans penis
- Assessment of the urethral meatus
- Assessment of the penile shaft
- Assessment of the scrotum and testes
- Assessment of the presence of hernias

Sexual Maturity. Assess the external genitalia for sexual maturity (see Chapter 45). Note the distribution and quantity of pubic hair. Pubic hair is absent in infants and children and is thick, extending onto the thighs, in adults. The density of growth and distribution of hair should be consistent with that expected for the client's age group. An abnormal quantity or distribution may indicate hormonal imbalances, chronic disease, dermatitis, or a response to medications. Hair loss may be symmetrical and nonscarring, or asymmetrical and scarring.

Penis. Note the shape and size of the penis. The penis attains adult size and shape after puberty. Note the size, color, and texture of the scrotum. The scrotum darkens and develops rugae after puberty. Assess the sexual maturity using Tanner's Sexual Maturity Rating (SMR) (see Chapter 45).

Part the pubic hair as necessary to facilitate thorough examination of the skin. Inspect and palpate the skin for color, temperature, lesions, rashes, masses, excoriations, lacerations, abnormalities, infestations, or lack of hygiene. Gently move and manipulate the penis and scrotum to allow visualization of their posterior sides. Palpate thoroughly and note the type and location of any lesions, macules, papules, ulcers, vesicles, rashes, lacerations, excoriations, or masses. Hot red skin may indicate cellulitis, infection, or inflammation. The presence of lesions may indicate dermatitis or sexually transmitted disease.

Inspect and palpate the prepuce and foreskin in uncircumcised males. Note any lesions, swelling, edema, lacerations, erythema, or ecchymosis. Gently retract the foreskin and inspect. Smegma, a whitish, pasty exudate, may be present normally. Pay particular attention to the junction between the

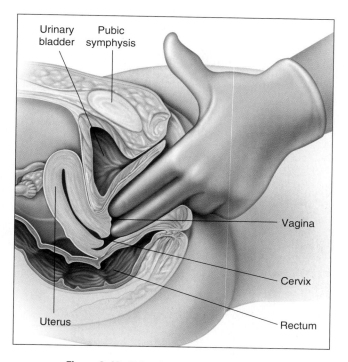

Figure 8-49. Palpating the uterus and cervix.

prepuce and the glans, as this is a common site for lesions of sexually transmitted diseases. Any difficulty in retracting or inability to retract the foreskin (phimosis), or difficulty in replacing or inability to replace a retracted foreskin (paraphimosis) is abnormal and should be noted and further evaluated.

Inspect and palpate the full surface of the glans. The glans normally appears moist and pink in uncircumcised males. Note the presence and exact location of any lesions, masses, swelling, edema, abnormalities, erythema, ecchymosis, or balanitis (inflammation of the glans with marked erythema and edema).

Note the location of the urinary meatus. It normally appears as a pink slitlike opening located in the center of the glans. Check for hypospadias, congenital displacement of the urethral meatus (usually found on the posterior side of the glans or penile shaft). Note the location and type of any lesions or abnormalities. Inspect for urethral prolapse, a perceivable small rosette of prolapsed membranes protruding from the meatus. Inspect also for fissures and fistulas. Open the meatus slightly by gently compressing the glans between your thumb and finger (or allow the client to do this). Inspect the color of the lining of the meatus and culture and describe any obvious discharge (e.g., yellow, white, clear, blood tinged), which may well indicate the presence of a urethritis. Discharge should be cultured for gonorrhea, chlamydia, and bacteria, and a potassium hydroxide and wet preparation should be performed at this time to assess for the presence of yeast and *Trichomonas,* respectively. If the client has complained of discharge and none is seen, you may need to gently "milk" the shaft of the penis to produce a bead of discharge for culture.

Inspect and palpate the shaft of the penis. Gently manipulate and lift the penis to allow inspection and palpation of the entire surface area. Note the exact location and type of lesions, masses, or abnormalities. Palpate for induration (hardness) and tenderness along the ventral surface of the penis. In infants and children, this may be omitted. Tenderness or induration along the ventral surface may indicate urethral stricture and periurethral inflammation, or carcinoma.

Scrotum and Testes.
Inspect and palpate the scrotum and testes. Gently palpate the testicles by grasping them between your thumb and forefinger. Palpate the epididymis, spermatic cord, and vas deferens. Note any lesions, masses, tenderness, or enlargement. Transilluminate the scrotum and testicle if a mass is suspected or an enlargement is observed. A fluid-filled mass will illuminate well, whereas a mass filled with blood, pus, or solid tissue will not.

Normally the scrotum consists of coarse, loose, rugate skin of slightly darker pigmentation than the rest of the body. The left testicle is normally lower than the right. When compressed gently between your two fingers, the testes are sensitive but not painful and should not feel much greater than 1 inch in diameter. Check for undescended testicles (cryptorchidism) and a poorly developed scrotum on one or both sides. Note any nontender swelling or masses such as hydrocele or spermatocele (fluid-filled cysts of the tunica vaginalis

and epididymis, respectively). Both hydroceles and spermatoceles transilluminate when a penlight is held up against the scrotal sac.

Palpate for testicular cancer, a hard, palpable, nontender nodule usually favoring the anterior side of the testes. Note any tender swelling or mass. This may be caused by scrotal edema (from congestive heart failure, chronic renal failure, or nephrotic syndrome), epididymitis (an acute bacterial infection of the epididymis), or testicular torsion (a painful swelling caused by torsion or twisting of the spermatic cord).

Palpate the vas deferens and spermatic cord. Note any thickening, which may occur with chronic infections and tuberculosis. Note the presence of a varicocele, a string of beadlike nodules or varicosities (which feel characteristically like a "bag of worms"), palpated usually on the left side.

Inguinal Canal.
Inspect and palpate the inguinal canal for hernias. Figure 8-50 illustrates the structures of the inguinal area. Ask the client to stand and bear down as though having a bowel movement. Inspect the inguinal areas and scrotum for any bulging or masses. With one finger, press inward on the loose skin at a low point on the scrotum. Follow the spermatic cord upward by invaginating loose scrotal skin until you can palpate the external inguinal ring. If possible, follow the inguinal canal to the internal inguinal ring.

Ask the client to bear down and again feel for any bulging or masses. If a hernia is palpable, apply gentle pressure and note whether it is reducible. Never force your finger into the inguinal canal. If you meet with resistance or the client complains of pain, discontinue the examination.

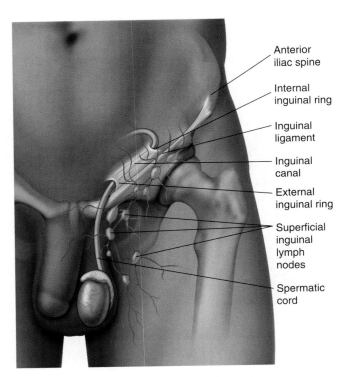

Figure 8-50. Structures of the inguinal area.

Identify any existing hernias. A direct inguinal hernia is palpated above the inguinal ring, bulges anteriorly, does not travel down the inguinal canal, and may, but rarely does, invade the scrotum. An indirect inguinal hernia is palpated above the inguinal ligament close to the internal inguinal ring; it travels down the inguinal canal and often invades the scrotum. A femoral hernia is palpated below the inguinal ligament and appears more lateral than an inguinal hernia and is often difficult to distinguish from an enlarged inguinal lymph node. All hernias may become painful if strangulation occurs either by torsion of the bowel or by compression by surrounding tissues.

Key Principles

- The physical examination is a systematic means of collecting objective assessment data.
- The four basic techniques used in physical examination are inspection, palpation, percussion, and auscultation, and they are performed in that order.
- In performing a physical examination, you rely heavily on the use of your five senses, particularly your ability to observe.
- Physical examination should be conducted following a regular pattern of examination and with the client positioned for the most accurate collection of data.
- The general survey provides information on the overall state of the client.
- The mental status examination provides a detailed description of the client's cognitive functioning at a given time.
- Good, preferably natural, light should be used to avoid distortion of color when inspecting the skin.
- A thorough description of a lesion is useful in determining if the lesion is a primary or secondary lesion and whether it is benign or malignant.
- Specific tests for hearing are performed only if gross hearing testing suggests a problem.
- Assessing the heart provides cues to the structure and function of the heart.
- Assessment of the peripheral vascular system focuses on the blood pressure and the pulses (and other signs of peripheral circulation) in relationship to cardiac function.
- Assessing the function of the veins is part of assessing venous return to the heart.
- Abdominal assessment determines function of the bowel and detects abnormalities of other organs and structures in the abdomen.
- Assessment of the musculoskeletal system detects abnormalities of the structure and function of bones, muscles, and joints.
- The physical assessment is focused on the areas and techniques used to detect problems as appropriate to the client's history and reason for seeking care.

Bibliography

Barkauskas, V., Baumann, L., & Darling-Fisher, C. S. (2002). *Health and physical assessment* (3rd ed.). St Louis, MO: Mosby.

Bickley, L. S., & Hoekelman, R. A. (1998). *Bates' guide to physical examination and history* (7th ed.). Philadelphia: Lippincott Williams & Wilkins.

Csokasy, J. (1999). Assessment of acute confusion: Use of the NEECHAM confusion scale. *Applied Nursing Research, 12*(1), 51-55.

Hines, S. E. (2000). Performing a focused physical examination. *Patient Care, 34*(23), 76.

Jarvis, C. (1999). *Physical examination and health assessment* (3rd ed.). Philadelphia: Saunders.

Leasia, M. S., & Monahan, F. D. (1997). *A practical guide to health assessment.* Philadelphia: Saunders.

Ludwig, L. M. (1998). Cardiovascular assessment for home healthcare nurses: Part II. Assessing blood pressure and cardiac function. *Home Healthcare Nurse, 16*(8), 547-554.

Mahon, S. M. (1998). Cancer risk assessment: Conceptual considerations for clinical practice. *Oncology Nursing Forum, 25*(9), 1535-1547.

Nicoteri, J. A. (1999). Rising above "soar" throats. Take a common-sense approach to assessing young adults with sore throats. *American Journal of Nursing, 99*(3), 18-20.

O'Hanlon-Nichols, T. (1998a). Basic assessment series: The adult pulmonary system. *American Journal of Nursing, 98*(2), 39-45.

O'Hanlon-Nichols, T. (1998b). Basic assessment series: A review of the adult musculoskeletal system. *American Journal of Nursing, 98*(6), 48-52.

O'Hanlon-Nichols, T. (1999). Neurological assessment. *American Journal of Nursing, 99*(6), 44.

Rice, K. L. (1998). Sounding out blood flow with a Doppler device. *Nursing98, 28*(9), 56-57.

Scott, A., & Hamilton, K. (1998). Nutritional screening: An audit. *Nursing Standards, 12*(48), 46-47.

Seidel, H. M., Ball, J. W., Dains, J. E., & Benedict, G. W. (1999). *Mosby's guide to physical examination* (4th ed.). St Louis, MO: Mosby.

Skillen, D. L., Anderson, M. C., & Knight, C. L. (2001). The created environment for physical assessment by case managers. *Western Journal of Nursing Research, 23*(1), 72-90.

Stevenson, C. (1998). Abdominal assessment clarifications. *Home Healthcare Nurse, 16*(6), 363.

Walton, J. (2001). Beat the odds. *Nursing, 31*(3), 54-59.

Nursing Diagnosis

9

Learning Objectives

After studying this chapter, you should be able to do the following:

- Discuss the classification of nursing diagnoses
- Describe the five components of a NANDA nursing diagnosis
- Compare and contrast four types of nursing diagnoses
- Describe the process of diagnostic reasoning
- Discuss several sources of diagnostic error and how to avoid them

In nursing diagnosis, the second phase of the nursing process, you make conclusions about the meaning of the assessment data (Figure 9-1). As you gather assessment data about a client through the nursing history and physical examination, you recognize interrelationships among pieces of data and group them into clusters to form nursing diagnoses. A nursing diagnosis implies that you have made decisions about the nature of a client's problems or needs and have given those problems names. It is the result of the analysis and synthesis of your assessment data.

Nursing diagnosis is identifying the client problems that are amenable to treatment with nursing care. Nurses treat human responses to illness or health needs rather than diagnosing and treating the illness or condition that created the response. Thus nurses may manage symptoms, response to treatment, attitudes, feelings, or changes in lifestyle associated with an illness. Nursing diagnoses focus on the client's problems rather than on the nurse's problems in providing the care.

In their strictest sense, nursing diagnoses are problems or needs for which you are accountable and that you are capable of diagnosing and treating *independently*. However, many client problems in a health care setting require collaboration with a multidisciplinary health care team. A **collaborative problem** is a clinical problem that cannot be solved by you alone (or by the nursing staff) but instead requires treatments or medications that you are unable to perform or not licensed to order.

Nursing diagnoses are a part of the nursing process. The phases of the nursing process are interlinked and function as a whole to help you make sound clinical judgments. Making a nursing diagnosis establishes a link between assessment and planning interventions. With accurate diagnoses, you will be able to select or design interventions to meet the client's individual needs or solve problems.

Making nursing diagnoses helps you think critically in nursing practice. Making a nursing diagnosis may be as simple as giving a name to an obvious problem or client need. At other times, complex thinking skills may be required to correctly identify the problem, its cause, and the factors that contribute to it. One of the most important skills that you must possess as a nurse is the ability to think through problems and make sound clinical judgments about the needs of clients under your care. In a constantly changing health care environment driven by economic constraints, providing quality care requires that you have strong skills in critical thinking (see Chapter 5). Nurses who can think critically about all aspects of nursing care increase their ability to be safe practitioners.

CONCEPT OF STANDARDIZED NURSING DIAGNOSIS LANGUAGE

A standardized language for nursing diagnoses means that all nurses are using the same words to describe the phenomena treated or managed by nurses. All sciences have a standardized language—when a microbiologist writes about *Staphylococcus,* all microbiologists understand what is meant. Nursing has borrowed language from medicine, physiology, and psychology but is only beginning to develop language for the human conditions that are uniquely responsive to nursing care.

The North American Nursing Diagnosis Association (NANDA) is the organization officially sanctioned by the American Nurses' Association as the body responsible for developing a system of naming and classifying nursing diagnoses. NANDA defines a **nursing diagnosis** as a clinical judgment about individual, family, or community responses to actual or potential health problems or life processes. A nursing diagnosis provides you with a basis for selecting nursing interventions to achieve outcomes for which you are accountable (NANDA, 2001).

Evolution

Making nursing diagnoses is a relatively recent trend in nursing practice. However, if nursing diagnosis is a technique for describing areas of human concern that nurses are qualified to help clients manage, then nurses have been making diagnoses since nursing practice began. Until the 1950s, nurses were reluctant to use the term *diagnosis* because it could create confusion between medical practice and nursing practice. Virginia Henderson and Faye Abdellah are credited with advancing nursing as a profession by providing the beginnings of a language that encouraged nurses to identify *client-centered problems* instead of nursing tasks as the focus of nursing practice. In Chapter 5 you learned about the human needs identified by these theorists.

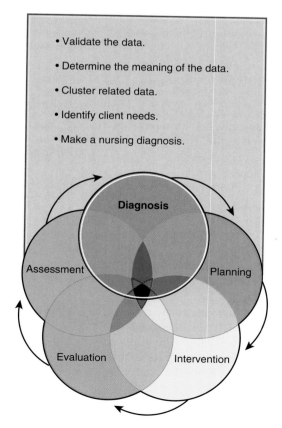

- Validate the data.
- Determine the meaning of the data.
- Cluster related data.
- Identify client needs.
- Make a nursing diagnosis.

Figure 9-1. Nursing diagnosis is the second phase of the nursing process.

Many other nurses then began writing about client problems, and some began calling them nursing diagnoses. By 1971, the American Nurses' Association included making a nursing diagnosis in its standards for nursing practice, and the term began to appear in nurse practice acts. Believing that the profession of nursing would benefit from the use of a common language, the faculty at St. Louis University organized the first national conference for the classification of nursing diagnosis in 1973. As a result of this conference, the North American Nursing Diagnosis Association was established in 1983. NANDA's purpose is to develop, refine, and promote a taxonomy of nursing diagnostic language that can be used by all professional nurses (Kim, McFarland, & McLane, 1984). This group continues to meet every other year to accomplish its ongoing work.

Rationales for Using a Standardized Nursing Language

A language of nursing diagnoses communicates the role of the nurse and the problems or conditions that are treated by nurses. Nurses, clients, and other members of the health care team benefit from clear communication about the phenomena treated by nurses and thus about the contribution of nursing to the client's welfare. Some of the benefits of a shared diagnostic language include the following:

- It fosters critical thinking by placing the emphasis on nursing care to solve the client's problem rather than on completing tasks.
- It provides a method for identifying the focus or goal of nursing activity.
- It increases the likelihood of using creative approaches to nursing rather than repetition of the usual interventions, especially when those interventions are not working.
- It provides a common language for nurses to communicate with one another and the health care team.
- It ensures that nursing care is documented in a manner that is recognizable and retrievable for quality improvement studies.
- It contributes to the autonomy and self-regulatory capacity of nursing.
- It defines the nursing body of knowledge and scope of practice.
- It facilitates nursing research by enabling retrieval of nursing data from a computerized medical record to document the effectiveness of nursing care.
- It paves the way for third-party reimbursement for nursing care that can be proven to be beneficial and cost effective.

The advent of computerized medical and health record systems has increased the need for a standardized nursing language that reflects nursing practice in the client's record. In agencies, such as home health, where nursing is the primary service offered, client record systems need to clearly document client problems treated by nurses. On the other hand, in hospital records, practitioners from multiple disciplines document in the same record. A multidisciplinary approach to documentation often subsumes nursing care into the care of other practitioners, particularly physicians, and as a result the contribution of nursing care is virtually invisible. The NANDA nomenclature is a systematic means of reflecting nursing practice in the client's record.

This issue is broader than issues found in providing care to a single client. When the system of naming problems does not reflect any options specific to nursing, the nurse is challenged to enter data into the system that shows the benefit of nursing care to the client. If these benefits cannot be named or identified, then they certainly cannot be controlled, financed, researched, or put into public policy (Clark & Lang, 1992).

Taxonomies

A **taxonomy** is a system of identifying, naming, and classifying phenomena. In nursing, the phenomena are human responses, physiological and behavioral, for which nursing care can be beneficial. A taxonomy is useful to nursing scientists in distinguishing various client problems and improving methods of nursing practice. There are three major taxonomies for nursing diagnoses. Taxonomies for nursing interventions and nursing outcomes are discussed in Chapter 10.

NANDA Taxonomy. NANDA began the process of developing a language of nursing diagnoses by listing the problems or conditions treated by nurses and classifying these conditions into categories of human responses. Taxonomies in any discipline evolve as the science develops. As nurses began using the system of nursing diagnoses, they recognized that additional nursing diagnoses were needed to completely capture the role of the nurse, and both nurse scientists and practicing nurses submitted new diagnoses to NANDA. As these diagnoses were added to the taxonomy, some weaknesses were recognized in the classification system. One major weakness was the lack of diagnoses at the wellness end of the health-illness continuum. NANDA then researched the best method of classifying client problems and introduced Taxonomy II in 2000.

Taxonomy II. Taxonomy II is a multiaxial system of naming nursing diagnoses. With more than one axis, the diagnosis can capture up to seven parameters to make the diagnosis specific to the individual needs of the client. The seven axes are as follows:

- Axis 1: The diagnostic concept. These concepts are classified in 13 domains (Box 9-1).
- Axis 2: Time (acute [less than 6 months] to chronic [more than 6 months], intermittent, continuous, long term, short term). Time may not be relevant to all diagnostic situations.
- Axis 3: Unit of care (individual, family, community, target group). When the unit of care is the individual, it need not be specified.
- Axis 4: Age (fetus, infant, toddler, child, adolescent, young adult, middle adult, older adult).
- Axis 5: Potentiality—the health axis (actual, risk for, opportunity [or potential] for growth or enhancement). This axis indicates the health status as the position on the health illness continuum.
- Axis 6: Descriptor (limits or specifies the meaning of the diagnostic concept). Examples include compromised, delayed, ineffective, effective, readiness, desires.
- Axis 7: Topology (parts or regions of the body).

Box 9-1   Domains of the Diagnostic Concepts

DOMAIN 1: HEALTH PROMOTION. The awareness of well-being or normality of function and the strategies used to maintain control of and enhance that well-being or normality of function
- Class 1: Health awareness—Recognition of normal function and well-being
- Class 2: Health management—Identifying, controlling, performing, and integrating activities to maintain health and well-being

DOMAIN 2: NUTRITION. The activities of taking in, assimilating, and using nutrients for the purpose of tissues maintenance, tissue repair, and the production of energy
- Class 1: Ingestion—Taking food or nutrients into the body
- Class 2: Digestion—The physical and chemical activities that convert foodstuffs into substances suitable for absorption and assimilation
- Class 3: Absorption—The act of taking up nutrients through body tissue
- Class 4: Metabolism—The chemical and physical processes occurring in living organisms and cells for the development and use of protoplasm, production of waste and energy, with the release of energy for all vital processes
- Class 5: Hydration—The taking in and absorption of fluids and electrolytes

DOMAIN 3: ELIMINATION. Secretion and excretion of waste products from the body
- Class 1: Urinary system—The process of secretion and excretion of urine
- Class 2: Gastrointestinal system—Excretion and expulsion of waste products from the bowel
- Class 3: Integumentary system—Process of secretion and excretion through the skin
- Class 4: Pulmonary system—Removal of by-products or metabolic products, secretions, and foreign material from the lungs or bronchi

DOMAIN 4: REST/ACTIVITY. The production, conservation, expenditure, or balance of energy resources
- Class 1: Sleep/rest—Slumber, repose, ease, or inactivity
- Class 2: Activity/exercise—Moving parts of the body (mobility), doing work, or performing actions, often (but not always) against resistance
- Class 3: Energy balance—A dynamic state of harmony between intake and expenditure of resources
- Class 4: Cardiovascular/pulmonary—Cardiopulmonary mechanisms that support activity/rest

DOMAIN 5: PERCEPTION/COGNITION. The human information-processing system including attention, orientation, sensation/perception, cognition, and communication
- Class 1: Attention—Mental readiness to notice or observe
- Class 2: Orientation—Awareness of time, place, and person
- Class 3: Sensation/perception—Receiving information through the senses of touch, taste, smell, vision, hearing, and kinesthesia, and the comprehension of sense data resulting in naming, associating, and/or pattern recognition
- Class 4: Cognition—Use of memory, learning, thinking, problem solving, abstraction, judgment, insight, intellectual capacity, calculation, and language
- Class 5: Communication—Sending and receiving verbal and nonverbal information

DOMAIN 6: SELF-PERCEPTION. Awareness about the self
- Class 1: Self-concept—The perception(s) about the total self
- Class 2: Self-esteem—Assessment of one's own worth, capability, significance, and success
- Class 2: Body image—A mental image of one's own body

DOMAIN 7: ROLE RELATIONSHIPS. The positive and negative connections or associations between persons or groups of persons and the means by which those connections are demonstrated
- Class 1: Caregiving roles—Socially expected behavior patterns by care-providing persons who are not health care professionals
- Class 2: Family relationships—Associations of people who are biologically related or related by choice
- Class 3: Role performance—Quality of functioning in socially expected behavior patterns

DOMAIN 8: SEXUALITY. Sexual identity, sexual function, and reproduction
- Class 1: Sexual identity—The state of being a specific person in regard to sexuality and/or gender
- Class 2: Sexual function—The capacity or ability to participate in sexual activities
- Class 3: Reproduction—Any process by which new individuals (people) are produced

DOMAIN 9: COPING/STRESS TOLERANCE. Contending with life events/life processes
- Class 1: Posttrauma responses—Reactions occurring after physical or psychological trauma
- Class 2: Coping responses—The process of managing environmental stress
- Class 3: Neurobehavioral response—Behavioral responses reflecting nerve and brain function

DOMAIN 10: LIFE PRINCIPLES. Principles underlying conduct, thought, and behavior about acts, customs, or institutions viewed as being true or having intrinsic worth
- Class 1: Values—The identification and ranking of preferred modes of conduct and status
- Class 2: Beliefs—Opinions, expectations, or judgments about acts, customs, or institutions viewed as being true or having intrinsic worth
- Class 3: Value/belief/action congruence—The correspondence or balance achieved between values, beliefs, and actions

DOMAIN 11: SAFETY AND PROTECTION. Freedom from danger, physical injury, or immune system damage; preservation from loss; and protection of safety and security
- Class 1: Infection—Host response following pathogenic invasion
- Class 2: Physical injury—Bodily harm or hurt
- Class 3: Violence—The exertion of excessive force or power so as to cause injury or abuse
- Class 4: Environmental hazards—Sources of danger in the surroundings
- Class 5: Defensive processes—The processes by which the self protects itself from the nonself
- Class 6: Thermoregulation—The physiologic process of regulating heath and energy within the body for purposes of protecting the organism

DOMAIN 12: COMFORT. Sense of mental, physical, or social well-being or ease
- Class 1: Physical comfort—Sense of well-being or ease
- Class 2: Environmental comfort—Sense of well-being or ease in/with one's environment
- Class 3: Social comfort—Sense of well-being or ease with one's social situations

DOMAIN 13: GROWTH/DEVELOPMENT. Age-appropriate increases in physical dimensions, organ systems, and/or attainment of developmental milestones
- Class 1: Growth—Increase in physical dimensions or maturity of organ systems
- Class 2: Development—Attainment, lack of attainment, or loss of developmental milestones

North American Nursing Diagnosis Association. (2001). *Nursing diagnoses: Definitions and classification, 2001-2002.* Philadelphia: Author.

Box 9-2	Nursing Diagnoses Grouped by Functional Health Pattern

HEALTH PERCEPTION–HEALTH MANAGEMENT PATTERN

Disturbed Energy field
Ineffective Health maintenance
*Health-management deficit**
Risk for Health-management deficit
Health-seeking behaviors
Risk for Infection
Risk for Injury
Risk for perioperative-positioning Injury
Noncompliance
Risk for Noncompliance
Risk for Poisoning
Ineffective Protection
Risk for Sudden infant death syndrome
Risk for Suffocation
Effective Therapeutic regimen management
Ineffective Therapeutic regimen management
Ineffective community Therapeutic regimen management
Ineffective family Therapeutic regimen management
Readiness for enhanced Therapeutic regimen management
Risk for ineffective management of Therapeutic regimen

NUTRITIONAL–METABOLIC PATTERN

Latex Allergy response
Risk for latex Allergy response
Risk for Aspiration
Risk for imbalanced Body temperature
Effective Breastfeeding
Ineffective Breastfeeding
Interrupted Breastfeeding
Impaired Dentition
Adult Failure to thrive
Readiness for enhanced Fluid balance
Deficient Fluid volume
Excess Fluid volume
Risk for deficient Fluid volume
Risk for imbalanced Fluid volume
Hyperthermia
Hypothermia
Ineffective Infant feeding pattern
Nausea
Readiness for enhanced Nutrition
Imbalanced Nutrition: less than body requirements
Imbalanced Nutrition: more than body requirements
Risk for imbalanced Nutrition: more than body requirements
Impaired Oral mucous membrane
Pressure ulcer
Impaired Skin integrity
Risk for impaired Skin integrity

Impaired Swallowing
Ineffective Thermoregulation
Impaired Tissue integrity

ELIMINATION PATTERN

Bowel incontinence
Constipation
Perceived Constipation
Intermittent Constipation pattern
Risk for Constipation
Diarrhea
Functional urinary Incontinence
Reflex urinary Incontinence
Stress urinary Incontinence
Urge Incontinence
Risk for urge urinary Incontinence
Total urinary Incontinence
Impaired Urinary elimination
Readiness for enhanced Urinary elimination
Urinary retention

ACTIVITY–EXERCISE PATTERN

Activity intolerance
Risk for Activity intolerance
Ineffective Airway clearance
Autonomic dysreflexia
Risk for Autonomic dysreflexia
Ineffective Breathing pattern
Decreased Cardiac output
Risk for delayed Development
Developmental delay: self-care skills
Risk for Disuse syndrome
Deficient Diversional activity
Fatigue
Impaired Gas exchange
Risk for disproportionate Growth
Delayed Growth and development
Impaired Home maintenance
Disorganized Infant behavior
Readiness for enhanced organized Infant behavior
Risk for disorganized Infant behavior
Decreased Intracranial adaptive capacity
Risk for Joint contractures
Impaired bed Mobility
Impaired physical Mobility
Impaired transfer Mobility
Impaired wheelchair Mobility
Risk for Peripheral neurovascular dysfunction
Bathing/hygiene Self-care deficit
Dressing/grooming Self-care deficit
Feeding Self-care deficit
Toileting Self-care deficit
Total Self-care deficit
Delayed Surgical recovery
Ineffective Tissue perfusion

Impaired spontaneous Ventilation
Dysfunctional Ventilatory weaning
Impaired Walking

SLEEP–REST PATTERN

Sleep deprivation
Delayed Sleep onset
Disturbed Sleep pattern
Sleep-pattern reversal
Readiness for enhanced Sleep

COGNITIVE–PPERCEPTUAL PATTERN

Attention-concentration deficit
Risk for Cognitive impairment
Impaired verbal Communication
Readiness for enhanced Communication
Decisional Conflict
Acute Confusion
Chronic Confusion
Impaired Environmental interpretation syndrome
Deficient Knowledge
Readiness for enhanced Knowledge of (specify)
Impaired Memory
Uncompensated Memory loss
Unilateral Neglect
Acute Pain
Chronic Pain
Pain self-management deficit
Sensory deprivation
Sensory overload
Disturbed Sensory perception
Disturbed Thought process

SELF-PERCEPTION–SELF-CONCEPT PATTERN

Anxiety
Anticipatory Anxiety (mild, moderate, severe)
Death Anxiety
Mild Anxiety
Moderate Anxiety
Severe Anxiety (panic)
Disturbed Body image
Reactive Depression
Fear
Hopelessness
Disturbed personal Identity
Risk for Loneliness
Powerlessness
Readiness for enhanced Self-concept
Chronic low Self-esteem
Risk for situational low Self-esteem
Situational low Self-esteem
Risk for Self-mutilation

ROLE–RELATIONSHIP PATTERN

Risk for impaired parent/infant/child Attachment
Weak parent/infant Attachment

Modified from Gordon, M. (2000). *Manual of nursing diagnoses* (9th ed.). St Louis, MO: Mosby; and NANDA International (2002). *NANDA nursing diagnoses: Definitions and classifications, 2002-2003.* Philadelphia: Author.

Box 9-2   Nursing Diagnoses Grouped by Functional Health Pattern—cont'd

ROLE–RELATIONSHIP PATTERN—cont'd

Caregiver role strain
Risk for Caregiver role strain
Parental role Conflict
Developmental delay
Developmental delay: communication skills
Dysfunctional Family processes: alcoholism
Interrupted Family processes
Readiness for enhanced Family processes
Anticipatory Grieving
Dysfunctional Grieving
Unresolved Independence-dependence conflict
Impaired Parenting
Readiness for enhanced Parenting
Risk for impaired Parenting
Ineffective Role performance
Parent/infant Separation

Social isolation
Impaired Social interaction
Chronic Sorrow
Relocation Stress syndrome
Risk for Violence
Risk for other-directed Violence
Risk for self-directed Violence

SEXUALITY–REPRODUCTION PATTERN

Rape-trauma syndrome
Rape-trauma syndrome: compound reaction
Rape-trauma syndrome: silent reaction
Sexual dysfunction
Ineffective Sexuality patterns

COPING-STRESS–TOLERANCE PATTERN

Impaired Adjustment
Avoidance Coping

Compromised family Coping
Defensive Coping
Disabled family Coping
Ineffective Coping
Ineffective community Coping
Readiness for enhanced community Coping
Readiness for enhanced Coping
Readiness for enhanced family Coping
Ineffective Denial
Posttrauma syndrome
Risk for Posttrauma syndrome
Support system deficit

VALUE–BELIEF PATTERN

Spiritual distress
Readiness for enhanced Spiritual well-being
Risk for Spiritual distress

You can choose the diagnostic concept or the human response that explains the individual's situation, and you can choose the descriptor from the descriptor axis. And you have five more axes to help make the diagnosis specific.

Diagnoses have not been developed or approved for testing with all possible combinations of axes, and some combinations would not make sense. As you begin to use NANDA nursing diagnoses, you should start with the list of approved diagnoses (Box 9-2). Although you are free to create diagnoses using the axes in any combination, you should carefully consider the logic of your decision and whether or not your diagnosis clearly communicates the client's problem.

Omaha System.
The Omaha System is a classification system developed by the staff of the Visiting Nurse Association (VNA) of Omaha, Nebraska, as a documentation and data management system that conveys the autonomy of community health nursing practice. The project to develop the system represents 15 years of research. The system includes a problem classification scheme that is a taxonomy of nursing diagnoses valuable to community health nurses. Thus the domains within the scheme reflect the home and community practice setting. For example, diagnoses within the environmental domain address material resources, physical surroundings, and the client's community. This system has the advantage of having been developed from what visiting or home health nurses actually do within the framework of reimbursable nursing practice (Martin & Scheet, 1992).

Saba System.
The Saba Nursing Diagnoses for Home Health Care: Classification and Coding Scheme was developed through a project that reviewed 8961 clients of home care agencies. The system consists of nursing diagnoses and interventions that serve as a framework for home health nursing practice. Like the Omaha System, the Saba system is closely linked to services that can be provided under Medicare. The Saba system also has the advantage of communicating what home health nurses actually do. Many of the Saba nursing diagnoses are identical to those of NANDA.

Psychiatric Nursing Diagnoses.
Because psychiatric nurses felt that the list of NANDA diagnoses did not capture the client problems managed by psychiatric nurses, a task force was formed in 1984 under the American Nurses' Association to develop psychiatric nursing diagnoses. In 1994, this group turned its work over to NANDA for further refinement and development. Because psychiatric nurses find the *Diagnostic and Statistical Manual of Mental Disorders* useful, the psychiatric group has proposed that some of the diagnoses from this manual be recognized as nursing diagnoses. That group of nursing diagnostic labels is listed in the 1999-2000 NANDA manual as undergoing development (NANDA, 1999).

COMPONENTS OF A NURSING DIAGNOSIS

A NANDA nursing diagnosis has five components: a label, a definition, a set of defining characteristics, a group of related factors, and risk factors (Box 9-3, p. 182). The label and related factors are documented in the client's plan of care. Applicable defining characteristics are documented as assessment findings.

Label
The **diagnostic label** is the name of the nursing diagnosis. It is a concise term or phrase that represents a pattern of related cues that are characteristics, signs, or symptoms. It may include a **descriptor,** or a judgment that modifies, limits, or specifies the meaning of a nursing diagnosis, such as *decreased, deficient, excessive,* or *readiness* (NANDA, 2001).

Definition
The *definition* of the diagnosis provides a description of the pattern of signs and symptoms, delineates the meaning of the label, and helps to differentiate it from similar or related diagnoses.

Box 9-3	Components of a Sample NANDA Nursing Diagnosis

DIAGNOSTIC STATEMENT

Urge urinary incontinence

DEFINITION

Involuntary passage of urine occurring soon after a strong sense of urgency to void.

DEFINING CHARACTERISTICS

Urinary urgency
Bladder contracture/spasm
Frequency (voiding more often than every 2 hours)
Nocturia (more than two times per night)
Voiding in small amounts (less than 100 ml) or in large amounts (more than 550 ml)
Inability to reach toilet in time

RELATED FACTORS

Alcohol, caffeine, decreased bladder capacity (e.g., history of pelvic inflammatory disease, abdominal surgeries, indwelling urinary catheter), increased fluids, increased urine concentration, irritation of bladder stretch receptors causing spasm (e.g., bladder infection), overdistention of bladder.

From NANDA International (2002). *NANDA nursing diagnoses: Definitions and classification, 2002-2003.* Philadelphia: Author.

Box 9-4	Questions to Consider When Identifying Related Factors

ETIOLOGY

- What is the cause of the problem?
- Do the related factors allow me to understand the etiology, or cause, of this client's human response?
- Is the cause of the problem clear?
- Will removing or ameliorating the cause solve the problem?
- Can a nurse treat the etiology?

CONTRIBUTING FACTORS

- What client behaviors contribute to the problem?
- Are there client behaviors that can be changed to reduce or eliminate the problem? Examples: health habits, knowledge.

PROVIDING DIRECTION TO NURSING CARE

- Do the related factors help me decide which interventions are most appropriate?
- Can nursing care change the related factors?
- If so, which factors can be changed by nursing care?
- Does the information make a difference in the interventions that will be performed for this client?
- Will changing the related factors solve the problem, manage the problem, or help the client tolerate the problem until a definitive solution can be found?

Defining Characteristics

Defining characteristics are descriptions of a client's behavior that determine whether a nursing diagnosis is present and whether a particular diagnosis is appropriate or accurate. Defining characteristics are either directly or indirectly observable clinical cues. **Cues** are the indicators of the presence or existence of a problem or condition that represents a client's underlying health status. Subjective and objective data (symptoms and signs) of a problem provide the clinical cues that a problem is present.

Related Factors

Related factors show some type of patterned relationship to the nursing diagnosis. The related factor may be antecedent (prior) to, associated with, contributing to, or abetting the nursing diagnosis. These specific related factors help direct how the problem should be managed. The related factors may be an etiology or causative factor; therefore the treatment is to remove the cause. However, the etiologies of nursing diagnoses are often medical diagnoses that a nurse cannot treat. The nurse can help the client manage the medical treatment or manage the symptoms until the medical treatment becomes effective. The nurse can also manage factors that contribute to the problem. By identifying a related factor, nursing management focuses on treating responses and thus supporting the medical treatment. Writing the "related to" part of the nursing diagnostic statement is often a creative process based on understanding of the medical condition and the client's patterns of behavior (Box 9-4).

Risk Factors

Risk factors are factors in the internal or external environment that increase the vulnerability of a person, family, or community to an unhealthful state or event. A significant part of nursing practice is preventive, thus nursing language must be able to express client problems that require prevention.

THE HEALTH AXIS

The health axis helps you identify the client's position on a continuum from health to illness. Because nursing care focuses on prevention, restoration of health, and maintaining wellness, nursing diagnoses can be described as actual, risk, or wellness diagnoses that represent these different spheres of nursing care. Nurses also help to manage problems where collaboration with the physician is necessary.

Actual Nursing Diagnoses

Actual nursing diagnoses describe human responses to health conditions/life processes that exist at the present time (NANDA, 2001). Thus they describe a client's current problem. When a client has an actual diagnosis, you can identify the signs and symptoms (defining characteristics) that indicate the presence of the diagnosis. For example, if your client is unable to completely empty urine from the bladder, you would make an actual diagnosis of *Urinary retention.*

"Risk for" Nursing Diagnoses

A "**risk for**" **nursing diagnosis** describes human responses that *may* develop in a vulnerable person, family, or community. Risk-for diagnoses are supported by risk factors that contribute to increased vulnerability (NANDA, 2001). These nursing diagnoses are used when the client does not have a sufficient number of defining characteristics present to justify making the actual nursing diagnosis. Thus risk-for diagnoses are used to help you plan nursing care aimed at *preventing* the problem.

For instance, an elderly woman in a nursing home might have a risk for impaired skin integrity. The client does not actually have any broken skin or abraded areas visible. Nonetheless, she is thin, eats poorly, is confined to bed, is not using pressure-relieving devices, and sometimes wets the bed at night. All of these factors predispose her to skin breakdown. The nursing diagnosis *Risk for impaired skin integrity* alerts the nursing home staff that preventive measures should be taken to reduce the risk of skin breakdown.

Although the current NANDA taxonomy lists individual risk-for nursing diagnoses, risk is an element of Axis 5 and may be used with any nursing diagnosis for a client who does not actually have the problem but is at risk. Making diagnoses that define the client's risk communicates this important information to clients and suggests a plan of preventive care. Some agencies prefer that nursing diagnoses be made only when actual problems exist, and thus they make the assumption that preventive nursing care is provided.

Wellness Nursing Diagnoses

A **wellness nursing diagnosis** is a human response to a state or level of wellness in an individual, family, or community that has the desire to move toward a higher state of being healthy; it is usually the result of deliberate action (Carpenito, 2001; NANDA, 2001). The client is functioning effectively but desires a higher level of wellness.

For example, the nursing diagnosis *Health-seeking behavior* related to a request for information about birth control might be used with a young woman who is engaged to be married. This diagnosis reflects that the woman desires information to maintain health in the future.

Collaborative Problems

In some client situations, the problems to be resolved require the interventions of more than one member of the health care team. In such cases, health team members share the responsibilities associated with solving those problems. There is overlap between medical and nursing diagnoses and problems identified by such others as physical therapists, nutritionists, and social workers. Carpenito (2001) calls these *collaborative problems,* because the solutions require interventions from several members of the team (Figure 9-2). However, many nursing diagnoses represent problems treated or managed by both the physician and the nurse. Some aspects of the care are independent nursing interventions, and other aspects are dependent nursing interventions.

A collaborative problem suggests that you are working interdependently and cooperatively with all health team

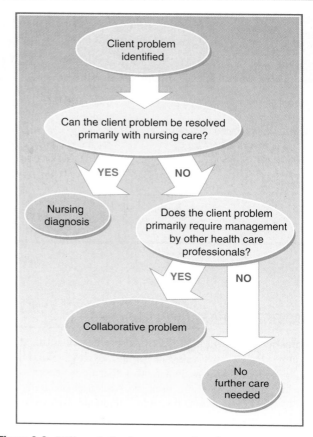

Figure 9-2. Differentiating between nursing diagnoses and collaborative problems.

members needed to solve the problem. This is in contrast to your independent functioning, when you work alone or with other nursing colleagues to solve the problem, and to your dependent functioning, when you follow someone else's orders (usually those of a physician). In the dependent function, you do not write the order, but you are responsible for carrying it out in a safe and competent manner.

A case example may illustrate how medical, nursing, and collaborative problems require the use of dependent, independent, and interdependent functions, respectively. Table 9-1 (p. 184) organizes the data from this example into diagnoses. Note that the medical, nursing, and collaborative diagnoses may have exactly the same labels, but the focus of care for each type of diagnosis is specific to the specialty.

John Chase breaks his leg in football practice. A physician sets the bone, puts a cast on the leg, and orders physical therapy and pain medication. The physical therapist must decide the physical therapy needed on the basis of the type of cast applied and the length of the cast and must then teach John the proper method for getting around on crutches or i a wheelchair. The nurse must administer the pain medic tion, teach John how to use the medication at home, ass his knowledge of broken bones and bone healing, enh; this knowledge as needed, and help him decide how he manage his daily activities while in the cast.

Table 9-1   Examples of the Relationships Between Medical, Collaborative, and Nursing Problems and the Functions of the Health Care Team Members

Collaborative Medical Problem/ Dependent Function	Problem/Interdependent Function	Nursing Problem/Independent Function
Pain: Physician orders pain medication. Nurse administers medication safely.	*Pain:* Physician orders pain medication. Nurse teaches client how to use medication at home.	*Pain:* Nurse teaches relaxation techniques and positioning methods to reduce the need for pain medication.
Impaired physical mobility: Physician orders physical therapy. Physical therapist carries out orders.	*Impaired physical mobility:* Physical therapist determines types of therapy needed and initiates a treatment plan. Nurse helps client understand how to do exercises at home.	*Impaired physical mobility:* Nurse helps client decide how client will manage daily activities at home and in school while the cast is on.
	Knowledge deficit: Physical therapist teaches client how to ambulate on crutches. Nurse encourages client to practice crutch walking in the corridor before going home.	*Knowledge deficit:* Nurse assesses client's knowledge about bone healing and provides information about the relationship between diet and bone growth.

DIAGNOSTIC REASONING PROCESS

Diagnostic reasoning is professional problem identification. It requires logical, but value-laden and flexible, thinking to identify problems and related factors that both accounts for individual client needs and uses the strengths of client and nurse to the fullest extent possible. Diagnostic reasoning in nursing is somewhat different from diagnostic reasoning in medicine. Although the steps are similar for both, the contexts and the factors under consideration are different. The task of medical diagnosis is one of assessing, identifying, and labeling disease states. The physician generates hypotheses on the basis of signs and symptoms that are part of a well-defined and widely shared vocabulary. The steps in medical diagnostic reasoning include the following:

- Assess the signs and symptoms present.
- Generate several hypotheses about what the disease state might be.
- From a mental set of descriptors, evaluate and differentiate potential diseases.
- Select the disease that best describes the client's set of signs and symptoms.
- Select the best treatment for the disease on the basis of the underlying cause(s) of the disease.

Even though experienced nurses can often identify specific disease states in some clients, the nurse's function is not to diagnose disease. However, the process of diagnostic reasoning in nursing requires the same clear, logical steps in thinking that are required for medical diagnosis. The difference, however, is that nurses diagnose the *human responses* to actual and potential health problems that *result from* or have *an impact on* disease, lifestyle, and life situations. Human responses include physiological, cognitive, emotional, and social changes that have to do with the meaning of health and illness to the person as well as how the person is able to function.

Because you must take into account the psychosocial and life circumstances of the client (in addition to the medical di-

agnosis) when making any nursing diagnoses, nursing diagnosis often requires both complex and creative critical thinking. In contrast to medicine, making a nursing diagnosis does not necessarily limit the possibilities for treatment to a narrow choice of known protocols. Diagnostic reasoning in nursing takes into account both the assets and the deficits of each client, and it occurs in cycles that are repeated until the problem is resolved.

Critical Thinking

Critical thinking links the idea of rationality, reasonableness, and reflection to the practical decision making necessary in nursing. Additionally, critical thinking in nursing must be done within the context of the nurse–client interaction, the client's value system, and the interdisciplinary health care system.

The level of critical thinking needed to make clinical judgments about a client's life and health requires that you have a high level of ability in diagnostic reasoning and clinical judgment. You will use steps similar to those used for diagnostic reasoning in medicine.

- Assess the client and analyze the data.
- To identify patterns of responses, cluster cues that are logically related.
- Form hypotheses about the meaning of the client's human responses.
- Select and evaluate potential nursing diagnostic labels that reflect the cue clusters.
- Select the labels that best describe the client's human responses.
- Determine the causes or related factors for each diagnosis chosen.
- Plan interventions on the basis of the related factors to meet the goals of correcting or impacting the diagnosis.

The hardest parts of the process for the beginner are clustering client assessment data into meaningful sets and generating hypotheses about the client's human responses. Clustering cues is harder when you have little clinical experience and are just beginning to learn about the effects of illness and medical treatments. As you study the health patterns in this textbook, learn about specific diseases, and practice making nursing diagnoses on the basis of your assessment of clients, you will learn patterns of cues that commonly occur together.

Nursing diagnoses, then, are the labels you apply to the cue clusters generated from your assessment of the client. All of the defining characteristics do not need to be present for you to make a diagnosis. However, there should be a good match, or "fit," between the actual client data and the defining characteristics of the diagnosis. The diagnoses are then linked to the factors that caused or are related to the diagnoses. Nursing interventions are planned on the basis of those causal or related factors.

Sometimes one cue is sufficient to make a diagnosis, but generally a diagnosis is made from a cluster of cues. Recognizing the complete cluster of cues will help you plan care. Once you can recognize common patterns of cue clusters, your diagnostic reasoning ability will improve rapidly.

When you make a diagnosis, you are making a clinical judgment. A **clinical judgment** is a conclusion or an opinion that a problem or situation requires nursing care and that determines the cause of the problem, distinguishes between similar problems, or discriminates between two or more courses of action. Additionally, clinical judgments involve making decisions about what to observe, how to observe, prioritizing problems, and deciding what to do in a clinical situation. Clinical judgment encompasses both critical thinking and diagnostic reasoning.

As a novice, you cannot expect to have the same clinical judgment abilities as an experienced nurse; however, even a novice is capable of quite sophisticated judgments given practice, time, and good supervision. The more experience you have with a particular client population, the more sensitive, specific, and expert your clinical judgments will be about the clients under your care.

Steps in the Diagnostic Process

The process of arriving at a nursing diagnosis involves several interrelated steps; no step exists in isolation from the whole. The process is also ongoing: each step is repeated until you are satisfied that the plan of care is the best one possible on the basis of the data available.

In the initial contact with the client, often on admission to a facility or service, the emphasis is on gathering assessment data and generating tentative diagnoses. Making the first set of nursing diagnoses for a client takes more time and effort than updating and changing the care plan. Schedule extra time to generate the initial care plan, because the data are new. A carefully constructed initial care plan will ultimately save you time. It is easier to update and revise a good care plan than to create the care plan on an ad hoc basis.

In the following paragraphs, we discuss the steps in the diagnostic reasoning process. Box 9-5 (p. 186) illustrates an example of how to use the diagnostic reasoning process.

Reviewing the Assessment Data. The first step in making a nursing diagnosis is to review all the assessment data available about the client. This includes the client and family information, medical history and physical examination data, laboratory and other diagnostic tests, as well as data obtained from the nursing history and physical assessment. The amount of information may seem overwhelming at first, but as you review the data, you will be able to make distinctions between relevant and irrelevant data by asking two questions: What is the significance of these data for nursing care? What problems could the client have on the basis of this information?

As you review the assessment data, you are looking for subjective and objective cues. Some examples of cues may be a cough, a pattern of bruises, or a client's report of stress caused by an impending divorce.

Clustering the Data. A single cue often alerts you to a problem. However, it is almost never enough to make a definitive diagnosis, and it is certainly not enough to associate the diagnosis with a related factor. Thus the next step in generating nursing diagnoses is to mentally organize the data into clusters of cues that seem to fit logically together and lead to insights or inferences about the client's condition. For example, a cough could be a cue to a number of nursing diagnoses. If the client also has wheezing, dyspnea, cyanosis, and a history of asthma, an experienced nurse would consider the nursing diagnosis *Impaired gas exchange related to airway obstruction secondary to asthma.*

Remember that not all data are useful as cues and may not fit into any meaningful clusters. On the other hand, some important cues may not be available. Thus you may have to reassess the client or review the database to obtain the missing information at a later time.

Before moving on to the next step, review the clusters you have generated. Do they make sense conceptually and logically? Do they provide insights into the client's condition? Do the clusters indicate probable nursing diagnoses?

Selecting Possible Nursing Diagnoses. After answering these questions, review each potential problem represented in a data cluster. Think critically about which nursing diagnoses might be relevant to the situation. Remember that diagnoses cannot be selected in isolation from the goals of care. When you understand the client's reason for seeking service, goals for health, preferences in managing care, and lifestyle, you will be more likely to choose a diagnosis that is appropriate for the individual client and that is realistically manageable within the care setting. For example, the hospital nurse probably does not often use the diagnosis of *Impaired home maintenance management,* and the school nurse may have little use for *Decreased cardiac output.*

Differentiating Among Possible Diagnoses. Finding the most useful nursing diagnosis involves ruling out several possible diagnoses. Once you have identified possible nursing diagnoses for your client, you will need to narrow the possibilities until you identify the most appropriate diagnosis for each problem. **Differential diagnosis** is the term used to describe the process of deciding among several possible diagnoses to most accurately describe the client's problem. This process involves comparing the client's assessment data with the defining characteristics of possible diagnoses to determine which one has the best fit. The following questions and steps are useful in differentiating between diagnoses:

- Does the cluster of cues match one of the diagnoses better than the others? If so, this is probably the correct diagnosis.
- If the cluster of cues does not match perfectly any of the diagnoses under consideration, where does the problem lie? Perhaps there are not enough data available to choose appropriately.
- If not enough data are available, determine which data you need to make a decision. Then collect the data.
- Review the defining characteristics and data again to find the best match. Perhaps there is now a high probability of two or more diagnoses being correct.
- If data cannot be found to help make a decision, you can keep both diagnoses in the care plan until the situation becomes clearer, and you can consult with the client about which diagnosis is correct.

Identifying Appropriate Diagnoses. After selecting possible diagnoses and undertaking the process of differentiating between them, you will reach the point of identifying the nursing diagnosis or diagnoses most appropriate for your client. It is at this point that you will need to exercise clinical judgment; not all of the nursing diagnoses may be amenable to immediate intervention at this time. Not all possible diagnoses may be relevant to the current situation. Consequently, they need not be included in the care plan. Finally, some diagnoses will be of lower priority than others. Exercise your judgment when prioritizing diagnoses, setting goals for care, and planning nursing interventions to meet those goals.

Determining Related Factors. Next, complete the diagnosis by determining what the "related to," or etiologic (causal), factors are for the diagnoses you have selected. The related-to or etiologic statement is important because it gives direction to nursing care, guiding your choice of nursing interventions to alleviate the client's health concern.

When selecting a related factor, it might be helpful to ask yourself, "Does this information help me decide which interventions are most appropriate?" For example, selecting the diagnosis *Risk for infection related to postoperative care* is neither desirable nor useful. It focuses on nursing actions, not the client's problem. A better choice would be *Risk for infection related to shallow breathing, use of indwelling catheter, and surgical incision.* Selecting the more specific and client-focused factors makes determining interventions more efficient.

Box 9-5   Making a Nursing Diagnosis: A Case Example

Mrs. Brown is a 45-year-old woman who was admitted to the hospital with a medical diagnosis of "moderately severe vaginal bleeding secondary to fibroadenoma." She was sent directly to the operating room, where she underwent an abdominal hysterectomy. She was transferred to the surgical nursing unit from the postanesthesia care unit (PACU). She had an IV of D_5 lactated Ringer's solution running in her left arm, a surgical dressing on her abdomen that was clean and dry, and an indwelling catheter in her bladder. She responded to verbal commands but was still sedated when she arrived on the nursing unit. Her color was pale. Her vital signs were as follows: blood pressure, 126/78; pulse, 88; temperature, 97.8° F.

Step 1: Review the Assessment

When the nurse, Janine Cole, comes on duty 2 hours later, she reviews Mrs. Brown's chart. She finds that Mrs. Brown began bleeding suddenly and heavily the night before and was driven to the hospital by her husband. Her estimated blood loss before surgery was 500 ml. Blood loss during surgery was estimated at less than 500 ml. In the PACU her hemoglobin was 9.0 and hematocrit, 32%. She received one unit of blood.

When Janine enters Mrs. Brown's room, she finds Mrs. Brown awake but drowsy. Her husband is in the room with her. He looks tired and worried. The client's vital signs are as follows: blood pressure, 110/76; pulse, 78; and temperature, 98.6° F. Her color is pink. Her capillary refill rate is less than 3 seconds. The dressing has a 5-cm circle of pink drainage but is otherwise dry. Her urine output was 50 ml in the last hour.

Mrs. Brown is restless and complains of discomfort. She is reluctant to move or to have Janine touch her or the bed because she says it hurts when the bed is jostled. Aside from her discomfort, she seems to be primarily worried about her husband. She keeps asking him if he is all right and encouraging him to go home and rest. She tells Janine that he has been up all night and has had no sleep.

Step 2: Cluster the Data

Janine clusters data under the appropriate functional health patterns. She does not have data on some of the health patterns, so she uses only the ones that are appropriate at this time.

- *Health perception–health management:* 4 hours postoperative state (abdominal hysterectomy)
- *Nutritional–metabolic:* NPO last night and until 9 AM this morning, IV 5% R/L at 20 gtt/min, now taking small sips of clear liquids. Temperature is 98.6° F, abdominal wound present, dressing slightly pink in one 5-cm spot but otherwise dry.
- *Elimination:* Indwelling catheter drainage is 50 ml in the last hour, intake from IV was 1200 ml, no bowel sounds on auscultation.
- *Activity–exercise:* Has been immobile in OR, still recumbent and inactive as a result of IV catheter, sedation. Pulse is 78, blood pressure is 110/76.
- *Cognitive–perceptual:* Drowsy but alert to surroundings. Restless, complains of discomfort, reluctant to move or have bed touched.
- *Self-perception–self-concept:* No data on how she feels about hysterectomy and impact this will have on her sense of self as woman.
- *Role–relationship:* Husband is present and concerned. She is more concerned about him than about her own discomfort.

Step 3: Select Possible Nursing Diagnoses

Janine considers the data clusters and makes the following list of possible nursing diagnoses: *Impaired skin integrity, Risk for infection, Pain, Altered urinary elimination, Impaired physical mobility, Bathing/hygiene self-care deficit,* and *Anxiety.* Some of these diagnoses may be ruled out when Janine compares the actual data about Mrs. Brown with the defining characteristics of the diagnoses initially selected (see Table 9-4, p. 190).

| Box 9-5 | Making a Nursing Diagnosis: A Case Example—cont'd |

STEP 4: DIFFERENTIATE AMONG POSSIBLE DIAGNOSES

Janine then compares the defining characteristics of the possible diagnoses with the actual data she has about Mrs. Brown.

STEP 5: IDENTIFY APPROPRIATE DIAGNOSES

Janine compiles the final list of nursing diagnoses and arranges them by priority:

- Pain
- Risk for infection
- Impaired physical mobility
- Impaired skin integrity
- Bathing/hygiene self-care deficit
- Risk for altered urinary elimination

Anxiety was removed from the list as not valid. The highest priority is to help Mrs. Brown get comfortable and become free of pain. When she is no longer uncomfortable, it will be easier to help her groom herself and get out of bed.

STEP 6: DETERMINE RELATED FACTORS

Janine now links the nursing diagnoses with their "related to" factors or etiologies and comes up with the following final list of diagnoses:

- Pain related to inflammatory response in abdominal incision
- Impaired skin integrity related to abdominal surgical incision
- Impaired physical mobility related to pain from abdominal incision, sedation, IV in arm
- Risk for infection related to impaired skin integrity, history of blood loss, and presence of indwelling catheter and IV site
- Bathing/hygiene self-care deficit related to presence of IV in one arm, indwelling catheter in bladder, pain, and sedation due to recent operative procedure
- Risk for altered urinary elimination related to edema secondary to pelvic surgery

STEP 7: DISCUSS THE DIAGNOSES WITH THE CLIENT

Janine returns to Mrs. Brown's room to administer her pain medication and to verify the other nursing diagnoses she has made. Although the diagnoses of Impaired skin integrity, Risk for infection, and Bathing/hygiene self-care deficit are based on objective evidence and might not require validation from the client, Janine discusses them with Mrs. Brown to establish mutual goals. Mrs. Brown recognizes the need to manage her wound, prevent infection, accept assistance with bathing, and walk to prevent postoperative complications. Mrs. Brown says that she is not anxious about anything, just worried that her husband has been up all night and has not had any sleep. Once Mrs. Brown has validated the nursing diagnoses, Janine enters them into the nursing care plan.

STEP 8: PLAN THE NURSING CARE

Janine plans her nursing care for Mrs. Brown on the basis of the etiologies of the nursing diagnoses. Because the highest priority was Mrs. Brown's pain, Janine gave the prescribed pain medication and repositioned her for comfort. The diagnoses Impaired skin integrity and Risk for infection share "related to" factors: the abdominal wound and the catheter. In addition to maintaining strict asepsis with dressing changes and catheter care, Janine plans to urge Mrs. Brown to deep-breathe frequently to reduce the risk of postoperative pneumonia. A third intervention she plans will be to ambulate Mrs. Brown as soon as possible to increase bowel peristalsis, reduce the risk of paralytic ileus, and prevent pneumonia.

Janine also plans to assist Mrs. Brown with her bath today to alleviate the Bathing/hygiene self-care deficit diagnosis; the presence of an IV in one arm, a painful abdominal wound, and a catheter significantly reduce Mrs. Brown's ability to manage her own hygiene. Finally, Janine will help Mrs. Brown get out of bed and move around several times during the day to help her increase her physical mobility.

Janine will continue to monitor Mrs. Brown's progress and will alter, delete, or add to the list of nursing diagnoses as needed throughout Mrs. Brown's hospital stay. Reviewing the nursing process steps frequently (at least once a shift, and more often if needed) during a client's stay is crucial to maintaining an accurate picture of the client's needs and giving the best possible care on the basis of those needs.

A second question to ask yourself is "Does this information make a difference in the interventions that will be performed for this client?" For example, for a client who has had a total joint replacement and must learn to walk again, you would select the diagnosis Impaired physical mobility related to pain. This diagnosis reflects your knowledge that pain management will be a major factor in helping the client begin to walk. It therefore focuses nursing care on pain management. The diagnosis Impaired physical mobility related to a total hip replacement fails to reflect your knowledge that the hip is stable and that the client can walk but does not want to because of the pain.

In some cases, nursing interventions are methods of implementing medical therapy for a specific medical diagnosis. For example, given the diagnosis Impaired thought processes related to stage three Alzheimer's disease, you must recognize that neither you nor the physician can change the client's advanced Alzheimer's disease. This diagnosis tells you that the change in thinking is irreversible, so the plan of care focuses on helping the client manage within the limitations imposed by the illness. Now consider the same label with a different etiology: Impaired thought processes related to lithium toxicity. This diagnosis reveals that the client has a reversible problem. The nursing interventions, therefore, focus on the client following the physician's treatment plan for hydration, helping the client cope, reducing the client's anxiety, and maintaining the client's safety.

Validating Nursing Diagnoses With the Client. Finally, discuss your nursing diagnoses with the client and family (Figure 9-3, p. 188). Does the client agree with your inferences? If so, set nursing care goals with input from the client. This is a sound method for validating your nursing diagnoses and ensures that your goals and those of the client match. Table 9-2 (p. 188) summarizes the diagnostic reasoning process.

Writing the Nursing Diagnostic Statement

Writing a useful nursing diagnosis means identifying the client's problem clearly so that all nurses who use the nursing care plan have the same understanding of the client's

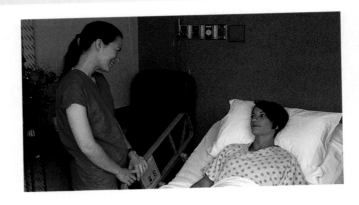

Figure 9-3. Discussing nursing diagnoses with the client and family ensures that your goals and those of the client and family match.

Table 9-2	Applying the Diagnostic Reasoning Process*		
Actual Client Data	**Possible Nursing Diagnosis**	**Defining Characteristics**	**Nursing Decision**
Client has broken skin and traumatized tissue due to abdominal surgery. Indwelling catheter is inserted in bladder.	Impaired skin integrity	Present: Disruption of skin surface; invasion of body structures Not present: Destruction of skin layers	This is a valid diagnosis. Two out of three of the following characteristics are present.
Client has broken skin and traumatized tissue due to abdominal surgery. Indwelling catheter is inserted in bladder. Altered bowel peristalsis due to general anesthesia and abdominal surgery; hemoglobin is decreased, surgery is an invasive procedure, and no antibiotics ordered at present.	Risk for infection	Present: Inadequate primary defenses (broken skin, traumatized tissue), inadequate secondary defenses (decreased hemoglobin, altered peristalsis), tissue destruction and increased environmental exposure (invasive procedure) Not present: Inadequate primary defenses (decrease in ciliary action, stasis of body fluids, change in pH secretions); inadequate secondary defenses (leukopenia, suppressed inflammatory response) and immunosuppression; chronic disease; malnutrition; pharmaceutical agents; trauma; rupture of amniotic membranes; insufficient knowledge to avoid exposure to pathogens	This is a valid diagnosis for most postoperative clients for at least the first few days, especially for those who are not receiving antibiotics. The client is at risk for wound infection, respiratory infection (since abdominal surgery may decrease ability to breathe deeply), paralytic ileus (intestinal paralysis caused by handling of the bowel during surgery), and urinary tract infection owing to a catheter.
Verbalized discomfort, expressed concern about movement causing pain, reluctance to let anyone touch the bed, and restless behavior.	Pain	Present: Verbal or coded reports; protective behavior; expressive behavior, such as restlessness Not present: Observed evidence; antalgic position and gestures; guarding behavior; facial mask; sleep disturbance. Self-focus; narrowed focus; distraction behavior, autonomic alteration in muscle tone; autonomic responses; changes in appetite and eating	This is a valid nursing diagnosis. There are several defining characteristics present.
A hysterectomy results in edema in the pelvic region, which may result in difficulty in passing urine. Preventive measure (an indwelling catheter) is in place.	Urinary retention	Present: Retention; risk for inability to pass urine without Foley catheter	The diagnosis is valid. Write the diagnosis as Risk for urinary retention and institute preventive measures when indwelling catheter is discontinued.
Client is reluctant to move, intravenous catheter in arm, indwelling urinary catheter in bladder, abdominal incision, pain.	Impaired physical mobility	Present: Inability to purposefully move within the physical environment, including bed mobility, transfer, and ambulation; reluctance to move; imposed restriction of movement Not present: Limited range of motion; decreased muscle strength, control, or mass	This is a valid diagnosis. The client will very likely need help to get out of bed and to ambulate the first time or two. However, this diagnosis will very likely be valid only for a short time because the client will be encouraged to be out of bed as soon as possible.

*This table shows a comparison between actual client data, possible diagnoses, defining characteristics of possible diagnoses, and nursing decisions about the validity of

Table 9-3	Examples of Legally Inadvisable Nursing Diagnostic Statements	
Inadvisable Diagnosis	**Problem**	**Appropriate Diagnosis**
Ineffective airway clearance related to infrequent suctioning	Suggests negligence	*Ineffective airway clearance* related to shallow breathing
Risk for infection related to improper aseptic technique	Implies lapse in standards of care	*Risk for infection* related to operative incision in abdomen
Ineffective infant feeding pattern related to poor mothering	Judgmental and derogatory	*Ineffective infant feeding* pattern related to poor suck/swallow rhythm
Bathing/hygiene self-care deficit related to poverty	Judgmental	*Bathing/hygiene self-care deficit* related to lack of running water in home
Ineffective breastfeeding related to maternal self-absorption	Implies mother is neglectful	*Ineffective breastfeeding* related to maternal uncertainty and anxiety

problems. How a problem is stated focuses nursing care and provides a basis for evaluating the effectiveness of the chosen care. As noted earlier, the related factor is especially important in providing needed clarity. The following paragraphs provide some useful tips for writing diagnostic statements that are meaningful and useful.

Identify the Client's Needs. The diagnosis should identify client needs or problems rather than nursing problems. One of the advantages of using NANDA diagnoses is that they focus on client problems and human responses. You may be tempted to write the related-to statement in terms of services or procedures; however, stating the need for services as a nursing diagnosis will not help you make decisions about how to provide those services.

You may also be tempted to write the related-to statement in terms of the technology being used. Again, the management of technology is your problem, not the client's. Asking yourself why the technology is being used may help you identify the client's problem. Likewise the medical diagnosis may be part of the cue cluster, but it should not be the related factor because a nurse is not licensed to treat it. Instead, focus on the associated factors that impact the client's ability to function.

Avoid Legally Inadvisable Statements. State all of your nursing diagnoses in a manner that meets the legal guidelines for entries into the health record. Your related factors should not place a value judgment on the client's behavior or make a judgment that could be construed as libel in a court of law. Also avoid statements suggesting that nursing care has been or is potentially negligent. Table 9-3 gives examples of legally inadvisable nursing diagnostic statements.

SOURCES OF DIAGNOSTIC ERROR

Naturally, it is possible to make errors during the process of making a nursing diagnosis. Errors can occur during data collection, clustering, or interpretation. It is also possible to overdiagnose or underdiagnose the client's problems.

Errors in Data Collecting

You may be tempted to begin with a medical diagnosis and anticipate a client's problems on the basis of that diagnosis. Although this may be a good way to begin identifying possible nursing diagnoses, additional assessment is always needed. Relying on the medical diagnosis may lead to premature termination of data collection and analysis, thus reducing the likelihood of a comprehensive assessment. As a result, client problems unrelated to or unexpected from the medical diagnosis may be missed.

A second error in data collection occurs if you fail to collect adequate data from which to make inferences. This leads to two potential problems. The first problem is making an inferential leap to the wrong diagnosis on the basis of insufficient data. Table 9-4 (p. 190) gives some examples of this type of error. The second problem is that you may fail to make a needed diagnosis because you lack the necessary clinical cues (see the following paragraph). Except in an emergency situation, always take the time to do an adequate assessment.

Errors in Cue Clustering

Errors in cue clustering often result from inadequate data, poor critical thinking, or lack of familiarity with either the clinical population or the nursing diagnosis language. If cues from assessment data are incorrectly clustered, you may name the cluster incorrectly and choose the wrong nursing diagnosis. Choosing the wrong diagnosis results in ineffective interventions. This does not serve the client well because the problem does not get resolved. It does not serve you well either, because your time and energy are wasted on ineffective nursing care.

Another error in cue clustering made frequently by novices is making a nursing diagnosis on the basis of a single cue. Only rarely are accurate diagnoses based on a single cue. Almost always, more data are needed before inferences can be drawn. Validate or confirm your diagnoses with the client as one means of avoiding cue clustering errors.

Errors in Interpretation

A frequent source of error is interpreting cues inappropriately. In some cases, assessment data may be ambiguous and difficult to interpret, or the data may lead you to infer two or more equally possible diagnoses. The best solution is to verify the possible diagnoses with the client or the client's family.

Failure to identify and include client health strengths in your analysis of cues is another source of inappropriate interpretation. Clients have strengths and resources that nurses may not know about. These strengths can have a significant impact on their health status and their ability to

Table 9-4	Selected Sources of Diagnostic Error			
Cues Used to Form Diagnosis	Incorrect Diagnosis	Diagnostic Error	Cues Ignored in Forming Diagnosis	Correct Diagnosis
Heart rate 50 beats per minute	*Decreased cardiac output*	Inferential leap; failure to consider all significant cues	Skin warm and dry, blood pressure 125/80, color pink, usual heart rate 52.	None needed; cue reflects normal function
Client asks to be left alone	*Social isolation*	Inappropriate interpretation of cues	Client did not sleep last night and needs a nap.	*Fatigue*
Urine output 30 ml per hour	*Fluid volume deficit*	Insufficient cues	Client has a history of renal failure and is developing edema.	*Fluid volume excess*
Client appears uncomfortable and is restless after surgery for a fractured hip.	*Pain*	Inaccurate cue grouping	Further assessment reveals that the bladder is full and the client needs a bedpan.	*Self-care deficit (toileting)*
The client has not had a bowel movement in 3 days.	*Constipation*	Use of a single cue as the basis of the diagnosis	The client normally has a bowel movement every 3 days.	None needed; cue reflects normal function
Client has not monitored blood glucose levels for last 10 days and expresses frustration and anger with managing diet and insulin.	*Ineffective management of therapeutic regimen*	Inconsistent or ambivalent cues	Client has been well controlled and able to manage in the past. Client separated from spouse last week.	*Ineffective individual coping*
Client is immobilized from a fractured leg and has a long-leg cast in place.	*Impaired home maintenance management*	Inferential leap from insufficient data	Family has housekeeper, but all bedrooms are located upstairs.	*Impaired physical mobility*

cope with health problems and life processes. Failure to assess for strengths as well as problems often leads to misinterpretation.

Underdiagnosis and Overdiagnosis

An underdiagnosis can occur because of problems in the client assessment. To ensure comprehensive care and avoid missing problems, you need a systematic method of assessing and documenting the client's health status. If the documentation method lacks a sufficient number of categories, important areas may be subsumed in a larger category and be overlooked. Broad categories should have subcategories. For example, if one category is physiological, the body systems can be used as subcategories to make sure the physical assessment is complete.

If you have an insufficient knowledge base, you may miss the significance of important cues. The more you know about the client's medical problem and responses to that problem, the more specific and sensitive your nursing diagnoses will be.

Overdiagnosis occurs when you anticipate possible problems and fail to validate their actual existence. This approach suggests inadequate assessment. A second kind of overdiagnosis occurs when you simultaneously attempt to diagnose every problem the client has now, may have soon, and could have at any time in the future. This practice results in a long list of diagnoses, many of which are irrelevant to the client's immediate problem or the setting for care. Determine which problems have priority, represent the immediate concerns, or

are important to the client. Always validate nursing diagnoses and goals with the client.

Key Principles

- As the second phase of the nursing process, nursing diagnosis is the end product of assessment.
- A nursing diagnosis is a clinical judgment about individual, family, or community responses to actual or potential health problems or life processes. It provides the basis for selecting nursing interventions to achieve outcomes for which you are accountable.
- Nursing diagnoses are human responses—the way clients respond to the life- and health-related conditions. Nursing diagnoses are not problems that *nurses* have but that *clients* have.
- Making a nursing diagnosis is the link between making an assessment and planning interventions. Without accurate diagnosis of the client's problems, you cannot determine appropriate interventions.
- Nursing diagnoses identify problems the management of which nurses may be held accountable for.
- There are five components of a NANDA nursing diagnosis: a label, a definition, a set of defining characteristics, a group of related factors, and risk factors.
- Diagnostic reasoning consists of collecting and reviewing client assessment data, generating clusters of cues and forming hypotheses about what the client's human responses might be, evaluating probable nursing diagnosis labels that reflect the cue

clusters generated, selecting the best labels to describe the client's human responses, determining the related factors for each diagnosis, and planning interventions on the basis of each diagnosis and its related factors.

- Common errors in nursing diagnosis occur when data are incorrectly collected, clustered, or interpreted.
- Underdiagnosing or overdiagnosing the client's condition is an impediment to quality care.

Bibliography

*Aquilino, M. L. (1997). Cognitive development, clinical knowledge, and clinical experience related to diagnostic ability. *Nursing Diagnosis: The Journal of Nursing Language and Classification, 8*(3), 110-119.

*Avant, K. (1990). The art and science in nursing diagnosis development. *Nursing Diagnosis: The Journal of Nursing Language and Classification, 1*(2), 51-55.

Carpenito, L. J. (2001). *Nursing diagnosis: Application to clinical practice* (9th ed.). Philadelphia: Lippincott-Raven.

Clark, J., & Lang, N. (1992). Nursing's next advance: An internal classification for nursing practice. *International Nursing Review, 39*(4), 109-112.

Cox, H. C., Newfield, S. A., Ridenour, N. A., Slate, K. L., Sridaromont, M. D., Hinz, M. D., Lubno, M. A., & Slater, M. M. (2001). *Clinical applications of nursing diagnosis: Adult, child, women's, psychiatric, gerontic, and home health considerations* (4th ed.). Philadelphia: Davis.

Cutler, L. (2000). The diagnostic domain of nursing. *Nursing Critical Care, 5*(2), 59-61.

*Asterisk indicates a classic or definitive work on this subject.

*Feinstein, A. R. (1967). *Clinical judgment.* New York: Robert Krieger.

Gordon, M. (2000). *Manual of nursing diagnosis.* St Louis, MO: Mosby.

*Hamers, J. P., Huijer Abu-Saad, H., & Halfens, R. J. (1994). Diagnostic process and decision making in nursing: A literature review. *Journal of Professional Nursing, 10*(3), 154-163.

Harbison, J. (2001). Clinical decision making in nursing: Theoretical perspectives and their relevance to practice. *Journal of Advanced Nursing, 35*(1), 126-133.

*Kim, M. J., McFarland, G. K., & McLane, A. M. (1984). *Classifications of nursing diagnoses: Proceedings of the second national conference.* Philadelphia: North American Nursing Diagnosis Association.

Kirkley, D. (2001). Words on standardized languages. *American Journal of Nursing, 101*(1), 14.

Lavin, M. A., Maas, M., Gordon, M., Warren, J., Avant, K., Sparks, S., Perry, A., & Whitley, G. G. (2001). Words on standardized languages. *American Journal of Nursing, 101*(1), 13.

Lewis, E. P. (2001). Words on standardized languages [Discussion]. *American Journal of Nursing, 101*(1), 13.

*Martin, K. S., & Scheet, N. J. (1992). *The Omaha system: Applications for community health nursing.* Philadelphia: Saunders.

North American Nursing Diagnosis Association. (1999). *Nursing diagnoses: Definitions and classification, 1999-2000.* Philadelphia: Author.

North American Nursing Diagnosis Association. (2002). *Nursing diagnoses: Definitions and classification, 2002-2003.* Philadelphia: Author.

*Tanner, C. A. (1993). *Rethinking clinical judgment.* NLN Publications, Apr. (14-2511), 15-41. New York.

Planning, Intervening, and Evaluating

Key Terms

care plan conference

case management

clinical pathway

collaboration

computerized care plan

consultation

discharge planning

evaluation

expected outcome

goals

individualized care plan

long-term goal

nurse-initiated
  intervention

nursing care plan

nursing intervention

Nursing Intervention
  Classification

Nursing Outcomes
  Classification

nursing-sensitive client
  outcome

physician-initiated
  intervention

short-term goal

standardized care plan

standards of care

Learning Objectives

After studying this chapter, you should be able to do the following:

- Describe types of planning for individual clients
- Identify the process of planning expected outcomes and interventions
- Discuss the categories and types of interventions to individualize care for each client
- Describe the development of a nursing care plan
- Describe the process of evaluating expected outcomes

Planning is the third phase of the nursing process (after assessment and nursing diagnosis), and it is during this phase that you will identify the goals of nursing care and the actions you will take to attain those goals (Figure 10-1). Planning includes two steps: (1) identification of the outcome criteria the nurse will use to determine if the goal has been met, and (2) the interventions the nurse will use to effect changes to achieve these outcomes. The American Nurses' Association (ANA) supports planning as a means to use theoretical and research-based understandings to prescribe interventions to attain expected outcomes (ANA, 1995a).

The result of the assessment and planning process is a **nursing care plan** (NCP). The NCP is a guide for health care that identifies client problems in need of nursing care (specified by nursing diagnoses), predicts outcomes that are sensitive to nursing care, and lists interventions that will result in the expected outcomes. The client problem is stated as a nursing diagnosis. The diagnostic label, or stem, of the diagnosis helps establish a broad goal. The related factor gives direction to the expected outcomes and interventions. An **expected outcome** is the desired result from nursing care expressed in terms of measurable client behaviors (criteria). A **nursing intervention** is "any treatment, based upon clinical judgment and knowledge, that a nurse performs to enhance [client] outcomes" (McCloskey & Bulechek, 2000, p. xix). The nursing care plan is recorded in the client's health record and serves as a tool to communicate the plan of care to all members of the health care team.

Planning is essential for determining and providing optimal nursing care. As health care resources become more limited, planning becomes even more important. Systematic planning allows you to make the best use of the resources available while avoiding use of ineffective—and therefore wasted—resources.

Although planning is the third phase of the nursing process, it does not take place in isolation. Indeed, planning is interwoven with all phases of the nursing process. You will begin planning and continue doing so throughout the process of gathering assessment data and identifying client problems.

PLANNING FOR INDIVIDUALS

Planning applies both to individual clients and to groups or client populations that are served by a health care agency. For an individual client, planning involves identifying the person's health problems and developing a plan of care to address them. For a group, planning involves identifying characteristics common to the population and making decisions about the services to be offered, the environment in which care will take place, and the staffing needed to accomplish that care.

Nurses plan care both independently and together with other members of the health care team. For each client, you will begin planning for nursing care at or even before your initial contact. You will continue planning throughout the client's stay in the hospital or other health care facility, and you may plan for home or community care after the client's discharge.

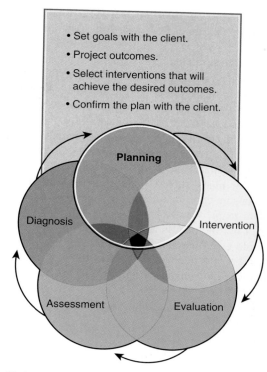

Figure 10-1. During the planning phase of the nursing process, you will set goals with the client, project expected outcomes, select interventions to achieve the desired outcomes, and confirm the plan with the client.

As the client's condition changes, plans must be reviewed and modified, sometimes together with other members of the health care team. Planning for discharge begins during the initial contact with the client by establishing the expected outcomes and anticipating follow-up care that may be needed.

Initial Planning

Your first contact with a client allows you to begin assessing the client and the problems. You will complete a thorough history and perform a physical examination to gather data needed to identify and anticipate problems. While doing so, you will begin to form impressions about the client's most acute, immediate, or important problem. Naturally, you should also ask the client what he considers to be his most urgent or important problem. If his perception differs from yours, the two of you will need to work together to identify the real and perceived needs.

Next, you will develop an overall plan of care for the client that spans the length of stay or duration of services. The nursing plan includes steps needed to support the client during medical care and to help the client become independent in self-care.

Although the plan primarily addresses the reason for admission, it should also include strategies to manage other problems that could influence the resolution of the client's primary problem, or to manage other ongoing problems. Consequently, plans should include other members of the health care team and referrals to other settings for additional services.

As an example, consider an elderly client admitted to the hospital with fractured ribs and difficulty breathing after falling at home. When assessing her, the nurse immediately notices rapid respirations and shortness of breath. The client complains of severe pain. In this case, the nursing plan would include oxygen therapy and pain medication. The nurse calls a respiratory therapist to begin oxygen therapy while giving the client her prescribed pain medication. At the same time, the nurse begins to formulate a plan to investigate reasons for the fall and to prevent future falls—in other words, discharge planning is initiated.

All initial plans should be documented in the client's record to ensure coordination of care among members of the health care team. However, remember that planning occurs whether or not the plan is recorded in the client's record. In the example given, the nurse would record the interventions applied and results attained rather than the plan to treat pain and administer oxygen, because the interventions were begun immediately. However, the plan to assess why the client fell and ways to prevent future falls would be recorded.

Ongoing Planning

During a client's stay in a health care facility, planning is ongoing because the client's health condition may change. These changes must be monitored, and interventions must be altered and implemented as appropriate. Some diagnoses may be resolved and others added.

In an acute care setting, a client's condition may change rapidly, thus altering your initial plan. For example, you may plan to check a client's vital signs twice daily, only to find that the client has become weak and dizzy in the interim. If you determine that the vital signs must be checked more often than originally planned, you will need to revise the written plan in the client's record so other members of the health care team are aware of the change.

In a long-term care setting, where changes are often gradual and sometime subtle, ongoing planning may be more formal. If a client's functional abilities decline in two areas, a change-of-status assessment and a revised care plan must be initiated. For example, if your client's mental function declines and his ambulation changes from steady to unsteady, you would need to create a new plan of care. Prompt revisions to the client's plan of care not only ensure the correct care but also help maintain funding for the client's care, especially from Medicare.

Discharge Planning

At the moment a client enters the health care system, you will begin planning for his discharge. **Discharge planning** means "preparation for moving a client from one level of care to another within or outside the current health care agency" (McCloskey & Bulechek, 2000, p. 258). Although discharge planning is an independent nursing activity, the prudent nurse seeks input from many members of the health care team. Activities for discharge planning appear in Box 10-1.

Discharge planning addresses client needs that will continue after the present services end. Such planning may include arranging for home care to help the client recover fully

---

Box 10-1   Discharge Planning Intervention

DISCHARGE PLANNING

Definition: Preparation for moving a client from one level of care to another within or outside the current health care agency

Activities

- Help the client, family, and significant others to prepare for discharge.
- Collaborate with the physician, client, family, significant others, and other health team members in planning for continuity of health care.
- Coordinate efforts of different health care providers to ensure a timely discharge.
- Identify the client's and the primary caregiver's understanding of knowledge or skills required after discharge.
- Identify what the client should be taught for care after discharge.
- Monitor readiness for discharge.
- Communicate the client's discharge plans, as appropriate.
- Document the client's discharge plans, as appropriate.
- Document the client's discharge plans in the chart.
- Formulate a maintenance plan for follow-up after discharge.
- Assist the client, family, and significant others in planning for the supportive environment necessary to provide the client's care after leaving the hospital.
- Develop a plan that considers the client's health, social, and financial needs.
- Arrange for evaluation after discharge, as appropriate.
- Encourage self-care, as appropriate.
- Arrange discharge to the next level of care.
- Arrange for caregiver support, as appropriate.
- Discuss financial resources if the client needs health care after discharge.
- Coordinate referrals relevant to linkages among health care providers.

Modified from McCloskey, J. C., & Bulechek, G. M. (2000). *Nursing interventions classification (NIC)*. St Louis, MO: Mosby.

---

after hospital discharge. It may include rehabilitation services for a client recovering from a stroke, being fitted for an artificial leg, or learning to walk on an implanted hip joint.

In addition to specifying which services a client will need, discharge planning also addresses the setting in which those services should be delivered. Typical settings include inpatient facilities, outpatient facilities, and the client's home. The client's support system, home environment, and transportation options are all important considerations in planning for safe ongoing care after discharge.

Collaborative Planning

Collaboration is the act of two or more health care professionals performing work cooperatively to achieve a common goal. It implies a partnership of professionals, each of whom recognizes and acknowledges the expertise of the other members of the health care team. Authority in a collaborative situation is derived from professional knowledge, sphere of activity, and responsibility rather than from a hierarchical relationship.

Collaborative planning occurs in every clinical setting and may involve other nurses, physicians, dietitians, respiratory therapists, social workers, and other team members. Collaborative planning ensures continuity and coordination of care.

Consultation

Consultation is the act of two or more health care professionals, one of whom is an expert or specialist solicited to offer an opinion, deliberating for the purpose of making decisions. When the nurse lacks the knowledge or expertise to solve a problem or determines that a plan of care is not effective, it is appropriate to consult with a person who has more experience in the problem area. Nurses working in institutional settings have multiple nursing resources available for consultation. Head nurses, charge nurses, supervisors, and clinical nurse specialists all provide consultation in the planning process. Consultation may occur during all phases of the nursing process, but it is very important in the planning process.

Consulting with specialists and experts provides optimal care for each client by helping to solve difficult problems. Each consultant brings a different viewpoint and area of expertise to the development of the care plan. For example, an enterostomal therapist could provide information on a special paste that facilitates adhesion of a stomal wafer to the skin for bag attachment. A physical therapist could discuss the benefits of using a transfer board instead of a lift for moving a client from bed to chair.

Successful consultation has five major elements. First, the nurse identifies an appropriate person with expertise in the problem area. Second, the nurse provides the consultant with factual information about the client and the nature of the problem. Third, the nurse allows the consultant to make an independent judgment about the nature of the problem and possible solution. Fourth, after the consultant has made a judgment, the nurse and consultant discuss the differences in their findings. Fifth, the nurse and consultant decide who should implement the care recommended.

Care Plan Conferences

A **care plan conference** is the action of a group conferring or consulting together to plan care for the client (Figure 10-2). Various members of the health care team may organize a care plan conference to review the client's problem list and to plan further strategies to achieve the outcomes established for the client. Typically, the client, family members or significant others, and any team members involved in the client's recovery are invited to the care plan conference.

The frequency and attendees of care plan conferences vary with the setting and the client's situation. A conference may include a nurse, a physician, and a family member who meet in the hall to discuss the client's care. Or a conference may be a formal meeting in which all persons involved in the client's care agree to meet at a specific place and time.

In long-term care, formal care plan conferences are held when the client is admitted to the facility, at 3-month intervals, and when the client's condition changes. Health care professionals who usually attend these meetings include the nurse, activity director, social worker, dietitian, and other therapists, such as a physical therapist or speech therapist. The client has the right to be included in the conference or may be represented by a family member. The physician may also be involved.

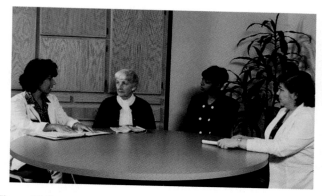

Figure 10-2. A care plan conference allows members of the health care team to discuss and revise the client's care plan as needed. Often, the client or a family member is invited to attend.

In the hospital setting, formal conferences are less common but may occur in special situations. For example, in some hospitals, interdisciplinary teams work together to plan for the treatment of child abuse and neglect. The composition of these teams varies but may include nurses, social workers, psychiatrists, abuse counselors, physicians, and teachers.

Teamwork is needed to facilitate these conferences. The group leader can facilitate the interdisciplinary team meeting by keeping the group focused on important issues and concluding the meeting in a reasonable amount of time. Consultation with team members during the meeting ensures that outcomes are consistent with the plans of the entire team.

THE PLANNING PROCESS

Planning for individual client care includes establishing priorities, making decisions about the desired results of care, and selecting the interventions most likely to achieve those results. The client's care must be organized on the basis of the priority of activities essential for life and recovery. It also must consider the client's perceptions and self-care abilities.

Establishing Priorities

You must make decisions about which diagnoses need immediate attention, which can be safely postponed, and which should be treated in another setting. During the planning process, you will need to establish priorities.

Establishing priorities means that you rank the nursing diagnoses in order of importance. The meaning of *importance* varies with the setting, the client's condition, and the client's needs. Importance can mean the diagnosis that should be treated first or the diagnosis that should receive the most time and energy.

Maslow's hierarchy is a helpful tool for thinking about priorities (Figure 10-3). Abraham Maslow is credited with being one of the founders of the humanistic psychology movement. He hypothesized that human needs motivate behavior on the basis of a hierarchy of the potency of these needs. He arranged human needs in a pyramid that suggests both the order in which we satisfy the needs and the order in which

Nursing Priorities from Maslow's Hierarchy

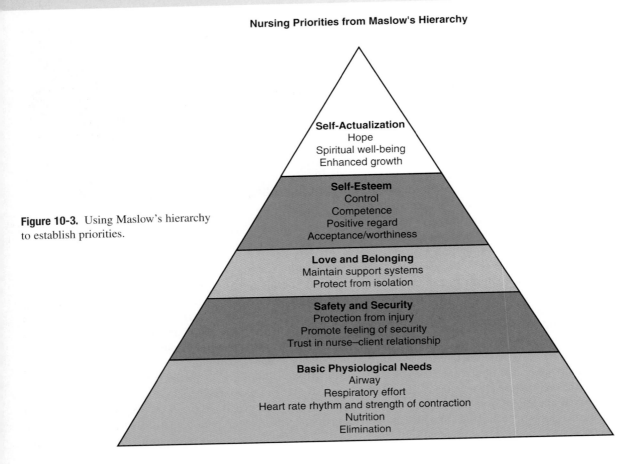

Figure 10-3. Using Maslow's hierarchy to establish priorities.

which these needs contribute to development over a lifetime. Albeit imperfect as a framework for establishing nursing priorities, Maslow's hierarchy of needs is useful in giving general guidance.

Threats to Physiological Integrity. When a client has a threat to physiological integrity, physical needs demand highest priority. The degree of the threat may influence how completely the client screens out other needs. Basic human needs include air, water, and food. Related to these basic needs, the first priority is any threat to the vital functions of breathing, heartbeat, and blood pressure. A person having difficulty breathing will not want a nurse to discuss his sense of self-worth. The immediate need is to relieve the difficult breathing.

Imagine a client with lung cancer, who is struggling to breathe, nauseated from chemotherapy, too weak to rise from bed unassisted, and aware that she will die in a short time. The following is a prioritized list of diagnoses for this client:

- Ineffective breathing pattern related to obstructed airway
- Altered nutrition: less than body requirements, related to nausea and vomiting
- Impaired physical mobility related to generalized weakness
- Hopelessness related to coping with the diagnosis of a terminal illness
- Bathing/hygiene self-care deficit related to generalized weakness

All of the problems listed are important, but breathing is basic to life. If the breathing pattern is life threatening, this diagnosis will have the highest priority. Getting enough to eat is secondary in importance at that moment. When vital functions are stable, attention can be turned to the other physiological systems.

> *Action Alert!* Give top priority to basic survival needs when your client has a threat to physiological integrity.

Ensuring safety and security is the second level of need. Although you might forgo safety for physiological integrity on a rare occasion, the principle that safety is a priority second only to physiological integrity is apparent from Maslow's hierarchy. Making the client feel secure through a trusting nurse–client relationship is also important.

Another nursing goal is to help clients satisfy their need for love and belonging through their relationships with significant others. In Chapter 47 you will learn about the concept of the family as a client. In addition, clients' relationships with the health care team can be valuable in helping them meet the need for belonging. Strive to help the client feel like an important member of the team.

Self-esteem develops when the need for love and belonging is met; it develops out of successful relationships or interactions with others. A high level of self-esteem is positively correlated with compliance with a treatment regimen and with taking affirmative actions to improve health. When the need for self-esteem is satisfied, clients are free to pursue self-actualization, or to become whatever they are capable of becoming.

When planning care, be prepared to shift priorities as the client's condition and needs change. Indeed, only rarely are priorities clear and stable. You must consider the strong interrelationships among nursing diagnoses when establishing priorities, and be aware that higher-level needs can drive the needs on the lower levels of the pyramid. For example, feeling a deficit in love and belonging, a person may seek self-esteem in other ways. Then, it may be that finding self-esteem separate from others is the force that drives this person to self-actualization.

The interrelationships may also have effects in the other direction. In the nursing diagnoses listed earlier for the client with lung cancer, hopelessness was placed low on the list of priorities. However, hopelessness may need to be treated before the client is interested in food. Recognizing that one diagnosis has priority does not mean the remaining diagnoses are ignored or delayed.

You will often find yourself meeting several needs at once. For example, while suctioning a client, you can monitor an intravenous feeding and give hope and comfort through your touch and tone of voice.

The Health Care Setting. Priorities also tend to vary with the health care setting involved. In an intensive care unit, for example, the nursing diagnosis *Ineffective breathing pattern* may be the top priority of nurses working to sustain the client's life. After discharge, the client may have the same diagnosis. However, the diagnosis *Knowledge deficit related to inexperience with managing a medical condition* may become the higher priority because the client's breathing pattern has stabilized and the focus of home care shifts to health education.

For the hospital nurse, priorities are more likely to involve physiological diagnoses, and care typically addresses physical needs. The priorities in the care plan can change daily or even hourly as the person's condition improves or worsens. As physical needs are stabilized, other problems can be managed.

In a long-term care setting, where the client's physical needs are stable, quality-of-life issues may take on greater importance than physical care. Consider a care plan in a long-term care setting that addresses the following nursing diagnostic concepts:

• Altered thought processes
• Bathing/hygiene self-care deficit
• Dressing/grooming self-care deficit
• Impaired physical mobility

Responding to each of these diagnoses requires increasing the client's independence, which becomes your priority for care. Being well groomed may not be as important as the client's being able to manage self-care. Thus, a plan that seeks to improve the altered thought processes and impaired mobility would help to accomplish the main priority—independence.

Client's Perception of Need. Another consideration in planning priorities for nursing diagnoses is the client's perception of the situation. If a client has just come to a nursing unit after an emergency appendectomy and complains of pain, you

would place a high priority on his physical safety and would respond to his concern by establishing pain as a priority diagnosis. Alternatively, a long-term-care client who prefers not to participate in social activities would not choose *Social isolation* as a diagnosis to receive high priority.

Clearly, considering a client's input helps you to provide care that is individualized and satisfying to the client. However, the planning process also allows you to help clients recognize problems and accept help.

Client's Self-Care Ability. For the client able to provide self-care, some diagnoses will have a lower priority in your plan. For example, *Bathing/hygiene self-care deficit* may have a high priority for a postsurgical client but not for a client who can manage self-care independently. (If surgery involved the arms or shoulders, the client may not have adequate self-care abilities, which would raise the diagnosis to a higher priority.)

Determining which nursing diagnoses take precedence over others is a decision-making process that may change repeatedly depending on the client's condition. Learning to set priorities appropriately, however, will reap many benefits as you plan your client's care.

Establishing Outcomes

As part of the planning process, you will establish the desirable end result—the expected outcome—of nursing care for each nursing diagnosis. By devising an expected outcome, you express a reasonable expectation that nursing care can produce the intended result. In other words, you can be held accountable for the results of the care you planned. The following paragraphs discuss the criteria that you should apply when deciding whether your expected outcomes qualify as appropriate results of nursing care.

The expected results should be *realistic* or *achievable.* Realistic expectations are based on a review of the entire database and the nursing diagnoses relevant to a particular client to determine if the outcome can be expected for this client. Carefully evaluate the person's disabilities, resources, and unique life circumstances. Logical reasoning should verify that nursing care can achieve the result predicted.

Ideally, your expected outcomes will describe results of nursing care that are *measurable* and can be directly observed. Another member of the health care team should be able to read the outcomes and have the same image of the expected results as you did when you developed them.

Use two components to describe what you want to accomplish in measurable terms: an action and a qualifier that describes the health state to be achieved. Choose verbs to describe cognitive, affective, and psychomotor actions (Box 10-2).

For example, if the nursing diagnosis is *Knowledge deficit related to lack of experience in giving insulin,* you would expect your nursing care to result in the client knowing how to self-administer insulin. However, if you phrase the expected outcome as "The client knows the steps needed to self-administer insulin," you have no way to measure the client's behavior (i.e., the client's knowledge). Therefore, use a measurable action verb. In cognitive terms, your outcome could say, "The client

Box 10-2 Verbs for Writing Measurable Outcome Statements

COGNITIVE DOMAIN

Knowledge: Defines, describes, labels, lists, matches, names, outlines [the information being taught]

Comprehension: Converts, distinguishes, estimates, explains, gives examples of [the information being taught]

Application: Applies (in a different situation), computes, demonstrates, discovers, manipulates, predicts, shows [behaviors on the basis of the information]

Analysis: Diagrams, discriminates, illustrates, infers, outlines, relates

Synthesis: Categorizes, combines, compiles, organizes, plans, rearranges, revises

Evaluation: Appraises, compares, concludes, critiques, interprets, relates

AFFECTIVE DOMAIN

Receiving: Asks questions, chooses, attends to

Responding: Answers, assists, helps, demonstrates, presents, reads, reviews, describes intention to act

Valuing: Acts, completes task, differentiates among behaviors, explains value, joins a support group, justifies behavior, proposes, reads

Organization: Consistently adheres to behavior, alters, arranges, combines, defends, integrates, or otherwise modifies behavior

Characterization by a value: Displays the value of, influences others, proposes the value to others

PSYCHOMOTOR DOMAIN

Perception: Chooses, detects, distinguishes, isolates, relates, selects, separates

Set: Begins, displays, explains, moves, proceeds, reacts, responds, shows, starts

Guided response: Assembles, builds, calibrates, constructs, dismantles, measures

Mechanism: Assembles, builds, calibrates, constructs, dismantles, measures

Complex overt response: Assembles, builds, calibrates, constructs, dismantles

Adaptation: Adapts, alters, changes, rearranges, reorganizes, revises, varies

Origination: Arranges, combines, composes, constructs, creates, designs, originates

Modified from Gronlund, N. E. (2000). *How to write and use instructional objectives* (6th ed.). Upper Saddle River, NJ: Prentice Hall.

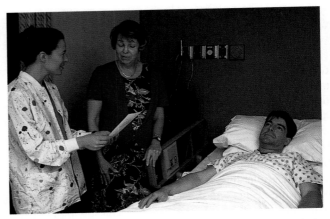

Figure 10-4. Planning is done not only *for* the client and family but *with* the client and family. Mutual goal-setting ensures that the nurse, client, and family are working together.

portunity to be more actively involved in decision making. Including the client's family and friends in setting goals and outcomes may be helpful as well. Significant others are often responsible for carrying out the nursing plan after discharge. They may be more willing to continue the therapeutic regimen at home if they understand its rationale and have had input into the decision-making process.

Finally, your planning should include decisions about the *time frame* during which the intended results will be achieved. The time frame may reflect short-term goals or long-term goals. A **short-term goal** suggests that the resolution of the nursing diagnosis can be accomplished in an hour, a day, or a week, and it is sometimes an intermediary goal that shows progress toward the longer-term goal. A **long-term goal** suggests that the expectation for resolution of the nursing diagnosis will take place in small measurable steps but may take a few weeks or months. Especially in a rehabilitative or long-term care setting, a long-term goal may be ongoing.

It is essential that you be able to determine realistic time frames for attaining expected outcomes. Specifying the date for achieving an expected outcome reflects your best judgment about the time needed. This judgment is based on knowledge about the problem, the person's condition, the support systems available, and the necessary nursing interventions.

For example, consider the expected outcome that the client will no longer have hard, dry stools. If the client takes a cathartic medication, the time frame for evaluation of the expected outcome could be 3 days. If the client prefers to resolve the problem by a diet change and activity increase rather than medication, the time frame may be 2 weeks.

In a general sense, setting appropriate time frames can provide benefits beyond those inherent in achieving an expected outcome. For example, setting time frames can accomplish the following:

- Motivate the client to strive toward resolution of the problem
- Provide the client (and nurse) with a sense of accomplishment

will state the steps to follow in self-administering insulin." In terms of psychomotor performance, your outcome could say, "The client will correctly administer insulin to himself."

The expected results should be *acceptable* to the client. Always remember that planning is done not only *for* the client but also *with* the client (Figure 10-4). Establishing expected results in collaboration with the client could favorably affect treatment results and client satisfaction. Although you can help a client by setting realistic expectations, the client must participate actively in planning to be a full partner in care.

To elicit a client's enthusiastic participation in the program of care, listen to his concerns, talk frankly, negotiate, and sometimes compromise. Many people welcome the op-

- "Pace" nursing care and encourage focus on continued progress
- Prompt the nurse to evaluate the achievement of the outcome

If an expected outcome is unmet, it means that the time frame must be reconsidered, the expected outcome must be modified, or new interventions must be devised. Of course, expected outcomes must be revised as the client's health status changes.

Defining Outcomes. The term *outcome* has come into popular use from the idea that nurses should be able to demonstrate the results of care in specific, measurable terms. The best of nursing care may not be worthwhile if it fails to result in measurable changes in the client's behavior or condition.

A *goal* describes something that you expect to happen or that you desire as a result of nursing care. Commonly, however, **goals** are broad, general statements about the desired results of nursing care; *expected outcomes* offer specific criteria for measuring results. The goal is derived from the stem of the diagnosis.

For example, if the nursing diagnosis is *Activity intolerance related to ineffective breathing secondary to emphysema,* the goal would be to increase the client's activity tolerance. To meet that broad goal, you would devise a set of expected outcomes that allow you to measure the improvement in activity tolerance. The outcomes are derived from the methods to make the breathing pattern more effective as well as from the goal itself. Specific outcomes might include the following:

- Client takes bronchodilator on a regular schedule.
- Client correctly uses inhaler before attempting exercise.
- Client can walk one block without shortness of breath.

The overall goal comes from the client's description of the problem and could be something like, "I want to be able to walk to the park to visit with my friends." The expected outcomes in this case illustrate specific ways to accomplish-and measure the accomplishment of—that goal.

Regional and institutional differences in the use of terminology and documentation systems may determine your use of goals, outcomes, and other terms. The important idea that remains, however, is that concrete descriptions of client behaviors are used to demonstrate when the plan of care has been successful. The outcomes or goals that you devise should be linked to your nursing diagnoses and direct interventions to achieve the desired changes.

Types of Outcomes. Ways to measure health care outcomes have developed over time. Early in the twentieth century, common outcome measurements included morbidity, mortality, length of client stay, and infection rate. However, as the health care industry has become more sophisticated and the consumer more knowledgeable, these measures of success have been deemed inadequate to capture the complexity of health care and measure the specific outcomes produced.

Now, client satisfaction forms an important outcome measure as well. Global multidisciplinary measures describe the client's satisfaction with care, the hospital stay, activities of daily living, and cognitive function. Other outcome measurements may include structural or process characteristics that judge the effectiveness and efficiency of a health care setting. Such outcomes in this situation may be cost, profit, unscheduled readmissions, unscheduled repeat surgeries, and unnecessary procedures. Global measurements are adequate for assessing the effectiveness of a health care system but are not specific for measuring the results of nursing care or specific outcomes for individual clients.

Discipline-specific outcomes can be influenced and changed by the discipline involved. A **nursing-sensitive client outcome** is "a measurable client or family caregiver state, behavior, or perception that is conceptualized as a variable and is largely influenced by and sensitive to nursing interventions" (Johnson et al., 2000, p. 24). In your nursing care plans, you would choose only outcomes that are sensitive to nursing interventions when describing the client's state.

Nursing Outcomes Classification System. The **Nursing Outcomes Classification** (Iowa Outcomes Project, 1997) is a standardized language for measuring the effects of nursing care using indicators sensitive to nursing intervention. Increasingly, nurses and facilities are recognizing the benefits of using a standardized outcome classification system. The research-based Nursing Outcomes Classification (NOC) system from the Iowa Outcomes Project is the best known and most highly developed system available.

The NOC outcomes follow the principles just discussed, but they have several distinguishing features. The NOC outcomes are one-word or two-word generalizations that describe the results of nursing care, followed by measurement criteria for each one. Think of the outcome label as reflecting the goal, and the indicators as being the specific measurable outcome criteria. Additionally, the NOC introduces the element of being able to measure success on a scale. Table 10-1 (p. 200) illustrates NOC outcomes for vital sign status.

The NOC project describes outcomes as client states, behaviors, or perceptions at a particular point in time as a result of or in response to a nursing intervention (Johnson et al., 2000). Outcomes (the labels) are at a higher level of abstraction than the measurement criteria to help you link the outcome to the client's problem or nursing diagnosis. For each outcome, you can select indicator behaviors (criteria) for an individual client.

The NOC system offers a list of expected outcomes that allow you to evaluate whether a nursing diagnosis has been resolved. Examples of outcomes include bowel elimination, cognitive orientation, compliance behavior, coping, fear control, grief resolution, respiratory status, gas exchange, and vital sign status.

NOC outcomes have several advantages. The language is understandable to all health care professionals. The outcomes are measured on a scale that allows negative and positive changes and a lack of change resulting from nursing interventions (Johnson et al., 2000).

The indicators define the client outcome and list aspects of a client state that are needed to measure the outcome. You are

Table 10-1	Example of Nursing-Sensitive Client Outcomes—Vital Signs Status				
Indicator	Extreme Deviation From Expected Range	Substantial Deviation From Expected Range	Moderate Deviation From Expected Range	Mild Deviation From Expected Range	No Deviation From Expected Range
Temperature	1	2	3	4	5
Apical pulse rate	1	2	3	4	5
Radial pulse rate	1	2	3	4	5
Respiration rate	1	2	3	4	5
Systolic blood pressure	1	2	3	4	5
Diastolic blood pressure	1	2	3	4	5
Other (specify)	1	2	3	4	5

Johnson, M., Maas, M., & Moorhead, S. (2000). *Nursing outcomes classification (NOC)*. St Louis, MO Mosby.

Definition: Temperature, pulse, respiration, and blood pressure are within the expected range for the individual.

not required to use all the indicators to assess the outcome state in every circumstance; which you use depends on the nursing diagnosis, the interventions, and the care setting. Indicators can be modified, deleted, or added in different clinical situations. In other words, you choose the indicators that are pertinent to your client.

INTERVENTION

Intervention is the action phase of the nursing process—the phase in which you provide the services to reach the goals of supporting and protecting your client (Figure 10-5). Having recognized an actual or potential health problem, you plan interventions to change the client's level of physical, psychosocial, or spiritual functioning in the context of the family. An intervention may help the client make lifestyle changes, support physical function, support homeostasis, support psychosocial well-being, support the family unit, and make effective use of the health care delivery system to solve problems. Effective intervention in each of the domains requires the use of nine skills, which will be described here.

Identifying nursing interventions involves selecting actions that enable the client to achieve outcomes and to resolve the related factors in nursing diagnoses. These actions may be called nursing orders, nursing activities, or nursing approaches. When communicated to the nursing team, the intervention should contain elements that clearly explain the action to be performed.

Skills of Intervention

The skills you will need to intervene are used in all the domains of intervention. These skills involve being able to function in the areas of cognitive (thinking) processes, technical (psychomotor) activities, and interpersonal relationships (affective).

Teaching. Highly developed teaching skills are a most important asset for a nurse. In this information age, clients expect to be kept well informed about the treatment plan and to participate in the decision-making process. Both the client and the providers benefit when this goal is accomplished. For example, safety improves when the client has knowledge of

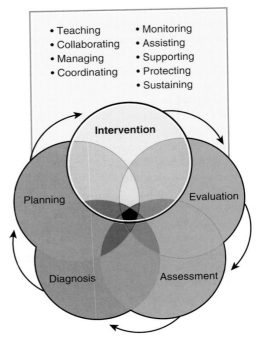

Figure 10-5. Intervention is the action phase of the nursing process. During the intervention phase, you provide the services identified during the planning process to support and protect your client. Intervention involves teaching, collaborating, managing, coordinating, monitoring, assisting, supporting, protecting, and sustaining.

the benefits and risks of care. Likewise, complications are fewer when the client knows how to manage a disorder or monitor a recovery period at home.

Collaborating. Sometimes you will intervene for your clients by collaborating with colleagues. Collaboration is the professional method of asking for and receiving assistance to ensure the best possible care for your client.

Managing. You can intervene for a client by managing care provided by others, and parts of your nursing care plan can be delegated to other health care workers. For example, a nursing assistant may intervene by bathing the client. Although the intervention is delegated, you are still accountable for the activity. You need to know that the intervention was completed; the nursing assistant needs to report any irregularities that arose during the intervention.

Coordinating. When multiple health team members are involved in the client's care, intervention involves coordination of the client's care. Commonly, a nurse takes charge of that coordination. Nurses have broad general knowledge of the roles and functions of the health care team and are in the best position to coordinate the various services that might be needed by the client.

Monitoring. Surveillance or monitoring is a primary nursing intervention, particularly in acute care settings. Monitoring the client's status and reporting changes to the physician is a major component of nursing. It ensures that the physician receives the information necessary to accomplish the client's health goals and to prevent complications. The purposes of monitoring are to detect complications, to evaluate the effectiveness of the interventions, and to ensure that the interventions are carried out correctly.

Assisting. Assisting is providing direct physical care when the client is unable to perform self-care. Interventions may involve assisting a client who is partially or fully unable to care for himself. The client may be disabled and need assistance to perform the basic activities of daily living, or he may lack the manual dexterity to perform medical treatments. You would provide assistance when the client needs help to take medications, seek health-related services, or plan for the management of a health problem.

Supporting. Interventions may be primarily supportive when the client has the ability and the knowledge but lacks willpower, resilience, or the motivation to self-care. Supportive care makes the client feel able to face adverse circumstances, find inner strength, and believe in self-efficacy. To give supportive care you do not necessarily change your client's methods of self-care; rather, you strengthen the client to get needs met.

Care is also classified as supportive when a client's physiological processes are marginally functional, and care is needed to maintain life functions. Physiological support involves implementing the physician's plan. You may give intravenous fluid or blood to maintain blood pressure, or medications to strengthen the heart or control arrhythmias.

Protecting. Nurses play a major role in protecting clients from harm. The hospital (or other health care institution) environment should be the safest environment possible, whether the client is critically ill, having surgery, learning to walk after a stroke, learning to cope with blindness, or needs protected living in old age. However, medical treatment always involves some degree of risk, which means that clients need constant surveillance and intervention to prevent harm. For

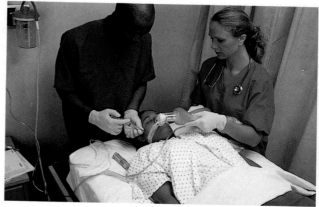

Figure 10-6. In today's health care environment, nurses must be prepared to accomplish highly technical direct care interventions. Remember, however, that a highly technical setting makes sensitive psychosocial interventions more important than ever.

example, you may act to prevent the complications of bed rest, adverse effects of medications, and injuries.

Sustaining. Nursing interventions sustain life and physical function when the client's condition is critical. The most obvious example is the implementation of cardiopulmonary resuscitation when the heartbeat or respiration has stopped. Critical care, recovery room, and emergency room nurses are involved in life-sustaining procedures.

Types of Interventions

Nursing interventions can be direct or indirect and may originate with a nurse, a physician, or another type of health care provider.

Direct Care Nursing Interventions. A direct care intervention "is a treatment performed through interaction with the client(s)" (Iowa Intervention Project, 1996, p. xvii). Direct care interventions include both physiological and psychosocial nursing actions designed to improve the client's health or modify the environment in a way that is conducive to health or that prevents disease.

Examples of physiological direct care nursing interventions include bowel training, cast care, cardiac precautions, constipation/impaction management, ambulation, eye care, and self-care assistance (toileting, for example). Examples of psychosocial direct care nursing interventions include counseling, emotional support, hope instillation, humor, and presence. Figure 10-6 shows a nurse performing a direct care intervention.

Indirect Care Nursing Interventions. The term *indirect care intervention* is unique to the Nursing Intervention Classification further discussed later. Nursing includes many activities intended to maintain a safe environment and to coordinate the client's care. Even though these activities are not at the client's bedside and may not even be specific to an individual, they are necessary for client welfare. An *indirect*

Box 10-3   Example of an Indirect Care Nursing Intervention

SHIFT REPORT

Definition: Exchanging essential client care information with other nursing staff at change of shift

Activities

- Review pertinent demographic data, including name, age, and room number.
- Identify chief complaint and reason for admission, as appropriate.
- Summarize significant health history, as necessary.
- Identify key medical and nursing diagnoses, as appropriate.
- Identify resolved medical and nursing diagnoses, as appropriate.
- Present information succinctly, focusing on recent and significant data needed by nursing staff assuming responsibility for care.
- Describe treatment regimen, including diet, fluid therapy, medications, and exercise.
- Identify laboratory and diagnostic tests to be completed during the next 24 hours.
- Describe health status data, including vital signs and signs and symptoms present during the shift.
- Describe nursing interventions being implemented.
- Describe client and family responses to nursing interventions.
- Summarize progress toward goals.
- Summarize discharge plans, as appropriate.

From McCloskey, J.C. & Bulechek, G. M. (2000). *Nursing interventions classification (NIC)*. St Louis, MO: Mosby.

Box 10-4   Example of a Nurse-Initiated Nursing Intervention

DRESSING

Definition: Choosing, putting on, and removing clothes for a person who cannot do so independently

Activities

- Identify areas where client needs assistance in dressing.
- Monitor client's ability to dress independently.
- Dress client after personal hygiene completed.
- Encourage participation in selection of clothing.
- Dress affected extremity first, as appropriate.
- Dress in nonrestrictive clothing, as appropriate.
- Dress in personal clothing, as appropriate.
- Change client's clothing at bedtime.
- Select shoes or slippers conducive to ambulation.
- Offer to launder clothing, as necessary.
- Continue giving assistance until the client can assume full responsibility for dressing.

From McCloskey, J.C. & Bulechek, G. M. (2000). *Nursing interventions classification (NIC)*. St Louis, MO: Mosby.

---

care intervention is administrative or collaborative activity performed on behalf of the client or for the client's general welfare, but not directly with the client. (McCloskey & Bulechek, 2000). Examples of indirect care nursing interventions include delegation, emergency cart checking, shift report, and telephone consultation. Box 10-3 shows an example of an indirect care intervention needed for continuity of care in an acute care facility. Including indirect care interventions in a record-keeping system captures nursing activities that help the client but do not directly involve the client.

Nurse-Initiated and Physician-Initiated Nursing Interventions. Nurses provide two types of care for their clients. Independent nursing care is within the scope of nursing practice and does not require a physician's order. Interdependent nursing care is within the scope of nursing practice but is carried out only as part of a physician's treatment plan. Both types of actions are correctly described as nursing care because these actions require a nurse's expertise to ensure the client's safety.

A **nurse-initiated intervention** is within the scope of nursing practice and is prescribed by the nurse independent of the physician. It is "an intervention initiated by the nurse in response to a nursing diagnosis; an autonomous action based on scientific rationale that is executed to benefit the client in a predicted way related to the nursing diagnosis and projected outcome" (McCloskey & Bulechek, 2003). Helping the client to dress is an example of a nurse-initiated intervention or independent action (Box 10-4).

A physician-initiated intervention is within the scope of nursing practice but requires a physician's order for the nurse to implement. A **physician-initiated intervention** is "a treatment initiated by a physician in response to a medical diagnosis but carried out by a nurse in response to a 'doctor's order.' Nurses may also carry out treatments initiated by other providers, such as pharmacists, respiratory therapists, or physician assistants" (McCloskey & Bulechek, 2003). An example of a physician-initiated intervention is management of the client's diet when the client is recovering from an illness that has caused a medical need for dietary limitations (Box 10-5).

Elements of an Intervention

Nursing interventions should be written clearly enough that all nurses involved in the client's care can implement the care in the same manner. Planning involves making decisions about the *who, what, where, when, why,* and *how* of client care (Table 10-2). *Who* refers to the person providing care. The best person to provide care may be a physical therapist, a nurse, a nursing assistant, a family member, the client, or another practitioner. *What* refers to the care that will most effectively meet the client's needs. *Where* could be the client's home, a clinic, or a hospital. *When* refers to the time that the care is delivered or to the sequence of events required. The time may be before the client is admitted to a hospital, during a hospital stay, after discharge, during a clinic or office visit, or at a particular time of day. *Why* provides the rationale for care and includes evidence that the care is important, will work, or will meet individual client needs. *How* defines the methods of intervention required and may specify measures needed to individualize a client's care.

Box 10-5	Example of a Physician-Initiated Nursing Intervention

DIET STAGING

Definition: Instituting required diet restrictions with subsequent progression of diet as tolerated

Activities

- Determine presence of bowel sounds.
- Institute NPO status, as needed.
- Clamp nasogastric tube and monitor tolerance, as appropriate.
- Monitor for alertness and presence of gag reflex, as appropriate.
- Monitor tolerance to ingestion of ice chips and water.
- Determine if client is passing flatus.
- Collaborate with other health care team members to progress diet as rapidly as possible without complications.
- For adults and children, progress the diet from clear liquid to full liquid to soft diet to regular or special diet, as tolerated.
- For babies, progress the diet from glucose water or oral electrolyte solution to half-strength formula and then to full-strength formula.
- Monitor tolerance to diet progression.
- Offer six small feedings rather than three meals, as appropriate.
- Post the diet restrictions at bedside, on chart, and in care plan.

From McCloskey, J.C. & Bulechek, G. M. (2000). *Nursing interventions classification (NIC)*. St Louis, MO: Mosby.

Table 10-2	Individualized Nursing Interventions: Specify Who, What, When, Where, How, Why*
Physician's Order	**Nursing Intervention**
Ambulate tid	Encourage client to walk at 0900, 1300, 1800; 20 steps in the room with a walker.
	ALTERNATIVE
	Encourage client to walk 4 lengths of the hall morning, afternoon, and evening, before discharge.
	ALTERNATIVE
	Walk with physical therapy tid using a gait belt, progressing from standing at bedside to walking the length of the hall before discharge. Give Vicodin on request at the onset of pain (to prevent severe pain).
Vicodin DS, 1 tablet prn q 4-6h	**ALTERNATIVE**
	Give Vicodin 30 minutes before ambulating with physical therapy (to enable to walk).
	ALTERNATIVE
	Give Vicodin q4h until pain is controlled.

*Note: "Client will" is assumed; the "why" is in parentheses because it is not necessarily stated in writing interventions.

Nursing Intervention Classification System. The words that describe nursing interventions are as much a part of the language of nursing as are nursing diagnoses. For nurses to communicate with each other and to describe nursing to the health care team, the language of nursing needs to be standardized so that it has a common meaning among nurses. Standardized communication can be used for care-plan development, research, staff education, or curriculum development, for example. The **Nursing Intervention Classification** (NIC) system, developed at the University of Iowa, is a standardized language appropriate for computerized client information systems to describe the component of client care that is nursing practice. It is useful to assist nurses in documenting care. With the NIC system, the nurse can use a few words, rather than writing a sentence or two, to describe an array of activities on the client's behalf.

Most of the NIC interventions are appropriate for use in any health care setting or specialty area. Common core interventions across specialties are active listening, emotional support, infection control, vital-signs monitoring, infection protection, and medication management. By classifying nursing interventions into broad categories, the NIC taxonomy describes the scope of nursing practice.

Although the NIC taxonomy is useful for describing the nursing management of a client, it does not prescribe interventions for particular nursing diagnoses. The nurse makes the judgment about which interventions will most effectively manage a diagnosis. Sometimes several interventions may be required to plan care for a nursing diagnosis. As with the outcome classification, the label is a category and the nurse selects the activities for the individual client.

THE NURSING CARE PLAN

The nursing care plan consists of three components: client problems (nursing diagnoses), expected outcomes, and interventions. The list of client problems may be common, including input from the entire health care team, or it may contain problems identified only by nurses. The use of a common list facilitates a multidisciplinary team approach. The advantage of a separate list is that it clearly identifies the contribution of nursing to client care.

The problem list may identify nursing diagnoses using the North American Nursing Diagnosis Association (NANDA) taxonomy, or it may adopt another system for naming problems treated by nurses. NANDA diagnoses are more likely to appear when nurses write a separate list; however, some agencies use NANDA language even in a common problem list.

The nurse who writes the care plan may develop outcomes statements, or the nurse might use NOC language to identify outcomes on the care plan. The language for interventions can be taken from the NIC system, the Omaha system, or the Home Healthcare Classification system (McCloskey & Bulechek, 2003; Martin & Scheet, 1992; & Saba et al., 1991). Interventions should be written specifically enough that care can be administered consistently by all nurses assigned to the client's care over a period of time.

The use of the NIC and NOC systems is rapidly growing in computerized record-keeping systems and may become the standard for documentation, along with NANDA diagnoses.

Guidelines for Developing Care Plans

The plan of care establishes priorities and guides the efforts of the client, the nurses, and other members of the health care team. As these decisions are made, the care plan is written to provide documentation for all health care personnel who will be caring for the client.

The traditional nursing care plan is formatted in three columns, with additional columns for the date and signature of the person who developed the plan and for the dates when outcomes are achieved. When the problem is resolved, it is documented on the nursing care plan. Evaluation data are charted in nursing progress notes, or, in student care plans, they may be written in an additional column.

Purposes of a Written Care Plan

The written care plan has evolved as a tool for providing current information for client care. The purpose of a nursing care plan is to communicate the planned care to the health care team, thus ensuring continuity of care. A written plan should be concise to communicate information efficiently. On the other hand, it should provide enough information to ensure that everyone providing the care will provide the same care. The purposes of a care plan can also include the following:

- Identify all problems being treated
- Provide a detailed guide for nursing care
- Individualize the care provided
- Set priorities
- Coordinate care among all health care workers
- Guide evaluation of care
- Provide for individual and family participation in planning
- Document current nursing practice

Types of Care Plans

There are different types of care plans in practice today, each with advantages and disadvantages. These types of care plans have varying degrees of individualization and standardization.

Individualized Care Plans. An **individualized care plan** is one written specifically for each client who enters a health care facility (Box 10-6). This type of care plan is developed

---

Nursing Care Plan   SAMPLE NURSING CARE PLAN USING STANDARDIZED LANGUAGE   Box 10-6

Mrs. Worden tripped over her space heater at home and fell. She burned her left anterior thigh on the space heater and fractured her right hip. Her frail elderly husband called the emergency number (911), and an ambulance responded. Mrs. Worden was admitted to the local hospital, where she underwent an open reduction and internal fixation to repair the fractured right hip. Treatment was also started for the second-degree burn on her left thigh. After 4 days on the inpatient surgical unit, she was ready for discharge but not independent enough in mobility or activities of daily living to return home. She was discharged to a skilled unit in a local nursing home.

Admission data included the following:
- White female, age 84. Height 5 ft. 3 in. Weight 128 pounds.
- BP 148/72, T 97.6, RP 68 and regular, R 18.
- Wound anterior thigh measured 4 cm × 3 cm with a depth of 0.5 cm.

- Incision right hip measured 9 cm in length with 13 sutures intact. Skin was pink with no signs of infection. Skin edges approximated.
- Range of motion: all extremities within normal limits except right hip abduction was only 20 degrees and right knee flexion was only 45 degrees. Pain noted on movement of right leg during range of motion.
- Ambulated 4 yards with pain and fatigue.
- Is continent of bladder and bowel.
- Oral intake has been a regular diet with intake of 75% to 100% at each meal.
- Last known bowel movement was 2 days prior with a usual routine of daily defecation.
- Oriented to time, person, and place.
- Very upset that she could not go home for physical and occupational therapy rather than going to the nursing home.

NANDA Nursing Diagnosis	NOC Expected Outcomes With Indicators	NIC Interventions With Selected Activities	Evaluation Data
PAIN	PAIN LEVEL:	ANALGESIC ADMINISTRATION:	24 HOURS AFTER ADMINISTRATION:
Related Factors: • Second-degree burn on left thigh from contact with space heater • Reports pain 6/10 during dressing change • Appears tense and jerks away from nurse when dressing removed	• Report of pain will decrease to moderate (3-4/10). • Physiological signs of pain will be slight to moderate.	• Check medical order for drug, dose, and frequency of analgesic prescribed. • Check for history of drug allergy. • Administer analgesic (morphine in this case) 30 minutes before dressing change. • Advise that drowsiness can occur. Put side rails up and call light within reach. • Document response.	• Morphine administered IM 30 minutes before dressing change. • Reported pain of 2/10 with dressing change. • Appeared to sleep through most of dressing change. No change in facial expression, restlessness, or muscle tension with dressing change. • Side rails up and call light within reach.

Nursing outcome and intervention labels from Johnson, M., Bulechek, G., McCloskey Dochterman, J. M., Maas, M., & Moorhead, S. (2001). *Nursing diagnoses, outcome, and interventions: NANDA, NOC, and NIC linkages.* St Louis, MO: Mosby.

from the admission history, physical and functional assessment, and problems anticipated on the basis of the physician's treatment plan.

Individualized care plans allow you to identify the unique problems of each client, to decide on the outcomes to be achieved, and to identify which nursing interventions will be appropriate to achieve those outcomes. These plans contain only the applicable nursing diagnoses, outcomes, and interventions. The disadvantage of individualized care plans is the time required to write them.

Standardized Care Plans. **Standardized care plans** are typically written by a group of nurses who use their collective expertise to produce a plan to direct nursing care for clients with specific medical diagnoses (such as myocardial infarction) or nursing diagnoses (such as *Pain* or *Anxiety*). They are also developed for clients undergoing special procedures (such as cardiac catheterization).

These care plans are duplicated and made available to the appropriate units in the health care facility. The format is designed with extra space so you can individualize the plan by filling in specific client characteristics, related factors associated with the nursing diagnosis, deadlines for the outcomes, and additional details in the interventions. For example, you can individualize interventions by adding frequencies, amounts, times, and client preferences.

Standardized care plans have the advantage of saving you time by reducing the amount of writing required. They are also particularly helpful to nurses working in unfamiliar areas. The main disadvantage of standardized care plans is the lack of individualization. Not all of the nursing diagnoses, outcomes, and interventions listed on the standardized care plan pertain to every client. Using a standardized care plan requires you to critically analyze its applicability to an individual.

Computerized Care Plans. A **computerized care plan** is a care plan created by a computer program. Many software vendors have developed computerized care plans written by expert clinicians.

A computerized care plan has nursing diagnoses, client outcomes, and nursing interventions, and it also allows for the relevant dates to be inserted. You choose the appropriate nursing diagnoses, outcomes, and interventions for the individual client.

Advantages of computerized care plans include their legibility and the ease with which they can be changed or updated. They also allow nurse researchers to collect data about groups of clients. The disadvantage is that, like standardized care plans, they lack individualization. However, computerized care plans can be simpler to individualize than standardized forms.

A prerequisite for computerized client records is a health care vocabulary that can be coded for a computer. The NANDA, NIC, NOC, Omaha, and Home Healthcare Classification systems are the most widely recognized standardized languages for nursing (McCloskey & Bulechek, 2003; Johnson, Maas, & Moorhead, 2000; Martin & Scheet, 1992; NANDA, 1999; & Saba et al., 1991).

The basic goal of the medical informatics community is the development of information systems that facilitate useful retrieval of biomedical information. Ideally, nursing would have a unified, single language system that could be used throughout the country. All nurses could communicate the function of nursing in a unique language. Nursing information could be retrieved from large, distributed information spaces, and nursing would be able to articulate with classifications from other disciplines.

Case Management Plans. The concept of case management has been developed to reduce costs while ensuring quality of care. **Case management** is a care delivery system that focuses on the management of client care across an episode of illness. The goals of case management are to do the following:

- Coordinate needed care and services across disciplines to reduce fragmented or duplicated care
- Achieve satisfactory clinical outcomes
- Reduce cost per case
- Reduce the length of hospital stay and use resources effectively
- Reduce readmission rates (Bower, 1994).

The case manager works with the client, family, health care team, and payers to develop client goals. The case manager then designs plans to reach those goals. Once a plan is formulated, the case manager carries out the plan, revises the plan if it is ineffective, and coordinates all care.

Case management is a model of nursing practice that gives one person the responsibility for overseeing the client's care over the course of an illness. The case manager ensures that the client's care is well coordinated, with no gaps or overlaps in service.

Case management may describe many different entities in different health care settings. It may be a group of activities that nurses perform in one setting, a client care delivery system, a professional practice model, or a separate service performed by independent practitioners or insurance companies. Case management is used across the health care continuum from home health to long-term care to hospitals.

Indeed, case management models exist on a continuum from working with an individual client to managing a system of service delivery. At the client end, a hospital case manager may be responsible for client care from before admission to after discharge. In another model, the case manager may focus on services provided to groups of clients, and on planning a system that controls costs and reduces the length of hospital stay. At the extreme business end of the spectrum is outcome management. An outcome manager's function is similar to that of a case manager but is more focused on researching and analyzing cost-effective ways to produce desired outcomes among large groups of clients.

Nursing case management was introduced in the acute care setting in 1985 to respond to the prepaid health movement, which seeks to ensure quality care in a health care system focused on cost control. In most settings, case management is still performed by nurses. Case management involves health assessment and planning for services to meet the comprehensive needs of the client. The case manager arranges for the services, coordinated delivery, and monitors the care (Bower, 1992).

Nurses who are case managers use both nursing terminology and the terminology of other disciplines to develop plans of care for clients in multiple settings over a period of time. For example, a client with chronic obstructive pulmonary disease may have home health services, be admitted for an acute exacerbation of the disease, and be discharged to long-term care before being able to go home again. The nurse case manager would plan this entire span of services.

Clinical Pathways. A **clinical pathway** is a standardized multidisciplinary care plan that projects the expected course of the client's treatment and progress over the hospital stay. It is a method for describing the plan of care by predicting the course of the client's hospital stay and prescribing the care and outcomes on a day-by-day basis. Clinical pathways are guidelines for health professionals in hospitals, home care, and long-term care.

You may hear clinical pathways called care maps, clinical paths, critical paths, critical pathways, collaborative care plans, and multidisciplinary care plans. All have the commonality of containing all the critical elements of the client's care. No matter which name is applied to it, a clinical pathway is a plan of care with a predictable time table for the client to achieve the goals. This type of plan is seen by many as a way to maintain quality care and coordinate services while controlling costs.

Most clinical pathways are written on a grid that lists the client's problems, outcomes, and interventions by multidisciplinary staff along a specified time line. Figure 10-7 shows an example of a clinical pathway. Usually, the facility's pathway is developed by a group of multidisciplinary clinicians who care for clients with specific illnesses. In fact, the pathway's primary value lies in its multidisciplinary approach. Ideally, the clinical pathway should include each discipline's standardized language.

Clinical pathways are available for procedures, conditions, illnesses, and diagnosis-related groups. Time lines can range from a few hours or days to a period covering weeks or months, depending on the condition or procedure for which the pathway was developed. For example, a clinical pathway for a client having a sigmoidoscopy would cover just a few hours. A clinical pathway for a client having a total hip replacement may include a 3- to 4-day acute care phase after surgery, followed by another 4 days of skilled nursing care before discharge.

EVALUATION

Evaluation is a systematic and ongoing process of examining whether expected outcomes have been achieved and whether nursing care has been effective (Figure 10-8, p. 211). However, evaluation must also examine the quality of nursing care delivery and link positive client outcomes to quality care.

To evaluate the client's progress toward attaining expected outcomes, you will first need to review the expected outcomes for each diagnosis. The purposes of expected outcomes are to direct nursing interventions, to maintain continuity of nursing care, and to measure the effectiveness of nursing interventions. Keep in mind that accurate, meaningful evaluation relies on expected outcomes that are measurable, realistic, and attainable in relation to a client's capabilities and available resources.

Standards are established to evaluate the quality of care and to guide nursing practice. Nurses must agree on the standards and consistently practice according to the standards if nursing care is to be identified as the cause of positive outcomes. This chapter introduces evaluation by outcomes and by standards of practice.

Evaluating Client Outcomes

The process of evaluating nursing care reconsiders each phase of the nursing process. Was assessment accurate and thorough? Was the nursing diagnosis derived correctly from the data, and did it accurately identify the problem? Were the expected outcomes measurable, realistic, and appropriate? Were the interventions appropriate and appropriately implemented? During the evaluation phase, ask yourself the following key questions:

- What are the client's responses to interventions in relation to expected outcomes? Are the responses desirable or undesirable?
- Are the interventions effective in meeting expected outcomes? If not, why are the interventions ineffective? Is it necessary to revise outcomes or interventions?
- Is the nursing diagnosis still active? Is it necessary to revise it or to add new nursing diagnoses?

Examining the Client's Responses to Interventions. As you are intervening, you should evaluate the client's physical and psychosocial responses, and document the responses as desirable or undesirable. Desirable responses indicate that the purposes of interventions are achieved and the client is progressing toward expected outcomes. Undesirable responses indicate poor progress toward expected outcomes or the occurrence of complications or side effects. Your evaluation may include responses to both medical and nursing interventions.

To assess physical and psychosocial responses to medications or treatments, you evaluate whether the purposes of medications or treatments are being achieved, the occurrence of complications or side effects, and the client's understanding of the medications or treatments. Through the process of continuous evaluation, you may identify problems that need additional attention. For example, some clients stop taking antibiotics or antihypertensives when their symptoms have subsided. When you evaluate the client's psychosocial responses to medications, you identify the problem of lack of understanding of medications.

Evaluating responses to diagnostic tests or procedures is another important aspect of nursing care. Throughout tests or

Text continued on p. 211

VALLEY BAPTIST MEDICAL CENTER
Harlingen, Texas

ADMISSION ORDERS - PNEUMONIA

1. ☐ Admit to medical floor.　　☐ Other _____

2. ☐ Admit to the service of Dr. _____

3. Diagnosis _____

　 _____

4. ☐ Initiate Pneumonia Restorative Care Path.

5. LAB:　☐ ER Profile (CBC w/diff, Chem 14)
　　　　☐ Blood cultures X 2, 15 minutes apart - separate sticks
　　　　☐ Aminophylline Level, if patient taking.
　　　　☐ Sputum C&S / Induction p.r.n. by RT.
　　　　☐ UA
　　　　☐ If SpO_2 <92%, collect ABG
　　　　☐ _____

6. ☐ Chest X-ray

7. ☐ O_2 at _____ LPM via _____　　☐ Follow O_2 Protocol

8. ☐ Respiratory Treatment: _____

　 ☐ Bronchodilator Protocol　　☐ Suction p.r.n.

9. ☐ Diet: _____

10. ☐ IV: _____

11. ☐ Antibiotic Therapy: _____

　 _____

　 ☐ Initial Dose NOW

12. ☐ Acetaminophen gr X, 1 suppository or 650 mg P.O. for Temp >100.6F° q 4 hrs p.r.n.

13. ☐ Old charts to the floor.

14. ☐ Vital signs q 4 hours until stable, then routine.

15. Activity: ☐ Ambulate at least BID　☐ Bathroom with assistance　☐ Bed rest

16. ☐ Social Service to evaluate.

17. _____

　 _____

Date _____ Time _____　_____ M.D.
　　　　　　　　　　　　　　　　　　　　　Physician Signature

VBMC 1965-129-0396

Figure 10-7. An example of a clinical pathway for a client with pneumonia.

Continued

VALLEY BAPTIST MEDICAL CENTER
Harlingen, Texas

RESTORATIVE CARE PATH
PNEUMONIA > 17 Years of Age

KEY: Initials=Completed; N/A = Not Applicable; 0 - Variance

Page 1 of 2   VBMC 1620-005-0196

DRG: 79 and 89

Special Considerations:

☐ ER ☐ PATT ☐ Direct Adm

	Day 1: RN Review	Day 2: RN Review	Day 3: RN Review	Day 4: RN Review	Day 5: RN Review	EXPECTED OUTCOMES
Consults	___ Call Internal Medicine or primary MD to admit	If not improved 48 hrs after admission, consider pulmonary consult	___ All consults notified	——→ ——→	——→ ——→	All consults notified
Tests	___ ER Profile ___ Blood Culture X 2 (separate sticks) 15 min. apart ___ Aminophylline Level (if taking) ___ UA ___ Sputum C&S / Induction p.r.n. by RT ___ CXR ___ If O₂Sat <92, collect ABG	___ Call MD for abnormal labs ___ ABGs p.r.n. ___ Swab for MRSA for nursing home patients or transfers ___ If sputum not collected, in 4 hrs, notify MD	___ Call MD for abnormal labs ___ In 48 hrs, if no clinical improvement, consider CBC, CXR, alternate means of sputum collection	——→ ——→	——→ ——→	All labs WNL or stable for patient.
Assessment & Evaluation	___ Initiate Database ___ Vital signs q 1 hr or as indicated ___ F/C if unable to void ___ I&O ___ Assess for TB risk factors	___ Vital signs q 4 hrs ___ Check voiding ——→	——→ ——→ ——→ ——→	——→ ——→	——→ ——→	Pt afebrile, consider disch Voiding adequate I&O WNL
Activity / Safety	___ Bed rest with BRP ___ Raise HOB 30°	——→ Activity as tolerated ——→	——→ ——→	If pt afebrile X 24 hrs, consider disch ——→ ——→	——→ ——→	Return to previous activity level
Treatments	___ O₂ ___ L/min (NC / Mask / Trach) ___ Resp. Tx: ___ O₂ Sat Monitor ___ Suction p.r.n.	___ O₂ protocol ——→ ——→ ——→	——→ ——→ ——→ ——→	——→ ——→ ——→ ——→	——→ ——→ ——→ ——→	Respiratory status stable
Diet	___ Assess nutritional status ___ Dietitian? ☐ Yes ☐ No	Diet ___	Diet ___	Diet ___	Diet ___	Patient tolerates prescribed diet

Date: ___   Date: ___   Date: ___   Date: ___   Date: ___

Initial / Signature/Status / Initial / Signature/Status / Case Manager / Initial / Signature/Status

Figure 10-7, cont'd. An example of a clinical pathway for a client with pneumonia.

VALLEY BAPTIST MEDICAL CENTER
Harlingen, Texas
RESTORATIVE CARE PATH
PNEUMONIA > 17 Years of Age

Page 2 of 2

VBMC 1620-005-0196

	Date: Day 1: RN Review	Date: Day 2: RN Review	Date: Day 3: RN Review	Date: Day 4: RN Review	Date: Day 5: RN Review	EXPECTED OUTCOMES
Meds / IV Fluids	__ Start IV __ Start Antibiotic Protocol __ IV @ __ hr __ List Home meds __ ER Fever Protocol __ Continue IV antibiotics __ Adjust antibiotics per culture results.	Reevaluate antibiotic therapy if no clinical improvement ------>	__ Consider Saline lock __ Consider P.O. antibiotics	------> ------>	------> ------>	D.C. with P.O. antibiotics
Pain Management	__ Medicate as ordered; document effect. ------>	------>	------>	------>	------>	Prescription for pain meds as needed.
Patient/Family Education	__ Explain procedures, meds & equipment. __ Provide educational materials __ Provide opportunity for questions. __ Reinforce teaching __ Return demo & document progress __ Provide patient pathway	------> ------>	------> ------>	------> ------>	------> ------>	Pt/family verbalize understanding of D/C instructions, follow-up appointment/classes.
Psychosocial	__ Allow verbalization of feelings __ Consider referral to Pastoral Services.	------> ------>	------> ------>	------> ------>	_____ No anxiety ------>	No anxiety noted
Discharge Planning / Continuum of Care	__ Social Service Consult __ Obtain old chart & send to floor with patient. __ Discharge Planning Assessment __ Discharge home __ Admit (consider STO)	------>	------>	------> __ Consider discharge	------>	Discharge: □ Home □ NHP □ Home Health □ Transfer □ Rehab □ Other □ Records faxed □ Report called □ D.C. instructions given.
Signatures 7 - 3						
Signatures 3 - 11						
Signatures 11 - 7						

Figure 10-7, cont'd. An example of a clinical pathway for a client with pneumonia.

Continued

	EMERGENCY ROOM	DAY 1	DAY 2	DAY 3	DAY 4	DAY 5
Activity	• You will be on bed rest. • Your nurse will raise the head of your bed to help you breathe easier.	• Activity will be encouraged, however, **PLEASE ASK** for assistance to prevent a fall or injury.	• Your activity level will be increased daily. • If you need assistance, please use the call bell.	• Your activity level will be increased daily. • If you need assistance, please use the call bell.	• Your activity level will be increased daily. • Use the call bell if needed.	• Your activity level will be increased daily.
Treatments	• Nurses or Respiratory Therapist (RT) may start oxygen. • RT will check the oxygen level by either a blood test or monitor. • You will be expected to try to produce some sputum for lab testing. • If you are unable to produce sputum, RT may be asked to help you.	• Your nurse will be checking blood pressure, heart rate, temperature and respirations. • Your nurse may measure your fluid intake and urine output. • RT will continue to check your oxygen level.	• Nurses will continue to check blood pressure, heart rate, temperature and respirations. • RT will continue to check your oxygen level.	• Nurses will continue to check blood pressure, heart rate, temperature and respirations. • Oxygen checks continued. You will be slowly taken off oxygen. • Continued monitoring of intake & output.	• Nurses will continue checking blood pressure, heart rate, temperature and respirations. • You will be slowly taken off oxygen.	• Nurses will continue to check blood pressure, heart rate, temperature and respirations.
Tests	• Your doctor may order urinalysis, blood tests, chest x-rays and respiratory treatments. • Your family doctor may be called to admit you. If you do not have a doctor, one will be provided for you.	• If you were unable to cough up any sputum, you will be asked to try again. • If you were unable to urinate, a tube called a foley catheter may be inserted into your bladder.	• You may have more blood tests, another chest x-ray, and possible re-collection of sputum.			
Medications	• Your nurse will start an IV in a vein to administer antibiotics. • The doctor may order medication for pain or fever. • If you have a list of your home medications, please give it to your nurse.	• Your nurse will continue to monitor your IV on a regular basis. • You may be started on some of your own home medications given by the nurses.	• The nurse will continue monitoring your IV or you may begin taking antibiotics by mouth.			
Teaching	• Your doctor or nurse will explain procedures, medications and equipment. • You will be given an opportunity to ask questions. • Instructions will be reviewed with you and your family.					
Diet		• A dietitian may be asked to visit with you about your eating habits.				
Discharge Planning	• You should expect to stay in the Emergency Room for a limited period of time, then be taken to a room in the hospital.	• A social worker and/or case manager will meet with you to discuss any discharge needs.	• Social services will continue to provide referrals and/or arrangements as needed.	• Social Services continues referrals/arrangements. • If your condition has improved sufficiently, you may be discharged.	• Discharge plans/referrals completed. • If improved sufficiently, you may be discharged.	• Referrals and all arrangements completed. • Discharged to home.

Figure 10-7, cont'd. An example of a clinical pathway for a client with pneumonia.

procedures, the client may have many questions or concerns and may develop complications. Care can then be provided to ease the client's anxiety, increase the client's understanding, or detect complications or side effects at an early stage.

After providing nursing interventions, you should evaluate responses of the client and family members. After the client or family members have received health teaching, evaluate their understanding of the teaching. They may not understand the information completely or may have some misunderstanding. Some families may need further information. Others may need reinforcement to perform appropriate health behaviors.

Evaluating the client's and family members' perceptions of care provided is also important. You may perceive that good nursing care has been provided, but the client or family members may think otherwise. The client's perceptions of nursing care influence the satisfaction with nursing care, which is often used as a *quality indicator* of care by health care agencies. Therefore, feedback from the client or family members needs to be sought to understand their perceptions of the care received and to help improve client satisfaction with nursing care. If a client or family member is dissatisfied with the care, you will need to identify the causes of this dissatisfaction and seek ways to reduce or alleviate it.

Appraising the Success of Interventions.

After evaluating the client's responses to interventions, you must judge the success of the interventions in achieving expected outcomes. Continue effective interventions and try to determine why others are ineffective. Interventions that are inappropriate or insufficient to meet the goals need to be discontinued or revised.

Outcomes may be completely met, partially met, or not met. When the client responds as expected, outcomes are completely met. When client's responses indicate some progress toward the goals, outcomes are partially met. When client's responses do not show any progress toward attaining goals, none of the outcomes are met. If the expected outcomes were not appropriately customized to the client's health status, for example, they may need to be revised.

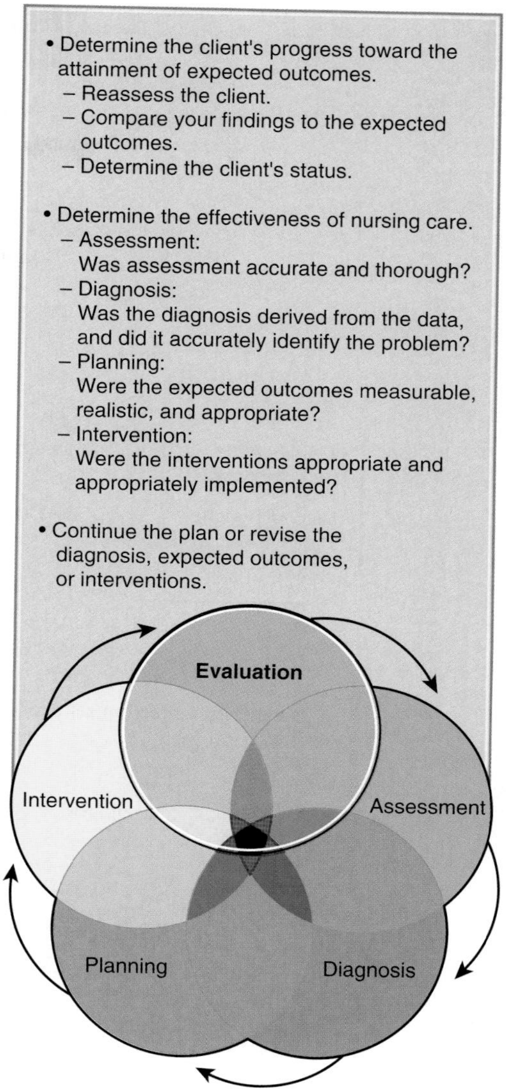

Continuing, Revising, or Resolving the Care Plan.

After evaluating the success of interventions in achieving the outcomes, you will need to decide whether the nursing care plan should be continued or revised (Figure 10-9, p. 212). If the client attained the expected outcomes, the nursing diagnosis is said to be resolved. If the expected outcomes were only partially attained, you may need to revise interventions, add new ones, or discontinue others (Box 10-7, p. 213). However, there may be justification for continuing interventions when the problem is not resolved. For example you may determine that more time is needed and thus continue the interventions.

When your evaluation identifies new problems, you will need to revise the client's existing care plan to address those problems. For example, acute pain is a common problem after surgery, and narcotics usually control surgical pain. However, because these clients commonly develop constipa-

- Determine the client's progress toward the attainment of expected outcomes.
  - Reassess the client.
  - Compare your findings to the expected outcomes.
  - Determine the client's status.

- Determine the effectiveness of nursing care.
  - Assessment:
    Was assessment accurate and thorough?
  - Diagnosis:
    Was the diagnosis derived from the data, and did it accurately identify the problem?
  - Planning:
    Were the expected outcomes measurable, realistic, and appropriate?
  - Intervention:
    Were the interventions appropriate and appropriately implemented?

- Continue the plan or revise the diagnosis, expected outcomes, or interventions.

Figure 10-8. The process of evaluation.

tion, your care plan needs to address reducing or preventing constipation.

Factors Affecting Outcomes Attainment

Many factors affect the attainment of client outcomes. Evaluate yourself frequently to see if you are enhancing or impeding outcome attainment.

Facilitators.

Stated clearly, realistic outcomes facilitate evaluations. A clear understanding of the client's illness and treatments will help you to select reasonable expected outcomes. After thoroughly identifying the client's problems and gathering adequate supporting data, you will be able to establish individualized and realistic outcomes.

Thinking of evaluation as a continuous process facilitates evaluation (Figure 10-10, p. 214). It requires frequent monitoring to gauge the client's progress in attaining an expected outcome. Observe for signs that progress is being made or that the client's condition is conducive to progress.

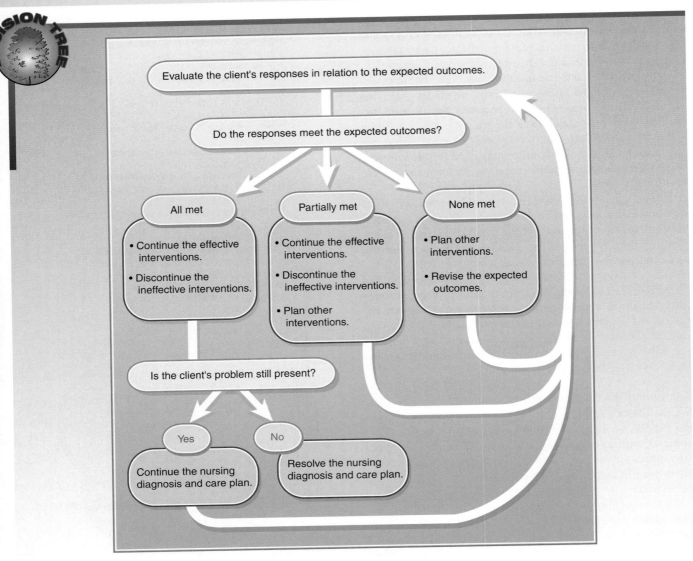

Figure 10-9. The process of evaluating a care plan.

Maintaining continuity of care facilitates outcome attainment. Because all of a client's health problems may not be resolved with one episode of care, document all pertinent information about the client's problems, care plans, and progress toward expected outcomes. That way, the client's care plan can be continued, and the progress toward attaining the expected outcomes can be continuously assessed.

Collaborating with other health care professionals is also crucial for facilitating outcome attainment. You should not only work closely with physicians but also recognize the client's need for other health professionals. Using an interdisciplinary approach to meet the client's needs will expedite recovery.

Client participation facilitates attaining outcomes. Clients who understand what you seek to accomplish through the interventions applied are more motivated to reach the goals. Box 10-8 (p. 213) summarizes factors that facilitate outcome attainment.

Barriers. Barriers that impede the attainment of expected outcomes need to be evaluated as well. Barriers involve you and your colleagues more than the client and his condition. For example, a lack of critical thinking can leave you unaware of the client's problems and uncertain about why the goals are not being attained. Avoid focusing on routine tasks, such as taking vital signs or giving medications and treatments. Instead, think critically as you work through the nursing process to identify and solve the client's problems. Ask yourself wide-ranging questions as you evaluate the success of the nursing process in your client's care (Box 10-9, p. 214).

Lack of knowledge about client care, diseases, and treatments is another barrier that affects outcome attainment. To think critically, you need to equip yourself continuously with knowledge relevant to client care. You can use many methods to keep your knowledge current and comprehensive.

Fragmented nursing care is another factor that hinders outcome attainment. In today's fast-paced clinical settings,

Nursing Care Plan AN EXAMPLE OF REVISIONS FOR AN UNMET EXPECTED OUTCOME

Box 10-7

CLIENT DATA

A 72-year-old man with deep vein thrombosis in the left leg and a history of a brain tumor was hospitalized for 3 days.

NANDA Nursing Diagnosis	NOC Expected Outcomes With Indicators	NIC Interventions With Selected Activities	Evaluation Data
IMBALANCED NUTRITION: LESS THAN BODY REQUIREMENTS	NUTRITION STATUS:	NUTRITION MANAGEMENT:	
Related Factors: • Poor appetite • Decreased oral intake	• Client will eat 75% or more of each meal. • Explain the importance of proper nutrition and fluid intake in avoiding further blood clots and facilitating recovery. • Encourage intake of high-protein, high-calorie foods.	• Explore causes of poor nutrition. • Monitor intake and output daily. • Identify favorite foods and drinks and assist client to obtain them. • Explain the importance of proper nutrition and fluid intake in avoiding further blood clots.	• 0800. Refuses to eat breakfast; has no appetite. • Oral intake has been less than 25% of meals. Last 24-hr intake 900 ml, and output 800 ml. Has had poor appetite for 1 month since radiation. Mouth dry, lips cracked. • Likes to drink chocolate milk and eat orange sherbet. Drank 50 ml milk and half cup of sherbet. • Explained importance of nutrition and hydration. States he has no appetite but will try. • Discussed setting goal of 25% of meals and a cup of favorite fluid q2h while awake. Agreed to try. • 1000. Does not want to drink chocolate milk anymore. Offered cranberry juice. Drank 20 ml. • 1200. Ate 10% of lunch. States feeling tired.

REVISIONS

Continues to have poor nutrition; will revise plan. Change expected outcome to Client will increase oral intake by eating 25% of meals.

ADD NURSING DIAGNOSIS

IMPAIRED ORAL MUCOUS MEMBRANE	ORAL HEALTH:		
• Dryness, dehydration	• Client will have moist, pink mucous membranes.	• Contact physician about dehydration and adding protein drink to diet. • Assess oral membranes daily. • Provide oral baking soda and saline mouth rinse before each meal.	

Nursing outcome and intervention labels from Johnson, M., Bulechek, G., McCloskey Dochterman, J. M., Maas, M., & Moorhead, S. (2001). *Nursing diagnoses, outcomes, and interventions: NANDA, NOC, and NIC linkages.* St Louis, MO: Mosby.

interventions may not be consistently implemented, documented, and reassessed from shift to shift. Consequently, client problems may take longer than necessary to be resolved (Figure 10-11, p. 214).

To avoid fragmented care, you need to improve the team's working relationship and to maintain continuity of care. Strive to develop a system to facilitate verbal and written communication among the staff regarding each client's care. Some health care institutions use clinical care guidelines and computerized client records to facilitate continuity of care.

Lack of communication among professionals in different disciplines can also deter outcome attainment. When health

Box 10-8	Factors Facilitating Outcome Attainment

- Understand clearly the expected outcomes for each problem.
- Understand the client's disease and treatments.
- Assess the client accurately and thoroughly.
- Identify all pertinent problems.
- Formulate realistic and individualized outcomes.
- Revise outcomes and interventions when necessary.
- Maintain the continuity of care.
- Work as a team with other health care professionals.
- Encourage the client's participation in identifying problems and setting goals.

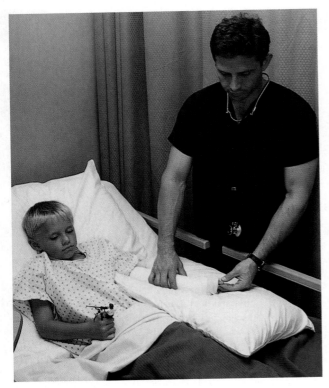

Figure 10-10. Evaluation is a continuous process. This nurse evaluates the circulation in a child's casted arm in an ongoing, regular manner.

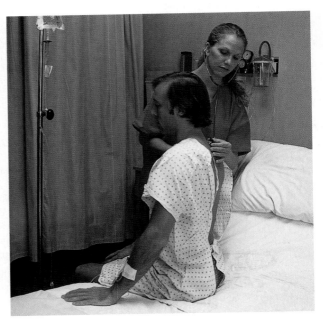

Figure 10-11. Avoidance of fragmented nursing care is critical to the achievement of expected outcomes. This nurse continuously reassesses and documents her client's respiratory status.

Box 10-9   Evaluating the Success of the Nursing Process

ASSESSMENT

- What is the pathophysiology of my client's medical diagnoses? What is the relationship between the client's diagnoses and treatments?
- What are my client's physical and psychosocial responses to the present illness, diagnoses, and treatments?
- What diagnostic tests has the client had? What are the relationships between abnormal results, the client's responses, and treatments?
- What are my client's treatments (e.g., diet, routine and PRN medications, activity, and so on)? Why are these prescribed? What are the client's responses to these treatments?

DIAGNOSIS

- What actual and potential problems can I identify from assessment data?
- What is the priority of these problems?
- How do I describe these problems with nursing diagnoses approved by the North American Nursing Diagnosis Association?
- Do I have sufficient evidence (contributing factors, signs, symptoms) to confirm the diagnoses?
- Do I need to seek further data from current or past medical records, other health team members, family members, or other references to confirm or to rule out the nursing diagnoses?

PLANNING

- Are these outcomes client-focused? Is my client aware of the expected outcomes? Is my client ready to participate in setting specific goals (outcome criteria)?

- Are these outcomes measurable and achievable in the short term or the long term?
- Are these outcomes aimed to restore, maintain, or promote my client's health?

INTERVENTION

- What interventions can be implemented to achieve expected outcomes?
- Do these interventions conform to professional standards and organizational standards and protocols?
- How should I implement these interventions safely and effectively?
- What can I do to maintain the continuity of care?

EVALUATION

- What are the client's responses to interventions in relationship to the expected outcomes?
- Are outcomes all met, partially met, or not met? Is it necessary to revise some outcomes to make them attainable?
- Are these interventions effective toward achieving the expected outcomes? Are there problems with interventions? Are there better ways to implement these interventions?
- Are there alternative approaches to reach the goals?
- Should I continue, revise, or discontinue these interventions?
- Should I continue or resolve these nursing diagnoses?
- Has evaluation identified any new problems that require a nursing response?

Box 10-10 Barriers to the Attainment of Expected Outcomes

- Lack of critical thinking to understand the client's problems
- Lack of logical reasoning in connecting diagnoses, expected outcomes, and interventions
- Lack of adequate validation with client
- Inadequate assessment of the client's responses to interventions
- Fragmented care, in nursing or across the health care team
- Lack of collaborative work with other health care professionals
- Lack of client's involvement

professionals fail to communicate or to make adequate referrals, the client's problem may not resolve appropriately.

Lack of involvement by the client himself is another barrier to outcome attainment (Box 10-10). Usually, that lack of involvement stems from a lack of adequate information. Most clients want to be informed about their condition, their treatment, and what they can do to improve their health or prevent problems. Most clients also want to be involved in making decisions about their care. To help a client reach the expected outcomes, explain the plan of care and encourage the client to participate in it. Encourage questions and clarify anything that is confusing to the client.

Standards for Evaluation

The standards established by the ANA are the most influential in the profession. Many specialty nursing professional organizations, such as those of pediatric clinical nursing, gerontological nursing, acute care nursing, and oncology nursing, derive their standards from those created by the ANA. Professional standards are not legally binding; however, the nurse practice act and regulations adopted by each state do have the power to be legally binding.

The ANA defines **standards of care** as "authoritative statements that describe a competent level of clinical nursing practice demonstrated through assessment, diagnosis, outcome identification, planning, implementation, and evaluation" (ANA, 1998, p. 2) (see Appendix A). These standards emphasize the nurse's practice in caring for the client regardless of the nurse's educational background. In other words, every nurse is expected to demonstrate competent practice in these standards.

The ANA outlines six standards of care: assessment, diagnosis, outcome identification, planning care, implementation, and evaluation. The organization also lists criteria to measure the nurse's practice in each standard (see Appendix A). Competent practice of these standards reflects competent use of the nursing process. The criteria to measure competent practice of the standards are called indicators (ANA, 1998).

Standards of care (internal and external) are used in court cases to evaluate the quality of care delivered and the competence of the nurses delivering it. When the evidence indicates that nurses failed to meet these standards, the duty of care has been breached. The nurse or nurses involved are then guilty of malpractice. Thus nurses are responsible for performing—and documenting—competent care that meets all internal and external standards.

Key Principles

- The planning phase of the nursing process is used to set priorities, develop outcomes, designate deadlines, and identify nursing interventions.
- Planning for individuals is initiated with entry to the health care system, continues throughout the time of service, and ensures ongoing care through discharge planning.
- Planning for individuals is a team effort through collaboration, consultation, and care plan conferences.
- Planning for groups of clients with a common set of needs involves designing services for the population being served, determining the level of staffing, and designing the environment of care.
- The planning process involves setting priorities on the basis of the client's physical needs, the services expected in the setting, the client's perception of need, and the client's ability to provide self-care.
- Predicting the outcomes of nursing care implies that nursing can be held responsible for nursing-sensitive outcomes, not just for the provision of nursing care.
- The Nursing Outcome Classification system is a standardized language for stating nursing-sensitive outcomes, developed at the University of Iowa.
- The skills required for successful intervention are cognitive, technical, interpersonal, and ethical/legal.
- Implementation always includes reassessment and the continuation of the planning phase.
- Intervention is not complete until the care is documented.
- Nurse-initiated and physician-initiated interventions treat the related factors to resolve the signs and symptoms that define the nursing diagnosis.
- The Nursing Intervention Classification system is a standardized method of identifying nursing interventions.
- A nursing care plan is a guide to client care that coordinates the actions of the nursing team and improves continuity of care over the course of an illness.
- A nursing care plan includes nursing diagnoses, expected outcomes, and interventions.
- The type of nursing care plan is less important than the goal of providing comprehensive care designed to meet the needs of the individual client.
- Evaluation is a systematic and ongoing component of the nursing process to determine if the client's progress toward expected outcomes is achieved, if interventions provided are effective in meeting expected outcomes, and if nursing care is provided according to standards of practice.
- Expected outcomes should be established before evaluation. Outcomes should be measurable and individualized and have an estimated time frame.
- After interventions are implemented, the client's physical and psychosocial responses to the interventions are evaluated. Desirable and undesirable responses are noted, and interventions for undesirable responses are made.
- The success of interventions should be appraised and a determination made to continue, revise, or resolve care plans.

- Nurses should evaluate themselves frequently to ensure that they are facilitators of, and not barriers to, outcome attainment.
- ANA standards consist of standards of care and standards of professional performance. Standards of care describe competent practice of nursing process. Standards of professional performance depict competent professional behaviors.

Bibliography

*American Nurses' Association. (1985). *Code for nurses with interpretive statements.* Kansas City, MO: Author.

*American Nurses' Association. (1994). *Guidelines on reporting incompetent, unethical, or illegal practices.* Washington, DC: Author.

*American Nurses' Association. (1995a). *Implementation of nursing practice standards and guidelines.* Washington, DC: Author.

American Nurses' Association. (1995b). *Nursing's social policy statement.* Washington, DC: American Nurses Publishing.

American Nurses' Association. (1998). *Standards of clinical nursing practice,* (2nd ed.). Kansas City, MO: Author.

Bower, K. A. (1992). *Nursing case management.* Publication number NS-32. Washington, DC: American Nurse's Publication.

Bower, K. A. (1994). Case management and clinical paths: Definitions and relationships. In P. L. Spath (Ed.), *Clinical paths: Tools for outcomes management* (pp. 25-32). Chicago: American Hospital.

Carroll, D., & Seers, K. (1998). Relaxation for the relief of chronic pain: A systematic review. *Journal of Advanced Nursing, 27*(3), 476-487.

Castle, N. G., & Mor, V. (1998). Physical restraints in nursing homes: A review of the literature since the Nursing Home Reform Act of 1987. *Medicare Residents Review, 55*(2), 139-170.

Cimino, J. J., & Clayton, P. D. (1994). Coping with changing controlled vocabularies. In *Proceedings Eighteenth Annual Symposium on Computer Applications in Medical Care.* Philadelphia: Hanley & Belfus.

Denehy, J. (1998). Integrating Nursing Outcomes Classification in nursing education. *Journal Nursing Care Quality, 12*(5), 73-84.

Forsyth, T. J., Maney, L. A., Ramirez, A., Raviotta, G., Burts, J. L., & Litzenberger, D. (1998). Nursing case management in the NICU: Enhanced coordination for discharge planning. *Neonatal Network, 17*(7), 23-24.

Gronlund, N. E. (2000). *How to write and use instructional objectives* (6th ed.). Upper Saddle River, NJ: Prentice-Hall.

Haag-Heitman, B., & Kramer, A. (1998). Creating a clinical practice development model. *American Journal of Nursing, 98*(8), 39-43.

*Ignatavicius, D., & Hausman, K. (1995). *Clinical pathways for collaborative practice.* Philadelphia: Saunders.

Johnson, M., Maas, M., & Moorhead, S. (2000). *Nursing Outcomes Classification (NOC),* (2nd ed.). St. Louis, MO: Mosby.

Johnson, M., Bulechek, G., McCloskey Dochterman, J. M., Maas, M., & Moorhead, S. (2001). *Nursing diagnoses, outcomes, and interventions: NANDA, NOC, and NIC linkages.* St Louis, MO: Mosby.

Joint Commission on Accreditation of Healthcare Organizations. (1994a). *Framework for improving performance: A guide for nurses.* Oakbrook Terrace, IL: Author.

Joint Commission on Accreditation of Healthcare Organizations. (1994b). *Accreditation manual for hospitals: Vol. I. Standards.* Oakbrook Terrace, IL: Author.

Kobs, A. E. (1998). Getting started on benchmarking. *Outcomes Management in Nursing Practice, 2*(1), 45-48.

Maas, M. L., Specht, J. P., Weiler, K., Buckwalter, K. C., & Turner, B. (1998). Special care units for people with Alzheimer's disease: Only for the privileged few? *Journal of Gerontology Nursing, 24*(3), 28-37.

*Martin, K. S., & Scheet, N. J. (1992). *The Omaha System: Applications for Community Health Nursing.* Philadelphia: Saunders.

*Maslow, A. (1954). *Motivation and personality.* New York: Harper & Row.

McCloskey, J. C., & Bulechek, G. M. (2000). *Nursing Interventions Classification (NIC).* St Louis, MO: Mosby.

Moorhead, S., Clarke, M., Willits, M., & Tomsha, K. A. (1998). Nursing Outcomes Classification implementation projects across the care continuum. *Journal of Nursing Care Quality 12*(5), 52-63.

North American Nursing Diagnosis Association. (1999). *Nursing Diagnoses: Definitions and classification, 1999-2000.* Philadelphia: Author.

Parsley, K. (1998). In search of pathways. *Nursing Times, 94*(32), 40-41.

Prophet, C. M., & Delaney, C. W. (1998). Nursing Outcomes Classification: Implications for nursing information systems and the computer-based patient record. *Journal of Nursing Care Quality, 12*(5), 21-29.

Reed, L., Blegen, M. A., & Goode, C. S. (1998). Adverse patient occurrences as a measure of nursing care quality. *Journal of Nursing Administration, 28*(5), 62-69.

Rosenberg, M. L. (1998). Developing behavioral health clinical guidelines for depression: Emerging standards for guiding care. *Nursing Case Management, 3*(5), 204-207.

*Saba, V. K., O'Hare, P. A., Zuckerman, A. E., Boondas, J., Levine, E., & Oatway, D. M. (1991). A nursing intervention taxonomy for home health care. *Nursing and Health Care, 12*(6), 296-299.

Timms, J. A., & Behrenbeck, J. G. (1998). Implementing the Nursing Outcomes Classification in a clinical information system in a tertiary care setting. *Journal of Nursing Care Quality, 12*(5), 64-72.

---

*Asterisk indicates a classic or definitive work on this subject.

Documenting Care

Learning Objectives

After studying this chapter, you should be able to do the following:

- Understand the purposes of documentation
- Identify the methods of implementation of the principles of documentation
- Identify content pertinent to various types of nursing entries, special populations, and facilities
- Differentiate among documentation formats and the usefulness of various types of flow sheets
- Apply the principles of documentation to computerized documentation systems

Geraldine Peters, age 88, lives alone and was working in her garden when she fell and fractured her left hip. She was taken to the emergency department of a hospital nearby, where she was evaluated. She was admitted to an orthopedic nursing unit and placed in traction until she could be prepared for surgery. The next morning she was transferred to the operating room for an open reduction and internal fixation of her left hip (ORIF). From the recovery room she went to the ICU for an overnight stay to monitor her heart and then she was transferred back to the orthopedic unit. Ms. Peters's care and her responses to that care are documented in each department to ensure communication among the members of the health care team and coordination of care across multiple services. This chapter addresses the purposes, principles, and methods of documenting client care.

Documentation is the recording of information relevant to assessment, planning, implementation, and evaluation (client response); it is a legal record that is permanent and retrievable for future purposes. Record-keeping systems are either handwritten or computerized, and the format varies among health care agencies. Although the primary purpose continues to be creating a record of the client's health problems, treatments, and results, documentation systems have evolved in an effort to adjust to changes in health care delivery, to reflect changes in nursing practice, and to incorporate requirements of regulatory agencies.

PURPOSES OF DOCUMENTATION

As you saw in the case study of Ms. Peters, a health record is used to communicate to multiple members of the health care team. If Ms. Peters is admitted to the same hospital next year, the record may be retrieved to review her history. If an untoward event occurs and she decides to sue the hospital, her record will be used in court. The hospital may use her record to review the quality of care given on the orthopedic unit. The Joint Commission on Accreditation of Healthcare Organizations (JCAHO) may retrieve her record to examine compliance with standards of care. Effective documentation will meet the requirements of all these uses of the client's record.

Communication

The primary purpose of documentation of a client's care is communication among health team members to promote continuity of care among departments, throughout 24 hours of care, and during the entire hospital stay. It is essential that all personnel provide written documentation of anything they have observed or done with a client to ensure coordination of activities and continuity of care. Proper documentation informs appropriate personnel about a client's condition and response to illness, the care that has been given, and the results of care.

For example, the operating room personnel would examine Ms. Peters's chart for information relevant to surgery. Among other things, they need to know that she is allergic to penicillin, has a history of heart disease, and fell after becoming dizzy.

Quality Assurance

A second purpose of documentation is to provide substantiation of quality of care. As part of a quality assurance program, health care agencies periodically conduct chart audits to determine whether or not the care provided meets established standards for care. In addition, health care accrediting agencies, such as JCAHO, require regular quality assurance audits of client care.

The client record must show evidence of compliance with standards of care. Standards of care are guidelines that represent generally accepted practice and are derived from a variety of sources including the American Nurses' Association (ANA), the nurse practice act, JCAHO, and agency policy or procedure. For example, the ANA *Standards of Clinical Nursing Practice* (1999) require the use of the nursing process in providing care to clients. Communication of the use of this process is primarily through documentation in the client's medical record. ANA Standards of Care relevant to documentation are summarized in Appendix A.

Good documentation serves as the basis for collecting this quality assurance data. The record provides evidence that professional and agency standards have been incorporated into the client's care. The record should reflect initial and ongoing assessment, the problems identified through assessment, expected outcomes of care, interventions, and evaluation of progress toward expected outcomes. Data that evaluate care are critical in monitoring for quality assurance in client care and are necessary to ensure that standards of care are met. Currently in quality assurance auditing, an emphasis is placed on client outcomes as the measure of quality, and these are monitored through complete and accurate documentation.

Legal Accountability

The third purpose of documentation of care is to provide legal evidence through which nurses are held accountable for their actions. Legally, nurses can be held accountable for failure to practice within the applicable standards of care. Documentation should, therefore, verify the need for interventions, verify the type of care given, and allow examination of progress toward expected outcomes.

Common liability issues for nurses include protection from avoidable injury, monitoring and reporting changes in condition, and performing interventions correctly. The record should document assessment of clients at risk and safety measures implemented. The use of restraints is a safety factor that requires a physician's order (including a time limit). Specific agency policy should be followed for documentation.

In the event of an error, document your assessment of the client, notification of the physician, and any follow-up care.

For example, a medication error is usually noted on the medication administration record (MAR). An example of suggested documentation of a medication error follows:

SAMPLE CHARTING

| 7/16/02 | 4:30 P.M. | Awake, alert, and oriented X3. Resp. 18, BP 110/72. Dr. Johnson notified of administration of M.S. 10 mg IM. C. Larsen, RN |
| | 5:00 P.M. | Awake, alert, and oriented X3. Resp. 16, BP 112/76. C. Larsen, RN |

Additionally, an *incident form* is usually required for documentation in the event of a client fall, accident, or error. Incident forms are not part of the legal client record; rather these forms are used to track incidents for the purpose of discovering methods of prevention. Documenting in the legal record that an error was made and that an incident form was completed is not necessary and is never recommended.

Action Alert! Remember that the chart is a legal record and protects the client, the nurse, and the health care agency.

Reimbursement

The fourth use of the information documented in a client's record is reimbursement by third party payors. Cost awareness has become important in health care. Reimbursement for client care by Medicare, Medicaid, health maintenance organizations (HMOs), or insurance companies is often decided by a review of the client's record. As cost-containment efforts intensify, documentation of nursing care is used to determine and justify the need for services. Utilization review committees monitor lengths of stay and need for services.

Action Alert! Document the client's condition, nursing activities, and treatments and procedures completely. Reimbursement for services may be denied if documentation is inadequate.

Cost awareness has increased the emphasis on what care is necessary and how care is to be implemented. Clear, concise, and accurate documentation is essential for capturing scarce resources for client care. Complete data related to admission, supplies used, monitoring activities, follow-up, education, and discharge planning are necessary for appropriate reimbursement.

Research

Finally, documentation is used to provide data for nursing research. Nursing research results in new approaches to client care, and it increases professional knowledge. The value of this research depends on complete and accurate documentation of client data. Research has led to development of standardized formats for collecting and recording data and allows researchers to detect trends that predict health care needs of the individual and the community. In addition, research questions are often generated through review of data trends obtained from health care records.

PRINCIPLES OF DOCUMENTATION

Whether documentation is computerized or handwritten, the principles are the same. These principles imply rules for legibility, brevity, sequence, corrections, omissions, signing, and confidentiality. Proper charting should follow the principles of effective documentation, and it uses correct terminology as well as abbreviations. Charting too quickly may lead to incomplete entries or statements that do not communicate the intended meaning.

The client's chart is a legal record and therefore must conform to certain legal standards. Because the record is a permanent legal record, ink is used in handwritten records. Black ink allows the chart to be duplicated with adequate readability for long-term storage. Documentation that is clear, accurate, and legally sound requires following certain rules of charting (Box 11-1).

Terminology

Terminology should be commonly understood by the health care team and should communicate clearly and concisely. Entries in clients' records include standard medical and nursing terminology and commonly recognized abbreviations to facilitate communication. Standard abbreviations and certain symbols are consistently used in the health professions to

---

Box 11-1	Do's and Don't's of Charting

- DO be sure to know the agency policies and procedures about documentation.
- DO check the name on the chart before making an entry.
- DO chart brief, concise, and complete entries. Eliminate all unnecessary words.
- DO sign each entry or follow agency policy for initialing entries.
- DO use objective, measurable terms.
- DO use black ink.
- DO write neatly and legibly.
- DO use standard abbreviations whenever necessary and only those acceptable to the agency.
- DO use quotes whenever appropriate to relate what the client actually said.
- DO write entries logically and sequentially.
- DO make addendums as needed.
- DO make entries about nursing care as close to the time of delivery as possible.
- DO report failure of client to follow treatment regimens and to take medications or receive treatments, and the rationale given by the client.
- DON'T sign anyone else's entry or document for someone else.
- DON'T skip lines or spaces.
- DON'T use the word "client" or "patient" throughout the document.
- DON'T write opinions or biased statements.
- DON'T make entries suggesting an error or unsafe practice.
- DON'T repeat narratively if flow sheets and other forms are used for the same information.

communicate in an abridged format. Consistency in their use saves time and space without interrupting communication. Health care facilities compile lists of acceptable abbreviations and symbols that are used in that facility. It is your responsibility to become acquainted with accepted abbreviations in a particular agency. (See the inside back cover of this book for common abbreviations.)

What may be an acceptable medical abbreviation in one geographical or specialty area may be unheard or used differently in another area. For example, PAT is a fairly common abbreviation for paroxysmal atrial tachycardia, but this term may also be used on obstetrical units to abbreviate pregnancy at term or on other units to indicate preadmission testing.

Action Alert! Use only approved abbreviations.

Symbols and medical terms that represent root words, prefixes, and suffixes are used to condense charting entries. When you break down words into root words and understand prefixes and suffixes added to root words, it helps you to decipher what unfamiliar words mean. Knowledge of these word parts will assist you in building a good medical vocabulary, and they should be committed to memory (Table 11-1).

Legibility

Legibility is essential when documenting in the health care record. Entries may be made in script or print—whichever is more legible. Proper use of terms and correct spelling are extremely important. Poor handwriting and spelling reflect negatively on you and could be translated by a jury as inadequate nursing care.

Action Alert! Consider the consequences of trying to interpret charting that is not readable. Recalling information from illegible entries may be difficult or even impossible if the record is requested in a court of law several years after the entries were made.

Brevity

Charting entries should be as brief as possible. Sentences are stripped to essential components, eliminating all words that can be stripped without changing the intended meaning of the entry. This includes articles such as "a" and "the" as well as the subject of the sentence.

SAMPLE CHARTING		
7/16/02	0700	Dentures removed/cleaned with Polident. Oral mucous membranes smooth, pink, s̄ lesions. Assisted c̄ bed bath, linens changed.
		C. Lott, RN

Note that neither the client's name nor the word *client* or *patient* was charted because *all* entries are about the client. If necessary, the name of the person notified when the client

is admitted, results of laboratory work, or any important detail that is to be reported by orders of the physician may be used in the charting. Using an actual name should be followed by the title or position of the person. This is not absolutely necessary but it does eliminate confusion if the physician did not receive the information requested. An example would be the following:

SAMPLE CHARTING		
7/16/02	0940	Report of STAT CBC called to Jane Doe, RN at Dr. Smith's office.
		C. Lott, RN

Completeness

Although brevity is essential, you should document all information necessary to explain the events of a shift. Anyone reading the documentation should have a clear picture of what took place or is being described. If necessary, direct quotes can be used to describe what a client said. The need for complete entries is critical when a record is used in a court of law. Remember that charting may be read or audited years later by various people including nurses, physicians, peer-review organizations, lawyers, and others who have never seen the client (Raymond, 2001).

Action Alert! Always chart each significant event with the time it occurred. Entries do not have to be made on the hour but when they occur. From a legal perspective, entries not made in a client's record imply actions not taken or treatments not given. It may be helpful to remember the saying, "If you didn't chart it, you didn't do it."

Sequence and Timeliness

Recording of information on the client's record must be sequential. Noting the time and date is important for evaluating client care and for legal purposes. Every charting format has a single place for the year, month, and date to be recorded, thus eliminating the need for documenting the date with every entry. However, the exact time for every event must be included with each entry and should include A.M. or P.M. unless military time is used.

The exact time events occur during the shift and the amount of time between events becomes critically important when special medication is given, follow-up care is necessary, a client's condition changes, or vital procedures, such as organ transplants, are being planned. Inaccurate times or prolonged time between entries may indicate poor implementation of standards of care.

Charting statements should be logically organized according to time (0800, 0840, 0915, 0935, and so on) and content. Just as you must use an organized sequence so that you do not omit any information when assessing a client, documentation of data collection should also be organized and logical in sequence. The statement is also more easily read when written

Table 11-1 Symbols, Root Words, Prefixes, and Suffixes Used in Documentation

Term	Meaning	Term	Meaning
SYMBOLS		**ROOT WORDS—CONT'D**	
>	greater than	thora	chest
<	less than	uro	urine
↑	increase	vaso	vessel
↓	decrease	veno	vein
Δ	change		
~	approximately	**PREFIXES**	
+	positive	a- or an-	without
−	negative	anti-	against
M	murmur	bi-	twice, two
2°	secondary to	bio-	life
✔	check on	brady-	slow
		chole-	bile; gall
ROOT WORDS		di-	double
		dys-	difficult, painful
adeno	gland	ecto-	outside
angio	vessel	endo-	within
arterio	artery	hemi-	half
arthro	joint	hyper-	above; excessive
cardio	heart	hypo-	decreased
cerebro	brain	leuko-	white
cyst	bladder	noct-	night
cyto	cell	olig-	deficiency
derma	skin	para-	beside
hemo	blood	peri-	around
hepato	liver	poly-	many; multiple
hystero	uterus	retro-	backward
lith	stone; calculus	supra-	above
meningo	meninges	tachy-	fast
myelo	bone marrow, spinal cord	trans-	across
myo	muscle	uni-	one
nephro	kidney		
neuro	nerves	**SUFFIXES**	
-oma	tumor	-cele	swelling, protrusion
ophtha	eye	-ectomy	removal
ortho	straight	-emesis	vomiting
osteo	bone	-emia	blood
oto	ear	-graph, -gram	tracing
-oxia	oxygen	-itis	inflammation
patho	disease	-ostomy	artificial opening
phlebo	vein	-otomy	incision of; cutting into
pnea, pneum	breathing; lungs	-penia	deficiency; lack of
pyelo	renal pelvis	-plasty	repair of
pyo	pus	-rhea	discharge
pyro	heat	-uria	urine
reno	kidney		
thrombo	blood clot		

in a logical pattern. Entries should be logical according to the format of charting being used (e.g., head-to-toe approach, body systems).

Corrections

The two types of corrections commonly made to a record are correcting a written entry and adding an entry later. Individual agency policies may vary for the correct format to use when correcting an entry. Common policies include drawing a single line through the entry alone or drawing a single line and writing the word *void* or *error* in the space above the incorrect entry, followed by the initials of the writer. The word *error* may still be used by some agencies, but it is no longer recommended because it implies a wrong. A single line instead of multiple lines is required to keep the incorrect entry legible.

Action Alert! Never attempt to obscure original entries. Erasing, whiting out, or blackening the entry is not permitted because of the implication of covering up an error or mistake.

In the event an entry needs to be made on the client's record for 0830, but another nurse has already made a notation for 0915, making the entry out of sequence, an addendum must be written. It would be incorrect to avoid entering the note on the chart. This information must be noted as an addendum. Consider the following example:

SAMPLE CHARTING		
7/16/02	0910	Abdominal dressing changed per Dr. Jones. Suture line intact with small amt. serosanguineous drainage noted at proximal edge. C. Lott, RN
	0935	Addendum 0830 Assisted to chair per P.T. c̄ assistance X2 and use of walker. c/o weakness and instructed not to weight bear on Ⓛ leg. C. Lott, RN

Note that in the previous example, the time of each entry remains sequential (0910, then 0935). The event time of the late entry (0830), however, is made after the word *addendum.* The time 0830 is when the nursing action actually occurred. Addenda should be avoided as much as possible. Charting in a timely manner throughout the shift instead of once or twice toward the end of the shift usually prevents entries from being out of sequence. Timely documentation also promotes adequate detail and helps with overall time management of the shift in the event of emergent transfer of a client.

If information that is omitted is recalled a day or several days later, it should be noted in the current notes with the current date and time, followed by "addendum to nurse's notes of [month, day, and year]," followed by the entry. Agency policy will specify if the term *late entry* rather than *addendum* should be used.

In rereading an entry, you often discover that certain words needed to clarify an entry have been accidentally omitted. An omitted word or phrase must not be squeezed between words in small letters or inserted above or below a written line. An addendum would need to be made to clarify the entry with the necessary description.

Omissions

Blank spaces are not to be left on the chart. As much as possible, you should write to the end of a line instead of leaving the space blank. Avoid writing outside of the lines (in the margin) of the charting form. A horizontal line is drawn through any empty space to the right margin to prevent later entries from being made in front of a signature.

Consider the following correct example:

SAMPLE CHARTING		
7/16/02	0910	Penrose drain intact, compressed, & draining 400 ml serosanguineous fluid. Reports no discomfort. Foley draining clear, yellow urine with 300 ml output. C. Lott, RN

If a part of a page is blank at the end of the 24-hour time period, an X should be drawn through the remainder of the page. Notes should flow from shift to shift, and a new set of notes should be started after 24 hours.

If it is necessary to recopy a page of the chart, the person copying the page should date and time the entry and write "Copied by . . ." followed by his or her signature. Copying a chart usually requires written consent by the client or responsible party.

Signatures

The correct way to sign a notation in the client's record is using the first initial and full last name, followed by the abbreviation of the health care worker's position title (RN, LPN, SN). Some agencies require the full first and last names followed by an abbreviation of the individual's current position. You usually sign to the far right of the entry once it is complete.

Traditionally, SN has been the accepted abbreviation for student nurse. Even if the student has another title such as LPN (licensed practical nurse), he or she is to use the abbreviation for student nurse when functioning in that capacity. The student nurse may also be required to write the initials of the school affiliation along with the title SN. A written signature must follow every entry into a client's record. In this way, institutions provide a guarantee that the right person gave the care. It is also how an agency would determine who gave the care, if a record is reviewed at a later date.

The correct format would be as follows:

SAMPLE CHARTING		
7/16/02	1530	Awake & oriented to time, place, & person. Skin warm and dry. C. Lott, RN
	1600	CBC drawn per lab. C. Lott, RN
	1645	To radiology via wheelchair for CXR. C. Lott, RN

When a form has only enough space for initials, there will always be a signature key for the professional to sign, to identify the initials.

Confidentiality

All client records are confidential files that require written permission of the client to be copied. Information within the chart is often of a personal matter as well as legal evidence of the care provided and should be available to the necessary health team members only. Client records are not accessible to insurance companies, significant others, research teams, or third parties (including payors) without the written permission of the client. Clients themselves must sign and submit a request for the information from their medical file.

> *Action Alert!* Safeguard all client information. It is the responsibility of the nurse and other health team members to maintain confidentiality concerning medical records within any medical facility. This includes being sure that no documents are left unattended in public areas.

CONTENT OF DOCUMENTATION

Although agencies vary in their specific requirements about what needs to be charted, you should develop a systematic approach to documentation of client care. The system may be a head-to-toe, body-systems, problem-oriented, human-needs, functional health patterns, or any other organized approach for deriving significant data to be documented. Regardless of your choice of organizational method, there are guidelines that should be followed. All significant client care should be documented either in narrative (progress) notes or on **flow sheets** (forms used to document data that can be more easily followed in graphic or tabular form).

On admission to a facility, most health care agencies require a health history to be completed, followed by a current needs assessment. These may be combined or on separate forms. The format and degree of detail will vary according to the health care agency. The registered nurse on the unit usually completes the initial health history form, which then becomes a permanent part of the chart. The person who took the health history or the person assuming responsibility for care of the client may complete the current needs assessment. Some forms for this process are more structured, such as a checklist format with which you can easily check or circle observations. Other forms are unstructured but usually list areas to be assessed, with room for you to write narrative observations. If no specific form is used by the agency for this purpose, write narrative notes. After completing these admission forms, document the client's arrival and subsequent care needs.

Types of Entries

Various types of entries may be made in a chart. Among these are admit notes for a newly admitted client, change-of-shift notes, assessment findings, interval or progress notes, transfer and discharge notes, client teaching notes, and descriptions of observations.

Admit Notes. On assuming responsibility for a new client who just entered the facility, you usually record an admit note. An **admit note** (or admission note) is the first nurse's note acknowledging the arrival of a new client. Following the admit note, a narrative entry noting the complete assessment is made, and this is followed by notes describing the client's

current status at appropriate intervals, with notations of any changes in the client's condition. On arrival, documentation of the client's orientation to the facility should be made. If the admission history or assessment form provides a place for this information, an additional narrative note is not necessary.

The admit note usually includes the following: time of arrival, age, sex, how the client arrived, where the client came from, medical diagnosis, chief complaint, general appearance, treatments in progress, allergies, vital signs (if required by the agency or if abnormal), notification of physician, and stat (from the Latin *statim,* meaning immediately) laboratory work or orders that have been completed (Figure 11-1).

Change-of-Shift Notes. At the change of shift, you do not need to document an admit note for a client who has been in the facility for a period of time. Instead, you usually begin each shift with documentation of the client assessment made on rounds. Any format is acceptable, but the documentation should include a thorough assessment of the client's current status, followed by interval notes describing any change in the client's status related to expected outcomes. It may be a requirement of the facility to note that a report was received or given and by whom.

SAMPLE CHARTING		
7/16/02	0834	Shift report received from S. Smith, RN. Awake & alert on rounds. [continue note with current assessment data]

| 7/14/03 | 1400 | 68-year-old female admitted to room 268A via stretcher from ER with dx. Fx. (L) hip. P 92, BP 142/89, R 21, T 98.8. c/o pain to (L) hip from mid-thigh to greater trochanter area, marked bruising noted in same area s̄ edema at present. Stated fell while gardening and unable to "get up again," lives alone, neighbor called 911. IV of D5W infusing at TKO rate to (R) upper arm s̄ signs of infiltration or inflammation c̄ 950 cc TBA. Nursing history and assessment noted, NKA, Dr. Parker notified of admit, new orders noted. ———— |
| | | *C. Lott, RN* |

Figure 11-1. Example of an admit note.

Assessment Notes. After an admit note or a beginning shift note, a complete assessment of the current status of the client should follow. Documentation of the complete assessment may be entered using different formats: narrative, flow chart, charting by exception, or a combination of various formats. Various methods for charting any entry narratively are acceptable: head-to-toe assessment, body systems, functional health patterns, or nursing diagnosis (Figure 11-2).

Interval or Progress Notes. After the complete assessment is made, interval notes should be entered. Agencies use one of the following terms: *interval notes, progress notes,* or *daily notes.* **Interval notes** or **progress notes** are nursing notes entered at various times during a shift; they reflect any aspect of change in client condition or anything affecting the client such as tests, stat or prn (as needed) medications, and procedures. Content to include in an interval note is determined by you and by the condition of the client, but it may include the following: treatments, medications, new orders, ambulation, periods of rest, presence of visitors, special tests, and client symptoms.

When you make rounds on clients, the status of their condition is noted. Documentation at intervals usually means every 2 to 4 hours. This will vary depending on the agency policy and perhaps the policy on a unit within the agency. In more critical situations, or whenever a client's condition warrants, entries may be required more often than every 2 hours and they should include who was notified and if orders were obtained. Charting more frequently than the agency requires is a nursing judgment as long as the agency guidelines are followed for the minimal amount of documentation needed.

If the interval is too long between notations or there is lack of sufficient explanation leading up to a serious change in status, the documentation is not acceptable. The status of the client may remain unchanged on rounds and can be noted as such by you.

Transfer and Discharge Notes. When a client is transferred to another facility or to another unit, whether temporarily or permanently, you should write a transfer note. A **transfer note** is a nursing note that reflects the movement of a client from one unit to another within the agency, or to another agency. Policies should exist on every unit for specific content to include in a transfer note. Generally, the notation includes the reason for transfer, method of transportation, person giving and receiving the report, notification of physicians or family members, and the condition of the client, including vital signs and treatments in progress (Figure 11-3).

7/14/03	1430	Awake, alert, oriented x3. PERRLA. Stated feels "tired and exhausted from experience." Resp. even, non-labored. Lungs clear in all lobes. Heart sounds normal S1 and S2, regular rhythm. Radial pulses equal, regular, and palpable + 2/3. IV to (R) upper arm of D5W infusing at TKO rate c̄ 900 cc TBA s̄ signs of infiltration or phlebitis. Finger capillary refill <3 sec. bilaterally. Abdomen soft c̄ active bowel sounds in all 4 quadrants. Denies difficulty c̄ bowel or bladder. (L) hip bruised, non-edematous, painful to touch. Trochanter roll in place to keep leg aligned. Peripheral pulses palpable, +2/3, equal. No edema to extremities. Feet warm and dry c̄ toe capillary refill <3 sec. SR up x2, neighbor at bedside. ————— C. Lott, RN

Figure 11-2. Example of an assessment note.

7/18/03	0900	Transfer arrangements to Heritage skilled facility for services of Dr. Warren complete. Hospital chart copied, to be sent with client. ————— C. Lott, RN
	1110	Transferred to Heritage skilled facility by stretcher per AST Ambulance Service. Neighbor, Sandy, present, copy of hospital chart given to ambulance attendant, J. Wild. No treatments in progress. No acute distress, skin warm and dry. Color flesh-toned. (L) hip incision clean and dry s̄ irritation or redness. Denies pain at present. Peripheral pulses palpable, + 2/4, and equal. T 98.9, P 76, R 18, BP 132/78. ————— C. Lott, RN

Figure 11-3. Example of a transfer note.

A similar notation should be made when a client is sent for a test within the same facility, but less information is usually required. Information to be included depends on the client's condition and may include place (e.g., laboratory, x-ray), method of transfer (e.g., wheelchair, stretcher), persons accompanying the client, attachments (e.g., drainage tubes), level of consciousness, and vital signs.

When the client returns to a unit, a note should be made that includes appropriate assessment of the client's condition, time of arrival, method of transfer, and attachments. Depending on the reason for the absence from the unit, specific assessment findings may be required in this entry, such as vital signs, level of consciousness, and ability to swallow.

When a client is discharged from the hospital, a discharge note should be made to close the chart. A **discharge note** is a nursing note that reflects the circumstances around the release of a client from a facility. This entry should not be made until all other necessary entries have been completed. The specific information needed for a discharge note may vary according to the type of facility. Some agencies require a summary of the client's stay showing improvement or reason for discharge, client teaching, and a note addressing the client's understanding of the self-care needed. Like the transfer note, a discharge summary should generally include preparations for the discharge, the time of departure, method of transportation, family members present, condition of the client, vital signs, community resources to assist the client, client teaching, prescriptions, and any other necessary paperwork given to the client (Figure 11-4).

Client Teaching Notes.
Instructions given to a client need careful documentation. If the client is unable to understand or prefers, a family member or significant other should be taught. An assessment should be conducted to determine the learning method preferred by the client or family member.

Client teaching may include medications, wound care, diabetic care, activity restrictions or progression, or diet. The method of teaching may include videos, discussion, reading, demonstration, and return demonstration. The content that is taught needs to be documented, as does the method of teaching. In addition, the time frame, person responsible for teaching, client's readiness to learn, and the results of the teaching need to be charted. If more than just the client is involved, noting who attended the teaching session is important. If pamphlets or booklets are given to the client for further reading, they (along with title and date of publication) should be noted.

How the client responds to the teaching must be documented. To evaluate the teaching, it is essential to determine whether clients or family members can return-demonstrate a skill such as wound care or explain the information in their own words.

All teaching that occurs should be noted, including reinforcement of information already taught. Special teaching forms may be required in an agency by staff assigned to this responsibility. When client educators teach the client or family, you should note that in the narrative.

Descriptions of Observations.
Nurses' notes should be recorded objectively. State observations rather than opinions. Furthermore, if you believe that a client is less alert today than yesterday, you should describe the client's state of awareness today rather than stating "not as alert today."

Subjective data presented by the client are included in the nurse's notes and should be clearly labeled as such. Precede the subjective data by "States," indicating that the client is relating the information, or by using quotation marks around the client's exact words.

Vague documentation should be avoided at all times. Words such as "seems to be" or "apparently" should not be used. It is more descriptive to document the behavior that led to a conclusion. Similarly, adjectives such as *good, some, a little, bad,* and *better* should be avoided, because these terms are relative and may have different meanings for people using them.

Although the term *normal* may be used to describe some physical assessment, it is usually not the best choice for most entries. Of course, unflattering adjectives that characterize the client's behavior (e.g., obnoxious, ignorant) should never be used.

Action Alert! Write nurse's notes to convey an accurate, objective picture of the client or the facts pertaining to a client situation.

7/30/03	1320	Dr. Warren visited c̄ orders to d/c current meds. Home health nurse S. Beil, RN, notified of discharge and arrangements for first visit made. PT notified of D/C and need for education. ——————— K. Smith, RN
	1400	PT visited concerning walker and reinforced proper use. ——— K. Smith, RN
	1430	Neighbor notified and on her way. ——— K. Smith, RN
	1500	Neighbor present. HL in Ⓡ upper arm discontinued. Site s̄ redness or warmth. T 98⁶, P 68, R 22, BP 110/72. No complaints. Skin warm and dry. Ⓛhip incision healing, intact s̄ inflammation or irritation. Pedal pulses + 2/3, equal, feet warm and dry. Discharge instructions given c̄ prescription for Lasix and Lanoxin. Neighbor stated she would pick up her prescriptions on the way home. ——— K. Smith, RN
	1525	Discharged per wc s̄ distress. ——— K. Smith, RN

Figure 11-4. Example of a discharge note.

Symptoms and Complaints. Any symptom or complaint should be documented in detail. These may include subjective or objective data and should be specific in terms of location, duration, intensity, amount, size, and frequency. With any complaint noted, there should be evidence of care given and the client's response to the care.

Dressings, Tubes, or Attached Devices. Observations of tubes should be documented in the initial entry of each shift and at least every 2 hours thereafter. Documentation should be more frequent when the condition requires it. Notations about dressings should include the location of the dressing, the nature of the secure attachment of the dressing to client, and the amount as well as a description of any drainage observed. If a dressing is removed, the condition of the skin under it should be described (e.g., edges are approximated; any redness, edema, drainage, sutures, or staples) (Figure 11-5).

Tubes providing intravenous (IV), nasogastric, or gastrostomy feeding should be observed for the fluid being administered, the rate of flow, and correct placement, and to ensure that devices are secured with tape or holder. In addition, the infusion site should be noted for any tenderness, redness, edema, or warmth. An IV site is usually assessed at least every 2 hours. Notation of the IV site may be included on a flow sheet. The type and condition of any feeding or gastrostomy tube (e.g., Levin, Keo-feed, PEG) should also be recorded, along with documentation of patency and proper placement. Use of an infusion pump and the reason for it must be noted (see Figure 11-5). If an agency policy requires the use of a pump for certain age groups or for clients with specific conditions, this can be noted as "IV D_5W 50 cc to R arm per pump."

Notations concerning any drainage tubes should include the location and patency of the tube, attachment to any drainage or suction system, and a description of any drainage. The description of drainage should include color, character, odor, and amount. Specific amounts are recorded on the intake and output (I&O) flow sheet at specified intervals (see Figure 11-5). Agencies may use flow sheets rather than narrative notes for documenting all data related to attachments.

Medications and Treatments. Most agencies maintain a medication administration record (MAR) for the purpose of documenting all medications and treatments. Sometimes a medication or treatment is directed to be given stat (immediately). When the direction is to give the medication or treatment prn (as needed), with the decision based on your judgment, a statement should be charted in the progress notes about the events that led to your decision. For example, if you give a client a medication that has been ordered prn for pain, you should document when you gave it by entering the time you gave it and your initials on the MAR. In the progress notes write why you gave it, and include an adequate description of the pain (e.g., location, type, intensity). A follow-up note must be recorded at an appropriate interval to evaluate the effectiveness of the medication or treatment. When documenting the effects of a medication or treatment, take care to record all the information objectively (see Figure 11-5).

> *Action Alert!* Documentation should include a follow-up note related to the client's response to prn medications at appropriate time intervals, to show an acceptable standard of care.

There are times when a medication or treatment is not given as ordered. This may be because, in your judgment, it would be harmful for the client at that time, or because the client refuses the treatment or is off the floor when it should be done. In any case, the withholding of the treatment should be documented, along with the explanation for the action. It is also appropriate to notify the physician if any routine medication is withheld, and this too should be documented. An example for Mrs. Geraldine Peters might be as follows:

Dressing	7/15/03	2030	Dressing on ⓛ hip c̄ red 2 cm area of drainage. Dressing changed. Staples present, incision c̄ 2 cm area of redness noted at lateral end. ——— S. Richards, RN
Tubes	7/15/03	2030	IV D5W in ⓡ antecubital space infusing at 50 cc/hr c̄ 300 cc TBA. Site free of redness or edema. Hemovac to ⓛ hip intact, depressed c̄ 50 cc red drainage. ——— S. Richards, RN
Attached Devices	7/15/03	2030	Foley catheter to GU bag patent and draining 300 cc clear, amber urine. ——— S. Richards, RN
Medication and Treatment	7/15/03	2030	Holding ⓛ leg and C/O constant throbbing pain at incision area. Tylox tabs ii given PO. SR up x4, instructed not to get OOB s̄ assistance, call bell in reach. ——— S. Richards, RN
		2245	States "feels much better." No nonverbal expression of discomfort noted. ——— S. Richards, RN
Valuables	7/14/03	1430	Jewelry and keys placed in folder #2396, sent to admit office c̄ J. Zimmerman, clerk. Client provided receipt. ——— S. Richards, RN

Figure 11-5. Descriptions of observations.

SAMPLE CHARTING		
7/16/02	0910	C/O sharp, constant pain in ⓡ hip, requesting pain medication. BP 98/50, P 62, RR 10. Oriented X3. Responds to verbal stimuli but easily returns to sleep. Explained the need to wait for pain medicine due to

	SAMPLE CHARTING, CONT'D
	low BP & resp. and length
	of time since last injection
	3 hours (order is for q4
	hrs). Will reassess in 15
	minutes. C. Lott, RN———
0920	Continues to c/o pain in Ⓛ
	hip. Pain a level 7 on 1-10
	scale with 10 being most
	severe. VS unchanged. Pain
	medication not lasting be-
	tween ordered frequency.
	Dr. Smith notified of com-
	plaint of pain. New orders
	noted. C. Lott, RN———

Observations of Psychosocial Status. In addition to physical needs, you should document significant data related to psychosocial status. Assess the client's sensorium in relation to level of consciousness and orientation to time, place, and person. Any confusion or change in consciousness is significant and should be documented specifically.

The safety and security needs of clients seeking health care are frequently threatened, resulting in anxiety. Any evidence of fear or anxiety should be documented in the client's record. If a client decides to leave the facility against the advice of the physician (unless ordered by law to be admitted), note the same information as a routine discharge but chart "left AMA" (i.e., against medical advice). If the client states a reason for leaving, this should be included in the narrative. The physician should be notified of any AMA situation and an entry made in the chart as to this notification. Any additional agency policies should also be followed.

Activities of Daily Living. Activities of daily living (ADLs) are often documented primarily on flow sheets and should be recorded by the person administering care. If a flow sheet is not available, ADLs should be noted in narrative format. Information recorded related to ADLs includes type of bath, oral hygiene, change of linen, and type of assistance needed. The type of assistance and the number of health care workers needed to move a client from place to place should also be included. Examples of ways to note transfer needs include independent, minimal supervision and/or assistance, continuous supervision and/or assistance of one person, continuous assistance of two persons, or total care. ADLs can also be charted using terminology that indicates the client's degree of independence.

Valuables. When a client enters a facility with jewelry or valuables that need to be secured during the stay, an entry should be made that these items were sent to the appropriate department. The detailed description of specific items such as jewelry, and the amount of money in the wallet, should be included with the belongings, usually on the outside of the folder in which they are placed, rather than charted (see Figure 11-5). Describe any valuables such as jewelry in general terms. Instead of "solid gold, one-carat diamond ring," a better description might be "yellow ring with clear stone." Agencies may require the signature of two health care professionals on any documentation of valuables, with a copy placed in the client's chart. If valuables are sent home with a family member, it is important to document the name of the person who took the valuables and the relationship to the client.

Spiritual Care. Spiritual care is often neglected in documentation, but it is an important entry for complete documentation of client care. Entries may need to be included that describe signs and symptoms of spiritual distress, symbols or articles of spiritual meaning, rituals practiced, source of hope, expressions of grief, and notification of chaplain or spiritual advisor.

Safety Concerns. A significant area needing detailed and complete documentation is that of safety issues for the client, particularly the older adult or immobile client. Although flow sheets now include many of these safety concerns, narrative charting may still be needed. Regardless of where the information is written, documenting safety measures taken for each client while in a facility is essential. Examples of important safety concerns include side rails, unsteady gait, assistance needed with ambulation, past medication or surgery, ability to use call lights, knowledge of emergency call lights, use of restraints, offering toiletry if immobile, history of falls, mental changes, and transporting clients. Client teaching about safety should be adequately documented.

Many facilities have special guidelines for including safety concerns, and these are usually required for every client. However, you have the right and responsibility to note safety issues in a factual manner as often as needed (Table 11-2, p. 228).

Significant Notations for Special Populations

Documentation entries need to be made for special groups, such as older adults, children, and culturally diverse clients. Life span considerations in older adults as well as in children are a part of the charting that may not be as necessary for other clients. Issues specific to a client, such as language barriers or dietary customs of a specific culture, should be noted.

Older Adult Clients. Special care should be taken to include accurate and complete descriptions of the skin, ADLs, mobility, mental status, and the behavior of older adult clients. Accurate and descriptive documentation of the physical assessment of these clients on admission is crucial, especially if abuse is suspected. Notes should include how prepared older adults are to go home, the type of assistance needed at home (or, if they are unable to go to their own home, discharge planning—beginning on the day of admittance), and any emotional needs. Throughout older clients' stay in a health care facility, it is essential to document progress in their ability to carry out ADLs so that, if possible, it can be shown on discharge that they are sufficiently able to perform self-care.

Table 11-2	Necessary Charting Entries for Safety Concerns
Medication administration	SR placed up if sedating, instructions given not to get OOB without assistance.
Transporting client	SR placed up, attendant with client at all times.
Admit	Instructions given on using call light and the difference in regular and emergency light.
Restraints	Notation according to agency policy; offered water, meal, bathroom privileges; ROM and skin condition checked.
Ambulation	Assistance required, use of house shoes, use of assistive devices such as walker, cane.
Change in LOC or sensorium from a recent major event such as surgery	Instructions given not to get up the first time without health care assistance. VS taken if dizziness experienced or change in LOC. SR up if disoriented, notification of doctor if status changes, presence of sitter or family member.
Falls	Actual facts as reported by client, family, and health care workers should be included. Actual assessment findings on first discovering the accident, including the position client was in when found; notification of physician, family, or house supervisor. Also specific accounts leading up to the event. Report what was done, such as x-rays and notification of physician. Note the history of falls during last hospitalization or at home when admitting the client.

| 7/14/03 | 0800 | Remains alert, oriented x3. Assist c̄ AM care on a daily basis, dresses self. Attends activity 1 or 2x per month, joins in c̄ other residents. Likes to visit Mrs. Brown in room 112-A. Family visited 3x this month and took her on pass for a day. Seemed to enjoy the visit. Eating in the dining room and assists others c̄ their trays. No change in overall condition. (L) hip incision healed, uses (L) hip c̄ assist of walker. Physical therapy visits 2x per week, tolerates P.T. s̄ any problems. Continent of bowel and bladder. Sleeps uninterrupted for 6-8 hours per night. —— S. Richards, RN |

Figure 11-6. Example of an entry in a long-term care facility.

Box 11-2	Guidelines for Extended and Long-Term Care

- Know the requirements of the regulating body of the agency; read quarterly reviews, know when to document.
- Know policies and procedures of the facility.
- Note phone calls, visits by relatives, interactions with other clients.
- Verify how nurses spend their time with the client on a visit; be aware of issues concerning reimbursement.
- Be specific in indicating progress or lack thereof (e.g., ambulated 10 feet on 7/21/99, progressed to 15 feet on 7/22/99).
- Record supplies used.
- Note activities performed by nurses for other departments on the weekends: continuous passive motion machines, physical therapy, electrocardiography, and so on.
- Describe a clear picture that includes fine details: could not open milk carton or use utensils; after meat cut and packages opened, self-fed without problems.
- Include entries that reflect progress or lack of progress toward the goals and objectives on the client's plan of care.
- Include the client's response to drug therapies.

Pediatric Clients. Special attention should be paid to document observations about the relationship between parents and child, dependence of the child on the parent, developmental level of the child (related to age), ability of the child to play, language used by child and parents, and any additional emotional needs for children. Examples might include the following: mother rocks child and reads a book; child speaks in complete, simple sentences; or child able to stack blocks, play hide-and-seek, and self-entertain with colors. Accurate and descriptive documentation of the physical assessment of children on admission is crucial, especially if abuse is suspected.

Clients From Varied Cultures. Suggested areas for documentation for culturally diverse clients include native language, fluency of English, ability to read and write, beliefs about cause of illness, dietary differences (foods excluded or preferred), special concerns related to religious beliefs, and individual needs, such as for uninterrupted time for meditation.

Extended and Long-Term Care

Extended-care facilities may have additional forms that are used for documentation. The use of a classification system to show acuity and specifications of the amount or type of equipment or supplies is often included in documentation for extended-care and long-term-care facilities. Group sessions with family members, planning a home visit in preparation for discharge, or visits with social workers to discuss discharge options are also included. Long-term-care facilities may require weekly or monthly charting in a summary manner as opposed to daily or shift notations. Narrative entries are usu-

ally made about such items as the client's abilities, progress, or degenerative changes (Figure 11-6). Box 11-2 is a list of guidelines for documentation in these types of facilities.

Home Health Guidelines

Documentation in a home health care setting is often different from documenting in an acute care facility because of the need to justify the visit by a professional nurse. Home health nurses usually document an initial assessment with a complete database. Visits thereafter are usually progress notes for each visit and include direct care, teaching or instructions given, performance of skills, and evaluation of homebound status. Home health nurses use progress notes written in narrative format that should be consistent with other disciplines charting on the same client. With each visit, the need for the help of a professional health care worker must be noted. Reimbursement for the visit is directly related to the accuracy and wording of the documentation showing a need for profes-

Table 11-3 — Guidelines for Beginning Nurses in a Home Health Setting

DIRECT SKILLED CARE

Diverse and involved care that can be provided only by trained professionals	• Catheter changes, catheter care • Wound care • Treatments/administering medications • Injections/administering medications • Ostomy care • Aseptic technique • Heat treatments • Tube feedings

CLIENT TEACHING

A part of any skill done	• Inclusion of client and family • Response to information • Ability to perform activity independently • Verbalizes understanding of the instruction • Booklets or educational material left for client or family

HOMEBOUND STATUS

Inability to leave home to obtain similar health care services at a clinic, doctor's office, or outpatient clinic	• Reason for status on admit, and weekly thereafter • Support of other disciplines • Evaluation

SAMPLE CHARTING—CONT'D

No change in size of Ⓛ heel pressure ulcer. Family turning client q 2 hours and keeping heels clear of mattress as directed. Family still unable to perform wound care.
K. Hobson, RN

Table 11-4 — Examples of Charting Entries for Medications

Irritating medications such as hydroxyzine (Vistaril) or iron	Must chart IM "Z-track"
Antiarrhythmics	Change in the cardiac rhythm
Pain medication	Safety measure after administered, VS, relief obtained
Antianginals/ antihypertensives	VS
Insulin administration	Glucose value before administration, condition of client during peak times
Diuretics	Recent electrolyte values, signs or symptoms of electrolyte loss
Heparin or anticoagulants	Coagulation laboratory tests; PT, PTT
Allergies	What specific response the client has

sional assistance. General guidelines are offered for beginning nurses in a home health setting (Table 11-3).

Additional suggestions for effective charting in a home health situation include the following:

- Leave out extraneous information that could affect reimbursement.
- Record all equipment and supplies used at the visit. Know which medical equipment can be provided and document why.
- Avoid vague statements like "doing better" or "no acute distress."
- Monitor new procedures to ensure that all personnel are doing the same thing.
- Note safety concerns such as "throw rugs removed from path to BR."

Key terms in home health include *assessment, instructions,* and *skilled care.* Home health nurses must be especially confident in knowing definitions and in medication administration. All charting should be made with the assumption that the documents will probably be audited. Following is an example of home health charting:

SAMPLE CHARTING

7/16/02	0905	Wound area remains open, wound edges irregular; sacral wound area intact, stage 2 has decreased in size: 2 cm L and 2 cm W.

Problem areas frequently identified in charting for home health care clients include the following:

- Lack of a clear picture of what is going on with the client
- Discrepancies between what went on with the client and what appeared in the chart
- Difficulty in determining the client's status, functional limitations, current level of activity, or homebound status
- Why the nurse is seeing and needs to continue seeing the client
- Failure to document for Medicare reimbursement

Special Entries

Finally, several situations require special notations in which you should make complete and accurate explanations. First, notification of physicians should include the time they were notified, how they were notified (e.g., direct call, beeper), and why. When the physician responds, note the time and the action taken as a result of the phone call. Failure on the part of the physician to respond should be noted as well. Second, any follow-up entry should emphasize what actions were taken, why, and the client's response.

Third, charting results of specific laboratory tests or nursing actions when administering certain classifications of medications is generally expected (Table 11-4). For example, adjusting a heparin drip according to a sliding scale order would include noting the partial thromboplastin time (PTT) value and the adjusted rate of the heparin. Documentation of a blood pressure or pulse is required for many classes of cardiac medications such as digoxin (Lanoxin) or antihypertensives.

DOCUMENTATION FORMATS

Types of Records

Health care records have traditionally been organized in one of two ways: problem oriented or source oriented. The emergence of case management has introduced critical/clinical pathways as another method of organizing client care information.

Problem-Oriented Records.
Problem-oriented medical records are a form of documentation originally designed to organize information according to identified client problems, with all members of the health team documenting information sequentially. Problem-oriented records consist of four components: the database, the problem list, initial plans for each problem, and progress notes for each problem. All members of the health care team make entries on the same record using the same problem list. Problems are added to the list using the language appropriate for the health care provider making the entry. For example, physicians would add medical diagnoses, whereas nurses would use nursing diagnoses. The primary advantages of this system are the inclusion of a common problem list and the ease with which all members of a health care team can monitor progress related to each problem.

Source-Oriented Records.
Source-oriented medical records are a type of medical record with separate divisions according to health discipline (e.g., medicine, nursing, laboratory, respiratory care). These records include information about care given, the client's response to care, and other events documented chronologically and sequentially in a specific location in the record designated for the particular health team member making the entry.

Documentation Format

Regardless of the organization of the medical record itself, health care agencies may choose from a variety of formats for documentation. The format chosen depends on the type of agency, the primary purposes of documentation, and the types of health care workers involved. Regardless of the format, the principles, the mechanics, and generally even the content remain the same. How the content is recorded, however, depends on the format chosen. This discussion addresses several formats currently used including the use of flow sheets for documenting relevant data.

The format for documentation may be a free-style narrative, it may be problem focused or process focused, or it may be a combination of these. Source-oriented records that separate parts of the chart by discipline might still use a problem-oriented approach to document nursing care. Additionally, flow sheets are used to document routine daily care.

Narrative Charting.
Narrative charting is a method of charting that provides information in the form of statements that describe events surrounding client care. It is often relatively unstructured, providing you with flexibility in determining how information is recorded, or the format may be structured and problem focused. Free-style narrative charting allows anyone reading the record to easily follow a sequence of events. Medical as well as nursing interventions may be included and may relate to more than one identified problem at the same time. It also allows inclusion of significant events related to the client that might not be directly related to an identified client problem.

The method is, however, time consuming and makes retrieval of information and tracking of progress and outcomes more difficult. In addition, the lack of specific prompting of notations in terms of times or identified problems often leads to entries that fail to sufficiently address client problems. Entries may also include unnecessary or meaningless notations simply because you feel compelled to write *something* at periodic time intervals. You should avoid duplication of content already included on the record to reduce discrepancies in data.

Narrative documentation can easily be combined with flow sheets to retain the advantage of complete descriptions when desirable, together with the brevity of the flow sheet when descriptive data is not needed. Examples of narrative charting have been used throughout this chapter.

Problem-Focused Charting.
APIE (PIE), focus, and **SOAP formats** for charting allow documentation using the nursing process. Advantages of problem-focused formats include easy reference to specific problems and use of the nursing process. One disadvantage cited by nurses is that all entries must relate to a specific problem on the problem list, making it difficult to document events unrelated to an identified problem. Most systems require charting about problems periodically, even if unchanged. Therefore, this format may not be the most efficient for some settings, particularly long-term care. If several problems are included on the problem list, documentation may be lengthy. Regardless of the format used, the problem list must remain current and accurate.

APIE (PIE) Charting. The acronym APIE stands for the following:

A   Assessment
P   Problem identification
I   Interventions
E   Evaluation

The process begins with an admission assessment that is usually completed on a separate form, and the initiation of a problem list (which may be in the form of a nursing diagnosis or a problem statement) that is based on the initial assessment. An example of a problem list for Ms. Peters is found in Figure 11-7, and Figure 11-8 shows examples of data entries using the APIE format.

Some agencies include data to support the problem identified, by adding AEB (as evidenced by) to the diagnosis. For example, *Pain related to surgical incision AEB guarding of incision and verbal complaints of pain.* Some problem lists may also include goals or expected outcomes for each problem.

Documentation of client care is focused on interventions and evaluation related to problems listed. Each entry in the

Date/Initials	Problem #	Nursing Diagnosis	Date Resolved/Initials
7/15/03 BSM	#1	Pain related to surgical incision.	
7/15/03 BSM	#2	Risk for infection related to surgical incision.	
7/15/03 CRT	#3	Impaired home maintenance related to impaired mobility	

Figure 11-7. Example of an APIE problem list.

progress notes is preceded by the date, time, and problem number, and it indicates whether the entry relates to implementation or evaluation (see Figure 11-8).

Each problem should be evaluated at least once per shift (and some agencies may require more frequent entries). Only information related to implementation or evaluation of problems on the problem list is included in the progress notes. Once the initial or admission assessment is complete, routine assessment is recorded each shift on a flow sheet. An "assessment" entry is not required in the progress notes unless there is a change in the client's status. For example, if the client introduced earlier with the nursing diagnosis of *Pain related to surgical incision* complains later of constipation, this would be noted as in Figure 11-8. Problem number 4 would also be added to the problem list. As problems are resolved, the date is indicated on the problem list.

FOCUS CHARTING. **Focus charting** is a method of charting that addresses client problems or needs and includes a column that summarizes the focus of the entry. It does not necessarily require the use of a nursing diagnosis (some agencies use nursing diagnoses for the focus; others do not). This focus can include a nursing diagnosis, activities or concerns of the client, or other incidents. The format requires using the acronym DAR or the acronym DAE:

DAR	DAE
Data	Data
Action	Action
Response	Evaluation

Data should include all subjective and objective observations, whereas *action* indicates any interventions resulting from the observations. *Response* or *evaluation* entries document the effect of the intervention on the client and may be recorded immediately or at a later time if appropriate. For example, if medication is given for pain, the response will not likely be assessed until sufficient time has been allowed for the medication to be effective. This format also employs flow sheets for documentation of routine observations and interventions. Figure 11-9 (p. 232) is an example of focus charting.

Date	Time	Problem #	Remarks
7/16/03	1600	#1	I = Tylox i given PO for c/o incisional pain. —S. Richards, RN
	1630	#1	E = Sitting in chair at bedside. States pain relieved. —S. Richards, RN
		Assessment	States she feels constipated. Last BM 7/12. Abdomen firm.
		P#4	Constipation related to decreased activity and change in diet.
		I#4	Dr. Alvarez notified. Stool softener adm. as ordered. Encouraged to ↑ fluid intake. Nutrition consult for foods with fiber. —S. Richards, RN

OR

Date	Time	Problem #	Remarks
7/16/03	1600	IP#1	Tylox i given PO for c/o incisional pain. —S. Richards, RN
	1630	EP#1	Sitting in chair at bedside. States pain relieved. —S. Richards, RN
		Assessment	States she feels constipated. Last BM 7/12. Abdomen firm.
		P#4	Constipation related to decreased activity and change in diet.
		IP#4	Dr. Alvarez notified. Stool softener adm. as ordered. Encouraged to ↑ fluid intake. —S. Richards, RN

Figure 11-8. Example of APIE data entries.

Advantages of focus charting include flexibility, easy data retrieval, and close alignment with the nursing process. One disadvantage is the possibility of inconsistency in the labeling of problems.

SOAP CHARTING. **SOAP charting** is used to record progress notes with problem-focused charting. The progress notes include narrative notes as well as flow sheets, and they are used by all members of the health team. The

Date	Time	Focus	Notes
7/16/03	1600	Pain	D = c/o pain at incision site Ⓛ hip. Requests pain medication. ——— S. Richards, RN
			A = Tylox ii given PO. ——— S. Richards, RN
	1600	Dressing	D = Abd. dressing c̄ mod. amt. serous drainage. ——— S. Richards, RN
			A = Dsg. reinforced. ——— S. Richards, RN
	1630	Pain	R = States pain relieved. ——— S. Richards, RN
		Dressing	R = Dsg. dry and intact. ——— S. Richards, RN

Figure 11-9. Example of focus charting.

Date/Time	Problem	Progress Notes
7/16/03 1600	#1 Pain related to surgical incision	S = States discomfort in Ⓛ hip. ——— O = Grimaces c̄ movement to Ⓛ side. Requests pain medication q3h. ———
		A = No change. ———
		P = Continue pain meds prn. ——— S. Richards, RN

Figure 11-10. Example of a progress note in SOAP charting.

narrative notes are specifically related to a problem list and are numbered and titled accordingly. For example, a reference made to a client's surgical incision would be preceded by the number of the problem (from the problem list) and/or the name of the problem (e.g., No. 1, Open reduction and internal fixation).

The format contains four parts, remembered by the acronym SOAP, which stands for

Subjective data
Objective data
Assessment
Plan

Subjective data describe the client's problem as the client sees it; neither measurable nor observable, subjective data must be related to the health care provider by the client. *Objective data* are those items of information that are measurable or observable by another person—for example, laboratory findings. In the *assessment* component of the note, conclusions are summarized on the basis of the data presented, whereas the *plan* outlines actions that will address the identified problem. For example, the plan may include further diagnostic tests, therapeutic medical or nursing interventions, or client education. Often the plan is simply to continue the previously outlined plan.

Sometimes, not all SOAP elements are present or appropriate. For example, if there are no objective data to support a problem, "none" is written by the "O" in the SOAP note. One example of a progress note in the SOAP format is found in Figure 11-10. Advantages of the SOAP format include a uniform problem list used by all personnel and easy reference to data related to specific problems. Disadvantages include lack of flexibility (as seen in the APIE method), as all documentation is directed toward a specific problem.

Charting by Exception.

Charting by exception provides documentation only if data are significant or abnormal. This format reduces lengthy and repetitive charting and allows client progress to be followed more easily. This system pro-

vides comprehensive flow sheets for documentation of both medical and nursing orders. If assessment is within normal limits or unchanged from the previous assessment, no narrative progress notes are necessary. Charting by exception is predicated on establishment of norms for assessment, with forms varying by agency. For example, the 24-hour assessment example included in Figure 11-11 and the entry made in Figure 11-12 (p. 236) are examples of charting by exception.

The flow sheet provides a column for each hour in a 24-hour period. You simply place a check mark (√) or initials in each block to indicate findings at a given time. If assessment findings are normal, no other documentation is needed. Specific notations can be included in the block that indicate specific observations. In Figure 11-11, the notation of 100% is included under diet to indicate the proportion of food consumed. An arrow (↓) is placed in the block indicating bed position. If the nurse initials findings considered abnormal, a detailed description is then required in the progress notes.

Although charting by exception is time efficient and reduces duplication, it is more difficult to identify omissions in care, and details are often limited. It is also more difficult to follow the nursing process using this format. Charting by exception may be misleading when defending care from a legal point of view (Higginbotham, 2001).

Flow Sheets. Regardless of the format, flow sheets are often used to document data that can be more easily followed in graphic or tabular form. They are used in many agencies to facilitate documentation of routine assessment data and nursing interventions in checklist format. Trends related to ADLs, body systems review, and other nursing observations and activities can be easily followed using flow sheets. Checklists and flow sheets provide a method for summarizing client progress in an abbreviated manner, which saves time and often improves the quality of documentation ("Charting tips," 1998). Not only are flow sheets often more legible but they facilitate consistent documentation of assessment and interventions.

The format of the flow sheet may be relatively unstructured, with the nurse adding categories as needed, or it may be very structured, requiring checks in appropriate columns. Structured formats remind you of certain data that should be included at regular intervals, reinforcing standards of care. All flow sheets require date and signature of the person who is making the observation. Some observations will require further description in narrative progress notes.

DATE: 7/15/03 DIAGNOSIS ORIF Ⓛ hip
ALLERGIES NKDA
SIGNATURES:

	7a - 7p	Initials	7p - 7a	Initials
NURSE	C Lott, RN	(CL)		( )
NURSE		( )		( )
TECH/ASST		( )		( )
OTHER		( )		( )

NURSING 24 HOUR ASSESSMENT

SYSTEM

NEUROLOGICAL	7A	8	9	10	11	12P	1	2	3	4	5	6	7	8	9	10	11	12A	1	2	3	4	5	6
NORMAL — ALERT-APPROP. FOR AGE										CL														
ORIENTED X3										CL														
MAEW										CL														
ABNORMAL — LETHARGIC																								
DISORIENTED																								
UNRESPONSIVE																								
PAIN SCALE (Rate 1-10)										8	4													

Discharge Outcome: Patient will demonstrate optimal contact with reality; maintains usual reality orientation; regains/maintains usual level of consciousness free of adverse neurologic symptoms/complications.

CARDIOVASCULAR	7A	8	9	10	11	12P	1	2	3	4	5	6	7	8	9	10	11	12A	1	2	3	4	5	6
NORMAL — HEART RATE (WNL For Age)										CL														
CAPILLARY REFILL (2-3 SEC)										CL														
RAD. PULSES EQUAL & STRONG R, L, Bil.										CL														
PED. PULSES EQUAL & STRONG R, L, Bil.										CL														
ABNORMAL — IRREGULAR RATE																								
WEAK PULSES																								
ABSENT PULSES																								
EDEMA																								
ECG RATE																								
ECG RHYTHM																								

Discharge Outcome: Patient displays vital signs within patient's normal range. • Patient demonstrates adequate perfusion as individually appropriate.

PULMONARY	7A	8	9	10	11	12P	1	2	3	4	5	6	7	8	9	10	11	12A	1	2	3	4	5	6
NORMAL — B.S. CLEAR: R, L, Bil.										CL														
B.S. EQUAL BILATERALLY										CL														
RATE REGULAR (WNL for Age)										CL														
Pulse Ox O₂ Sat.																								
Probe Placement Site																								
O₂ Device																								
FiO₂ or l/m																								

**Call MD if O₂ Sat. is 92% or less, unless otherwise ordered by physician. If patient's O₂ Sat. is <93% - - assess patient which would include B.S., respiratory effort, vital signs, and the need for respiratory treatment.

ABNORMAL																								
COUGH																								
SHALLOW RESP.																								
LABORED RESP.																								
IRREGULAR RESP.																								
SPUTUM-DESCRIBE:																								
ADVENTITIOUS BREATH SOUNDS																								
DECREASED BREATH SOUNDS																								

Discharge Outcome: Patient will maintain effective breathing pattern with respiratory rate within normal range for patient.

GASTROINTESTINAL	7A	8	9	10	11	12P	1	2	3	4	5	6	7	8	9	10	11	12A	1	2	3	4	5	6
NORMAL — ABDOMEN SOFT										CL														
BOWEL SOUNDS ALL QUADRANTS										CL														
FLATUS																								
ABNORMAL — FIRM																								
TENDERNESS																								
DISTENDED																								
BOWEL SOUNDS ABNORMAL																								
STOOL ABNORMAL																								
NAUSEA &/OR VOMITING																								

Discharge Outcome: Patient will establish/maintain normal patterns of bowel functioning for patient.

#035

1808.4 • 9/08/97

Figure 11-11. Nursing 24-hour assessment. (Courtesy North Oaks Health System, Hammond, LA.)

Continued

DATE: 7/15/03

SIGNATURES: 7a - 7p   Initials   7p - 7a   Initials

NURSE ___CLott, M___ (CL) _____ (   )
NURSE _____ (   ) _____ (   )
TECH/ASST _____ (   ) _____ (   )
OTHER _____ (   ) _____ (   )

NURSING 24 HOUR ASSESSMENT

GENITOURINARY (NORMAL)	7A	8	9	10	11	12P	1	2	3	4	5	6	7	8	9	10	11	12A	1	2	3	4	5	6
INDWELLING FOLEY																								
URINE CLEAR										CL														

GENITOURINARY (ABNORMAL)	7A	8	9	10	11	12P	1	2	3	4	5	6	7	8	9	10	11	12A	1	2	3	4	5	6
INCONTINENT																								
CLOUDY URINE																								
BLOODY URINE																								

Discharge Outcome: Patient will maintain/regain effective pattern of elimination.

SKIN (NORMAL)	7A	8	9	10	11	12P	1	2	3	4	5	6	7	8	9	10	11	12A	1	2	3	4	5	6
WARM, DRY										CL														
INTACT																								
GOOD TURGOR										CL														
MUCUS MEMBRANES MOIST																								
COOL																								

SKIN (ABNORMAL)																								
FLUSHED, HOT																								
GRAY, CYANOTIC																								
DIAPHORETIC																								
RASH/LESION																								
ABRASION, BRUISES																								
COLD																								
CLAMMY																								

Braden Scale: Circle Appropriate Score
1. If Braden score is 17-23, pressure ulcer prevention precautions will be implemented.
2. If Braden score is 12-16, moderate pressure ulcer prevention precautions will be implemented.
3. If Braden score is 0-11, strict pressure ulcer prevention precautions will be implemented.
Previous Score:_____   Today's Score:_____

SKIN INJURY/WOUND ☐ YES ☐ NO
IF YES, REQUIRES SKIN INJURY/WOUND ASSESSMENT FLOWSHEET AND NARRATIVE DOCUMENTATION.

CLINICAL CONDITION PARAMETERS

SENSORY PERCEPTION: RESPONSE TO PRESSURE-RELATED DISCOMFORT
- Completely Limited (unresponsive, quad, coma) — 1
- Very Limited (Responds only to painful stimuli, paraplegic, semicoma) — 2
- Slightly Limited (Responds with some sensory impairment CVA) — 3
- No Impairment (No limiting sensory deficit) — (4)

MOISTURE DEGREE TO WHICH SKIN IS EXPOSED TO MOISTURE
- Constantly Moist (Always incontinent, 2 or more linen changes every 8 hours) — 1
- Moist (Often Incontinent, linen change every 8 hours) — 2
- Occasionally Moist (Seldom incontinent, linen changes 2 every 24 hours) — 3
- Rarely Moist (Skin is dry, routine linen change) — (4)

ACTIVITY: DEGREE OF PHYSICAL ACTIVITY
- Bedrest (Confined to bed) — (1)
- Chairfast (Minimum weight bearing, ambulatory w/assist) — 2
- Walks Occasionally (Ambulatory short distance, sits mostly) — 3
- Walks Frequently (Ambulatory outside room, BID) — 4

MOBILITY: ABILITY TO CONTROL, CHANGE BODY POSITION
- Completely Immobile (Cannot move self) — 1
- Very Limited (Makes insignificant movements) — 2
- Slightly Limited (Makes slight changes independently) — (3)
- No Limitation (Makes major, independent changes) — 4

NUTRITION: USUAL FOOD INTAKE PATTERN
- Very Poor (NPO, IV > 5 days, < 1/3 meals) — 1
- Probably Inadequate (Needs assistance, < 1/2 meals) — 2
- Adequate (TPN, enteral needs met, > 1/2 meals) — 3
- Excellent (No supplement, eats most meals) — (4)

FRICTION AND SHEAR: ABILITY TO MAINTAIN BODY POSITION
- Problem (Requires complete assist., slides down in bed/chair) — 1
- Potential Problem (Requires maximum assist., sometimes slides down in bed/chair) — 2
- No Apparent Problem (Moves independently, maintains good position in bed/chair) — (3)

Discharge Outcome: Patient will display timely wound healing; maintain intact skin or regain skin integrity; maintain circulation to skin; or the patient will be free from skin impairments or decubitus ulcers.

NUTRITION	7A	8	9	10	11	12P	1	2	3	4	5	6	7	8	9	10	11	12A	1	2	3	4	5	6
DIET (% EATEN)											100%													
SNACKS (% EATEN)																								
DIET/SNACKS OFFERED																								
FLUIDS REFUSED																								
NOURISHMENT REFUSED																								

Discharge Outcome: Patient will demonstrate stable weight/or progressive weight gain with normalization of lab values and free of signs of malnutrition. Obesity assessed.

Figure 11-11, cont'd. Nursing 24-hour assessment. (Courtesy North Oaks Health System, Hammond, LA.)

NORTH🍂OAKS

DATE: 7/15/03

SIGNATURES:	7a - 7p	Initials	7p - 7a	Initials
NURSE	C Lott, RN	(CL)		( )
NURSE		( )		( )
TECH/ASST		( )		( )
OTHER		( )		( )

NURSING 24 HOUR ASSESSMENT

	PSYCHOSOCIAL	7A	8	9	10	11	12P	1	2	3	4	5	6	7	8	9	10	11	12A	1	2	3	4	5	6
NORMAL	COOPERATIVE										CL														
	APP. EMOTIONAL RESPONSE																								
	APP. SOCIAL INTERACTION																								
	AWAKE										CL														
	ASLEEP																								
	DROWSY/RESTING																								
ABNORMAL	RESTLESS/ANXIOUS																								
	WITHDRAWN/DEPRESSED																								
	UNCOOPERATIVE																								
	HOSTILE/COMBATIVE																								
	NONCOMPLIANT																								
	CRYING																								
	HALLUCINATIONS																								
	CONFUSION																								
	CURSING																								
	THREATENING																								

Discharge Outcome: Patient will maintain/regain bio-psychosocial homeostasis.

HYGIENE	7A	8	9	10	11	12P	1	2	3	4	5	6	7	8	9	10	11	12A	1	2	3	4	5	6
COMPLETE BATH																								
ASSISTED BATH										CL														
SELF																								
SHOWER/TUB/SITZ BATH																								
PERI-CARE/CATHETER CARE																								
ORAL-CARE																								
LINENS CHANGED										CL														

Discharge Outcome: Patient will resume/perform self-care activities within level of own ability or if unable, patient will receive help to maintain personal hygiene.

SAFETY	7A	8	9	10	11	12P	1	2	3	4	5	6	7	8	9	10	11	12A	1	2	3	4	5	6
PATIENT SAFETY CHECK q2H										CL														
ID BAND CHECKED q SHIFT										CL														
SIDE RAILS UP X 2										CL														
FAMILY (F), SITTER (S), OTHER (O)																								
BED POSITION ↑↓										↓														
BED WHEELS LOCKED										CL														
SEIZURE PRECAUTIONS																								

Discharge Outcome: Patient will remain free of injury during hospital stay.

ACTIVITY	7A	8	9	10	11	12P	1	2	3	4	5	6	7	8	9	10	11	12A	1	2	3	4	5	6
TURN: R, L, B, A																								
UP IN CHAIR																								
AMBULATED																								

Discharge Outcome: Patient will be able to perform schedule of activities appropriately for condition and mental readiness.

IVs, TX, & DRESSINGS	7A	8	9	10	11	12P	1	2	3	4	5	6	7	8	9	10	11	12A	1	2	3	4	5	6
IV SITE CHECKED: (WNL)										CL														
INFUSION PUMP																								
IV SITE ROTATED																								
Dressing Ⓒ hip										CL														

Discharge Outcome: IV/wound sites will be free of S/S of complications/infections; patient will receive parenteral therapy safely and comfortably; patient will regain fluid and electrolyte balance; patient will be free from preventable complications of IV Therapy.

MD VISIT	TIME		TIME		TIME		TIME		TIME	

Figure 11-11, cont'd. Nursing 24-hour assessment. (Courtesy North Oaks Health System, Hammond, LA.)

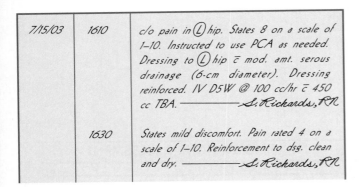

| 7/15/03 | 1610 | c/o pain in Ⓛ hip. States 8 on a scale of 1–10. Instructed to use PCA as needed. Dressing to Ⓛ hip c̄ mod. amt. serous drainage (6-cm diameter). Dressing reinforced. IV D5W @ 100 cc/hr c̄ 450 cc TBA. ————S. Richards, RN |
| | 1630 | States mild discomfort. Pain rated 4 on a scale of 1–10. Reinforcement to dsg. clean and dry. ————S. Richards, RN |

Figure 11-12. Example of charting by exception.

Box 11-3   Characteristics of Computerized Records

- Meets the legal criterion of legibility
- Automatically enters the time of the entry; the time of care must be added
- Recorder is identified by password-protected entry, rather than by a signature
- Entered data cannot be changed; incorrect entries must be noted by entering a correction entry
- Requires keyboarding skills
- Employs security systems to protect confidentiality
- Can force charting to address problem list, the nursing process, or other specific needs of the agency
- Allows reduction of keyboarding required by using a menu option list or forced choice system
- May limit the ability to adequately convey meaning if the forced choices are not well constructed
- Allows for late data entries
- Allows retrieval of information for specific problems across multiple records

Graphic Records. Graphic records are used to record vital signs in most agencies. Graphs vary among agencies, and Figure 11-13 is but one example. Some forms also provide a graph for documentation of pulse and respiration, but most simply provide a space to write the number values for pulse, respiration, and blood pressure. Some agencies use tabular forms for recording *all* vital signs, and some use such forms only when vital signs are recorded at more frequent intervals than the graph allows.

Other Types of Flow Sheets. Other flow sheets commonly used for recording data include the following:

- Intake and output (I&O) (see Figure 11-13)
- Wound assessment (Figure 11-14, p. 238)
- Medication administration records
- Intensive vital signs
- Neurological checks
- Peritoneal dialysis
- Fetal monitoring

Clinical Pathways. **Clinical pathways,** also called **critical pathways** or **care maps,** may be recorded using an interdisciplinary approach or organized by health care discipline. Outcomes of care and planned interventions are derived collaboratively by all members of the health team and reviewed and updated regularly. Any exceptions (variations) are documented, along with suspected causes for the variance and actions taken in response.

DOCUMENTATION BY COMPUTER

Computer-based records (electronic medical records) are used in many health care settings to facilitate delivery of client care and support the data analysis necessary for strategic planning (Harris & Bleich, 2001). Computer-based records contain information that is identical to that found in traditional records, but they eliminate repetitive entries and allow more freedom of access to the data base (Box 11-3).

Confidentiality and security of the computer system are major concerns. To keep the client's record confidential, the person who enters data into a computer logs on to the system using a secure password, which should be changed monthly to maintain security. The network is protected by a firewall. Some computer systems provide on-line access from remote sites, but this increases the problems with security.

A second issue is training of personnel. Despite the considerable time often invested in training personnel in the use of electronic medical records, studies have shown that computerized systems can increase time efficiency, consistency, and accuracy in record keeping (McCarger, Johnson, & Billingsley, 2001). The nurse enters assessment data by selecting from a list; thus the accuracy and pertinence of the data depends on the naming conventions entered into the system.

A third issue is the language used to name the nursing problems, the lists of data for assessment, and anything else that is entered by picking from a list. The field of medical or nursing informatics is constantly evolving, which requires updating of software programs to stay abreast of changes in terminology.

The use of computer systems for documentation in health care agencies varies in scope depending on the agency. Most health care agencies have incorporated information systems for management of admissions; billing; and communication of orders for diet, pharmacy, and diagnostic tests. Use of these systems allows departments within an institution to interact, and it provides a database for research and quality assurance. In addition, agency-wide computer information systems are more efficient because information entered in the system can be automatically transferred to other areas (Thede, 1998). Many agencies have incorporated software for documentation of client care. Systems may include options for generating individualized care plans, automated Kardex, and acuity levels, as well as providing a mechanism for recording ongoing assessment data.

Although some systems provide computer input only at the nurses' desk, bedside systems—including hand-held systems (Figure 11-15, p. 239)—are becoming more common. Bedside

NORTH🌿OAKS
12-HOUR GRAPHIC AND I&O RECORD

		7A-7P			7P-7A			7A-7P			7P-7A			7A-7P			7P-7A			7A-7P			7P-7A			7A-7P			7P-7A		
Date																																	
Hour		8	12	4	8	12	4	8	12	4	8	12	4	8	12	4	8	12	4	8	12	4	8	12	4	8	12	4	8	12	4

Temperature graph grid with values 105, 104, 103, 102, 101, 100, 99, 98, 97

		7a-7p	7p-7a	7a-7p	7p-7a	7a-7p	7p-7a	7a-7p	7p-7a	7a-7p	7p-7a
	Pulse										
	Respiration										
	Blood Pressure										
	Weight										
	Bowel Mov't										
Intake	Parenteral										
	Oral										
	Blood/Plasma										
	Piggy Back										
	Tube Feeding										
	G.U. Irrigant										
	12 Hr. Total										
	24 Hr. Total										
Output	Catheter										
	Emesis										
	Suction										
	Voiding										
	Drain										
	12 Hr. Total										
	24 Hr. Total										
	Meals	B____% L____% D____%		B____% L____% D____%		B____% L____% D____%		B____% L____% D____%		B____% L____% D____%	

Instock #001

3132.2 • 11/9/98

Figure 11-13. Example of a graphic record. (Courtesy North Oaks Health System, Hammond, LA.)

NORTH OAKS

Attachment D: Skin Injury/Wound Assessment Flowsheet

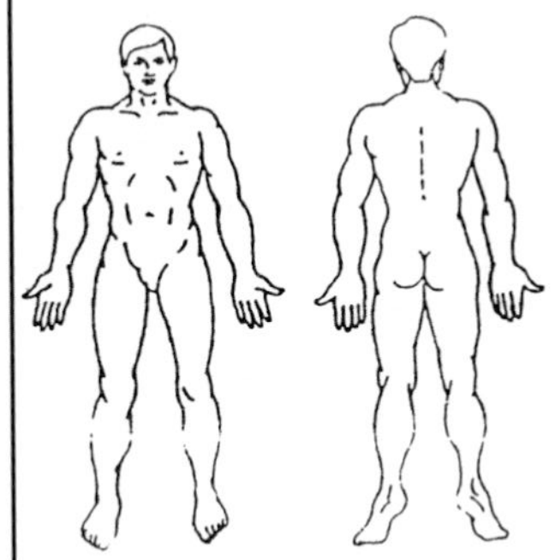

STAGE 1: Nonblanchable erythema of intact skin.

STAGE 2: Partial thickness skin loss involving epidermis and/or dermis.

STAGE 3: Full thickness skin loss involving damage or necrosis of subcutaneous tissue that may extend down to, but not through, underlying fascia.

STAGE 4: Full thickness skin loss with extensive destruction tissue necrosis or damage to muscle, bone or supporting structures.

Unable to stage due to eschar covering wound. **Complete a full row of information for each injury/wound.**

(Addressograph)

R   L   R

Number each injury/wound on the diagram.

Injury/Wound Types

Stasis Ulcer
Pressure Ulcer
Arterial Ulcer
Surgical Wound
Laceration

Bruises
Skin Tear
Rash
Hematoma
Other: Specify.

Drainage	Odor	Color
Serous Purulent None Other: Specify.	Mild Foul None Other: Specify.	Pink Red Black Eschar Other: Specify.

Date	Site#	Injury/Wound Type (Specify)	Stage	Length Width cm	Depth cm	Tunneling Yes/No	Color	Drainage Amt/Type	Odor	Culture Date	Treatments & Comments	Signature & Title

JOB#2841.4+(2/18/98)

Figure 11-14. Example of a skin injury/wound assessment flow sheet. (Courtesy North Oaks Health System, Hammond, LA.)

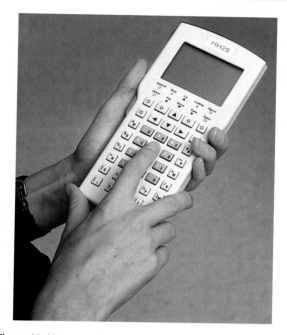

Figure 11-15. A hand-held computer documentation system.

charting systems, also referred to as point-of-care (POC) systems, often include prompts for data to be entered, which results in records that are more accurate and complete. In addition, charting at the bedside saves you time and allows current information to be immediately available to all who need it. Some systems automatically retrieve and record information (e.g., vital signs) from electronic devices and simultaneously enter the data in more than one place on the record, avoiding duplication of effort. Legibility of information is an added benefit from computer documentation systems.

Although charting by computer is an efficient method of documentation, concern about protecting client rights with regard to the security of the information has increased. Major concerns include confidentiality, access to information, and inappropriate alterations in client records. Documentation on the client's computerized record requires the individual charting to have a log-in and password for entering the computer record system. It is imperative that this password not be shared with anyone. Anything entered will be credited to the person to whom the password or signature is assigned. In addition, you should log off the computer before leaving the terminal to ensure that information about a client is not displayed on the monitor for others to view. Computer-generated printouts should also be protected so that information about clients is not indiscriminately duplicated or distributed. Most agencies using computer charting incorporate a system for logging and tracking computer printouts.

Charting procedures for computer records systems vary by agency. Data are often recorded in flow-sheet format for easy storage and retrieval. Systems can also be designed to record standard phrases such as nursing diagnoses, interventions, or outcomes classification systems. Many incorporate the use of free-text narratives in addition to standardized phrases, to al-

low specific and relevant documentation. The ANA's Nursing Information and Data Set Evaluation Center (NIDSEC) developed guidelines for nursing information systems. The standards provide a framework for evaluation on nomenclature, clinical content, storage and retrieval of data, and confidentiality and security components (ANA, 1997).

Nursing Informatics. Informatics is the science of identifying, collecting, storing, and processing information. It is concerned with providing an economical, efficient data management system that is useful to the users of the system. To design nursing informatics systems, information specialists are concerned with the development of a common language for nursing assessment, diagnosis, outcomes, and interventions.

Nursing informatics has an important role in ensuring that nursing's data and knowledge are structured in such a way that they can be understood and used by other members of the health care team. However, because nursing utilizes information for purposes different from those of other clinical disciplines, it may require programs and information management tools that are tailored to the unique goals of clinical nursing.

Thus the practice of nursing informatics includes the following:

- The development and evaluation of applications, tools, processes, and structures that assist nurses with the management of data required to take care of clients and to support the practice of nursing
- Adapting or customizing existing informatics technology to the requirements of nurses
- Collaboration with other health care and informatics professionals to develop informatics products and standards for nursing and health care informatics

The Future. Nursing informatics does not involve just storing data; it involves storing data in a way that is clinically useful. Examples of possible clinical uses include the following:

- Nursing care planning: You enter the client's signs and symptoms and the computer generates a list of possible nursing diagnoses, outcomes, and interventions. The accuracy of this list would of course depend on your accuracy in entering the data, and on the program used to transform that data into a care plan.
- Access to knowledge: Your client is having a possible drug reaction. You enter data about the reaction. The computer already knows what medications the client is taking and is connected to a database of medication information. It generates a list of possible medications that could have caused the reaction.
- Promoting continuity of care: You access your client's chart and are alerted to pertinent information—for example, the client has received pain medication every 4 hours for the past 24 hours, has not had a bowel movement in 4 days, or is due for an IV site change.

Building a computer program to automate or even support such transformations requires an understanding of the nature and structure of the information to be processed, the transformations that will be uniquely useful in nursing, and the algorithms (decision trees) and heuristics (rules of thumb) used by expert nurses for decision making.

We do not yet know the best way to implement these tools in the clinical environment or how to make them fit naturally into the clinician's workflow. When clinicians see that the benefits of a new system outweigh the burden of changing their documenting methods, they will make the effort. Whatever system is implemented must be carefully integrated into an institution's workflow processes.

Key Principles

- The purposes of charting involve communication, quality assurance, legal accountability, reimbursement, and research.
- All documentation entries should include standard medical terminology and approved abbreviations.
- Common principles of good documentation include legibility, brevity, sequence, making corrections appropriately, omitting blank spaces, signing properly, and using black ink.
- All medical records are confidential.
- Content can be documented using several types of entries: admit note, change-of-shift note, assessment findings, interval notes, and discharge note.
- Special notations should be made when a client is transferred or discharged, or when client teaching is conducted.
- All objective and subjective observations should be documented completely, accurately, and specifically.
- Significant data concerning psychosocial status, ADLs, valuables, spiritual care, and safety concerns should be documented as directed by agency policy.
- Older adults, children, and culturally diverse clients require specific documentation particular to their population.
- Documentation for extended-care, long-term, and home health agencies should include life span issues, support for reimbursement, and key terms specific to the various types of agencies.
- Entries can be made using various formats for documentation.

- Flow sheets, used to document data in an abbreviated form, allow quick reference for specific data.
- Computerized records allow systematic data entry and retrieval and facilitate consistency for purposes of quality assurance and research.

Bibliography

American Nurses' Association. (1997). *NIDSEC standards and scoring guidelines.* Washington, DC: Author.

*American Nurses' Association. (1999). *Standards of clinical nursing practice* (2nd ed.). Washington, DC: Author.

Buchauer, A., Pohl, U., Kurzel, N., & Haux, R. (1999). Mobilizing a health professional's workstation: Results of an evaluation study. *International Journal of Medical Informatics, 54*(2), 105-111.

Charting tips: Using flow sheets correctly. (1998). *Nursing, 98*(6), 76.

Griffiths, J., & Hutchings, W. (1999). The wider implications of an audit of care plan documentation. *Journal of Clinical Nursing 8*(1), 57-65.

Harris, M., & Bleich, M. (2001). Design and evaluation of electronic medical records. In C. Chang, S. A. Price, & S. K. Pfoutz (Eds.). *Economics and nursing: Critical professional issues* (pp. 442-465). Philadelphia: Davis.

Higginbotham, E. (2001). Documentation. In O'Keefe, M. E. (Ed.). *Nursing practice and the law* (pp. 163-176). Philadelphia: Davis.

McCarger, P., Johnson, J. E., & Billingsley, M. (2001). Practice applications. In V. K. Saba & K. A. McCormick (Eds.). *Essentials of computers for nurses: Informatics for the new millennium* (3rd ed.). New York: McGraw-Hill.

Raymond, L. (2001). How to chart for peer review. *RN, 64*(6), 67-70.

Thede, L. Q. (1998). *Computers in nursing.* Philadelphia: Lippincott Williams & Wilkins.

Weintraub, M. I. (1999). Documentation and informed consent. *Neurologic Clinics, 17*(2), 371-381.

*Asterisk indicates a classic or definitive work on this subject.

The Nurse–Client Relationship

Learning Objectives

After studying this chapter, you should be able to do the following:

- Understand the nature of a therapeutic relationship based on the phases of the relationship, elements of the relationship, theories about the relationship, and elements of the communication process

- Describe verbal and nonverbal behaviors that affect communication

- Identify and give examples of therapeutic communication techniques

- Identify and give examples of nontherapeutic communication techniques

Jane Smith, RN, was dispensing bedtime medications in a busy medical–surgical unit. As Mr. Lewis took his pills, he quietly commented, "I feel pretty scared about my operation tomorrow." Ms. Smith looked at him condescendingly. "That surgery is a piece of cake," she said. "You have nothing to be afraid of." Mr. Lewis didn't respond, but when Ms. Smith came to work the next day she learned that her client had had a sleepless night. "We all *tried* to talk to him about what was bothering him," reported the day nurse, "but he said nobody at this hospital cared enough to talk to him." What went wrong?

Had Ms. Smith been more aware of therapeutic communication techniques, she might have avoided upsetting her client. What could she have done better? What did she do that she should not have done? How might she have responded in a more sensitive and empathetic manner? The answers to these questions lie in an understanding of therapeutic communication.

This chapter will orient you to beginning theories, principles, and techniques of therapeutic communication related to the nurse–client interaction. Because you will be expected to use therapeutic communication techniques throughout your professional life, it is vital that you begin to learn these techniques early in your student experience. As with most skills you learn in nursing, you will continue to develop competence and gain mastery of these techniques as you practice them in the clinical setting. Also, the more you practice, the more confident you will be, and the better the outcomes will be.

THE THERAPEUTIC RELATIONSHIP

A **therapeutic relationship** is a helping relationship. Nurses are helpers, and clients are those seeking help. A therapeutic relationship is personal, focused on the client, and aimed at realizing mutually determined goals.

In a therapeutic relationship, people who are seeking help bring their own life experiences, intelligence, achievements, values, beliefs, feelings, and motivations for change to the relationship. You bring experience, understanding, and skills. You and your client can be viewed as unique systems that intersect on a common ground: the therapeutic nurse–client relationship.

Although it is true that people often help each other in social relationships, this kind of help differs from that occurring in therapeutic relationships. Social relationships may involve an infinite range of nonspecific helping activities, such as walking the neighbor's dog or helping a person who is using a walker to cross the street safely. The interaction involved in social helping may give the helper more satisfaction than the person being helped. In contrast, the help provided in the therapeutic relationship is the main reason for the relationship; it is focused on the client and has a specific purpose.

Action Alert! Focus on eliciting the client's feelings, thoughts, and values, and center on achieving the client's goals.

Another difference between social and therapeutic relationships is that the social relationship is more reciprocal, with both persons sharing personal beliefs, feelings, and opinions with each other. This is not true of the therapeutic relationship. You may share feelings with the client but only when such sharing is appropriate for the benefit of the client.

Phases of the Therapeutic Relationship

Therapeutic relationships develop and evolve over time. This time may be brief, or it may extend over weeks, months, or even years. Regardless of the length of time, there are three distinct phases to the relationship: the orientation phase, the working phase, and the termination phase. Because relationships are fluid, the phases flow into each other; nevertheless, each phase may be recognized by the tasks associated with it.

Orientation Phase. In the orientation phase of the therapeutic relationship, you and the client make a verbal agreement to work together to solve one or more of the client's problems. This agreement initiates a working relationship and forms the basis for the work you will do together.

As you enter into a relationship with a client, it is helpful to be aware of the personal feelings that can arise at these times. Both of you may be anxious and uncomfortable during this phase. You may feel inadequate, and the client may feel unsure about you and may need to know that you are willing and able to help.

A primary goal of the orientation phase is the establishment of trust (Figure 12-1). Trust is enhanced when you connect with the client in a respectful and nonintrusive manner that conveys personal consideration and concern.

Honesty and enthusiasm help to establish trust. You can convey these two traits in such responses as "I don't know the answer right now, but I will find out and let you know in an hour," or "I cannot promise I can help solve your problem, but I can listen and I do care."

Action Alert! Do not pretend to know an answer to a client's question if you do not. This deception will erode the client's trust. Your candor is necessary to promote client confidence.

Trust is also promoted when you establish confidentiality as a ground rule for the relationship. Confidentiality is an ethical obligation to share a client's health care information only with those who have a professional need to know it. You may safely promise your clients that you will respect their privacy and will share information only when there is a medical need to do so. It is important to tell your clients that you cannot maintain confidentiality if doing so would endanger their health and well-being or that of others. Unrealistic promises could create an ethical dilemma for you if the client confides something that must be revealed to others for the client's

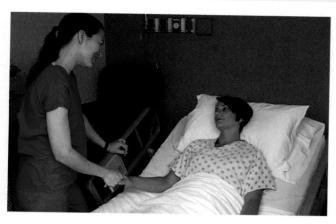

Figure 12-1. Establishing trust with the client is a key goal of the orientation phase of a therapeutic relationship. You can do this by conveying respect, personal consideration, and concern for the client's needs.

protection or for the protection of others. Consider the following example. What would you do if you had pledged unconditional confidentiality to a client, only to have him confide that he has active tuberculosis and works with AIDS patients? If you do not report this information, you risk the possibility of an infectious disease catastrophe. If you do reveal it, you have broken your word and violated the client's trust.

For reasons such as these, it is unrealistic to promise a client absolute confidentiality about the communications between you. In summary, maintaining appropriate levels of confidentiality should make clients feel that you will protect them and will not allow them to hurt themselves or others. If clients feel safe, they will feel a sense of trust, and the therapeutic relationship will be reinforced.

Besides establishing trust, you should establish other ground rules for the relationship. If you will be meeting with a client frequently, be sure to specify clearly where, when, and for how long each meeting will be. For example, a primary nurse might say, "I will be teaching you how to care for your Hickman catheter. We will meet here for an hour tomorrow at 10:00 A.M. so that I can assess your current knowledge. After tomorrow, we will work together 30 minutes a day for 5 days while you are hospitalized until you can comfortably and safely take care of your catheter."

As you establish meeting times and places, honesty and achievability are paramount. Do not promise what you may not be able to do. It is better if the client can rely on meeting with you 15 minutes each day than for you to promise 30-minute sessions that you may not have the time for.

At any time in the relationship, you may begin to feel a bond with your client. **Therapeutic rapport** is a special bond that exists between a nurse and a client who have established a sense of trust and a mutual understanding of what will occur in their relationship.

Working Phase. Once rapport has been established and the relationship has been structured, the working phase (middle phase) of the therapeutic relationship begins. In this phase the nurse performs additional client assessment and analyzes the resulting data. The client's feelings, values, beliefs, and attitudes are sought out and examined.

Often during this phase, initial nursing diagnoses are corrected, or additional nursing diagnoses are formulated. However, the working phase is mainly a time for completing nursing interventions that address expected nursing outcomes. You respond to clients mainly by presenting information and by validating and clarifying their understandings. Rather than directing clients, you attempt to help them become self-directed. It is a time when clients can formulate and test solutions to their problems. Evaluation also occurs in this phase of the relationship and, when necessary, the care plan is revised.

Termination Phase. The termination phase of the therapeutic relationship occurs near the end of the relationship, when the work of the client and nurse is coming to a close. The termination itself should not be abrupt or unexpected and should be acknowledged from the beginning of the relationship by both you and the client.

Recall the example given earlier, in the discussion of the orientation phase of the therapeutic relationship. The primary nurse clearly stated she would work with the client on catheter care for a certain time each day for a specified number of days. No one should have interpreted her offer to meet with the client as extending beyond the hospital stay. She was saying, in effect, "I will be meeting with you only until you are discharged." Clear communication helps to clarify expectations from the start of the relationship.

Even when the termination is thoughtfully planned, it may still be difficult to end a meaningful interaction. You and the client are aware that this phase precedes a permanent separation, and you both may feel anxiety, sadness, and a sense of loss.

How the client reacts to the termination depends on the meaning assigned to it, the length of the relationship, and the extent to which outcomes were achieved. Some clients may display denial and regret and may engage in acting-out behaviors. **Acting-out behaviors** are inappropriate or unexpected client behaviors that communicate the client's true or subconscious feelings and concerns. A client who is acting out during termination may refuse to talk when meeting with you, fail to keep appointments, and become more forgetful. At such times, you may help the client to recognize feelings about parting while emphasizing positive changes that have occurred during the relationship. It may be helpful to offer support and express optimism for the future. At the same time, it is important to be clear about ending the relationship without offering false hope for continuation. Although this process can be uncomfortable for you, it provides the client with clear boundaries and expectations.

Elements of the Therapeutic Relationship

Three elements are present in all phases of the therapeutic relationship: you, the client, and the communication between the two of you. You are a helper trained in skills that facilitate client growth, whereas the client is seeking help with personal growth in the areas of health promotion or adaptation to or recovery from illness. Communication is the meaningful interaction between the two of you that leads to such growth.

The Communication Process. Communication is the basic element of human interactions, and it includes both verbal and nonverbal messages. Each message consists of several components (Heery, 2000). A widely accepted model for the communication process consists of the following six elements (Figure 12-2):

- **Encoder (sender):** This person initiates a transaction to exchange information, convey thoughts and feelings, or engage another person.
- **Message:** This is the content a sender wishes to transmit to another person (the receiver) in the process of communication. The message must be encoded in a language of symbols or cues that are understandable to both sender and receiver.
- **Sensory channel:** This is the means by which a message is sent. The three primary channels are visual, auditory, and kinesthetic. Using these three channels, a wink, a tone of voice, and a hand gesture can all effectively convey a message without benefit of words.
- **Decoder (receiver):** This is the person to whom a message is aimed. This person must be able to decode the message sent to understand it clearly. If the message that the sender transmits is what the receiver understands, then clear and effective communication has occurred.
- **Context:** This is the condition under which a communication occurs.
- **Feedback:** This is the process by which effectiveness of communication is determined.

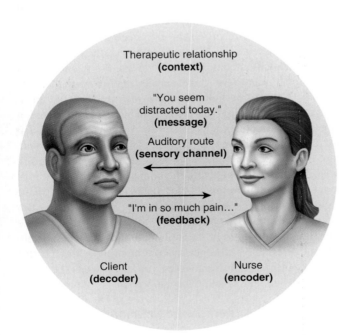

Figure 12-2. This diagram shows the six elements of communication within the therapeutic relationship: the encoder (sender), the message, the sensory channel, the decoder (receiver), feedback, and context.

The feedback process is such an important element of communication that it warrants further discussion. There are four types of feedback: internal, external, positive, and negative.

Internal feedback is a mechanism of self-perception. When you communicate, you automatically assess what you have said or done. For example, if you make a verbal blunder, you react self-consciously after realizing your mistake. If, however, you feel you have communicated clearly what you meant, you are pleased and satisfied with the effort.

External feedback is received from another or others in the form of visual, auditory, or kinesthetic information. The response to the message sent gives information about how effectively you transmitted the message.

Positive feedback affirms your efforts to communicate by rewarding and reinforcing successful communication. If your messages are met with a smile or exclamation of relief, you feel good and continue to use those communication behaviors.

Negative feedback is a response that tells you your original message was poorly transmitted or received and needs to be modified. However, there is more to negative feedback than just a message telling you that the original message was garbled. Negative feedback may also be judgmental and indicate that the receiver disagreed with your message.

It is important to note that both sender and receiver can seek feedback and clarify and qualify the message as needed. For example, consider the following interaction between Mrs. Herbert and Rick Jones, RN, after Mr. Jones completes Mrs. Herbert's diabetic teaching:

> Mrs. Herbert: "I think I understood the procedure better yesterday."
> Rick Jones, RN (*insulted by an unfavorable comparison to another nurse and seeking clarification*): "Are you thinking that I have confused you with today's teaching?"
> Mrs. Herbert (*realizing that Mr. Jones misunderstood*): "I wasn't saying it was your fault. I was just more with it yesterday."

Had Mr. Jones not clarified what Mrs. Herbert meant, he might have left the interaction with negative feelings about Mrs. Herbert and about his own ability to do diabetic teaching.

With this example, you can see how disruptive it could be to an interaction, and even to a relationship, if an unclear message is not clarified by seeking and receiving feedback or correction. It is unfortunate in this situation that the client had to be the one to seek feedback and to clarify, because this should have been done by the nurse. A more helpful question by Mr. Jones might have been, "Can you tell me more about why you feel more confused today?" This would have allowed Mrs. Herbert to clarify her statement without having to be burdened by considering the effect of her statement on Mr. Jones.

Action Alert! Clarify understanding of a message to ensure communication is both clear and therapeutic.

Theories About the Nurse–Client Relationship. Several theorists have provided us with a better understanding of the nurse, the client, and communication, and of the interaction among these elements in a therapeutic relationship. Selected examples follow:

PEPLAU'S THEORY. Hildegard Peplau, a psychiatric nurse and one of the first nurse theorists, identified six roles that are assumed by the nurse in a therapeutic relationship with a client (Peplau, 1952):

- *The stranger:* This role is shared by both the nurse and the client entering the therapeutic relationship. The nurse offers the client respect, interest, and acceptance in a nonpersonal manner. The client is assumed to be emotionally intact unless conflicting evidence arises.
- *The resource:* The nurse assumes the role of a resource person, helping the consumer–client to negotiate the health care system by providing care and offering answers to specific questions.
- *The teacher:* The nurse assumes the role of teacher to help educate the client and to help the client understand and use experiences within the health care system to attain health goals.
- *The leader:* The nurse assumes the leadership role to help the client–follower contribute to and participate in a democratic nursing process.
- *The surrogate:* The nurse assumes the role of surrogate parent to help the client resolve interpersonal problems that need to be safely worked out in the presence of an understanding other and to give the client a corrective interpersonal experience.
- *The counselor:* The nurse assumes the counselor role to help integrate reality and the client's emotional responses to illness into the total life experience.

Peplau believed that nurses who related with clients in a healthy way could provide corrective interpersonal experiences for them; that is, if clients had positive relationships with nurses, they could then have healthier relationships with others. She encouraged nurses to promote trust in their relationships by relating to their clients in an authentic manner. For Peplau, relating in an authentic manner meant sharing feelings and thoughts appropriately. For example, note how Mrs. Lyons, a renal nurse, shares her feelings with Mr. Little when he learns his second kidney transplant is failing. His eyes are red and he is clenching his fists, but he is unable to verbalize his feelings.

Mrs. Lyons *(making eye contact with Mr. Little):* "This is a hard piece of news for you."
Mr. Little *(silent, but starts to cry)*
Mrs. Lyons: "I feel sad too, Mr. Little. Having two transplants fail is very hard."

Peplau noted that closeness in a therapeutic relationship builds trust, increases the client's self-esteem, and leads to new personal growth for the client.

TRAVELBEE'S THEORY. Joyce Travelbee, another noted nurse theorist, pointed out that the nurse is a human being

who is vulnerable to stereotypes, labels, and generalizations (Travelbee, 1966). Travelbee noted that it is not possible for a stereotype (of a nurse) to relate to another stereotype (of a client) in a human way. In the following example, Miss Lane is a nurse working with paralyzed adults. In Miss Lane's stereotyped view, paralyzed clients have enough problems and should not be overly challenged. She also believes she is overworked and underpaid and that her clients should be grateful for the care she gives. Miss Lane is assigned to work with Lisa Simmons, a 28-year-old woman recovering from a devastating car crash. Lisa is alert, bright, and highly motivated.

Miss Lane: "Good morning, Lisa. Let me cut up your breakfast for you."
Lisa: "My arms are fine, it's my legs that don't work."
Miss Lane *(to herself):* You poor thing, you need all the help you can get. You're lucky I'm your nurse today. *(to Lisa)* "No sweetie, let's do it my way, I don't have all day for this."

Not only has Miss Lane not related to Lisa as another human being who is deserving of respect and consideration, but she has also given Lisa a reason to view nurses as callous, rude, and insensitive.

Travelbee noted that one nursing goal is to change the distorted beliefs others have about nurses and nursing. According to Travelbee, the client is the help-seeker whose overt and covert needs are the focus of the therapeutic relationship. She proposed that understanding the individual client's experience is paramount and that people cannot be known if their uniqueness is not appreciated. Your task, then, is to see the individual "with fresh eyes" and without labeling or stereotyping.

An important component of Travelbee's theory concerns the process of *human reduction*. This term, a synonym for dehumanization, refers to viewing the client as other than a human being. Viewing the client as an illness ("the heart attack in Room 210"), a task ("the bed-bath-and-dressing-change on Team B"), or a stereotype ("all amputees") are three examples of human reduction. It is only in overcoming assigned labels that you and the client can relate on a human level and establish a therapeutic relationship.

Like Peplau, Travelbee conceptualized the communication process as a means of fostering the development of human relationships. She believed that the human-to-human relationship allows the nurse to help clients and their families cope with illness and find meaning in the experience. She believed communication to be reciprocal, dynamic, and influential. Travelbee recognized that each interaction has differences and similarities, which prohibits the forming of rigid rules of action but does permit the nurse to develop skill as a communicator.

KING'S THEORY. Imogene King (1981) developed a nursing theory based on interacting personal, interpersonal, and social systems. Individuals involved in an interactive process mutually identify goals and the means by which to achieve them. In the nurse–client relationship, it is the nurse's responsibility to establish an interpersonal relationship, with the interaction focused on meeting the client's needs. Communication is viewed as the vehicle by which human relationships are developed and maintained, and it requires an atmosphere of mutual respect. The nurse uses knowledge of communication to observe client behavior and accurately interpret the meaning of the behavior. According to King, communication is verbal, nonverbal, situational, perceptual, transactional, and irreversible (King, 1981).

WATZLAWICK'S THEORY. Paul Watzlawick, a noted communication theorist, wrote extensively about the pragmatics of communication. He believed communication to be inevitable (Watzlawick, Jackson, & Bandas, 1967). He noted the following:

- All behavior has message, value, or meaning.
- You are always behaving. You cannot fail to behave.
- Inasmuch as you cannot stop behaving, you cannot stop communicating.
- Therefore, communication is inevitable.

TYPES OF COMMUNICATION

There are generally two types of communication: verbal and nonverbal. Each type has several components.

Verbal Communication

Verbal communication involves the use of words to convey messages. This type of communication is achieved by speaking or writing in a code that is mutually understood by sender and receiver. The tool of verbal communication is language. **Language** is a set of words that have meanings that are comprehensible within a group. Because a word has a definition, however, does not guarantee that its meaning will be interpreted in the same way by all group members. For example, in the English language, the word *hot* could refer to something very warm, something stolen, or something sexually attractive. It is important, therefore, to validate meaning between you and the client.

Talking. Talking is the act of verbalizing symbols to convey thoughts, feelings, or ideas. It is a skill so taken for granted that it is almost impossible to communicate without it. A sense of helplessness can be overwhelming for clients who are intubated, who do not speak the dominant language, or who are rendered speechless by surgery or a neurological disorder.

Writing. Written communication transfers a thought or spoken symbol into printed form. Being able to communicate accurately and clearly in writing is critical for you (e.g., when documenting nursing care). It can be especially useful in communicating with clients who are unable to hear or speak clearly or at all. If you communicate with clients by writing, you should communicate as clearly as if you were speaking to the person. For example, it is important that you use clear language, use an appropriate vocabulary, and speak at the client's level of understanding. Correct spelling is vital to clear written communication.

When communicating with clients in writing, you should ensure that your printing is large enough and dark enough to be legible, that the room lighting is conducive to reading, and that the client is wearing reading glasses, if needed.

Nonverbal Communication

Nonverbal communication is a set of behaviors that conveys messages either without words or by supplementing verbal communication. Nonverbal communication consists of body language, paralanguage, and any other means by which one communicates with others without the use of words. As a health care professional, you are very concerned with body language and paralanguage.

Body language refers to nonverbal communication behaviors that are accomplished by the movement of our bodies or body parts, by the presentation of ourselves to the world, and by the use of our personal space (see later). Common body language behaviors include personal appearance, conscious and unconscious changes in facial expressions, body posture and gestures, the distance maintained from others, and how others are touched by us (Figure 12-3). **Paralanguage** refers to nonverbal components of spoken language. These components give speech its rhythm and humanness and include stress, accent, pitch, pause, intonation, rate, volume, and quality.

> *Action Alert!* Carefully observe a client's nonverbal behavior. Because it is unconscious, it often provides a more reliable indication of the person's true message.

Body Language. Clients typically communicate a great deal using body language; therefore, messages sent by this means can be important in the overall assessment of the client. A few examples of the general areas you may assess in this way follow.

PERSONAL APPEARANCE. A rapid assessment of the client's general appearance gives an initial impression of factors as varied as social standing, self-esteem, and emotional status. Because most persons are aware of being judged by their general appearance, they usually take steps to alter their appearance to create a more favorable impression, even in a health care setting.

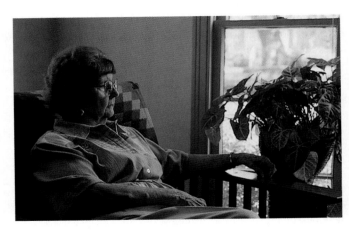

Figure 12-3. Body language is one important form of nonverbal communication. What might this woman's body language be saying?

You can obtain useful information about a client's condition by observing whether the client has attended to good grooming. A client's neglected personal appearance may be caused by a variety of reasons including lack of bathing facilities, physical handicap, lack of appropriate socialization, lack of energy (resulting from severe depression, physical weakness or handicap, or disease), or lack of time. At the same time, you must be careful not to make judgments about a client on the basis of external appearance. To provide professional and appropriate care to clients, avoid hasty judgments and validate initial impressions with additional data.

FACIAL EXPRESSIONS. Assessing a client's eyes and facial movements can also yield valuable information. When you assess these areas, note whether the movements are voluntary or involuntary (winks or smiles versus tics or twitches). Note whether the client can focus and maintain eye contact. Observe the eyes for redness, clarity, and tearing, and the face for the raising and lowering of eyebrows or the presence of a smirk, smile, or frown.

A client can communicate pain, fear, anger, sadness, happiness, contentment, or excitement with the eyes and with facial muscular activity. Do not be too quick to assign meaning to facial expressions alone, however, because reading body language is not an exact science. For example, if you note a client's eyes are red-rimmed and teary and that he has difficulty making eye contact with you, further investigation is warranted. It may be that the client is embarrassed that he has been crying, or he may be a bashful person who is suffering from a seasonal allergy. Other possibilities exist to explain these few observations. Use your observations of facial expressions as cues to alert you to instances in which further assessment might be needed.

BODY POSTURE. As is true of facial movement, body posture and stance can also provide cues to a person's physical and emotional state. To assess body posture, note whether the person is standing straight, is slumped, or is hunched over. An erect posture usually signifies a feeling of fitness and confidence. Slumping often occurs in persons who are physically exhausted, weak, emotionally depressed. Hunching can signal a desire to be left alone. A client who is hunching with forearms crossed over the abdomen may be guarding a painful abdomen. A more severely hunched posture, with head down, forearms brought up across the chest, and knees brought up to guard the abdomen (a fetal position), may indicate extreme fear or depression.

GESTURES. Observe the types of gestures used by clients. Some clients talk with their hands by gesturing while they speak. Emphatic gestures often convey messages of urgency. The urgency may be accompanied by distress, great happiness, or excitement. Urgent hand gestures may represent the conversion of pent-up emotional energy into physical energy that can be released. Thus, urgent hand gestures can be a sign that the client has strong needs to be heard (and perhaps assisted). They may also be a means of client coping when the person is unable to adequately convey urgent messages verbally. It is also important to understand what gestures mean within different cultures to avoid misunderstanding when communicating with clients from diverse backgrounds.

PERSONAL DISTANCE. We all have a **personal space,** a private zone or "bubble" around our body, that we believe is an extension of ourselves. We carry this personal space around with us at all times. A select number of people are allowed to enter this space at certain times, and we tend to be uncomfortable if others enter this space at all. Therefore, we behave in ways to prevent this from happening. At certain times and in certain situations, we expand our personal space, and to maintain our comfort, we need most people to stay even farther away from us than usual.

The size of this space appears to be culturally determined, at least in part, and it can vary considerably from culture to culture. People within each culture respect others' personal spaces and use culturally determined body language signals to help maintain appropriate distances from each other. In Western culture, most people maintain similar distances from each other according to their relationships and to the activities involved. As an example, two men who are strangers on opposing teams might grapple together on a football field when they would never think of allowing their bodies to come into contact in the shower after the game.

TOUCHING. Nurse–client touching is an issue that requires great sensitivity. Because nursing is a hands-on profession, it is daily practice to touch clients often and intimately. However, be constantly aware that touch conveys many meanings to clients. It may indicate agreement, caring, loving, or even sexual desire.

Many clients are hungry for a handclasp or other form of human touch and will demonstrate this by reaching out to you (Figure 12-4). Most clients desire or feel neutral about a casual touch such as a pat on the arm during the course of normal conversation. However, clients who have been physically or sexually abused tend to see uninvited touch as a boundary violation.

If a client has not indicated a specific desire to touch or be touched, assess the client's feelings about touch before using it. A rule of thumb is to ask permission before touching. It is

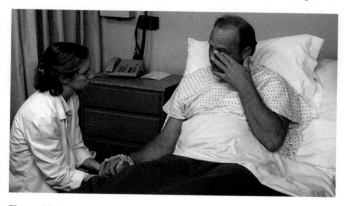

Figure 12-4. Many clients are hungry for a handclasp or another form of human touch. By touching the client when appropriate, you can convey warmth and empathy. However, if the client feels touch is inappropriate, draw back and respect the person's feelings. Otherwise, you risk undermining your attempt to communicate.

easy to ask, "May I touch your arm?" Asking can help avoid possible problems. In certain settings it is appropriate to say, "I'd like to give you a hug. May I?"

Touch may be accepted more or less readily in different situations. For example, a hug may be greeted with relief by a family member in a hospice when support is needed most, but it would probably be perceived as a violation of personal space in an initial meeting with a client in a clinic. Touching can soothe or disturb people to their very depths. Therefore, it must be used judiciously, on the basis of an assessment of the client's needs and wishes.

Paralanguage. Clients may communicate a great deal with verbal messages as they attempt to relate the content of their thoughts. Even better communication can occur when appropriate use is made of nonverbal components of speech, or paralanguage. An understanding of paralanguage can help you grasp the content of the client's message, and it can sometimes help you become attuned to the emotional component of the message—the client's mood.

STRESS. *Stress* refers to the part of a word, phrase, or sentence that is highlighted by changing pitch or elongating the syllable. Words that are stressed are generally the more important words. For example, the following statements have slightly different meanings because of the way stress is used:

"Nice to meet you." (with no particular stress)
"*Nice* to meet you."
"Nice to *meet* you."
"Nice to meet *you.*"

ACCENT. *Accent* refers to the different pronunciation of syllables used by nonnative speakers of a language. Accent alone can cause a loss of clarity that can result in a breakdown in communication. Do not pretend that you understand what someone has said when you do not. Seek to clarify what has been said by asking the person to repeat what was said, to use different words, or to write out the troublesome phrase.

PITCH. *Pitch* refers to whether the voice is high or low. Pitch results from the speed of vocal cord vibrations. Pitch is related to gender in that most men's voices are pitched lower than most women's voices. It is also related to age in that children's voices are usually pitched higher than adults' voices. In any individual, changes in pitch can alter the meaning of the content of a message. For example, pitch rises at the end of a question (interrogative sentence) and stays the same or becomes lower in making a statement (declarative sentence). Thus, the meaning of the interrogative "You have tuberculosis?" is very different from the meaning of the declarative "You have tuberculosis."

PAUSE. *Pauses* punctuate speech with periods of silence or non–word sounds, such as "Let me see . . . " or "Hmm, I believe you are right." Often a pause indicates that the person is still considering something, is considering whether to share something, or is searching for the words to encode properly what is to be told. At other times, pauses are used for effect as part of varying intonation. In any event, the pause should be respected and the person given adequate time to complete the communication interrupted by a pause.

INTONATION. *Intonation* is the variety of stress and pause patterns within a phrase or sentence. For example, people often use one intonation when giving a formal speech and other intonations when communicating with a superior at work or with a close friend.

RATE. The *rate* of speech refers to how many syllables are spoken per unit of time. Rate also takes into account the number of pauses made. Increased rate of speech may indicate nervousness or agitation. It is sometimes possible to control anxiety by focusing on a rapid speech rate and slowing it.

VOLUME. *Volume* comprises the loudness and intensity associated with the speaking voice. Intensity is a measure of forcefulness and can convey a message about the speaker's emotions. Generally, a loud voice indicates anger or frustration, and the speaker uses it as if loudness could somehow increase the power of the words to control the listener or others. Changes in volume (either up or down) may also occur in anxiety.

QUALITY. Voice *quality* is a measure of clarity, hoarseness, or nasality in the speaker's voice. Physical and emotional conditions can cause a change in voice quality. For example, the voice often becomes husky with deeply felt emotions, harsher with anger, and more nasal with a cold.

FACILITATING EFFECTIVE THERAPEUTIC COMMUNICATION

Nursing Attitudes That Promote Communication

The term *patient-centered communication* has been used to describe strategies and behaviors that promote mutual understanding and shared decision making between the nurse and the client (Brown, 1999). Therapeutic communication is enhanced when you adopt helpful attitudes to indicate interest in and regard for the client. Before entering into the nurse–client relationship, it is useful to know about these communication-enhancing strategies. These nursing attitudes are sometimes referred to as *responsive attitudes*.

Awareness. Awareness of clients is necessary before human relationships with them are possible. In showing awareness, you acknowledge the presence of the client. It is important to introduce yourself and call the client by name ("How to build," 2000). **Attending behaviors** show that you are paying attention and listening to what the client is saying. Examples of attending behaviors that can be used to facilitate communication include facing the client, leaning toward the client, using appropriate eye contact, keeping your eyes open with eyebrows raised, and maintaining an *open body posture*, a body position in which the arms and legs are uncrossed.

Acceptance, Respect, and Unconditional Positive Regard. Acceptance is an openness to the unique qualities and attributes of individual clients. Acceptance does not mean condoning inappropriate client behaviors. It means that clients are accepted for who they are, even if their behavior is undesirable. Respect is more than an attitude of acceptance. It also includes valuing, highly regarding, or esteeming clients for who they are.

Unconditional positive regard, a term coined by the psychologist Carl Rogers (1951), describes respect for the client that does not depend on the client's behavior. You learn to value and care for clients simply because their humanity warrants your care.

You avoid being critical, derogatory, or judgmental. You understand that the client's imperfections are part of the total picture; the imperfections may be undesirable behaviors, but they are coping mechanisms the client needs at the time. Many clients struggle with the dehumanizing aspects of illness and dependency. You empower clients by showing respect and by appreciating their humanness without ridiculing or demeaning them.

Another reason to avoid judging a client is simply that a client should not view you as a judge. If this type of relationship should occur, the client may seek to please you, which diverts attention from the objective of focusing on the client's needs.

Empathy. Empathy is the accurate perception of the client's feelings. It is the ability to "be in the other person's shoes" without taking on the client's feelings or thoughts. Empathy is not sympathy, wherein you feel pity or compassion for the client. Rather, it is a sense of understanding or "being with" the client. Evans, Witt, Alligood, and O'Neil (1998) identify two types of empathy, *basic* and *trained*. Basic empathy is a raw "feeling for" sense of where and how the client is emotionally. Not everyone is born with equal amounts of basic empathy, but it is possible to learn trained empathy. This is based on learning a role and a way to respond to clients in the nurse–client relationship. It is possible to learn to assess and respond to clients' feelings empathetically even if you are not a "natural" at it. During your nursing career, you will experience both empathy with and sympathy for clients, but empathy will help you build important bridges in communicating with clients.

Relatedness. Relatedness is the recognition of similarities between you and the client and the forging of emotional connections based on those similarities. Relating to clients helps to establish human-to-human ties that make communication possible. Common experiences enable you and the client to be more readily known to each other.

Caring. Caring is taking an emotional risk to feel a personal interest in the client's welfare. By investing yourself in the client, you consciously decide to take emotional risks and give of your skills, compassion, and experience. Such concern can be draining, and you must continually assess personal psychic energy and emotional resources to prevent exhaustion and burnout.

Objectivity. Objectivity is an unbiased, reality-based stance that allows you to assess the facts of a client's situation without being emotionally pulled into the client's difficulties. You can be objective and still have warm feelings for the client and attend to the client's thoughts and feelings. Thinking about the client objectively allows you to understand client experiences and to identify areas of difficulty in order to guide the client toward developing appropriate problem-solving skills.

Protectiveness. Protectiveness leads you to shield the fragile and vulnerable client during the person's recovery from illness. There is a fine line between protectiveness and fostering dependence. Protectiveness is a caring attitude that should be used judiciously while you continue to evaluate the client's capacity to defend the self.

Genuineness. Genuineness is your ability to be honest, open, and sincere in self-presentation. The phrase "what you see is what you get" describes the demeanor of a genuine person. It is important not to confuse being genuine with being totally self-disclosing or casually spontaneous, as one would be with friends or family. For example, you may share a family's joy on the birth of a baby and demonstrate it with warm congratulations for the parents and admiration for the baby. For a client with a new baby, a warm, encouraging smile might be sufficient.

Openness. Being open with a client reflects your ability and willingness to be real, genuine, and emotionally accessible. Openness does not mean that boundaries are violated. It means that you choose what to share with the client and share it in an authentic manner. When you are open with a client, the client tends to lower defenses and to relate more honestly to you.

Professional Closeness or Distance. The nurse–client relationship is characterized by professional boundaries. In this relationship, there is a delicate balance between maintaining objectivity and professional distance, and the warmth, openness, and availability associated with professional closeness. You should be accessible to the client while maintaining an awareness that the therapeutic relationship is not a friendship or other social relationship. At the same time, be careful not to be impersonal and not to treat clients with indifference.

Professional closeness and stance vary throughout the relationship as you and the client come together as strangers, work on mutual goals, and proceed to termination. New nurses may feel uncomfortable with attempts at maintaining professional closeness and stance. A good rule to follow is to become invested without being engulfed. This means that you care about clients and allow yourself to know their concerns, but it does not mean taking their thoughts, feelings, or attitudes as your own.

Sense of Humor. Many have questioned the appropriateness of using any form of humor in a therapeutic relationship. Certain types of humor must be avoided, such as morbid humor, humor based on sarcasm, or humor that degrades anyone. These are inappropriate and unprofessional. However, you must be able to laugh at yourself and at humorous situations that can arise. Being a role model of this openness and demonstrating the appropriate use of humor can be therapeutic for clients just as it is for you.

An appreciation of the humorous side of life can be a desirable attitude in nurses. However, the ability to use humor therapeutically is a talent that not all nurses possess. When you are comfortable with the sensitive use of humor, you can sometimes use it to put clients at ease, defuse emotionally loaded situations, or simply inject a light note into an otherwise difficult day. You must assess each client's readiness for humor. If the client is likely to perceive any levity as a put-down, it is much better to maintain a more serious demeanor. Although clients can appreciate wit as much as anyone, they must first feel that you are trustworthy, dependable, and invested in their well-being.

Respecting Differences

You must develop effective communication skills to enhance your work with clients of different groups, of different cultures, and at different stages of health.

Developmental Differences. Communication techniques must be appropriate for the client's stage of development; otherwise, communication can be diminished. Examples of how to apply therapeutic techniques to children, adolescents, and adults of all ages have been provided in the tables appearing later in this chapter.

Cultural Differences. Whether or not clients from different cultures speak your language, they often have different customs, values, mores, and social structures, all of which can affect communication. Clearly, the more you understand about your client's culture, the better you will be able to communicate. It is helpful to learn crucial words and sentences in the client's language or to have a translator write out cards with commonly used bilingual sentences. However, understanding the nonnative client requires more than just learning a few new phrases. You must be aware of any personal biases to avoid stereotyping and labeling these clients. Respect for the client's experience and acceptance of the differences that exist between you can help establish a safe, therapeutic environment in which maximal communication can occur.

Sex Differences. Men and women communicate differently, and understanding these differences enhances therapeutic relationships. A number of experts have studied differences in communication styles between men and women. According to Tannen (1990), men seek dominance in a hierarchical structure to be independent; women avoid being dependent and subordinate but do not need to dominate. Intimacy to women means a free sharing of thoughts, hopes, and feelings. Men avoid such sharing to preserve personal freedom.

Tannen's theories can help you to negotiate hierarchy and power issues delicately when talking with persons of both sexes. For example, Tannen referred to *rapport talk* and *report talk*. Rapport talk, more comfortable to women, is a way of connecting with others and negotiating relationships. Examples of rapport talk are the techniques of offering self, suggesting collaboration, exploring, and focusing. Report talk, the demonstration of knowledge and skill, is the preferred conversational style of men. Examples of report talk are presenting reality, encouraging formulation of a plan, and summarizing. In short, women speak to connect; men speak to preserve status and independence (Tannen, 1990). You must recognize the validity of both styles. A respectful awareness that sex affects style, as well as a willingness to "read between the lines," promotes more effective communication with clients of both sexes.

TECHNIQUES THAT ENHANCE THERAPEUTIC COMMUNICATION

To maximize therapeutic communication it is important to use techniques that encourage clients to open up and speak more freely. A number of techniques of therapeutic communication that are generally considered helpful to use are listed in Table 12-1. Like any other tools, if they are used inappropriately, they can impede communication instead of enhancing it. It is helpful to know what to do and what not to do when using them. Here are some guidelines:

- Individualize each technique to the client's level of understanding. For example, you might tell a 40-year-old man, "I will demonstrate the correct technique for injecting your insulin," but to a 6-year-old girl you might say, "I will show you how to give your doll a shot."
- Vary the communication technique. Avoid using a single technique repeatedly. For example, saying "Tell me more" shows interest in what the client is saying and is therapeutic. But if you say "Tell me more" after everything the client says, it demonstrates that you are not giving a thoughtful response to each of the client's answers. Too many repetitions of the same response can be counterproductive.
- Use paralanguage appropriately to convey your intended meaning. For example, you may say something generally considered to be therapeutic, such as "I see," and say it sarcastically, icily, or in some other tone that is nontherapeutic. Another nurse may say something generally considered to be nontherapeutic but say it so warmly and with such caring that it is actually therapeutic for the client. Two nurses may say the same words and one will be seen as helpful and the other as condescending. In such cases, paralanguage may make the difference.
- If you are using therapeutic techniques correctly, your client will be doing most of the talking as you listen and guide the interaction. If you find you are doing most of the talking, something is wrong, and you need to pause and reflect about how to get back on track.
- You will probably make mistakes in talking with clients, and you will say some things that are not the best possible responses. In fact, there may be times that you will be angry with yourself because you said something so nontherapeutic. However, if you have a genuinely therapeutic relationship with the client, the relationship will survive an error or two.
- As you enter the clinical area to talk with a client for the first time, relax and realize that most clients want very much to talk to you.

Table 12-1   Therapeutic Communication Techniques

Technique	Description/Definition	Example
Offering self	The nurse offers to stay with the client and either talk or just sit quietly.	*Nurse with child:* "Let's sit in the playroom together and play for 10 minutes." *Nurse with adolescent:* "Let's have juice or soda together." *Nurse with adult:* "I'll be back in 15 minutes to sit with you."
Providing broad openings	The nurse invites the client to select a topic.	*Nurse with child:* "What will we talk about today?" *Nurse with adolescent:* "Tell me what I can teach you about your dialysis." *Nurse with adult:* "What shall we cover next?"
Providing silence	The nurse allows the verbal conversation to stop to provide a time for quiet contemplation of what has been discussed, for formulation of thoughts about how to proceed, or to reduce tension.	(Silence)
Focusing	The nurse selects one topic for exploration from among several possible topics presented by the client.	*Nurse with child:* "Tell me your favorite food for breakfast before you tell me about lunch." *Nurse with adolescent:* "You mentioned several things you like about school. What do you like best?" *Nurse with adult:* "You mention several advantages to your hip surgery. What is the single greatest improvement you have noticed?"
Asking for clarification	The nurse lets the client know that what was said was unclear. If necessary, the nurse asks for clarification or suggests ways to make the message clearer.	*Nurse with child:* "I did not understand that you said. Would you say it again for me?" *Nurse with adolescent:* "Maybe you would explain more about what you mean so I can be more helpful." *Nurse with adult:* "Let me tell you what I heard you say to me."

Reflecting	The client asks a question, and the nurse turns the question around and reflects it back to the client, or the client makes a statement, and the nurse selects one or more words to reflect back to the client for consideration. This technique strengthens the client's confidence.	*Nurse with child:*
		  Child: "Should I wear blue or green?"
		  Nurse: "Which would you like to wear?"
		Nurse with adolescent:
		  Adolescent: "My mom won't let me pierce my tongue."
		  Nurse: "What would it be like to have a pierced tongue?"
		Nurse with adult:
		  Nurse: "What should I tell the doctor?"
		  Nurse: "What would you like to tell the doctor?"

Placing events in time or sequence	The nurse asks the client to explain more about when an event occurred (placing the event in time) or to explain the sequence of events (placing events in the order in which they occurred) to clarify for the nurse.	*Nurse with child:* "Did you get sick before or after you ate?" *Nurse with adolescent:* "Tell me the steps you followed in changing your dressing." *Nurse with adult:* "Did your blood sugar go up after breakfast today or yesterday?"

Restating	The nurse paraphrases what the client has said. This paraphrased message may be fed back to the client in the form of a statement or a question to provide the client the opportunity to agree or disagree and clarify further.	*Nurse with child:*
		  Child: "I want my blankie."
		  Nurse: "You would like your blankie."
		Nurse with adolescent:
		  Adolescent: "I just puked."
		  Nurse: "You were sick to your stomach."
		Nurse with adult:
		  Adult: "It's no use."
		  Nurse: "You are pretty discouraged."

Seeking consensual validation	The nurse attempts to verify with the client that a certain term means the same thing to both parties.	*Nurse with child:* "You want Baby Lisa? Is she your doll?" *Nurse with adolescent:* "When you say you were high, did you mean you had just taken some drugs?" *Nurse with adult:* "Tell me if I understand your meaning correctly."
Encouraging descriptions of perceptions	The nurse asks the client to describe perceptions and associated emotions. This is particularly useful in understanding a client's experiences during hallucinations.	*Nurse with child:* "Tell me what you saw when I turned off the light." *Nurse with adolescent:* "How do you think the other kids feel about you?" *Nurse with adult:* "Describe what it is like when you hear the messages from God."

Continued

Table 12-1	Therapeutic Communication Techniques—cont'd	
Technique	Description/Definition	Example
Presenting reality	When a client has had an unrealistic perception of reality, the nurse accepts the fact that the client has misperceived something but indicates that the nurse did not have a similar perception. When something in the environment is stimulating the misperception, the nurse attempts to point this out.	*Nurse with child:* "I think that shadow on the wall might look like a monster to you." *Nurse with adolescent:* "The other kids tell me they worry that you don't seem to like them." *Nurse with adult:* "I have heard that God usually speaks to our hearts instead of our ears."
Summarizing	The nurse briefly states, in an orderly manner, what has been discussed. The purpose is to help ensure that client and nurse are in agreement about what went on, what decisions were made to help ensure that nothing was omitted, and to bring the relationship to a close.	*Nurse with child:* "Tomorrow we will do your bath before breakfast and cartoons." *Nurse with adolescent:* "Let me review the steps for coughing and deep-breathing exercises." *Nurse with adult:* "You have told me all the appropriate things to do to take care of that wound. I think you are ready to do it by yourself from now on."

- Any specific techniques of communication might be used at any time, according to the client and the situation, but some techniques tend to be more helpful at the beginning of an interaction, and some tend to be more helpful in the middle or at the end of an interaction.

Beginning the Interaction
Offering Self. Offering self is a technique in which you offer to stay with the client and either talk or just sit quietly. In offering self, you need to clearly establish parameters for the amount of time offered. For example, "I have 30 minutes available to talk with you at 10 o'clock today" or "I will stay with you while you wait for your family." Additional examples are found in Table 12-1.

In some cases, it is therapeutic to give the client a choice about your offer. Say, for example, "Would you like to meet with me for 20 minutes at 1 o'clock today?" However, some clients, such as those who are depressed, very much need to have you with them but will tend to reject your offer. Others should not be asked to make decisions about anything, because it raises their anxiety level. As you learn more and more about your clients and their individual needs, you will learn who can be asked and who should just be told that you are there for them. Until you do know, or if you are ever in doubt, it is always safe to offer self without allowing a choice.

Offering self can be very helpful when you are talking with those clients who seem unable to express their thoughts or who do not want to talk at the moment. You can say something like, "It is okay if you don't feel like talking right now. I'll just stay here with you for 20 minutes." If you make this time commitment, be sure to honor it for as long as you indicated. This helps establish that you are someone who can be trusted.

Providing Broad Openings. Early in a meeting with a client, it may be useful to provide a broad opening. In this case, you invite the client to select a topic for discussion. Here, too, it is therapeutic to set some parameters concerning what you are willing to discuss. For example, in most instances, it would not be helpful for the client to discuss your personal information or for you to engage in social-level small talk with the client. Therefore, it is not always appropriate to say, "We can talk about anything you like." It is better to say, for example, "We can discuss the issues that are bothering you." The latter is a very broad, client-focused opening.

Making Observations. In making observations, you acknowledge that something or someone exists or has changed in some way. Make observations without appearing to judge either positively or negatively. For example, you may observe that your client is distracted and pacing nervously. Sharing your observation by commenting "You seem distracted and nervous" may provide the opportunity for the client to discuss what has led to this behavior.

Suggesting Collaboration. Suggesting collaboration is a technique in which you offer to work together with the client. This technique is useful at the beginning of a relationship with a client because it establishes that you and the client will work together as a team. Initially, the work may involve discussing some of the issues of concern to the client. Later, as problems are identified and nursing diagnoses are made, the work may shift to establishing and meeting client outcomes. At all times, the work focuses on the client.

Action Alert! Begin any therapeutic interaction with clarity, and focus on the client.

Continuing the Interaction
Providing Silence. Providing silence in a therapeutic manner allows the verbal conversation to stop and provides a time for quiet contemplation of what has been discussed or for formulating thoughts about how to proceed. The silence can also provide an opportunity for reducing tension when the

interaction has been concerned with powerful issues and when emotions have been particularly deep.

Many people (nurses as well as clients) are uncomfortable with silence and will talk continuously about nothing in particular just to avoid it. This is clearly not a therapeutic approach to take. If you find that you are uncomfortable with silence, think about what has been going on during the silence, and use it constructively to think about what you will say next. You will find that, with practice, you can become more and more comfortable with silence.

Accepting Messages. Accepting messages is a way of providing feedback to acknowledge to the client that you have heard and understood what the client said. The acknowledgment is done in a manner that is neutral in tone, without agreeing, disagreeing, or providing any judgments about the message. The accepting may be done verbally or nonverbally. Your method of accepting messages should be brief and should allow the client to continue on with a train of thought without any real interruption.

Providing General Leads. In ordinary social communications, people take turns communicating. After your clients have spoken for awhile, they may hesitate because they are uncertain about whether it is appropriate to continue or whether they should try to draw you into the conversation. It is your task to keep clients focused on their own issues and to ensure that they continue to feel comfortable discussing them. To do this, you may use the technique of providing general leads. General leads are brief interjections ("Yes, I see" or "And then what happened?") that let clients know that they are on the right track and should continue. The leads provided should not cause real interruptions in the train of thought as they urge clients forward.

Exploring. As clients talk, they may mention something that you believe is significant enough to warrant further attention. If they have introduced the subject and have not indicated that further discussion is undesirable, it is appropriate to attempt to delve into the matter in greater detail. To do this, you use the technique of *exploring*. To explore, ask the client to describe something in more detail or to discuss it more fully. However, be careful not to use the nontherapeutic technique of *probing*. If your client gives an indication that further discussion is off-limits, honor this, and use another technique, such as providing a general lead to get the client to continue with what he was saying. For example, if your client says, "I won't discuss what that doctor told me," it is counterproductive and disrespectful to ask further questions about that subject.

Focusing. When clients are talking with you, they may bring up many different topics or concerns at once. These may all be worth exploring further, but you cannot explore them simultaneously. When this happens, it is best to select one subject to explore further while keeping others in mind for future discussion. Selecting one subject for exploration from among several is termed *focusing*.

For example, an adult client may say, "Things really fell apart after my second heart attack. I knew if I didn't control my diabetes that I would wind up near dead. You know, diabetics can lose their kidneys if they are not careful. I have two uncles who went bad from too much sugar. I think I'm a goner." How do you decide which point to explore? You may choose to focus on how the client feels about being diabetic, about the possible effects of diabetes, about having had two heart attacks, or about mortality.

If you focus on one point, you can always return to other issues later on. You might prepare the client for this by making an observation, focusing, and then requesting further exploration in the future. For example, you might say, "You have given me a great deal to think about, and much of it seems worth talking about *(making an observation)*. For now, I would like to know more about your most recent heart attack *(focusing),* and later on, perhaps we can discuss your other concerns *(requesting further exploration in the future)."*

Action Alert! Use these techniques to give the client permission to discuss concerns. Keep the interaction client centered, and clarify without speaking for the client.

Active Listening. Listening is the process in which spoken and other auditory information is received. Listening is an integral part of therapeutic communication. **Active listening** is understanding not only the words spoken but the feeling and intent behind the message (Klagsbrun, 2001). Active listening plays a role in helping the client communicate thoughts, feelings, and beliefs. You take an active part in listening by eliciting details from the client and by inviting the client to think more about what is being said.

Active listening is a means of "being with" the client and indicating acceptance and agreement, using verbal and nonverbal cues. It is an art and the key to therapeutic interaction. To use active listening, you must understand and be able to use all of the other therapeutic techniques of communication. Compare the following examples:

Passive listening:
    Client: "I just learned I have cancer."
    Nurse: "I see."
    Client: "I'm afraid I will die."
    Nurse: "Hmm."
Active listening:
    Client: "I just learned I have cancer."
    Nurse *(with concern in voice and turning to face client):*
      "I wonder how you're feeling about this."
    Client: "I'm afraid I will die."
    Nurse: "Dying feels like a real possibility to you."
    Client: "My mother died of cancer when I was eight, and I
      have an eight-year-old."
    Nurse: "This really hits close to you."

Note how active listening brought out information not available to the passive listener. This is truly the basis for therapeutic interaction.

Action Alert! Actively listening to what the client says and responding to it in a considered way demonstrates your care and concern for the client and the client's message.

Keeping Communication Clear

ASKING FOR CLARIFICATION. Sometimes clients say things that are unclear, that have more than one specific meaning, or that are simply vague. These garbled messages can impede communication. When this occurs, you can use several techniques to help clarify the message for both you and the client. The most straightforward technique is asking for clarification. Simply let the client know that you are not certain about what was said and, if necessary, request that the client clarify anything that is obscure. If you are unsure of the meaning you could say, "I'm not sure I follow what you mean." If the client does not understand what was unclear, you may have to tell the client how it could be clarified for you.

RESTATING. Another way to clarify is to use the therapeutic technique of *restating,* or paraphrasing, what the client has said. To do this, you alter the client's words to express your understanding of the client's meaning. You send this back to the client in the form of a statement or in the form of a question, and you provide the client the opportunity to agree or disagree that this was the intended message and, if necessary, to clarify further.

SEEKING CONSENSUAL VALIDATION. Sometimes, when a certain term used by a client has been unclear, you can use the technique of seeking consensual validation to help ensure that both you and the client agree on the meaning of the term. For example, at the end of a lesson about insulin injection, a client might say, "I'm through." You may interpret this in one of three ways: the client has learned the information well enough to self-inject insulin, the client is feeling tired after intense teaching, or the client is feeling discouraged and needs extra support. Focus on one of these three, and seek to verify whether or not that is what the client meant. You might ask, "When you say you are through, I understand that you are tired. Is that correct?" This gives the client the opportunity to agree or disagree and clarify further.

PLACING EVENTS IN TIME OR SEQUENCE. Often in describing an event or a series of events, clients fail to relate the story in strict chronological order. This can make the client's message about the occurrence difficult to follow. When this happens, you can ask the client to explain more about when the event occurred (placing the event in time) or to explain the sequence of a series of events (placing events in sequence).

Helping the Client Increase Self-Awareness

VERBALIZING THE IMPLIED. With the technique of *verbalizing the implied,* you understand the words the client has said but believe the words have an underlying meaning that was hinted at but not voiced specifically. You may need to verbalize this underlying message. The client may then verify that the message you received was indeed true. This frees the client to discuss with you some underlying feelings that were not voiced before. On the other hand, it is possible that the client did not mean to imply anything more than the actual words expressed. In this case, verbalizing the implied allows the client to verify that you have an inaccurate perception of the message.

ENCOURAGING ASSESSMENT OF EMOTIONS. It is important for people to be in touch with their own feelings. Too often, to cope with overwhelming feelings, clients wall themselves off from all emotions. This can be very unhealthy. To help clients get back in touch with their feelings, use the technique of encouraging assessment of emotions. To do this, ask clients to focus on their feelings, and ask them how they feel.

TRANSLATING INTO FEELINGS. Sometimes clients find it difficult or impossible to express their feelings verbally by using appropriate terms for common emotions. You can help clients by translating their messages into verbal expressions of feelings. However, you should always be open to correction if the client finds the translation inaccurate.

REFLECTING. In this technique, you reflect questions and statements back to the client to help the client to think about them and come to a conclusion. This helps the client gain confidence in making assessments and decisions and encourages the client's self-reliance.

There are two forms of reflection. One form is used when clients ask a question and the question is turned around and reflected back to them. For example, the client might ask, "How am I doing with my physical therapy?" and you might reflect back with, "How do you think you're doing?" This demonstrates that you value the client's opinion.

The second form reflects back to clients some of their own words and is referred to as selective reflection. This should not be confused with *parroting,* in which all of the client's words are directed back without thought on your part. With reflection, however, you think about the message and select the word or words that are important for the client to think about. This requires active involvement by both you and the client. For example, the client might say, "I'm scared about my surgery tomorrow." With reflection, you might ask, "Scared?" and suggest that the client consider and further discuss the feeling of being scared.

ENCOURAGING COMPARISON. To help clients integrate new experiences into what they know of life and to help them learn, you can encourage comparison. To do this, you may ask the client to compare or contrast a certain life experience with another.

Helping the Client Maintain Contact With Reality

ENCOURAGING DESCRIPTIONS OF PERCEPTIONS. Sometimes clients perceive things that others do not. It can be helpful for the client to describe such perceptions and the emotions attached to them. This technique of encouraging descriptions of perceptions is suitable when working with clients who have hallucinations of various types. It is not recommended that you attempt to communicate with a client who is actively hallucinating. If you know this is happening, wait until the hallucination has ended before attempting to elicit the client's perceptions and emotions.

PRESENTING REALITY. If you are with clients when a misperception of reality occurs, you can be the person who can help them identify what is real and what is not. This technique, called *presenting reality,* can be very reassuring to some people. Similar to the technique of voicing doubt, you accept the fact that the client has perceived something that you have not perceived, but you let the client know that you did not have a similar perception. You might say, for example, "It must be very frightening for you to hear sirens wailing, but I don't hear anything."

Concluding the Interaction

Encouraging Formulation of a Plan of Action. Once you enter the working phase of the relationship, and once you and the client have identified problems, diagnoses, and desired outcomes, you need to encourage formulation of a plan of action. This technique calls for encouraging the client to formulate the plan. It is more therapeutic and more likely to be successfully carried out if the plan comes from the client rather than from you.

To encourage formulation of a plan of action, ask the client to consider what might be the best thing to do in a future situation. This future situation might be one that the client has never experienced, or it might be one that the client has experienced but was not able to handle successfully. This allows the client to think things out in advance and to be prepared.

This technique may also be used near the end of a relationship in which the client has had an opportunity to try out a plan and has not been successful. After evaluating with the client what went wrong, you might suggest formulation of a new plan of action. This helps the client to see that new approaches can always be tried.

Summarizing. One therapeutic technique that might be done at intervals is summarizing. In this technique you summarize by briefly stating, in an orderly manner, what you and the client have discussed to that point in the interaction. This is usually thought of as a final activity, but if a client presents a great deal of data to you, it is often helpful to stop and summarize briefly at opportune times. This helps ensure that you and the client agree about what went on and what decisions were made. It also helps to ensure that you covered all of the information you both wanted to discuss. Of course, summarizing can help bring closure in the termination phase of a therapeutic relationship.

TECHNIQUES THAT IMPAIR THERAPEUTIC COMMUNICATION

Just as there are techniques that facilitate communication, there are also barriers to therapeutic communication. Nontherapeutic communication techniques impair the flow of communication in what would otherwise be a progressive movement toward client growth. Some nontherapeutic techniques thwart communication by undermining you, such as by calling into question your honesty or diminishing the client's trust in you. Other nontherapeutic techniques thwart communication by undermining the client. Nontherapeutic techniques that undermine the client are those that are demeaning, those that reinforce or strengthen irrational ideas or beliefs, those that tend to raise client anxiety levels, and those that tend to make the client dependent on you. Still other nontherapeutic techniques block the flow of ideas between the client and you. Some nontherapeutic techniques block communication in more than one way. Table 12-2 describes many nontherapeutic communication techniques along with selected examples that might be used with pediatric, adolescent, and adult clients.

Table 12-2 Nontherapeutic Communication Techniques		
Technique	**Description/Definition**	**Example**
Belittling feelings expressed	The nurse minimizes the degree of the client's distress or discomfort, thereby implying that the client's feelings are insignificant.	*Nurse with child:* Child: "I hate shots." Nurse: "You are not the only one." *Nurse with adolescent:* Adolescent: "There is no reason to go on." Nurse: "Aren't you being a little dramatic?" *Nurse with adult:* Adult: "My life means nothing." Nurse: "If you take a walk, you will feel better."
False reassurance	The nurse implies that the anxious client has no cause for worry or concern.	*Nurse with child:* "No need to fuss over such a small needle." *Nurse with adolescent:* "One day you will look back at this and laugh." *Nurse with adult:* "Your chest pain isn't a heart attack."
Parroting	The nurse mechanically repeats the client's words without evaluating what has been said and without helping the client to think things through. It indicates a lack of interest, respect, and relatedness on the nurse's part.	*Nurse with child:* Child: "My mommy left." Nurse: "Your mommy left." *Nurse with adolescent:* Adolescent: "I am not going for dialysis." Nurse: "You are not going for dialysis."

Continued

Table 12-2	Nontherapeutic Communication Techniques—cont'd	
Technique	**Description/Definition**	**Example**
Parroting—cont'd		*Nurse with adult:* Adult: "I do not see any options for treatment." Nurse: "You do not see any options for treatment."
Disapproving	The nurse makes a negative value judgment about the client's behavior or thinking.	*Nurse with child:* "Shame on you!" *Nurse with adolescent:* "I cannot believe you did that." *Nurse with adult:* "Why don't you stop all this foolishness?"
Disagreeing	The nurse opposes the client's thinking. The nurse's disagreement implies the client is wrong and must defend the position.	*Nurse with child:* "I think you are wrong about this." *Nurse with adolescent:* "You can say what you like, but it does not make it right." *Nurse with adult:* "I definitely disagree with you."
Rationalizing feelings expressed	The nurse provides a seemingly rational (but untrue) excuse for the client's expression of emotions to avoid an emotional reaction to the client's feelings or to avoid having to respond appropriately to the client. This rationalization of feelings robs affective material shared by the client of its power.	*Nurse with child:* Child: "I'm mad." Nurse: "Maybe you are just tired." *Nurse with adolescent:* "Jack, crying because you hurt will only make it worse." *Nurse with adult:* Adult: "Now I am just a heart patient." Nurse: "Wouldn't you be worse off if you had AIDS?"
Interpreting	The nurse attempts to tell the client the meaning of the client's experience by seeking to make conscious that which is unconscious.	*Nurse with child:* "What you really mean is . . . ." *Nurse with adolescent:* "Your true feelings are . . . ." *Nurse with adult:* "On a deeper level, you believe . . . ."
Advising	The nurse literally tells the client what to do. This implies that the nurse knows best and the client is incapable of independent problem solving.	*Nurse with child:* "Tell the doctor how much better you feel today." *Nurse with adolescent:* "Stop eating sweets and you will lose weight." *Nurse with adult:* "I would choose option A."
Blaming	The nurse inappropriately expresses feelings of anger or impatience with the client as a means of faulting the client because the nurse–client relationship is not progressing well. This is a therapeutic dead-end that negates the nurse's role as a client advocate, destroys trust, and takes away client motivation to work with the nurse to identify and explore sensitive topics.	*Nurse with child:* "Well, you can't expect a sticker when you cry every time I come near you." *Nurse with adolescent:* "Get your act together, and things will go better for you." *Nurse with adult:* "Nobody told you to pull your back out, did they?"
Patronizing	The nurse treats the client in a condescending manner, thereby demeaning the client. This makes acceptance, respect, and mutual decision making impossible.	*Nurse with child:* "Just go play somewhere now." *Nurse with adolescent:* "Of course your ideas are important to me, sweetie." *Nurse with adult:* "Let's put on our slippers before we fall."
Making stereotypical comments	The nurse makes empty conversation using trite phrases and cliches, thereby encouraging the client to do the same rather than honestly exploring issues.	*Nurse with child:* "You will thank me later." *Nurse with adolescent:* "Pretty is as pretty does." *Nurse with adult:* "Let a smile be your umbrella."
Introducing an unrelated topic	The nurse changes the subject when the client brings up material the nurse prefers not to discuss.	*Nurse with child:* Child: "What is sex?" Nurse: "Finish your lunch before it gets cold." *Nurse with adolescent:* Adolescent: "What is my diagnosis?" Nurse: "Did you see the game last night?" *Nurse with adult:* Adult: "The doctor says that I am dying." Nurse: "Time for a bath."
Using jargon	The nurse excludes the client and makes the interaction incomprehensible by using nursing jargon (the specialized language used by a group).	*Nurse with child:* "Do not regurgitate your nutritional supplement." *Nurse with adolescent:* "Your increased sexual preoccupation indicates progression toward full maturation." *Nurse with adult:* "Coronary abnormalities are indicated on the angiogram."

Table 12-2 Nontherapeutic Communication Techniques—cont'd

Technique	Description/Definition	Example
Giving literal responses	The nurse responds to the client's figurative statement as though it were factual. The nurse misses a chance to explore material with the client.	*Nurse with child:* Child: "My insides are exploding." Nurse: "That sounds messy." *Nurse with adolescent:* Adolescent: "I am losing my mind." Nurse: "Find it." *Nurse with adult:* Adult: "My world is ending" Nurse: "The world is not ending."
Requesting an explanation	The nurse asks "why" of the client, thereby asking for a reason for feelings and behaviors when the client may not know the reason.	*Nurse with child:* "Why don't you stop crying?" *Nurse with adolescent:* "Why are you upset?" *Nurse with adult:* "Why can't you fall asleep?"
Probing	The nurse digs for information or persistently questions the client even after the client indicates unwillingness to discuss the issues.	*Nurse with child:* Nurse: "Tell me about the test." Child: "I do not want to." Nurse: "Tell me anyway." *Nurse with adolescent:* "Tell me more about that terrible event." *Nurse with adult:* "I cannot help you if you do not give me all the information about your drug habit."

Key Principles

- The three phases of the therapeutic relationship are the orientation phase, the working phase, and the termination phase. Each phase has certain tasks associated with it.
- The six elements of communication are encoder, message, sensory channel, decoder, feedback, and context.
- Two types of communication are verbal and nonverbal.
- Verbal communication includes using words through talking or writing.
- Body language is a form of nonverbal communication that consists of human communication by alterations in personal appearance, changes in facial expressions, changes in body posture, use of gestures, maintenance of personal distances, and use of touching.
- Paralanguage is a form of nonverbal communication that consists of the elements of stress, accent, pitch, pause, intonation, rate, volume, and quality.
- Nursing attitudes that facilitate effective therapeutic communication include awareness, acceptance, respect, unconditional positive regard, empathy, relatedness, caring, objectivity, protectiveness, genuineness, openness, appropriate professional closeness or distance, and a sense of humor.
- It is vital to recognize nontherapeutic communication techniques in order to avoid using them as you begin to learn and practice therapeutic communication techniques.
- Inappropriate use of therapeutic communication techniques can change them from therapeutic techniques into nontherapeutic techniques.
- Although any specific therapeutic technique might be used at any time, some techniques tend to be more helpful at the beginning, the middle, or at the end of an interaction.

Bibliography

Arnold, E., & Boggs, K. U. (1999). *Interpersonal relationships: Professional communication skills for nurses* (3rd ed.). Philadelphia: Saunders.

Brown, S. J. (1999). Patient-centered communication. *Annual Review of Nursing Research, 17,* 85-103.

Evans, G. W., Witt, D. L., Alligood, M. R., & O'Neil, M. (1998). Empathy: A study of two types. *Issues in Mental Health Nursing, 19*(5), 453-461.

Heery, K. (2000). Straight talk about the patient interview. *Nursing 2000, 30*(6), 66-67.

How to build rapport with patients. (2000). *Nursing 2000, 30*(9), 73.

*King, I. M. (1981). *A theory for nursing: Systems, concepts, process.* New York: Delmar.

Klagsbrun, J. (2001). Listening and focusing: Holistic health care tools for nurses. *Nursing Clinics of North America, 36*(1), 115-129.

*Peplau, H. (1952). *Interpersonal relations in nursing.* New York: McGraw-Hill.

Riley, J. B. (2000). *Communication in nursing* (4th ed.). St Louis, MO: Mosby.

*Rogers, C. R. (1951). *Client-centered therapy.* Boston: Houghton Mifflin.

*Tannen, D. (1990). *You just don't understand: Women and men in conversation.* New York: Ballantine Books.

*Travelbee, J. (1966). *Interpersonal aspects of nursing.* Philadelphia: Davis.

*Watzlawick, P., Jackson, D. D., & Bandas, J. B. (1967). *Pragmatics of human communication: A study of interactional patterns, pathologies, and paradoxes.* New York: Norton.

*Asterisk indicates a classic or definitive work on this subject.

Client Teaching

Learning Objectives

After studying this chapter, you should be able to do the following:

- Discuss the rationale for client teaching, including its purpose and benefits
- Describe the teaching and learning process, including domains of learning and principles of effective teaching
- Describe factors that affect client teaching
- Discuss the nursing diagnosis *Deficient knowledge*
- Develop a teaching plan for a client
- Discuss strategies for effectively implementing client teaching
- Discuss methods for evaluating teaching and learning

Charlotte Avery is an 82-year-old Jamaican-American woman who lives in Boca Raton, Florida. Mrs. Avery is a retired restaurant manager. She lives alone in the home she shared with her third husband, Charles, who passed away 2 years ago. Mrs. Avery was recently diagnosed with insulin-dependent diabetes mellitus. She needs information about her condition and self-care. The nurse makes the diagnosis of *Deficient knowledge* (see below).

KEY NURSING DIAGNOSIS FOR Teaching and Learning

Deficient knowledge (specify): State in which a person lacks skills or information to successfully manage his or her own health care

CONCEPTS OF CLIENT TEACHING

Public access to health care information has never been greater. Bookstore shelves are crowded with self-help books and medical reference texts. The latest medical research findings are published in newspapers and magazines and even reported on the evening news. Pharmaceutical companies advertise prescription drugs in television commercials, encouraging consumers to ask their family health care providers for more information. Via the internet, consumers can retrieve information from around the world on any topic within minutes.

At the same time, the public need for health care teaching has also continued to rise. Hospitals that discharge clients earlier than ever must make sure that those clients can care for themselves at home. Current trends in health care require that clients and their families quickly assume responsibility for self-care management, and the focus on outcomes dictates that nurses be accountable for care that includes education.

Client Rights and Nursing Standards

Client education has been considered an integral part of nursing practice since it was first recognized as a discipline. In addition, the role of the nurse in client education is now legally mandated through the nurse practice act in each state (Bastable, 2003). The Joint Commission on Accreditation for Healthcare Organizations (JCAHO), which accredits hospitals, has included client education in its nursing standards since 1993, and more recently it has expanded that expectation to include interdisciplinary participation and documentation of client understanding (Davidhizer & Brownson, 1999).

In addition to legal and accreditation mandates for client teaching, the American Hospital Association (AHA) published the *Patient's Bill of Rights* in 1975 and the *Patient Care Partnership: Understanding Expectations, Rights, and Responsibilities* in 2003. This document established the rights of clients to receive complete and current information concerning diagnosis, treatment, and prognosis in terms they can understand (AHA, 1975). More recently, the federal government has published *Healthy People 2010: Objectives for Improving Health,* which outlines national objectives for health promotion and disease prevention (U.S. Department of Health and Human Services, 2000). These objectives call for the development of programs that educate the public about reducing risk behaviors and that promote positive health practices.

Benefits of Client Teaching

The benefits of teaching are well documented. Benefits of health teaching and learning include positive client outcomes and decreased readmissions to the hospital (Box 13-1). Client teaching also helps to control costs and maintain quality care.

Cost Control. Client teaching has become an important factor in controlling costs within health care systems. Education helps control costs by means of the following:
- Preventing illnesses that may require expensive care
- Enabling the client to manage a prescribed treatment regimen after discharge from an acute care facility
- Promoting client safety, which may decrease or prevent complications, and which ultimately reduces costs
- Preparing the client to anticipate and recognize complications, to seek help early, and to prevent hospital readmission
- Increasing the care that can be given at home, including high-technology care and diagnostic testing
- Increasing compliance with the treatment regimen, thus reducing the need for more costly medical procedures

Quality Control. Client teaching has also become a critical component of maintaining quality of care. Education helps maintain quality by means of the following:
- Encouraging the client and family to be active partners in the delivery of health care, thus improving the outcome
- Increasing client satisfaction by helping the client understand what can reasonably be expected from the health care system
- Increasing the client's sense of control, which is derived from knowledge
- Ensuring that clients have the knowledge they need to provide self-care
- Increasing communication between the client and provider
- Increasing client satisfaction through a mutually respectful relationship

THE TEACHING AND LEARNING PROCESS

Teaching and learning are mutually dependent aspects of a dynamic, interactive process. **Teaching** is a set of planned activities performed to influence knowledge, behavior, or skill. To teach effectively, you must understand the subject to be taught, accurately assess the client's learning needs, control

A PATIENT'S PERSPECTIVE   Box 13-1
"The Clinic Nurses Have Taught Me So Much About How to Manage Diabetes"

When I was 48, I began to feel like my body was shutting down. I was tired all the time, I had no energy, and I was losing weight. But my doctor didn't seem concerned, so I just chalked it up to stress. And there was plenty of that. My dad was dying of a brain tumor, my mother had been diagnosed with Alzheimer's, and, as the oldest daughter, I was the primary caregiver.

After Dad died in 1991, I took my mother to Vermont to visit my brother and his family. One afternoon as we were walking through the woods, I slipped and grabbed onto a nearby tree branch to keep from falling. Unfortunately, a thorn on the branch pierced my hand. It wasn't terribly painful, so I just put some ointment and a bandage on it and thought nothing more about it. The next morning, my arm was twice its normal size! A local doctor gave me a shot of antibiotics and a prescription and told me to check in with my regular doctor as soon as I got home, which I did. He couldn't explain why I had experienced such an extreme reaction but thought that maybe I had multiple sclerosis. A few months after that, however, he came up with the real diagnosis: diabetes.

As soon as my doctor figured out what the problem was, he put me on 130 units of insulin a day. Almost immediately, I began to gain weight, even though I was walking three to five miles a day. Eventually, I gained a hundred pounds. My vision began to deteriorate, because the blood vessels in my eyes were hemorrhaging. So the doctor sent me to a specialist who did laser treatments to stop the hemorrhaging, at a cost of $1500 per treatment. My vision loss made it impossible for me to work, so it wasn't long be-

fore I ran out of money and was forced to go to a public clinic for all my medical care. Ironically, that turned out to be the best thing that could have happened to me.

The clinic is run by nurses, and it is wonderful. I can't say enough good things about the way they treat you. Everyone there is friendly. They always call you by name. They take time to listen. They make sure that you're scheduled for routine screenings, such as Pap smears, mammograms, and so on. They recognize that people's circumstances change, and they don't punish you because you don't have money. What's more, I get better care now than when I did have money!

The doctors who work at my clinic are all volunteers, and they are excellent. My endocrinologist is a woman, and she keeps up on all the latest research. My former doctor was not good at controlling my diabetes. Over a period of time, my clinic doctor has gotten me totally off insulin and onto oral medications. My diet was pretty good, but she fine-tuned it. She also suggested that I find an additional caregiver for my mother. Those changes have made a huge difference in my life, in my weight, and in my blood sugar.

The clinic nurses have taught me so much about how to manage diabetes. And every three months I have tests for long-term blood sugar control and liver function because of the oral medications I'm taking. So far, my diabetes is under really good control.

the learning environment, and use methods appropriate for the client's needs.

Learning is the acquisition of knowledge, behavior, or skill through experience, practice, study, or instruction. It is an all-encompassing experience that involves acquiring new knowledge, information, and skills, and thus changing one's behavior. Learning may cause people to change their attitudes, perceptions, habits, and methods of problem solving.

Coherence With the Nursing Process

The teaching and learning process correlates with the nursing process (Table 13-1). In the assessment phase, you gather subjective and objective data related to the client's knowledge base and learning needs. In the diagnosis phase, you identify specific learning needs. Then you develop a plan, take appropriate actions to implement the plan, and evaluate the teaching and learning processes. If needed, modify, on the basis of your evaluation, the plan to improve client understanding.

Domains of Learning

Learning theorists have identified three primary domains of learning that include the following:

- Cognitive domain: the ability to make sense of and use information
- Affective domain: the feelings and values associated with information
- Psychomotor domain: manipulative and motor skills

A taxonomy used to categorize levels of behaviors according to complexity within each domain is useful in developing learning objectives. Although each domain is described separately, it is understood that cognitive, affective, and psy-

chomotor behaviors do not occur in isolation but are interdependent processes that occur simultaneously. By integrating all of these domains into your teaching plans, you will improve the quality of your teaching and promote client learning. We will now explore each of the domains in more detail.

Cognitive Domain. The **cognitive learning domain** is considered the "thinking" domain. It includes acquiring knowledge, comprehending, and using critical thinking skills (Figure 13-1). Learning takes place at several levels in the cognitive domain and Bloom and his associates (1956) describe them as follows:

- **Acquisition:** To acquire knowledge, the client obtains information, commonly by memorizing terms, facts, principles, and procedures.
- **Comprehension:** Comprehension implies understanding of new information. When people comprehend new information, they can repeat the content back in their own words, relate the information to something already known, or attach meaning to the information.
- **Application:** Application of knowledge is the intellectual ability to use acquired information in similar but different situations.
- **Analysis:** Analysis, the fourth level of cognitive learning, is the ability to separate information into components of the whole.
- **Synthesis:** Synthesis is reassembling parts to identify a new whole. The client uses the information that you provide and communicates a creative and unique use of the information.
- **Evaluation:** Evaluation involves making judgments about the effects of the treatment.

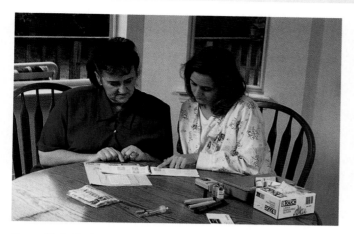

Figure 13-1. In the *cognitive* domain, the client is able to discuss the signs and symptoms of low blood glucose.

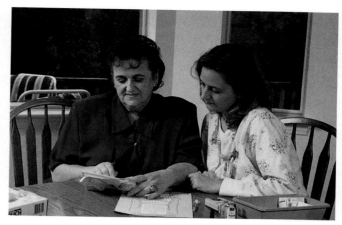

Figure 13-2. In the *affective* domain, the client commits to performing daily self-injections.

Table 13-1	Comparison of the Nursing Process and the Teaching Process	
Step	**Nursing Process**	**Teaching Process**
1	• Collect and analyze data.	• Collect and analyze data about client's knowledge.
2	• Assess client needs.	• Identify learning needs.
3	• Label needs with nursing diagnoses.	• Make an educational diagnosis, such as *Deficient knowledge, Ineffective health maintenance,* or *Health-seeking behaviors.*
4	• Identify desired outcomes. • Plan nursing interventions.	• Prepare a teaching plan by writing objectives, content, time frame, teaching format, and how to teach content, such as by using audiovisual equipment.
5	• Implement nursing care. • Evaluate client's outcomes. • Reassess as needed.	• Implement the teaching plan and delivery of content. • Evaluate client learning on basis of objectives. • Reassess as needed.

Synthesis and evaluation represent the highest levels of cognitive ability. Although nurses routinely synthesize and evaluate information at these levels, clients—especially sick clients—are not always able to reach this level of attainment. Clients may be only able to comprehend the steps of a carefully prescribed routine; they may not be able to analyze or modify that routine. When teaching such a client, limit yourself to essential information, such as the cause of an illness, lifestyle changes needed to prevent complications, basic symptom management, and specific skills as needed, such as how to irrigate a colostomy. Usually, the client can function when given this amount of information; in-depth explanations can be added as the client asks questions.

Affective Domain. The **affective learning domain** includes the ethics, principles, and reasoning that determine and guide moral or "right" behavior. The affective domain includes values, beliefs, feelings, and attitudes (Figure 13-2). Thus teaching in the affective domain can address a client's health-seeking behaviors and choices at a deep and powerful level.

Emotions are also addressed in the affective domain. Feelings that arise in response to health care situations need to be recognized and managed. Anger, frustration, relief, and joy are often experienced as part of obtaining health care, being diagnosed with an illness, or even receiving a clean bill of health. Helping a client understand and manage feelings is essential to integrating new learning into activities of daily living.

Within the affective domain, five levels of learning were identified by Krathwohl, Bloom, and Masia (1964). These levels are described in terms of behavior that you can assess:
- **Receiving:** Affective learning begins with the process of receiving. The person names the feeling or emotion and recognizes that the emotion may be interfering with action.
- **Responding:** Responding occurs when the client can freely discuss feelings.
- **Valuing:** Valuing occurs when a person freely chooses a particular action from among several alternatives.
- **Organizing:** Organizing integrates a value into everyday life.
- **Characterizing:** Characterizing refers to the client's ability to internalize values into a philosophy of life, making it possible to behave consistently in accordance with those values.

You can promote a client's health and well-being by facilitating high-level learning in the affective domain. To do so, you must accomplish the following three personal goals:
- Understand your own value system, and provide information to clients in a manner that minimizes your own biases.
- Respect the validity and uniqueness of each individual's personal, cultural, and religious value system, even when it differs from yours.
- Provide accurate and complete information about health and illness, thereby setting the stage for affective learning.

Learning in the affective domain can be difficult to evaluate and typically must be an ongoing process. Some clients

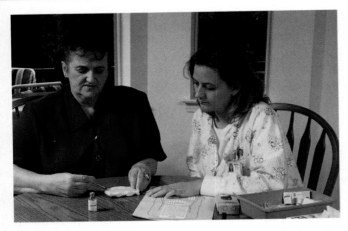

Figure 13-3. In the *psychomotor* domain, the client manipulates the equipment to perform self-injection.

may take years to internalize feelings and values fully enough to change their behavior.

Psychomotor Domain. The **psychomotor learning domain** includes physical and motor skills, such as giving injections (Figure 13-3). These skills may require varying levels of dexterity, coordination, and the ability to manipulate equipment and objects. Development of psychomotor skills involves integration of the other two domains as well. Psychomotor learning also includes perceptual processes that some theorists consider a separate domain. Incorporating the perceptual processes, Simpson (1972) identified the following levels of learning in the psychomotor domain:

- **Perception:** Ability to receive, respond, and connect meaning to sensory cues associated with a task to be performed.
- **Set:** Set is the level in which the client shows a readiness to take on a particular skill or task.
- **Guided response:** At this level, the client tries to imitate the behavior portrayed by the nurse.
- **Mechanism:** At this level, the client has successfully achieved a task or skill. This skill will then become a habit and a change from previous behavior.
- **Complex overt response:** Here, the client can perform the task or skill independently, without having to give attention to the task.
- **Adaptation:** At this level, the client has mastered the skill so proficiently that the task can be adapted to varying physical conditions or situations.
- **Origination:** This level of the psychomotor domain challenges the client to create new ways or acts of manipulating the skills or abilities.

Proficiency at each level of the psychomotor domain is necessary to master many manual skills. Once mastered, the psychomotor skill then becomes a means to the end.

A clear understanding of the interdependence of cognitive, affective, and psychomotor domains of learning will enable you to assess each client's learning needs with confidence. When those needs are accurately identified, learning objectives can be mutually negotiated and teaching in all domains implemented.

FACTORS AFFECTING CLIENT TEACHING

Many factors can influence the effectiveness of your teaching, including you, your client, the family or significant others, and the situation. Additionally, time to teach is a factor. You will have limited interaction with clients. Therefore you must maximize your teaching effectiveness to compensate for the short teaching time available.

Client Characteristics

Many characteristics can influence a client's approach to learning, such as age, race, gender, medical diagnosis, and clinical progress. Likewise, religious beliefs and cultural background may alter the client's learning needs and therefore affect the methods by which you present materials in particular content areas. Other important assessment factors include literacy, education, developmental level, and learning style.

Literacy Level. You may encounter clients who cannot read or who cannot read English. Clients who can read will have varying abilities, from very basic to very advanced. Many clients will be embarrassed to admit their inability to read educational materials. Consequently, you must determine each client's ability to read and comprehend educational materials. The number of years in school is often an inaccurate measure of literacy. It is more useful to observe client behavior for clues of illiteracy, including confusion, nervousness, making excuses, or irrelevant statements that indicate lack of communication.

Several standardized tests are available to measure reading skills. In addition, there is also an instrument available to assess the readability of instructional materials for a given population (Doak, Doak, & Root, 1996). Be prepared to provide privacy and the educational methods that complement each client's learning ability.

Level of Knowledge. Before you begin teaching a client, assess general health knowledge, perception of current illness, and the type of teaching that will be most helpful and easily understood. To make this assessment, you most likely will want to consider the client's level of formal education. However, you cannot assume that a well-educated person is a well-informed person when it comes to health education. You should determine how much a client knows or how well he can perform a skill before initiating a teaching plan.

In addition to assessing a client's knowledge level, determine the following:

- What he has been told by a physician or has learned from media sources
- What he knows about his illness
- What his previous experience is with illness, the health care system, or hospitalization

These factors may influence his knowledge level and readiness to learn.

Developmental Level. Learning can also be influenced by whether the client is a child, an adolescent, an adult, or an older adult. Additionally, a client who is developmentally delayed will need particular attention so that teaching, if appropriate, is done at an optimal level.

CHILDREN. For children, the teaching and learning process can be fundamentally different than that used by adults. You must adjust the complexity and volume of information taught to each child's age and cognitive level. You also must carefully choose terms and examples to keep them appropriate for the child's age level.

For example, young children may learn best by playing games, drawing, or watching video-modeling of behavior. The use of dolls, stuffed animals, or other toys may be helpful. Many children are receptive to instruction that involves role-playing. This type of interaction may be therapeutic as well as educational. Children and their parents may require specialized teaching approaches (Box 13-2). Note that parents may need affective domain assessment for their emotional reactions to their children's problems.

ADOLESCENTS. The first approach to effective teaching with adolescents is to develop a trusting relationship. Privacy is essential when discussing personal matters, such as self-esteem. How a teen "looks" to his peers is of utmost importance because peers play a vital role in the life of teenagers.

Adolescents expect honesty, openness, and the truth about their illness. Thus you will want to allow adolescents to have as much control as possible in the health care arena. This includes letting them choose what they want to wear and eat, within reason. If possible, let them visit with friends.

ADULTS. Knowles (1980) identified four assumptions that characterize adult learning. Of course, people differ, and not all of the following assumptions may apply to any one client, but by sensibly integrating the principles into the learning process, you can create a successful and supportive learning environment.

LEARNING IS SELF-DIRECTED. As people mature, their learning becomes increasingly self-directed, largely because changes in self-concept take the learner from a state of dependency to a state of increasing independence. In general, adults identify their learning needs and then take action to acquire the knowledge they know they need.

LEARNING IS BUILT ON PREVIOUS KNOWLEDGE. The adult learner brings a lifetime of accumulated learning to each new learning experience. Indeed, as adults, we define or characterize ourselves largely by our experiences. The older we become, the more ingrained our previous experiences become. Therefore, to facilitate adult learning, you should make use of previous learning and experiences as resources to enhance present learning.

LEARNING IS PRACTICAL. Learning is more likely to happen when an adult is ready to learn. That readiness results in part from an adult's realization that a certain knowledge is needed to perform effectively in a chosen role. Health education receives attention, and learning becomes meaningful, when the adult needs the information and is aware of the need. Therefore health education is more effective when the person has signs and symptoms of an illness.

LEARNING IS PURPOSEFUL. Closely related to readiness to learn is the fourth assumption, that learning is purposeful.

Box 13-2 Tips for Teaching Children

- Trust is essential to a therapeutic relationship with a child.
- In general, the younger the child, the shorter the attention span.
- Children are exposed to various levels of information about health care. Be sure to assess the child's knowledge.
- Children form misconceptions easily. A child's imagination may create greater fear than the truth, told directly and simply.
- Parents can often provide cues to the child's emotional response and capacity for understanding information. However, some parents may underestimate or overestimate their child's capacity.
- Children may regress developmentally in a situation of illness.
- Children may better manage uncomfortable information through role-playing with dolls and models.

Adult learning is often based on real-life problems, and it is most effective when immediate results are obtained. (This problem-centered learning differs from the subject-oriented learning done in school, which has a delayed application.) When you are teaching adults, it is helpful to make sure they understand the purpose of learning.

ELDERLY ADULTS. Although intelligence may actually increase as a person ages, the capacity to learn is affected by functional changes. These changes may not appreciably affect performance until a person's eighties or nineties. However, chronic and debilitating diseases often alter intellectual abilities.

Reaction time, or the amount of time required for a response to a stimulus, slows with age. An older person needs more time to process information and perform psychomotor skills. It may take longer to make decisions, especially if the decision requires thinking about multiple aspects of a problem. Instructions need to be free of unnecessary detail and explanations. A person can become confused by paying too much attention to irrelevant detail. If this occurs, redirect the client to the main learning points.

Although memory may not be severely impaired, an older person is often slower in acquiring, storing, and recalling new information. To compensate, the person uses selective attention to screen out extraneous information, thus sometimes missing information that is actually important. If you slow the pace of teaching new information, you can help older persons compensate for their decreased ability.

The capacity to learn is affected by stress and fatigue. The older person often fatigues more easily and thus has more difficulty paying attention to new information. Additionally, stress is associated with multiple stimuli or trying to think about a number of things at the same time. When the activities of daily living require more thinking time and energy, the older adult may be less able to screen out extraneous thoughts and concentrate on learning new information. If the older adult becomes overwhelmed by the information provided, prioritize the key or "survival" points as a lesson summary. This will enhance client safety by identifying what is necessary to promote health.

Remember that changes with aging are highly variable. Older adults have written a first novel, taken up painting, and otherwise developed new skills. Do not underestimate their learning ability.

Learning Styles. Every client has a preferred learning style, a way of processing information that works best. Research on learning styles has been well documented in the literature (Kolb, 1984). You can enhance the effectiveness of your teaching by discovering this style for each client early in the course of teaching. Unfortunately, many nurse educators use the teaching strategy that is most comfortable for themselves, rather than individualizing their strategy to accommodate the client's style of learning.

Some clients prefer to hear you talk about a topic. Others prefer to read a pamphlet or handout and then to ask questions after studying independently. To increase your effectiveness, ask your clients how they most enjoy learning new information; then adapt your teaching strategy to their preference.

Nurse educators agree that education is a process. Meaningful interactions provide creative ways for mutual understanding, problem solving, and decision making. Adapting yourself into the nurse educator role means that you find the learning style that is best for your client and that you adapt the teaching material to accomplish a behavior change (Bastable, 2003). When the spouse, significant other, or family is the actual target of health teaching, assessment of their readiness to learn and of their motivation becomes important.

Factors That Facilitate Learning

To teach effectively, you must understand and use factors that facilitate learning. These factors—readiness and motivation—can guide your decisions about teaching children, adults, families, groups, and communities.

Readiness. The client must be both physically and emotionally ready to learn. Health status may have a profound effect on readiness to learn, as it may affect both cognitive ability and energy level. Readiness to learn often depends on the concern generated by illness or the threat of illness. Clients who are acutely ill are generally focused on short-term needs. As recovery progresses, more attention can be devoted to prevention.

Motivation. Clients learn more if they have a genuine desire or motivation to learn. Motivation is greatest in clients who recognize their learning needs and perceive the available teaching as meaningful. Motivation depends on acceptance of self-responsibility for health. As clients become more independent, learning becomes more self-directed.

Motivation can be difficult to measure and, usually, you must rely on indirect signs. Strategies to assess motivation include asking questions or engaging the client in a conversation about the topic. An unmotivated client will become distracted, change the subject, or otherwise show signs of not paying attention. Some clients will suggest that you give the information to their spouse or significant other.

People differ in the amount and type of information they can tolerate concerning their illness or behavior. Some people become anxious if they feel uninformed about their illness, including its cause, prevention, and treatment. Others become anxious if you try to talk about their disorder. When anxious clients resist instruction, wait until they begin asking questions or show other signs of readiness. At this point, their anxiety may have lessened, and they may be more receptive to new information.

The motivation to learn increases in an atmosphere of acceptance. Clients need to feel that you are genuinely interested in helping them learn. They also need time to assimilate ideas and develop new skills. They have the right to make mistakes and even to fail at a task without "losing face." You can increase their motivation by acting as a facilitator, not as a judge.

Factors That Inhibit Learning

Barriers to learning may include physiological, psychological, cultural, environmental, socioeconomic, and teaching factors.

Physiological Factors. Clients who are critically ill, in severe pain, restless, oxygen deprived, fatigued, weak, deaf, or vision-impaired face physical obstacles to learning. These obstacles interfere with readiness to learn because they reduce the person's ability to concentrate, and they deplete energy. All but the simplest information must be postponed until the client is able to attend to learning, and any information provided during a serious illness should be repeated as the client recovers. Box 13-3 examines the effects that teaching has on clients who will be undergoing invasive procedures.

Physiological barriers include perceptual problems. Always assess hearing and visual acuity. If the client has a sensory deficit, consider this when selecting visual aids or teaching strategies.

Psychological Factors. Psychological barriers are related to motivation. Attitude often changes throughout the course of a serious illness and also when a person moves from being well to being ill. It is helpful to understand what the client's personality and self-image were like before the onset of the present illness. Clients sometimes experience a personality change as a result of a real or perceived threat to their self-esteem or present lifestyle.

Teaching content may be altered by the medical or nursing prognosis. A client who is terminally ill may have different learning needs and capabilities than those of a client not facing death. Unfortunately, because the learning needs of the dying client are different, often they are ignored altogether.

Psychological stresses also interfere with concentration. People who feel anxious, fearful, and angry about their illness may have difficulty learning. Those who have trouble adjusting to a new diagnosis may experience denial, which postpones their readiness to learn.

Cultural Factors. Teaching and learning can be complicated when clients speak languages that are different from yours or have cultural or ethnic backgrounds and values that differ from yours. In all cases, you and your clients will benefit from your awareness of cultural differences

THE STATE OF NURSING RESEARCH: Preparing Clients for Invasive Procedures

Box 13-3

What Are the Issues?

Undergoing invasive diagnostic procedures is a stressful experience for clients. Privacy concerns, pain, and anxiety about possible results occupy clients' minds. Medications are often administered to help reduce the anxiety. Pre-procedure preparation by the nurse also helps decrease clients' anxiety. In the past, clients admitted to the hospital for diagnostic tests were often given ample time for the nurse to provide information and answer questions. Since the advent of outpatient treatment centers, new approaches to preparing clients for procedures are necessary.

What Research Has Been Conducted?

Two groups of researchers investigated the experiences of clients undergoing gastrointestinal diagnostic procedures in outpatient settings. One group looked at how clients received information about the procedures (Clements & Melby, 1998). They discovered that both nurses and written material were sources of information for the procedure. They found age differences: older people used nurses for information, and younger people used written sources.

More recently, Salmore and Nelson (2000) went one step further and looked at the effects of preparation on actual client outcomes. They used a combination of interventions including relaxation, imagery, and music. The client outcomes measured were blood pressure, pulse, and pulse oximetry. People in their study were scheduled for a gastrointestinal examination (either colonoscopy or esophagogastroduodenoscopy). The intervention included a home visit to obtain informed consent and baseline data on vital signs. The experimental group also received verbal and printed information on relaxation and imagery and tapes of relaxation music. They were encouraged to use the materials at home. Vital sign measurements were obtained on all clients on admission, during the procedure, and prior to discharge. Clients received standard medications. Clients in the treatment groups had significantly lower blood pressure readings during the procedures.

What Has the Research Concluded?

Giving people information about diagnostic procedures, and encouraging them to practice relaxation and imagery can have a calming effect on clients, as evidenced by decreases in blood pressure.

What Is the Future of Research in This Area?

Pre-procedure teaching is just one area where nurses can share information to help clients cope more effectively. Nurses need to develop new teaching approaches that can be used in outpatient settings. The telephone, email, and the internet may offer new ways to teach people in their homes.

References

Clements, H., & Melby, V. (1998). An investigation into the information obtained by patients undergoing gastroscopy investigations. *Journal of Clinical Nursing*, *7*(4), 333-342.

Salmore, R. G., & Nelson, J. (2000). The effect of preprocedure teaching, relaxation instruction, and music on anxiety as measured by blood pressures in an outpatient gastrointestinal endoscopy laboratory. *Gastroenterology Nursing*, *23*(3), 102-110.

and your willingness to obtain assistance with teaching when needed.

Some ethnic groups follow unique beliefs and practices, many of which involve diet, nutrition, health, and illness. Certain foods may be forbidden; certain health rituals may be required. At all times, consider cultural and religious values when assessing overall teaching and learning needs. However, avoid stereotyping clients by their ethnic or cultural background. Lack of cultural sensitivity may result in lost investment of teaching time and in distancing of those who most need education about health promotion practices (Price & Cortis, 2000).

Also recognize that the values you hold may—and probably do—vary from those of your clients. For example, you may value self-care and independence; the client may not. You may have trouble identifying with a client who says, "Just tell my wife. She gives me all my pills." Yet you must regard each client as a unique individual with valid wishes about teaching and learning.

Environmental Factors. Learning is facilitated in a pleasant, quiet environment, free from distractions. The teaching area should be well lit, comfortably warm, and (if possible) away from the hub of activity.

Noise, interruptions, and lack of privacy can seriously disrupt teaching sessions. When the room is too hot or cold, the client may be too uncomfortable to concentrate. In group teaching sessions, some clients may be distracted by the movements and noises of others in the room.

Distractions from the teaching process may arise in a variety of settings. Imagine the distractions possible in a homeless shelter or in a client's cluttered home with barking dogs, small children, and a loud television. Even a hospital room does not always offer the privacy and quiet needed for teaching, because visitors, physicians, and other nurses enter the room to complete their roles. Reducing stimuli to gain your client's full attention may challenge you to be creative for your teaching and learning sessions.

Socioeconomic Factors. When teaching clients about their illness and the care required, it helps to consider their home situation, living arrangements, and usual activities. Evaluate their relationships with significant others to determine the strength of their personal support system. Assess the type of work they do as well as their level of stress. Knowing their financial situation enables you to plan cost-effective health and maintenance care when possible. Keep in mind, however, that some clients are very private about their financial matters. Be prepared to explain your need to know about their financial condition.

 What factors might affect Mrs. Avery's ability to learn?

IMPLEMENTING THE TEACHING–LEARNING PROCESS

Health teaching involves assessment of client learning needs, determining learning objectives, planning appropriate teaching strategies, implementing the teaching plan, and evaluating the outcomes of the instruction. The process closely parallels the nursing process.

Assessment

For a client with learning needs, you will follow the phases of the nursing process just as you would for a client with physiological needs. Assessment should include client characteristics as well as factors present that facilitate or inhibit learning. Several nursing diagnoses can be applied to clients with learning needs, but *Deficient knowledge* is the most common. In certain client situations, a related diagnosis—such as *Noncompliance, Ineffective health maintenance,* or *Self-care deficit*—may be more appropriate. *Deficient knowledge* is defined as "the absence or deficiency of cognitive information related to [a] specific topic" (NANDA, 2001).

Focused Assessment for *Deficient Knowledge.*

Any client can have a need for health-related knowledge; however, several factors may increase the risk of *Deficient knowledge.* Clients at greatest risk include those with chronic illnesses that require complex treatment regimens, those needing special procedures, and those for whom preventive measures are important, such as pregnant clients, elderly clients with respiratory disease, and clients with impaired immunity.

Generally, the uneducated client is thought to be at greater risk, but highly educated clients often do not have experience with or understanding of medical or health problems. Family members, including children, also need information, as does anyone who acts as the client's caregiver.

DEFINING CHARACTERISTICS. Verbalization that a client has no knowledge, incomplete knowledge, or incorrect knowledge is a defining characteristic for the nursing diagnosis *Deficient knowledge.* Clients may tell you directly that they need knowledge, or they may ask questions that indicate the specific knowledge sought. Look for objective clues that they do not have appropriate knowledge or do not understand. The evidence may be indirect, as when they fail to follow instructions accurately or perform poorly on tests or return demonstrations.

RELATED FACTORS. Related factors may give direction to your choice of interventions. These factors may require you to modify your teaching to minimize the effect of a factor or remove it before implementing the teaching plan. Related factors for *Deficient knowledge* include the following:

- Cognitive limitation
- Information misinterpretation
- Lack of interest in learning
- Lack of motivation
- Lack of readiness to learn
- Lack of recall
- Limited exposure to information (specify)
- Limited practice of skill
- Unfamiliarity with information resources

 Think again about Mrs. Avery. What questions would you ask her to elicit information about her teaching-learning needs?

Diagnosis

Although teaching is an appropriate intervention for almost all nursing diagnoses, *Deficient knowledge* is the nursing diagnosis identified most often for clients with learning needs. You must consider the goal of client teaching before selecting the diagnosis. If the goal of teaching is to maintain health, the diagnosis should be *Ineffective health maintenance.* If the goal of teaching is to ensure compliance with the treatment regimen, the diagnosis should be *Ineffective management of therapeutic regimen.* If the goal of teaching is to convince the client of the value of continuing with treatment, the diagnosis is *Noncompliance.*

The diagnosis can be *Deficient knowledge* when there is a barrier to learning that needs to be removed—for example, limited vision that interferes with reading labels, or situational depression that interferes with the client's desire to learn about illness. When the goal of care is to help the client learn, it is appropriate to identify the diagnosis as *Deficient knowledge.*

Action Alert! Determine the highest priority nursing diagnosis before developing the plan for meeting learning needs.

Related Nursing Diagnoses. *Ineffective health maintenance* is closely related to *Deficient knowledge.* Assess the client's ability to identify an adaptive behavior, manage a health-related behavior, or seek assistance (NANDA, 2001). Client teaching is a pertinent intervention when you identify the related factor as a lack of material resources, a lack of (or significant alteration in) communication ability, or a lack of effective individual coping. All affect the teaching and learning process.

Assess the client for *Health-seeking behaviors.* Determine if the client needs assistance to actively seek ways to alter personal health habits and/or the environment to move toward a higher level of health (NANDA, 2001). Assess the client's knowledge of ways to achieve his health goals or change unhealthy behaviors.

Assess for *Ineffective coping.* Identify adaptive behaviors and abilities of the client to meet life's demands and roles (NANDA, 2001). Teaching may be needed to develop good nutrition habits, to manage stress, and to develop coping strategies.

Planning

After selecting the appropriate nursing diagnosis, you must decide what the client is expected to accomplish. Expected outcomes depend on the individual assessment, and they might include the following examples:

- Expresses interest in learning new information
- Repeats the key facts or principles to be learned
- Applies the information in a novel situation
- Demonstrates correct use of the information by selecting foods correctly, performing psychomotor skill, or other action

Goals and objectives provide a framework for reaching desired outcomes. Goals are broad, multidimensional, long-term expectations. They are derived by identifying what the client wants to achieve, and they take into consideration the resources available to attain the expected outcomes.

Learning Objectives. Learning objectives are essential tasks to be accomplished in order to achieve goals. A **learning objective** is a statement that describes the intended results of learning rather than the process of instruction. It documents in a clear, realistic, and measurable manner the performance that demonstrates a client's competency in a certain area. It must be client centered and stated in behavioral terms to allow measurement and evaluation of the client's progress. A well-written learning objective includes the following elements:

- The expected performance
- Conditions in which the behavior will be performed
- Criteria by which the performance will be evaluated
  Compare the following learning objectives:
- *Objective 1:* Mrs. Avery will understand about diabetes mellitus before discharge from the health care facility.
- *Objective 2:* By the end of the second teaching session, Mrs. Avery will be able to state the signs and symptoms of hyperglycemia (high blood glucose) with 100% accuracy.

The first objective is vague and ambiguous and therefore difficult to evaluate. The second objective is specific and measurable, with a clearer statement of the desired outcome. It incorporates the characteristics of a well-written objective. It lists all the necessary characteristics, including the following:

- *Performance:* State the signs and symptoms of hyperglycemia
- *Condition(s):* By the end of the second teaching session
- *Criterion:* 100% accuracy

A clear objective that includes measurable terminology allows you to evaluate whether the desired learning has occurred. Additionally, Mrs. Avery will know the goals of your teaching sessions, and she will be able to focus her efforts on meeting those goals. Because the management of diabetes mellitus requires a number of procedures, you may need several learning objectives (in a variety of domains) to help Mrs. Avery learn to assume the responsibility for self-care. Such objectives might include the following:

- By the end of the first teaching session, Mrs. Avery will correctly explain the pathophysiology of diabetes in terms appropriate to her level (cognitive domain).
- By the end of the first teaching session, Mrs. Avery will verbalize the importance of adhering to her prescribed diet (affective domain).
- Each morning before breakfast, Mrs. Avery will correctly measure her blood glucose level, using the fingerstick method, sterile technique, the proper equipment, accurate interpretation of the results, and correct documentation of the findings (psychomotor domain).
- On the day before discharge, Mrs. Avery will use a list provided to her to choose appropriate foods and plan a sample breakfast, lunch, and dinner menu with 100% accuracy (cognitive domain).

What to Teach. After determining expected learning outcomes, you must decide what to teach the client, when to teach it, and how to teach it. Together with the client, develop a spe-cific teaching plan that (1) builds on the client's present knowledge base, (2) provides new information, and (3) increases the client's level of understanding about the health status. Topics selected should be based on the client's learning needs and specific, measurable learning objectives. Learning needs may vary according to client location. For example, the hospitalized client might have learning needs related to an unfamiliar environment, whereas a client at home might have learning needs related to self-care and available resources.

> *Action Alert!* Continually assess clients' learning needs and identify other areas of interest unique to each client. Ask clients for input into the teaching plan to ensure that the content is interesting and relevant to their needs.

TEACHING PLAN. A **teaching plan** is an organized, individualized, written presentation of what the client must learn and how the instructions and information will be provided. It should be outcome oriented, with individualized goals set by the nurse and the client. Like a nursing care plan, it follows the steps of the nursing process. A standardized teaching plan may be designed for groups of clients, such as clients newly diagnosed with diabetes or clients who have had coronary bypass surgery; however, each plan should be individualized for the specific client. A sample teaching plan is prepared for Mrs. Avery, who is beginning insulin therapy for her diabetes (see Box 13-4, p. 271).

In general, clients will be more successful in remembering and assimilating information if you begin with the simple and proceed to the complex. In a well-developed teaching plan, each concept presented is based on a broader and more fundamental concept. Clearly, a person cannot understand abnormalities of function without first understanding normal function. Likewise, a client will not comprehend the treatment and prevention of a disease without first learning about its cause. Thus, when teaching someone about illness and therapy, you should begin with a broad discussion of the normal anatomy and physiology of the diseased organ or system. Then proceed to describe factors that cause the disease, and end the discussion with a presentation of how the client can take part in the treatment and rehabilitation program.

When to Teach. Keep in mind that teaching can take place at any time. It can be scheduled or unscheduled. For example, instruction can be given at specific times that are formally designated and spaced throughout the day, or informally when a person asks questions or encounters new experiences. Environment and timing can be very important determinants of success in the teaching-learning process. If possible, the client should choose the best time and place for teaching and the environment should be quiet, with good lighting, and relatively stress free. In general, try to avoid noisy, hectic times or other times when clients are distracted (such as during meals or after administration of pain medication). Involvement of family and significant others is usually beneficial, as their support will be helpful in achieving outcomes (Arnold & Boggs, 1999).

How to Teach. Many avenues are available for making the best use of your teaching time. Depending on the client's needs and the resources available, you can use one-to-one instruction, group lectures, printed materials, programmed instruction, computerized teaching, other teaching aids, and other expert teachers. Sometimes clients will benefit from more than one mode of instruction.

INDIVIDUAL OR GROUP INSTRUCTION. One-to-one instruction, whether formal or informal, allows you to pace and customize your teaching to the client's learning rate. It also allows more flexibility in considering the client's comfort level and variations in ability to absorb content.

Group instruction requires a meeting place, handout materials, a meeting agenda and lesson plan, and seating that facilitates group interaction (chairs placed in a circle, for example). You must deliver a prepared lecture on the chosen topic, lead a discussion, review major points covered in the discussion, and arrange for the next meeting.

The three major advantages of group meetings are the economy of teaching time, the possibility of delivering a large amount of factual information, and the opportunity for clients with similar problems to share experiences, viewpoints, and opinions with each other. Two disadvantages are the lack of ability to pace your teaching to individual learning rates and the possibility that some clients will be too intimidated to ask questions in front of the group.

PRINTED MATERIALS. Printed materials—such as pamphlets and brochures—allow clients to read and study at their own pace. They are affordable, portable, and can be used to teach or reinforce a learning experience. Also, clients can share the materials with family and significant others so that all have similar information.

Action Alert! Be sure to assess reading level prior to distributing printed materials.

PROGRAMMED OR COMPUTER-ASSISTED INSTRUCTION. Programmed instruction involves a prepared program of study that lists learning objectives and provides activities to meet those objectives. It may include a pretest and posttest for self-evaluation. Computer-assisted instruction (CAI) is similar to programmed instruction, except that the learner uses a computer program. It allows self-study and self-pacing, and it may also provide an interactive component that printed materials cannot. Computerized learning packages are finding increased use at all educational levels. They are likely to enjoy broader usage as client education software becomes more common. This teaching method requires self-direction on the part of the client and is usually more effective with highly motivated clients.

AUDIO AND VISUAL INSTRUCTIONAL AIDS. Teaching can be enhanced by the proper use of aids, such as drawings, models of organs, charts, graphs, audiotapes, a bulletin board, a blackboard, posters, pictures, an overhead projector, slide shows, films, videotapes, closed-circuit television, flash cards, programmed instruction, and games (Gaberson & Oermann, 1999). Increasing numbers of websites are also available for on-line instruction. Clients should be cautioned to establish credibility by determining the source of the information.

HUMAN RESOURCES. The use of a specialized resource person can be extremely helpful to a client's learning process.

For example, when teaching about a special diet, you could have a dietitian attend your session and share information as needed. Physicians, physical therapists, and occupational therapists all make significant contributions to teaching and learning.

Other clients can help as well, especially those who have successfully managed a similar condition. These experienced people can help a client know that it is possible to change behaviors and manage difficult disorders. For example, someone who has successfully managed lifestyle changes after having cardiac bypass surgery might be called to talk with a client preparing for the surgery.

Intervention

To implement teaching, you will need to use effective strategies and appropriate learning activities. Teaching content and methodology is documented in the health record as a part of nursing interventions.

Strategies for Effective Teaching Intervention. As the teacher, your behaviors have a profound influence on the client's ability to learn. By employing the following strategies for effective teaching intervention, you can maximize the learning process.

SELECT APPROPRIATE TEACHING METHODS. The teaching method selected depends on the subject matter and on the client's background, personality, and needs. Teaching may involve formal lectures and demonstrations. However, informal individual or group discussions are more appropriate for most clients in a health care setting.

When using adjunct methods, it is wise to be available afterward to answer questions and evaluate what clients have learned. Before using print or video teaching aids, verify their content and assess the comprehension level of your audience. For general audiences, a reading level between grade 4 and grade 6 is best. For each client, do your best to provide accurate, current, and relevant information at the level and in the style most likely to fulfill the person's unique learning needs.

REWARD POSITIVE BEHAVIORS. Rewards for correct behaviors reinforce learning. Behaviors that are rewarded are more likely to be repeated. For ill clients, rewards tend to involve the following:
- Reduced pain or other symptoms
- Return of a normal or near-normal lifestyle
- Avoidance of complications
- Positive regard from a nurse or physician

Immediate rewards from you provide better reinforcement than delayed rewards.

Action Alert! Compliment immediately when a client asks a thoughtful question, demonstrates something learned about the illness, or performs a procedure satisfactorily.

ENCOURAGE ACTIVE PARTICIPATION. People learn more effectively when they participate in their health education program. Active participation generates interest; lack of participation generates boredom.

You can encourage participation in a number of ways. For instance, when presenting written material, make sure the client understands it. Clients who are merely handed a list of instructions may or may not follow them. Most instructions require discussion about why they are important. After demonstrating a procedure, ask the client to work through each step with you rather than waiting for a return demonstration.

REPEAT KEY FACTS AND CONCEPTS. Repetition of key facts and concepts reinforces learning. Likewise, practice reinforces new skills. Reviewing materials presented earlier prepares the client for receiving new materials. Encourage your clients to repeat, practice, and review.

ENCOURAGE IMMEDIATE PRACTICE. Clients retain new information and skills longer when they put them into practice right away. For example, in many obstetric units, it is common practice for new mothers to begin caring for their infants almost immediately. Under supervision, mothers learn how to bathe, feed, and diaper. New mothers are encouraged to practice skills right away, under supervision, instead of being sent home to flounder alone. In contrast, when clients cannot use their knowledge right way, they tend to forget what they have learned.

Action Alert! If a client does not have an opportunity to use newly acquired information or skills soon after learning, be sure to provide written information that the client can refer to later.

HELP THE CLIENT SURMOUNT LEARNING PLATEAUS. Clients occasionally reach learning plateaus, where it may appear that they have lost interest. The person may even seem discouraged. Remember, however, that learning plateaus are normal. To surmount them, use visual aids, movies, or other stimulating methods of presentation, which give the client a break from structured learning until the previous level of enthusiasm returns.

NEGOTIATE. By actively involving clients in the decision-making process, nurses stimulate clients' motivation to learn. Clients are more apt to be enthusiastic about learning the information that they have identified as important to them. Combining client interests with content necessary to reach health care goals makes the teaching and learning process mutually gratifying.

Some clients resist learning. Perhaps they are still in denial about the disease process, or they feel angry at the adjustments they must make in their lifestyle. They may also resist for other reasons: they "don't have time," are presently asymptomatic, or lack family support, for example. For these individuals, contracting may be an effective way to elicit their participation. In a **learning contract,** much like any business contract, each party (nurse and client) agrees to contribute certain things to the agreement. The nurse provides information, and the client agrees to use that information.

Mager (1975) states that instruction is effective to the degree that it succeeds in changing behavior in the desired direction. The learning contract helps the client commit to goals to achieve the desired outcomes in the learning situation. The nurse prioritizes the most essential aspects of care within the contract. As times goes by, the contract helps the client experience the satisfaction or reward of accomplishment in learning, and the contract can be changed to include other learning needs.

Learning Activities. Clearly, teaching and learning can take place in many settings. Three of the most important activities for any form of learning are discussion, demonstration, and role-playing.

DISCUSSION. Discussion encourages clients to participate actively in the health education program. You can draw clients into a discussion by asking for a response to something you just taught. For example, you might ask clients to share ways in which the information applies to their life, such as examples of personal experiences or related opinions. In a class for clients receiving radiation treatment, for example, you might ask how they coped with hair loss.

DEMONSTRATION. Demonstrations provide the best method for teaching motor skills, such as how to give a self-injection or how to transfer safely from a bed to a wheelchair. To prepare for a demonstration, complete the following steps:
- Make notes, and organize your thoughts so you can narrate your demonstration clearly.
- Obtain the needed equipment, and make sure it works.
- Outline the procedure on a handout so your client can follow along with you.
- Practice the demonstration until you can do it skillfully.

When giving the demonstration, make sure clients can see it clearly. Proceed slowly, allowing questions as you go. Afterward, immediately reinforce learning by having the clients return the demonstration to the best of their ability.

ROLE-PLAYING. Role-playing is a creative learning activity in which a person can act as different people (physician, nurse, spouse, employer) in a variety of real-life situations to help learn new behaviors or solve problems. Initially, some people may feel shy or embarrassed about role-playing. As they become comfortable, however, they discover that it can be a very effective strategy for gaining new insights in a safe environment. Role-playing can be effective in teaching, parenting, and other interpersonal skills.

Documentation of Teaching. Use documentation to record the progress when teaching is done in multiple sessions. Additionally, documentation records the cost effectiveness of your teaching for quality evaluation, confirms the outcomes of the teaching and learning process, and provides legal material that could be considered in a court of law. As in other areas of nursing, accurate and complete documentation of your teaching is crucial.

When Mrs. Avery is discharged from the hospital, the nurse writes the following discharge note:

SAMPLE DOCUMENTATION FOR MRS. AVERY

Discharged per wheelchair with granddaughter to automobile. Able to walk in the hall. Has given self insulin with supervision. Referred to home health for follow-up teaching. Has appointment with physician in 1 week.

Evaluation

Evaluating how well the nurse and the client have met teaching and learning goals is an important part of the teaching and learning process. Remember that it is important to develop learning objectives in terms of behaviors and measurable outcomes *before* beginning the teaching and learning process. Then, after the program, you can evaluate the success of the teaching and how well the client has made positive life changes. Ideally, evaluation should determine that *learning has occurred* and that you were effective as a teacher. If discrepancies exist between the desired and actual outcomes, systematic problem solving can help to rectify them and strengthen the teaching and learning process even more (Box 13-4).

Action Alert! Be aware that, to ensure that the client's learning needs are met, you may need to modify the original teaching plan on the basis of the evaluation results.

Evaluation of Teaching. Evaluation of the teaching process measures whether the short-term learning goals have been met and whether the knowledge results in long-term behavioral changes. Evaluation also examines the effects of the change in behavior on health status and whether resources used to produce the change in health status are the most cost-effective method of treatment.

   SHORT-TERM GOALS. Ask yourself a variety of questions to determine whether short-term learning has occurred and is being acted on. These may include the following:

- Has the client been given the necessary information for a safe discharge?
- Has the client accomplished the learning objectives?
- Can the client demonstrate proficiency in the skills needed to maintain self-care?
- Is there a measurable difference in the client's attitude about the highest level of health attainable?
- Can the client cope with limitations imposed by the illness?
- Does the client show a willingness to make necessary lifestyle changes?
- Do the client's significant others understand the client's problems and demonstrate readiness to provide appropriate support?

   LONG-TERM GOALS. If you focus only on the evaluation of short-term learning (i.e., what a client learns before discharge), you will neglect the importance of long-term changes in behavior. The client, the facility staff, the outpatient nurse, and the physician all share responsibility for reinforcing long-term learning and evaluating its success over time.

   Long-term evaluation may involve follow-up questionnaires or telephone calls at selected intervals after discharge. This method allows clients to demonstrate the success of learning in a real-life situation. Many times, when clients are in a health care facility and away from the demands of everyday living, they assume that a behavioral change will be easy to implement. However, the ideal is seldom encountered at home or in the workplace. Additional learning, problem solving, and creativity may be necessary to integrate the desired change at home. In contrast, in the relaxed and familiar home environ-

ment, the person may discover a readiness to learn that was not present during the stress of the institutional environment.

   The fact is that short-term outcomes may differ from the long-term reality. Clients may "know" what is needed at the time of discharge, but they may forget or neglect that need over time, especially if they lack support or reinforcement. Long-term follow-up can renew information learned in the hospital. By reinforcing what is learned in institutional teaching programs, the primary care nurse in the community provides continuity and promotes retention of learning.

   Feedback received from clients after they have been discharged also provides tremendous benefits to the nurses responsible for the original teaching. Feedback allows nurses to evaluate the effectiveness of hospital teaching by identifying relevant content and effective teaching strategies.

Evaluation of Learning. Helpful methods to evaluate a client's learning include discussion, oral tests, written tests, and return demonstration. Testing should be fun, easy, and nonthreatening. It should give the client positive reinforcement that learning has occurred, rather than focusing on what needs to be learned. In client education, testing is more a teaching tool than it is an evaluation process.

   DISCUSSION. In the evaluation process, the discussion method is used to review what has been learned. Review three or four main points. Ask the client questions to evaluate whether learning has occurred. Observe the client's comfort level with the information and evaluate the client's ability to apply the information to the health care concern and, as a result, change the behavior.

   ORAL TESTS. Oral testing requires preparation on your part and can be quite time consuming because it is accomplished one-to-one with the client. Large-group oral testing may be ineffective because not all clients are able to answer. If a client has trouble articulating answers, outcomes are difficult to evaluate.

   Oral testing can be beneficial when a reading level cannot be matched to a written test or the client has visual deficits. The desired outcome is for the client to verbalize the key points and to apply the knowledge.

   WRITTEN TESTS. Written tests prepared for individuals or groups require that clients be able to read. They can be in the form of multiple choice, true-or-false, matching, or essay questions. They require a space that is quiet, comfortable, and conducive to thinking, because they ask the client to recall teaching. The goal of written testing is to reflect what the client has learned and give the client a sense of satisfaction. Written test items should be piloted and analyzed for clarity and relevance prior to administration to the client. This reduces the likelihood of confusion and frustration for the client and increases the validity of test results.

   RETURN DEMONSTRATION. Return demonstration is an excellent means of evaluating a skill or task. You demonstrate the skill or task and then ask the client to return, or mirror, the skill. Written steps or instructions supplied along with the demonstration enhance recall when the demonstration is finished. The desired outcome is for the client to perform all the steps independently without error.

Nursing Care Plan TEACHING PLAN FOR A DIABETIC CLIENT BEGINNING INSULIN THERAPY   Box 13-4

ADMISSION DATA

Charlotte Avery is an 82-year-old Jamaican-American woman who lives in Boca Raton, Florida. After Mrs. Avery's parents died, she became the proprietor of her family's restaurant business. Mrs. Avery retired 7 years ago. Her son now runs the restaurant, and she cares for two great-grandchildren. When Mrs. Avery fainted in her home 3 days ago, her 9-year-old great-grandchild called 911. It was later found that Mrs. Avery's diabetes was out of control. Her physician told her that she would no longer be able to control her diabetes with diet and oral medications alone. She must now learn to monitor her blood glucose and self-administer insulin. The nurse developed the following teaching plan for Mrs. Avery.

NANDA Nursing Diagnosis	NOC Expected Outcomes With Indicators	NIC Interventions With Selected Activities	Evaluation Data
DEFICIENT KNOWLEDGE: DIABETES MANAGEMENT (AFFECTIVE)	**KNOWLEDGE: DIABETES MANAGEMENT**	**TEACHING: INDIVIDUAL**	**AFTER 1 MONTH OF CARE**
Related Factor: • Readiness to learn	• Client will discuss her feelings about taking insulin. • Client will accept the need for insulin and dietary change. • Client will articulate confidence in her ability self-administer insulin injections. • Client will make a commitment to keep daily records of glucose monitoring and insulin injections and reactions.	• Provide a quiet environment that supports discussion of feelings. • Assess client's desire to self-administer injections. • Provide constructive and positive feedback in the learning process. • Provide a record book for recording.	• States has survived birth of five children, death of 3 husbands and loss of first restaurant by fire. This seems like minor problem in comparison. • States need to remain healthy to care for 2 great-grandchildren. • States she knows she can learn but information confusing. • Records sample data accurately in record book.
Related Factor: • Seeking knowledge	**KNOWLEDGE: MEDICATION** • Client will complete a multiple choice test of knowledge of insulin and its effects. • Client will list the differences between regular and intermediate-acting insulin.	**TEACHING: PRESCRIBED MEDICATION** • Provide video explaining effects of insulin and mechanism of action. • Provide multiple choice test and provide instructions. • Describe difference in types of insulin and provide handout.	• Observed video twice and asked appropriate questions. • Correctly answered 90% of questions. Indicated understanding after discussion of incorrect items. • Listened and read information about insulin. • Stated, "NPH will last all day. Regular is only good for one meal."
Related Factor: • Lack of experience with injectible medications	**KNOWLEDGE: TREATMENT** • Client will inject accurate dosage of insulin using correct technique. • Client will demonstrate correct procedure for monitoring blood glucose.	**TEACHING: PSYCHOMOTOR SKILL** • Demonstrate correct procedure for drawing medication and subcutaneous injection. Observe return demonstration. • Demonstrate procedure for fingerstick and use of glucometer. Observe return demonstration.	• Withdrew amount accurately. Hesitant to inject self. Injected correctly on second attempt. • Used appropriate technique for fingerstick. Initially confused about use of glucometer. Completed procedure with coaching.

CRITICAL THINKING QUESTIONS

1. The following is documented during a follow-up visit to the clinic: *Verbalized that she had an episode of low blood glucose last weekend. Action taken was to check her blood glucose level (which was 42), drink a glass of orange juice, eat two peanut butter crackers, and rest. Repeated her blood glucose 30 minutes later; reading was 96. Stated she felt better and continued her housework.* From this documentation, how would you evaluate the effectiveness of the teaching plan for Mrs. Avery?

2. Considering the change in learning ability that can occur with aging, how many teaching sessions would you need before Mrs. Avery self-injects her insulin? Can Mrs. Avery be expected to administer her insulin independently? How would you explain the pathological changes associated with diabetic complications?

Nursing outcome and intervention labels from Johnson, M., Bulechek, G., McCloskey Dochterman, J. M., Maas, M., & Moorhead, S. (2001). *Nursing diagnoses, outcomes, and interventions: NANDA, NOC, and NIC linkages.* St Louis, MO: Mosby.

Key Principles

- Nursing standards for practice include client education. They assume that clients have a right to information and that nurses have a legal mandate to provide client education.
- In addition to the client's right to information, client education benefits health care through cost control and quality control.
- The purposes of client education are to promote health, prevent illness, restore health, and help clients cope with illness.
- Learning theorists have identified three primary domains of learning: cognitive, affective, and psychomotor.
- Client characteristics affecting teaching are literacy, level of education, developmental level, and learning style.
- Readiness to learn and motivation facilitate learning.
- The client must be physically and psychologically able to learn.
- Cultural and environmental factors can inhibit learning.
- The ability of the nurse as an educator affects learning positively or negatively.
- *Deficient knowledge* is diagnosed when the client lacks knowledge of health management practices that are necessary to achieve or maintain health.
- Other nursing diagnoses commonly used for client education are *Ineffective health maintenance, Health-seeking behaviors,* and *Ineffective coping.*
- Planning to teach includes selecting topics, developing a teaching plan, and writing learning objectives.
- Although most client teaching is one-to-one instruction, many teaching methods are available to maximize efficiency and effectiveness.
- Strategies for effective implementation include selecting appropriate teaching methods, rewarding positive behaviors, encouraging active participation, repeating key factors and concepts, encouraging immediate feedback, helping the client surmount learning plateaus, and negotiating.
- Evaluation of learning requires evaluating both the short-term goal of acquiring knowledge and the long-term goal of changing behavior.
- The method of evaluation should reinforce learning.

Bibliography

*American Hospital Association. (1975). *A patient's bill of rights.* Chicago: Author.

American Hospital Association. (2003). *Patient care partnership: Understanding expectations, rights, and responsibilities.* Chicago: The Association.

Arnold, E., & Boggs, K. U. (1999). *Interpersonal relationships: Professional communication skills for nurses* (3rd ed.). Philadelphia: Saunders.

Bastable, S. B. (2003). *Nurse as educator* (2nd ed.). Boston: Jones and Bartlett.

Beggs, V. L., Willis, S. B., Maislen, E. L., Stokes, T. M., White, D., Sanford, M., Becker, A., Barber, S., Pawlow, P. C., & Downs, C. (1998). Patient education for discharge after coronary bypass surgery in the 1990s: Are patients adequately prepared? *Journal of Cardiovascular Nursing, 12*(4), 72-86.

*Bloom, B. J. (1956). *Taxonomy of educational objectives, Book 1. Cognitive domain.* New York: Longman.

*Bloom, B. J., Englehart, M. S., Furst, E. J., Hill, W. H., & Krathwohl, D. R. (1956). *Taxonomy of educational objectives: The classification of educational goals, Handbook 1. Cognitive domain.* New York: David McKay.

*Brown, C., Wright, R., & Christensen, D. (1987). Association between type of medication instruction and patients' knowledge, side effects and compliance. *Hospital and Community Psychiatry, 38*(1), 55-60.

Clayton, M. (1998). Encouraging children to use cycle helmets. *Paediatric Nursing, 10*(3), 14-16.

Davidhizer, R. E. & Brownson, K. (1999). Literacy, cultural diversity, and client education. *Healthcare Manager, 18*(1), 39-47.

*Doak, C. C., Doak, L. G., & Root, J. E. (1996). *Teaching patients with low literacy skills* (2nd ed.). Philadelphia: Lippincott.

Ellison, G. C., & Rayman, K. M. (1998). Exemplars' experience of self-managing type 2 diabetes. *Diabetes Education, 14*(2), 325-330.

Gaberson, K. B. & Oermann, M. H. (1999). *Clinical teaching strategies in nursing.* New York: Springer.

*Johnson, J., Rice, V., Fuller, S., & Endress, M. (1978). Sensory information: Instruction in a coping strategy and recovery from surgery. *Research in Nursing and Health, 1*(1), 4-17.

Johnson, M., Bulecheck, G., McCloskey Dochtermann, J., Mass, M., & Moorhead, S. (2001). *Nursing diagnoses, outcomes, & interventions: NANDA, NOC, and NIC linkages.* St Louis, MO: Mosby.

*Knowles, M. (1980). *The adult learner: A neglected species* (2nd ed.). Houston: Gulf.

*Kolb, D. (1984). *Experiential learning: Experience as the source of learning and development.* Englewood Cliffs, NJ: Prentice-Hall.

*Krathwohl, D. R., Bloom, B. J., & Masia, B. B. (1964). *Taxonomy of educational objectives: The classification of educational goals, Handbook II. The affective domain.* New York: David McKay.

Lightfoot, J., & Bines, W. (1998). Keeping children healthy: Role of the school nurse. *Nursing Times, 94*(21), 65-68.

*Mager, R. F. (1975). *Preparing instructional objectives* (2nd ed.). Belmont, CA: Fearon-Pitman.

North American Nursing Diagnosis Association. (2001). *NANDA nursing diagnoses: Definitions and classification, 2001-2002.* Philadelphia: Author.

Posel, N. (1998). Preoperative teaching in the preadmission clinic. *Journal of Nursing Staff Development, 14*(1), 52-56.

Price, K. M., & Cortis, J. D. (2000). The way forward for transcultural nursing. *Nurse Education Today, 20,* 233-223.

Richards, B., Colman, A. W., & Hollingsworth, R. A. (1998). The current role of the Internet in patient education. *Internet Journal Medical Information, 50*(1-3), 279-285.

Ryan, J. M., & Southern, J. (1998). A & E nursing and the Internet. *Accident & Emergency Nursing, 6*(2), 106-109.

Salmore, R. G., & Nelson, J. (2000). The effect of preprocedure teaching, relaxation instruction, and music on anxiety as measured by blood pressures in an outpatient gastrointestinal endoscopy laboratory. *Gastroenterolog Nursing 23*(3), 102-110.

*Simpson, E. J. (1972). The classification of educational objectives in the psychomotor domain. In M. T. Rainier (Ed.), *Contributions of behavioral science to instructional technology: The psychomotor domain* (3rd ed.). Englewood Cliffs, NJ: Gryphon Press, Prentice-Hall.

U.S. Department of Health and Human Services. (2000). *Healthy people 2010: Objectives for improving health,* Vol. II. Washington, DC: U.S. Government Printing Office.

*Asterisk indicates a classic or definitive work on this subject.

Managing Client Care

Learning Objectives

After studying this chapter, you should be able to do the following:

- Describe the impact of organizational philosophy, structure, and methods of communication on nursing practice in a complex health care agency
- Distinguish between nursing as a leadership role and as a management role in a health care agency
- Describe the organization of nursing service as a means to provide quality client care
- Describe the issues of managing change, risk management, and conflict management
- Identify the role of the nurse in a collaborative health care team

Because approximately 60% of nurses are employed in acute care hospitals, the major setting for nursing practice is a complex, business-oriented health care organization. In this setting, nursing is challenged to fulfill the professional values associated with caring for other people. Nursing is a service profession that gives care through providing one-on-one practical help and meeting the unique and holistic health needs of the client. To be effective in providing quality nursing care in a health care organization, nurses need to understand the system and use it effectively to provide leadership in meeting the needs of the clients.

Nursing is a leadership role in a health care agency whether the nurse manages care by working one-to-one with the client, by coordinating the care with other providers, by delegating aspects of the care to others, or by providing leadership to a team of providers. Nursing leadership derives its power from nurses' unique role in the health care setting: they have a 24-hour relationship with the client and are concerned with the client's comprehensive needs. They have overall **responsibility** for care (the obligation to act or direct to accomplish a goal). Additionally, nursing leadership includes the role of an advocate for clients and families.

The leadership role of nursing in the health care organization is perhaps most visibly identified with the role of the nurse manager. **Nurse manager** usually refers to a nurse's role in organizational management as nurse executive, middle manager, and first-line manager of nursing services (Table 14-1). First-line managers are identified with the actual delivery of care (Figure 14-1). However, all nurse management roles share the goal of providing quality service to meet the client's needs. Nurse managers have **accountability** for their respective units; that is, they are answerable for personal actions and the action of other staff.

Management can be thought of as the implementation of strategies that promote effective and efficient use of resources to meet goals. The goal at all levels of nursing service is to provide high-quality nursing care in a cost-effective manner. This definition of management can also be applied to managers of direct client care—for example, the staff nurse.

The leadership and management roles involved in a staff nurse position are evident when the nurse is working with a nursing team, coordinating with other departments, delegating to team members, collaborating with the physician and other health care providers, and being an advocate for the client. The staff nurse is the person who most directly influences the quality of care received by the client.

Therefore you need to understand the context of the health care organization, what it means to be a leader, the qualities needed by nurses who manage client care, the role of the nurse manager at the organizational level, and the organizational patterns of nursing units.

THE HEALTH CARE ORGANIZATION

Nursing care is usually delivered within a health care agency that has an organizational structure for the delivery of health services. In addition to nursing services, the health care agency provides pharmacy services, diagnostic services, medical services, food services, and housekeeping services.

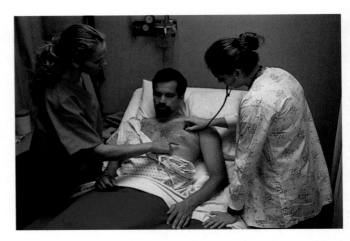

Figure 14-1. First-line managers are identified with the actual delivery of care. Here, a first-line manager works side-by-side with a staff nurse, giving direct care to a client.

Table 14-1	Characteristics of Nurse Managers at Different Levels		
Level of Management	Title	Educational Preparation	Tasks
First-line manager	• Team leader • Case manager • Charge nurse	• RN • 1 to 2 years of nursing experience	• Manage client care • Supervise team members • Know status of all clients • Know all team members' roles
Middle manager	• Unit manager • Supervisor	• RN • BSN or MSN preferred • 1 to 5 years of nursing experience	• Supervise nurses and ancillary staff • 24-hour accountability • Manage resources • Motivate others • Act as change agent • Manage quality • Manage risk
Nurse executive	• Director of nursing • Vice president for nursing • Nursing CEO	• RN • MSN or PhD in allied health preferred • Management experience	• Operationalize nursing • Provide resources • Facilitate quality care • Facilitate efficiency

A complex organizational structure, or social system, exists for the purpose of coordinating these departments to ensure that the client receives needed services in a timely manner. The structure varies with the services provided and the size of the organization. Whether the agency is a hospital, nursing home, clinic, or home care agency, a nurse plans and delivers care within an organizational framework designed to effectively and efficiently meet the needs of its clients.

Nursing care is delivered within the context of the philosophy of the institution; how the philosophy is translated into goals, policies, and procedures; and the management style of its leaders. Quality of care within an agency begins when a health care organization defines itself and the product it intends to deliver. This definition is reflected in the agency's philosophy and goals.

Philosophy and Mission

The philosophy of an organization comprises its values and beliefs and underlies the way it goes about its work. When a philosophy is effectively implemented, it is reflected in the services provided and the methods of providing services; it permeates the organization from the top down and from the bottom up. The philosophy may be communicated through a mission statement that makes clear to the public what the agency is committed to providing. Institutional philosophies may be developed from the rationale for establishing an agency. These may be concerned with providing access to care, providing quality care, meeting community needs, or making a profit (cost effectiveness).

Access to care means that services are available and accessible to the clients to be served. A hospital may be established to provide access to health care in a town where the residents would otherwise have to travel far to receive services, or to provide services for an indigent population. For example, a small rural hospital may decide that its role is to provide basic services, but it provides links to larger metropolitan hospitals for more advanced levels of care.

Quality can mean the latest technology, personalized care, well-coordinated services, or high standards for care. For example, a heart hospital may be established to provide all cardiac care services at one location, thus improving the quality of cardiac care in the community. On the other hand, the mission statement of a home health agency may express the value of maintaining independence and functional ability of elderly residents in the community.

The philosophy of a health care organization may be to meet a community need. For example, a hospital may be established to provide for the specific needs of women. Or a community with a problem of overcrowded emergency departments might establish minor emergency or urgent care facilities to serve clients who do not need full emergency department services.

Regardless of the values that underlie a health care agency's philosophy, in today's environment of managed care, cost and quality care are both driving forces. An institution may include in its philosophy that health care is a business, and that cost efficiency is an important component.

Some hospitals are **for-profit,** meaning that the agency exists to make a profit. In a competitive marketplace, a for-profit institution can be expected to provide quality care. A **not-for-profit** hospital may make a profit but does not exist for that purpose. The profit is often returned to the institution to maintain or upgrade equipment or to meet other needs. A **nonprofit** hospital does not make a profit and may be supported by charitable donations or taxes. However, any of these types of agencies is concerned with cost control.

The philosophy of a department of nursing reflects the values of the institution and the values of nursing. It directs nursing behavior and serves as the basis for determining the means to accomplish nursing services (Tuck, Harris, & Baliko, 2000). The inclusion of nursing values in the institutional philosophy demonstrates a commitment to professional values and the development of nursing.

Goals and Objectives

Goals are the means to ensure that the expressed values are upheld in the delivery of services. In other words, goals express the philosophy in more specific terms. For example, the home health agency designed to maintain independent living for older adults may have a goal of increasing the independence of its clients. A tertiary care hospital's goal is to provide state-of-the-art technology to improve the survival of certain client populations. Objectives are more specific plans to implement goals. A specific objective would be to obtain or develop the technology to improve the survival of burn victims.

Policies and Procedures

Objectives become the guidelines for establishing policies and procedures. Organizations develop policies and procedures on the basis of standards of practice and standards of client care. A **policy** is a set of rules and regulations that govern nursing practice and nursing care. Policies may pertain to clients, such as the client's bill of rights, or to the nursing staff, such as the staff's employment, deployment, and assignment; staffing patterns; staff mix (the number of registered nurses, licensed professional nurses, and nursing assistants); attendance; sick leave; chemical dependency; incident reports; and floating to other units.

A **procedure** is a detailed description of a specific method of performing nursing care. Procedural guidelines, such as medication administration, insertion of nasogastric tubes or urinary catheters, and isolation, are published in a procedure manual. The procedure manual describes who is responsible for performing the procedures, what equipment or supplies are necessary, and what information should be assessed and documented.

Protocols. A **protocol** contains detailed guidelines for nursing care for clients with specific conditions. For example, protocols may be developed for alcohol withdrawal, cardiac catheterization, fall risk, skin risk, restraints, surgical client management, and chest pain. Protocols are also developed to allow nurses to perform procedures beyond the legal scope of nursing practice. For example, the critical care unit may develop a protocol that allows the nurse to treat life-threatening arrhythmias before the physician arrives. This protocol defines life-threatening arrhythmia, the dosage and frequency of medications or treatments to be used, the staff responsible for administering the medication or treatment, and the assessment and documentation to be done.

Nurse managers have an important role in developing and implementing policies, procedures, and protocols, as well as in monitoring and measuring the success of carrying out the institutional mission. Nurses must justify their importance in the provision of health care by demonstrating that nursing care is appropriate, safe, effective, and efficient.

JCAHO Standards. Policies and procedures are often derived from the standards of the Joint Commission on Accreditation of Healthcare Organizations (JCAHO). JCAHO accredits health care organizations, which is not only prestigious but also necessary for them to continue to receive federal funds, for example. Although JCAHO is a voluntary accreditation organization, federal and state regulatory agencies and insurance carriers require that health care organizations be accredited by JCAHO to be certified, to be licensed, or to receive reimbursement.

JCAHO evaluates each health care organization every 3 years. The extent of an organization's compliance with JCAHO standards determines the organization's accreditation status. In the past, accreditation indicated that an organization had the capability to provide quality care. However, the public demands the evaluation of actual performance, or outcome information, instead of potential capability. Thus JCAHO continuously improves and revises its standards so that an organization's accreditation reflects its actual performance of quality care (JCAHO, 2002).

During the accreditation process JCAHO examines the organization's performance in *doing the right thing* and *doing the right thing well*. The characteristics of doing the right thing are efficacy and appropriateness. The characteristics of doing the right thing *well* are availability, effectiveness, timeliness, safety, efficiency, continuity, respect, and caring. JCAHO believes that the organization demonstrating these characteristics is more likely to provide high-quality care with optimal client outcomes and efficient resource use.

ANA Standards. The American Nurses' Association (ANA) published the first standards of practice for the nursing profession in 1973. They defined the nursing professional's accountability to the public and described the nursing professional's responsibilities. To clarify the nature and scope of nursing practice, the ANA revised and elaborated on the original standards in 1991, 1998, 2003 (in draft) (see Appendix A). The revisions addressed two dimensions: standards of care and standards of professional performance.

Standards of professional performance are defined as "authoritative statements that describe a competent level of behavior in the professional role, including activities related to quality of care, performance appraisal, education,

collegiality, ethics, collaboration, research, and resource utilization" (ANA, 1998). Appendix A lists behaviors that demonstrate the standards of professional performance (ANA, 1998).

NURSES AS LEADERS AND MANAGERS

All nurses should strive to be leaders in the health care setting. However, only a few nurses are interested in a management role in the organization.

Leadership

Leadership shapes the future through influencing others. It includes activities or interactions that provide a sense of direction toward goal achievement, coaching and mentoring, and demonstrating proactive behaviors. A leader on a nursing unit will listen to the concerns of colleagues and provide feedback to help the person manage stressful situations or improve nursing care. Role modeling is also a leadership strategy that can involve dress, language, and social skills as well as excellence in nursing techniques and communication with clients (Fox, Fox, and Wells, 1999). You do not have to be a nurse manager to be a leader in providing quality care.

Effective managers incorporate leadership strategies to further an organization's objectives by using interpersonal interactions that inspire others to work toward those goals. Whereas management involves implementing strategies to accomplish organizational goals, **leadership** involves showing others the way, directing others in a course of action, going ahead of others, or going with and inspiring others. Successful nurse managers employ leadership skills to increase their effectiveness as managers.

Theories of leadership incorporate communication skills, understanding of group process, and a strong vision for health care as the means to effect group movement in a specific direction. Leaders use open, honest, clear, and concise communication. They listen actively and use group process to build consensus and stimulate enthusiasm for projects. Nurse leaders understand the importance of their work, and they incorporate the values of the profession in all aspects of it.

Because the position of a nurse manager involves inspiring others to work, all nurse managers should be leaders. However, leaders can do the work of inspiring others from any position. A nurse may be a leader among a group of peers, influencing the way the group goes about the daily activities of providing for clients. Leaders work to create change that benefits clients throughout the health care industry. Leadership qualities are an essential component of the effective nurse's storehouse of strategies for promoting health.

Leadership style can be either transactional or transformational (Table 14-2). Transactional leadership "pursues a cost-benefit, economic exchange to meet subordinates' current material and psychic needs in return for contracted services rendered by the subordinate." Transactional leaders use a contingent reward for a desired behavior approach to management. Workers are given clear expectations of the desired behaviors and the rewards for those behaviors. In transformational

Table 14-2	Styles of Leadership Communication
Transformational	**Transactional**
• Empowers and trusts employees • Focuses on goal attainment • Shares responsibility and accountability • Facilitates participation • Encourages discussion • Encourages staff input • Uses data to solve problems • Delegates • Listens • Observes • Communicates beliefs • Communicates expectations • Gives factual messages • Has positive attitude • Rewards contributions • Builds consensus	• Views giving reward for expected behaviors as motivation • Focuses on expected behaviors • May be authoritarian • Demands or coerces • Tells • Makes rules, and rewards compliance • May punish • Talks • Monitors and watches • Imposes rules • Demands results • Dictates • Encourages dependency

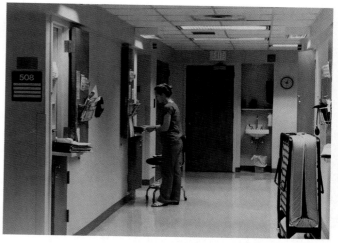

Figure 14-2. Employees who feel trusted will behave more responsibly. This nurse is working independently to help accomplish the organization's mission.

leadership, the leader shares a vision and a sense of mission and shows respect and confidence by trusting the employee to act in a way consistent with the mission (Figure 14-2). Transformational leadership motivates by inspiration. Furthermore, the transformational model stimulates intellectual growth to understand the problems of the nursing unit and considers individual needs for support, encouragement, and developmental experiences (Morrison, Jones and Fuller, 1997).

Empowerment is one of the most important influences transformational leaders have on followers. Retention rates for nurses are higher when there is shared leadership or shared governance (Ohman, 1999). Shared leadership is a form of stewardship based on trust and uses shared authority, control, decision making, and accountability. Shared leadership can increase unit personnel participation, point-of-service decisions, and job satisfaction levels when compared to traditional arrangements. It enables nursing staff to generate a sense of co-ownership of core work processes necessary for quality client care (Fox, Fox, and Wells, 1999).

Roles of Managers

The roles filled by a nurse manager result largely from the responsibilities incurred at various levels of the organization's hierarchy. In general, however, those roles involve managing quality of care, budgets, and personnel.

Managing Quality. **Quality assurance** refers to the process of achieving excellence in the service rendered to every client. A quality assurance program is based on a clear definition of quality and the reliable and valid outcomes used to measure it. Although the current trend in health care is toward cost containment, the goal is to achieve this without reducing the quality of client services. Managing quality means accentuating positive outcomes as well as avoiding negative outcomes.

Three main steps are involved in quality assurance activities. First, each nursing unit selects aspects of care to represent the standards for care, criteria for achievement of the standards, and methods of monitoring. Second, the nursing department analyzes the data to determine potential causes of poor compliance. Third, the unit seeks ways to improve compliance with the standards.

Retrospective audits and concurrent audits are used to conduct quality assurance activities. The **retrospective audit** is an evaluation method to inspect the medical record for documentation of compliance with the standards. This method requires less time than a concurrent audit and thus is used most often by the health care organization. The **concurrent audit** is an evaluation method to inspect the nursing staff's compliance with predetermined standards and criteria while the nurses are providing care. The auditor compares the performance against other nurses' performance and over time.

Generally, each organization designates responsibilities for conducting an audit to the quality assurance staff, the head nurse, the charge nurse, or the nurse educator. However, a peer review approach in which every member of the nursing staff is involved in auditing for quality of care is a growing trend (Figure 14-3, p. 278).

Using the retrospective audit method, every member of the nursing staff randomly selects and examines three charts per month to determine if the documentation complies with the criteria. This unit predetermines that 90% of the selected charts must comply with the standard. Thus, if less than 90% of the charts comply with the standard, the unit will analyze the causes of substandard performance. The staff members who did not perform according to the criteria will be identified and advised by the head nurse or charge nurse. Reasons for not performing according to the standards, and ways to improve compliance, will be identified.

The concurrent audit method is often used for members of a nursing staff during their orientation period. When new nurses are performing intravenous therapy, for example, they are expected to find the nurse educator or a mentor nurse who

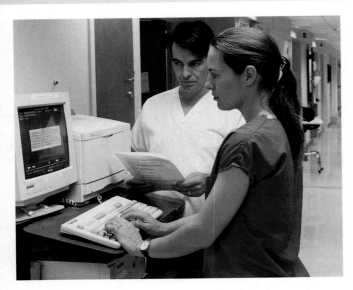

Figure 14-3. Recently, nursing staff members have become involved in auditing the performance of other staff members through the review of client records.

can observe their performance and ensure that it meets the standard of intravenous therapy.

Because quality assurance activities require tedious, comprehensive evaluation of documentation to show compliance with standards, they may have a delayed impact on quality of care. Thus quality assurance activities have been gradually replaced with continuous quality improvement activities. **Continuous quality improvement** (CQI) is a systematic approach to control and improve quality from the perspective of both professionals and clients. It is also called *total quality improvement* or *total quality management*. It incorporates professionals' and clients' perspectives of quality to set desirable outcomes. It uses statistical methods to measure processes of care and outcomes. And it requires relevant health care personnel to continuously improve processes of care to achieve predetermined outcomes. CQI is based on two main assumptions: (1) quality can always be improved, and (2) the health care delivery system often prevents health care providers from providing quality care. Thus CQI works on the system to improve the quality of care. When predetermined outcomes are not achieved, all relevant health care personnel work together to identify the problems and to seek ways to improve the system until desirable outcomes are achieved.

Managing Budgets.
Cost containment is a major goal in health care today and affects all health care practitioners. The challenge for nurses is to balance the value of nursing and the quality of care with the cost of providing care, while continuing to fulfill our obligation to be client advocates.

Nurse managers strive to ensure the highest quality care at the lowest possible cost. As health care costs have risen, government agencies, and now insurance companies, have become more careful about seeking justification for expenditures. Private for-profit health care agencies are in business to make a profit and must answer to investors when they do not

realize that profit. Therefore, they are extremely cautious about the expenditures that they are willing to incur while providing care.

Agencies that pay for health care (such as insurance companies) also expect health care providers, and nurses in particular, to carefully document and justify the necessity of all services provided to a client. Nurses must understand all factors that influence a unit's operation to be able to mount effective arguments for or against changes that influence the unit's function. Nurse managers also must justify staffing patterns by projecting the number and types of staff needed to produce quality health care. They also must project and justify the supplies and equipment needed. In short, they must provide a reasoned argument that quality nursing care is being delivered in the most efficient way possible.

Managing Personnel.
Nurse managers are responsible for evaluating performance and possibly for hiring and firing as well. They not only evaluate but they coach or counsel health care providers. They assume responsibility for staff development and education, and for the implementation of standards of care. They collaborate with other departments and disciplines in the interest of client care management. And nurse managers represent the health care institution and nursing as leaders. All of these tasks require that nurse managers be capable leaders who can communicate, organize, and delegate.

A **performance appraisal** is an organized and uniform method of evaluation of a nurse's job contribution, quality of work, and potential for advancement, made by the nurse's supervisor. Performance appraisals focus on each staff member's consistent compliance with standards. They may be used formally or informally to identify performance strengths and areas for improvement. Often the results of a performance appraisal are used to determine promotion, selection, termination, or pay raise. When appraisals indicate that a nurse consistently fails to comply with standards, this nurse becomes a problem employee and requires disciplinary action and frequent evaluation.

The process of performance appraisal varies with each organization. The organization defines a job description for its staff on the basis of its institutional standards, and then it conducts regular reviews of employees based on the job description. The process of performance appraisal must be described in the policy and procedure manual (JCAHO, 2002).

Each organization determines how each staff member should be evaluated. In general, nurses are expected to perform self-evaluation according to the institution's performance appraisal form. The nursing supervisor uses the same form to evaluate nurses' performance. Some organizations may also require each nurse to perform peer reviews. A **peer review** is the evaluation of the performance of one staff member by another staff member to judge the quality of care provided.

Managing Through Communication.
Communication is a key element of an empowering, democratic leadership style; it facilitates all other management activities. It is a process of giving and receiving messages for the purpose of transmitting

Table 14-3 Empowering Communication Techniques

Effective Messages	Less Effective Messages
"I observed that you were able to manage your clients' care today, but that you have to stay past work hours to complete your nurse's notes most days. I believe that work assignments should be set up in a way that lets us complete all of our duties within the scheduled work time. Is there something that we can do to help you accomplish that goal?"	"You never get your nurse's notes written during your shift. You need to get organized so you can get them done on time. I won't pay you overtime for notes any more." OR "I'll have Mary Jane change your assignment since you always have to stay overtime to finish your nurse's notes."
"Our client census is at a peak right now with some acutely ill clients. We are going to need one more nurse than usual for the next three shifts. These are the options available to us. . . ."	"I need three nurses to work overtime with the way the census is running. This is the new staffing schedule." OR "Can anybody work an extra shift to cover the increased census? My husband told me that he won't tolerate my covering all of the extra shifts for the unit any more."
"The team worked well together on this project. Through your efforts, we accomplished the changes in client outcomes that we needed."	"Lucky for you guys we met our goals somehow."

or exchanging information. An empowering nurse manager can communicate goals, delegate responsibilities and authority, coach, and inspire others through words and actions. Table 14-3 provides examples of empowering communication.

An empowering manager can also obtain information by being an active listener and an acute observer. Rather than accusing, empowering nurse managers state an observation and discuss alternatives. They listen to complaints and concerns and discuss alternative solutions without becoming defensive.

An empowering communicator uses messages that indicate personal ownership of beliefs, values, and needs. For example, the person says, "I want" or "I need" rather than "you must" or "you didn't." An empowering manager also communicates beliefs and expectations about values and goals. This approach promotes group participation rather than imposing values and coercing work.

An empowering communicator structures messages to make them more understandable and to facilitate clear communication. Avoid jargon and abbreviations, especially when communicating with people from other disciplines, because they can lead to misinterpretation or confusion. Keep messages factual, using appropriate details rather than global metaphors to present information. Also, empowering managers avoid the use of emotions when communicating about work.

In summary, transformational nurse managers actively seek employee input about policies and procedures rather than imposing rules without regard for their applicability. They maintain a positive attitude toward work and try to create a satisfying work environment. Responsibilities are shared rather than imposed. They trust that others are motivated to produce and capable of achieving a quality product. And they can risk their sense of control, or authority, in the interest of promoting a cohesive work unit.

ORGANIZATION OF NURSING UNITS

When you start to work on a nursing unit you need to understand the pattern of organizing the work of the unit. Each unit has its own method of organizing and working together as a team. The best method is the one that is efficient and produces the outcomes of quality client care as defined by the nurses on that unit. Three basic methods of organizing exist: functional assignments, team assignments, and total client care assignments. All methods are some variation on these three forms.

Patterns of Work

Perhaps the most efficient form of nursing unit organization is also the oldest method—functional nursing. It focuses on getting the work done in a timely manner. Using this method, tasks are assigned to the individual members of the team who possess the knowledge and skill to accomplish them. One nurse may give medication; another may change dressings and administer treatments. Usually, giving baths and making beds is assigned to the least skilled member of the team. Although this method of making assignments is efficient in terms of getting the tasks done, it has fallen into disfavor because it tends to fragment care: no one person assumes responsibility for total client care.

Team nursing overcomes some of the disadvantages of functional nursing while retaining the ability to effectively use multiple levels of personnel. **Team nursing** is more a concept than a specific pattern for organizing a work group. A team is created when a group of clients is assigned to a group of nursing personnel, which often consists of a combination of registered nurses, vocational or practical nurses, student nurses, and nursing assistants who work together and share responsibility for the care of the clients. A registered nurse is the team leader and makes assignments to team members on the basis of the abilities of the team members. All persons on the team are expected to feel responsible for the care of the group of clients. A team results in a small group, which facilitates communication. The registered nurse coordinates the team (perhaps planning care and administering medication).

One of the potential problems with team nursing is that the work group can easily lose the concept of working as a team. For the sake of efficiency, the work is divided and each member of the team performs specific tasks on the basis of that member's level of skill, thus creating a work group with a functional structure.

A **total client care** assignment avoids the possibility of care being fragmented. One nurse is assigned to provide comprehensive care to a small group of clients. A nurse is assigned to a client by matching the nurse's expertise to the client's needs. In this system, it becomes difficult to make assignments where personnel have widely different levels of skill.

Using **primary nursing** further enhances comprehensive care. Primary nursing gives the client a nurse who is at the bedside and responsible for the client's care over a 24-hour period. This method reduces the problems encountered when coordinating the activities of a team to provide comprehensive care. Primary nursing is more likely to be used in hospitals staffed entirely by registered nurses. However, some institutions use vocational or practical nurses as primary nurses when the client's care is within the knowledge and scope of practice for these nurses. Responsibility for 24-hour care is difficult to implement because nurses need days off, it is a difficult role for night shift nurses to implement, and changes often need to be made in the care plan when the primary nurse is not available. Thus primary nursing is often modified so that assignments of total client care apply to the period of time the nurse is on duty.

With the increased use of unlicensed assistive personnel, many hospitals are returning to the concept of team nursing. However, the size of the team has been reexamined. Using a work pattern of only two or three people working together is expected to improve communication and reduce the time it takes to keep the team working together. The **dyad** could be a registered nurse and an unlicensed assistive person. The **triad** could be two nurses with one nursing assistant, or some other combination depending on the skills required to meet the client's needs. The registered nurse will spend more time at the bedside than when a larger team is used, but an assistant will do tasks that do not require the registered nurse's skill.

There are two ways of working on a team. In one method, the work is divided and all members work independently to accomplish the tasks. In the other method, nurses are physically next to each accomplishing the same goal together. In the second method, the team members do not feel alone. Each member of the team is sharing the work with the others, and each makes a unique contribution to accomplishing the work. Each member is more likely to be attuned to the thinking of the others and thus they are all more likely to coordinate their actions to accomplish the shared goal. The nursing assistant learns in direct contact with the professional nurse, is more likely to continue to work within the same plan of care when working alone, and is more likely to communicate appropriate information to the professional nurse.

However, team nursing does not simply mean professional nurses working with personnel who have less training or education; it also means professional nurses working with other professional nurses to improve nursing care. Team nursing improves the quality of nursing care by allowing all levels of personnel to learn from the more experienced and knowledgeable members of the team. Team nursing provides the opportunity to see alternatives and discover new solutions to old problems. It causes nurses to look at themselves and one another both critically and supportively.

Communication

Communication is a key element of well-coordinated care when multiple caregivers are involved in that care. Because nursing care in a hospital setting is provided 24 hours a day and 7 days a week, many people must be involved in the care of any single client. Many methods and levels of communication are necessary to ensure that all personnel have the information necessary to provide care that is comprehensive and coordinated.

Physicians are the only members of the team who admit clients to a hospital. The client is admitted for a medical or surgical problem that requires nursing care to manage. The physician communicates the medical treatment plan by writing orders.

Nurses are responsible for the implementation of the physician's orders and for nursing care the client needs both in connection with the medical treatment plan and otherwise. The nurse writes a nursing care plan to communicate the

Table 14-4 **Change of Shift Report**	
Information to Be Exchanged	**Rationale/Hints**
Name, room number, physician, date of admission or date of surgery	Orient the listener to who and what you are talking about. For example, if the client is 1 day after surgery, the nurse will listen with a different mind-set than if the client is 5 days after surgery.
Medical diagnosis or surgery performed. A *brief* medical history of the current problem may be useful.	Experienced nurses will form a mental picture of what problems to anticipate and will begin to ask themselves questions about what needs to be done.
Surgery, tests, or procedures scheduled for the next 24 hours	Give this information early in the report. It is usually the priority and helps plan the day.
Vital signs, abnormal findings, information to report to physician	Identifies client's current status.
Tubes and equipment; include status (e.g., IV rate, amount left in bag, I&O, amount of drainage)	Identifies essential nursing activities.
Treatments	Identifies essential nursing activities.
General information: bath, activity, physical and mental impairments, assistance needed	Describes client's personal needs.
New orders, special problems, needed teaching, client–family dynamics	Describes client's personal needs.

needed nursing care to all nursing personnel over a 24-hour period and to ensure that the care is a well-coordinated effort.

Nursing care is then documented in the client's chart or record. Changes in the client's condition are also documented in the record. Through written communication, any nurse can review the chart to know what has been done for the client, whether the client's condition has changed, and whether the nursing care has been effective. Additionally, the chart serves as a permanent legal record of the client's hospital stay.

In addition to the written record, communication occurs through oral reports. When a nurse gives an oral report at the end of a shift to the next nurse who will assume responsibility for care of the client, it is called an **change-of shift report.** The nurse's work is not done until responsibility for the care of a client is passed to another nurse. This form of passing responsibility also occurs when a client is transferred from one unit to another. For example, the client may be moved to a more intensive care nursing unit or to a lower level of care.

Reporting in a manner that very quickly and efficiently provides another nurse with an overview of the client's condition, treatment plan, and needs in a manner that can be stored in an easily retrievable fashion in the mind of another person is an art. The reporter can err on the side of not supplying enough information, thus leaving out an element that is essential to the client's safety and well-being. On the other hand, too much detail overwhelms the listener and important information is lost amid the deluge of sometimes interesting but insignificant facts.

A good report always begins by orienting the listener to what is to come, proceeds in a systematic manner, and highlights essential events and findings. When reports are given in a consistent order, it is easier for the listener to mentally store and manage the information. Table 14-4 summarizes information to be provided in a report.

Nurses also provide verbal reports to the physician and to nursing supervisors. The same principles apply to these reports. When giving a report to a physician, anticipate the questions you might be asked and have the information readily available. For example, if the client becomes suddenly short of breath, before calling the physician you should take the vital signs, assess the lungs, and gather information about the onset of the shortness of breath. When you assess the client at the beginning of the shift, you are gathering information that may need to be reported to the physician.

Organizing Your Day

Nurses employ organizational skills to implement processes that lead to quality outcomes. They do so because nurses must manage multiple tasks to accomplish their mission. Thus they must use time effectively and maximize productivity. Time management requires organization and judicious delegation of tasks (Box 14-1).

Organization requires the nurse to identify tasks, obligations, and activities that must be accomplished in a given period of time. Then the nurse must estimate the time required by each task and rank the tasks, obligations, and activities in priority order. In general, the order should follow the institu-

tion's goals and objectives. Activities essential to achieving a goal must take place sooner than activities less essential to achieving the goal. Once the nurse has identified times and priorities, the next step is to establish a plan for accomplishing the tasks and activities.

A nurse's workday is both a series of anticipated events and a chaotic environment of constant change. Any shift has certain events that recur on a regular basis, such as meals, visiting hours, bedtime, and medication schedules. Other events are scheduled on a daily basis and thus can be anticipated. Diagnostic testing by other departments, surgery, and special procedures are often scheduled in advance. However, many events cannot be anticipated: the client's condition changes, the physician writes new orders, family arrives from out of town, or a nursing assistant is called to cover another unit, leaving you without help. Use a work sheet to make a general plan for the day. Box 14-2 shows a typical pattern of work for a day shift (7 A.M. to 3 P.M.).

Box 14-1   Time Management Tips

- Identify tasks, obligations, and activities.
- Write a list of tasks using a work management sheet, make a tentative schedule, and mark off as they have been accomplished. List tasks by clients and by time.
- Add notes to your work management sheet as needed throughout the day.
- Focus on the task at hand; complete each task before moving on to the next one.
- Control interruptions.
- Identify which tasks must be completed in specified time frames. Work ahead, not behind.
- Prioritize according to importance. Work on the most important first.
- Delegate tasks that don't require your expertise. Remember to give specific directions and to follow up on progress regularly.
- Do not accept assignments that you are not capable of completing.
- Avoid the need to be perfect.

Box 14-2   Typical Structure of the 8-Hour Day Shift

0645	Receive report from the night shift; nursing assistant takes vital signs
0700	Make rounds and assess assigned clients; nursing assistant starts baths
0730	Administer medications scheduled before meals; help nursing assistant serve trays; nursing assistant feeds clients if needed
0830	Prepare and administer medications due at 0900; baths by nursing assistant; physicians are making rounds (from 0600 to 1000); check for new orders; update physicians on clients' status
0930	Break
0945	Dressing changes, other treatments, 1000 medications; catch up on physician orders, charting; nursing assistant has a break, then does more baths
1130	Lunch; nursing assistant takes noon vital signs
1200	Noon medications; help nursing assistant with lunch trays
1230	Charting, 1300 medications; nursing assistant has lunch
1400	Intake and output calculations, charting, make rounds for final assessment, prepare for report to next shift
1445	Give report to next shift

Delegation

Some tasks need not be done specifically by the nurse and can be delegated. **Delegation** involves assigning responsibility for certain tasks to other people, thereby allowing the manager to concentrate on higher-level activities—tasks that can be accomplished only by a registered nurse. Box 14-3 lists strategies for effective delegation.

When a nurse delegates a task to another member of the health care team, the nurse must communicate all aspects of that task to the person charged with accomplishing it. A clear understanding of the nurse's expectations will help the person accomplish the task independently and successfully. The person to whom the task was delegated should have the freedom to decide on a course of action for accomplishing the task. Therefore, that person should have ability, knowledge, and motivation to accomplish the delegated task.

The nurse must know each employee's capabilities and the constraints dictated by licensure and education level. No nurse should delegate responsibility to ancillary personnel who lack the ability, education, or licensure to make appropriate nursing decisions. If the task requires nursing judgment, either the task should not be delegated, or the individual to whom the task was assigned should be instructed to report specific information back to the delegating nurse.

For example, a nurse may ask a personal care assistant—a nurse's aide—to take morning vital signs for all clients. However, although the assistant may be able to take and record blood pressures, this person does not have the ability to make judgments about the values obtained. Therefore, the delegating nurse must devise a specific mechanism for the assistant to report all morning vital signs to an identified nurse before delegating the task. The ultimate responsibility for a task lies with the person who delegated it.

In a general sense, work does flow more easily when shared with others. Consequently, nurses who use their knowledge of others, the work to be accomplished, and tasks appropriate for delegation will work more effectively and efficiently. In addition, they can accept responsibility and accountability for the work of others because tasks will have been delegated appropriately.

MANAGEMENT ISSUES

A major issue for nurse managers is managing change. The one constant in today's health care delivery system is change. Quality management programs are based on the ideal of continuously improving processes to continuously improve outcomes. To achieve that ideal, policies and procedures must be continuously evaluated and revised so institutions will function more effectively and efficiently. Deficiencies identified in quality indicators are viewed as opportunities for improvement and the impetus for change.

A second major issue is risk management. The public is highly aware of the possibility of injury or other untoward events in the health care environment and of the possibility of seeking reparation for damages through a lawsuit. The nurse manager has a responsibility for evaluating the risk and reducing it.

Managing Change

Nurse managers, acting as change agents, are obligated to influence the direction of change and maintain professional nursing standards. Change occurs more readily when it is planned and managed. Changes that happen without planning result in chaos. Consequently, effective nurse managers use steps similar to those in the nursing process to plan and accomplish changes in policies and procedures for their work units. Box 14-4 lists steps in the change process.

The Change Process. First, the manager identifies the need for change through assessment. Quality indicators, usually client outcome data, are assessed to detect trends that suggest a need for improvement.

In most cases, the nurse manager acts as a member of a process-improvement team. Staff nurses also participate in these teams in the interest of promoting democratic change. The planning phase of the process includes formulating how the policy or procedure should be rewritten, in keeping with professional standards, and how the rewritten version should be implemented. If the team decides that one more nurse is

---

Box 14-3   Steps in Effective Delegation

- **Identify the task.** Know whether the task can be legally delegated. You retain responsibility for assessment of the client's nursing care needs.
- **Analyze the skill and knowledge needed to accomplish the task.** Consider whether the task is within the scope of the assignee's education and ability, whether the circumstances are appropriate to delegate the specific task, whether directions and other communications have been sufficient, and how much direct supervision is needed. Know whether the person can properly and safely perform the task without jeopardizing the client's welfare, and whether the task requires professional nursing judgment. Instruct the unlicensed person in the delegated task or verify the competency to perform the nursing task through knowledge of individual characteristics, education, or training. Validate the person's understanding.
- **Assign the task.** Provide clear and concise details about the task, including the time frame and expected outcome, the purpose of the task, and any limitations in responsibility or authority for accomplishing the task.
- **Periodically evaluate the delegation of tasks.** Let the assignee complete the task with occasional follow-up and feedback. Adequately supervise the performance of the delegated nursing task. DO NOT delegate a task if you feel uncomfortable about someone else having control over how it will be completed.

Box 14-4   Steps for Managing a Planned Change

- Identify the need for change (assess).
- Identify the potential causes of a problem, or opportunity for improvement (analyze structures and processes).
- Identify potential actions (plan).
- Implement actions (implement).
- Evaluate outcomes (evaluate).
- Incorporate new behaviors into new structures or processes (evaluate).

needed to cover a certain number of calls, the process must also involve budget analysis to justify the expense of hiring another nurse, plans for advertising and hiring a new nurse, instituting policies and procedures for orienting the new nurse once hired, and staffing patterns for the entire team once the new nurse is oriented.

Once the plans are made, the next step is to implement them. In this example, the new nurse is hired. The change process does not end with implementation of the new policy or procedure, however. The next step entails evaluating the effectiveness of the planned change. And in the final step, further evaluation reveals either the need for more planning if the new process fails to improve the outcome, or the means to incorporate successful new behaviors into practice. Theoretically, when employees see the value of a planned change, they are more likely to accept it and incorporate the new behaviors it represents.

Controlling Anxiety. Nurse managers understand that change, even when planned carefully, causes anxiety, Indeed, the natural response of employees—virtually everyone, in fact—is to resist change. As the change agent, the nurse manager can initiate changes successfully by soliciting input from staff affected by the change, implementing the plan in stages, and demonstrating the effectiveness of the change through evaluation, thereby decreasing anxiety related to the change.

Several theories have been proposed to address resistance to change and ways to overcome that resistance. Change is effectively brought about in systems or organizations when the need for a change is recognized and accepted by those affected by the change: the employees. The first steps of the change process (assessment and analysis) help the manager raise the employees' awareness of a need for change. This starts the process of overcoming resistance.

Once employees have begun to recognize and accept the need for change, the nurse manager seeks input from them about how to implement the change. By facilitating employee involvement in the process, the nurse manager allows resistance to be addressed directly. People involved in the change process are more likely to become invested in the new process and accept the change when their concerns are heard and addressed as part of the planned change. Instituting changes in a stepwise manner also makes the process less threatening and therefore more acceptable. Finally, changes are most likely to be accepted and incorporated into new behaviors when evaluation shows the new plan to be effective.

The nurse manager is responsible for implementing the change, but the change itself requires the cooperation of everyone involved. It also requires the understanding that change is continuous. To help accomplish changes peacefully, the nurse manager needs leadership skills, communication skills, and education to influence acceptance of the change. Trusting relationships that result from a democratic, empowering leadership style and a consensus-building outlook form the basis for effective change.

Managing Risk

Risk management is the process of identifying, evaluating, and reducing or financing the cost of predictable losses. These losses include losses from litigation (lawsuits). Although risk management can be performed at the individual level to prevent personal lawsuits, the nurse manager implements risk management strategies at the institutional level.

The nurse manager must be keenly aware of competing professional, legal, and ethical claims. Nurse managers must evaluate all new programs, policies, and procedures in terms of their potential for doing good, causing harm, or both (Figure 14-4).

Malpractice and Negligence. The major legal issues faced by bedside nurses involve avoiding malpractice or negligence claims. Nurse managers are responsible for overseeing the legal practices of the health care providers they manage. They also must consider the legal implications of client care decisions and management practices when delegating care to other providers. Box 14-5 lists steps taken by nurse managers to minimize legal risk. The best protection comes from following professional standards of safe care when instituting policies and procedures used to guide nursing practice.

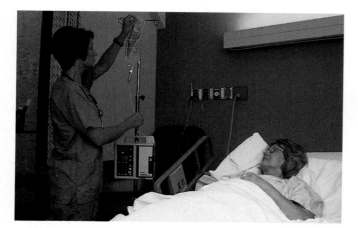

Figure 14-4. This nurse manager is evaluating a client's intravenous therapy to validate the effectiveness of her institution's policy for intravenous therapy.

Box 14-5	Risk Management/Quality Assurance Strategies

- Determine quality indicators essential to client care in this institution.
- Determine methods for measuring those indicators.
- Implement measurement strategies (measuring indicators and mapping trends).
- Assess and analyze variations from expected norms.
- Plan and implement strategies for improving performance.
- Gather data related to occurrences (indicators of potential problems, such as medication errors or employee injuries) and follow procedures to assess, analyze, plan, and implement strategies to alter the causes of the unusual occurrences.

Managing the legal risks in client care is closely tied to quality management activities.

Litigation can result from problems in performing technical skills or from problems in interpersonal communication. Therefore the nurse manager is responsible for creating an environment in which clients perceive both technical competence and an ethic of caring. Nurse managers have to assume a proactive stance in monitoring, evaluating, and correcting the services provided by other health care providers. They must ensure that providers have the tools (education, supplies, policies, and procedures) that enable them to provide the best possible care, technically and emotionally.

Discrimination and Safety. In their agency advocacy role, nurse managers also must act to avoid litigation brought by employees. Indeed, they are obligated to abide by federal, state, and local laws governing health care. The Equal Employment Opportunity Act, Americans With Disabilities Act, and Family Leave Act all provide guidelines that help to ensure fair and impartial treatment to all employees.

Most institutions have human resource departments that help nurse managers resolve issues related to gender, race, age, or disability discrimination. Nurse managers who are proactive about maintaining quality health care, and who use empowering communication styles to manage employees, will be more effective in avoiding legal problems related to infringement of an employee's rights.

Nurse managers must know and abide by Occupational Safety and Health Act (OSHA) regulations regarding maintenance of a safe work environment. That includes implementing policies about infection control, the use of chemical and biological agents, and the use of special equipment.

Licensure and Certification. It is often easy to think of potential good and harm only in terms of the effect on clients. However, nurse managers must promote good and avoid harm for the institution as well when implementing policies and procedures. Loss of revenue is only one type of harm that could befall the institution. Other issues can reduce the longevity of any health care agency. For example, governmental rules and regulations must be followed to maintain licensure or certification.

Nurse managers are obligated to abide by regulations imposed by those who pay for health care, such as the Health Care Financing Agency (HCFA) of the federal government. HCFA regulates Medicare and Medicaid as well as payment for services provided under those programs. Each insurance program, health maintenance organization, preferred provider service, and so on also imposes rules regarding allowed services and the means by which they are provided.

Agencies such as the Joint Commission for Accreditation of Health Care Organizations (JCAHO) also impose stringent guidelines regarding the provision of client care services. Nurse managers must know all of these regulations and the influence they have on practice in each environment. Any health care agency found to be out of compliance with these regulations could lose the license or certification that is required to do business.

Therefore nurse managers utilize leadership strategies to help other health care providers understand the rules and regulations and incorporate strategies to promote compliance. In an overall sense, they must use their knowledge of professional standards, legal implications of nursing practice and management, and ethical models to balance their obligation to act as client advocates with their obligation to promote the health care agency.

COLLABORATIVE HEALTH CARE TEAMS

Regardless of the type of health care facility involved, nurses are expected to participate in collaborative (multidisciplinary or interdisciplinary) health care teams as managers and as leaders. Client care is no longer the domain of one or two health care disciplines. Today, more people are living with chronic health conditions than ever before. And they require more assistance than that provided by physicians and nurses.

Collaborative health care teams have evolved as the means to ensure coordination of services and successful outcomes for clients. Box 14-6 lists the essentials of a multidisciplinary health care team. Each discipline is responsible

---

Box 14-6   Multidisciplinary Health Care Teams

Goal—To facilitate client's achievement of therapeutic goals, to improve client services, and to avoid overlap of client care services.

Membership—Those participating in the care of a single client or a group of clients being served by an institution or by a unit within an institution.

Purpose—Planning client care. Each discipline shares data of their care plan: client's progress toward therapeutic goals, response to individualized interventions. The entire team evaluates progress and plans future interventions.

Roles—Team members have a clear knowledge of their professional roles and the standards that guide their practice, which they share with the other team members in planning client care.

Nursing role—Nurses share nursing processes, nursing theories, and nursing research that influence their choice of interventions. They offer input regarding the standards and regulations that affect their practice in each unique client care setting.

ESSENTIAL COMPONENTS FOR A SUCCESSFUL TEAM EFFORT

- Shared goals
- Shared commitment to client care
- Shared accountability for client outcomes
- Open communication about interventions (care plans)

COMMON MEMBERS OF A MULTIDISCIPLINARY TEAM

- Nurse
- Physical therapist
- Occupational therapist
- Speech therapist
- Social worker
- Pastoral care provider
- Dietitian
- Physician
- Client
- Client's family

and accountable for the outcomes of its specific interventions. No one discipline has the power or right to negatively influence work being done with a client by another. Therefore it is extremely important that all providers work together to avoid overlapping services. They need a shared goal to produce the best client outcome efficiently and effectively.

Health care organizations have adopted collaborative team models that promote and protect professional autonomy for each discipline. In these models, all disciplines meet and confer about client care. Each member has an equal part but a different role in the client's care. No member of a team is more important than another, although, depending on the client's problem, one team member may be more involved at a given time. Members of collaborative health care teams share their expertise with other group members to plan, implement, and evaluate care strategies. Clients are involved as equal participants in the process.

Nurses have the opportunity to function as health care leaders in collaborative teams. Nurse managers, in the facilitator role, can provide education and guidance. They can model the behaviors that enhance communication and group cohesiveness. And they can evaluate the performance of nurses on these teams and coach them in improving communication and group participation. Nurse managers may also provide expert views on reimbursement, legal issues, professional standards, and organizational issues that affect team activities. Nurse managers make use of all the elements of management—quality, budgets, people, change, and risk—as tools to facilitate nurse participation and leadership in collaborative teams and all areas of practice.

Key Principles

- The philosophy and mission of an institution affects the performance of the organization from the top down; the goals, objective, policies, and procedures flow from the philosophy.
- Leadership is a quality of nursing practice regardless of the nurse's role within the organizational structure of a health care agency.
- Accomplishing multiple complex functions in a transformational management environment is a leadership style that empowers others and encourages their participation.
- Successful nurse managers have the characteristics of responsibility, accountability, leadership, and commitment to quality.
- Nurse managers are responsible and accountable for quality assurance, budgets, and personnel.
- The internal standards of each health care organization are influenced by external standards, such as ANA standards and standards of federal, state, and private regulatory agencies.
- The JCAHO surveys health care organizations to assess certain dimensions of the organization's performance. The demonstration of these characteristics indicates that the organization is likely to provide high-quality care.
- An organization develops internal standards to guide and standardize nursing practice, such as standards of practice, standards of client care, policies, procedures, protocols, case management, and clinical pathways.

- Change theories direct nurse managers through processes in which they recognize the need for change, plan for change, implement strategies for change, and motivate employees to embrace change.
- Nurse managers know and use ethical and legal models as they implement nursing care within the limitations of professional practice standards.
- In collaborative health care teams, client care is never exclusively the domain of any single health care discipline.

Bibliography

American Nurses Association (1998). *Standards of clinical nursing practice* (2nd ed.). Washington, D.C.: American Nursing Publishers, Pub. No. 9801ST.

American Nurses Association. (2003). Scope and standards of practice (draft). Washington, D.C.: American Nursing Publishers.

Anderson, C. A. (2001). From the editor: A culture of excellence and achievement. *Nursing Outlook, 49*(5), 209.

Anderson, K. (2001). Career path: Leadership skills—Be more than a voice in the crowd. *Nursing, 31*(6), 73.

Beecroft, P. C. (2001). Quality improvement and error rates. *Clinical Nurse Specialist, 15*(1), 1.

Bond, G. E., & Fiedler, F. E. (2001). Professional issues: The effects of leadership personality and stress on leader behavior: Implications for nursing practice. *Journal of Nursing Administration, 31*(10), 463-465.

Boykin, A., & Schoenhofer, S. (2001). The role of nursing leadership in creating caring environments in health care delivery systems. *Nursing Administration Quarterly, 25*(3), 1-7.

Brown, C. L. (2002). A theory of the process of creating power in relationships. *Nursing Administration Quarterly, 26*(2), 15-33.

Byram, D. A. (2000). Leadership: A skill, not a role. *AACN Clinical Issues: Advanced Practice in Acute & Critical Care, 11*(3), 463-469.

Chuong, B. (2001). Leadership lessons learned: Helping to develop leaders is our legacy! *AACN News, 18*(10), 12.

Coughlin, C. (2001). Care centered organizations. Part 2: The changing role of the nurse executives. *Journal of Nursing Administration, 31*(3), 113-120.

Crow, G. (2001). Caring and professional practice settings: The impact of technology, change, and efficiency. *Nursing Administration Quarterly, 25*(3), 15-23.

Curtin, L. (2001). Ethics & nursing administration: Part 1. *CurtinCalls, 3*(6), 4-5, back cover.

Curtin, L. L. (2001). The final Curtin: The trouble with teams. *Seminars for Nurse Managers, 9*(2), 132-135.

Dawes, B. S. G. (2001). The diversity of caring in the lives of patients and peers. *AORN Journal, 74*(6), 800-802.

Doherty, C., & Hope, W. (2000). Shared governance: Nurses making a difference. *Journal of Nursing Management, 8*(2), 77-81.

Drenkard, K. N. (2001a). Creating a future worth experiencing: Nursing strategic planning in an integrated healthcare delivery system. *Journal of Nursing Administration, 31*(7/8), 364-376.

Drenkard, K. N. (2001b). Team-based work redesign: The role of the manager when you are NOT on the team. *Seminars for Nurse Managers, 9*(2), 90-97.

Edick, V. W., & Whipple, T. W. (2001). Managing patient care with clinical pathways: A practical application. *Journal of Nursing Care Quality, 15*(3), 16-31, 75-76.

Ferguson, S. L., & Brindle, M. (2001). Perspectives in leadership: Nursing leadership—Vision and the reality. *Nursing Spectrum 13A,* NJ6, (New York/New Jersey Metro ed.), Jan 8.

Fox, R.T., Fox, D.H., & Wells, P. J. (1999). Performance of first-line management functions on productivity of hospital unit personnel. *Journal of Nursing Administration, 29*(9), 12-18.

Fralic, M. F. (2000). Consider this: What is leadership? *Journal of Nursing Administration, 30*(7/8), 340-341.

Frisina, M. E. (2001). Lead outside your comfort zone. *Nursing Management, 32*(11), 22-26.

Hagenow, N. R. (2001). Care executives: Organizational intelligence for these times. *Nursing Administration Quarterly, 25*(4), 30-35.

Harris, J. (2001). President's message: Shaping the system and culture of health care. *Dermatology Nursing, 13*(2), 86.

Hawkins, A. (2002). Self-awareness a key skill in influencing and leading others. *AACN News, 19*(1), 14.

Holder, P. (2001). Leadership circle: Leading from the rear. *SCI Nursing, 18*(1), 41-42.

Holle, M. L., & Blatchley, M. E. (2000). Teaching leadership with role theory. [First appeared in *NursingConnections, 2*(4).] *NursingConnections, 13*(4), 41-49.

Horton-Deutsch, S. L., & Mohr, W. K. (2001). The fading of nursing leadership. *Nursing Outlook, 49*(3), 121-126.

Iacono, M. (2000). Leadership/management: Managing conflict/ employee counseling. *Journal of Perianesthesia Nursing, 15*(4), 260-262.

Janney, M. A., Horstman, P. L., & Bane, D. (2001). Promoting registered nurse retention through shared decision making. *Journal of Nursing Administration, 31*(10), 483-488.

Joint Commission on Accreditation of Healthcare Organizations (JCAHO). (2002). Comprehensive Accreditation Manual for Hospitals (CAMH): The Official Handbook. Oakbrook Terrace, IL:. Author.

Kerfoot, K. (2001a). On leadership: From motivation to inspiration leadership. *Nursing Economics, 19*(5), 242-243.

Kerfoot, K. (2001b). On leadership: The art of raising the bar. *Dermatology Nursing, 13*(4), 301-302.

Kerfoot, K. (2001c). On leadership: The leader as synergist— Nursing economics. *Dermatology Nursing, 13*(2), 135-136.

Kline, J. (2000). Team commitment to achieving common goal. *OR Manager, 16*(8), 25-26.

Langston, N., & Corcoran, R. D. (2001). President's & CEO's message: The power of shared leadership—Promoting a way of being that will endure. *Nursing & Health Care Perspectives, 22*(5), 218.

Laschniger, H. K. S., Shamian, J., & Thomson, D. (2001). Impact of magnet hospital characteristics on nurses' perceptions of trust, burnout, quality of care, and work satisfaction. *Nursing Economics, 19*(5), 209-219.

Manthey, M. (2001). Creative Healthcare Management, Minneapolis, MN. Staffing issues: A core incremental staffing plan. *Journal of Nursing Administration, 31*(9), 424-425.

Marion, L. (2001). AAN news & opinion: The nursing leadership pipeline. *Nursing Outlook, 49*(5), 244-245.

McQueeney, M. (2000). Perspectives in leadership: Do you have what it takes to be a manager? *Nursing Spectrum 13*(10), 18, May 15 (Greater Chicago/NE Illinois & NW Indiana Edition).

Mintzer, B. (2001). Management forum. The power of a vision: A leader's journey. *Caring, 20*(7), 40-41.

Mohr, W. K., Deatrick, J., Richmond, T., & Mahon, M. M. (2001). A reflection on values in turbulent times. *Nursing Outlook, 49*(1), 30-36.

Morrison, R. S., Jones, L., & Fuller, B. (1997). The relationship between leadership style and empowerment on job satisfaction of nurses. *Journal of Nursing Administration, 27*(5), 27-34.

Narayan, M. C., Rea, K., Cressy, M. M., Rogers, J., Preuss, B. C., Drenkard, K., & Maklancie, M. (2002). Searching for nursing's future? Here's how to turn your vision into reality. *Nursing Management, 33*(1), 26-30.

Ohman, K. (1999). Nurse manager leadership. *Journal of Nursing Administration, 29*(12), 16, 21.

Olsen, J., & Coleman, J. R. (2001). Using continuous quality improvement techniques to determine the causes of hospital readmission. *Critical Care Nurse, 21*(2), 52-54, 57, 59-61.

Perkins, S. B., Connerney, I., & Hastings, C. E. (2000). Outcomes management: From concepts to application. *AACN Clinical Issues: Advanced Practice in Acute & Critical Care, 11*(3), 339-350.

Pesut, D. J. (2001a). Future think: Deep change. *Nursing Outlook, 49*(3), 118.

Pesut, D. J. (2001b). Future think: Spiral dynamics—Leadership insights. *Nursing Outlook, 49*(2), 70.

Schroeder, P. (2001). From the editor: Assessing effectiveness in improving performance. *Journal of Nursing Care Quality, 15*(4), vi.

Smith, A. P. (2001). Leadership roundtable: Removing the fluff— The quality in quality improvement. *Nursing Economics, 19*(4), 183-185, 188.

Triolo, P., Kazzaz, Y., & Sherwood, G. (2000). Caring leadership: Essential during turbulence. *Excellence in Nursing Administration, 1*(2), 1, 3.

Tuck, I., Harris, L. H., & Baliko, B. (2000) Values expressed in philosophies of nursing services. *Journal of Nursing Administration, 30*(4), 180-184.

Walker, J. (2001). Developing a shared leadership model at the unit level. *Journal of Perinatal & Neonatal Nursing, 15*(1), 26-39.

Wooten, L. (2001). Research corner: Focus is on continuous quality improvement process. *AACN News, 18*(1), 4, 6.

Zangwill, M. (2001). On the path to quality improvement: Nurses guide the team. *On-Call, 4*(7), 18-21.

Nursing Research

Learning Objectives

After studying this chapter, you should be able to do the following:

- Describe the importance of nursing research
- Identify the types of ethical dilemmas in nursing research and the mechanisms for the protection of human subjects
- Describe the types of research personnel, types of studies, and the parts of a typical research study
- Discuss the steps of the research process
- Identify ways of implementing nursing research findings in your nursing practice

Imagine that you are in the library, and you take a break from studying your fundamentals text. In the study carrel you find a nursing research journal and, as you flip through the journal, you come upon the following text:

> The purpose of this study was to determine the accuracy and reliability of three types of thermometers: IVAC (IVAC Corp., San Diego, CA), TempraDOT (PyMaH Corp., Somerville, NJ), and an off-the-shelf mercury thermometer used to take oral temperatures. Roy's adaptation model provided the theoretical basis for the study. The convenience sample consisted of 35 adults who volunteered for the study. Information was collected by two registered nurses following the manufacturers' recommendations required for an accurate reading. Results indicated no differences in the validity and reliability of the three types of thermometers.

Just then, your instructor stops by your carrel and says, "I see you're reading the study about thermometers." She asks you the following questions:

- Do you think a sample of 35 adults is large enough that you could use this research with all adult clients?
- If you were working in pediatrics, could you use this study to guide your practice with children?
- Do other factors besides the recommendations made by the manufacturer affect the accuracy of temperature measurement?
- How would you know which of the temperature readings was the correct one if the readings varied from one thermometer to another?
- If you were going to take rectal or axillary temperatures, would an IVAC and a mercury thermometer be equally accurate?

How would you answer?

Welcome to the world of nursing research. It shapes your daily practice in ways you never imagined. Indeed, it forms the basis for most of the nursing knowledge you will use in your nursing career and for many of the facts and concepts presented in your nursing courses.

Research improves nursing practice. However, before you can begin to incorporate research successfully into your practice, you must be able to evaluate it. Questions such as those just asked and many others need to be answered before you can accept any research study as a valid basis to change your practice. The purpose of this chapter is to help you ask the right questions and evaluate the answers before you use the results of nursing research in your practice.

IMPORTANCE OF NURSING RESEARCH

Nursing research is the method used to develop knowledge about issues important to nursing practice today and in the future. More than ever before, nurses are being asked to determine their role in the delivery of health care and to document the effectiveness of that role. To define a distinct nursing role in health care delivery, nurses need a body of knowledge that separates nursing from other health professions. The body of knowledge developed through nursing research will help nurses articulate what they do and how their actions improve the health of their clients.

Additionally, research can provide a guide for decision making in nursing practice. Research can help you answer important questions, such as the following: What should I assess? Which clients can reach the goal of self-care? Which interventions produce the best client outcomes? When should evaluation take place? Nursing research also has the potential to identify the importance of the caring component of health care delivery in achieving the outcome of a healthier society.

The National Institutes of Health recognizes the importance of nursing research. To support nursing research, the National Institute of Nursing Research (NINR), a division of the National Institutes of Health, was established. The NINR mission is to establish a scientific basis for the care of individuals across their life span, to promote healthy lifestyles, to promote quality of life in those with chronic illness, and to care for individuals at the end of life (NINR, 2000). This mission is accomplished by supporting grants to universities and organizations and by research conducted at laboratories in Bethesda, Maryland. The NINR website, http://www.nih.gov/ninr/research/diversity/mission.html, lists specific goals and objectives as well as strategic plans for the 21st century.

Contributions to Society

Nursing research has improved the quality of life for many people. Through nursing research, new knowledge has been developed to improve nursing care for clients of all ages and cultures. For example, neonatal research has provided nurses with new methods for stimulating respiration in low-birth-weight infants. It has yielded new knowledge about the effects of parental touch and environmental lighting for preterm infants. Additionally, children and adolescents have benefited from studies about the psychosocial stress of being hospitalized or isolated because of a chronic illness. Adults have benefited from studies about spousal and elder abuse and about adaptation to pain.

Nurse researchers have addressed topics of concern to our clients. A rapidly growing body of nursing research knowledge exists to improve the physical and psychosocial well-being of clients with many types of illnesses or conditions. Many client teaching pamphlets and videos are based on the findings from nursing research studies.

Advancement of the Nursing Profession

In addition to contributing to society, nursing research also advances the profession of nursing by expanding the body of nursing knowledge. Nurse researchers develop and share knowledge with other nurses seeking answers to the same questions. Extension of the knowledge base is essential for the continued growth of the profession and for the improvement of nursing care. Through nursing research, nurses learn new ways to solve old problems and address current professional issues. Without nursing research, nurses would not have valid and reliable information to serve as the basis for nursing decisions.

Nursing research contributes to the profession by expanding the scientific basis for nursing practice. For example, through research, nurses have discovered personal characteristics related to compliance with therapeutic regimens, identified groups at risk for specific health problems, designed effective nursing interventions for particular types of clients, and demonstrated how cultural beliefs influence health care. Solutions to clinical problems are commonly found in nursing research.

Finally, nursing research contributes to the profession by developing theories of nursing practice. Although the accumulation of facts is important, the organization of facts into theories increases our understanding of these facts. Nursing theory is the way the nurse theorist views the world of nursing and its influence on client care.

ETHICS OF NURSING RESEARCH

Ethical standards are especially important in nursing research because studies of health patterns involve the use of human subjects whose rights must be protected. To protect research subjects from ethical violations, many professions have established their own codes of ethics for research. A code of ethics serves to guide researchers in protecting the rights of human subjects. Various professions and government agencies have published codes of ethics, which address the principles of ethical human research, but include particular concerns of the individual professions.

In addition to professional codes of ethics, the National Commission for the Protection of Human Subjects of Biomedical and Behavioral Research (1978) issued a code of ethics that formed the basis of regulations for research sponsored by the federal government. Known as the Belmont Report, this document identified the ethical principles of human subject research and required informed consent and institutional review.

Risk/Benefit Ratio

Conducting ethical research involving human subjects requires analyzing the risk/benefit ratio. This ratio measures whether the risks to research subjects outweigh the possible benefits to society and the nursing profession. The risk to subjects should never exceed the value to society. For nurse researchers, this principle can be interpreted to mean that the topic of the research should be significant *and* have the potential to improve client care. If the research topic does not have the potential to improve client care, then the research should not be conducted.

All research involves risk to the subjects. In most cases the risks are minimal, but researchers should always try to reduce even minimal risks. The most common types of risks to subjects include the following:

- Psychological factors, such as fatigue, anxiety caused by self-disclosure, and anger at the type of questions being asked or the loss of privacy
- Physical factors, such as physical harm, discomfort, or adverse effects

- Sociological factors, including the loss of time and financial costs for extra laboratory tests or transportation

In addition to the benefits to society and the nursing profession, the subjects themselves may benefit from participation in the study. These benefits may include increased knowledge about themselves, knowledge that they may be helping others, enhanced self-esteem, access to an intervention that may be available only through research, comfort in being able to discuss their concerns with a nonjudgmental researcher, and direct monetary or material gains. (Some researchers give study participants a small honorarium or other token rewards for their time.)

Review Boards

Hospitals, universities, and other institutions where research is frequently conducted have a review board to protect the rights of subjects. These review boards are formal committees with protocols for reviewing research proposals and plans. Review boards are sometimes called *human subjects committees.*

Research supported by federal funds is subject to strict guidelines concerning the use of human or animal subjects. An **institutional review board** (IRB) is a committee whose duties include making sure that proposed research meets the federal requirements for ethical research. The federal government mandates the committee if the institution is receiving federal funds for research (Code of Federal Regulations, 1983).

Because not all research receives federal support or is conducted in institutions with review boards, some studies may not undergo formal review. Regardless of the lack of a formal review process, all researchers have a responsibility to ensure that their research plans adhere to ethical guidelines. Many solicit an external review even when not required to do so.

When publishing research, most authors acknowledge that an IRB or human subjects committee has reviewed the study. When the author identifies a formal review by a committee, you can assume that the study was reviewed for ethical considerations.

Informed Consent

Informed consent means that the subjects have been given sufficient information about the research to enable them to consent voluntarily to participate or to decline to participate (Box 15-1, p. 290). Subjects must have the ability to comprehend the information they are given about the study. Violations of the informed consent rule exist when there is no consent, or when a consenting client is either not fully informed of the details of a research study or not continually informed of study changes or results (Karigan, 2001).

Most researchers provide subjects with a written consent form, which the researcher will ask the subject to sign before joining the study. The researcher keeps this document, and the subject retains a copy. A sample research consent form is shown in Figure 15-1 (p. 290).

The procedure as described protects the rights of most subjects, but sometimes researchers are interested in studying

| Box 15-1 | **Elements of Informed Consent to Participate in a Research Study** |

A participant in a research study has a right to the following information. This information should be included in the consent form to be signed by the participant, and the participant should be given a copy of the form.

1. What the researcher hopes to learn.
2. The type of information to be collected.
3. How the information will be used in the study.
4. The requirements of the participant (e.g., time, travel, invasive procedures).
5. How the information will be collected (e.g., drawing blood, answering a questionnaire, interview).

6. How participants are selected.
7. Potential physical or emotional harm or discomfort.
8. Potential benefits to the subject (e.g., better health, monetary payment for participation).
9. Potential benefit to others, individual, or society.
10. Names of researchers, institutional affiliation, whom to contact with questions or concerns about the study.
11. Information about the right to withdraw at any time without penalty.
12. Information about the methods to insure confidentiality of participants.

CONSENT TO PARTICIPATE IN A RESEARCH STUDY

In signing this consent form, I understand that I will be part of a research study that will focus on the effects of exercise on weight loss. I understand that I am agreeing to participate in the study for a total of six weeks, during which I will be asked to consume only prepackaged meals and snacks totaling 2000 calories per day. The foods and snacks will be provided for me free of charge, and I will be able to select the foods from a list that will be provided. I understand that I will keep a record of all foods and fluids consumed by me and will present this record weekly. I also understand that I will need to be present at the Tomlinson Health Sciences Center each Monday morning during the length of the study between 6:00 a.m. and 6:30 a.m., where I will be weighed without clothes, after emptying my bladder, and before I have consumed any food or liquids. I understand that I may or may not be asked to walk continuously for 30 minutes on Mondays, Wednesdays, and Fridays.

I have been informed that participation in the study is entirely voluntary, and that even after the study begins I can terminate my participation at any time. I have been told that my weight and records will not be given to anyone else and that no reports of this study will ever identify me in any way.

This study will help to develop a better understanding of the relationship between weight loss and exercise. I understand that the results of this research will be given to me if I ask for them and that Dr. Kathy Lauchner is the person to contact if I have any questions about the study or about my rights as a study participant. Dr. Lauchner can be reached by collect call at 1-800-555-1212.

Date: _____ Participant's Signature_____

Researcher's Signature_____

Figure 15-1. A sample research consent form.

special, vulnerable groups of subjects who may be incapable of giving fully informed consent. Vulnerable groups typically include infants, children, pregnant women, the terminally ill, institutionalized or hospitalized clients, and mentally, emotionally, or physically disabled individuals. With these vulnerable subjects, the researcher may be required to undertake additional procedures and be especially sensitive about protecting subjects' rights. The researcher should make sure that risks are minimal and possible benefits are pronounced.

Ethical Dilemmas in Nursing Research

Nurse researchers rarely decide purposely to violate the ethical principles of research. However, enthusiasm for conducting research may pose ethical dilemmas for the nurse researcher who comes to believe that the knowledge gained from research is more important and beneficial than the rights of subjects or ethical principles. Following are some examples of research questions and associated ethical dilemmas.

Research question: Do maternity clients discharged 24 hours after childbirth experience fewer complications when visited by a home health nurse? *Ethical dilemma:* If a home health nurse visits only some clients, other clients are not visited. If one group is receiving treatment, and the other group is not receiving treatment, are there potentially hazardous consequences to the group not receiving treatment? If the answer to this question is yes, the researcher is endangering the group not receiving treatment. How can this problem be resolved?

Research question: How do clients cope with the new diagnosis of an impending terminal illness? *Ethical dilemma:* Clients diagnosed with a terminal illness are very vulnerable. To answer the question, the researcher may need to ask intrusive questions. By asking these questions, the researcher may cause psychological trauma and increase the client's anxiety level. However, the results of this study may give nurses valuable insight into the coping mechanisms used by newly diagnosed terminally ill clients. Is this study fair to the subjects?

As these examples illustrate, nurse researchers frequently encounter ethical dilemmas. Ethical codes and IRBs help guide researchers in resolving these dilemmas and protecting the rights of subjects.

THE RESEARCH STUDY

The research project itself is usually called a study or an investigation. The tools that the researcher uses to conduct a study are called **instruments.** Instruments can be thermometers, laboratory tests, a list of questions, or a checklist. The term **data** is used to designate the information the researcher is interested in collecting. Data may take the form of words or may have numeric value.

The people being studied are called subjects, study participants, or informants. Subjects are enlisted from *populations,* the groups of individuals that the researcher is interested in studying. For example, if a researcher wants to understand the

Table 15-1	Types of Nonexperimental Research
Types of Design	**Characteristics**
Correlational	Examines the relationship between two or more variables to see if, when one variable changes, the other variable also changes without any active intervention
Descriptive	Accurately identifies and describes the characteristics of individuals, situations, or groups
Case study	Involves the detailed investigation of an individual, group, or institution to understand which variables are important to the subjects' history, care, or development
Historical	Examines events that have occurred in the past through systematic collection of data and critical evaluation
Needs assessment	Involves the collection of data to estimate the needs of a community or an organization so that decisions can be made
Survey	Collection of data from a sample of subjects who resemble the population in terms of variables being studied; studies to examine opinions, attributes, behavior, or characteristics of a population

reasons abused wives stay in relationships with their abusers, a sample of abused wives will be asked to participate in the study. If the sample truly represents the population of abused wives, the researcher can derive conclusions about the whole population from the sample.

Personnel

The person who undertakes a research project is usually called a researcher but is sometimes called an *investigator.* When a team of people undertakes a research project, the person directing the study is called the *principal investigator* or *project director.*

Types of Studies

The type of research depends on the questions asked by the researcher and the topic under study. Some research questions may be asked in different ways, which influences the type of research. Not all types of research lend themselves to all questions.

Research studies range from experimental to nonexperimental. **Experimental research** is a study in which the researcher manipulates a treatment or intervention, randomly assigns subjects to either a control or an experimental group, and has control over the research situation. Because nurse researchers study human subjects, often in health care situations, a true experimental design is difficult. Consequently, nursing research is most commonly quasi-experimental or nonexperimental research. **Quasi-experimental research** is a type of study in which the researcher manipulates a treatment or intervention but is unable to randomize subjects into groups or lacks a control group. **Nonexperimental research** is a type of study in which the researcher collects data without the introduction of a treatment or intervention. The major types of nonexperimental research appear in Table 15-1.

Effects of Exercise on Weight Loss

ABSTRACT: The purpose of this 6-week study was to determine the effects of 30 minutes of walking, three times a week, on weight loss. A random sample of 100 adult males and females, enrolled in a structured weight loss program, participated in the study. All of the subjects continued their normal activity levels, while one-half of the subjects agreed to increase their exercise level by walking three times a week. The Roy adaptation model served as the theoretical framework. Results indicated that those subjects who walked three times a week had a significantly greater weight loss than those subjects who maintained their normal activity.

Americans are increasingly striving to lose weight. The majority of the population is overweight, and Americans spend approximately $30 million each year on weight loss medications and dietary aids (Sampson, 1997). Obesity is a major health problem in the United States and one that influences the physical and mental health of the population. The purpose of this study was to determine the effects of 30 minutes of walking, three times a week, on subjects enrolled in a weight-loss program consisting of a 2000-kcal/day diet. The hypothesis was that people who walked 30 minutes three times a week would lose more weight than people who did not.

Several researchers have studied the effects of exercise on weight loss. Johnson (1995) studied 400 adults over the age of 65 who attended a 30-minute exercise class a minimum of once a week for a 6-month period. The results of that study indicated that subjects who attended the exercise class a minimum of three times a week lost weight, while those who attended less than three times a week did not lose weight. Likewise, Smith (1997) found that children who played baseball three times a week also lost weight, while children who played baseball less than three times a week did not lose weight.

The theoretical framework for the current study is the Roy adaptation model. According to Roy (Roy & Andrews, 1996), focal, contextual, and residual stimuli influence adaptation in the physiological, self-concept, role function, and interdependence modes. This study examined the need for nutrition and activity and rest in the physiological mode. The researchers viewed weight loss as an adaptation in the physiological mode, diet as a focal stimulus, and exercise as a contextual stimulus.

Methods

During the 6 weeks of the study, all 100 participants consumed prepackaged meals and snacks totaling 2000 kcal/day. On a flowsheet designed for this study, each subject was required to record all food and fluid intake immediately upon consumption. In addition, the subjects assigned to an exercise group were required to walk for 30 minutes on Mondays, Wednesdays, and Fridays for the 6 weeks of the study. Each participant in the exercise group was given a stopwatch to time the length of the walking. All participants were weighed using the same scale each Monday morning between 6:00 a.m. and 6:30 a.m. without clothes, after emptying their bladders and before consuming any foods or fluids.

Approval of the institutional review board was obtained for this study. All research data were collected by the researcher, who explained the study to each participant and procured informed consent.

Subjects for the study were solicited from an advertisement in a local newspaper. Of the 400 adults who responded to the advertisement, 150 met the criteria established by the researcher. These criteria included willingness to follow the study protocol, absence of physical or mental illnesses, and ability to pass a physical examination conducted by the researcher. Of the 150 respondents who met the criteria, 100 were randomly selected for inclusion in the study and randomly assigned to either the exercise or nonexercise groups. All of the subjects completed the study.

Subjects ranged in age from 22 to 64 and included 56 females and 44 males. The majority of the subjects, 82%, were employed outside the home, and education levels ranged from completion of the sophomore year of high school to a master's degree.

Instrumentation used to gather data included a Brice-Jones scale and Olympic stopwatches. The scale was calibrated by a technician from the state Bureau of Weights and Measurements each Monday morning prior to collecting the weight data. Between each subject the scale was reset at the 0 level. During the time of the study, the scale was not moved. New stopwatches were used for the study. Prior to the beginning and at the end of the study, each stopwatch was tested by a computer timing device to ensure accuracy.

Data Analysis

The data were analyzed using a t-test. The mean weight loss for the nonexercise group was 6 lb, while the mean weight loss for the exercise group was 9 lb. These results were significant ($p < .05$).

Results

The results of this study indicate that exercising three times a week for 30 minutes contributed to weight loss. The weight loss for the exercise group was

Figure 15-2. Example of a brief research article.

approximately one-third greater than for the nonexercise group. The flowsheets for both groups indicated that study participants adhered to the study protocol and consumed only the prepackaged meals. The amount of fluids consumed by the subjects varied from 1400 mL to 3200 mL, with the mean consumption being 2200 mL. One subject in the exercise group was unable to exercise on the specified day, but did exercise the following day.

Discussion of the Results
The findings from this study suggest that exercise does influence weight loss. These findings support the previous studies conducted by Johnson (1995) and Smith (1997). Exercise seems to increase weight loss in adults, as well as in children and older adults. These three studies may represent a beginning body of knowledge about the effects of exercise on weight loss.

The amount of fluids consumed by the subjects varied greatly, and may have influenced weight loss. The effect of fluid consumption on weight loss is an area for further study. In addition, the ability of the

subjects to adhere to the diet deserves further consideration. The researcher acknowledges that in most studies, the subjects do not report such strict adherence to the diet. The adherence in this study may be due to the limited time frame of the study or to the prepackaged meals. This too is an area for further research.

This study supports the Roy model. The exercising subjects lost weight, and the researcher viewed this weight loss as a physiological adaptation to the focal stimulus of diet and the contextual stimulus of exercise.

References
Johnson, K. N. (1995). Exercise and weight loss in children. *Journal of Pediatric Conditions, 65*(5), 332–336.
Roy, C., & Andrews, H. A. (1996). *The Roy adaptation model* (2nd Ed.). Norwalk, CT: Appleton & Lange.
Sampson, T. R. (1997). *American weight loss statistics.* Bluffs, MT: Sanderson.
Smith, P. T. (1997). Weight loss in older adults. *Journal of Gerontological Physiology, 6*(4), 11–28.

Figure 15-2, cont'd. Example of a brief research article.

Parts of the Study
The reading of a research report begins with an **abstract,** which is a short summary that contains brief information about the purpose of the study, the number of subjects, the methodology used to select subjects, the type of study conducted, and the major results obtained from the study. The reader uses the abstract to decide whether the study contains information of interest. Some nursing journals print only the abstract of a study along with a reference that readers use to locate the full study report. An example of an abstract and a brief research article appear in Figure 15-2.

If the entire study is included in the journal, you will typically find the following parts:

* *Introduction:* Usually, this section describes the research problem, presents the purpose of the study, reviews current literature, outlines the theoretical background, and explains the research questions.
* *Methods:* This section describes how the researchers sought to answer the research questions. This section also includes the sample size, how the sample was selected, how the data were collected, and the instruments used to collect data.
* *Data analysis:* Here you will see how the data were analyzed and which statistical tests were used to analyze the data. This section frequently includes tables, charts, or graphs.
* *Results:* This section describes the results obtained by the study, usually by addressing each research question individually.
* *Discussion:* This section includes the researchers' interpretation of the results, any conclusions drawn from the study,

the relationship of the study findings to the theoretical background, and suggestions for future research.
* *References:* Here you will find all the references used in the study.

Many of the research reports found in current nursing literature are primary sources. A *primary source* is the original research report written by the researchers. A *secondary source* is any other published material that reports on the study. When a research report or textbook cites a study, it becomes a secondary source. A secondary source is an adaptation of the primary source and may contain another person's interpretation of the research.

STEPS IN THE RESEARCH PROCESS

As you read nursing research, you will find that the research process follows a series of unique and essential steps. Although these steps may vary with the type of research conducted, a typical research study follows this order:

* Statement of the research problem
* Review of the literature
* Development of a theoretical construct
* Identification of variables
* Clarification of operational definitions
* Formulation of the research questions
* Selection of a research strategy
* Collection of data
* Analysis of data
* Interpretation of findings

These steps help the researcher address a problem in an orderly way. They also help consumers of research to understand and evaluate the study. Most research articles are organized and written according to these steps. The steps are common to all research, not only nursing research.

Statement of the Problem

A **research problem** is an observation, situation, occurrence, or even a hunch that an investigator chooses to research. Initially, it may simply be an area of interest that the researcher then further defines. Most problems begin with something the researcher has observed in practice. For example, if in clinical practice a nurse observes that some diabetic patients are better able to control their blood glucose levels than others, the researcher might question the reason for this difference.

In addition to the significance of the study, researchers must consider whether it is possible to design a study to research the problem. Not all problems are amenable to all research methods. For example, issues that are of a moral or ethical nature are not easily researchable.

Another consideration that researchers must address is the feasibility of conducting the research. All researchers face limitations, such as time, availability of subjects and resources (such as equipment), cooperation of institutions, financial support, and the facilities needed to conduct the research. Many researchers must change or limit their research problems on the basis of availability of resources.

The research problem or purpose of the research should be stated early in the research report. In the problem or purpose statement, the researcher should clearly identify what the study is about, any suspected relationships, and the population of interest. For example, a purpose statement might be, *The purpose of this study is to compare the effects of grief on the physiological health of women who experienced the death of a spouse within the preceding 12 months and the effects of grief on the physiological health of women who experienced the death of a child within the preceding 12 months.*

The researcher's use of verbs in the purpose statement often identifies the state of the knowledge about the subject or the manner in which the researcher sought to solve the problem. The verbs *explore* or *describe* usually indicate a topic about which little is known, whereas *test* or *compare* suggests a more thoroughly developed knowledge base. Verbs such as *show, prove,* or *demonstrate* indicate possible researcher bias and should not be used.

Review of the Literature

The researcher begins to study the problem by reviewing the current information about the problem. A literature review is essential to all types of research and serves as the foundation for the research study. The researcher conducts the review by thoroughly examining all available literature related to the research problem. The purposes of the literature review are to help the researcher identify or refine the research problem, strengthen the rationale for the research, develop a conceptual framework, and provide a useful approach for the study.

The researcher typically conducts the literature review using a computer search. Computer searches are used to reach bibliographic information stored in databases. A computer search may be completed at any computer that has access to the database. Library computers usually have access to databases, or the librarian can help you find access to the desired database. Table 15-2 identifies databases of interest to nurses. These are the same databases you would use to look for information about any nursing topic of interest.

In addition, many nursing journals can be accessed at www.nursingcenter.com from any computer with an Internet connection. This site provides full-text access to many articles and has its own search engine. There are other websites that provide free access to nursing journals worldwide. The major difficulty when using journal web sites is that web addresses change.

Researchers and nurses frequently read abstracts to determine the potential usefulness of an article. To fully evaluate the research, however, the entire article must be examined. At the end of the article, the reference list can be used to obtain further articles about the topic of interest.

Development of a Theoretical Framework

A **theoretical framework** is a logical but abstract structure that suggests the relationships among the variables in a research study. The framework allows for the organization and explanation of all the information included in the study. Working within a framework enables the researcher to tie the research to

Table 15-2	Computer Search Database Resources
Database	**Types of Listings**
CINAHL	Corresponds with the information in *Cumulative Index to Nursing and Allied Health Literature* from 1983 to present
MEDLARS/ MEDLINE	Corresponds with the information in *Index Medicus, International Nursing Index,* and *Index to Dental Literature* from 1966 to present
EMBASE	Corresponds with the information in *Excerpta Medica* from 1974 to present
HEALTH	Corresponds with the information in *Hospital Literature Index* from 1975 to present
ERIC	Corresponds with the information in *Resources in Education* and *Current Index to Journal in Education* from 1966 to present
SOCIAL SCISEARCH	Corresponds with the information in *Science Citation Index* from 1965 to present
PsycINFO	Corresponds with the information in *Psychological Abstracts* from 1967 to present
Sociological Abstracts	Corresponds with the information in *Sociological Abstracts* from 1963 to present
Dissertation Abstracts Online	Corresponds with the information in *Dissertation Abstracts International* from 1961 to the present
BIOETHICSLINE	Includes citations from 1973 to present concerning ethical questions in health care; housed at the National Library of Medicine and the Kennedy Institute of Ethics
CANCERLIT	Includes all cancer-related literature from 1963 to present

the body of nursing knowledge. Thus the study findings can be generalized to similar populations. All frameworks are based on key concepts and the relationships among those concepts.

For example, a researcher who wants to examine the effect of poor health on life satisfaction must recognize that both poor health and life satisfaction are abstract concepts. Such concepts are frequently organized into theories. In this example, the researcher might want to use the Roy adaptation model (Roy & Andrews, 1999) as the theoretical basis for the study. In this model, poor health would be viewed as a focal stimulus to trigger adaptation and lead to either life satisfaction or lack of satisfaction. Without the model, it might be tempting to look only at the negative effects of poor health. Using a theory helps researchers clarify relationships and explain relationships. In addition, theory use contributes to the testing of that theory, which increases nursing knowledge.

Identification of Variables

The concepts under investigation in research studies are called variables because they are expected to change or differ from one person to another or from one time to another. The researcher is often trying to study how variation in one concept produces change in another concept. Almost anything in people and their environments may vary and thus be considered a variable. If all humans were 5 feet tall and weighed 100 pounds, then height and weight would not be variables. Disease conditions are variables because not all people have the disease; those who do may have varying degrees of severity. Other examples of variables include temperature, weight, knowledge, nursing interventions received, self-concept, health, and grief.

Researchers talk about independent and dependent variables rather than about cause and effect because, even though a relationship may exist between two variables, the relationship does not prove cause and effect. An **independent variable** may change during the study, but the change is expected to remain constant or to cause change in another variable. A **dependent variable** is expected to change with the treatment—that is, it is expected to result from (or be caused by) an independent variable. Following are three easy ways to distinguish between dependent and independent variables:

- The independent variable is the cause, and the dependent variable is the effect.
- The independent variable is what the researcher will manipulate, and the dependent variable is the outcome of that manipulation.

- Changes in the dependent variable depend on changes in the independent variable.

Now apply these criteria to a research problem: Do clients who receive home nursing care after discharge experience fewer complications? *Home health nursing* is the independent variable, because home health nursing may be the cause of fewer complications, and it is what the researcher will manipulate. The dependent variable is *complications* or the effect. *Complications* depend on changes in the independent variable *(home health nursing)*. For more practice in determining independent and dependent variables, see Table 15-3.

Clarification of Operational Definitions

Research requires precision in measurement of the concepts. An **operational definition** is the precise meaning of the concept as it is being used in the study, defined in a manner that specifies how the concept will be measured. For example, if the researcher has identified height as a variable for a study, the operational definition may be the distance from the bottom of the feet to the top of the head as measured in inches using a specified measuring device. This definition specifies that information will be collected in inches, not centimeters. Also, this definition specifies to other researchers and readers exactly how this term is used in this study, allowing the replication of the study in the future.

Operational definitions are even more important when researchers are studying variables that are not as easily defined as height. Variables such as self-concept, pain, grief, stress, and adaptation may be very difficult to operationalize.

Formulation of a Hypothesis

A **hypothesis** is a tentative prediction of the relationship between two or more variables being studied. It includes independent and dependent variables. In a previous example, the research problem was to compare the effects of grief on the physiological health of women who had experienced the death of a spouse versus a child during the preceding 12 months. The hypothesis for this problem could be as follows: *Women who have experienced the death of a child in the past 12 months will report less grief and better physiological health than women who have experienced the death of a spouse in the past 12 months.* If the hypothesis fails to propose a relationship between two or more variables, it cannot be tested.

A hypothesis should be based on a thorough review of the literature or on previous research, or it could be deduced from

Table 15-3	Examples of Independent and Dependent Variables		
Research Question		**Independent Variable**	**Dependent**
Does involvement in health-promotion activities increase the level of adaptation?		Involvement in health-promotion activities	Adaptation
How does the client's culture affect the request for pain medication?		Client's culture	Request for pain medication
Do clients who receive pain medication frequently after surgery experience fewer postoperative complications?		Receiving pain medications	Experience fewer complications
Does cigarette smoking cause lung cancer?		Cigarette smoking	Lung cancer
Do mothers experiencing the birth of their second child feel less anxiety than mothers experiencing the birth of their first child?		Birth of the first or second child	Anxiety

a theory. The researcher should present a sound, justifiable, logical rationale for the study hypothesis.

Select a Research Design

A **research design** is a researcher's strategy for testing a hypothesis. The hypothesis should guide the design, but the researcher must decide what design would be best for the study. Research designs are categorized as either quantitative or qualitative. **Quantitative research** is a type of study that uses variables analyzed as numbers, and **qualitative research** is a type of study that uses ideas that are analyzed as words. Quantitative designs usually are best suited to studies that focus on determining relationships, whereas qualitative designs are best suited to studies that focus on discovery or exploration. Quantitative studies are considered to be more rigorous research, but qualitative studies are often more suited to the kinds of value-laden phenomena of interest to nurses.

Collection of Data

Data collection is the process by which the researcher acquires subjects and collects the information needed to answer the research question. It is the actual measurement of the study variables. Researchers use various instruments or tools—such as questionnaires, interviews, scales, observations, and physiological measurements—to collect data.

Any instrument used in research should be reliable and valid. *Reliability* is the degree of consistency and accuracy with which an instrument measures a variable. For example, if an instrument is used to measure temperature, that instrument (in this case a thermometer) should measure the temperature accurately each time it is used. With physiological measures, instruments are usually straightforward. Concepts, such as health or stress, can be difficult to measure. *Validity* is the ability of an instrument to measure what it is designed to measure. For example, a valid measure of self-concept must measure a person's perception of the self, not another person's assessment of the study subject's beliefs about self. One method of addressing validity is to ask experts to evaluate the instruments. To evaluate an instrument's validity, the reader of the research must decide if the experts are in fact experts, if the number of experts was sufficient, and if the author revised the instrument on the basis of input by the experts.

Sampling is the process of selecting the subjects from the population being studied. It is an economical and efficient means of collecting data when use of an entire population is not feasible. Sampling techniques and the criteria used to define the population affect whether the findings can be *generalized* as being true of the whole population. The sample should reflect the same variations as those of the population. Generally, the largest sample size possible is the best.

There are two basic sampling techniques used in nursing research: random (or probability) sampling, and nonrandom (or nonprobability) sampling. *Random sampling* is the only method of obtaining a representative sample. In a randomly selected sample, each member of the population has an equal chance of appearing in the sample. It reduces the possibility of researcher bias. *Nonrandom sampling* involves the selection of subjects using nonrandom techniques—for example, using clients who volunteer to participate in the study. It is less rigorous and results in a less representative sample. The major disadvantage of nonrandom samples is that they limit the researcher's ability to generalize from the study results.

Analysis of Data

The primary purpose of data analysis is to impose order on the quantity of data so that conclusions can be made and communicated. The researcher's choice of research design determines how the data should be analyzed. Quantitative research uses statistical computation to summarize the collected data, compare and contrast the data, test theoretical relationships, generalize about the population on the basis of sample findings, and evaluate possible cause-and-effect relationships. Most researchers use computers to help with statistical analysis.

Qualitative research should be analyzed through words and logic. It depends on intuitive and analytical reasoning to guide the organization, clustering, and reduction of data. *Reduction* is the organization of volumes of narrative data into concepts that allow the researcher to deduce meanings. After the data are reduced, they may be displayed using tables, graphs, and matrices. From the data display, the researcher draws conclusions and attaches meaning to the findings.

Interpretation of Findings

To interpret research findings, the researcher examines, organizes, and attaches meaning to the results obtained from the data analysis. Study findings should be drawn from the data analysis and related back to the theoretical framework.

The researcher forms conclusions from the current study coupled with information learned from previous research studies. When forming conclusions, the researcher must clearly state that the research supports or does not support a position; the researcher must not state that the research *proves* a position. No one study ever proves a hypothesis. Also, conclusions should result from a logical reduction of the data and not extended to include variables not addressed in the study. When formulating conclusions, the researcher should provide practical suggestions for implementing the findings in nursing. The areas of nursing where the findings can be implemented should be identified, as should implications for nursing education and further nursing research.

RESEARCH IN NURSING PRACTICE

The goal of nursing research is to improve nursing practice. Consequently, nurses must incorporate valid findings from nursing research into their practices. Nursing practice identifies areas for research, and nursing research helps solve clinical practice problems. This reciprocal relationship improves practice and provides new professional knowledge.

Research Functions According to Level of Practice

All nurses, including nursing students, share the responsibility for improving practice, and all can contribute to nursing research. Students and practicing nurses are commonly unsure of their role in nursing research. In an attempt to clarify this confusion, the ANA has identified the investigative functions of nurses at various educational levels (Table 15-4).

Nurses at all educational levels can contribute to nursing research by collecting data for an ongoing research study. It is important for all nurses to understand the factors that can affect research results and to make sure that the data collected will be as accurate as possible.

When assisting with research data collection, it is critical that you follow the research protocol. Slight differences in protocol may make significant changes in study results. If, for example, the research protocol states that blood must be drawn 30 minutes after the administration of a medication, and you draw the blood 60 minutes afterward, the study results may be invalid. If the study protocol cannot be followed, contact the principal investigator to determine what to do with the data. Never just assume that the 30 minutes (for example) makes no difference. The value of research depends on accurate, precise data collection.

Identifying Nursing Research Problems

Nursing research problems begin as questions that need to be answered or problems that need to be solved. The nurse's everyday experience provides a rich supply of problems for investigation. Student nurses and practicing nurses encounter occurrences or situations that are puzzling or problematic. As a student, you have probably asked such questions as, "Why is this procedure done this way?" "Is there a better way?" "Why did this happen?" "What would happen if . . . ?" These questions are frequently the beginning of research problems.

Research problems may also come from nursing literature. Most research articles include recommendations for further research, in which the author discusses areas of related research that, if conducted, would build on current knowledge. Also, inconsistencies in the findings of reported research often provide ideas for further study. Similar studies may yield conflicting results, possibly because of the different samples or different situations. Nursing knowledge benefits from the replication of studies with different samples and in different situations to establish the validity and generalizability of previous findings.

A third source of research problems comes from nursing theory. To be useful in practice, theories must be tested through research. When theory is used as a basis for research, deductions from the theory must be developed. The researcher would ask such questions as, "If I use this theory, what behavior would I expect in this situation under this condition?" "Can I predict what would happen using this theory?" "What study findings would provide support or nonsupport for this theory?"

Another source for identifying nursing research problems is external. Some organizations or government agencies sponsor funded research and may identify topics for research on the basis of current social concerns or problems. For example, in the last few years many government agencies have requested a variety of research projects affecting minority populations (NINR, 2000). In addition, many nursing specialty practice groups fund research related to the specialty area.

Evaluating Research Findings

Research in a practice profession, such as nursing, provides information needed to improve practice. For research to improve practice, researchers must study problems that have

Table 15-4 Educational Preparation for Participation in Nursing Research	
Educational Preparation	**Investigative Functions**
Associate Degree in Nursing	• Helping to identify clinical problems in nursing practice • Assisting in the collection of data within a structured format • In conjunction with nurses holding more advanced credentials, appropriately using research findings in clinical practice
Baccalaureate Degree in Nursing	• Identifying clinical problems requiring investigation • Assisting experienced investigators to gain access to clinical sites • Collecting data and implementing nursing research findings
Master's Degree in Nursing	• Being active members of the research team • Assuming the role of clinical expert • Collaborating with experienced investigators in proposal development, data collection, data analysis and interpretation • Appraising the clinical relevance of research findings • Providing leadership for integrating findings in clinical practice
Doctoral Education	• Contributing to nursing knowledge through the conduct of research aimed at theory generation or theory testing • Designing studies independently or in collaboration with other researchers or clinicians • Acquiring funding for research • Disseminating research findings to the scientific community, to clinicians and, as appropriate, to policy makers and the lay public

From the American Nurses Association Council. *Position statement on education preparation for participation in nursing research.* Reprinted with permission.

been identified by practicing nurses. The practicing nurse should have the skill to evaluate research findings and develop interventions that make appropriate use of the information. Nursing research has relevance for all nurses, not just the minority of nurses who are nurse researchers. The following sections offer an introduction to the evaluation of nursing research.

Tentative Nature of Research Findings.

The results of research never prove that a hypothesis or theory is true. Rather, all research results are tentative. A hypothesis tests only one small part of a theory, and researchers cannot even state that the small part of the theory tested by the hypothesis is true. The hypothesis may be faulty, the sample may be too small, the sample may not be representative of the population, or there may be another serious flaw in the study. For example, suppose that an undiscovered enzyme controls blood cholesterol levels, but researchers report that blood cholesterol levels have been proven to result from diet, exercise, metabolism, and family history. What the researcher considered proof would be false. The results of the study were not proof. They merely indicated that a relationship existed for this sample. Instead of indications of proof, watch for phrases such as *the data support* or *the data indicate* as you read studies. Research results are always tentative and are based on the sample and study involved.

Research Bias.

Bias is a factor that can change or distort the results of a study. In a good research study, you can feel confident that a change in the dependent variable occurs because of the independent variable. However, when a researcher does not attempt to control for bias, this relationship may not be true. Bias may result from the researcher's conscious or unconscious desire to demonstrate a relationship between variables. Bias is commonly introduced when studies are designed to elicit specific results.

Another source of bias is the difference among subjects in groups that are being compared. When groups are formed on a nonrandom basis, the risk of bias is always present. For example, in a study in which blood cholesterol level is the dependent variable and diet and exercise are the independent variables, a major concern is that individuals with high cholesterol may differ from those with low cholesterol in ways not connected with the independent variables. Other differences, like metabolism and family history, may cause high or low cholesterol. Unless these other differences, called extraneous variables, are controlled, the resulting biases make it difficult for the researcher to conclude that lower cholesterol levels are related to diet and exercise.

When study data are collected by observation, the researcher's beliefs may unconsciously bias objective collection. To prevent bias from occurring, a *double-blind* technique is often used. The double-blind technique removes observer bias because both the subject and the person collecting the data are "blind" to the research objective. If this technique cannot be used, many researchers use two or more independent observers to reduce or eliminate observer bias.

Threats to Validity.

If a study has validity, it actually measures what it was designed to measure. When evaluating research, you should examine factors within the design and factors external to the study that could affect the results. These two factors are called internal and external validity.

Internal validity depends on the extent to which a change in the dependent variable can be attributed to the independent variable. True experiments possess a high degree of internal validity because of the use of control groups and randomization. This enables the researcher to control for extraneous variables, thereby ruling out most alternative explanations for the study results.

Other research designs always have alternative explanations for the study results because extraneous variables, in addition to the independent variable, could cause a change in the dependent variable. These alternative explanations are called threats to internal validity and have been grouped into several classifications:

- *History:* Have any extraneous variables occurred during the time of the study? Were there any changes in the environment that could have influenced the study findings?
- *Maturation:* Has the passage of time since the beginning of the study affected the results? Are there any internal changes in subjects—such as aging, growth and development, or wound healing—that would affect the study results?
- *Mortality:* Did the loss of subjects from different groups during the study affect the results? Was the loss of subjects from each group approximately equal?
- *Selection:* If the subjects were not randomly assigned to groups, were there preexisting differences between groups?
- *Testing:* Were the pretests and posttests identical? Could the subjects remember the material from the pretest to the posttest?
- *Instrumentation:* If the pretest and the posttest were not identical, where they equal? If different observers were collecting data, how were these people trained to ensure that each used the same technique and scored the data in the same manner?

External validity refers to the extent to which findings can be generalized to other populations, samples, or situations. Researchers almost never conduct studies to use the findings with only one group of subjects. Researchers hope that other nurses in similar situations can use the study findings. There are several threats to external validity, two of which will be discussed here.

- *Sample inadequacy:* Does the sample represent the population? Is the sample large enough for the researcher to draw conclusions?
- *Hawthorne effect:* Did the study cause the subjects to act in a way that was different from how they usually acted?

Faulty Statistics.

Statistical analysis allows the researcher to make quantitative data meaningful. It allows the researcher to summarize, organize, compare, evaluate, and communicate numerical data. Without statistics, data would be a mass of numbers with little or no meaning.

Statistics are classified as either descriptive or inferential. Descriptive statistics are used to describe data. Examples of descriptive statistics include averages and percentages. Researchers use inferential statistics, on the other hand, to make inferences or draw conclusions about a population. The difference between the two is that descriptive statistics are concerned only with characteristics of the data obtained by the researcher, whereas inferential statistics are concerned with generalizations to a population.

When researchers use inferential statistics to generalize findings to a population, the statistical tests used have assumptions that should be met in order to use the test. If these assumptions are violated, then the results of the test may be questionable. If the researcher uses an inappropriate measurement level (e.g., rounding to the nearest tenth) or violates major statistical assumptions, then the study results may be invalid.

Implementing Research Findings

The responsibility for implementing research findings is shared by all nurses (Figure 15-3). In fact, nurses' behaviors and attitudes are critical to the success of any efforts to base nursing practice on research findings (Estabrooks, 1998). Individual nurses can contribute to implementing research findings by doing the following:

- Read and evaluate nursing research articles.
- Attend professional research conferences.
- Support nursing research projects.
- Participate in institutional research projects.
- Share research findings with other nurses.

Expanding Professional Knowledge Base. Nursing students and staff nurses who read research reports and look for opportunities to apply sound research findings make an important contribution to the expansion of nursing knowledge in addition to improving their own clinical skills. Nurse researchers are usually not interested in pursuing knowledge for its own sake but want their findings to improve practice.

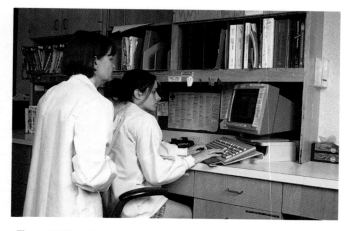

Figure 15-3. All nurses share the responsibility for implementing the findings of nursing research.

When research findings are incorporated into individual clinical practice, nursing knowledge expands. Nurses identify when particular findings seem to work or not to work. From this evaluation, new hypotheses are formed, ideas are generated, and the nursing profession is revitalized. Some of the new hypotheses and ideas may never be tested in a controlled research study, but, as nurses communicate new and different methods, nursing practice is improved and the knowledge base of nursing is expanded.

Every nurse has an important role to play in making use of nursing research. Research originates from questions being asked by practicing nurses. Every nurse has not only the right but also the responsibility to ask for evidence that practices and procedures are effective. Clinical decisions must be based on sound rationales. Practices and procedures must be challenged and changed on the basis of current knowledge rather than simply accepted because "it's always been that way."

The use of rationales for nursing practices and procedures has evolved into evidence-based nursing practice, which is the careful and practical use of current best evidence to guide health care decisions (Omery & Williams, 1999). Although the terms *evidenced-based nursing practice* and *nursing research* are frequently used interchangeably, evidence-based nursing practice may include nursing research, but it may also include the consensus of expert clinicians. Nursing research, on the other hand, is based on the steps of the research process. The outcome of nursing research is the generation of new knowledge, whereas the outcome of evidence-based practice is usually clinical guidelines for practice.

Making Clinical Decisions. There is tremendous potential for using nursing research to make clinical decisions. The nursing process requires nurses to make many decisions. What will be assessed? What are the priority nursing diagnoses? What plan of care will produce the best outcomes? What interventions are necessary? How will the results be evaluated? When will the results be evaluated? Nursing research plays an important role at each phase of the nursing process by helping nurses make informed decisions when carrying out the nursing process.

Research-based nursing decisions begin when clinical problems are identified. If the problem has minimal significance to nurses, or if making a change or introducing a new intervention will not benefit clients or nurses, there is little point in implementing the change. However, when an important problem has been identified, you can proceed by identifying and critiquing the current research literature for information that will help you make decisions in your practice situation.

Improving Quality of Care. The best way for you, as a student, to use nursing research to improve the quality of your practice is to identify an area of nursing where you have unanswered questions. Go to your library, and conduct a literature search using manual or computer techniques. Your reference librarian can help you locate the various indexes and provide information and assistance with computer searches. Once you have located several research articles of interest, consult the listing of periodicals for your library or access journal websites to select one or two journal articles. If your library does not have research journals or if you cannot access journal websites, the reference librarian may be able to help you obtain them through an interlibrary loan. After you have obtained the articles, it is helpful to photocopy or print them so that you can make notations in the margins.

As you read the articles, try to identify the positive and negative aspects of the articles and any flaws in the research. Pay particular attention to the implications for clinical practice. Then identify how you can use the research to improve the quality of care you provide to your clients. Incorporating nursing research into your clinical practice provides constant renewal of your nursing knowledge and that of the profession at large.

Key Principles

- Nursing research is important because it serves the public through improved health care, and it establishes a scientific basis for nursing practice.
- Ethical research protects study participants by rigidly following protocols that maintain the rights of subjects.
- Because of the nature of the issues studied, nursing research is often quasi-experimental rather than experimental.
- The steps of the research process follow a standard format that reflects the scientific method and produces rigorous, disciplined study that can be replicated.
- Every nurse has a role to play in advancing the profession of nursing through research, either by conducting research or by using interventions that are based on the research findings.
- Research problems ideally come from problems encountered in a clinical practice setting, the resolution of which would improve the outcomes of client care.
- A single research study can offer evidence that supports a position, fact, or belief about nursing care, but it cannot be used to prove the truth of a hypothesis.
- Research contributes to practice by generating ideas about the nature of human responses, naming and describing the human responses treated by nurses, validating methods of intervention, and demonstrating nursing-sensitive outcomes.

Bibliography

*American Nurses Association. (1975). *Human rights guidelines for nurses in clinical and other research.* Kansas City, MO: Author.

*American Nurses Association. (1997). *Education for participation in nursing research.* Retrieved January 24, 2002, from http://www.nursingworld.org/readroom/position/research/rseducat.html.

*Code of Federal Regulations. (1983). *Protection of human subjects: 45 C.F.R. 46* (revised as of March 8, 1983). Washington, DC: U.S. Department of Health and Human Services.

Dooks, P. (2001). Diffusion of pain management research into nursing practice. *Cancer Nursing, 24*(2), 99-103.

Dufalt, M. A., & Sullivan, M. C. (1999). Generating and testing pain management standards through collaborative research utilization. *Image: Journal of Nursing Scholarship, 31*(4), 355-356.

Dufalt, M. A., & Willey-Lessne, C. (1999). Using a collaborative research utilization model to develop and test the effects of clinical pathways for pain management. *Journal of Nursing Quality Care, 13*(4), 19-33.

Estabrooks, C. A. (1998). Will evidence-based nursing practice make practice perfect? *Canadian Journal of Nursing Research, 30*(1), 15-36.

Fellows, L. S., Miller, E. H., Frederickson, M., Bly, B., & Felt, P. (2000). Evidence-based practice for enteral feedings: Aspiration prevention strategies, bedside detection, and practice changes. *MEDSURG Nursing, 9*(1), 27-31.

Karigan, M. (2001). Ethics in clinical research: The nursing perspective. *American Journal of Nursing, 101*(9), 26-31.

*National Commission for the Protection of Human Subjects of Biomedical and Behavioral Research. (1978). *Belmont report: Ethical principles and guidelines for research involving human subjects.* Washington, DC: U.S. Government Printing Office.

National Institute of Nursing Research. (2000). About NINR. Retrieved January 20, 2002, from http://www.nih.gov/ninr/research/diversity/mission.htlm.

Omery, A., & Williams, R. P. (1999). An appraisal of research utilization across the United States. *Journal of Nursing Administration, 29*(12), 50-56.

Polit-O'Hara, D. F., Hungler, B. P., & Polit, D. (1998). *Nursing research: Principles and methods* (6th ed.). Philadelphia: Lippincott, Williams & Wilkins.

Roy, C., & Andrews, H. (1999). *The Roy adaptation model* (2nd ed.). Norwalk, CT: Appleton & Lange.

Schroeter, K. (1998). Impact of a 5-minute scrub on the microbial flora found on artificial, polished, or natural fingernails of operating room personnel. *AORN Journal, 68*(12), 880-884.

Smith, J. (1998). Are electric thermometry techniques suitable alternatives to traditional mercury in glass thermometry techniques in the paediatric setting? *Journal of Advanced Nursing, 28*(5), 1030-1039.

*Asterisk indicates a classic or definitive work on this subject.

Infancy Through Adolescence

Learning Objectives

After studying this chapter, you should be able to do the following:

- Compare and contrast significant theories of growth and development

- Identify developmental milestones from infancy through adolescence

- Describe environmental, socioeconomic, nutritional, and physiological factors affecting growth and development for the child from infancy through adolescence

- Describe the assessment of growth and development and health maintenance from infancy through adolescence

- Discuss assessment strategies to detect delayed growth and development and to promote health maintenance

- Select an appropriate related nursing diagnosis for the well infant, child, and adolescent with problems in growth and development and health maintenance

- Plan interventions to promote growth and development health maintenance from infancy through adolescence

- Evaluate outcomes from infancy through adolescence, for *Delayed growth and development* and for *Ineffective health maintenance*

- Assess, plan, and intervene with parents who exhibit alterations in parenting

Yung Hi is a 33-month-old Korean girl who has been in the United States for only 6 months. She and her mother, maternal grandmother, and brother joined her father, who has been employed as a physics professor at the local state university for more than a year. Dr. Kim speaks fluent English, but the rest of the family understands more English than they can speak.

Yung Hi fell while playing in the parking lot of their apartment complex. Her older brother tripped and fell on her outstretched leg as it extended over the curb. Yung Hi's mother witnessed the accident. When Dr. Kim attempted to move her and was unable to, he called for an ambulance.

Yung Hi is admitted to the hospital with a diagnosis of a displaced fracture of the right femur. She will be in Buck's traction for 8 weeks after closed reduction of the fracture and placement of Steinmann pins. Because of this long immobilization, there is concern that Yung Hi's normal developmental activities will be interrupted. Therefore the nurse considers the nursing diagnoses *Risk for delayed growth and development* and *Ineffective health maintenance*.

KEY NURSING DIAGNOSES FOR Growth and Development

Delayed growth and development: The state in which an individual demonstrates deviations from the norms for his or her age group

Ineffective health maintenance: Inability to identify, manage, or seek out help to maintain health

Risk for impaired parenting: Risk for inability of the primary caregiver to create, maintain, or regain an environment that promotes the optimal growth and development of the child

---

Every nurse should be aware of growth parameters and developmental milestones in clients. Knowledge of growth and development will help you in assessing whether or not the client is developing and growing normally. Assessment leads to planning and to implementing interventions to enhance these processes. You need to recognize when there are abnormalities of growth and development, and to provide nursing care accordingly.

CONCEPTS OF GROWTH AND DEVELOPMENT

The words *growth* and *development* have separate and distinct definitions even though they are often used together. Human growth and development is a dynamic process and continues through the life span. **Growth** is the physiological development of a living being and is the quantitative (measurable) change seen in the body. It refers to an increase in specific parameters, such as height and weight. Variations in growth occur with each person. Growth is often sporadic, with rapid spurts occurring at several points, such as the prenatal, neonatal, infant, and adolescent stages.

Development is a progression of behavioral changes that involve the acquisition of appropriate cognitive, linguistic, and psychosocial skills. Development is a qualitative change and refers to increasing competence in behavioral functioning. During each developmental stage, certain goals should be achieved. Attainment of these hallmarks of development indicates whether a child is progressing normally. The following principles about the basic processes of growth and development are important for you to know:

- Human growth and development follows predictable, continuous, and expected sequential patterns that are influenced by genes, environment, and positive and negative factors that are present or absent in a person's life.
- Each stage of development depends on adequate completion of the previous stage and is itself the foundation for the development of new skills.

- Neuromuscular growth and development starts at the head and moves toward the feet, a pattern called **cephalocaudal.** For example, infants first achieve head control and then shoulder and trunk control before learning to sit or walk.
- Skill development starts at the midline of the body and moves outward, a pattern called **proximodistal.** Infants begin to move their arms and then to use their hands together before using each arm separately or beginning to use the fingers to manipulate objects.
- Periods of time when a person has an increased vulnerability to physical, chemical, psychological, or environmental influences are called **critical periods.** Growth or development may stop temporarily or regress during stressful life events.
- Development becomes increasingly differentiated over time, starting with a generalized response and progressing to a skilled specific response. This is called **differentiated development.** For example, a newborn's initial response to a playful stimulus involves the total body, whereas a 3-year-old can respond more specifically with laughter.

THEORIES OF GROWTH AND DEVELOPMENT

Stages of physical growth usually correspond to certain developmental changes. A variety of theories have been proposed to explain how a person develops. Developmental theories related to specific age groups include the psychosocial, the cognitive, and the developmental task theories.

Psychosocial Theory

Psychosocial development involves subjective feelings and interpersonal relationships. Erik Erikson described a series of psychosocial stages to outline the emotional and social development of the personality. Each stage defines a task that must be achieved. The resolution of the task may be successful, partial, or unsuccessful. Successful completion or mastery of each stage is built on the satisfactory completion of the previous stage. Erikson believed that the greater the task achievement, the healthier the personality of the individual; failure to achieve a task influences the person's ability to achieve the next task (Erikson, 1968). Erikson's theory is useful to nurses, because it describes expected emotional behaviors from birth through later adulthood.

Erikson describes eight major psychosocial crises experienced by people as they progress in their development. The stages reflect both positive and negative aspects of the critical periods every person goes through. Resolution of the conflicts at each stage enables the person to function effectively in society. Newborns to children 3 years of age experience the first two stages, trust versus mistrust, and autonomy versus shame and doubt.

Cognitive Theory

The intellectual process of knowing characterizes cognition, which includes perception, judgment, use of language, and memory. Cognitive development represents a progression of mental abilities from illogical thinking to logical thinking, from simple to complex problem solving, and from understanding concrete ideas to understanding abstract ideas.

The theorist best known for exploring cognitive development is Jean Piaget. He described cognitive development as involving the increasing ability to think and reason in a logical manner. Piaget believed that intellectual development is an adaptive process that occurs as a regulatory function of both physiological and intellectual growth.

According to Piaget, a person uses three abilities during cognitive development: assimilation, accommodation, and adaptation. Assimilation is the process of learning from new experiences. People acquire knowledge and skills as well as insight into the world around them. Accommodation is a process of change, or modifying old ways of thinking to fit new situations. This adjustment is possible because new knowledge has been assimilated. Adaptation, or coping behavior, is the change that occurs as a result of assimilation and accommodation.

Developmental Task Theory

Robert Havighurst believed that living and growing are based on learning and that people must continuously learn to adjust to the changing society around them. He described these learned behaviors as developmental tasks. A developmental task is an important activity that arises at a certain period in life (Box 16-1). Successful achievement of these tasks leads to happiness and success in later tasks, whereas failure leads to unhappiness, societal disapproval, and difficulty with later tasks (Havighurst, 1972).

People progress from birth to death by working their way from one stage of development to the next while solving problems encountered at each stage. Tasks arise mainly from the biological nature of the human, but they can be derived from cultural patterns as well. Thus lists of developmental tasks will not be the same for all cultures. Infancy and early childhood represent the first of six life stages, each associated with essential developmental tasks. Havighurst's remaining five

Box 16-1	**Havighurst's Developmental Tasks of Infancy and Early Childhood**

- Learning to take solid foods
- Learning to walk
- Learning to talk
- Learning to control elimination of body wastes
- Learning gender differences and sexual modesty
- Achieving psychological stability
- Forming concepts of social and physical reality
- Learning to relate emotionally to others
- Learning to distinguish right from wrong and developing a conscience

life stages include middle childhood, pre-adolescence and adolescence, early adulthood, middle age, and later life.

DEVELOPMENTAL MILESTONES

Growth and development are evaluated by comparing an individual's characteristics with the range of growth and developmental characteristics expected for a person in the same age group. *Developmental milestones* are the predictable patterns of normal development according to age. Table 16-1 lists developmental milestones for newborns, infants, and toddlers. The following sections discuss growth and development characteristics from infancy through adolescence.

Newborns

A newborn is an infant born within the previous 28 days. The child's parents usually follow growth and development of the newborn intensely and enthusiastically. They may have many questions about the "normalcy" of their baby's behavior. Even so, they are often able to provide you with significant cues to the progression of the child's development.

Growth Parameters. At birth, the average weight for a European-American female is 7.5 pounds (3.4 kg), and for a male, 7.7 pounds (3.5 kg). Normal weights may range, however, from 5.5 pounds (2.5 kg) to 8.5 pounds (4 kg). Newborns of Asian and Native American descent are somewhat smaller. Because most (70% to 75%) of a newborn's weight is from water, the typical newborn loses 5% to 10% of the birthweight in the first few days after birth. This weight loss is normal, and newborns usually regain that weight in about 1 week (Pomerance, 1995).

A newborn's length is measured from head to heel (Figure 16-1, *A*). Average normal lengths range from 19 to 21 inches (48 to 53 cm). Female babies are, on average, smaller than male babies. For the most accurate measurement of length, newborns should be placed flat on their backs with at least one leg extended.

At birth, a newborn's head is about one-third the size of an adult's head. Measurement of head circumference is of particular importance in babies to determine the growth rate of the skull and the brain (see Figure 16-1, *B*). The usual newborn head circumference ranges from 12.5 to 14.5 inches

Table 16-1	Developmental Milestones for Newborns, Infants, and Toddlers	
Age	Developmental Milestone
0 to 1 month	• Differentiates between light and dark • Turns toward direction of sound • Responds to touch
1 to 3 months	• Supports upper body with arms when prone • Raises head and chest • Brings hand to mouth • Opens and shuts hands • Begins hand–eye coordination • Begins babbling and cooing
4 to 7 months	• Rolls from stomach to back • Sits with support and then sits independently • Finds hidden object • Babbles, laughs, and squeals • Performs social play (such as peek-a-boo)
8 to 12 months	• Rocks • Moves from sitting or crawling to a prone position • Makes initial walking effort • Uses pincer grasp • Mimics gestures • Shakes, throws, and drops objects • Drinks from cup • Responds to verbal cues
1 to 2 years	• Walks alone • Climbs • Scribbles • Sorts objects • Shows return of separation anxiety • Imitates others
2 to 3 years	• Runs • Peddles tricycle • Screws and unscrews jar lids or objects • Holds writing instrument • Begins to make circular and horizontal strokes

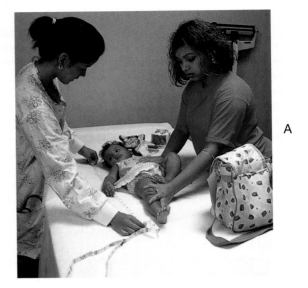

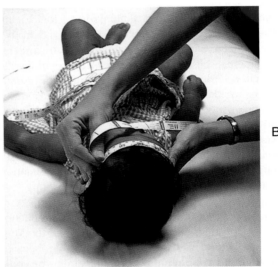

Figure 16-1. Measuring growth. **A,** Body length. **B,** Head circumference.

(32 to 37 cm). The head circumference should be about 1 inch (2.5 cm) greater than the chest circumference. A newborn who deviates from this normal range may have central nervous system anomalies (Pomerance, 1995).

Sensory Development. A newborn can smell at birth, as soon as the nose is cleared of mucus and other fluids. Newborns can recognize the smell of their mother's milk and respond to this smell by turning toward the mother.

Familiar sounds are recognizable, and the newborn often turns toward the sound. Newborns with intact hearing will react with a startle to a loud noise, referred to as the startle reflex, which disappears by age 4 months. Usually they can distinguish between their mother's voice and another woman's voice within a few days.

Newborns can follow large moving objects and blink in response to bright lights. A newborn's pupils respond very slowly, however, and the eyes cannot focus on close objects. Because color vision is not fully developed, newborns prefer to focus on black and white objects, especially geometric shapes and checkerboards.

A newborn's sense of touch is well developed at birth. The baby's positive response to the warmth and security of swaddling, holding, and touching demonstrates the importance of touch for healthy development. The newborn is also sensitive to temperature extremes and pain. Babies cannot isolate the discomfort, however, and they react with a generalized response.

Motor Development. The development of the newborn's ability to move and to control the body is called motor development. Initially, the newborn has uncoordinated body movement. A newborn's normal motor activity includes involuntary reflexes and turning the head from side to side when in a prone or supine position. As the baby obtains more muscle control, body movements become smoother and more purposeful.

Reflexes. Reflexes in the newborn are involuntary responses. The presence of these specific reflexes indicates normal nervous system development in the newborn. The natural progression of neural development is cephalocaudal, proximodistal, and general to specific. Also present at birth are the abilities to yawn, stretch, sneeze, burp, and hiccup.

Psychosocial Development. Erikson's stage of trust versus mistrust occurs from birth to age 1 year. The most important person for the infant at this stage is the mother or primary caretaker, and the quality of this relationship and the degree to which the infant's needs are met are extremely important to the development of trust. While building this relationship, an infant receives information through all the senses. **Sensory stimulation** is the activation and exhilaration of the senses. An appropriate amount of sensory stimulation enables the infant to develop trust. If the infant's needs are not met, either through overstimulation or neglect, then some degree of mistrust develops.

Psychosocial development in the newborn is initiated with the process of attachment. **Attachment** is the development of strong ties of affection of an infant with a significant other (mother, father, sibling, caretaker). This is a psychological rather than a biological process. Bowlby (1969) studied the process in which the infant or child forms an attachment by seeking proximity with a specific figure.

Recognizing that attachment occurs both from infant to parent and from parent to infant, researchers developed the concept of mutual bonding through observation of premature infants. Bonding is a process of forming an attachment between parent and newborn. Although bonding was initially studied as occurring during the first hours after birth, it continues to develop during the first year and possibly beyond.

The emotional bond between mother and newborn is developed and sustained through cyclical cues and communication from one to the other (Figure 16-2). Even at this early stage, newborns attempt to communicate and are consoled by gentle human touch. Crying is the primary means by which newborns make their needs and wants known. Parents are often able to distinguish between different types of cries, such as those of hunger and those of discomfort. The process of parent–child attachment is not instantaneous. Most parents require several months before they feel they know their newborn.

Cognitive Development. Cognitive development in the newborn is primarily reflexive. However, the newborn reacts socially to caregivers by paying attention to the face or voice and by cuddling when held. The baby is able to interact with the environment by responding to various stimuli, such as touch and sound. The newborn displays displeasure by crying and shows satisfaction by quieting and making soft vocalizations. According to Piaget (1950), newborns are active participants in learning through their senses. Additionally as motor function progresses from reflexes to purposeful activities, the child rapidly increases interactions with the environment.

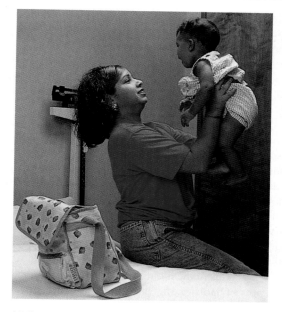

Figure 16-2. The emotional bond between mother and infant is developed and sustained trough cyclical cues and communication from one to the other.

Infants

Infant is the term given to a child from the age of 1 month to the end of 12 months. Infancy is a time of continuous and rapid growth and development. Most parents of infants carefully monitor their baby's height and weight throughout the first year and celebrate the achievements of numerous developmental milestones.

Growth Parameters. Height and weight are predictable along a growth curve. An infant usually gains 5 to 7 ounces weekly for about the first 4 to 6 months. By 4 to 7 months the birthweight doubles (Wong, Hockenberry-Eaton, Wilson, Winkelstein, & Schwartz, 2001). By 1 year of age, the normal infant weighs about three times its birthweight. The average male baby weighs 22 pounds (10 kg), and the average female baby weighs 21 pounds (9.5 kg) by the first birthday (Pomerance, 1995).

The rate of increase in height is largely influenced by the baby's size at birth and by nutrition. By the end of the infant's first year, recumbent length has increased 50% since birth, and the average range is 28 to 32 inches. Head growth begins to slow down between 8 and 12 months of age. By 10 months, head and chest circumferences are about the same. Head circumference is usually 18 inches (47 cm) by the end of infancy (Pomerance, 1995). Because the rate of growth for each child differs, these measurements should be compared with the percentile curves on a growth chart.

Sensory Development. The senses of smell and taste continue to develop throughout the first year. Many new smells and tastes are introduced with the taking of solid foods at 4 to 6 months of age. With each new food experience, the infant begins to show discrimination toward favorite tastes and smells.

Eyes begin to focus and fixate at 4 months. The infant can recognize familiar objects and follow moving ones. Most 9-month-old babies can recognize facial characteristics and often smile in response to a familiar face. By the end of the first year, depth perception has developed, and the infant will be able to recognize a change in level, such as the start and finish of a step or the edge of a bed.

At about 5 months, the infant will pause while feeding to listen to the mother's voice. A 9-month-old baby will locate the source of sounds and be able to recognize familiar sounds or voices. By 1 year of age, the infant listens to sounds, begins to distinguish words, and can respond to simple commands.

Touch remains important. Infants continue to demonstrate positive responses to the security of being held and cuddled. Touching different-textured fabrics and object shapes also positively stimulates babies. Exploration through touching and placing items in the mouth to further explore them begins at 3 months of age and may last through toddlerhood.

Motor Development. From 1 to 3 months of age, the infant attains additional physical skills and becomes more neurologically sophisticated. In the prone position, infants can raise their head and chest and support their upper body with their arms. By 4 to 7 months, the infant can roll from stomach to back and vice versa. By 5 months, an infant can sit with support. By the end of 7 months, most infants can sit without support.

From 8 to 12 months of age, infants make great developmental strides. They can get up on their hands and knees and rock back and forth on both knees. Crawling begins by the 10th month. Infants of this age can move from a sitting to a crawling to a prone position. The infant makes first efforts toward walking, such as pulling to stand, standing briefly with support, cruising along furniture, and walking two to three steps unassisted. The pincer grasp is developed, and the infant takes great pleasure in manipulating objects (Figure 16-3). Parents can encourage the development of this skill by offering items that promote grasping, such as cereal bits, and containers to put them in.

Reflexes. As the infant develops neurologically, the primitive or neonatal reflexes begin to disappear. Later infant reflexes develop at 3 months of age, beginning with the Landau reflex (lifts both head and legs when suspended prone with support under abdomen). Refer to a specialist if you are concerned about delays in development, such as head lag.

Psychosocial Development. Psychologically, the infant begins to communicate through body language. There are attempts to imitate some facial expressions and movements, such as a social smile, by the end of the second month. The 4-month-old infant enjoys interacting with people and will vocalize displeasure when left alone. Infants mimic gestures, babble with inflection, say "mama" and "dada," and try to imitate other words by about 6 months of age. The infant responds to simple verbal cues and uses simple gestures, such as shaking the head "no" and waving "bye-bye." Smiling,

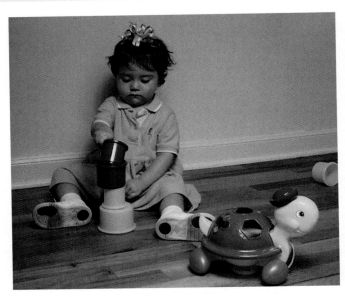

Figure 16-3. With development of the pincer grasp, the infant takes great pleasure in stacking objects and putting objects into containers and removing them.

laughing, waving, and reaching out to others are examples of purposeful interactive social behavior.

Self-esteem develops through trust and increasing control of the body. Trust develops when the parent or caregiver can be counted on to provide essential needs. However, by 6 to 9 months the infant begins to have a greater awareness of self as separate from mother or father. Separation anxiety emerges as crying when the infant is separated from parents or approached by strangers. Thus self-esteem requires the development of a sense of control.

Cognitive Development. Infants learn about their world through their activities. They anticipate feeding times and "going bye-bye." They become excited when they see their parents. They have an increasing ability to concentrate and to recognize and respond to a familiar environment or a friend of the family.

Rudimentary language skills are developing. Babies begin to coo and make sounds soon after birth, and by 12 months they can convey their wishes through several key words. Use of syllable repetition (ma-ma, da-da), early phonetic expression (babbling), and imitation of intonations and sounds are characteristic of the language development of infants.

Piaget's first stage of cognitive development, the sensorimotor stage, has six substages, four of which are related to infancy (Cowan, 1978). The first substage is reflexive, the emergence of directed behavior (birth to 1 month). The second substage is scheme coordination and early goal directions (1½ to 4 months). During this time, the infant discovers enjoyment of random behaviors, such as sucking a thumb, and repeats them. Piaget's third substage, intention, beginning independence of action and thought (4 to 6 months), is when infants relate their own behavior to change in the environment, such as intentionally shaking a rattle to hear the sound.

By 6 to 12 months, an infant can coordinate more than one thought pattern at a time to reach a goal, such as repeatedly throwing an object on the floor. Infants in this substage are also beginning to develop a sense of object permanence. **Object permanence,** the awareness that unseen objects do not disappear, is evidenced when the infant searches for an object that has been moved out of sight. This behavior is the first sign of object permanence.

Toddlers

Toddler is the term for a child aged 1 to 3 years. The term is derived from the pattern of locomotion of children in this age group. Toddlers walk with their feet several inches apart and their arms held out to maintain balance. The ability to walk is an important developmental milestone as toddlers move toward the increasing independence of childhood, leaving the dependency of infancy behind.

Growth Parameters. The most noticeable physical change during the toddler years occurs as head growth slows and the relatively short legs and trunk of an infant begin to lengthen. Baby fat begins to decrease. The abdomen continues to be prominent, as it was in infancy, but appetite changes. Physiological growth and development continues steadily, but the pace of the gains is considerably slower than during infancy. Weight gain is about 4 pounds (2 kg) yearly, with height increases averaging 2.2 inches (6 cm) yearly. By age 2, the female toddler is about 34 inches (86.4 cm) tall and weighs 27 pounds (12.2 kg). Boys average 34 inches (86.4 cm) and almost 28 pounds (12.9 kg) by age 2 (Pomerance, 1995).

Sensory Development. All the senses continue to develop and become more associated with each other during the toddler stage. Toddlers use all their senses to explore their environment. Walking enhances their ability to explore without relying on others. Vision is fairly well established by ages 1 and 2. Visual acuity is about 20/40. The ability to focus on near and far objects is fairly well developed by 18 months and continues to develop with age. Hearing is at adult levels by age 3.

The toddler's taste buds are sensitive to the natural flavors of food, and taste preferences begin to emerge. Toddlers are less likely to try a new food if the food has an unfamiliar appearance, smell, texture, or taste. Touch is also a very important sense to the toddler. A distressed toddler often uses tactile sensations as a self-comforting technique, such as stroking the satin ribbon on a favorite stuffed animal.

Motor Development. Fine muscle (fine motor) coordination and large muscle (gross motor) activity improve during toddlerhood. At 18 months of age, a toddler can pick up beads and put them in a cup. The toddler can also hold a spoon and a cup and walk up stairs with assistance. By age 3, fine motor skills have continued to improve and include turning the page of a book one at a time, screwing and unscrewing objects, turning handles, and making vertical, circular, and horizontal strokes with a writing instrument. Gross motor skills of the

3-year-old include climbing, walking up and down stairs unassisted, running easily, bending over without falling, peddling a tricycle, and kicking a ball.

Remember that Yung Hi is in the toddler stage of her growth and development. She had been running and playing with her brother when the accident occurred. What types of activities will Yung be able to accomplish while in traction? How can you help her maintain the developmental milestones she has already achieved?

Reflexes. Neural growth continues during the toddler years, with additional myelinization and cortical brain development. Neurological growth and musculoskeletal development allow the toddler to perform more complex physical tasks. The primitive reflexes of infancy must disappear before voluntary behaviors appear. By age 3, deep tendon reflexes (biceps, triceps, patellar, and Achilles) are well developed.

Psychosocial Development. Erickson's second stage, autonomy versus shame and doubt, applies to children from age 2 to 3. This stage is influenced by toddlers' maturing muscle systems, which gives them a sense of control over their body. This mastery enables the toddler to experience a sense of power and, thus, autonomy.

According to Erikson, toddlers enter the stage of autonomy versus shame and doubt. Independence increases and is demonstrated by the toddler's self-feeding, walking, talking, and toileting. Children who do not feel autonomous may be reluctant to explore and be fearful of activities and people. A major developmental gain for this age is the achievement of a sense of independence and autonomy. The struggle between choosing independence over dependence is a frustrating decision for the toddler. Toddlers tolerate their parents being out of sight in a comfortable setting and revel in their independence, but the return of separation anxiety can be a significant problem if the settings or people are unfamiliar. The fear of abandonment is great during early toddler years. Separation anxiety can be very traumatic for both parents and children and is frequently seen during these years.

Toddlers also begin to develop their sense of autonomy by asserting themselves with frequent use of the word "no." It may be used to refuse a request, to demonstrate lack of understanding, or to practice a word that the child notices has a dramatic effect on others. They can become very negative, practicing the power of "no" every day for months.

Temper tantrums usually make their appearance at about age 2. Tantrums stem from the child's striving for power and control and the sudden loss of both. There are so many activities toddlers want and struggle to do but that they are not developmentally ready to perform.

Toddlers enjoy playing near others, but they frequently do not share objects or engage in close interactive activities with other children. In parallel play, toddlers play beside but not with their friends. The types of play that appeal to toddlers are those that allow them to use large muscles, those that include repetitive and rhythmic motions, and those involving language. Play is a natural way to enhance the toddler's physical and psychosocial development.

Self-concept and body image are also part of psychosocial development. Toddlers develop their sense of self-esteem not only through others' responses to them but also through pleasure in their accomplishments. Mastering toilet training, gaining motor skills, and making choices all enhance a toddler's self-confidence. Sexuality is another aspect of toddler development. Toddlers begin to develop some gender-based expectations, can describe themselves as a girl or a boy, and can accurately apply gender labels to those around them. Havighurst's developmental task during toddlerhood shows the child learning to control the elimination of urine and feces (toilet training), learning gender differences, forming concepts, learning language, and distinguishing right from wrong.

Cognitive Development. According to Piaget, substage 5 is the search for knowledge through trial and error. In this substage (12 to 18 months) the toddler demonstrates solving problems by trial and error. Substage 6—mental combinations of symbolic schemes (15 months to 2 years)—is a culmination of sensorimotor stages and a transition to the next stage. For example, a toddler will not handle a toy immediately to see how it works but will look at it carefully to think about how it works. Toddlers are becoming more differentiated from the environment. They will search for a hidden object where they last saw it, showing increasingly thorough understanding of object permanence.

By the end of the second year, the toddler enters the first part of the preoperational stage with preconceptual thinking. This stage is characterized by the beginning use of symbols, mental imagery, and increased language skills. A toddler continues to be very concrete and self-centered in thinking, which is the source of many miscommunications between parent and child.

During this time, language skills increase tremendously. Toddlers engage in collective monologues by themselves or in groups of children. The understanding of language increases. Toddlers can follow a two- or three-word command and can understand many sentences. The understanding of physical relationships begins with concepts, such as "on," "in," and "under." A 3-year-old can say name, age, and gender and use four- to five-word sentences. Strangers are beginning to understand what the toddler is trying to say. The child at this age can recognize all common objects and pictures.

Yung Hi cries occasionally and remains nonverbal with the nurses. She speaks Korean with her parents and clings to her mother. Yung Hi's father has been attempting to explain the traction and hospital room to his wife and child. This may be a good time to have the father translate and assess for developmental data that will help you determine how to make Yung Hi's long stay less traumatic.

Preschoolers
Developmental Theory. A preschooler is a child between the ages of 3 and 5 years. Certain developmental changes take place throughout this time, particularly in the area of cognition, which is the act or process of knowing. Piaget's stages pertinent to the preschool- and school-age child are the preoperational stage (2 to 7 years), discussed here, and the concrete operational stage (7 to 11 years), discussed under School-Aged Children later.

The preoperational stage is divided into two phases: the preoperational phase, ages 2 to 4, and the phase of intuitive thought, ages 4 to 7. During the preoperational phase, children shift from totally egocentric thought to social awareness and the ability to consider others' viewpoints. They acquire language and learn that they can use thought to deal with the world symbolically. They use words to describe actions and mentally and symbolically accomplish actions through the use of words. They develop the ability to imagine an action without performing the act. For example, they can imagine pulling a toy even if they do not actually have the toy to pull.

As the phase of intuitive thought begins, at about age 4, preschoolers first begin to think about the future and start to plan what they will be doing later in the day or in a few days, instead of concentrating on the here and now. This reflects their increasing ability to think. Around age 5 they show an increasing ability to use language to describe their emotions. An important requirement for preschoolers' mental development is that they be reared in an intellectually stimulating environment.

Action Alert! Counsel parents to give their children age-appropriate materials and to encourage them to explore their environment. Maximum mental growth takes place when they are stimulated mentally, year after year.

Physical Development. During the preschool period, a significant change in body contour occurs. The prominent lordosis and protuberant abdomen characteristic of the toddler change to slimmer, taller, and more childlike proportions. The child's future body type becomes more apparent. Body types may be *ectomorphic* (lanky body build), *mesomorphic* (medium muscular body), or *endomorphic* (large build). Weight, height, and growth differentials depend on genetic factors (e.g., tall parents generally have tall children), cultural and ethnic characteristics, dietary habits, and the general health of the child. In the United States, African-American children tend to be taller than European-American children, who, in turn, are taller than Asian-American children (Rice, 1997).

Growth Parameters. The average preschool child gains weight slowly, only 4.5 pounds (2 kg) a year. It is not unusual for parents to perceive that the child is losing weight during this developmental period, whereas they are actually seeing age-appropriate changes in body contours. Preschoolers also grow slowly, gaining only 2 inches (51 mm) to 3.5 inches (89 mm) in an average year.

Physiological Changes. Preschool-age children undergo many physiological changes. Increased growth of lymphatic tissue increases the levels of antibodies in the child, so illnesses become more localized as in a runny nose with diminished systemic reaction such as fever. Heart murmurs may be heard on auscultation; this is because the heart changes its size in relation to the thorax, and murmurs at this stage are not normally a cause for concern. The heart rate decreases to about 85 beats per minute, and blood pressure stabilizes at about 100/60 mm Hg. The bladder is still quite small, so voiding occurs about eight to ten times daily; this explains why preschool children forget to use the toilet when they become absorbed in an activity and instead wet their clothes.

Dentition. Preschoolers generally have all 20 of their deciduous teeth by age 3 years. Rarely do new teeth erupt during this period. The American Academy of Pediatric Dentistry (2002) recommends initiating dental care when the first tooth erupts, with checkups twice a year thereafter.

Motor Development. Preschoolers experience tremendous improvement in large and fine muscle coordination. They can run well, walk up and down stairs, and learn to hop. By age 5 years, they can usually skip and throw and catch balls (Table 16-2). Improving fine motor skills and hand–eye coordination enables them to copy circles, squares, and triangles and to print letters and numbers. Their motor development depends primarily on overall physical maturation and is influenced by their opportunities for exercise and practice of activities such as skipping and hopping.

Table 16-2	Motor Skills of the Child 4 to 11 Years Old
Age	**Motor Skill**
4 years	• Walks on tiptoes • Alternates feet when descending stairs • Hops or jumps forward • Holds a pencil with control • Can cut and paste
5 years	• Skips • Throws overhand with some accuracy • Can catch a bounced ball • Handles scissors with skill • Rides a tricycle
6 years	• Ties own shoes • Runs, jumps, climbs • Skips • Rides a bike with training wheels • Learns to swim
7 to 8 years	• Can use inline skates • Rides a bicycle • Swimming improves • Continues to refine small muscle control • Is more graceful • Can throw and hit a baseball
9 to 11 years	• Can participate in most sports • Has good hand–eye coordination • Refines gross and fine motor skills • Can do craft projects • Can catch a ball in one hand

Language Development. By age 5, preschoolers have a vocabulary of more than 2000 words. They can use all parts of speech correctly. They tend to use more verbs than nouns. Their sentences average four to five words in length. They can define familiar objects, identify colors, and express their feelings. They understand the concepts of "under," "over," "up," and "down" and of opposites, such as "open" versus "closed." The pattern of asking questions is at its peak and they will repeat a question until they receive an answer.

Psychosocial Development. The psychosocial development of preschoolers is marked by an increasing sense of personal identity and willingness to work with others. Erikson identifies this third of his eight psychological stages as the tasks of "sense of initiative over guilt."

Peer Relationships. The development of peer relationships is one of the most important aspects of a child's social development. Four-year-olds continue to play in groups but may become involved in more arguments as they begin testing their roles in the group. The increasing conflict may cause parents to worry that their child is regressing, but it is really a forward movement. Five-year-olds begin selecting their "best" friends. They depend less on parents and more on peers for social interaction. They tend to offer approval, make demands on one another, and demonstrate the ability to show empathy when others are distressed (Rice, 1997).

Gender-Role Development. At ages 4 to 5, preschoolers develop gender-role identification and begin to assume the roles of persons of their own sex. Kohlberg (1966) states that the child's self-categorization as a boy or girl is the basic organizer of the gender-role attitudes that develop. Children act consistently in accordance with gender expectations communicated to them by family members and society. Boys and girls are socialized differently from birth. In the United States, boys are often expected to be more active and aggressive, whereas girls are expected to be polite and less aggressive. However, these behavioral tendencies are at least partially biological thus they will not entirely be suppressed by changes in socialization.

Play. Play promotes physical, social, and mental development of preschoolers. Five-year-olds continue to enjoy the rough-and-tumble play that they participated in at age 4, but they become more interested in group games, such as board games or sports such as soccer. This helps them learn to take turns and to be able to accept losing or winning and to cooperate with other children in a group. Active play is important for physical growth, refinement of motor skills, and releasing pent-up energy; the use of tricycles, wagons, sports equipment, and water play can help develop muscles and coordination. Playtime also helps them to learn to control their impulses and feelings and to express them in socially acceptable ways. Imaginative play is a healthy outlet for ill children because it allows them to think of creative solutions to their illness experiences and to develop problem-solving skills.

Action Alert! Inform parents that playtime is especially significant for the child who is ill. Through play, children can express and work out fears, anger, and misunderstandings about their illness.

Symbolic play is pretend or imaginative play that enables preschool children to recreate experiences and to try out roles (Figure 16-4). They create imaginary companions with whom they talk and play, and who become a regular part of their daily routines. Reassure parents that it is normal for their preschoolers to create imaginary playmates and that it helps the child differentiate between fantasy and reality.

Fears. Common fears that develop at this time include fear of the dark, separation from parents, and, in some cases, fear of bodily harm.
- *Fear of the dark:* The vivid imagination of the preschool-age child can turn a stuffed toy by day into a threatening monster in the dark. Parents must be prepared for this fear and understand that it is a normal phase of growth. They may need to reassure their child who is reluctant to go to sleep unless a light is on or who wakes up screaming from a nightmare.
- *Fear of separation or abandonment:* Fear of separation continues to be a concern for preschoolers because they do not have a sense of time. They are not comforted by mother's reassurances that she will return to preschool in 2 hours.
- *Fear of mutilation:* Some preschoolers have a fear of bodily harm that may make it difficult for them to cooperate with medical personnel and treatments, such as needlesticks or an otoscopic examination. They cry out not only from the pain but also from the sight of injury.

Action Alert! Encourage parents to thoroughly prepare their children for any separation experiences, such as being admitted to the hospital.

Moral Development. Piaget (1997) describes the development of moral judgment as a gradual cognitive process enhanced by the increasing social relationships of children. Early in their moral development, children are constrained by the "rules of the game." As children develop, they learn that rules are not absolute but can be altered by social consensus, and that adult rules are no longer sacred.

Preschoolers begin to have an elemental concept of God if they have been provided some exposure to religion. This belief in an outside force aids the development of conscience (Kohlberg, 1981), but preschoolers tend to do good out of self-interest rather than because of spiritual motivation. They enjoy the security of religious rituals, such as grace said before meals. Praying to God and observing religious traditions can help children through stressful periods such as hospitalization.

School-Age Children
Developmental Theory. According to Piaget (1980), school-age children are in the concrete operational stage of development. The cognitive developmental stage of **concrete opera-**

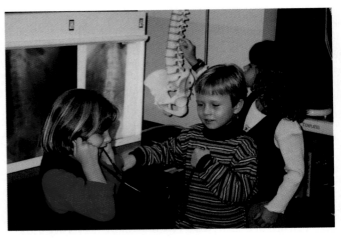

Figure 16-4. Symbolic play enables preschool children to recreate experiences and try out various adult roles.

tions occurs when children begin to project themselves into other people's situations and realize that their own way of thinking is not the only way. Decentering accommodation is a child's ability to adapt thought processes to perceive more than one reason for a person's actions.

At this time, children's thoughts become increasingly logical and coherent and they are able to classify, sort, and organize facts. However, they still lack the capacity to generalize or deal in abstract ideas. School-age children are able to increase their understanding of many concepts associated with objects. Class inclusion is a child's ability to understand that objects can belong to more than one group. The ability to group things into categories enables the child to expand knowledge through category-based indicators, which enables them to solve problems. **Conservation** is a child's ability to understand that changing the shape of a substance does not change its volume. Preschool-age children lack this perception (Figure 16-5). Understanding this concept helps limit sibling arguments over who has more milk when two different-shaped glasses of equal volume are presented.

Action Alert! Teach parents to understand that their school-age child may demonstrate varying abilities to handle problems and can most effectively handle one major problem at a time.

Language Development. At age 6, the child's vocabulary is quite large—about 10,000 words—and it reaches about 40,000 by adolescence. School-age children enlarge their vocabularies by analyzing the structure of complex words and thinking about them and using them more precisely. They appreciate the multiple meanings of words. Their conversational strategies become more refined. Children have generally mastered most of the grammar of their language when they enter school, and the use of complex grammatical constructions improves (Beck, 1998).

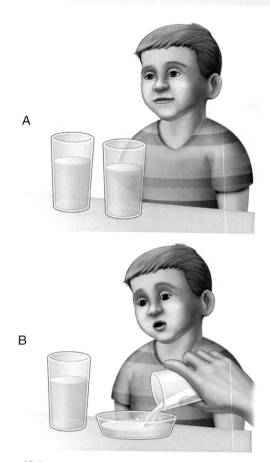

A

B

Figure 16-5. The preschool child does not yet understand the principle of conservation. **A,** The preschooler is able to understand that two glasses of the same size contain equal amounts of liquid. **B,** However, when the contents of one of the glasses is poured into a dish of equal volume, the child becomes perplexed because he does not understand that changing the shape of a substance does not change its volume.

Psychosocial Theory. According to Erikson's stages of development, the developmental task of the school years is the establishment of a sense of industry, in which the child is motivated to expend effort in a purposeful activity. During this stage, a child masters social and cognitive skills. However, there is a risk that the child will not gain competency at a chosen task and will develop a sense of inferiority rather than of industry. Successful completion of this stage of development enables children to recognize their abilities as well as their liabilities and to develop a sense of competence. Competition is also important; by comparing themselves to their peers, children can understand their own personal strengths and weaknesses.

Physical Development. A school-age child is a child between 6 and 11 years old. Although some girls begin puberty during the end of this period, most researchers consider these girls developmentally pre-adolescent despite their physical changes. During the school years, children's rate of physical

growth is steady but slower than at any time since birth; however, their motor, cognitive, and psychosocial development progresses rapidly.

Growth Parameters. On average, school-age children grow 1 to 2 inches (25 to 51 mm) and gain 3 to 5 pounds (1.36 to 2.27 kg) per year. Boys are slightly taller and heavier than girls during the early school years, but by age 9, girls experience an acceleration in skeletal growth and begin to be taller and heavier than boys. Boys experience an acceleration in growth around 12 years of age (Beck, 1998).

Physiological Changes. Cardiovascular function is usually stable in school-age children. Growth of the brain is complete around age 10, and this results in the refinement of fine motor coordination. Maturation of the respiratory system leads to increased oxygen–carbon dioxide exchange, increasing exertion ability and stamina. The frontal sinuses are developed, and sinus-caused headaches become a possibility.

Dentition. During the school-age years, all primary teeth are lost and the majority of permanent teeth have erupted. The timing is somewhat variable, depending on both heredity and nutrition (Figure 16-6, p. 312). Children need to brush and floss daily to maintain healthy teeth and gums. A dentist needs to be consulted about jaw malformations or misaligned teeth.

Action Alert! Remind parents that children should have a dental examination and teeth cleaning every 6 months.

Sexual Maturation. At about 10 years of age, the hypothalamus transmits an enzyme to the anterior pituitary gland to begin production of gonadotropic hormones, which activate changes in testes and ovaries (Cunningham, 2001). Timing of sexual maturity varies widely between 10 and 14 years of age. Puberty is occurring increasingly earlier, and it would not be unusual to find school-age girls already menstruating at age 11 or earlier.

Action Alert! Encourage parents to discuss sexual responsibility with the child. Children at this age should also be reminded that their body is their own to be used only in the way they choose.

Motor Development. As musculature increases in size, coordination continues to improve. Most 6- to 11-year-olds can learn to in-line skate; play baseball, soccer, or tennis; and do gymnastics. Fine-motor skills continue to develop as well. School-age children can sew, learn to use garden tools, handle a hammer and a saw, draw in proportion, and master penmanship in writing. Reaction time depends on brain maturation, which is why so many children aged 5 to 7 have trouble catching a ball. Any sport that requires quick reactions, distance judgment, and hand–eye coordination may be difficult for younger school-age children.

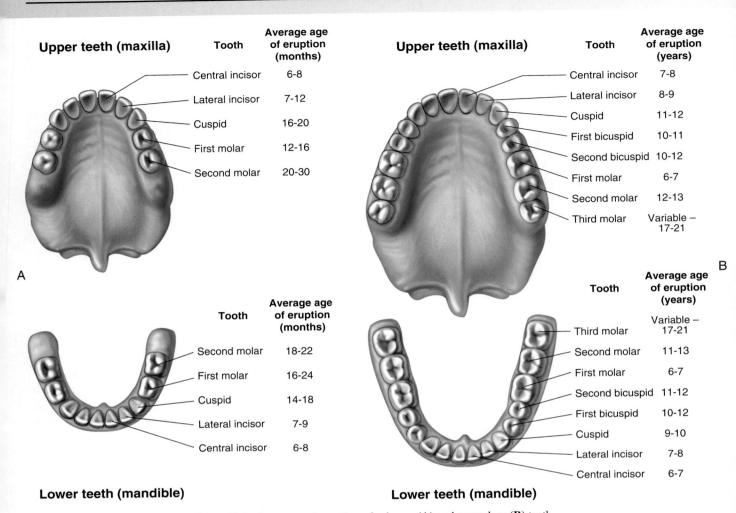

Upper teeth (maxilla)	Tooth	Average age of eruption (months)
	Central incisor	6-8
	Lateral incisor	7-12
	Cuspid	16-20
	First molar	12-16
	Second molar	20-30

A

Upper teeth (maxilla)	Tooth	Average age of eruption (years)
	Central incisor	7-8
	Lateral incisor	8-9
	Cuspid	11-12
	First bicuspid	10-11
	Second bicuspid	10-12
	First molar	6-7
	Second molar	12-13
	Third molar	Variable – 17-21

B

Tooth	Average age of eruption (months)
Second molar	18-22
First molar	16-24
Cuspid	14-18
Lateral incisor	7-9
Central incisor	6-8

Lower teeth (mandible)

Tooth	Average age of eruption (years)
Third molar	Variable – 17-21
Second molar	11-13
First molar	6-7
Second bicuspid	11-12
First bicuspid	10-12
Cuspid	9-10
Lateral incisor	7-8
Central incisor	6-7

Lower teeth (mandible)

Figure 16-6. Sequence of eruption of primary (**A**) and secondary (**B**) teeth.

Peer Relationships. Learning to understand and get along with children who are different from themselves are important developmental tasks; generally, school-age children prefer same-sex friends. Their acceptance by their peers is very important and influences their adjustment during adolescence (Box 16-2).

Gender-Role Development. Gender stereotypes are learned through parents, teachers, peers, and the media. Children's understanding of gender roles broadens, and their gender role identities change as they think more about people as personalities.

Play. During the school years, group activities dominate playtime. Through group dynamics, school-age children learn to work cooperatively toward a common goal. Success in physical and cognitive play is important.

Fears. As children explore the world around them, having new experiences and confronting new challenges, fears and anxieties are an unavoidable part of growing up. Children between the ages of 6 and 11 have many fears and concerns, such as fear of darkness, animals, high places, or thunderstorms. The death of a close friend or family member may cause them much anxiety about the health of those around them. Children

---

Box 16-2 Behavioral Characteristics That Promote Peer Acceptance

- Being outgoing, socially interactive
- Being physically attractive (girls); having athletic ability (boys)
- Having a high level of energy
- Participating early in social events
- Having a good sense of humor and being good natured
- Accepting others even when they are different from oneself
- Performing well in school
- Having the ability to communicate effectively

---

want to be reassured that these terrible things will not happen to them. It is important to let children talk about a frightening situation and to share what is on their minds.

Action Alert! Children may be concerned about what they see on TV or read in the newspaper. Encourage parents to reassure their children and provide them the perspective they need to understand what they are viewing. To handle terrifying and confusing situations, children take their emotional cues from the adults around them.

Moral Development. At age 6 or 7, children know the rules and behaviors that are expected of them, but they do not understand the reasons behind them. Rewards and punishments guide their judgments. Older school-age children are able to understand what prompts an action and therefore do not judge an action only on its consequences.

Adolescents

Adolescence is the period of transition between childhood and adulthood. It is a period of rapid growth and dramatic change, both physically and psychologically. For the purpose of discussion, this chapter defines adolescence as being between the ages of 12 and 21. Keep in mind, however, that children grow and develop at different rates, and any definition of adolescence should be flexible on both ends. The three stages of adolescence are the following:

- Early adolescence, from about age 12 to 14, when the adolescent has not entirely left the world of childhood
- Middle adolescence, from about age 15 to 17, when the adolescent undergoes a time of consolidation
- Late adolescence, from about age 18 to 21, when adolescents reach the threshold of adulthood and begin to establish themselves as independent persons

Developmental Theory. During early adolescence, most youngsters acquire the stage of thinking that Piaget and Infelder (1958) call **formal operations,** which is the ability to reason abstractly. For example, the adolescent can engage in "if, then" deliberations, recognizing that if one event has occurred, another will likely follow. For example, if Mom's car will not start in the morning and she says that the battery is probably dead, then the adolescent will realize that other accessories in the car—such as the radio and lights—also will not function.

Similarly, adolescents develop the ability to reason and question constructs that they previously took for granted, such as the belief that parents are always correct. They begin to question others. They also develop the ability to see another person's perspective. In addition, they begin to think about *thinking* and their own thoughts.

Another hallmark of adolescents' cognitive development is **egocentrism,** which refers to their tendency to spend so much time thinking about and focusing on their own thoughts and changes in their own body that they come to believe that others are focused on them as well. As a result, young adolescents construct what Elkind (1992) has termed the "imaginary audience." This is a belief that everyone in your proximity is deeply interested in your every thought and action. This leads adolescents to believe that they must be very special because everyone else is so fascinated by them. Several types of "typical" adolescent beliefs result from this type of thinking, such as "No one has ever experienced what I'm feeling" and "Other people will die, but not me." The belief in the uniqueness of oneself is referred to as the personal fable. Although most people never completely lose their personal fables, the fables decline in influence as adolescents grow older and share experiences with others.

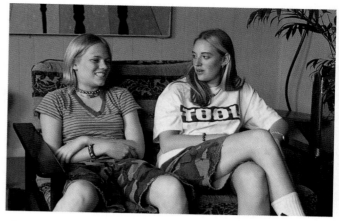

Figure 16-7. Peers have a strong influence on adolescents' clothes, hairstyle, and manner of speech.

Egocentrism similarly decreases from early through late adolescence.

Psychosocial Development. Erik Erikson, the foremost theorist on psychosocial development, describes the chief developmental task of adolescence as the development of identity versus identity diffusion. To achieve a sense of identity, the adolescent must be able to integrate past, present, and future selves. During this period, the adolescent gradually becomes less reliant on family and more reliant on the self and others. A sense of group identity becomes strong and may lead to specific behaviors, styles of hair and dress, and activities (Figure 16-7). However, the family still influences an adolescent's basic values and provides important emotional support, regardless of whether the adolescent consciously recognizes this influence. Gender identity also becomes consolidated during adolescence, and young people may begin to have heterosexual relationships, homosexual relationships, or both.

Physical Development. The hallmark of adolescence is a physical process known as puberty—the sequence of physiological events that cause the reproductive organs to mature, making conception and childbirth possible. In girls, menarche is the hallmark event of this change. **Menarche** is the time of the first menstrual period; it occurs at an average age of 12 years and 4 months, although the age may range from 9 to 17 years. In boys, the first nocturnal emission marks the transition to puberty. A **nocturnal emission** is a discharge of semen during sleep; it occurs at an average age of 13 years and 4 months, but the age may range from 11 to 15 years.

During adolescence, secondary sexual characteristics appear. These changes in bodily features, such as pubic hair, axillary hair, and fully developed breasts and penis, are induced by sex hormones. Secondary sexual characteristics develop in the same sequence in all adolescents, although the timing differs from person to person. The sexual maturity scale developed by Tanner identifies five stages of pubertal development that focus on breasts in girls and scrotal and penile development in boys (Figure 16-8). Pubic hair can be assessed in both sexes but offers less important information in the overall physical assessment.

Adolescents experience a rapid growth in height called the pubertal growth spurt. It begins before menarche or the first nocturnal emission and accounts for 15% to 25% of the final adult height. Body fat is also affected. In girls, the amount of adipose tissue increases, reducing the proportion of lean body mass. In boys, the lean body mass increases during this time.

Girls begin their growth spurt at an earlier age than boys but commonly reach a shorter adult height because of a lower velocity of growth and a shorter period of growth. The cardiorespiratory system grows at a disproportionate rate to the rest of the body, making aerobic activity at this age an important part of physical fitness.

Motor Development. During early puberty, many adolescents experience some awkwardness because the feet, legs, and arms begin the growth spurt before the height catches up. This gives many young teens a gangly appearance. The musculoskeletal system is also most vulnerable to injury during the period of peak height velocity, which occurs during Tanner stage III.

Moral Development. Adolescents must establish their own set of morals and values in order to gain autonomy from adults. Their decisions involving moral dilemmas are based

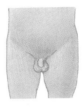

Stage I
Penis: Childhood size and proportion
Testes and scrotum: Childhood size and proportion
Pubic hair: None

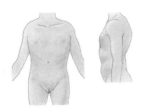

Stage I
Breasts: Pre-adolescent; elevation of the papilla only
Pubic hair: None

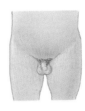

Stage II
Penis: Slight or no enlargement
Testes and scrotum: Enlargement; scrotal skin reddens, changes in texture
Pubic hair: Sparse growth of long, downy pubic hair mainly at the base of the penis

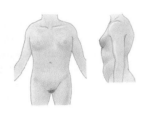

Stage II
Breasts: Breast budding (thelarche); small mound formed by elevation of the breast and papilla, with enlargement of the areolar diameter
Pubic hair: Sparse growth of long, downy pubic hair over mons veneris or labia majora; may occur with breast budding or several weeks or months later (pubarche)

Stage III
Breasts: Further enlargement of breast tissue and areola with no separation of their contours
Pubic hair: Increased amount of hair and changes in the character of the hair (darker, coarser, and more curly), spread sparsely over junction of pubes

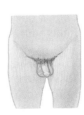

Stage III
Penis: Enlargement, particularly in length
Testes and scrotum: Further enlargement
Pubic hair: Darker, coarser, curlier hair spread sparsely over the pubic symphysis

A

B

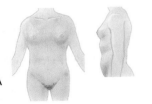

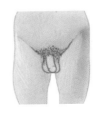

Stage IV
Penis: Further enlargement in length and breadth, with development of the glans
Testes and scrotum: Further enlargement
Pubic hair: Coarse and curly hair; greater area covered than in Stage III, but still less than in an adult, with no spread to thighs

Stage IV
Breasts: Double contour form: projection of areola and papilla form a secondary mound on top of breast tissue
Pubic hair: Adult appearance but less area covered; no spread to medial aspects of thighs

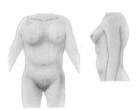

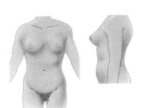

Stage V
Breasts: Larger, more mature breast with single contour form
Pubic hair: Adult distribution and quantity, with spread to medial aspect of thighs

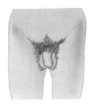

Stage V
Penis: Adult in size and shape
Testes and scrotum: Adult in size and shape
Pubic hair: Adult distribution and quantity, with spread to thighs but not to abdomen

Figure 16-8. Tanner stages of physical development. **A,** Female. **B,** Male. (From Bowden, Y. R., Dickey, S. B., & Greenberg, C. S. [1998]. *Children and their families: The continuum of care.* Philadelphia: Saunders.)

on an internalized set of moral principles, which enables them to evaluate the situation and plan a course of action consistent with their ideals. Late adolescence involves serious questioning of existing moral values and their relevance to the individual and society. This is consistent with Kohlberg's level III, postconventional morality.

FACTORS AFFECTING GROWTH AND DEVELOPMENT

Many factors, such as environment, socioeconomic status, nutrition, and physiological status, influence growth and development. In adolescence, as in other stages of development, lifestyle and psychological factors influence health behaviors. The interaction of these factors greatly affects response to everyday situations. These factors also influence the choices caregivers make regarding health care behaviors.

Environmental Factors
Family Dynamics. Family dynamics is the pattern of interpersonal relationships within a family. This pattern is affected by the structure, size, and composition of the family. A child's ability to feel secure about self and relate to others depends on how well identity is established and how supportive the family members are of the child. Parents who are nurturing, supportive, and consistent in enforcing rules will help to foster adolescent development.

Family Structure. Each individual has a position in the family structure and plays a defined role in interactions within the family group. Structure includes traditions and values that set standards for interaction within and outside the group. Family size and composition also influence child development. Parents treat children differently, and sibling interactions vary depending on the child's position within the family. Age differences between siblings affect the childhood environment. The arrival of a baby brother or sister has the greatest impact on the older child, and a 2- to 4-year difference in age appears to be most threatening.

Culture and Religion. Culture influences everything people do, produce, know, and believe in as they grow and develop as members of social groups. As children become familiar with the patterns of behavior associated with their culture, they also develop distinctive personalities, thoughts, and feelings,

as suggested in Box 16-3. Religious development refers to the acceptance of specific beliefs, values, rules of conduct, and rituals.

Discipline. The term *discipline* refers to adherence to a set of rules for conduct, and it also describes actions taken to enforce the rules after noncompliance. Limit setting means establishing guidelines for behavior. Children want and need limits. These limits must be clear and enforced consistently for children to adhere to the rules.

Community. Children and their families reside in a community in which residents share and are influenced by a common environment. The community can encourage a positive outcome for children or it can stunt it. Children living in high-risk neighborhoods have more social and behavioral problems than those in low-risk neighborhoods.

Socioeconomic Factors
Socioeconomic factors, such as income, educational level, and single parenthood, influence the growth and development of children. A child who grows up in an economically deprived home may have impairments in physical, psychosocial, and cognitive development. Inadequate educational resources can influence parenting skills, finances, and basic knowledge of a child's developmental needs. One of the most adverse influences on health is low socioeconomic status. People whose socioeconomic status is low suffer from more health problems at any one time than people in any other group. These families often have poor medical care, higher mortality rates, and higher rates of psychological and mental illnesses.

Nutritional Factors
Nutritional concerns for the child begin during pregnancy and continue after birth, when the parents decide what method of feeding to choose. Human milk is the most desirable for the first 12 months of life.

Solid foods are introduced gradually, beginning at about 4 months. Iron-fortified cereals are usually recommended by 6 months. After that, strained, pureed infant foods are gradually added, one at a time, usually one every 5 days. As each new food is added to the infant's diet, the parent should observe for signs of intolerance or allergy. The toddler's growth rate slows, decreasing slightly the need for calories, fluids, and protein. Most toddlers are eating the same food prepared for

Box 16-3

Cross-Cultural Care CARING FOR A KOREAN TODDLER

Yung Hi, the young client presented in this chapter, and her family are Korean and new to the United States. Koreans, like many Asian peoples, are of Mongolian-Tungus descent. Although each person is unique, Korean people are generally characterized as being generous, kind, and resourceful. The following behaviors also have been identified as culturally characteristic and valued by Korean people:
- Putting the family's welfare ahead of the individual's
- Viewing infants and young children as passive and dependent
- Having a strong sense of self-respect and self-control

- Maintaining a stoic demeanor and offering few complaints
- Being polite by giving a person the response she is expecting
- Avoiding physical contact
- Upholding men as authority figures, with women expected to be obedient
- Believing that education is important
- Viewing health as a balance between positive and negative energy forces (yin and yang)

the family and using a cup. Nutrition continues to be important as the child grows and develops.

Poor nutrition may cause a child to tire easily, have a poor appetite, experience slower growth, or become ill because of an inability to resist pathogens and infections. As children grow toward adolescence, poor eating habits can contribute to the development of obesity. Discuss with parents the importance of providing children and adolescents with nutritious, appealing foods.

Physiological Factors

Most children grow and develop without problems. However, a variety of physiological factors may influence a child's growth and development. One of the most difficult—and most costly—stems from preterm birth; these infants may experience developmental delay and chronic illness as complications. Physiological factors that impact on the child's growth and development may include respiratory ailments such as recurrent colds and asthma, as well as ear infections (most commonly otitis media). Other common childhood occurrences include enuresis (recurrent involuntary urination), head lice, and animal or insect bites.

Action Alert! When a child fails to startle at loud noises, does not always respond when called, or has delayed or difficult understanding of speech, there is a probability of a hearing deficit in one or both ears. Encourage parents to be aware of these signs.

Parents should encourage their children to exercise and become involved in enjoyable and vigorous activities that promote their physical development, preferably with other children at the same developmental level. Activities should help children develop motor skills that will enable them to reach their full physical potential and should provide them with basic skills and habits that will make fitness an enjoyable, lifelong activity.

The number of hours per day spent sleeping varies with individual children and with different age groups. The preschool-age child sleeps approximately 11 hours; this gradually decreases during the school-age years to 9 or 10 hours.

Physiological factors and acute or chronic illness may affect the adolescent's growth and development as well. As mentioned earlier, the average age of the onset of puberty is 12 years in girls and 13 years in boys. A delay of more than 2 or 3 years from this norm may cause adolescents tremendous anxiety. **Constitutional delay of puberty** is defined as an absence of early signs of puberty (Tanner stage II breasts by age 13 for girls or Tanner stage II genitalia by age 14 for boys). Constitutional delay of puberty is the basis of more than 90% of cases of delayed puberty; it does not indicate underlying pathology but simply that the adolescent is a "late bloomer."

Although benign and self-limiting, constitutional delay of puberty can cause psychological problems, such as body image disturbance, self-esteem disturbance, negative emotional reactions, long-term dependency on parents, and failure to acquire appropriate social skills. It is important to reassure adolescents and their parents that this condition is self-limiting

and that the adolescent is normal. Disorders that cause a pathological delay of puberty are all rare.

Action Alert! Reassure adolescents with constitutional delay of puberty that they are normal.

A common complaint of adolescent boys is **gynecomastia,** which is a benign increase in breast tissue associated with puberty. It results from an imbalance in circulating estrogens and androgens. Gynecomastia can be unilateral or bilateral, and the breasts are frequently tender when touched, even by clothing. Most cases resolve spontaneously within 12 to 18 months.

Action Alert! Assure boys with gynecomastia that the condition is a normal and relatively common part of puberty and that it usually goes away by itself within about 12 to 18 months.

Fortunately, most acute illnesses during adolescence are short-lived and easily treated. However, mononucleosis deserves special mention because it is most prevalent during the adolescent and young adult years. The vast majority of cases of mononucleosis are caused by Epstein-Barr virus. Transmission typically occurs through saliva during direct, prolonged contact with oropharyngeal secretions.

The number of adolescents living with chronic illness has increased, not because the incidence of disease has changed but because more children with chronic conditions are surviving. The most common are asthma, diabetes mellitus, congenital heart disease, sickle cell disease, chronic renal disease, epilepsy, and hemophilia.

Lifestyle Factors

Attention Deficit/Hyperactivity Disorder. Attention-deficit/hyperactivity disorder (ADHD) is a neuropsychological disorder associated with disturbances in attention, impulsivity, and hyperactivity. ADHD is estimated to affect 6% to 9% of children and adolescents, and it is more prevalent in boys. Children with ADHD are at risk for developing emotional and behavioral problems, such as misconduct or antisocial behaviors, substance abuse, depression, and anxiety disorders (Jellinek, 1998).

Learning Disability. According to the Learning Disabilities Association of America (1999), a learning disability is a lifelong disorder that affects the manner in which people of normal or above-average intelligence select, retain, and express information. It has been estimated that approximately 5% of public school children have a learning disability (Shaywitz, Fletcher, & Shaywitz, 1995). The deficiency usually occurs in specific areas such as reading, although related skills such as writing and mathematical concepts may also be affected. An evaluation may reveal that overall ability as measured by IQ tests is not abnormal, but standardized academic achievement tests may demonstrate areas of weakness.

Substance Abuse. When children begin to experiment with drugs, they often mistakenly think they can control their use. Children at risk for drug use are those who have poor self-concept or a strong need for acceptance and approval of their peers. Children who have school or family stresses may find relief in the use of controlled substances.

Substance abuse is a primary risk factor for altered growth and development in children and adolescents because it interferes with biological, psychological, and sociocultural integrity. It is a cofactor in the most common causes of deaths and injuries in this age group, including motor vehicle and other accidents, homicide, suicide, and the diseases that can result from unprotected sexual intercourse.

Tobacco Use. Cigarette smoking is another serious health problem among children and adolescents that has profound implications for their adult health. They may believe that the use of cigarettes is better than alcohol or marijuana, which is illegal. The prevalence of smoking remains high among all groups of adolescents.

Action Alert! Encourage parents to discuss the risks of tobacco, alcohol, and other drugs with their children.

Violence. Homicide is the second leading cause of death among 15- to 24-year-olds and the leading cause of death for African-American and Hispanic males. Risk factors for homicide include the use of alcohol or drugs, exposure to media violence, a personal history of child abuse, witnessing violence (particularly in the home), and poverty. A sense of helplessness pervades many young people who grow up in poverty (Neinstein, Juliani, & Shapiro, 2002).

Sexual Behavior. Another prominent cause of morbidity and mortality among adolescents is their sexual behavior. More than 7% of teens report having intercourse before age 13. Estimates vary, but most studies agree that at least half of adolescents in the United States engage in intercourse during their high school years, and 43.2% did not use a condom in the last sexual intercourse. Sixteen percent reported having intercourse with four or more partners. Adolescents are in the age group at greatest risk for acquiring sexually transmitted diseases (STDs). Adolescents are more likely to have multiple sexual partners and to engage in unprotected intercourse than their adult counterparts; both are risk factors for STDs (Neinstein & Anderson, 2002).

Provide teens with the information on the risks of sexual activity in a nonjudgmental and informative manner, including discussions of both abstinence and methods of birth control.

Obesity. Obesity is defined as body weight or body-fat percentage that exceeds a chosen reference point. Among adolescents aged 12 to 17 years, about 12% are overweight, a figure that represents a 6% increase from the 1980s to the 1990s (National Center for Health Statistics, 1998). These teens tend to eat very quickly and for emotional comfort, usually while engaged in other activities such as watching television. They overindulge in fast foods and skip breakfast and lunch only to consume many calories at night. Counseling should include

teaching nutrition as well as promoting exercise. Because adolescents are usually not the ones who buy and prepare food, it is helpful to involve the parents in treatment as well. Moran (as cited in Wong et al., 2001) states the current prevalence of childhood obesity in the United States is 25% to 30%. Recently there has been an increase in type II diabetes among adolescents who are obese.

Psychological Factors
Suicide. It is difficult to estimate how many adolescents commit suicide because of the number that go unreported—a single-car accident that actually was a suicide, for example. Adolescent girls make more suicide attempts than boys.

Eating Disorders. *Anorexia nervosa* is a complex disorder characterized by self-induced weight loss driven by a morbid fear of becoming fat. Of the adolescents suffering from this affliction, 90% are girls. These teenagers are preoccupied with food and weight and have a distorted body image. They have a revulsion for food that results in a weight loss of 25% or more of the normal body weight with no other apparent illness or psychiatric disorder. They may exercise compulsively to work off any food eaten. Anorexia is the third most common chronic condition among adolescent girls (after obesity and asthma). The syndrome can begin in children as young as age 9 years.

Bulimia nervosa is a disorder characterized by binge eating coupled with purging via emetics, laxatives, or self-induced vomiting. It may be a subtype of anorexia, and it has a similar etiological pattern. Although they may experience mild weight loss or gain, girls with bulimia often have a stable weight. They may suffer from gastric or esophageal rupture, parotid gland enlargement, hypokalemia, erosion of dental enamel from induced vomiting, scars on the knuckles of one hand, and amenorrhea or irregular menses.

ASSESSMENT

Assessment of the physical, cognitive, and psychosocial capabilities of the newborn, infant, toddler, preschool and school-age child, and adolescent is completed at initial and follow-up visits to the physician or advanced practice nurse. The purpose of these examinations is health promotion and disease prevention.

General Assessment
Newborns, Infants, and Toddlers. The examination for newborns, infants, and toddlers, called the well-baby examination, includes the health history and the physical examination. A comprehensive health history includes many components (Box 16-4, p. 318). Typically, the health care provider obtains a complete history during the initial health care visit and updates it on subsequent visits. For an ill child, the history focuses on the current complaint. The health history closes with a review of systems. Before beginning the physical examination, make sure the child is warm and comfortable. Proceed to examine each body system thoroughly and accurately, using inspection, palpation, percussion, and auscultation.

Box 16-4	Example of Health History Questions

- *Reason for contact:* Why did the child come to the health care provider? Was it for a health maintenance visit, or was there a complaint of illness?
- *Present illness, chief concern:* What are the signs and associated symptoms? What makes them better or worse? Which over-the-counter drugs were taken? How long did the symptoms persist? What was done for the problem?
- *Family history:* What is the health status of siblings, parents, and grandparents? Are there significant illnesses or genetic problems in the family? Any heart, kidney, or congenital diseases? Does anyone in the family have seizures, mental retardation, or mental illness? Is there a family history of tuberculosis, diabetes, or sexually transmitted disease? Do allergies run in the family? If they do, inquire further about specific symptoms.
- *Prenatal and childbirth history:* Were there any medical, surgical, or pregnancy problems? Has the mother had any miscarriages or still-births? Ask the mother about the pregnancy with this child. Did she use cigarettes, alcohol, or drugs while pregnant? If so, how much? Was this pregnancy planned? What was the labor like? How long was it? Were there any complications? What type of analgesia or anesthesia was used?
- *Neonatal history:* Were there any unusual circumstances during the newborn period? When did the baby sleep through the night? Was the baby unusually fussy? At what time of the day was the baby most fretful?
- *Social history:* What is the home situation like? Who are the significant others in the child's life? In what activities is the child engaged? Does the child attend day care? How does the child like it?
- *Nutritional history:* What type of infant feeding is or was being done? What is a typical menu for 24 hours? What foods does the child like or dislike? Are there any food allergies?
- *Developmental history:* Were typical developmental milestones achieved? When did they occur? Were there any significant developmental delays?
- *Immunization history:* What immunizations were given? Do they need to be updated? Were there any untoward reactions?

Instruments used to assess growth include a tape measure, a height marker, and a scale. Use a tape measure to obtain height (or length) and head circumference. At age 2 years, measure the child's standing height.

Weigh an infant or small child without clothing on a hygienic paper liner, because the weight of the diaper can add 10% or more to the child's weight. By age 3 years, the child, dressed only in underpants, should be weighed on a standing scale. Scales used for weighing children may be self-adjusting, or they may need to be balanced before each use.

Measure the head circumference of the newborn and until the child is 3 years old. Place the measuring tape around the largest circumference of the head, just above the eyebrows and the posterior prominence of the occiput. The tape should remain horizontal from front to back.

Compare the child's height and weight with growth charts to detect risks from slow or accelerated growth. Initial measurements are done immediately after birth and compared with a graph of the relationship between gestational age in weeks and birthweight to determine if the newborn is average, small, or large for gestational age. During frequent health vis-

its from the newborn through the toddler stage, the relationships between height and weight continue to be measured and recorded on charts to diagnose any disorders related to physical, emotional, environmental, or social deficiencies.

The simplest and most efficient method of assessing developmental milestones is to obtain a developmental history. Ask parents to recall when developmental events occurred in their child's life. Various methods and instruments are available to ascertain developmental milestones in children, such as the Denver Developmental Screening Test II.

Preschool and School-Age Children. Optimal childhood growth and development, and prevention of accidents and illness are the objectives of pediatric health supervision. The aim of the health history is to review the child's past physical and psychosocial history and to determine whether the parents or the child has any complaints or concerns. It includes a complete assessment of nutrition, exercise habits, sleep patterns, and growth and development milestones. Progress in school and the child's social interactions with family and peers should also be evaluated.

The depth and extent of a nursing health history vary with its intended purpose. The format used for history taking is usually a combination of direct and indirect techniques to elicit information about each of the functional health patterns. The school-age child should be able to cooperate fully with you, whereas the younger child may be more challenging.

Preschoolers and school-age children should have routine well-child examinations. The well-child examination involves several evaluations. The immunization history is reviewed to be sure the child is current. Measurements of the child's height, weight, and blood pressure are obtained, and vision and hearing are screened. A complete physical examination is performed.

Additional diagnostic tests may be performed, but there is some variability in the tests performed at each visit. The following are examples of such tests.

CHOLESTEROL SCREENING. Parents are becoming increasingly aware that risk factors for cardiovascular disease, particularly coronary artery disease related to dietary cholesterol intake, may be present in their children. However, there is no consensus regarding the efficacy of universal cholesterol screening in children.

> *Action Alert!* Advise parents of young children to provide diets low in cholesterol and saturated fat. Recommend an active lifestyle for children and the avoidance of smoking, including exposure to secondhand smoke.

BLOOD TESTING FOR LEAD POISONING. According to the Centers for Disease Control and Prevention (CDC), 890,000 American children aged 1 to 5 years have elevated levels of lead in their blood, and more than one fifth of African-American children living in housing built before 1946 have elevated blood lead levels. The major sources of lead exposure are deteriorated lead-based paint in older

Box 16-5	Sample Health History Questions for an Adolescent

HOME

- Where do you live and who lives there with you?
- Do you get along?
- Do you have privacy in your home?

EDUCATION

- What grade are you in?
- What are you good at in school? What is hard for you?
- What kinds of grades do you get?

ACTIVITIES

- What do you do after school?
- What do you do with your friends?

ALCOHOL

- Do you know anyone who has tried drugs, alcohol, or cigarettes?
- Have you ever tried drugs or alcohol?
- Do you drink alcohol? What do you usually drink, and how often? Alone or with friends?

SEXUAL BEHAVIOR

- Many young people become interested in sexual relationships at your age. Do you currently have, or have you ever had, a boyfriend or girl-friend? (Include both options for all clients.)

- Have you ever been worried that you had a sexually transmitted disease or that you were (or were responsible for someone becoming) pregnant?
- Have you used anything to prevent disease or pregnancy?
- What did you use?

SUICIDAL TENDENCIES

- Everybody feels sad or depressed sometimes. Do you think that you feel that way more often than other young people your age?
- Have you ever felt that life was not worth living?
- Have you ever wanted to kill yourself? (If yes:) Have you made a plan to kill yourself?

WEIGHT

- Do you feel that your weight is just right, too low, or too high?
- Have you ever tried to do anything to change your weight?
- Do you think about food a lot?

INJURIES

- Have you ever been the victim of violence or seen someone being assaulted?
- Do you or any of your friends drive a car? Do they ever drive after drinking?
- Have you ever gotten in a car with a driver who has been drinking?
- Do you ever drive after having had something to drink?
- Do you know students in your school who have guns or other weapons?
- Do you have a gun? Are there guns in your home?

housing and dust and soil that are contaminated with lead from old paint and from past emissions of leaded gasoline. Lead poisoning can cause learning disabilities, behavioral problems, and, at very high levels, seizures, coma, and even death. The CDC recommends that at-risk children undergo a blood test for lead (CDC, 1998a).

TUBERCULOSIS SCREENING. In the United States, tuberculosis (TB) occurs in less than 1% of children. However, all children should have a careful history to ascertain their risk and should be screened three times during childhood for TB: at 12 to 15 months of age, before entering kindergarten, and at 14 to 16 years of age. The multipuncture Mono-Vac is adequate for routine screening rather than the purified protein derivative (PPD) test. Children found to be at risk should be identified and screened yearly.

Adolescents. Most health problems encountered by well adolescents are caused by health-risk behaviors. If possible, interview an adolescent client without the parents present, and reassure the client that your conversation will be confidential (unless the teen is suicidal or homicidal). Most adolescents would prefer not to divulge certain information in front of their parents, such as grades, drug use, sexual behavior, and suicidal thoughts. You may want to interview the parents separately to determine their concerns.

Do not be afraid to ask adolescents about illegal, unsafe, or otherwise undesirable behavior. Research has shown that they will not interpret the question as tacit approval to engage in

that behavior. For example, asking adolescents whether they have ever had a sexual relationship will not encourage them to begin a sexual relationship.

Adolescents are more likely to be honest when respected and questioned honestly. They are very sensitive not only to what you actually say to them but to what they think your perceptions are of them. It is important for you to remain nonjudgmental. Teens who believe they are being criticized are unlikely to return for care.

When you assess adolescents, ask the least personal questions first to allow them to become comfortable talking with you. For example, ask about home, education, and other activities before you ask about drug use, sexuality, and suicide risk (Box 16-5). Ask teens about their perceptions of their own weight and their ideal weight, and what measures, if any, they have taken to alter their weight. Finally, question their risk for injury. Also assess adolescents' developmental level. Are they operating at an earlier cognitive level than you would expect? Are they more physically mature than the average teenager of the same age?

Make sure to assess the adolescent's physical, cognitive, and psychological functioning, beginning with a general assessment of appearance. Monitor the teen's vital signs, vision, and hearing, and obtain the results of any other diagnostic screening tests. Obtain height and weight, and assess for anorexia or bulimia if the client has a weight loss of more than 10% of previous weight or if the body weight is in the 5th percentile.

Pay particular attention to the adolescent growth spurt, which peaks in girls at about age 12 years and in boys at about age 14 years. During this period, adolescents experience many physical changes. Boys gain an average of 8 inches (20 cm) in height and more than 40 pounds (18.3 kg) in weight, whereas girls gain somewhat less height and weight. Boys' voices begin to deepen, and facial hair appears on the upper lip and then on the cheeks and lower lip. Pubic hair begins to develop, and the penis, testes, and scrotum enlarge. Some boys experience gynecomastia. Girls' breasts and pubic hair begin to develop. Menarche usually takes place during Tanner stage III or IV (see Figure 16-8).

Depending on the reason for your examination, you should pay particular attention to certain areas. For example, if the adolescent is undergoing a sports physical, you would assess the heart, lungs, and abdomen for any abnormalities, and you would test all the joints for range of motion, flexibility, strength, and reflexes.

Scoliosis is a structural lateral curvature of the spine. More than 60% of cases occur in girls. It often first appears during late childhood or adolescence, so all adolescents should be appropriately screened. Many states mandate scoliosis screening in the schools.

All teens should have hearing, vision, and blood pressure screenings annually and should be encouraged to have dental checkups and perform good dental care. They should be up to date with immunizations, including tetanus and diphtheria (every 10 years), hepatitis B, measles, mumps, rubella (the second inoculation), and varicella (if there is no history of chicken pox). They should also be screened for tuberculosis.

Iron deficiency anemia is a relatively common problem in adolescents, especially girls. This usually results from menstrual blood loss and lack of iron in the diet. All teens should have their hemoglobin or hematocrit level measured yearly to check for this condition. Adolescents whose parents have a serum cholesterol level greater than 240 mg/dL and adolescents who are over 19 years of age should be screened for total blood cholesterol level at least once (American Medical Association [AMA], 2001).

Testicular cancer is a disease of adolescents and young men. It is readily treatable when detected early. Adolescent males should be screened for this disorder and taught how to examine their testicles so they can perform a self-examination regularly.

Although breast cancer is exceedingly rare in adolescents, all girls who have reached Tanner stage II (see Figure 16-8) of breast development should have a breast examination as part of their regular physical. This also enables you to monitor breast development during puberty. All adolescent girls should be taught to perform a breast self-examination and to make it a routine part of their health behaviors.

All adolescents should be asked annually about involvement in sexual behaviors that may result in unwanted pregnancy and STDs, including infection with the human immunodeficiency virus (HIV). Sexually active adolescent girls should have a cervical culture and boys should have urine leukocyte esterase analysis to screen for gonorrhea. The frequency of screening for STDs depends on the sexual practices of the adolescent involved. All sexually active girls or any young women 18 years or older should be screened annually for cervical cancer with a Papanicolaou (Pap) test. Adolescents at risk for HIV infection should be offered confidential HIV screening (AMA, 2001).

Focused Assessment for *Delayed Growth and Development*

Assessment of growth and development is a routine part of a well-child assessment from birth through school age. It is based on knowledge of normal growth and development and the methods of eliciting information from the child and the parent.

Defining Characteristics. The defining characteristics related to the nursing diagnosis *Delayed growth and development* are observed behaviors that indicate that the individual is experiencing an alteration in growth and development. They include the following:

- Delay or difficulty in performing skills (motor, social, or expressive) typical of the child's age-group
- Altered physical growth (weight or height)
- Inability to perform self-care or self-control activities appropriate for the child's age

Related Factors. Children are at risk for problems of growth and development from both internal and external factors. Physical development requires health, nutrition, and exercise. Psychosocial development requires opportunities to complete developmental tasks with a warm, caring adult to guide the way. The particular risks that are common for children are illness, lead poisoning, substance abuse, TB, safety, home life, and school.

Children who have chronic illnesses, unstable family lives, teenage mothers, or multiple caregivers are at risk for *Delayed growth and development*. If you practice in a hospital, you will know that a child who is withdrawn or whose behavior is inappropriate for the age may be reacting to the hospital or may have a larger developmental problem. During the child's health maintenance visit in the clinic, you can pick up cues by listening to the parent's description of the child and by observing the child's behavior.

Related factors for *Delayed growth and development* can be divided into two categories: those of the parent and those of the child. You need to decide whether the problem of *Delayed growth and development* can best be solved by working directly with the child or with the parent. Parenting style and parenting skills are basic related factors for *Delayed growth and development*. Physiological factors should be considered if a disability or chronic disease is present. The care plan would then include modifications that take the disability into account.

If the parents lack the skills to provide a lifestyle conducive to healthy growth, or if they are just indifferent to the child's needs, development may be hampered. Consistency is important in parenting. Parents who respond sporadically to the child's needs or vacillate between positive and negative responses will not provide the child with a consistent pattern of caring that is needed to enable the child to choose healthy behaviors.

Related factors in the child category include the following:
- Environmental and stimulation deficiencies
- Prescribed dependence
- Separation from significant others
- Effects of physical disability
- Prematurity

Related factors in the parent or caregiver category include the following:
- Disadvantaged social environment
- Poor support system
- Inadequate caretaking
- Indifference
- Inconsistent responsiveness
- Multiple caregivers

Upon assessment of Yung Hi, you see many of the related factors characteristic of a child with *Delayed growth and development*. Yung is a toddler in a private room and is on complete bed rest, with 8 weeks of traction to endure. She must depend totally on others. She is separated from her home and usual routine. Yung's physical disability limits her level of activity, and she cannot speak English. Her mother spends most of the day with her; however, when her father comes to visit in the evenings, he takes Yung's mother home with him. Have you determined any other related factors?

Focused Assessment for *Ineffective Health Maintenance*

The nursing diagnosis *Ineffective health maintenance* refers to an inability to identify, manage, or seek out help to maintain health. It is a state in which a person experiences, or is at risk of experiencing, a disruption in wellness from an unhealthy lifestyle. An alteration in health maintenance is almost never under the control of infants or toddlers; therefore you will need to assess the parent or family. As the child grows, you will begin to do health teaching with the child and certainly with the adolescent.

Defining Characteristics. The defining characteristics for *Ineffective health maintenance* include demonstration of an unhealthy lifestyle, lack of interest in health maintenance, and reported or observed inability to take responsibility for meeting basic health needs in any or all functional areas. Other characteristics may include an inability to follow instructions, impaired cognitive functioning, and a lack of adaptive behaviors to internal or external environmental changes.

For the infant, toddler, and child, altered health maintenance is a reflection of family health practices. Parents who lack education, have a history of substance use or abuse, are single parents, lack support systems, have financial distress, or have a chronic illness may present problems for the child's health and wellness. You can pick up further cues when discussing child immunization schedules with the parent, such as the parent's inability to concentrate or follow instructions or a lack of interest in making the next scheduled well-baby visit that includes immunizations.

Although adolescents continue to be influenced by family health practices, they are beginning to make health decisions for themselves and should be encouraged to develop healthy practices. Adolescents have an increased risk for the diagnosis *Ineffective health maintenance* because of their high-risk health behaviors, such as substance abuse, poor nutrition, and reckless driving. They often have feelings of invulnerability, coupled with peer pressure to engage in high-risk behaviors, which puts them at risk for physical illness, psychosocial problems, or death.

Related Factors. Related factors for *Ineffective health maintenance* involve the parents and the child or adolescent and may include the following:
- Ineffective individual or family coping
- Perceptual/cognitive impairment (complete or partial lack of gross or fine motor skills)
- Lack of, or significant alteration in, communication skills (written, verbal, or gestural)
- Unachieved developmental tasks
- Lack of material resources
- Dysfunctional grieving
- Disabling spiritual distress
- Lack of ability to make deliberate and thoughtful judgments

Focused Assessment for *Impaired Parenting*

A health maintenance visit for the school-age child includes an assessment of the parent's ability to provide a constructive environment that nurtures the growth and development of the child. During the health maintenance visit, look for cues by observing the interaction between the child and the parent and by listening to their descriptions of developmental issues and concerns.

Defining Characteristics. The defining characteristics of the nursing diagnosis *Impaired parenting* are observed delays in growth and development, observed inappropriate parenting behaviors, or concern with parenting skills expressed by the parent. Evidence of child abuse is a clear defining characteristic of *Impaired parenting*.

Related Factors. Difficulties in parenting can be related to a lack of knowledge or lack of exposure to positive parenting practices. Situational or personal factors may contribute to parental role conflicts.

Diagnosis

Once the components of the assessment are completed, you will determine a nursing diagnosis, as demonstrated in Table 16-3 (p. 322). The choice of a nursing diagnosis involving a child's growth and development in the first 3 years after birth depends on the problems identified and the etiological factors of the diagnosis. When the history and physical examination

Table 16-3	*Clustering Data to Make a Nursing Diagnosis*	
GROWTH AND DEVELOPMENT PROBLEMS		
Data Cluster		**Diagnosis**
30-month-old boy admitted to hospital for malnutrition. Height and weight below 15th percentile on growth charts. Child is lethargic and nonverbal. Mother reports withholding food when he cries.		*Delayed growth and development* related to inappropriate caregiving and possibly parental indifference
Unemployed teenage mother of 2-year-old unable to present immunization health record. Mother expresses lack of knowledge about "kids needing shots." Toddler diagnosed with mumps.		*Ineffective health maintenance* related to lack of knowledge and possibly lack of financial resources
Parents make and meet each scheduled well-child appointment for their school-age child. Child's immunizations are complete.		*Health-seeking behaviors* related to desire to obtain higher level of wellness through prevention
Jose is a 16-year-old who had above-average grades until this year. When his friends made the football team, he started hanging out with a different group. He has been arrested for reckless driving and possession of marijuana. His physician referred him to a psychiatric nurse practitioner for counseling.		*Ineffective individual coping* related to establishing peer relationships through reckless behavior
Marie is 17. She has made straight A's throughout school. She is in the school choir and on the newspaper staff and the drill team. Marie is thin and appears underdeveloped for her age. The nurse records her height at 5' 8" and weight at 98 lbs in an exam gown. Marie says that she thinks a lot about how fat she is.		*Disturbed body image* related to a distorted belief about her weight
William has been cutting classes and not doing his homework. His affect is flat; he says he wakes up at 4 in the morning and is tired all the time. His mother is afraid he is using drugs and brings him to a nurse practitioner for a physical exam. William denies using drugs but admits to planning his death, probably by taking his father's medication.		*Risk for violence* related to suicidal ideation

reveal abnormal growth or development parameters resulting from environmental deprivation, physical disability, or an acute problem, *Delayed growth and development* is an appropriate choice for a nursing diagnosis.

Because parenting style and parenting skills are related factors for *Delayed growth and development,* you will need to distinguish between the diagnoses *Impaired parenting, Ineffective family coping,* and *Delayed growth and development.* If the problem involves family functioning, such as an alcoholic or abusive family, you may choose *Ineffective family coping.* The approach to treatment then becomes centered on the family.

If you are working primarily with the parent and indirectly with the children, the diagnosis is more likely to be *Impaired parenting.* The defining characteristics of *Impaired parenting* suggest that the diagnosis refers to the more serious behaviors that define a parent's inability to relate positively to the child.

The nursing diagnosis *Ineffective health maintenance* is directly related to growth and development, but it has a different focus. Positive health practices help to ensure that growth and development proceed normally. Although this diagnosis is typically used for a well child who has no obvious problems, family health practices may place the child at risk for growing up unhealthy or for contracting specific illnesses or health problems of childhood, such as measles or dental caries.

Deficient diversional activity may be the appropriate nursing diagnosis for a child experiencing a restriction in, or decreased stimulation from, recreational or play activities. *Deficient diversional activity* influences developmental growth. It is associated with any prolonged hospitalization—for example, it can be used for Yung Hi, whose fractured femur required 8 weeks of traction. It is also an appropriate diagnosis for a homebound child with a chronic or disabling condition. Defining characteristics include isolation with limited ability to leave the room; lack of age-appropriate toys at the bedside; physical limitations affecting participation in usual activities; and irritability, moodiness, and inactivity.

You may find that *Deficient diversional activity* is also a related factor for other nursing diagnoses.

PLANNING

Planning a comprehensive, consistent care plan for wellness will include elements of the nursing diagnoses *Delayed growth and development* and *Ineffective health maintenance.*

Expected Outcomes for *Delayed Growth and Development.*
The expected outcome criteria for a child with altered growth and development are an increase in the child's weight, height, or both, and a demonstration of social, language, cognitive, or motor activities appropriate for the child's age. Additional outcome criteria for children or parents are the following:

- Children's participation in daily physical activities is appropriate for their age.
- The child experiences no injuries (other than normal cuts and bruises) from play activities or other activities of daily living.
- Parents will bring their child to a dentist at least once a year, and the child brushes and flosses teeth (under adult supervision) at least once daily.
- Parents will bring their child for recommended screening tests at appropriate times.
- An older school-age child understands his growth and development patterns.

Expected Outcomes for *Ineffective Health Maintenance.*
The overall expected outcome criteria for a client with altered health maintenance are that the child is present for all scheduled health maintenance visits and maintains health status. Other outcomes for this diagnosis are the following:

- Parents describe an appropriate health maintenance program.
- Parents demonstrate behaviors needed to manage the child's health alteration.
- Parents identify health resources available, such as pediatric nurse practitioner, nutritionist, and dentist.
- Child receives all scheduled immunizations.
- Parents use appropriate safety measures, such as car seats and age-appropriate toys.
- Children progress to at least their average performance levels in schoolwork and activities.

Plan primary prevention strategies with adolescents, with the goal of discouraging them from participating in high-risk behaviors. When planning care for well adolescents, focus your teaching on specific high-risk behaviors while incorporating teaching about all risk behaviors in an effort to prevent them. Because adolescence is normally a time of risk taking, chronically ill teens may have the additional problem of engaging in risk-taking behavior by failing to comply with their treatment regimen. It is essential to include the adolescent as an active partner in developing appropriate responses to the risk situation.

*I*NTERVENTION

Newborns, Infants, and Toddlers

Implementation of your care plan to promote healthy growth and development as well as health maintenance will involve working closely with the child's parents. Education of parents is the primary choice of intervention for both diagnoses.

Interventions to Promote Growth and Development.

Nurses play an important role in promoting healthy growth and development through informing and teaching parents of newborns, infants, and toddlers. Appropriate parenting skills in relation to attachment, play, nutrition, toilet training, rest and sleep, caring for a sick child, and referrals are the realms of the interventions discussed.

PROMOTING ATTACHMENT. Attachment is an ongoing process that begins during pregnancy and intensifies during the months after birth. Once established, it is a constant and consistent relationship. Attachment is strengthened by intense communication between parent and child through eye-to-eye contact, touch, voice, odor, and reciprocal, synchronous activity.

TEACHING PARENTING SKILLS. These days there are fewer opportunities to teach parents basic baby-care techniques. Another opportunity for parent education occurs during each well-child visit. Take time to answer parents' questions about childcare and child-rearing issues, such as discipline, sleep disturbances, and nutritional needs. Suggest classes, support groups, literature, and other resources.

Table 16-4	Age-Appropriate Toys
Age	**Appropriate Toys**
0 to 3 months	• Mobiles
	• Soft toys
4 to 7 months	• Toys with sounds and fingerholds
	• Rattles
	• Vinyl books
8 to 12 months	• Toys that float, squirt, or hold water
	• Busy boxes
	• Different-size containers or cups
	• Books
1 to 2 years	• Kitchen and tool sets with large parts
	• Dress-up clothes
	• Trucks, cars, and dolls
	• Books
	• Sandbox
2 to 3 years	• Pegboards with large pegs
	• Shape sorters
	• Nontoxic paints, crayons
	• Simple jigsaw puzzles
	• Tricycle

CREATIVE PLAY. Each newborn, infant, and toddler is a unique individual. Encourage parents to respect and enjoy their baby's individuality. This will help parents establish the best possible foundation for their child's development, high self-esteem, and healthy relationships with others. Discuss with parents appropriate toys available to stimulate the infant's and toddler's nervous systems to achieve developmental milestones (Table 16-4).

FEEDING AND ELIMINATION. Instruct parents that an infant should have six to eight wet diapers a day, sometimes more. Whether their infant is fed at the breast or by bottle will determine how many bowel movements there are in a day: breast-fed babies have more frequent stools. Tell parents that they will begin to notice a regular pattern in bowel and bladder elimination at around 8 months.

Inform parents that, when their child reaches 12 to 18 months, the growth rate begins to slow, decreasing the child's need for fluids and calories. Because of this decrease in nutritional needs, most children exhibit a decrease in appetite. Toddlers begin to feel a need to be in control of their abilities. By about 18 months, most toddlers become more picky and fussy about foods. Inform parents that good eating habits are established in the first 3 years after birth. By giving their child nutritious meals and snacks, they will be helping to set the stage for future food consumption.

Inform parents that, as their infant becomes a toddler, they can begin to assess for toilet-training readiness. Not only does their toddler have to show signs of physical, mental, and psychological readiness, but the parents must also be ready. Toddlers show physical signs of readiness by having regular bowel movements, being able to remove their own clothes, and staying dry for at least 2 hours or waking up dry from a nap. Mental readiness consists of being able to recognize the urge to urinate or defecate and to communicate, either verbally or nonverbally, the need to use the toilet. Psychologically, the toddler will show curiosity about siblings' or adults' toilet habits. The toddler tends to become impatient with a soiled or wet diaper and wants to be changed immediately.

Besides recognizing the child's readiness for toilet training, the parents need to be willing to invest the time needed for toilet training. Parents should make this process as positive, natural, and nonthreatening as possible. Instruct parents that their toddler should be ready to begin between the ages of 18 and 24 months. Bowel training is usually accomplished before bladder training because it is more predictable and has a more regular pattern.

REST AND SLEEP. Inform parents that, at first, newborns sleep about 16 hours a day in 3- to 4-hour stretches between feedings. Parents should be instructed to position newborns on their backs at all times. Research has shown this position appears to prevent sudden infant death syndrome (SIDS). As they get older and their stomachs grow, they go longer between feedings. By 2 months, they are more alert and social and will be awake more during the day. Because of the increased stomach capacity, they may skip a night feeding. By 3 months, parents will be happy to know, their child may be sleeping through the night.

At 4 months, parents should expect their infant to need only two naps a day, each lasting 1 to 3 hours. A consistent bedtime routine will help their infant to wind down at the end of the day. Such a routine may consist of a warm bath, rocking, stories, or soft music.

As the infant approaches 8 months, separation anxiety begins to increase. The child may resist going to bed and may wake up more often, looking for a parent. This is the time to introduce a transitional object (such as a blanket or teddy bear) to comfort the child when parents are not present. Stress the importance of following a consistent pattern or bedtime ritual.

As the child becomes a toddler, delaying tactics may be used. Tell parents to stick to the bedtime routine. During this age, dreams begin. Cutting teeth, a change in routine, or illness can also make an infant or toddler awaken more frequently in the night. Encourage parents to give attention to children's distress, but to let the children know they are to keep to their bedtime routine.

At 2 to 3 years, the child may take a single 1- to 2-hour nap around lunchtime. Some children may give up naps entirely. Again, inform parents that their child may begin to resist going to sleep. Part of this is from separation anxiety and part from the negativity stage of development. Giving the child choices at bedtime helps. A night-light may become necessary. Nightmares may also awaken toddlers. Parents should hold and comfort their child until they are calm enough to fall back to sleep.

Interventions to Promote Health Maintenance.

Interventions related to health maintenance include assisting parents with scheduling health maintenance visits so their children can receive preventive healthcare. Also, teach parents about immunizations, child safety, and dental care. Again, education of the parents is the primary intervention.

IMMUNIZATIONS. One of your most important tasks is to inform parents of the reasons for routine immunizations. Children are susceptible to disease because they have an immature immune system. Immunization protects the child from being infected and prevents the infection of others at day care centers.

When administered properly, immunizations provide the most cost-effective contribution to the health of children worldwide. They are recommended in an established schedule for healthy infants and children (Figure 16-9). Instruct parents on the importance of completing all scheduled immunizations. Give them an immunization schedule. Inform them of the common side effects of each vaccine. Although most side effects are mild, the parents need to know what to expect. Mild discomfort is normal, with slight fever, rash, or soreness at the site of injection. Serious reactions to vaccines are rare. If the child is immunodeficient because of acquired immunodeficiency syndrome (AIDS), an organ transplant, or immunosuppressive therapy, the parents should consult their physician about vaccines.

Parents should retain a vaccination record and have it updated each time the child receives a scheduled vaccination. A vaccination and health record will help the parents when they move to a new area or have a change of health care provider, or when their child attends day care, preschool, or elementary school. Work closely with parents to establish and maintain a schedule of immunizations.

SAFETY. Accidents are a leading cause of death of infants and toddlers. Many accidents result from a child's natural curiosity and exploration of the environment. Some common accidents are aspiration, choking, falls, burns, car accidents, and drowning. A vital part of assessing for potential accidents is to ask parents about safety hazards in the child's environment. For example, do the parents ever leave their baby or toddler unattended in the bath?

To give yourself a baseline for educational interventions, determine the parents' knowledge about safety and accident prevention. Many parents are unaware of the potential dangers that can be found in a home. The potential for serious injury is ever-present. If parents are made aware of these dangers, they may be able to prevent devastating consequences.

Action Alert! Infants lying unattended on raised surfaces such as counters and beds are at risk for falling and suffering severe injury. Keep crib rails up at all times, and use barriers to block stairways to prevent injuries to toddlers.

Exploration plays an integral part in the psychological development of the infant and toddler. As soon as locomotion is established, the parents should use gates as a means to control the infant's access to various areas. Instruct parents about safety latches that can be applied to drawers and cupboards that contain dangerous materials. Give parents the telephone number of the local poison control center and emergency department, and tell them to post the number near the telephone. Also, tell parents to keep syrup of ipecac in the medicine cabinet, and give them guidelines for its use.

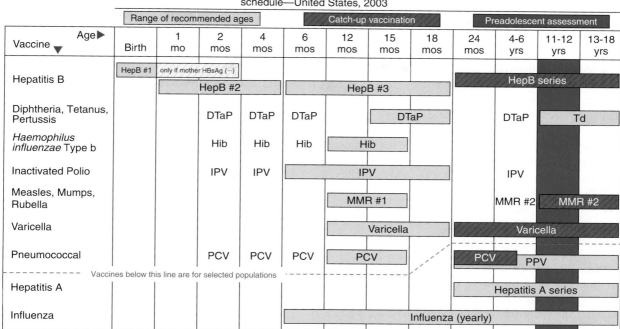

Figure 16-9. Recommended childhood immunization schedule, United Sates, 2003. (Redrawn from *American Academy of Pediatrics recommended childhood immunization schedule January-December 2001.* Available at www.aap.org/family/parents/immunize.htm.)

Playthings, although valuable in enhancing a child's development, may also cause injuries, accidents, or death. Teach parents to screen toys for age appropriateness. Children younger than age 3 should not have toys with small, removable parts on which they could choke. Instruct parents to check toys routinely for loose parts or sharp edges. All paints, crayons, molding clays, and other craft items should be nontoxic.

Accidents can occur when food is ingested too quickly or is too large to be swallowed safely. Therefore, food should also be age appropriate. As the infant progresses from liquids to solids, parents may mash, grind, or cook food until it is soft enough to swallow without chewing. When foods are prepared appropriately, toddlers can eat many of the same things their parents eat.

Action Alert! Prevent aspiration of foreign objects such as buttons, coins, and food (such as hot dogs) by not giving such small, hard objects to infants and toddlers. Choking can lead to respiratory arrest and death.

Accidental drowning is responsible for approximately 4000 deaths (including all age groups) per year in the United States. Males are affected 2 to 3 times more than females. Older infants and toddlers are disproportionately represented in these accidents. Warn parents that an infant or toddler can drown in only a few inches of water. Bathtubs, toilets, water buckets, and swimming pools are the usual sites of drowning (Baum, 2000).

Burns are another source of injury common to infants or toddlers. Instruct parents that they should never hold an infant or toddler when smoking, holding hot liquids, or cooking. Hot liquids or food should never be left near the edge of tables or counters. Tell parents to test bath water before putting a child into it. Also tell them to set their hot water heater at 120° F or lower.

Just as safety is important in the home, it is also important when traveling. A federally approved, properly installed car seat must be used at all times. Infants should sit facing backward in the car until they can sit independently. No infant or child should sit in the front seat of a car with a passenger-side air bag. A car seat should be used throughout the toddler stage of development.

DENTAL CARE. Dental health is important even for infants and young children. By age 3, some children already show alarming tooth decay. Neglected dental problems can lead to infection and subsequent tooth loss. Teach parents that healthy "baby teeth" influence the formation of healthy gums and permanent teeth. Ask the parents if the child has any history of dental problems or mouth pain. Ask if the infant or child is given fruit juice when put to bed. To prevent cavities, instruct parents to never let their child fall asleep with a bottle. This habit promotes decay because fluid pools around the teeth.

Action Alert! Inform parents that early childhood dental caries occur when a bottle of juice or milk is used as a pacifier at night.

Inform parents that dental hygiene is essential from the time of their child's first feeding. Even before the first teeth erupt, the child's mouth should be cleaned with a damp gauze or cloth after each feeding. On average, the first tooth erupts at 6 months. Some children show mild signs of drooling and increased finger sucking when teething. Other children become irritable and may refuse to eat. At the eruption of the first tooth, parents should begin to brush the tooth with a soft toothbrush and continue to assist their child with brushing through age 3.

Early screening for signs of caries or cavity development, starting during the first year after birth, could identify infants and toddlers who are at risk of developing early childhood caries. High-risk children include those with early signs of tooth decay, poor oral hygiene, limited exposure to fluorides, and frequent exposure to sugary snacks and drinks (Ismail, 1998).

Preschool and School-Age Children

Through the use of a thorough assessment process, you identify problems that affect children's growth and development. Your interventions will be based on establishing a trusting relationship with your clients and their families and incorporating their cultural beliefs in your interventions. The main interventions for *Delayed growth and development* and *Impaired parenting* are health education and counseling.

Interventions to Promote Health. Education and anticipatory guidance are the best preventive measures for parents of preschool and school-age children. Families need to understand normal growth and development and nurturing child care practices. Teaching parents how to determine when it is necessary to contact health care providers promotes good decision making about self-care. Box 16-6 lists selected reasons for parents to contact a health care provider.

- Teach parents the importance of teaching children to eat nutritious foods by using the food guide pyramid: milk and dairy products, lean meat, fish, poultry, fruits and vegetables, and breads and cereals.
- Parents should encourage their children in lifetime fitness activities such as walking, running, bicycling, and swimming.

| Box 16-6 | Reasons for Parents to Contact a Health Care Provider |

- Routine well-child examinations and immunizations
- Drastic changes in their child's behavior
- Severe pain
- Severe or worrisome injury
- Prolonged high fever (over 102° F [38.9° C])
- Persistent cough
- Foul-smelling drainage from the nose, eyes, ears, or anywhere else
- Persistent vomiting
- Unexplained persistent rash
- Prolonged diarrhea
- Blood in urine or stool

Action Alert! Encourage parents whose children are obese to participate in physical activities. Obese children tend to be less active, which reduces metabolism and increases fat accumulation.

- Parents are responsible for seeing that their children get 10 to 12 hours of sleep to function effectively during the day (American Academy of Pediatrics, 1998b). They must promote regular sleeping habits in their children.
- Antismoking efforts must begin before adolescence. It is important to talk with school-age children about the adverse health effects of smoking and how children can resist peer pressures. Instead of just going along with the crowd, the child needs the skills and confidence to make correct decisions.
- Children's early years are a critical time for the socializing effects of television, computer games, movie, and video game viewing habits. Encourage parents to set reasonable limits on the amount of time their children watch television, use a computer, or play video games. Encourage them to watch programs with their children.

Action Alert! Advise parents that when their children spend hours in front of a television, computer, or video game, they are missing the opportunity to develop their physical and social skills by playing with siblings or friends instead of being sedentary and solitary.

Interventions to Promote Effective Parenting. The purpose of discipline is to instruct children in proper conduct or action rather than to punish children. The ultimate goal of disciplinary action is to teach children to develop a sense of inner control so that they can follow generally accepted standards of behavior and live in accord with the rules and regulations established by the group (Blum, 1995). Disciplinary methods recommended by the American Academy of Pediatrics include showing children the natural consequences of their actions, as long as they do not place the child in danger. The Academy also recommends withholding privileges, and as a last resort, a time-out.

During the preschool years, it is important that a child have opportunities for peer interaction. A preschool child who has learned to be comfortable in groups is better able to learn in kindergarten. Explain to parents that interacting with older siblings is not the same as interacting in a group experience with peers.

The most important task for children in early school years is learning to read. Parents can serve as role models by reading books, magazines, and newspapers instead of watching television. Encourage parents to read aloud to their children at bedtime, to play word games with them, and to have them read simple directions to them. Some children may experience school phobia, the fear of attending school. Because fear is one of the most powerful negative human emotions, children may use physical symptoms such as vomiting, headache, or abdominal pain as an excuse to stay home from school. Explain to parents that they must determine the reason for their child's resistance to school before they can help the child to overcome the fear. Refer the child and family to a counselor if the phobia persists.

Interventions to Prevent Injury. No child can be considered free from risk of injury. Your awareness of some injury patterns may be helpful in counseling parents. The type of injuries to which a child is most vulnerable varies with personal circumstances and the child's age, size, and developmental ability. Parents of preschool-age children must realize that although their children's skills are becoming sophisticated, their judgment is not. Preschoolers cannot be relied on to recognize danger. In contrast, school-age children are less likely to experience unintentional injuries because they have developed more refined muscular coordination and have the cognitive abilities to avoid injuring themselves. It is often difficult for parents to maintain a balance between the level of supervision and restriction and their children's need for independence.

> *Action Alert!* Advise adolescents in early puberty to avoid collision sports and intense, prolonged physical training. Make their parents aware of the potential for harm.

PROMOTING HOME SAFETY. There are many safety tips you can share with parents during well-child visits to prevent future injury.

> *Action Alert!* Teaching parents about child safety should be part of every well-child visit. Most accidents occur because parents overestimate or underestimate their child's abilities.

Fires present a special danger to young children, who cannot be depended on to react quickly in an emergency. When a fire occurs, children who have not been trained for a fire emergency may mistakenly try to hide in a "safe place." Smoke detectors should be placed in all hallways adjacent to bedrooms as well as near the kitchen area and the garage. Children should be instructed to leave the house at once in the presence of smoke or fire, even if the fire is small. Calls to 911 can be made from another home. Ask the family if fire drills are held regularly so that children can plan and rehearse all possible escape routes. Children should be taught to "stop, drop, and roll" if their clothing should catch fire. House fires are not the only threat. Many children are burned when they accidentally upset a cooking pot, touch a hot grill, or play with fireworks. Portable heaters are another source of danger.

> *Action Alert!* Teach children to avoid playing with matches, to know fire escape routes, and to practice fire escape drills at home. Teach them to avoid hot stoves and to avoid playing with flammable substances.

Ask parents about whether they own guns. If so, instruct them that guns should be locked away unloaded and separate from the ammunition.

The term *latchkey children* describes children in elementary school who spend some part of their time before or after school without adult supervision. The name arose from children who carried keys to let themselves into their homes be-

fore the parents returned from work. Inform parents of community resources available to latchkey children.

PROMOTING SAFETY AT PLAY. Bicycling injuries begin to take their toll during the early school-age years. Children of this age are still not capable of making accurate judgments about speed and distance. To fit in with their peer group, these children may neglect to wear helmets. Children should demonstrate safe riding skills and understand traffic safety laws before being allowed to ride a bicycle on the street. Inform parents of community guidelines for bicycle safety. Pamphlets and videos can help parents teach bicycle safety to their children.

> *Action Alert!* Remind parents that they must select the proper equipment and see that their child learns and obeys traffic laws when riding a bicycle.

If a child uses a skateboard, scooter, or in-line skates, a helmet is mandatory because these activities take place on hard surfaces such as concrete and there is great risk of head injury. Wrists, knees, and elbows also need protective gear. Children under the age of 5 should not use skateboards or in-line skates because they are not developmentally prepared to protect themselves from injury.

> *Action Alert!* Advise parents to enforce safety guidelines such as prohibiting their children to use their in-line skates or skateboards on streets and highways.

Drowning is a leading cause of death among preschool and school-age children. Advise parents that their children should learn how to swim from an experienced and qualified swimming instructor. When children ride in a boat, they should always wear a personal flotation device. Remind parents that children learn by example, so it is important that adults also follow safety guidelines.

Adolescents
Interventions to Prevent Illness. Primary prevention is clearly a key issue in adolescent health because most of the morbidities of adolescents are behavioral and therefore preventable. Client teaching is important, but research has repeatedly shown that knowledge alone does not result in behavior change. You must also be skilled in the techniques of primary prevention (Box 16-7, p. 328).

> *Action Alert!* Consider the factors that motivate adolescents to change their high-risk behaviors as you develop your health education strategies.

Box 16-7   Primary Prevention for Adolescents

- Yearly health checkup, including complete blood count, blood pressure, height, weight, Tanner stage
- Immunizations, including tetanus and diphtheria every 10 years, hepatitis B series, measles, mumps, rubella, hepatitis A for high-risk persons (including those traveling to endemic areas), and tuberculosis
- Health education about the risks of weapons, dangers of alcohol and drug use, drunk driving

Interventions to Overcome Health Care Barriers.
A barrier to implementing care for adolescents is their perceived lack of access to health care providers. Some adolescents do not seek health care because they feel uncomfortable both in their pediatrician's office, where they were treated as a child, and in clinics that primarily serve adults. They may also be uncomfortable divulging personal information about a potentially embarrassing topic, such as a suspected pregnancy, to either their parents or health care providers. Some adolescents are unaware of where to obtain care. Others may not live where clinics are conveniently located. Still others have parents who may not be aware of the health needs or concerns of their adolescents.

An important goal of care for working with adolescents is to withhold judgments about teens' behaviors and to treat them with respect. Consult with them on treatment decisions instead of dealing only with their parents, because they are in the process of gaining independence from their families. They will be more likely to comply with the treatment regimen when they take part in the decision-making process.

Although an important goal is to help adolescents establish independence, you also need to consider the importance of parents in the care of adolescents and their concerns about their adolescents. Many parents are overly protective and very anxious. You can help them understand normal adolescent developmental needs so that parents can avoid impeding the teen's growth.

Interventions Through School-Based Clinics.
Studies have shown that school-based clinics are an effective means of providing care to adolescents. They are often an integral part of the school where adolescents seek care, and teachers and administrators often refer students with health problems to them.

Many clinics are multidisciplinary, with on-site social workers and health educators. In most clinics, primary care health services are provided by nurse practitioners who consult with physicians. They provide reproductive health services aimed at reducing rates of teen pregnancy and sexually transmitted diseases, and they often provide primary care health services, care for chronic and episodic illnesses (such as asthma and ear infections), health education, and mental health services. Most school districts mandate health education programs. In addition to one-to-one care, the group approach used in schools is very effective for teens because they are peer oriented.

EVALUATION

To objectively evaluate the degree of success in achieving a goal or outcome, assess the infant, toddler, child, or adolescent for the presence or absence of the desired behavior or response, and determine the level of agreement between the outcome criteria and the actual response. If the overall outcome is not met, reassessment and changes in the plan of care

---

Nursing Care Plan A CLIENT AT RISK FOR ALTERED GROWTH AND DEVELOPMENT   Box 16-8

ADMISSION DATA

Yung Hi is admitted from the postanesthesia care unit to the orthopedic unit. The unit nurse receives the following report:

33-month-old Asian female child admitted to ER with displaced fracture of the right femur. No known allergies or medical conditions. Toddler had been playing in playground of apartment complex when she fell, and her older brother tripped and fell on her outstretched leg. No reported loss of consciousness. Mother witnessed the fall and (through translation) said that the child did not hit her head. The father attempted to move the child and, when unable, called for an ambulance. Right thigh demonstrated deformity with apparent misalignment of femur and no break in skin integrity. Closed reduction and placement of Steinmann pins to right tibia for Buck's traction of right femur under general anesthesia in OR. Stable during procedure and while in recovery. Vitals: VP 92/48, pulse 146, respirations 38. Popliteal, posttibial, and pedal pulses present bilaterally with right pulses 12 and left 13. No other significant physical findings. Call in to physical therapy to place traction in room.

PHYSICIAN'S ORDERS

Admitting diagnosis: displaced fracture of right femur.
Surgical procedure: closed reduction right femur with Steinmann pin placement right tibia.
Bed rest with balanced suspension traction to Steinmann pins, 5 lb to each weight.
Do not elevate head of bed until further notice.
Neurovascular checks to right leg every 30 minutes × 4; every 1 hour × 4, then every 4 hours
Diet as tolerated.
Children's Tylenol with codeine 5 mL PO q3-4h PRN pain.
Colace elixir 30 mg PO every day.

NURSING ASSESSMENT

Drowsy and nonverbal. Mother at bedside. Mother reports no pain expressed. Vital signs stable. Traction in place to right leg with 5 lb to each weight. No redness, drainage, or swelling around pin sites at right tibia. Able to wiggle toes. Leg and foot pink and warm to touch, capillary refill approximately 2 seconds. Pedal and posttibial pulses strong (+2) bilaterally. Edema +1 noted to right leg and foot with large ecchymosis noted medial right thigh. Lung sounds clear bilaterally A & P. Positive bowel sounds, voiding adequate amounts clear, yellow urine in diaper. No skin breakdown noted over bony prominences at sacrum, heels, and scapulae.

Nursing Care Plan **A CLIENT AT RISK FOR ALTERED GROWTH AND DEVELOPMENT—CONT'D**   Box 16-8

NANDA Nursing Diagnosis	NOC Expected Outcomes With Indicators	NIC Interventions With Selected Activities	Evaluation Data
RISK FOR DELAYED GROWTH AND DEVELOPMENT **Related Factor:** • Diversional activity deficit and immobility secondary to traction	**PLAY PARTICIPATION** • Continue to demonstrate physical, psychosocial, and cognitive skills of previous stage of growth and development. • Maintain range of motion and strength. • Participate in age-appropriate play. • Demonstrate increased understanding of treatments. • Select and play with age-appropriate toys. • Express enjoyment in selected play activities. • Achieve developmental tasks appropriate to age.	**ACTIVITY THERAPY** • Ask family members to bring child's favorite toys, family pictures, and other objects from home to place at bedside. • Consult physical therapist (PT) for strength and range-of-motion exercises. • Consult play therapist and have therapist come when both parents present. • Provide child with opportunities for therapeutic play. • Place developmentally appropriate toys conductive to immobility at the bedside. • Schedule times to engage child in developmental play during day and early evening shift. • Monitor developmental status and progress at regular intervals.	**AFTER 24 HOURS OF CARE** • Parents brought in favorite stuffed bunny and blanket, pictures of each family member, and favorite book. • PT consulted. Will work with client T.I.D. Asked parents to be present to learn exercises and to help translate to client. • Play therapist met with parents and child. Favorite toys, music, and activities discussed. • Played nurse and doctor, with favorite stuffed rabbit as the client in traction. • Crayons, paints, pegboard, books, and stuffed animals at bedside. • Met with client and played at 10 A.M, 1 P.M, and 7 A.M. Parents, PT, and play therapist also with client and conducted play and physical activity. • Age-appropriate play, talks with mother and father, sings. Says "thank you" in English and nods head at same time.

CRITICAL THINKING QUESTIONS

1. Which developmental theory would you apply to Yung to assist you in caring for her? Why would you choose one theory over the other?

2. Yung wanted to keep her stuffed rabbit in traction after the therapeutic play session was over. Why do you think Yung wanted to do this?

Nursing outcome and intervention labels from Johnson, M., Bulechek, G., McCloskey Dochterman, J. M., Maas, M., & Moorhead, S. (2001). *Nursing diagnoses, outcomes, and interventions: NANDA, NOC, and NIC linkages.* St Louis, MO: Mosby.

would be warranted. It may be that another nursing diagnosis would be a better choice. Refer to Box 16-8 to see an example of nursing process in action. A discharge note for Yung Hi might look like this:

> **SAMPLE DOCUMENTATION NOTE FOR YUNG HI**
> Discharged with parent to return home per automobile. Able to walk bearing weight on leg. Happy to be going home. Behavior is age appropriate. Parents will encourage physical activity; expected to quickly resume normal physical activity for age. Has appointment with pediatrician in 1 week.

At this time you and the parents review the problems identified at the last visit and discuss whether and how they were resolved. It is not unusual for some problems to be resolved and replaced by new and different concerns. Finally, as part of the well child's annual evaluation, you should assess how the parents are adjusting to their changing role as their child grows and develops. It is important that the parents' expectations be realistic and that they promote their children's growth and development.

With many of the behavioral problems of adolescence, you will not have an objective, accurate measure of the outcome. For example, to evaluate a change in drinking habits, you will need to rely on the adolescent's report. However, if the adolescent does not feel completely comfortable with you, you may receive an inaccurate report. One objective way to look for a change in a teen's weekend drinking would be to check his attendance record on Mondays. Likewise, an objective way to evaluate an increase in condom use would be to check for a change in how often the client seeks treatment for sexually transmitted diseases.

Key Principles

• Although the terms *growth* and *development* are often used synonymously, they have separate and distinct definitions. Growth refers to a physiological process, whereas development involves the maturation of body organs and the acquisition of appropriate cognitive, linguistic, and psychosocial skills.

• Developmental theories attempt to explain how the human organism matures and acquires appropriate cognitive, linguistic, and psychosocial skills.

- Nursing process guides nursing care for the well infant, well child, and well adolescent.
- The use of nursing diagnoses guides the management of problems involving growth and development or altered health maintenance.
- Children progress through similar stages of growth and development, but the rate of progression and the behaviors observed vary with the individual.
- Understanding children's growth and development enables the nurse to individualize approaches to the child's health care needs on the basis of developmental variations in each stage.
- The nursing diagnosis *Altered growth and development* is appropriate for the infant, child, and adolescent who is not achieving normal physical growth or is not accomplishing the developmental tasks of the particular age-group.
- The nursing diagnosis *Altered parenting* is used when the family environment does not provide the basic needs for a child's physical growth and development.
- Evaluation of the well child is a systematic, ongoing process in which the nurse evaluates the child's progress toward attainment of goals. The nurse and the child's parents review the problems identified at the last visit, discuss their resolution, and make adjustments as needed.
- Substance abuse and cigarette smoking are serious health problems among children and adolescents and have profound implications for their adult health.
- Several principles should guide your assessment of the child, adolescent, and the parents: ensure confidentiality, order the questions from least personal to most personal, do not be afraid to ask, and be respectful and nonjudgmental.
- Primary prevention is a key issue to child and adolescent health.
- Look for objective measures of outcome attainment in adolescents.

Bibliography

*Allshouse, M., Rouse, T., & Eichelberger, M. (1993). Childhood injury: A current perspective. *Pediatric Emergency Care, 9*(3): 159-164.

American Academy of Pediatric Dentistry (2002). Dental care for your baby. Retrieved from www.aapd.org/publications/brochures/babycare.asp.

American Academy of Pediatrics. (1998a). *AAP recommends targeted lead screening, universal screening in high-risk areas.* Retrieved from www.aap.org/advocacy/archives/junpol.htm, April 8, 1999.

American Academy of Pediatrics. (1998b). In S. P. Shelov & R. E. Hanneman (Eds.), *Caring for your baby and young child* [rev. ed.]. New York: Bantam Books.

American Medical Association. (2001). *Guidelines for adolescent preventive services (GAPS): Recommendations for physicians and other health professionals.* Available from www.ama-assn.org/ama/pub/category/2279.html.

Baum, C. R. (2000). Environmental emergencies. In G. R. Flisher & S. Ludwig (Eds.), *Textbook of pediatric emergencies* (4th ed.) (pp. 943-963). Philadelphia: Lippincott Williams & Wilkins.

Beck, L. E. (1998). *Development throughout the lifespan.* Needham Heights, MA: Allyn & Bacon.

Bee, H., & Boyd, D. (2002). *Lifespan development* (3rd ed.). Boston: Allyn & Bacon.

Blum, N. J. (1995). Disciplining young children: The role of verbal instructions and reasoning. *Pediatrics, 96*(2), 336-341.

Bowden, Y. R., Dickey, S. B., & Greenberg, C. S. (1998). *Children and their families: The continuum of care.* Philadelphia: Saunders.

*Bowlby, J. (1969). *Attachment and loss.* New York: Basic Books.

Burstein, G. R., Gaydos, C. A., Diener-West, M., Howell, M. R., Zenilman, J. M., & Quinn, T. C. (1998). Incident *Chlamydia trachomatis* infections among inner-city adolescent females. *Journal of the American Medical Association, 280,* 521-526.

Centers for Disease Control and Prevention. (1998a). *CDC's lead poisoning prevention program.* Retrieved from www.cdc.gov/nceh/pubcatns/97fsheet/leadfcts/leadfcts.htm, April 10, 1999.

Centers for Disease Control and Prevention. (1998b). *Socioeconomic status and health chartbook in health, United States, 1998.* Available from www.cdc.gov/nchswww/products/pubs/pubd/hus/2010/98chtbk.htm, Feb. 1, 1999.

Cherow, E., Dickman, D. M., & Epstein, S. (1999). Organization resources for families of children with deafness or hearing loss. *Pediatric Clinics of North America, 46*(1), 153-162.

Cowan, P. A. (1978). *Piaget: With feeling.* New York: Holt, Rinehart & Winston.

Cunningham, F. G. (2001). *Williams obstetrics* (21st ed.). Norwalk, CT: McGraw-Hill

Desselle, D. D., & Pearlmutter, L. (1997). Navigating two cultures: Self-esteem and parents' communication patterns. *Social Work Education, 19*(1), 23-30.

Division of Adolescent and School Health, National Center for Chronic Disease Prevention and Health Promotion, CDC. *HIV Instruction and Selected HIV-Risk Behaviors Among High School Students: United States—1989-1991. Morbidity and Mortality Weekly Review, 41*(46), 866-868. Available at www.cdc.gov/epo/mmwr.

*Elkind, D. (1992). Cognitive development. In S. B. Friedman, M. Fisher, & S. K. Schoenberg (Eds.), *Comprehensive adolescent health care* (pp. 24-26). St Louis, MO: Quality Medical.

*Erikson, E. H. (1968). Childhood and society (2nd ed.). New York: Norton.

*Havighurst, R. J. (1972). *Developmental tasks and education.* New York: David McKey.

Hickey, J., & Goldberg, F. (1996). *Ultrasound review of obstetrics and gynecology.* Philadelphia: Lippincott-Raven.

Hoekelman, R. A. (1998). The physical examination of infants and children. In B. Bates (Ed.), *A guide to physical examination and history taking* (7th ed.) (pp. 555-625). Philadelphia: Lippincott.

Ismail, A. I. (1998). Prevention of early childhood caries. *Community Dentistry and Oral Epidemiology, 26*(1), 49-61.

Jellinek, M. (1998). Attention-deficit hyperactivity disorder. In R. A. Dershewitz (Ed.), *Ambulatory pediatric care* (3rd ed.). Philadelphia: Lippincott.

Johnson, M., Bulechek, G., McCloskey Dochterman, J. M., Maas, M., & Moorhead, S. (2001). *Nursing diagnoses, outcomes, and interventions: NANDA, NOC, and NIC linkages.* St Louis, MO: Mosby.

Jorde, L. B., Carey, J. C., Barnshad, M. J., & White, R. L. (2000). *Medical genetics* (2nd ed.). St Louis, MO: Mosby.

Keefer, C. H. (1998). The well child. In R. A. Dershewitz (Ed.), *Ambulatory pediatric care* (3rd ed.). Philadelphia: Lippincott.

Kenny, T. J., & Nitz, K. (2000). Mental retardation. In R. A. Hoekelman, S. B. Friedman, N. M. Nelson, M. L. Weitzman, & M. H. Wilson (Eds.), *Primary pediatric care* (4th ed.) (pp. 409-412). St Louis, MO: Mosby.

*Asterisk indicates a classic or definitive work on this subject.

*Klaus, M. H., & Kennell, J. H. (1982). *Parent-infant bonding* (2nd ed.). St Louis, MO: Mosby.

*Kohlberg, L. (1966). A cognitive developmental analysis of children's sex role concepts and attitudes. In A. Macroby (Ed.), *The development of sex differences.* Palo Alto, CA: Stanford University.

*Kohlberg, L. (1981). *Philosophy of moral development: Moral stages and the idea of justice.* New York: Harper & Row.

Krug, E. F., & Mikus, C. (1999). The preschool years. In M. D. Levine, W. B. Carey, & A. Crockers (Eds.), *Developmental-Behavioral Pediatrics* (3rd ed.) (pp. 51-68). Philadelphia: Saunders.

Kulin, H. E., & Muller, J. (1996). The biological aspects of puberty. *Pediatrics in Review, 17*(3), 75-86.

Landrigan, J., & Carlson, J. E. (1995). Environmental policy and children's health: The future of children. *Critical Issues for Children and Youth, 2*(5), 34-52.

Learning Disabilities Association of America. (1999). *When learning is a problem.* Retrieved from www.Idanatl.org/phamplets/learning.html, April 10, 1999.

Locker, D., Liddell, A., Dempster, L., & Shapiro, D. (1999). Age of onset of dental anxiety. *Journal of Dental Research, 78*(3), 790-796.

Lowdermilk, D., Perry, S., & Bobak, I. (2000). *Maternity and Women's Health Care* (7th ed.). St Louis, MO: Mosby.

MacKenzie, R., & Neinstein, L. S. (2002). Anorexia nervosa and bulimia. In L. S. Neinstein (Ed.), *Adolescent health care: A practical guide* (pp. 564-583). Baltimore: Williams & Wilkins.

Manning, F. (1995). *Fetal medicine: Principles and practice* (pp. 307-341). Norwalk, CT: Appleton & Lange.

Marcus, S. M. (1998). Lead poisoning. In R. A. Dershewitz (Ed.), *Ambulatory pediatric care* (3rd ed.). Philadelphia: Lippincott.

McFarland, G. K., and McFarlane, E. A. (1997). *Nursing diagnosis and intervention: Planning for patient care* (3rd ed.). St Louis, MO: Mosby.

McManaway, J. W. (2000). Visual problems. In R. A. Hoekelman, N. M. Nelson, M. L. Weitzman, & M. H. Wilson (Eds.), *Primary pediatric care* (4th ed.) (pp. 1148-1151). St Louis, MO: Mosby.

*Mercer, R. (1982). Parent infant interaction. In L. Sonstegard (Ed.), *Women's health and childrearing,* vol. 2. New York: Grune & Stratton.

National Center for Health Statistics. (1998). *Student use of most drugs reaches highest level in nine years: More report getting "very high, bombed or stoned."* PRIDE, Press Release, September 25, 1996. Available at www.cdc.gov/nchswww/default.htm.

Neinstein, L. S., & Anderson, M. M. (2002). Adolescent sexuality. In L. S. Neinstein (Ed.), *Adolescent health care: A practical guide* (pp. 627-639). Baltimore: Williams & Wilkins.

Neinstein, L. S., Juliani, M. A., & Shapiro, J. (2002). Suicide. In L. S. Neinstein (Ed.), *Adolescent health care: A practical guide* (pp. 1116-1123). Baltimore: Williams & Wilkins.

Neinstein, L. S., & Kaufman, F. R. (2002a). Abnormal growth and development. In L. S. Neinstein (Ed.), *Adolescent health care: A practical guide* (pp. 165-193). Baltimore: Williams & Wilkins.

Neinstein, L. S., & Kaufman, F. R. (2002b). Normal physical growth and development. In L. S. Neinstein (Ed.), *Adolescent health care: A practical guide* (pp. 3-39). Baltimore: Williams & Wilkins.

Neinstein, L. S., & Pinsky, D. (2002). Alcohol. In L. S. Neinstein (Ed.), *Adolescent health care: A practical guide* (pp. 1009-1017). Baltimore: Williams & Wilkins.

Neinstein, L. S., Rabinovitz, S. J., & Schneir, A. (2002). Teenage pregnancy. In L. S. Neinstein (Ed.), *Adolescent health care: A practical guide* (pp. 656-676). Baltimore: Williams & Wilkins.

Neinstein, L. S., & Zeltzer, L. K. (2002). Chronic illness in the adolescent. In L. S. Neinstein (Ed.), *Adolescent health care: A practical guide* (pp. 1173-1195). Baltimore: Williams & Wilkins.

North American Nursing Diagnosis Association. (2002). *Nursing diagnosis: Definitions and classification, 2001-2002* (4th ed.). Philadelphia: Author.

Petryshen, P., Stevens, B., Hawkins, J., & Stewart, M. (1997). Comparing nursing costs for preterm infants receiving conventional versus developmental care. *Nursing Economics, 15*(3), 138-145, 150.

*Piaget, J. (1950). *The psychology of intelligence.* London: Routledge and Kegan Paul.

*Piaget, J. (1980). Intellectual evolution from adolescence to adulthood. In R. E. Muuss (Ed.), *Adolescent behavior and society: A body of readings* (3rd ed.). New York: Random House.

*Piaget, J. (1997). *The moral judgement of the child.* Glencoe, IL: Free Press.

*Piaget, J., & Infelder, B. (1958). *The growth of logical thinking from childhood to adolescence.* New York: Basic Books.

*Piaget, J., & Infelder, B. (1969). *The psychology of the child.* New York: Basic Books.

Pomerance, H. H. (1995). Growth and its assessment. *Advances in Pediatrics, 42,* 545-573.

Resnick, M. D., Bearman, P. S., Blum, R. W., Bauman, K. E., Harris, K. M., Jones, J., et al. (1997). Protecting adolescents from harm. *Journal of the American Medical Association, 278*(10), 823-832.

Rice, F. P. (1997). *Childhood and adolescent development.* Englewood Cliffs, NJ: Prentice Hall.

Roye, C. F. (1995). How to care for your adolescent patient. *American Journal of Nursing, 9,*(12),18-23.

Santelli, J., Morreale, M., Wigton, A., & Grason, H. (1996). School health centers and primary care for adolescents: A review of the literature. *Journal of Adolescent Health, 18*(5), 357-366.

Shaywitz, B. A., Fletcher, J. M., & Shaywitz, S. E. (1995). Defining and classifying learning disabilities and attention-deficit/hyperactivity disorder. *Journal of Child Neurology, 10*(Suppl. 1), S50-S57.

*Singer, D., & Revenson, T. (1978). *A Piaget primer: How a child thinks.* New York: New American Library.

Spitz, A. M., Velebil, P., Koonin, L. M., Strauss, L. T., Goodman, K. A., Wingo, P., et al. (1996). Pregnancy, abortion, and birth rates among U.S. adolescents—1980, 1985, and 1990. *Journal of the American Medical Association, 275*(13), 989-994.

Steward, D. K. (1997). Nonorganic failure to thrive: A theoretical approach. *Journal of Pediatric Nursing, 12*(6), 342-347.

TV-Free America. (1999). *Television statistics.* Available from www.tvfa.org/stats.html, April 10, 1999.

U.S. Department of Health and Human Services. (1999). *YouthInfo Directory.* Available from www.youth.os.dhhs.gov/youthinf.htm, 1/31/99.

Warf, C. (2002). Youth violence. In L. S. Neinstein (Ed.), *Adolescent health care: A practical guide* (4th ed.). Baltimore: Williams & Wilkins.

*Winer, G. A. (1986). Cognitive and psychosocial development during adolescence. In C. S. Shuster & S. S. Ashburn (Eds.), *The process of human development* (pp. 527-546). Boston: Little, Brown.

Wong, D. L., Hockenberry-Eaton, M., Wilson, D., Winkelstein, M. L., & Schwartz, P. (2001). *Wong's essentials of pediatric nursing* (6th ed.). St Louis, MO: Mosby.

Yusuf, H., Averhoff, F., Smith, N., & Brink, E. (1998). Adolescent immunization: Rationale, recommendations, and implementation strategies. *Pediatric Annals, 27* (7) 436-444.

Zucke, B. S., Frank, D. A., & Augustyn, M. (1999). Infancy and toddler years. In M. D. Levine, W. B. Carey, & A. Crockers (Eds.), *Developmental-behavioral pediatrics* (3rd ed.) (pp. 24-37). Philadelphia: Saunders

The Young, Middle, and Older Adult

Learning Objectives

After studying this chapter, you should be able to do the following:

- Discuss the developmental tasks of adulthood
- Identify a variety of factors affecting adult development
- Describe the assessment of a well adult for normal function and risk factors
- Describe modifications of the health history and physical examination for the older adult
- Differentiate among the variety of nursing diagnoses appropriate for adults seeking knowledge or health care related to development or health maintenance
- Plan nursing interventions for health maintenance and reduce risk factors as appropriate to the adult's developmental level
- Evaluate the outcomes that describe progress toward the goals of health maintenance

Mr. Edward Biaggio, a 42-year-old obese Italian-American man, is married with two children who are in high school and living at home. He recently began working as a chief accountant at a large insurance company. The occupational health nurse began to monitor his blood pressure after he came in for a routine yearly health screening, because he was diagnosed with borderline hypertension. His blood pressure reading is 148/96. He is 5 feet 10 inches tall and weighs 227 pounds.

He has not had a physical examination since college. He smokes two packs of cigarettes a day and reports, "I don't eat many fruits and vegetables. I just never liked them." His diet is high in fat, and he has not exercised for "years." Mr. Biaggio says that he's surprised he has high blood pressure because he is not feeling bad. He knows he should lose a little weight, quit smoking, and get some exercise.

Possible nursing diagnoses for Mr. Biaggio's situation are defined below.

KEY NURSING DIAGNOSES FOR The Young, Middle, and Older Adult

Readiness for enhanced age-appropriate attainment of developmental milestones: Seeks assistance to manage age-appropriate developmental milestones

Ineffective health maintenance: Inability to identify, manage, and/or seek out help to maintain health

CONCEPTS OF ADULT DEVELOPMENT

Although physical growth is complete by the early 20s, the adult continues to develop. Each adult's development is unique and complex because genetics, socioeconomic status, ethnic group, religious faith, and social expectations influence it. Development refers to the progressive increase in skill and capacity to function.

Nurses need to be knowledgeable about human development to understand the client's health needs in relationship to the person's life stage. Human development is the scientific study of quantitative and qualitative ways adults change and do not change over time. These changes are influenced by internal (hereditary) and external (environmental) factors. By understanding adult development, you can help people cope with life's transitions and help them manage their health problems in a manner appropriate to their developmental stage.

Developmental Tasks

Young Adulthood. **Young adulthood** refers to the period of life from age 20 to 34. The 2000 U.S. Census Bureau (USCB) reported that approximately 59 million people, almost 21% of the population, were between the ages of 20 and 34 (USCB, 2002).

This developmental stage ranges from the end of adolescence to the beginning of middle adulthood. Young adults face a variety of developmental tasks that center around the assumption of adult roles and responsibilities (Figure 17-1, p. 334). During this period, most people are in search of self. They need to establish autonomy from parents or parent surrogates, develop philosophies of life and personal lifestyles, choose and prepare for employment, enter the workforce, marry or establish other types of significant relationships, develop parenting behaviors, and become participatory citizens. There is considerable variability in how and when different people accomplish these tasks. Young adults are expected to perform many roles, including those of parent, spouse or companion, son or daughter, citizen, civic leader, friend, and employee or employer.

Middle Adulthood. **Middle adulthood** refers to the period from age 35 to 64. In 2002, the USCB reported that more than 107 million people, more than 34% of the population, were between the ages of 35 and 64 (USCB, 2002).

During this period, generative activity (or generativity) expands. The adult focuses on creativity, productivity, and developing the capacity to care for others. This stage began early in adulthood, particularly with childbearing, child rearing, and establishing a career. Mature adults are concerned with establishing and guiding the next generation in their roles as parents, teachers, mentors, civic leaders, and guardians of the culture. If this is not accomplished, they may feel a sense of personal impoverishment.

Older Adults. Many people use the term *elderly* when describing an older person, especially when that person is frail, chronically ill, and in need of assistance from others. However, many people live healthy, productive lives well into their 80s and 90s. In this book, we prefer to use the term **older adult** to describe any person age 65 or older.

In 2002, the USCB reported that approximately 35 million people, 12.4% of the population, were age 65 and older (USCB, 2002) (Figure 17-2, p. 334). The fastest-growing segment of the U.S. population is the group who are over age 85. It is predicted that by 2050, the life expectancy for U.S. citizens will be 82.9 years (National Institute on Aging, 2000).

In their 60s, many healthy adults look forward to **retirement**—the permanent withdrawal from one's job—by making plans to travel, garden, learn new skills, and so on. Although grandparenting can be part of a person's life from the late 30s, an active relationship with grandchildren or great-grandchildren is common into the 60s and beyond. For people who can maintain their health, the 70s continue to provide opportunities for an active, fulfilling lifestyle, despite the increased likelihood of health problems. The 80s are more likely to be a time of slowing down, although the change is gradual and not necessarily significant for all people. Even the healthiest older people recognize a significant decline in physical function during their 90s, and they spend at least some time anticipating death. Typically, people in their 90s are the oldest living

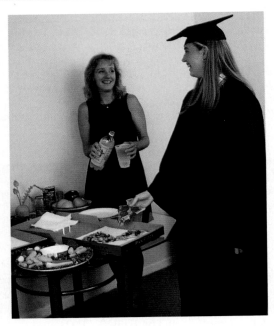

Figure 17-1. For many young adults, graduation from college is an important milestone that marks the end of adolescence and the beginning of adult roles and responsibilities.

relative in a family unit. Their quality of life is maintained through simple pleasures: the company of significant others, sharing life stories, dining with others, and maintaining an interest in the affairs of the world.

Developmental Theories

Biological. Examining the life span from the perspective of physical changes, biologists have divided it into the following three phases:

- Progressive growth from birth to age 25
- Stability almost to age 45
- A decline of physical capabilities after age 45

Other biologists have suggested the acquisition, possession, and loss of reproductive ability as the three stages of life. Additionally, biological theories hypothesize a finite end to increased longevity (in other words, although we see life spans as increasing, the maximum life span is estimated to be 120 years). However, the purely physical perspective does not capture the psychosocial changes in adult life.

Psychosocial. In his theory of psychosocial development, Erik Erikson (1963) identified eight stages of development from birth through death (Table 17-1). He believed that psychosocial development was a continuous process, and that

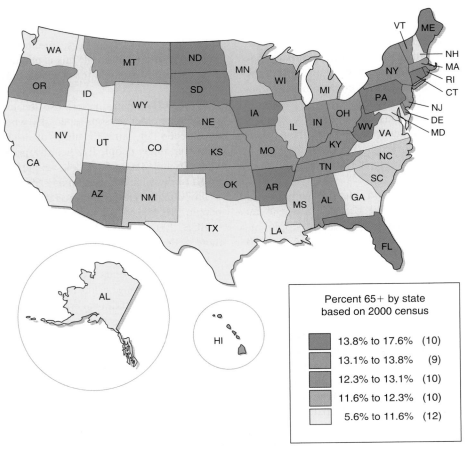

Figure 17-2. Percentage of Americans age 65 and over by state in 2000. Nationally, 12.4% of Americans are 65 or over. (Redrawn from Administration on Aging. *2000 census estimates for the older population.* Available at http://www.aoa.dhhs.gov/aoa/stats/2000pop/percentmap.html.)

delays or crises in one stage could delay or diminish the achievement of other stages. They also serve as an impetus to the next stage. In Chapter 16, you learned about the stages through adolescence. The adolescent makes a transition into adulthood and does not stop developing until death. Erikson's adult stages focus on intimacy versus isolation (young adult), generativity versus stagnation (middle adult), and ego integrity versus despair (older adult).

During the stage of intimacy versus isolation, young adults are in an intense search for self; they focus on developing their capacity for reciprocal love and close personal relationships based on commitment to others. They experience conflicting values as they try to sort out what life means to them. They must resolve the conflict of balancing independence and intimacy as they form significant relationships with partners, with the aim of providing a nurturing environment for children. These tasks are relevant in a variety of lifestyles, including heterosexual marriage, homosexual and heterosexual cohabitation, and voluntary childlessness.

Erikson's seventh stage of psychosocial development, generativity versus stagnation, is reached during middle adulthood. The person tends to assess generativity by focusing on creativity, productivity, procreation, and the development of a capacity to care for others. The individual must balance the feeling that life is personally satisfying and socially meaningful with the feeling that life is without meaning. If stagnation occurs, the person may become egocentric and self-absorbed (Figure 17-3).

In Erikson's eighth stage of psychosocial development, ego integrity versus despair, integrity is achieved by older adults who see themselves as having lived a productive life and having few regrets. Failure to achieve this can lead to feelings of hopelessness, despair, and fear of death (see Table 17-1).

Levinson (1978, 1986) conceived of development as a sequence of qualitatively distinct eras or seasons (Table 17-2, p. 336). Each of these eras in adult life has its own time and brings certain psychological challenges to the forefront of a person's life.

Cumming and Henry's disengagement theory (1961) pertains to adults past the age of 65. They proposed that in the normal course of aging, older adults gradually withdraw or disengage from social roles as a natural response to lessened capabilities and diminished interest, and to societal disincentives for participation. This theory argues that it is beneficial for both the aging individual and society that such disengagement take place, to minimize the social disruption caused at an aging person's eventual death.

Disengagement does appear to happen for some older adults; for example, some happy, healthy older adults disengage when they move to retirement communities, contentedly taking to a rocking chair or pursuing other solitary, passive activities while preparing for death. However, many older adults, even after retiring, remain highly involved in the life of their communities, their children and grandchildren, and friends, and the disengagement theory does not seem applicable to them.

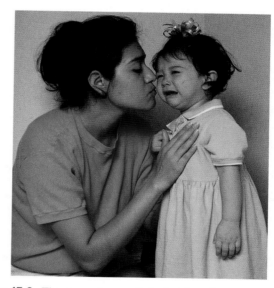

Figure 17-3. The stage of generativity involves the development of a capacity to care for others.

Table 17-1	Erikson's Stages of Development for the Young Adult, Middle Adult, and Older Adult Years	
Stage	**Age**	**Description**
VI	Young adult years	• Intimacy versus self-absorption, later called intimacy versus isolation. • Significant relationships are partners in friendship, sex, and competition and cooperation and ability to engage in a trusting fellowship. • The young adult seeks a permanent life partner with whom to give and receive love and support. • The primary issue is love.
VII	Middle adult years	• Generativity versus stagnation, which is a creative giving of the self to the world in a participatory way. Generativity is helping and guiding the next generation. • Unless such concern develops, the person focuses on self, stagnates, and commonly regresses. • Middle adults share tasks and divide necessary labor. • The primary issue is care.
VIII	65 years-death	• Ego integrity versus despair. • Reflects on and accepts one's life. • Feels a sense of fulfillment about life and accepts death as an unavoidable reality. • If unable to obtain a feeling of fulfillment and completeness, will despair and fear death.

Reprinted with permission from Erikson, E. H. (1963). *Childhood and society* (2nd ed.), New York: W. W. Norton & Company, Inc.; and by permission of The Random House Group Limited, London..

Table 17-2   Levinson's Development Phases

Approximate Age	Tasks
20 to 24	• Leaving the family. • Making the transition between adolescence and the adult world. • Those who go to college or military service have an intermediate experience.
25 to 29	• Getting into the adult world. • Building an initial life structure, deciding on an occupation, and working on intimacy versus isolation.
30 to 35	• A time of exploration and initial choice. • Age 30 transition. • Person either confirms earlier choices or may choose to modify or change the initial structure. • Person has vision of the future. • Person realizes extent to which he is dependent on and shaped by others, a deillusioning process. • A mentor can be very helpful at this stage.
35 to 39	• Settling down. • Person may build a second, and more stable, early adult life structure. • Becomes "one's own person." • Person moves from being mentored to being able to mentor.
38 to 42	• Midlife transition. • Person realizes that earlier choices cannot fulfill all of the self and that parts of the self were repressed or dormant. At some point, life must be restructured to express more of the self. • The adult reappraises, modifies, and rediscovers important neglected parts of the self and makes choices that provide for a new life structure. There may be a sense of compromise of the dream as person searches for what he really wants. • There is a sense of bodily decline and a need to confront one's mortality. The person recognizes that he is no longer young.
44 to 46	• Restabilization. • The fullest and most creative period of life. • Time represents both the possibility for further development and a threat to the self. • Person is building and living with a first provisional life structure for middle adulthood.
47 to 59	• Stable period of fulfillment.
60 to 65	• Preparing for retirement; work no longer the central focus. More time spent pursuing personal interests, such as travel, grandchildren, community services.
65-death	• Creates new life structure that suits person's retirement and health. Must deal with no longer being young and preparing for death.

Information from Levinson, D. J. (1978). *The seasons of a man's life.* New York: Knopf; and Levinson, D. J. (1996). *The seasons of a woman's life.* New York: Knopf.

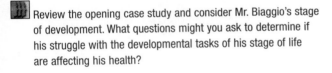 Review the opening case study and consider Mr. Biaggio's stage of development. What questions might you ask to determine if his struggle with the developmental tasks of his stage of life are affecting his health?

FACTORS AFFECTING ADULT DEVELOPMENT

Life expectancy in the United States has risen to 78.9 years primarily because of advances in public health, such as improved housing, sanitation, and immunizations. For those who reach the age of 65, life expectancy is longer. Today, risk factors that contribute to premature adult morbidity and mortality include high-risk lifestyle practices and other physiological, psychosocial, socioeconomic, and environmental factors.

Action Alert! Assist clients to live healthier and longer lives by avoiding behaviors that increase their risk for chronic diseases.

Lifestyle Risk Factors

Diet. In the United States, 23% of adults ages 20 and older (U.S. Department of Health and Human Services [USDHHS], 2000) are overweight, including 35% of men and 23% of women. Minority populations, especially women, are affected disproportionately: nearly half of African-American, Mexican-American, and Native American adults are overweight.

Several factors can contribute to poor nutritional status in the older adult. They include poor oral health; use of multiple medications, which can alter the absorption of vitamins and minerals; and reduced mobility, which makes obtaining and preparing meals challenging, especially for the older adult who lives alone.

Four of the ten leading causes of death in North America are linked to diet: heart disease, stroke, diabetes, and certain cancers, especially colorectal, endometrial, and ovarian cancer. The risks of developing hypertension or type II diabetes nearly triple for adults who are 20% or more overweight. Being overweight also increases the risk of gout, gallbladder disease, hip fractures, and osteoarthritis (USDHHS, 2000). Obese individuals may suffer from social stigmatization, discrimination, and lowered self-esteem.

Being too thin can also raise the risk of health problems. Anorexia nervosa, loss of appetite, and similar disorders are linked to menstrual irregularities and osteoporosis in women, and to a greater risk of early death in both women and men.

Our client, Mr. Biaggio, needs help with his diet. What do you know about the dietary patterns in the Italian culture? How could you find out more about Mr. Biaggio's pattern of eating? How can you motivate him to change?

> *Action Alert!* Clients should eat a diet with plenty of grain products, vegetables, and fruits—a diet that is low in saturated fat and cholesterol, moderate in sugars, and moderate in sodium.

Exercise. Regular physical activity is associated with lower death rates for adults of any age. It decreases the risk of death from heart disease, it lowers the risk of developing diabetes, and is associated with a decreased risk of colon cancer. It also helps prevent high blood pressure and helps reduce blood pressure in persons with elevated levels. Physical activity is an important factor in the adult's ability to maintain health and independence. Regular exercise promotes appetite, improves mental health, and decreases stress.

Rest and Sleep. Just as activity is important to the adult, so too is rest. According to the National Sleep Foundation (2001), adults need 8 hours of uninterrupted, quality sleep each night for optimum health, safety, and productivity. As age increases, so can the need for rest periods throughout the day.

Age-related changes that can affect a person's ability to sleep at night include nocturia, muscle cramps, and anxiety. The length of stage 4, the deep restful sleep, may decrease with age as well. To help increase sleeping time, the older person may benefit from avoiding physical exertion near bedtime, practicing effective toileting, avoiding stimulants (such as caffeine) after supper, and obtaining needed pain relief before trying to fall asleep.

Stress. Stress is the most common cause of illness in our society, and it is a major risk factor for the development of physical and psychological problems. It encompasses the negative cognitive and emotional states that result when clients feel that the demands placed on them exceed their ability to cope. It can be caused by external and internal influences. External stressors may stem from the following:

- The physical environment, such as loud noises, bright lights, excessive heat, and confined spaces
- The social environment, such as aggressiveness on the part of someone else
- The work environment, such as deadlines or "red tape"
- Major life events, such as the death of a relative, a lost job, a promotion, or a new baby
- Daily stressors, such as heavy traffic, misplaced keys, or a flat tire

Internal stressors commonly stem from lifestyle choices, such as drinking caffeinated beverages, getting too little sleep, or overloading the daily schedule. Stress may also stem from negative self-talk, such as pessimistic thinking and self-criticism, or from stressful personality traits, such as being a workaholic.

Only if clients cannot successfully handle situations alone do you step in to help them strengthen their weaknesses so they can overcome their restrictions and draw on a lifetime of experiences to meet current challenges. Allowing clients as much participation as possible ensures the success of this strategy.

 Think about Mr. Biaggio again. He has just taken a new job in an important position. Can you list possible stressors in his life?

> *Action Alert!* Reduce the negative effects of stress by reducing perceived pressures, increasing coping resources, or both.

Risky Behaviors

SMOKING. At least one in every five deaths in North America is related to cigarette smoking-related causes, such as lung cancer; cancer of the larynx, oral cavity, esophagus, pancreas, and urinary bladder; respiratory diseases, such as emphysema; and heart disease (Alberta Tobacco Reduction Alliance, 2002; USDHHS, 2000). Cigarette smoking is a major cause of death among Native Americans, Native Alaskans, blue-collar workers, and military personnel (USDHHS, 2000).

> *Action Alert!* Help your clients prevent premature death by helping them to stop smoking.

ALCOHOL ABUSE. The abuse of alcohol and other substances is a major health problem. Usually, it is difficult to detect alcohol abuse. Alcohol typically is metabolized more slowly in an older adult, resulting in a longer exposure time and a higher rate of tissue damage. Signs and symptoms of alcohol misuse may be similar to, or mistaken for, other clinical concerns. Often, however, alcoholism simply goes undetected by health care providers.

Adults who abuse alcohol increase their risk for hypertension, stroke, heart disease, certain cancers, accidents, violence, suicides, birth defects, and overall mortality. Alcohol abuse may cause cirrhosis of the liver, inflammation of the pancreas, damage to the brain and heart, and malnutrition. It may alter the effectiveness of medicines or increase the risk of toxic reactions. Some medications may increase blood alcohol levels or increase the adverse effect of alcohol on the brain.

> *Action Alert!* Help your client avoid drinking alcohol when taking any medications, because it can interact with medications and alter the way they are metabolized.

Alcohol and other substance abuse is also a problem because of effects on an unborn child. The incidence of fetal alcohol syndrome, a distinct cluster of physical and mental impairments caused by prenatal exposure to alcohol, has been estimated to range from 1 to 3 per 1000 live births (National Institute on Alcohol Abuse and Alcoholism, [USDHHS] 1999). Most experts agree that the incidence of partial presentations of fetal alcohol syndrome, including neurobehavioral anomalies, is much higher.

Action Alert! Educate pregnant women to avoid drinking during pregnancy, because major birth defects are linked to alcohol intake during pregnancy.

ILLICIT DRUG USE. Illicit drug use and its consequences threaten North Americans of every socioeconomic background, geographic region, educational level, and ethnic or racial identity. Accidents, crime, domestic violence, illness, lost opportunity, and reduced productivity are the direct consequences of substance abuse. Drug abuse and drug trafficking hurt families, businesses, and neighborhoods; impede education; and burden the criminal justice, health, and social service systems.

Chronic drug users are particularly susceptible to infectious diseases and are considered high-risk transmitters. They and their sexual partners have higher risks of contracting hepatitis, tuberculosis, gonorrhea, syphilis, and other sexually transmitted diseases. High-risk sexual behavior associated with crack cocaine and the injection of illegal drugs enhances the transmission and acquisition of human immunodeficiency virus (HIV).

Substance abuse is a common problem among families reported for child maltreatment. Researchers have found that 25% to 50% of men who commit domestic violence also have substance abuse problems. In addition, women with substance abuse problems are more likely to become victims of domestic violence. To make matters worse, North Americans who lack access to comprehensive health care and have smaller incomes may be less able to afford treatment to overcome drug dependence.

Developmental Risk Factors
Young Adults. Young adults who have difficulty in making adult choices and accepting responsibility for those choices are at risk for developmental delays. Young adults are expected to separate from their family of origin, establish viable careers, develop an intimate adult relationship with a significant other, marry, and become parents. Failure to achieve developmental tasks of young adulthood can result in a person living in isolation and/or dependent on their family of origin or society. A young adult unable to cope successfully with changing roles may experience high levels of stress, demonstrate substance abuse behaviors, or express unworthiness and depression.

Midlife Adults
MIDLIFE CRISIS. Some adults experience a midlife crisis, also called a midlife transition. **Midlife crisis** is a stressful life period during middle adulthood, precipitated by the review and reevaluation of one's past, including goals, priorities, and life accomplishments, during which the person experiences inner turmoil, self-doubt, and major restructuring of personality. Typically, a midlife crisis occurs in the early to middle forties, but it may not occur until the fifties.

As a group, middle-aged adults are commonly called the **sandwich generation.** They are caught between the needs of adjacent generations, caring for ill or frail parents while handling the competing demands of children and employment. Their responsibilities may range from financially supporting a retired parent to taking physical care of a frail, demented, dependent parent, while at the same time caring for their own children. Depending on the family's financial situation and the type of health insurance the elderly family member has, home health services can ease some of the middle-aged adult's caregiving tasks. Individual counseling and participation in support groups can help to relieve some of the family's stress and provide encouragement in difficult times.

All generations feel the effects of this sandwiching. For example, some elderly parents may feel that they have become a burden or inconvenience to their families, but they try to help their families any way they can (Figure 17-4). The children may feel neglected by their parents and resentful or jealous of their grandparents. The middle-aged adult is caught in the middle, trying to please everyone, but feels unsupported and unappreciated.

ONSET OF CHRONIC ILLNESS. Chronic illnesses, such as arthritis, hypertension, heart disease, and diabetes, can be major concerns for adults. An adult's level of hope, life satisfaction, and self-concept can be influenced by the adjustment to such a disease process. The goals for adults who have chronic illness are to maintain self-care, prevent complications, delay decline, and achieve the highest possible quality of life.

Older Adults
AGEISM. Self-concept in the older adult is dependent on self-concept throughout life. However, it is also affected by society's image of aging. **Ageism** is a stereotype, prejudice, or

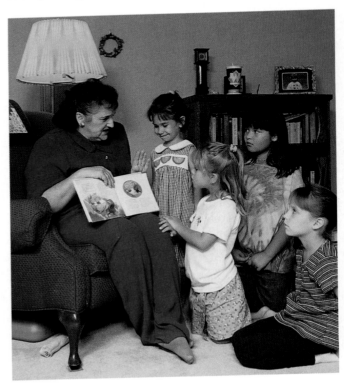

Figure 17-4. Although some older adults may feel that they have become a burden or an inconvenience to their families, they can still play an important role in the family by guiding the lives of future generations.

discrimination against people, especially older adults, based on their age and on a very narrow definition of how a certain age group is or lives. That definition is then used to view all members of this group as having the same characteristics, behaviors, or both.

Ageism is deeply embedded in Western culture. In a society that values youth and beauty to an obsessive degree, being old can be seen as a negative. Older adults, as they have aged, have been participants in their culture. As is true for victims of other prejudices, the effects of discriminatory thinking about being old can damage self-esteem. It is not uncommon to have ageist thinking present in older adults who are successfully adjusting to developmental changes but who see themselves as disconnected from their age cohort.

PERSONAL LOSS. For the older adult, the role of the spouse changes from earlier configurations. Although long marriage may result in a strong relationship, age-related health changes can bring new challenges for a couple. The death of a spouse is a common consequence of a long life; it is one of the most stressful passages for the older adult, causing profound loss and sense of change.

Living alone because of the death affects more women than men, both because women have a longer life span and because most men remarry. Men and women adjust to the loss of a spouse in different ways. The wives may have been in charge of monitoring their husbands' care and of making social arrangements, so the widower might be prone to isolation. Most men remarry (often with women younger than themselves). For a woman, the loss of a spouse may mean learning to manage finances, less income, and home repairs. It also means the loss of a companion and caretaker.

> *Action Alert!* Assess the ability to cope with loss. A bereaved widow or widower who feels unable to live without the deceased spouse may be suffering from dysfunctional grieving.

DEPRESSION. About one in four women and one in ten men suffer from depression at some point in life. Only about a third of these seek medical help (American Psychiatric Association, 2000; Thobaben & Buxton-Blake, 2002). Depression is a potential killer: as many as 15% of those who develop it commit suicide each year. The Centers for Disease Control listed suicide as the eighth leading cause of death in the United States (USDHHS, 2001). Most researchers, however, believe this number is too small.

Depression, although not a normal part of aging, is the most common problem in older adults. Estimates claim that 10% to 65% of people over age 60 have depressive symptoms at some time during their old age. The incidence is higher among nursing home residents than among older adults who live in the community (USDHHS, 2000).

Because depression commonly coexists with medical conditions and, in particular, dementias, it can be misdiagnosed or overlooked. Also, depressive disorders may cause or contribute to medical illnesses. Rates of depression for older persons hospitalized with medical conditions such as hip fracture or heart disease is 12%, and for those living in nursing homes

it ranges from 15% to 25% (USDHHS, 2000). Increasingly, findings indicate that severe depression heightens the risk of dying after a heart attack or stroke and reduces the quality of life for clients who have cancer and might reduce their survival time.

Another possible source of depression is drug therapy. The type of drug an adult may be taking, or a number of drugs taken to treat multiple problems, can contribute to depression. Several drugs taken for high blood pressure, heart disease, and insomnia are known to cause depression in some people. When assessing for depression and its causes, make sure you take a thorough drug history.

Clients who are depressed experience a great deal of functional impairment, resulting in lost work time, decreased job performance, and decreased family and social functioning. The stigmatization association with misunderstanding of mental illness prevents many people from seeking help. Encourage clients to seek treatment for depression; effective treatment is available.

Socioeconomic Risk Factors

Poverty. Poverty is associated with limited access to heath care, poor nutrition, substandard housing, and inadequate prenatal care. If clients have no health insurance, they tend to receive substandard medical care, putting them at risk for medical problems. In 2000, more than 31.1 million people in the United States (about 11.3% of the population) lived below the poverty line (USCB, 2001b). Better-educated and more affluent clients can afford a healthier diet, better preventive health care, and more prompt medical treatment. However, these advantages do not mean that their lifestyle practices will prevent chronic diseases and premature morbidity and mortality.

Health Insurance. Adult clients in the United States may have health insurance coverage through their employer, by private pay, or by federal or state health plans.

Most of the U.S. population (64.1%) was covered by a health plan related to employment. An estimated 14.0% of the population was without health insurance coverage during the entire year of 2000. Among the general population between ages 18 and 64, full-time and part-time workers were more likely to be insured than nonworkers. Among the working poor, however, there was less probability of being insured than among nonworkers. The primary reason was either that the employer failed to provide health insurance, or that the financial burden on employees to buy their company's plan was prohibitive. Canada is looking at similar issues resulting from the high cost of health care in relation to the gross national product. Cheaper health care insurance alternatives are being sought.

Native Americans and Native Alaskans were the least likely of all racial groups to have health insurance. Despite the Medicaid program, 29.5% of all poor people in the United States had no health insurance of any kind during 2000 (Kuttner, 1999; USCB, 2001a). Medicare covered 99.3% of people age 65 and over (USCB, 2001a). In spite of this, health care for older adults is becoming increasingly expensive and complex. The levels of health care deductibles are increasing, making it more difficult for even employed older adults to pay them. For those not working, paying the deductibles takes a larger percentage of their income. For both groups, the rising cost and use of medications is unpredictable. Older adults who now live in poverty will have a more difficult time meeting their basic survival needs, as well as their health care needs. Increasingly, working older adults are discovering that more of their after-tax dollars are spent on health care.

Housing Safety. People who are more affluent can afford better housing than those with lower incomes. In addition, if the neighborhood around the home declines as the house and the adult age, the person's safety may suffer. Without any hope of an increase in income, however, the person may be forced to remain in that area. Older adults may be forced to stay indoors more if they fear moving about in the neighborhood. Some have begun to share housing to address the problems of aging on fixed or decreasing incomes. This can be accomplished by home sharing—renting portions of the home to other older adults who have similar needs and interests. Some older adults sell their houses and move in with family members. If the husband dies first, the wife may be forced to sell the home and move to another, cheaper location or apartment.

As adults age, they may spend more time at home because of retirement or altered health and mobility. Age-related changes and the increased amount of time spent at home make it increasingly important to ensure the safety of an older adult's environment. Often, safety can be enhanced simply by encouraging the use of health aids already in place. Your goal is to mitigate the effects of age-related changes while helping the older client maintain as much independence as possible. For example, regular battery replacement in smoke and carbon monoxide detectors will improve warning systems to support safety. Encourage the older client to wear a hearing aid and glasses, if needed, to increase sensory awareness. Ensure that the home environment is free of hazards, such as throw rugs, that contribute to falls.

Employment. In 2000, the U.S. Department of Labor's Bureau of Labor Statistics (2001) reported that 83.2% of U.S. families had at least one employed member. Both parents were employed in 64.2% of married-couple families with children under 18; the father, but not the mother, was employed in 29.2% of these families. The proportion of "traditional" families—that is, families in which the father, but not the mother, is employed—is much larger among couples with preschool children (under 6 years of age) than among families whose youngest child was 6 to 17 years old.

The U.S. Department of Labor's Bureau of Labor Statistics (2002) reported that the unemployment rate was 5.6%. The unemployment rate for unmarried mothers—those who were single, widowed, divorced, or separated—with children under 18 was 7.5%. Among the families with unemployment, white and Hispanic families were more likely than black families to have at least one employed member.

Work-Related Injuries and Deaths. The National Institute for Occupational Safety and Health (NIOSH) estimates that over 50,000 people die annually from work-related illnesses, most of which go unreported. Every year, 6.3 million workplace injuries and over 500,000 work-related illnesses were reported to the federal government (Office of Disease Prevention and Health Promotion [ODPHP], 2002). Many others remain unreported. Those that often go unrecognized include musculoskeletal disorders of the upper extremity, irritant or allergic dermatitis, asthma, chronic obstructive lung disease, reproductive abnormalities, hearing loss, and cancers of the lung, skin, and bladder. Identification and remediation of causal or exacerbating workplace factors is necessary to prevent the recurrence of these disorders (ODPHP, 2002).

Physiological Risk Factors

Leading Causes of Death. The leading causes of death for adults younger than 25 are unintentional injuries, suicide, and homicide. For adults between the ages of 25 and 44, they are unintentional injuries, cancer, and heart disease (ODPHP, 2002). The leading causes of death for midlife adults between the ages of 45 and 64 are cancer, heart disease, and unintentional injuries (ODPHP, 2002). For adults 65 and older, they are heart disease, malignant neoplasm (lung, colorectal, breast), cerebrovascular disease, chronic obstructive pulmonary disease, pneumonia, and influenza (ODPHP, 2002).

> *Action Alert!* Living healthfully and avoiding behaviors that increase the risk of chronic disease will result in longer, healthier lives and lower health care costs.

Major Health Problems. Older adults must adapt to a number of physiological changes associated with aging (Figure 17-5). These changes include chronic illnesses, sensory

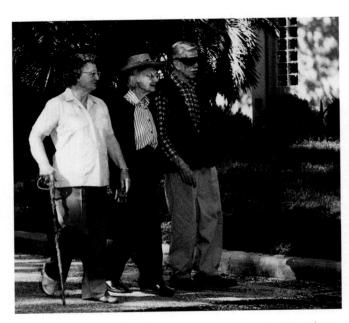

Figure 17-5. These older adults demonstrate some common adaptations to the physiological changes of older adulthood.

deficits, cognitive and intellectual changes, and changes in mobility. Chronic diseases account for 70% of all deaths in the United States, more than 60% of total medical care expenditures, and decreased quality of life for millions of Americans (National Center for Chronic Disease Prevention and Health Promotion, 2000).

For people in their 70s, chronic disease becomes more probable. If they have not yet had cataract surgery or a need for hearing aids, this decade carries a high likelihood that these aids will be needed. However, because cataract surgery has become relatively simple and hearing aids more effective, their lifestyle is not necessarily hampered.

Major surgery is common at this time, with such procedures as total hip and knee replacement, coronary artery bypass, and endarterectomy being used to help extend the period of active living. A change in motor coordination is noticeable, and the incidence of Alzheimer's disease and related dementias increases. For many, the 80s are associated with the giving up of driving a car, a major loss of freedom and independent living.

As people grow older, activities and the contribution to the family's general welfare, at least in terms of physical labor, gradually become more limited. Maintaining mobility and activity becomes more difficult. Major surgery is performed successfully on people in their 90s, but a decision to manage a health problem conservatively is more likely. Maintaining independent healthy living in the 90s requires the use of alternative strategies for managing the tasks of daily living, such as housekeeping, grocery shopping, cooking, and obtaining medical care.

HEART DISEASE. High blood cholesterol is an important modifiable risk factor for coronary artery disease, which is the leading cause of death for men and women in North America. Risk factors include a family history of very high cholesterol levels, premature coronary artery disease in a first-degree relative (before age 50 in men or age 60 in women), diabetes, smoking, and hypertension. Annually, about 1.5 million Americans have a new or recurrent myocardial infarction; about a third of these people die (ODPHP, 2002). In addition, obesity and sedentary lifestyle add to the risk factor.

HYPERTENSION. Nearly 2% of Canadians aged 20 to 34 have been diagnosed with high blood pressure. However, for each successive age group, prevalence increases, to a high of 36% for seniors aged 65 or older (Statistics Canada, 2002b). About 50 million Americans need monitoring or medication because they have elevated blood pressure (ODPHP, 2002). They are at increased risk for coronary artery disease, peripheral vascular disease, stroke, renal disease, or retinopathy. Treatment of hypertension is generally effective, although it must commonly be tailored to meet individual needs and responses.

Mr. Biaggio is advised to lower his blood pressure with diet and exercise. How often would you suggest that he have his blood pressure checked?

SENSORY DEFICITS. Visual changes with aging include a decrease in visual acuity and accommodation (the ability to focus at various distances). This loss of accommodation is called presbyopia, and it results from a loss of flexibility in the lens. Commonly, it begins to appear in 40-year-olds, when reading glasses become necessary. A variety of techniques can help you interact most effectively with an adult who has a visual or other sensory deficit (Box 17-1).

Other visual changes may occur as well. For example, older people's pupils may become less responsive to light, reducing their ability to see well in dimly lit areas or at night. They may need more light for reading and fine work. Difficulty in seeing at night can change or decrease the older adult's level of independence. If night driving becomes too challenging, for example, the person may need to make plans, or alter them, to avoid driving at night.

Action Alert! Teach your clients to position a 300-watt bulb so that it shines forward from behind their shoulder if they have difficulty reading.

Cataracts, or clouding of the lens, are a common age-related change. They can cause blurring and decreased light and color perception. Correction of this condition, the surgical removal of the clouded lens, commonly can be performed as same-day surgery. Afterward, the person may receive a lens implant or wear corrective lenses.

Glaucoma, also common in the older adult, is a degenerative disease of increasing intraocular pressure that arises when the aqueous humor is unable to drain properly from the anterior chamber of the eye. Glaucoma can lead to optic nerve damage if untreated. Yearly checks of intraocular pressure should be encouraged for all people age 40 and older, but especially for African Americans, who have a high risk for this condition. Medication commonly controls the disease process, but careful monitoring is essential for the rest of the person's life.

Box 17-1 Tips for Interacting Effectively With Adults Who Have Sensory Deficits

THE VISUALLY IMPAIRED ADULT

- Identify yourself each time you enter the client's space.
- Tell the client when you are leaving.
- Maximize available lighting.
- Use color-contrasted toiletries and kitchen utensils as visual cues.
- Do not move objects in the client's space without permission.
- Verbally cue the client before you hand him/her an object.
- Describe objects, such as food on a plate, as if they were on a clock face, to enhance communication.
- Make sure the client's glasses are clean and positioned properly.

THE HEARING-IMPAIRED ADULT

- When talking with the client, face him/her at his/her level. Make sure the area is well lit and keep your hands away from your face.
- Eliminate as much competing noise as possible.
- Speak at a moderate speed, articulate clearly, and use short sentences.
- Pause between sentences.
- Make sure that only one person speaks at a time.
- Use creative facial and hand gestures.
- Assess the use and function of hearing aids.
- Do not shout.

Modified from Ebersole, P., & Hess, P. (1998). *Toward healthy aging,* St Louis, MO: Mosby.

Loss of hearing is not a normal part of aging. However, it is not uncommon to gradually lose the ability to hear high-frequency sounds. Because of the gradual nature of this change, many older adults adapt to it without much difficulty. However, reduced hearing in older adults can also result from secretion of a drier type of cerumen than was produced when they were younger. These secretions can be more difficult to remove and, if they accumulate, can cause difficulty in hearing. Many individuals at this time have been exposed to unacceptable noise levels during their working years and are presently experiencing hearing deficits because they failed to use appropriate safety apparel.

Action Alert! Face the hearing-impaired person and use short, direct phrases while you assess hearing acuity. The failure of an older adult to answer your questions appropriately may indicate hearing loss.

COGNITIVE AND INTELLECTUAL DEVELOPMENT. It has been documented that healthy older adults do not demonstrate a decline in such intellectual abilities as wisdom, judgment, and common sense. They may have a slight, gradual decline in short-term memory, calculation ability, word fluency, and abstraction, beginning at about age 60. Older adults can learn new skills, but it may be at a slower pace. Sensory deficits and lack of relevance to their daily life must be factored into the teaching plan when working with older adult clients. Cognitive performance remains difficult to predict because of the many factors that can affect cognition in the older adult.

When tests are judiciously chosen and test-taking conditions are conducive to the older adult, the results typically show that intelligence does not decrease with age. Two of the more reliable and validated tools for assessing cognitive function in the older adult are the Mini-Mental State Examination developed by Folstein, Folstein, and McHugh (1975), and the Short Portable Mental Status Questionnaire developed by Pfeiffer (1975).

MOBILITY CONCERNS. Normal aging does not necessarily limit mobility. The extent to which age-related changes affect movement is often determined by movement patterns established before entering old age. Thus remaining active throughout life is a way to maintain healthy movement in old age (Figure 17-6).

As a person ages, gait changes can result from changes in muscles and joints. Muscle strength, flexibility, stability, and cognition are factors that contribute to mobility. When illness affects any of these factors, mobility may decline and the risk of falls may rise. Hip fracture is the most common fall-related injury leading to hospitalization in older adults. Roughly half of all persons sustaining hip fractures never regain full function; many must then walk with assistance or assistive devices. Falls are the second leading cause of injury death for adults between 65 and 84 years and the leading cause of injury death for those 85 years and older. Therefore, prevention of falls has a great influence on keeping older persons healthy. Through public health or community agencies, many communities have a falls-prevention program in place, which helps to support older adults living at home.

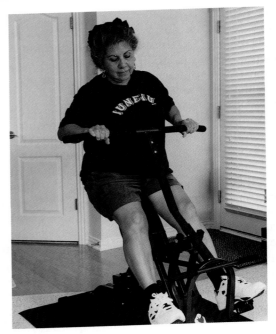

Figure 17-6. Remaining active throughout life is a way to maintain healthy movement in old age.

Cultural Risk Factors

Culture and ethnic origin are likely to be important influences on adults, especially when the person is a first-generation North American. The beliefs and norms of the groups to which each client belongs have shaped ideas about health, diet, education, illness, pain, silence, symptom reporting, family support, death, health care providers, and the elderly and aging. Within the context of the assessment, you need to determine the strength of the client's affiliation to an ethnic group, health practices, and beliefs about health care. Unless you incorporate these belief patterns into your care plans, you may create a conflict between your nursing interventions and your clients' cultural backgrounds.

Chronic disease has an increased impact on racial and ethnic minority groups. For example, the prevalence of diabetes among African Americans, Hispanics, Native Americans, and Native Alaskans is significantly higher than for white U.S. Americans (National Center for Chronic Disease Prevention and Health Promotion, 2000). The cancer survival rate among African Americans, American Indians, Native Alaskans, and Hawaiian Natives is lower than for white Americans. It is about 44%, compared with 59% for white U.S. Americans. This difference can be attributed largely to late diagnosis in minority groups (Clegg, Li, Hankey, Chu, & Edwards, 2002).

No single factor negatively affects the growth and development of people in racial and ethnic minority groups. Growth and development result from a complex interaction of factors, such as socioeconomic status, cultural characteristics, acculturation, stress, biological elements, targeted advertising, and varying capacities of communities to promote healthy lifestyle practices (National Center for Chronic Disease Prevention and Health Promotion, 2000).

ASSESSMENT

General Assessment of the Well Adult

Assessment of the well adult is a process of holistic assessment across all functional health patterns. Well adults are assessed for many reasons and in many settings: at a physician's office, community health clinic, nursing center, college health center, or occupational health center, to name a few.

Some clients need a preemployment examination before starting a new job. Others need physical examinations to participate in college sports. Women who wish to use contraception usually need annual physical examinations, and those who are pregnant are encouraged to seek prenatal and postnatal care. As adults age, they often seek care to learn how to maintain their health or to adjust to the physical changes they are experiencing. By assessing a well adult, you can help to prevent acute illness or manage chronic diseases.

Gerontologists have been concerned about the assessment of older adults because of some important differences between responses of younger and older adults. Older adults need a quiet, well-lit, and temperate environment, with no distractions. The testing environment should also be emotionally nonthreatening to reduce the client's anxiety. Before testing, it may be beneficial to both you and the older adult to have some relaxed time together to get to know one another. Under these conditions, the test taker can be motivated to work to maximum capacity.

A printed assessment form will help you be organized, and it will conserve the client's energy. Being efficient and client centered helps build trust between you and your client (Figure 17-7). The purpose of the assessment is to identify strengths and limitations so you can plan nursing interventions to optimize function and independence. For older adults, focus your assessment on function, not on the changes of aging. Structure your questions to elicit functional data. Make sure that older clients understand the purpose of the assessment; their understanding is vital to the success of your assessment. At the end of the assessment, allow time for them to ask questions and clarify any confusing aspects of your conversation.

Health History. Any nursing assessment normally begins with a health history. It includes the client's biographical data, past health history, chief complaint, and present health status, and it may include a family history and dynamics. For older adults, structure questions to gather information in a focused manner, and help them concentrate on events that might influence their current health. You can create a balance between allowing clients to talk and gathering relevant data.

The completeness of the health history is determined by the clients' health status, their ability to answer your questions, and their trust in the relationship they have with you. Start by asking them to describe their health. In their opinion, is it poor, good, or excellent? Assess for past health history that is relevant to understanding their current health status. Take a history of their lifetime health-seeking behaviors. Ask how much control they believe they have over their own

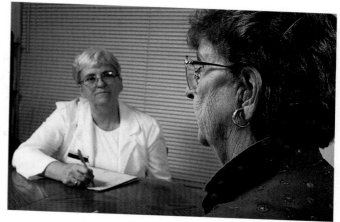

Figure 17-7. Establishing a trusting relationship with the client is an important component of assessing the older adult. This nurse takes the time to develop a relationship with the client before beginning the assessment.

health. Inquire about any illnesses within the past year that have prevented them from pursuing normal activities. Ask what they do to keep healthy. Specifically mention breast or testicular self-examinations. Ask whether they use alcohol or other drugs, and how much. Ask whether they smoke, how much, and for how long.

Medication History. Assessment of the clients' medication history should begin with a review of their current medications, times taken, purpose, and side effects. You should look at the medications in their containers to confirm drug name, dosage, and times per day. Encourage clients to talk with you about their prescriptions and any over-the-counter medications they take. Doing so will help you determine their level of understanding and beliefs about the drugs they take. This will help you identify potential, as well as actual, problems.

Functional Assessment

With older and disabled adults, you will need to do a functional assessment to identify their strengths and weakness in the activities of daily living (ADLs). These include the activities involved with eating, grooming, dressing, toileting, mobility, social interaction, and problem solving. You can use Gordon's functional health patterns as a framework to obtain the client's specific health history (see Chapter 6).

Physical Examination

TECHNIQUES FOR AGE DIFFERENCES. The type of physical examination you perform for a well adult depends largely on the reason for the examination and on the age of the person. For example, when you give a person a sports physical, you will screen for previous and current injuries, sexually transmitted diseases, and alcohol and other substance abuse. You would assess all joints for range of motion, flexibility, strength, and reflexes. You would listen to the person's heart and lungs and examine the eyes, ears, and abdomen for any abnormalities.

An annual physical examination for a woman of child-bearing age would include questions about possible domestic violence and increased risks for sexually transmitted diseases. You would take her vital signs, including an accurate height for osteoporosis prevention. You would assess her heart, lungs, thyroid gland, breasts, abdomen, and genital and rectal areas for any abnormalities. She would need a Papanicolaou test (the Pap test) if it has been 3 years since her last test—or fewer if she has an increased risk for cervical cancer.

For all well adult clients, you should also assess general health and cognitive and emotional functioning. Begin by assessing their appearance. Observe their behaviors and apparent mental status. Measuring cognitive function in older adults should be done carefully because some potential problems are caused by physical needs. For example, if the older adult tires easily, it may be advantageous to perform the testing in several sittings at different times.

> *Action Alert!* Do not assume confusion is a normal part of aging. For example, confusion in an older adult can signify the presence of an infection even before body temperature changes.

AGE-RELATED CHANGES. By their mid twenties, most adults are fully developed and at peak functioning. From then on, they will experience a gradual decline in touch sensitivity and in respiratory, cardiovascular, and immune system functions. You need to be familiar with the expected physical changes in the older adult.

GENERAL APPEARANCE. Skin changes, especially lines and sagging, become more pronounced in the forties and fifties. Age spots begin in the fifties and sixties. Hair begins to gray and thin in the early forties, a process that continues throughout adulthood. An adult's height begins to decline in the thirties and forties; because of compression of disks in the spinal column, height may drop an inch during the fifties and sixties.

VISION AND HEARING. During the thirties and forties, vision and hearing begin to change. The accommodative ability of the ocular lens declines; by the fifties and sixties, it no longer exists. Color discrimination declines as well, and most people have an increased sensitivity to glare during their forties and fifties. Hearing begins to decline in the thirties and forties, initially involving mostly high frequencies. By the fifties and sixties, hearing loss may include all frequencies, although it is still most pronounced at high frequencies.

HEAD AND NECK. As you perform the examination of the head and neck, you may see age-related changes, such as retraction of the gingivae, shrinkage of the roots of teeth, and atrophy of taste buds. These changes can lead to degeneration of tissues around the teeth, leading to loss of teeth and loss of taste discrimination. Determine the client's ability to swallow without choking.

CARDIOVASCULAR FUNCTION. Age-related changes that occur in the cardiovascular system include thickening and stiffening of the heart valves. More time is needed for the maximum heart rate to return to its resting rate. Cardiac output may be reduced during stress.

RESPIRATORY FUNCTION. Age-related changes in the older adult include increased airway resistance, a decreased exchange of oxygen and carbon dioxide (caused by diminished pulmonary circulation), and decreased strength in the respiratory accessory muscles, which causes rigidity in breathing. These changes can lead to other changes:

- A decrease in vital capacity, which is the maximum amount of air that can be expired after maximal inspiration
- A decrease in residual volume, which is the volume of gas left after maximal expiration
- A decrease in functional capacity, which is the amount of air left in the lungs after normal expiration

MUSCULOSKELETAL FUNCTION. Age-related changes in bones include a loss of bone mass and density, increased bone reabsorption, and decreased calcium absorption. As they age, muscles become smaller and have decreased numbers of muscle fibers, which presents as less muscle mass. Cell membrane deterioration results in a loss of fluid and potassium from cells. Slower movements are the result of prolonged contraction and relaxation time. Whether these changes are age related or result instead, or in part, from inactivity is still under investigation.

GASTROINTESTINAL FUNCTION. Age-related gastrointestinal changes may include inflammation of the gastric membrane from drug treatments. This can lead to ulcers or gastritis. Diverticulitis can result from obesity or from straining at bowel movements, a problem typically caused by the intake of too many refined, low-fiber foods. An age-related contributing factor can be a decrease in the colon's muscular strength.

BOWEL FUNCTION. Assessment of the abdomen may reveal loss of abdominal muscle tone, and decreased muscle tone in the colon may result in hypoactive bowel sounds. Loss of muscle tone increases the risk for constipation. Weakness of the internal anal sphincter may be a factor in controlling intestinal elimination. Assess for an abdominal mass in the left lower quadrant suggesting constipation. The elderly are also more prone to diverticulitis.

URINARY FUNCTION. Keep in mind that urinary incontinence (involuntary urination) is not a normal age-related change in the older adult. There are several types of urinary incontinence. They can be identified through a good health assessment and history, including a drug history. When taking the health history, check the client's daily pattern of urinating, including amount, times, frequency, and whether incontinence occurs. If it does occur, assess precipitating factors, time of day, and presence of blood in urine. If the older adult takes a medication with diuretic effects that could contribute to the risk of incontinence, consult with the physician who prescribed the medication.

SEXUAL FUNCTION. Include an assessment of the adult's sexual activity and function. Sexuality and interest in sexual intercourse do not necessarily decrease as a person ages. Important to a wellness lifestyle is having a relationship that meets the adult's sexual needs. Sexual activity and mental health are the most important predictors of sexual satisfaction.

Sexual activity increases during the twenties and thirties and begins to decline in the thirties and forties. Men experience a decrease in the quality of semen and sperm after age 40. The inability to obtain an erection can occur at any age, but it becomes more common in midlife. Fertility problems for women increase sharply in their forties. As basal metabolism declines in the forties and fifties, weight increases, and muscle and bone mass decline. This process accelerates in women after menopause. **Menopause** is the stage in the female climacteric during which hormone production is reduced, the ovaries stop producing eggs, and menstruation ceases. The woman's reproductive ability has now ended. Menopause usually occurs between ages 50 and 55, although the range is from 40 to 59. After menopause, the rate of osteoporosis increases. Nursing research has found that older adults are as interested in sexual activity as they were throughout their life, and that patterns remain constant into old age.

Diagnostic Tests. A key to wellness for the adult is appropriate screening, especially for clients in high-risk groups. You may be directly involved in screening or in teaching clients about the importance of screening tests (Table 17-3).

Coronary artery disease is the leading cause of death in the United States and Canada. Consequently, clients should be screened regularly, at least every 5 years for men between the ages of 35 and 65 and for women between 45 and 65, for elevated cholesterol level, a major modifiable risk factor for heart disease (ODPHP, 2002). If the total cholesterol level is increased, then the client should be tested for other lipid abnormalities as well.

Hypertension is a risk factor for coronary artery disease, congestive heart failure, stroke, ruptured aortic aneurysm, retinopathy, and renal disease. All adults should be screened for hypertension at least every 2 years. If the diastolic reading is 85 and the systolic reading is 140 or below, screening every

Table 17-3 Health Screening Guidelines for Well Adults

Test	Young Adulthood (Age 20 to 35)	Middle and Older Adulthood	Comments
Body measurement	Measure height and weight periodically.	Measure height and weight periodically	Obesity is a major public health problem.
Blood pressure	At least every 2 years for normotensive adults or annually for borderline hypertension. Others should seek the advice of a physician.	At least every 2 years for normotensive adults or annually for borderline hypertension. Others should seek the advice of a physician.	About 50 million Americans have hypertension that warrants monitoring or drug therapy.
Breast examination	Every 3 years. More frequent for high-risk groups.	Mammography and clinical breast examination every 1 to 2 years (age 50 to 75). Breast self-examination alone is useful but not reliable.	Breast cancer is the most common type of cancer in women and the second leading cause of death.
Cholesterol level	Should seek the advice of a physician. High-risk groups may need screening	Periodic screening for men ages 35 to 75 and women ages 45 to 75. High-risk groups should seek the advice of a physician.	High blood cholesterol is a modifiable risk factor for heart disease.
Papanicolaou test	All women who are age 18 or older or sexually active and who have a cervix should have a Pap test every 3 years.	All women who are age 18 or older or sexually active and who have a cervix should have a Pap test every 3 years.	The major risk factor for cervical cancer is sexually transmitted infection with human papillomavirus.
Prostate-specific antigen test		Annual test together with rectal examination beginning at age 50; earlier for men at high risk.	Prostate cancer is the second leading cause of cancer death in men.
Sigmoidoscopy		Every 3 to 5 years beginning at age 50 (age 40 for those with a family history of colorectal cancer, along with fecal occult blood tests, sigmoidoscopy, colonoscopy, or barium enema).	Colorectal cancer is the third leading cause of cancer death in the United States, most often among people older than age 40.
Tuberculosis	Skin testing for all persons at high risk.	Skin testing for all persons at high risk.	Control depends on screening high-risk populations and providing preventive therapy.
Vision	Comprehensive eye and vision examination every 2 to 3 years; more often if increased risk factors present.	Comprehensive eye and vision examination every 2 years; more often if increased risk factors present.	Vision loss is common in adults, especially with advancing age.

Based on recommendations from U.S. Department of Health and Human Services, Public Health Service, Office of Disease Prevention and Health Promotion. (1998). *Clinician's handbook of preventive services* (2nd ed.). Retrieved from http://text.nlm.nih.gov/ftrs/tocview Jan. 18, 1998; Report of the U.S. Preventive Services Task Force. (1996). *Guide to clinical preventive services* (2nd ed.). Baltimore: Williams & Wilkins.
NOTE: Recommendations of other groups will differ.

2 years is sufficient. Hypertension is never diagnosed on the basis of a single reading.

> Mr. Biaggio, from our case study, was being monitored by the occupational health nurse after he was diagnosed with borderline hypertension. He is self-monitoring his blood pressure and has obtained readings of 140/90, 160/88, and 150/92 in a single day. He says, "See, it isn't too bad for a man my age." How would you respond?

The annual incidence of breast cancer increases with age. Screening for breast cancer is recommended every 1 to 2 years for women over the age of 50. Screening includes a breast examination by a health practitioner and a mammogram. Screening in younger women is recommended when there is a family history of breast cancer, especially premenopausal breast cancer. All women should be encouraged to do breast self-examination every month.

All people older than age 50 should annually have a fecal occult blood test done for colorectal cancer, and a sigmoidoscopy every 3 to 5 years beginning at age 50 (or 40 if they have a family history of colorectal cancer) (ODPHP, 2002). When the finding is positive, a colonoscopy may be performed. Other screening methods include a digital rectal examination and a barium enema. For people who have first-degree relatives with colorectal cancer, a more thorough screening may be recommended.

Screening for cervical cancer is recommended for all women with a cervix who are sexually active or have reached age 18, whichever comes first. A Papanicolaou test should be performed every 1 to 3 years for women with a cervix (ODPHP, 2002). Risk factors of multiple sex partners, an early onset of sexual intercourse, low socioeconomic status, and HIV infection suggest the need for more frequent screening.

All men should have an annual prostate-specific antigen test and an annual rectal examination beginning at age 50, or earlier if at high risk.

Rubella contracted during the first 16 weeks of pregnancy causes serious complications, including miscarriage, abortion, stillbirth, and congenital rubella syndrome. All women of childbearing age should have either a documented history of rubella or a rubella titer. Offering nonpregnant women the rubella vaccine is an acceptable alternative.

All adults should be screened for problem drinking of alcohol. Heavy drinking is defined as more than five drinks per day, five times per week. Medical problems due to alcoholism include hepatitis, cirrhosis of the liver, cardiomyopathy, withdrawal syndrome, mental changes, and, in older adults, a dementia observed during the last stages of severe chronic alcoholism. Heavy drinking and alcoholism (dependency) have dire social consequences as well, including suicide, divorce, depression, domestic violence, unemployment, and poverty.

All clients should be screened for tobacco use, and those who use tobacco products should be advised to quit and encouraged to develop a plan to quit. Many methods are used to help tobacco users quit the habit, but success is directly related to the person's determination to quit rather than to the method itself. Most people try more than once before actually quitting.

All clients should be assessed for their immunization status. All clients need a diphtheria-tetanus vaccination every 10 years. Adults who have not had chicken pox should receive the varicella (chicken pox) immunization. Adults 65 and older should have a pneumococcal immunization once in their lifetime and an influenza vaccination annually. Seniors should be screened for tuberculosis because of its increasing incidence and their more vulnerable status.

Vision loss is common in adults, and the prevalence increases with advancing age. Young, normal-risk adults should have a comprehensive eye and vision examination every 2 to 3 years. Middle-aged and older, normal-risk adults should have such an examination every 2 years.

High-risk clients should be screened for tuberculosis. These include people who have close contact with someone known or suspected to have tuberculosis, people infected with HIV, people who inject illicit drugs, people who live or work in high-risk group settings (such as a nursing home or child care center), and people who are medically underserved. Controlling tuberculosis depends on thorough screening of high-risk populations and on providing preventive therapy.

Focused Assessment for *Readiness for Enhanced Age-Appropriate Attainment of Developmental Milestones*

Defining Characteristics. When a client seeks help with psychosocial development, you should consider the diagnosis of *Readiness for enhanced age-appropriate attainment of developmental milestones.* The reasons a person might seek assistance include a history of difficulty with a previous developmental stage or task or the potential for a transitional crisis, such as one associated with childbirth, parenting, midlife, or retirement.

However, this is highly individualized; therefore your assessment should include the client's perception of appropriate behavior and whether or not the behavior is causing difficulty in the person's life.

Related Factors. For the adult, a primary related factor in failure to attain developmental milestones is lack of knowledge. The diagnosis *Readiness for enhanced age-appropriate attainment of developmental milestones* assumes the client is seeking help; thus you can ask the client to identify the cause of this need for help. Related factors could include lack of knowledge, lack of motivation, ineffective coping skills, or inadequate role models.

However, the client could also have environmental or physical factors, such as a chronic illness, physical disability, or mental disability, that have prevented achievement of an adult task. In this case, the related factors would include prescribed dependence (such as protected living), or physical or mental disability (such as mental retardation or a mental illness), deficiencies of environment (such as homelessness), or inadequate caretaking.

Focused Assessment for *Ineffective Health Maintenance*

A focused assessment for clients with *Ineffective health maintenance* includes looking at their ability to identify, manage, or seek help to maintain health (NANDA, 2001). Ask questions that will provide cues to their ability and motivation to take responsibility for their own health. For example, "Have you engaged in a healthy lifestyle in the past? For what reasons did you seek health care in the past? Did you adopt the recommended interventions? Why or why not? Do you receive support from your family or significant other? How do family members or friends make it easy (or difficult) to maintain good health practices? To what extent do you believe that maintaining and improving health is possible? Do you need financial assistance to obtain medication?"

Review common causes of adult illness and injury, and discuss ways to reduce their risks. Determine the clients' level of interest in improving their health and reducing their risks. This will also help you assess their level of knowledge. Assess whether the clients face barriers to taking effective health actions, such as finances or health care resources.

Keep in mind the common causes of illness and death for adults. They include the following:
- Accidents, acquired immunodeficiency syndrome (AIDS), homicide, and suicide
- Substance abuse that interferes with productivity and relationships and raises the risk of injury, especially domestic violence, and death
- Unsafe sexual practices, which raise the risk of unwanted pregnancies and sexually transmitted diseases, including HIV infection
- Family, lifestyle, or occupational risk factors for cancer or heart disease (such as obesity, a sedentary lifestyle, tobacco use, alcohol abuse, and poor nutrition)
- History of a lack of health-seeking behaviors

Defining Characteristics. Defining characteristics for *Ineffective health maintenance* include the following:
- History of a lack of health-seeking behaviors
- Expressed interest in improving health behaviors
- Demonstrated lack of knowledge regarding basic health practices

- Reported or observed lack of equipment, finances, or other resources
- Reported or observed impairment of personal support systems
- Reported or observed inability to take responsibility for meeting basic health practices in any or all functional pattern areas
- Demonstrated lack of adaptive behaviors to internal or external environmental changes
- History of high-risk lifestyle behaviors, such as smoking or substance abuse, or exposure to environmental or occupational risk factors

Related Factors. Factors related to the onset of *Ineffective health maintenance* include the following:
- Ineffective individual or family coping
- Perceptual or cognitive impairment
- Impaired gross or fine motor skills
- Lack of or significant alteration in communication skills
- Unachieved developmental tasks
- Lack of material resources
- Dysfunctional grieving or disabling spiritual distress
- Lack of ability to make deliberate and thoughtful judgments

*D*IAGNOSIS

Keep in mind that the diagnosis *Delayed growth and development* is a broad category applicable to a client with multiple issues. Often, however, a single issue is the focus of nursing care. When this is the case, you will want to use a more specific nursing diagnosis. Group the client's diagnostic cues to help determine the best nursing diagnosis, as described in Table 17-4.

When the client needs to make dietary modifications (for example, to improve health), the diagnosis *Imbalanced nutrition: more than (less than) body requirements* is used. When the person needs knowledge to accomplish a change in lifestyle, the diagnosis *Deficient knowledge* is used. When the person is a parent who needs help with parenting skills, use the diagnosis *Impaired parenting*. When the person is overwhelmed with the stress of caring for a dependent person, the diagnosis is *Caregiver role strain*. When the person is not

Table 17-4 *Clustering Data to Make a Nursing Diagnosis*	
HIGH-RISK LIFESTYLE CHOICES	
Data Cluster	**Diagnosis**
A 52-year-old male client smokes two packs of cigarettes daily. He has not exercised regularly since he was in college, and he cannot remember when he last had a physical examination.	Ineffective health maintenance related to lifestyle/habits
A 64-year-old female client has had three consecutive blood pressure readings above 140/90. She says she feels fine and finds it hard to believe that anything is wrong.	Knowledge deficit regarding causes of hypertension related to perception
A 36-year-old male client, 5 feet 10 inches in height, weighs 237 pounds. He reports eating fast food every day for breakfast and lunch. He says that he eats fresh vegetables and fruits about three times a week.	Imbalanced nutrition: more than body requirements related to lifestyle management

managing an acute or chronic illness effectively, the diagnosis is *Ineffective therapeutic regimen management*. There may be justification for more specific nursing diagnoses of problems that will require management to be able to effectively resolve *Ineffective health maintenance*. Examples include *Ineffective coping, Disabled family coping, Dysfunctional grieving,* and *Spiritual distress*.

PLANNING

Each plan of care must be individualized to a client's needs, age, and culture. Address the client's concerns first. Then, together with the client, develop a care plan that includes achievable short- and long-term goals designed for success. For clients at risk for *Ineffective health maintenance,* the goal is for them to demonstrate the knowledge they need to improve their health behaviors and take action to change the behavior. For example, for middle-aged adults who are sedentary, the goal would be to engage regularly, preferably daily, in moderate physical activity for at least 30 minutes per day.

Some examples of expected outcomes for the well adult are the following:

- Outlines a realistic plan for increasing healthy behaviors (specify: exercise, diet, weight loss)
- Includes positive social interactions in daily schedule
- Establishes a target date for beginning a healthy behavior
- Seeks health-related information from valid sources
- Describes strategies to eliminate unhealthy behavior
- Performs activities of daily living consistent with energy and tolerance

Explore options with clients to help them achieve goals by changing behaviors (reducing weight, stopping tobacco use, increasing exercise, preventing unwanted pregnancy, and so on). With your assistance, clients should prioritize their goals and specify time frames for achieving them.

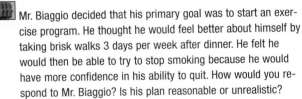
Mr. Biaggio decided that his primary goal was to start an exercise program. He thought he would feel better about himself by taking brisk walks 3 days per week after dinner. He felt he would then be able to try to stop smoking because he would have more confidence in his ability to quit. How would you respond to Mr. Biaggio? Is his plan reasonable or unrealistic?

INTERVENTION

Client interventions are based on trusting relationships. Your client relationships must be based on honesty, acceptance, respect, empathy, and cultural sensitivity. First, assess your own cultural beliefs, and become aware of regional, ethnic, and religious beliefs as well as of practices of groups in the area where you work. This aids you in the development of culturally specific interventions. Your interventions are to help clients improve their quality of life, maintain function, and delay or prevent age-related conditions.

The selection of interventions will depend on clients' cognitive and perceptual abilities as well as on the level of gross and fine motor skills needed to engage in health maintenance behaviors. If they are forgetful, they may need strategies to remind them about medications, meals, or exercise. Their communication skills (written, verbal, or gestural) are important in selecting health maintenance strategies.

Educating for Lifestyle Changes

When teaching clients about interventions to change lifestyle choices, give specific, informational instructions to help maximize compliance. Fully explaining the regimen and its rationale, demonstrating it clearly, and writing down the instructions will enhance behavior change. Providing clients with written pictorial material for them to keep and review reinforces the teaching session and will build on their ability to retain information (visually and auditory). For example, explain the purposes and expected effects of the interventions you recommend to the clients, and tell them when to expect these effects. This is especially important if the benefits of an intervention will not be immediate (for example, the benefits of a regular exercise program may not be apparent for several months). Otherwise, clients may become discouraged and abandon the intervention.

Suggest small changes rather than large ones. Ask clients to do only slightly more than they are already doing. By achieving a small goal, clients initiate a positive change that will encourage them to continue; this helps to avoid noncompliance.

Successful persuasion involves not only increasing clients' belief in their capacities but also structuring interventions so that they are likely to be successful. Sometimes, rather than eliminating established behaviors, it is better to add new ones. For example, it might be better to suggest to overweight clients that they add exercise to their day rather than that they eat less. Also, link clients' new behaviors with old ones. For example, if clients forget to take their daily medication, you might suggest that they take their medication in the morning while brushing their teeth (ODPHP, 2002).

Finally, use a combination of strategies to help educate clients, such as oral and written instructions, audiovisual aids, individual and group counseling, and community resources. Multiple techniques are more likely to foster success than single strategies. Refer clients to community agencies, voluntary health organizations (such as the American Heart Association), instructional references (such as books, videotapes, or the internet), or to support groups for clients with similar problems (ODPHP, 2002). Nursing interventions that can help homebound adults include connecting them with community services that can provide transportation to shopping areas, or with agencies that deliver prepared meals, such as Meals on Wheels.

If Mr. Biaggio succeeds in taking brisk walks three times a week for a month but makes no other changes, he is not likely to lose much weight. However, he may have achieved other benefits. Can you think of any?

Once clients fully understand the intervention, ask them for a specific commitment. Ask them to describe specifically what they plan to achieve. Doing this encourages them to begin thinking about how to integrate a new behavior into their daily schedule.

Also, ask clients if they are willing to carry out the commitment. Clients with a high degree of certainty are more likely to follow through. If your clients express uncertainty, you can explore the problems that they might be encountering in carrying out the regimen (ODPHP, 2002).

Diet. Nutritional assessments ascertain whether adults, particularly older adults, are able to obtain and prepare food and whether they consume adequate protein, calories, minerals, and vitamins. For adults, cultural influence on diet usually does not change with aging. Older adults who have followed dietary laws throughout their lives will continue to choose foods according to that diet. Decrease in taste and smell can reduce appetite. Additionally, decreased income, difficulty getting to the market, and decreased mobility can affect an adult's eating habits. Once the clients' concerns and an understanding of their issues are apparent, you can appropriately focus your teaching (ODPHP, 2002).

Exercise. An appropriate exercise program for adult clients should take into consideration their current level of mobility, which is determined by careful assessment. Even chair-bound older adults can do range-of-motion exercises. Adults who are more mobile can benefit from more advanced exercise programs that have been adapted to their needs. They should engage regularly, preferably daily, in moderate physical activity for at least 30 minutes.

Rest and Sleep. Clients and their family members should keep a regular sleep schedule, which means going to bed and getting up at the same time each day, even on weekends. Encourage clients to make their bedroom conducive to sleep, such as cool, quiet, and dark. It is better if they read or watch television in another room. Encourage clients to engage in a relaxing, nonstimulating activity at bedtime such as reading or listening to music. A warm bath or hot tub may promote sleep. Encourage clients not to bring their problems to bed and to avoid eating and drinking before bedtime (National Sleep Foundation, 2001).

Stress. Because stress is associated with increased disease susceptibility, stress management is an important component of health promotion activities. Daily stressors are associated more with health problems than are stressful life events because they result in a high level of stress being maintained over a long period.

Estate planning can be a source of stress for an older person who has spent a lifetime accumulating wealth or possessions and feels that it is important to leave something of value to others. It is important to be remembered, and, if the amount of money or property is small, it is important that it not have to go to pay for lawyers and court costs. Planning and making advance arrangements for burial or cremation, and so on, is another important topic.

The threat of an illness that results in hospitalization is a source of stress. Hospitalization is disruptive and frightening, and it has the potential to significantly reduce any savings that may have been accumulated. Even though private health insurance, Medicare, and supplemental health insurance pay a significant portion of medical expenses, hospitalization is expensive. Perhaps the greatest source of stress associated with hospitalization is the vulnerability to death or the loss of independence. Hospitalization for a fractured hip is particularly frightening, because most older adults know someone who sustained a fracture and had to enter a nursing home. The concept of loss of independence is a threat, and nursing homes are associated with death in their thoughts.

Exercise can be successfully used not only to maintain activity but also to decrease stress. Physical activity is an important factor in the adult's ability to maintain health and independence. Regular exercise promotes appetite, mental health, and balance. Adults quickly realize the benefits of a program of activity and exercise because the change in energy level can be quick and dramatic.

For older adults who live alone or even with another person, loneliness can be a problem. Supportive relationships and friendships are critical to well-being. Developing support systems can be a beneficial effect of health promotion groups.

Action Alert! Talking only of failures in life is a sign of possible despair.

Home Safety. Collaboratively, you, the client, and the client's family can increase home safety, often without much cost, through environment assessment. Teaching adults to use their spaces wisely is often all it takes for them to focus on current needs and age-related changes. Controlling clutter, using available lights, and repositioning electrical cords may be a change from how they are used to thinking about moving through their space, and it can be the start of placing a higher value on safety. The client might need teaching about the use of nonslip shoes and slippers, as well as the importance of protecting the feet by wearing shoes.

Educating for Health Management
Medication Management. Many of the nursing interventions for adults involve education about medications. At home, adults need to be assessed by the visiting nurse regarding their understanding about their drug regimen and compliance with it. After performing an assessment, you must educate clients about any misconceptions they might have about prescribed medications. Teach them about the interactions of prescribed drugs, and about the effects of taking them concurrently with over-the-counter drugs. Teach clients how to avoid medication errors and interactions, as outlined in Box 17-2 (p. 350).

Teach clients to drink plenty of fluids when taking medications. Explain that with aging, there is decreased absorption, and it takes longer for drugs to take effect. In addition, kidney function decreases, so drugs take longer to leave the body. In addition, because albumin (protein) levels are decreased, there is less protein for drugs to bind to, so there may

Teaching for Wellness
Helping an Adult Maintain Health
Box 17-2

Purpose: To maintain a healthy lifestyle.

Expected Outcome: The client will maintain his/her present level of functioning.

Client Instructions

Your client can do many things to maintain his/her health well into old age. You can help him/her by offering these suggestions:

- Maintain your social relationships. Use the telephone to call your family and friends. Attend family functions, church, activities, and senior citizen events in your community.
- Exercise every day. Walking is one of the best exercises. Wear sturdy shoes and work up to walking three to four times a week for 20 minutes each time.
- Relax. Take deep breaths and practice relaxation exercises. Visualize a peaceful outdoor scene or a happy family event. Decrease stressors in your life and share problems with a trusted person, such as your clergy.
- Eat sensibly. Eat from the five food groups. It may be easier—and better—to eat six small meals and one or two snacks than three meals each day. Drink plenty of fluids, especially water.
- Stop smoking. Do not be afraid to seek help, such as a smoking cessation class or a nicotine replacement plan, to help reduce the need for smoking. See your physician for help.
- Sleep well at night. To do so, try not to nap in the late afternoon or evening. Do not eat right before bed. Limit fluids in the evening hours to reduce the need to urinate during the night. If you wake up at night and do not fall back to sleep right away, get up and read or watch television until you become sleepy.
- Avoid constipation. Eat fruits and vegetables, drink fluids, and maintain a walking program, if possible. A stool softener, if suggested by your physician, can help with gentle elimination of stool.
- Maintain a comfortable environment. Use your heating and cooling system for adequate warmth in winter and a cool environment in very hot, humid weather.
- Practice health maintenance. Take medication as ordered. Schedule and keep appointments with your physician. Comply with suggested standards for screening tests, flu shots, and so on. Be alert to changes in your body, and seek help from your health care provider as soon as possible.

be more of the drug floating in the blood, which may lead to drug toxicity.

Instruct adults to carry a complete list of all the medications they are taking (prescription and over-the-counter), so that all health care providers stay informed about the medication regimen. Work with them to monitor their medications and, when possible, help them to use the least amount for the greatest effect. This takes effective communication between you, the client, the client's family, and the client's physician.

Make sure clients are aware of their allergies and that they communicate this information to all health care providers. When you care for a client in a short- or long-term facility, you will work together with pharmacists, physicians, and the other members of the multidisciplinary team to identify interactions, adverse reactions, and duplication of drug effects. If there is a possibility that clients will experience side effects from an intervention, such as those of medication for depression, tell the clients what to expect and under what circumstances they should stop the intervention and consult a health care provider (ODPHP, 2002).

The presence and use of support systems is directly related to the success of health maintenance activities. For the well older adult, belonging to a group of senior citizens who are experiencing similar problems in maintaining health can be a major source of support.

Health Maintenance Visits. Plan with clients for regular visits with a primary health care provider for screening and evaluation, including vision checks, physicals, immunizations, and foot care. Teaching clients to arrange annual checkups and immunizations at the same time yearly helps them remember their immunizations. Consistent scheduling helps clients arrange appointments in advance, making it possible for them to take advantage of support services provided by the community; this in turn improves client compliance in keeping appointments.

Counseling for Risky Behaviors. Research suggests that clients have only a few important beliefs about any one subject. To persuade clients to change their behavior, it is first necessary to identify their beliefs that are relevant to the high-risk behavior and to provide information based on this foundation. Counseling is used to help clients with problems related to illicit drugs and alcohol abuse, smoking, personal loss, and stress.

Changing a client's high-risk behaviors involves more than giving information. Knowledge is necessary but not sufficient to change health behaviors. One set of interventions is not effective for all clients; you will need to adapt your teaching and recommendations to each client's perceptions of health and ability to change. The best way to improve clients' health status and health behavior is by enhancing their self-efficacy (that is, their conviction that they can carry out a recommended action) (ODPHP, 2002).

Use the power of your profession. Research studies have indicated that your individual attention and feedback to the client are more useful than news media or other communication media in changing the client's knowledge and behavior. Most clients respect nurses and believe that what you say is important. However, some clients lack confidence in their ability to make lifestyle changes. Be empathic and supportive while providing firm, definite recommendations for changing high-risk behaviors. For example, you can say, "I want you to quit smoking." The message is simple and specific. You also need to monitor the client's progress through follow-up contact, either by appointment or telephone call, within a few weeks, to evaluate progress, reinforce successes, and identify and respond to problems (ODPHP, 2002).

Many barriers exist to making a change in unhealthy lifestyle behaviors. The client may feel unwilling to take responsibility for accomplishing day-to-day preventive behaviors for many reasons. Such unwillingness may result from lack of motivation, lack of readiness, inadequate health care teaching, lack of support, and lack of financial resources.

In clinics and other health care settings, barriers to implementing a preventive health program include an emphasis on curing illness and injury rather than prevention. You or your agency may not have an adequate system for tracking, monitoring, and following up on a client's progress. Your clients may lack health insurance, or their insurance may not pay for preventive services.

Other barriers may be related to you and other health care providers. You may lack training in preventive health services, or you may be confused over conflicting recommendations for adult health screening tests, personal beliefs, values, and assumptions. You may not have confidence that prevention interventions work. Additionally, you may lack time in the face of competing demands to do follow-up care with essentially well adults (ODPHP, 2002).

Development Issues. The main interventions for *Delayed development* are counseling and health education. Counseling is entering into a therapeutic relationship to help the client achieve personal development and avoid a crisis. The goals are to help clients solve their problems and to assist them in mobilizing their resources and regaining equilibrium. Their usual coping mechanisms do not work, and counseling can help them develop new coping mechanisms, such as identifying relatives or friends they can talk with about their problem. Education can provide information to enable the client to gain a better understanding of their developmental issues. For example, having a new mother take parent classes can give her confidence to be a parent.

Long-Term Care

Long-term care is a broad spectrum of nursing, medical, and other services for clients with functional limitations resulting from a chronic illness or condition that is expected to be ongoing. It is designed for the client who is not capable of independent living.

If clients have periods of confusion, totally independent living may not be possible. The lack of ability to make deliberate and thoughtful judgments is a determining factor for independent living. Clients may need to be referred for long-term care services. The types of services available in most communities include assisted living, adult day care, respite care, home care, subacute care/rehabilitation, and nursing home care.

Assisted Living. Assisted living communities are designed for older adults who are no longer able to live safely on their own, but who do not require the high level of care provided in a nursing home. They can receive assistance with medications, activities of daily living, meals, and housekeeping. The older adults live in their own private apartments that frequently have a limited kitchen area. Staff is available 24 hours a day for additional safety, and licensed nursing services are often provided on a limited basis. The staff provides social activities and scheduled transportation for doctor office visits, for example.

Adult Day Care. Adult day care (ADC) programs are community-based group programs designed to meet the needs of functionally impaired adults through an individual plan of care. The clients have difficulty taking care of themselves at home but wish to maintain their independence. The goals of these programs are to assist them in restoring or maintaining their capacity for self-care while under the direct supervision of professional staff.

Respite Care. Respite care provides a temporary respite for family caregivers by allowing ill family members to have a short-term stay in an assisted living community or a nursing home designed to keep them on a short-term basis. Generally, the older adults remain a week to a month, depending on their situation. They receive the services available at the facility, such as meals, medication monitoring, and assistance with bathing, that are available to the long-term residents.

Home Care. Home care refers to any of a variety of services provided to clients and families in their own residence for the purpose of treating illnesses, restoring health, rehabilitating, promoting health, and palliation.

Subacute Care/Rehabilitation. Subacute care/rehabilitation is inpatient care designed for adults who have an acute illness, injury, or exacerbation of disease process. Adults may be moved to a rehabilitation hospital for specific therapies expected to increase their function, or to a subacute unit in a nursing home. It is generally more intensive than traditional nursing home care but less so than acute care.

Nursing Home Care. For residents who require a high level of medical care and assistance, nursing home care provides 24-hour nursing care by licensed nurses. Residents generally have high functional care needs and multiple medical problems. Some nursing homes provide short-term rehabilitative stays for clients recovering from injuries or illnesses, and some have a separate unit for residents with Alzheimer's disease. Still other nursing homes provide nursing care for residents with Alzheimer's disease and other dementias only.

*E*VALUATION

Evaluation is a systematic, ongoing process of evaluating the client's progress toward the attainment of goals, as suggested in Box 17-3 (p. 352). Before evaluating altered development in the adult, you need to have set long-term goals that are in keeping with the clients' abilities and lifestyle. Also, the expected outcomes that you have chosen need to let the clients experience progress toward the long-term goals. Clients and their families, when appropriate, should be involved in the process. If the expected outcomes are not achieved within the defined time frame, reassessment is needed to examine the impediments to the progress. The ongoing assessment data you gather are used to revise nursing diagnoses, outcomes, and the plan of care, in consultation with clients and significant others. Evaluate the effectiveness of your interventions

Nursing Care Plan A MIDDLE-AGED ADULT WITH BORDERLINE HYPERTENSION   Box 17-3

ASSESSMENT DATA

After performing an assessment at the client's worksite, the occupational nurse records the following report: *"Mr. Biaggio is a 42-year-old obese Italian-American man, who is married with two children who are in high school and living at home. He works as an accountant at a large insurance company, smokes two packs of cigarettes/day, eats a diet high in fat, and has not exercised for "years." "I don't many eat fruits and vegetables. I just never liked them." Mr. Biaggio states he does not understand why he has high blood pressure and that he is not feeling bad. He knows he should lose a little weight and get some exercise. He knows that smoking is not good for him, but he has been unable to quit in the past. BP is 148/96. Height is 5'10", and weight is 227 lb."*

NURSING ORDERS

Health teaching about hypertension, low-salt diet, and weight reduction
Recommendations for smoking cessation and exercise
Follow-up appointment in 1 month
Refer to private physician for follow-up care

NANDA Nursing Diagnosis	NOC Expected Outcomes With Indicators	NIC Interventions With Selected Activities	Selected Evaluation Data
INEFFECTIVE HEALTH MAINTENANCE **Related Factors:** • Wt. 227 lbs • Ht. 5'10" • BP 148/96 • Smokes 2 packs cigarettes/day • 0 fruits/vegetables	**HEALTH PROMOTING BEHAVIORS** • Client will have appropriate screenings and immunizations done within the next 6 months. • Client will eliminate high-risk behaviors within 1 year. • Client will be knowledgeable about health promotion activities within 1 month exercise program.	**COUNSELING** • Review appropriate screening tests and immunizations for client's age-group. • Counsel client on recognizing high-risk behaviors and understanding their connection to chonic illness. • Review Mr. Biaggio's eating habits, including who cooks and how the food is prepared.	• Client has scheduled an appointment for a physical examination with his private physician. • Client can describe connection between smoking, high-fat diet, lack of exercise, and hypertension, heart disease, cancers, and other chronic diseases.

CRITICAL THINKING QUESTIONS

1. How might the family affect Mr. Biaggio's compliance with the treatment regime?
2. What other resources might be useful for him?
3. What approach would you use to help Mr. Biaggio stop smoking?
4. How is smoking related to Mr. Biaggio's hypertension?

Nursing outcome and intervention labels from Johnson, M., Bulechek, G., McCloskey Dochterman, J. M., Maas, M., & Moorhead, S. (2001). *Nursing diagnoses, outcomes, and interventions: NANDA, NOC, and NIC linkages.* St Louis, MO: Mosby.

by considering your clients' responses to them as well as the attainment of the goals.

The nurse in Mr. Biaggio's primary care clinic calls him 1 week after his appointment and records the following evaluation information in his chart.

> **SAMPLE DOCUMENTATION NOTE FOR MR. BIAGGIO**
> Reports that he has reduced his smoking to 1 pack a day for the week since his visit. Has continued to walk 3 times a week. His wife wants him to go with her to a nutrition class, but he is not sure about that.

Key Principles

• The developmental tasks of adults are partially related to age, but are influenced by genetics, socioeconomic status, ethnic group, religious faith, and social expectations.

• Biological development in the adult includes the periods of stability and decline.
• Erikson's stages of psychosocial development of the adult are centered around developing adult relationships, contributing to society, and developing satisfaction.
• Lifestyle risk factors for the adult are poor diet, lack of exercise, inadequate rest and sleep, stress, and engaging in risky behaviors.
• Each psychosocial stage of adulthood is associated with choices that can lead to health problems.
• Socioeconomic factors create risk for illness and injury at any developmental stage.
• The risk for illness increases with physical decline and is related to lifestyle choices.
• Assessment of the well adult is a process of holistic assessment of all functional health patterns.
• Cognitive function should be assessed carefully, in an environment that supports maximum function, using tools that are specifically designed for accuracy with older adults.

- Medication history is a part of health assessment.
- Problems of adult development are diagnosed as *Delayed growth and development* or a more specific diagnosis to address individual problems.
- Planning for the well adult is centered on the goals of maintaining health and preventing illness.
- Intervening with well adults to enable them to maintain health requires education for change in lifestyle.
- Intervening with the adult with health problems includes education for health management.
- Evaluation is a systematic, ongoing process.

Bibliography

Alberta Tobacco Reduction Alliance. (2002). *Smoking-related deaths.* Available from http://www.tobaccotruth.com/tobaccobasics/deaths.htm.

American Psychiatric Association. (2000). *Diagnostic and statistical manual of mental disorders* (4th ed.) [text revision, DSM-IV-TR]. Washington, DC: American Psychiatric Association.

Clegg, L. X., Li, F. P., Hankey, B. F., & Edwards, B. K. (2002). Cancer survival among U.S. whites and minorities. *Archives of Internal Medicine, 162,* 1985-1993.

*Cumming, E., & Henry, W. E. (1961). *Growing old: The process of disengagement.* New York: Basic Books.

*Erikson, E. (1959). Growth and crises of the healthy personality. *Psychological Issues, 1,* 50-100.

*Erikson, E. H. (1963). *Childhood and society* (2nd ed.). New York: Norton.

*Erikson, E. H. (1982). *The life cycle completed.* New York: Norton.

*Folstein, M. E., Folstein, S. E., & McHugh P. R. (1975). Mini-mental state: A practical method for grading the cognitive state of patients for the clinician. *Journal of Psychiatric Research, 12,* 189-198.

Johnson, M., Bulechek, G., McCloskey Dochterman, J. M., Maas, M., & Moorhead, S. (2001). *Nursing diagnoses, outcomes, and interventions: NANDA, NOC, and NIC linkages.* St Louis, MO: Mosby.

Kuttner, R. (1999). The American health care system: Employer-sponsored health coverage. *New England Journal of Medicine, 340,* 3. Available from http://www.nejm.org/content/1999/0340/0003/0248.asp.

*Levinson, D. J. (1978). *The seasons of a man's life.* New York: Knopf.

*Levinson, D. J. (1986). A conception of adult development. *American Psychologist, 41,* 3-13.

*Levinson, D. J. (1996). *The seasons of a woman's life.* New York: Knopf.

*Levinson, D., Darrow, C., Klein, E., Levinson, M., & McKee, B. (1986). Periods in the adult development of men: Ages 18-45. *Counseling Psychologist, 6*(12), 21-25.

MediResource. (2000a). *Depression.* Available from http://www.mediresource.net/canoe/health/PatientInfo.asp?DiseaseID=43.

MediResource. (2000b). *Suicide.* Available from http://www.mediresource.net/canoe/health/PatientInfo.asp?DiseaseID=206.

National Center for Chronic Disease Prevention and Health Promotion (U.S. Department of Health and Human Services, Public Health Services, Centers for Disease Control and Prevention). (2000). *Chronic diseases and their risk factors: The leading causes of death—A report with state-by-state information.* Available from http://www.cdc.gov/nccdphp/statbook/statbook.htm.

National Clearinghouse for Alcohol and Drug Information (U.S. Department of Health and Human Services, Substance Abuse and Maternal Health Services Administration). (1998). *The national drug control strategy, 1998.* Available from http://www.health.org/ndc98/contents.html.

National Institute on Aging (U.S. Department of Health and Human Services [USDHHS]). (2000). *Life expectancy in G-7 industrialized nations may exceed past predictions, study suggests.* Available from http://www.nia.nih.gov/news/pr/2000/06%2D14.htm.

National Institute on Alcohol Abuse and Alcoholism (U.S. Department of Health and Human Services). (1999). *Report of a subcommittee of the National Advisory Council on Alcohol Abuse and Alcoholism on the review of the extramural research portfolio for prevention.* Available from http://www.niaaa.nih.gov/extramural/prevention.htm.

National Sleep Foundation. (2001). A New Year's resolution for Americans from the National Sleep Foundation: Make time for sleep! Available from http://www.sleepfoundation.org/PressArchives/resolution.html.

North American Nursing Diagnosis Association. (2001). *Nursing diagnoses: Definitions and classification, 1999-2000.* Philadelphia: Author.

Office of Disease Prevention and Health Promotion (U.S. Department of Health and Human Services, Public Health Services). (2002). *Guide to clinical preventive services, 2000-2002* (3rd ed.). Available from http://www.ahrq.gov/clinic/uspstfix.htm.

*Pfeiffer, E. (1975). A short portable mental status questionnaire for the assessment of brain deficits in elderly patients. *Journal of the American Geriatric Society, 23,* 433-441.

Statistics Canada. (2002a). *Changes in unmet health care needs 2000/01.* Available from http://www.statcan.ca/Daily/English/020313/d020313a.htm.

Statistics Canada. (2002b). *High blood pressure.* Available from http://www.statcan.ca/english/freepub/82-221-XIE/00502/high/canada/cblood.htm.

Statistics Canada. (2002c) *Labour force characteristics by age and sex.* Available from http://www.statcan.ca/english/Pgdb/People/Labour/labor20a.htm.

Statistics Canada. (2002d). *Population by sex and age.* Available from http://www.statcan.ca/english/Pgdb/People/Population/demo10a.htm.

Thobaben, M., & Buxton-Blake, P. (2002). *Honor society of Sigma Theta Tau international nursing's online case studies for nursing: Ms. Florence Luke's road to recovery from a major depressive episode—Case Study LB0003.* Available from http://www.nursing-society.org/education/case_studies/cases/LB0003.html#issues.

U.S. Census Bureau (U.S. Department of Commerce). (2001a). *Health insurance coverage: 2000.* Available from http://www.census.gov/hhes/www/hlthin00.html.

U.S. Census Bureau (U.S. Department of Commerce). (2001b). *Poverty: 2000 highlights.* Available from http://www.census.gov/hhes/poverty/poverty00/pov00hi.html.

U.S. Census Bureau (U.S. Department of Commerce). (2002). *DP-1: Profile of general population characteristics.* Available from http://factfinder.census.gov/servlet/QTTable?ds_name=D&geo_id=D&qr_name=DEC_2000_SF1_U_DP1&_lang=en.

U.S. Department of Health and Human Services. (2000). *Healthy People 2010: Understanding and improving health* (2nd ed.). Washington, DC: U.S. Government Printing Office.

U.S. Department of Health and Human Services (Public Health Services, Centers for Disease Control and Prevention). (2001). *Suicide.* Available from http://www.cdc.gov/nchs/fastats/ suicide.htm.

U.S. Department of Labor, Bureau of Labor Statistics. (2001). *Employment characteristics of families summary.* Available from http://stats.bls.gov/news.release/famee.nr0.htm.

U.S. Department of Labor, Bureau of Labor Statistics. (2002). *The employment situation: January 2002.* Available from http://www.bls.gov/news.release/empsit.nr0.htm.

---

*Asterisk indicates a classic or definitive work on this subject.

Health Perception

Key Terms

disease
etiology
health goals
health-illness continuum
health perception
health promotion
health within illness
illness
population health
preventive health care
primary health care
primary prevention
secondary prevention
tertiary prevention
well-being
wellness

Learning Objectives

After studying this chapter, you should be able to do the following:

- Describe the perception of health for individuals, families, and communities
- Compare factors that affect health for individuals, families, and communities
- Understand the focus of assessment of health in the individual, family, and community
- Identify health goals and expected outcomes when planning for individuals, families, and communities
- Discuss the use of the nursing diagnosis *Health-seeking behaviors*
- Identify methodologies of intervention for improving the health of individuals, families, and communities
- Evaluate health outcomes in individuals, families, and communities

An advertisement appearing in a local newspaper invites citizens to a public forum organized by the local health council and regional health board. The purpose of the forum is to identify local and community health goals. The community, called Delta, is a local division of a Canadian province, but it could be anywhere in the United States. The community has a population of 46,000 and consists of a mix of farming and light industry. Many residents work in a nearby city.

At the public forum, 30 interested citizens gather. They include health professionals, municipal politicians, and lay citizens. The chairperson of the health council outlines the evening's agenda. First, participants will review individual and family health perceptions and how they relate to community health goals. Next, participants will be introduced to government health initiatives that are currently under development. These documents will serve as a resource and basis for discussion.

The group is beginning a process that will include assessing the perception of health in the community and identifying community needs, identifying local health goals and priorities, identifying expected outcomes of community health actions, determining the methodology (programs and services) to achieve identified outcomes, and evaluating the results.

The nurses involved in this group contribute their perception of health to the planning process. If they identify a nursing diagnosis for the community with which they were working, it might be *Health-seeking behaviors*.

KEY NURSING DIAGNOSES FOR Health Perception

Health-seeking behaviors (specify): Active seeking (by a person in stable health) of ways to alter personal health habits and/or the environment in order to move toward a higher level of health

Readiness for enhanced community coping: Pattern of community activities for adaptation and problem solving that is satisfactory for meeting the demand or needs of a community but can be improved for management or improvement of current and/or future problems or stressors

CONCEPTS OF HEALTH

Health is important to individuals, families, and communities. It is important to individuals to feel good, to be able to perform needed work, and to enjoy life. It is important to families to meet the needs of their members by providing love, belonging, food, shelter, and safety and by helping family members achieve their highest potential. Health is important to the community, from the standpoints of both quality of life and the economic well-being of its citizens. Additionally, health has been described as the bedrock on which social progress is built. Healthy people can do things that make life worthwhile, and as the level of health increases, so does the potential for happiness. **Health perception** is the knowledge and experience of one's state of wellness and well-being.

Nurses are involved in health care planning and decision making for individuals, families, and communities. To fulfill the nursing role at any of these three levels, you will need to understand the meaning of health to the individual, the family, and the community. As you begin to study this chapter on the perception of health, consider your own perception of health. Ask yourself important questions about health, such as these: What does it mean when I say I am healthy? Could I be healthier? How could I make that happen? Is it worth the effort? What would I need to sacrifice to become healthier? Are there factors in my environment that would hinder me from becoming a healthier person?

Also think about your family and community. What factors would you use to describe a healthy family? A healthy community? What would need to change in your community to increase the health of the people with whom you live and work? To answer these questions, you need to consider the influences of biology, behavior, physical environment, social environment, and public policies and interventions (Figure 18-1, p. 356).

Our ideas about health and illness changed over the past century. At the beginning of the twentieth century, society thought in terms of a dichotomy of health or illness. Health care was focused on conquering the most prevalent diseases. Around the middle of that century, the death rate from acute disease declined below that of chronic illness. Thus it became more important to identify the risk factors of chronic illnesses and to change lifestyle factors to prevent them. In the 1980s, the emphasis in health care shifted to changing behaviors and health habits as a way to prevent illness and prolong life. Today, the importance of a comprehensive program of health promotion is recognized as a means of managing all the factors that determine whether or not we are healthy and live in a healthy community. **Health promotion** is the advancement of health through the encouragement of activities that enhance the wellness of individuals, families, and communities.

Health as a National and an International Goal

As citizens of the world, we can no longer view health only from an individual or a local community perspective. A global economy and growing international mobility suggest that all countries must share the health concerns of any one country. The industrialized nations of the world look to each other for ideas about how to improve the health of their citizens and those in less developed countries. They also must monitor the threat of pathogen transmission across international boundaries.

The World Health Organization (WHO) has defined health as a state of complete physical, mental, and social well-being, and not merely as the absence of illness. This holistic definition recognizes that being healthy involves more than simply physiological functioning. The need for comprehensive health goals to address these determinants of health has been well recognized. **Health goals** outline broadly what needs to be done to achieve health for individuals, families, and communities.

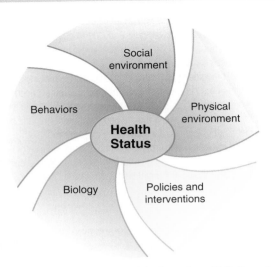

Figure 18-1. Determinants of health. (Data from U.S. Department of Health and Human Services. [2000]. *Healthy People 2010* [2nd ed]. Washington, DC: U.S. Government Printing Office.)

Box 18-2	Focus Areas for *Healthy People 2010*
Access to quality health services	Immunization and infectious diseases
Arthritis, osteoporosis, and chronic back pain	Injury and violence prevention
Cancer	Maternal, infant, and child health
Chronic kidney disease	Medical product safety
Diabetes	Mental health and mental disorders
Disability and secondary conditions	Nutrition and overweight
Educational and community-based programs	Occupational safety and health
Environmental health	Oral health
Family planning	Physical activity and fitness
Food safety	Public health infrastructure
Health communication	Respiratory diseases
Heart disease and stroke	Sexually transmitted diseases
Human immunodeficiency virus (HIV)	Substance abuse
	Tobacco use
	Vision and hearing

Box 18-1   *Healthy People 2010*: What Are Its Goals?

Healthy People 2010 is designed to achieve two overarching goals:

GOAL 1. INCREASE QUALITY AND YEARS OF HEALTHY LIFE: To help individuals of all ages increase life expectancy *and* improve their quality of life.

GOAL 2. ELIMINATE HEALTH DISPARITIES: To eliminate health disparities between different segments of the population.

The WHO also declared that health is a fundamental human right and established a social goal to attain the highest possible level of health by all people by the year 2000 (WHO, 1978). This goal was subsequently adopted by many nations, including the United States (Box 18-1). WHO further promoted primary health care as the key to attaining the target of health for all by the year 2000.

In 1995, the U.S. Public Health Service released updated target health objectives for the United States in a document entitled *Healthy People 2010: National Health Promotion and Disease Prevention Objectives*. This document outlined 28 priority areas and established scores of specific health objectives for the country (Box 18-2).

A consortium of more than 300 organizations worked with local, state, and federal government agencies to develop national goals for a preventive health agenda. Box 18-3 lists some facts that form the basis for the targets of *Healthy People 2010*. The first year of *Healthy People 2010* was a time of listening, and it began a broad consultation process for a decade-long agenda. The overarching goal of *Healthy People 2010* is "increasing the quality and years of healthy life," but the agenda also strengthened the *Healthy People 2000* goal of "reducing health disparities" to read "elimination of health disparities."

Definitions of Health

Whether a client is an individual, a family, or a community, your understanding of different perspectives of health will help you to manage health and health care from the client's perspective. The client's goals for health are derived from the definitions of health.

Health as the Absence of Disease. Health and illness can be viewed as a dichotomy, with health being defined as the absence of disease. A **disease** is a specific disorder characterized by a recognizable set of signs and symptoms and attributable to heredity, infection, diet, or environment. A disease is an interruption in the continuous process of health. A disease may disrupt the person's ability to function, and it may even shorten life.

Using this definition of health, health care is the diagnosis and treatment of disease based on identification of a specific disorder and its etiology. **Etiology** is the cause of the disease. If the cause of the disease can be removed, the person will often be cured of the disease. For example, using antibiotics to remove the cause of a disease will cure an infection caused by bacteria. Etiologies of diseases include the following:

- Biological agents, such as viruses, bacteria, fungi, rickettsia, protozoa, and helminths
- Chemical agents, such as metals, poisons, and strong irritants
- Physical agents, such as heat, cold, radiation, and electricity
- Stress
- Genetically transmitted defects
- Wear and tear on the body

However, the paradigm of treating the disease by removing the etiology works only for certain diseases. Function may be irreversibly altered before the etiology is removed. Thus not all diseases can be cured.

| **Box 18-3** | **Facts About Health Indicators** |

- Regular physical activity throughout life is important for maintaining a healthy body, enhancing psychological well-being, and preventing premature death. In 1999, 65% of adolescents engaged in the recommended amount of physical activity. In 1997, only 15% of adults performed the recommended amount of physical activity, and 40% of adults engaged in no leisure-time physical activity.
- Cigarette smoking is the single most preventable cause of disease and death in the United States. Smoking results in more deaths each year in the United States than AIDS, alcohol, cocaine, heroin, homicide, suicide, motor vehicle crashes, and fires—all combined. Tobacco-related deaths number more than 430,000 per year among U.S. adults, representing more than 5 million years of potential life lost. Direct medical costs attributable to smoking total at least $50 billion per year.
- Alcohol and illicit drug use are associated with many of this country's most serious problems, including violence, injury, and HIV infection. The annual economic costs to the United States from alcohol abuse were estimated to be $167 billion in 1995, and the costs from drug abuse were estimated to be $110 billion.
- Unintended pregnancies and sexually transmitted diseases (STDs), including infection with HIV, which causes AIDS, can result from unprotected sexual behaviors. Abstinence is the only method of complete protection. Condoms, if used correctly and consistently, can help prevent both unintended pregnancy and STDs.
- Nearly 700,000 cases of AIDS have been reported in the United States since the HIV/AIDS epidemic began in the 1980s. The latest estimates indicate that 800,000 to 900,000 people in the United States are currently infected with HIV. The lifetime cost of health care associated with HIV infection, in light of recent advances in HIV diagnostics and therapies, is $155,000 or more per person.
- Depression is associated with other medical conditions, such as heart disease, cancer, and diabetes, as well as with anxiety and eating disorders. Depression has also been associated with alcohol and illicit drug abuse. An estimated 8 million persons aged 15 to 54 years had coexisting mental and substance abuse disorders within the past year. The total of the estimated direct and indirect costs of mental illness in the United States in 1996 was $150 billion.
- More than 400 Americans die each day from injuries due primarily to motor vehicle crashes, firearms, poisonings, suffocation, falls, fires, and drowning. The risk of injury is so great that most persons sustain a significant injury at some time during their lives. Motor vehicle crashes are the most common cause of serious injury. In 1998 there were 15.6 deaths from motor vehicle crashes per 100,000 persons. In 1995 the cost of injury and violence in the United States was estimated at more than $224 billion per year. These costs include direct medical care and rehabilitation as well as productivity losses to the nation's workforce. The total societal cost of motor vehicle crashes alone exceeds $150 billion annually.
- An estimated 25% of preventable illnesses worldwide can be attributed to poor environmental quality. In the United States, air pollution alone is estimated to be associated with 50,000 premature deaths and an estimated $40 billion to $50 billion in health-related costs annually. Two indicators of air quality are ozone (outdoor) and environmental tobacco smoke (indoor).
- Vaccines are among the greatest public health achievements of the twentieth century. Immunizations can prevent disability and death from infectious diseases for individuals and can help control the spread of infections within communities.
- In 1998, 73% of children received all vaccines recommended for universal administration.
- In 1998, influenza immunization rates were 64% in adults aged 65 years and older—almost double the 1989 immunization rate of 33%. In 1998, only 46% of persons aged 65 years and older had ever received a pneumococcal vaccine.
- More than 44 million persons in the United States do not have health insurance, including 11 million uninsured children. Over the past decade, the proportion of persons under age 65 years with health insurance remained steady at about 85%. About one third of adults under age 65 years and below the poverty level were uninsured. For persons of Hispanic origin, approximately one third were without health insurance coverage in 1997. Mexican Americans had one of the highest uninsured rates at 40%.

From U.S. Department of Health and Human Services. (2000). With understanding and improving health and objectives for improving health. In *Healthy People 2010* (2nd ed.). Washington, DC: U.S. Government Printing Office. Retrieved from http://www. health.gov/healthypeople/Document/html/uih/uih_bw/uih_4.htm.

An acute condition is one with a sudden onset and, usually, a short duration. If the disease cannot be cured, it may become chronic. A chronic disease is one that lasts for an extended time, often for the person's lifetime. The definition of a chronic disease frequently specifies that it lasts 6 months or longer. Chronic diseases can have periods of remission in which symptoms disappear or are minimal, and periods of exacerbation in which symptoms reappear or become worse.

Chronic illness makes us less comfortable with a definition of health as an absence of disease. People with chronic illnesses may define themselves across a continuum of health from very poor health to even excellent health. The definition of health becomes less a matter of "Do I have a disease?" and more a matter of "How well can I function?" People with arthritis, muscular dystrophy, psoriasis, and even heart disease may believe themselves to be healthy and may describe themselves as ill only during an exacerbation of the disease.

That is why **illness** refers to the personal experience of feeling unhealthy, caused by changes in a person's state of well-being and social function.

Health as a Continuum. If health is not merely the absence of disease, then perhaps we should think of it as a continuum. A **health-illness continuum** ranges from high-level wellness—an optimal state of mental and physical well-being—to premature death (Figure 18-2, p. 358). In the center of the continuum is a neutral state in which the person cannot be considered either healthy or ill. From the neutral state to the limits of the continuum, there exist wide variations in levels of health and illness. Every person exists at some point on the continuum and may move back and forth between the two extremes. A person at any point on the continuum can be focused in the direction of wellness (Ryan & Travis, 1988).

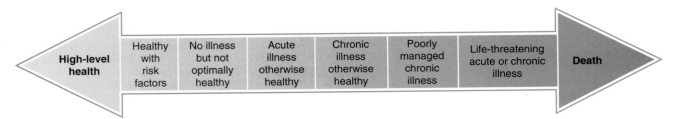

Figure 18-2. Health as a continuum.

Thinking of health as existing on a continuum has several advantages. For one, the health-illness continuum recognizes that few people are in an optimal state of health, thus providing the philosophy of optimal health as a goal and health care as a way of helping people move toward this goal. For another, the continuum discounts the notion that disease and health are dichotomous terms.

The health-illness continuum recognizes that more than one factor is necessary to determine a person's state of health. A person with arthritis who walks 3 miles a day, eats a well-balanced diet, and has a positive outlook on life may be closer to optimal health on the continuum than a person with no identifiable illness but with a sedentary lifestyle, a junk-food diet, a lack of energy, and a fear of the world.

The health-illness continuum makes room for health within illness. **Health within illness** is an event that can expand human potential by providing an opportunity for personal growth and well-being despite having an illness. The outcome of an illness is that the person becomes stronger as a human being, even though the disease may not be cured. Many people who suffer from chronic illness or life-threatening acute illness can develop a heightened sense of self and of personal potential, can feel greater spiritual inner peace, and can discover new meaning and purpose in life.

Health as Wellness and Well-Being. Health as high-level wellness includes both positive physiological function and a sense of well-being. **Well-being** is a subjective perception of a good and satisfactory existence in which the individual has a positive experience of personal abilities, harmony, and vitality. Like illness, well-being is a relative, changing state experienced in the course of everyday living.

Wellness is a state of optimal health or optimal physical and social functioning. Wellness includes optimal physical function, successful and satisfying relationships with others, emotional stability, managing feelings comfortably, intellectual growth, and a spiritual element that gives meaning and purpose to life (Figure 18-3). Additionally, several assumptions underlie the concept of wellness to give it meaning as a framework for health care (Ryan & Travis, 1988).

Individuals possess their own optimal level of functioning, which represents the best state of well-being that is possible for them. Each person sets individual goals that are compatible with body build, age, and physical state. Not everyone can jog 5 miles a day, nor would everyone enjoy the benefits associated with long-distance jogging.

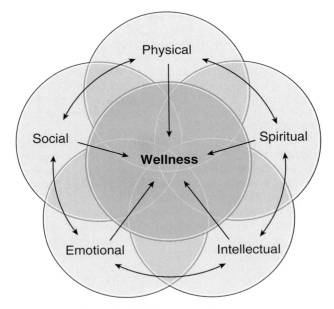

Figure 18-3. Dimensions of wellness.

Wellness is a choice that cannot be passively achieved. To achieve optimal health, a person must choose to engage in positive health actions and behaviors to achieve wellness. A person purposefully engages in actions to attain and maintain health. These actions can be in response to internal drives, stressors, or bodily functions, or they can be in response to environmental risk factors that threaten health and well-being.

Wellness is a process; thus the achievement of wellness is ongoing. Wellness is not a finite state to be achieved in the future, with the present being a time of constant struggle to attain this utopian state. Rather, the process itself is wellness when the person recognizes and experiences the possibility for health and happiness in each moment.

Wellness is an efficient channeling of energy received from the environment, transformed within you, and sent on to affect the world outside. Wellness is the integration of body, mind, and spirit, the appreciation that everything you do, think, feel, and believe has an impact on your state of health. Wellness is holding yourself in high esteem. Accepting yourself as a worthwhile person and recognizing the value in your personal attributes is necessary for high-level wellness. High-level wellness is associated with a good feeling about yourself in relationship to other people.

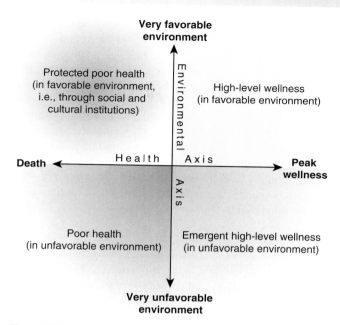

Figure 18-4. Dunn's concept of well-being. (Redrawn from Dunn, H. L. [1959]. High-level wellness for man and society. *American Journal of Public Health,* 49[6], 786-792.)

Box 18-4   The Population Health Approach

A population health approach has two major differences from an individual health approach.

RANGE OF HEALTH DETERMINANTS: Health problems cannot be totally explained by individual characteristics and behaviors. Individual health is also determined by factors that affect populations as a whole. Population health strategies address the entire range of factors that determine health.

POPULATIONS AS TARGET: Individual health care solves health problems or improves health one person at a time. Population health strategies are designed to affect the entire population.

Knowledge of the environment in which wellness is achieved is necessary to understand wellness. Dunn (1959) uses a grid to depict a concept of wellness (Figure 18-4). The horizontal axis is the continuum from peak wellness to death. The vertical axis is the environment, from very favorable to very unfavorable. The four quadrants in the grid represent the interactions of the state of wellness with the environment.

- *High-level wellness in a favorable environment.* This quadrant represents a person who is in an optimal state of health. The environment supports the person's efforts to achieve high-level wellness.
- *Emergent high-level wellness in an unfavorable environment.* This person has the knowledge, motivation, and physical stamina to achieve high-level wellness. Nonsupportive environmental factors could be demanding role responsibilities, a lack of financial resources, an unclean water supply, or an unsafe environment. High-level wellness is possible but would require more planning and effort.
- *Protected poor health in a favorable environment.* This person has one or more health problems but is able to manage them because the environment is supportive. The person has access to high-quality medical care, nursing services, and social services. Financial resources allow the person to engage home maintenance services as needed.
- *Poor health in an unfavorable environment.* This person has one or more health problems—such as old age, diabetes, and obesity—and an environment unfavorable to wellness. For example, the person might live in a rural farming community without medical services, might lack health insurance to pay for medicine, and the diabetes may frequently be uncontrolled, making complications likely.

Health in Populations. Health in a community is defined by the parameters of population health (Box 18-4). **Population health** considers health problems encountered as a result of being a part of a group and focuses intervention on the population rather than on the individual. A population can be a subgroup within a community, such as teenage mothers in the local high school, or a larger group, such as men at risk for heart disease. Population health addresses the five determinants of health: biology, behaviors, physical environment, social environment, public policies and interventions (U.S. Department of Health and Human Services, 2000).

Physical environment can be thought of as that which can be seen, touched, heard, smelled, and tasted. However, the physical environment also contains less tangible elements, such as radiation and ozone. The physical environment can harm individual and community health, especially when individuals and communities are exposed to toxic substances, irritants, infectious agents, and physical hazards in homes, schools, and worksites. The physical environment can also promote good health—for example, by providing clean and safe places for people to work, exercise, and play.

Our understanding of these determinants and how they relate to one another, coupled with our understanding of how individual and community health affects the health of the national community, is perhaps the most important key to achieving our *Healthy People 2010* goals of increasing the quality and years of life and of eliminating the nation's health disparities.

FACTORS AFFECTING HEALTH

When planning for health care, we must consider multiple factors that affect health. Some factors have greater impact on the types of services needed than others. The following factors are commonly considered in community health planning.

Biology

Biology refers to the individual's genetic makeup (those factors with which one is born), family history (which may suggest risk for disease), and the physical and mental health problems acquired during life.

Heredity, or genetic makeup (in this case, predisposition to specific illnesses), raises known health risks. Family histories of diabetes mellitus, cancer, and coronary artery disease are examples of known genetic risk factors. The methods of managing genetically transmitted disease include case-finding and treating the manifestations of the illness. However, genetics as a cause of disease is not clear-cut. The onset of many genetically transmitted diseases requires an interplay of environmental and lifestyle factors with heredity.

Social Environment

Social environment includes interactions with family, friends, co-workers, and others in the community. It also encompasses social institutions, such as law enforcement, the workplace, places of worship, and schools. Housing, public transportation, and the presence or absence of violence in the community are other components of the social environment.

Individual, family, and community health is affected by a variety of intellectual factors. In individuals, cognitive abilities, educational level, and past experience all play a role in shaping a person's attitude toward health care. A family's knowledge about health and illness influences its members' ability to understand disease patterns, factors involved in health and illness, and the importance of personal health practices. Likewise, the community's health status is influenced by the knowledge of its citizens. As citizens become more informed through modern communication and technology, more communities are calling for improved health standards and practices.

Social networks have a profound influence on the health status of individuals, families, and communities. The organization of the community and health care system can determine how clients can access and obtain health care. Recreational facilities, churches, and social organizations are part of the community social network that affects health and health status. You, along with other individuals, families, and communities, need to work toward shared values and collective actions that will ensure equitable health practices and treatment for all citizens.

Behaviors

Behaviors are individual responses or reactions to internal stimuli and external conditions. Behaviors can have a reciprocal relationship to biology; in other words, each can react to the other. Personal choices and the social and physical environments surrounding individuals can shape behaviors. The social and physical environments include all factors that affect the life of individuals, positively or negatively, and many may not be under their immediate or direct control.

In recent years, lifestyle factors have received major attention for their influence on health. Lifestyle includes diet, exercise, stress level, health practices, coping skills, education, work, interpersonal relationships, and cultural practices. They are the sum of a person's life experiences.

Family health practices play an important role in the health of individuals and communities. Families can promote a positive perception of health by providing a supportive environment, by promoting positive health practices, by appropriate use of health services, and by seeking safety and security for family members.

Cultural factors influence individual beliefs and values. Established customs influence entry into the health care system and personal health practices. In 1989, a study on health education practices of African Americans showed that most did not have access to health education as a means of primary prevention (Airhihenbuwa, 1989).

Additionally, factors such as income, layoffs, the cost of housing, the cost of health services, community design, education and training, social services, and public policy can all affect health status. In fact, these economic factors affect individual, family, and community health status in many ways. Thus economic factors must be addressed if citizens are to achieve improved health.

Physical Environment

Physical environmental factors contribute to the health status of individuals, families, and communities. The quality of one's work life, safety and security factors, and environmental ecosystem issues are examples of the many possible environmental factors that can influence health. It is important for you to assess the client's physical environment, recognize possible risk factors, and work with other health disciplines and team members to address the health risks identified.

Public Policy and Intervention

Public policies and interventions can have a powerful and positive effect on the health of individuals and the community. Examples include health promotion campaigns to prevent smoking; policies mandating child restraints and safety belt use in automobiles; disease prevention services, such as immunization of children, adolescents, and adults; and clinical services, such as enhanced mental health care. Policies and interventions that promote individual and community health may be implemented by a variety of agencies, such as transportation, education, energy, housing, labor, justice, and other venues, or through places of worship, community-based organizations, civic groups, and businesses.

The health of individuals and communities also depends greatly on access to quality health care. Expanding access to quality health care is important to eliminate health disparities and to increase the quality and years of healthy life for all people living in the United States. Health care in the broadest sense includes not only services received through health care providers but also health information and services received through other venues in the community.

Good health depends on equitable access to all necessary and appropriate health services. These consist of prevention and health promotion services, services to reduce pain and suffering and restore health, and services to enhance quality of life for those with chronic diseases and limitations. For example, adequate perinatal care can result in healthier babies.

ASSESSMENT

 The public forum for the citizens of Delta continues. Participants have searched for a definition of health that applies to their community. They now have a better understanding of the many related factors that contribute to a definition of health. They are ready to begin the process of assessing the health needs of the community, diagnosing problems, setting goals, and planning strategies to improve the health of individuals, families, and the community.

The Delta planning group is concerned with health primarily from the broad perspective of the needs of the community. A health assessment of an individual, family, or community shares a common definition of health but requires different data. Notice the differences in data used for assessment for the dimensions of health for individuals, families, and communities.

Individual Health

Assessment of individual health includes physical, social, emotional, intellectual, and spiritual dimensions. Specific individual health assessment is addressed throughout this book and may include characteristics of individual health such as these:

- Coping skills
- Capacity for making healthy lifestyle decisions
- Physical, mental, social, and emotional limitations
- Education and training
- Quality of work life
- Positive and supportive interpersonal relationships and social networks

Family Health

Assessment of family health includes physical, social, emotional, intellectual, and spiritual dimensions. Family strengths and problems are identified to provide a basis and direction for further assessment of individual family members (Figure 18-5).

Your nursing care plan for family health may address many factors that relate to family health. Those factors may belong to broad characteristics such as these:

- Positive and supportive interpersonal family relationships
- Consequences of family employment opportunities
- Consequences of family level of poverty
- Consequences of lower-status occupations
- Impact of job loss
- Safety and security issues
- Access to and appropriate use of health care services

The many other factors that relate to family health and function are addressed in other areas of this text.

Community Health

Assessment of community health includes physical, social, emotional, intellectual, and spiritual dimensions.

Community health assessment commonly uses statistics on populations and uses data to compare community needs with available services. Some examples include mortality and morbidity studies, annual health reports from multiple agencies, and health inventories and resource reports. Traditional methods of measuring the health of a community have centered on mortality (death rate), longevity (life expectancy), and morbidity (illness).

 An example of a community working together to assess the current social planning practices of its area can be found in the work program set up by the Corporation of Delta. Participants defined

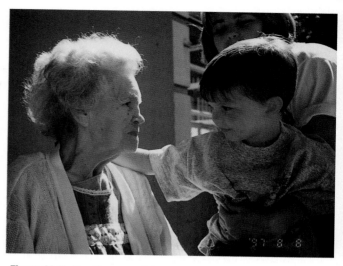

Figure 18-5. Family strength is seen in the contribution of a great-grandmother to the emotional development of a child. (Courtesy David A. Zerr.)

social planning at the community level as "a local, democratic system of planning and taking action toward community social needs and interests in support of community well-being."

When assessing community health, your plan may address broad social issues of community health, such as the following:

- A safe environment
- Affordable housing
- Community design
- Social services and public policy
- Cost-effective health services
- Preventive health practices
- Joint action for minority and cultural health issues

Community health is complex and specific to the community involved. No one pattern of community health can be understood without knowing the multitude of relevant environmental, social, and economic factors that affect it.

Focused Assessment for *Health-Seeking Behaviors*

The nursing diagnosis *Health-seeking behaviors* is observed in individuals, families, and communities. The key element of *Health-seeking behaviors* is choice. The individual, family, or community expresses the desire to seek a higher level of wellness, or you may observe behaviors that indicate a motivation to attain a higher level of wellness. Additional defining characteristics include the following:

- Expressed or observed desire for increased control of health practices
- Expression of concern about the effects of current environmental conditions on health status
- Stated or observed unfamiliarity with community wellness resources
- Demonstrated or observed lack of knowledge about health promotion behaviors

You will need to look for specific indicators of health-seeking behaviors in individuals, families, and communities to recognize opportunities to support health promotion activities and provide teaching (Box 18-5, p. 362).

Box 18-5 Examples of Health-Seeking Behaviors

INDIVIDUALS

- Having periodic physical examinations
- Seeking counseling for weight loss
- Requesting a health evaluation before starting an exercise program
- Using a seat belt
- Using a bicycle helmet
- Using sunscreen
- Using condoms
- Joining a support group to help break an addictive behavior pattern, such as the use of nicotine, alcohol, or illicit drugs
- Participating in recreational, social, and cultural community activities

FAMILIES

- Obtaining a family membership at a fitness center
- Seeking family therapy to manage addictive behavior in a teenager
- Making a commitment to reduce the incidence of colds and flu in the family
- Asking for assistance in managing the care of an elderly family member
- Expressing a need for information about caring for a new infant
- Expressing a need for information about making the home safe for all family members, especially children and older adults
- Seeking opportunities to enhance an employment situation

COMMUNITIES

- Petitioning of the city council by a neighborhood association for a new park in the area
- Organizing a group of concerned citizens to form a health clinic in a neighborhood with poor access to health care
- Seeking volunteers for a community action group to reduce violence in the public schools
- Initiating a public outcry over an incidence of hepatitis in the community and organizing a petition for better testing of community water supplies
- Attending a public hearing to discuss the provision of health services by schools
- Forming a committee in a community action group to study the need for affordable housing for disadvantaged groups
- Meeting to explore the possibilities of providing an education program to young parents about the importance of prenatal care and parenting skills
- Working with the community to address problems of low-income families, single-parent families, and gender-gap inequities in the labor force

---

DIAGNOSIS

The North American Nursing Diagnosis Association (NANDA) recognizes the need for both wellness nursing diagnoses and risk nursing diagnoses for individuals, families, and communities. Wellness nursing diagnoses describe human responses to levels of wellness in an individual, family, or community that have a potential for enhancement to a higher state (NANDA, 2001). Risk nursing diagnoses describe human responses to health conditions or life processes that may develop in a vulnerable individual, family, or community.

Nursing diagnoses can occur along the entire health-illness continuum. The individual, family, or community can be described as having a deficiency, dysfunction, or decrease in health behaviors that creates risk for diminished health. Additionally, the individual, family, or community can be recognized as having a potential for enhancing a state of wellness. The client—whether individual, family, or community—starts from a state of wellness and has the desire to increase that level of wellness.

PLANNING

Participants of the public forum can now move on to identify their community's health priorities. The goal of this community planning group is to meet the identified needs of individuals and families within the group, as well as the needs of the community as a whole. Planning will include identifying community resources to meet the health needs of individuals, families, and the community.

A statement of health goals, such as that in the preceding paragraph, flows from the perception of health. An understanding of related factors that contribute to the concept of health provides the assumptions that underlie health goals. Explicit goals provide guidelines for implementation. Thus planning includes designing interventions that can realistically be expected to achieve the goals.

INTERVENTION

Designing interventions to improve health requires both health promotion and preventive health care. Although, from a philosophical perspective, these two concepts are different, they are not mutually exclusive. As mentioned earlier, health promotion is the advancement of health through the encouragement of activities that enhance the wellness of individuals, families, and communities. **Preventive health care** is the recognition of the risk for disease, and the actions taken to reduce that risk.

Interventions to Promote Health

Health is a part of everyday living, and health care is an essential dimension to enhance the quality of life. Health in the context of health promotion is a dynamic rather than a static state, in which individuals and communities strive to maintain or regain a positive state of physical and psychological being. It is a basic force in daily life, influenced by circumstances, beliefs, culture, and the social, economic, and physical environment. Health promotion is the process of enabling people to be responsible for improving their health in keeping with its personal meaning.

Designing Health Promotion Activities. Health promotion is often described as educational techniques to help people take control of their lives and their health. However, it is more properly described as including educational, political, organizational, regulatory, and environmental supports for actions and conditions of living conducive to the health of individuals, families, and communities. Health promotion includes modifying the individual and collective lifestyle, modifying environments to support health, strengthening community action, reordering health services, and using public policy to enhance health. The activities that can be labeled as health promotion recognize the interrelationship of the person and the environmental, biological, social, and political determinants of health. The expected outcomes perhaps better define health promotion than the methods used to achieve the outcomes.

The outcomes for health promotion have little to do with the absence of disease. Health is expected to result in an improved quality of life. Quality living is in part being able to do what you want to do, do it well, and derive a sense of satisfaction from the effort. It is described in terms of effective functioning in areas of life that are important to each person. Through improved health, people can have the opportunity to maintain vigor and stamina throughout their life span. Additionally, better health will contribute to an increase in both individual and social productivity.

The outcomes for health promotion are described in practical, situation-specific results. For an occupational health effort, the expected outcomes include increased worker satisfaction, increased productivity, and a lower cost of employee health care. In a school setting, the expected outcomes are decreased absence from school, improved learning, increased motivation, and increased self-esteem.

The paradigm for health promotion recognizes the potential impact of the self-care movement that has been occurring since the 1970s. An activity can be labeled *health promotion* if it provides people with tools or knowledge to take control of their own health. The paradigm describes self-reliance, person-centered activities, and client participation.

The paradigm for health promotion, by its very nature, must include decisions about who is responsible for decision making in primary health care. The philosophy of health promotion places the responsibility for health on the individual and family rather than on the professional. However, if individuals are solely responsible for their own health, there is a danger that the biological, social, political, and environmental determinants of health may be ignored.

Considering these broad determinants of health, society as a whole bears some responsibility for the health of its members. The question is, then, whether health promotion is a responsibility of the public or private sector. If it is society's responsibility, and the public sector assumes some or all of the responsibility, should the decision making and program support lie with the local, state, or national government? To the extent that health is a national resource serving a common national interest, perhaps the responsibility is best placed in the federal government. To the extent that health needs reflect lo-

cal conditions and interests, the responsibility may be best held at the local and state level.

Health promotion is expected to provide the means to revolutionize public health as a means to manage chronic illness in the same way infection control practices revolutionized public health in the first half of the twentieth century.

Primary Health Care. Primary health care focuses on prevention and health promotion but with a much broader perspective than just medical and nursing care. **Primary health care** means all care necessary to people's lives and health, including health education, nutrition, sanitation, maternal and child health care, immunizations, prevention, and control of endemic disease (WHO, 1978).

Primary health care, although related to the common term *primary care* used when referring to a primary care physician, has a broader scope. Primary medical care refers to care provided at the point at which a client first enters the health care system. It is the first contact for the provision of coordinated care for a wide range of health concerns within a sustained relationship with a health care provider. If the range of concerns truly encompasses a comprehensive view of health care, it can be labeled primary health care.

In the definition of primary health care created by WHO (Box 18-6), there are five principles:

- Equitable accessibility of health services to all populations
- Maximum individual and community involvement in the planning and operation of health services
- Increased emphasis on services that are preventive and promotive rather than only curative
- Use of appropriate technology
- Integration of health development with social and economic development (Stewart, 1995)

The essence of the WHO definition integrates many of the associated factors. It combines a focus on individuals and families with a focus on the health of a defined population within a community. Primary health care is delivered by a variety of health professionals and providers working

---

Box 18-6   World Health Organization Definition of Primary Health Care

Primary health care is "essential health care based on practical, scientifically sound and socially acceptable methods and technology made universally accessible to individuals and families in the community through their full participation and at a cost that community and country can afford to maintain at every stage of their development in the spirit of self-reliance and self-determination. It forms an integral part both of the country's health system, of which it is the central function and main focus, and of the overall social and economic development of the community. It is the first level of contact of the individual, the family, and the community with the national health system bringing health care as close as possible to where the people live and work, and constitutes the first element of a continuing health care process."

From World Health Organization. (1978). *Primary health care: Report on the international conference on primary health care,* p. 21, Alma Ata, USSR, 6-12 September 1978. Geneva: Author.

collaboratively with clients to maintain health, support wellness, and treat illness. Full participation of clients and accountability to clients and the community for high-quality comprehensive services are essential features of primary health care.

These definitions indicate an important shift from a "medical" focus to a "health" focus in health care. The WHO definition identifies the multidisciplinary nature of the primary health contact, the collaborative nature of relationships between consumers and health care workers, and the accountability of consumer and community to strive for a high level of health.

The need for changes to primary care is fundamental to a reform of the health care system in both the United States and Canada. Nursing as a profession has the expertise to play a vital role in this change. Emerging roles and expanded nursing functions are part of this reform.

Interventions to Prevent Illness

Health promotion and illness prevention can be best understood in terms of health activities on the primary, secondary, and tertiary levels.

Levels of Preventive Care. **Primary prevention** consists of actions that are considered true prevention because they precede disease or dysfunction and are applied to clients considered physically and emotionally healthy to protect them from health problems. Activities are aimed at decreasing the probability of specific illnesses or dysfunction. They may include health education programs, immunizations, and physical and nutritional fitness activities. Primary prevention can be applied to an individual or to a general population, or it can focus on individuals at risk for developing specific diseases. An example is a public health nurse providing health education programs in high schools to inform teenagers about sexually transmitted diseases.

Secondary prevention consists of actions that focus on the early diagnosis and prompt treatment of people with health problems or illnesses and who are at risk for developing complications or worsening conditions. Activities are directed at diagnosis and prompt intervention to reduce the severity of the disease and to enable the client to return to normal function as quickly as possible. Secondary prevention includes nursing care delivered at home, at a hospital, or at a nursing center for screening techniques and treatment of early stages of disease. An example is a public health nurse who carries out screening tests for postpartum depression on mothers attending well-baby clinics.

Tertiary prevention involves minimizing the effects of a permanent, irreversible disease or disability through interventions directed at preventing complication and deterioration. Activities are directed at rehabilitation rather than diagnosis and treatment. Care at this level is aimed at helping the client achieve as high a level of functioning as possible, despite the limitations caused by illness or impairment. The term *preventive* is applied to this level of care because it involves prevention of further disability or reduced functioning. An example includes a nurse working in a geriatric care center who refers a diabetic client to a foot-care education program.

Methods of Prevention. The concept of disease prevention is based on identifying risk factors and using those factors to identify persons at risk for a specific disease. The value of prevention is a reduction in morbidity or mortality rates for the specific disease. However, not all diseases can be prevented. Hence prevention is often aimed at early detection of the disease to prolong life and reduce suffering.

The decision to implement widespread prevention strategies requires that multiple factors be considered: the prevalence of the disease, whether the disease can be prevented, the degree of devastation resulting from the effects of the disease, and the availability of treatment options that can eradicate the disease or prolong the client's life.

Another consideration is the availability and accuracy of methods to screen for risk factors and for the disease. If prevention demands major lifestyle changes or requires costly, risky, toxic, or unpleasant preventive measures, the benefits of prevention may not outweigh the risks. Additionally, screening tests need to have an acceptable margin of error. That is, the tests should produce a low number of false-positive or false-negative results. False-positive results can cause unnecessary worry and, sometimes, unnecessary procedures. False-negative results give a false sense of security that the disease is not present and may delay treatment.

Preventive measures can be difficult to administer. If clear cost savings cannot be shown, reimbursement for prevention may not be available. Additionally, a well-coordinated system of health care delivery is needed to ensure optimum use of money available for prevention.

Disease prevention is derived only in part from the hard sciences. Clinical interventions should address personal health practices and engage the client in joint decision making. Chapter 19 discusses the methods of promoting lifestyle changes. Although a one-to-one relationship with a clinician gives the client and clinician the opportunity to selectively make choices about screening tests, some problems may be more effectively prevented through prevention strategies at the community level. Examples include sexually transmitted diseases, acquired immunodeficiency syndrome (AIDS), teenage pregnancies, and child abuse.

$\mathcal{E}$VALUATION

After much discussion and debate, the workshop participants arrived at eight health priority/action statements for Delta: (1) promote a perception of health for individuals, families, and community, (2) pursue a process to gather and analyze health data, (3) promote collaborative planning and coordination of health promotion decisions and strategies, (4) promote education on health issues and community involvement with the issues identified, (5) make an effort to break down established stereotypes that hinder health promotion, such as multicultural issues, aboriginal issues, and youth issues, (6) foster initiatives that address child and youth health issues, (7) foster initiatives that address women's health issues, and (8) promote efforts to provide adequate resources for preventive health initiatives.

The last step for the workshop participants is to work toward measurable outcomes for the health priorities identified. The hour is late, and participants have exhausted their energies with the identification of health priority/action statements. They agree to draft action plans for each of the eight statements. Plans are made for the next meeting, when future steps in the quest to develop health goals for the citizens of Delta will be addressed.

The case situation that appears throughout this chapter provides the community context that illustrates the significance of health promotion. The importance of a perception of health for establishing goals and actions for individuals, families, and communities emerged as the top health priority in the workshop scenario.

To evaluate health goals fully, those goals must be explicit, and they must provide specific implementation guidelines and evaluation criteria. For example, consider the goal of improving nutrition by reducing saturated fat intake. During the planning process for a community, you might establish as an expected outcome that community members would reduce their fat intake by reading food labels properly. As one step of the evaluation process for this outcome, you could demonstrate by survey that foods available in the community's grocery stores have fat content listed on their labels. If the survey finds that foods are not clearly labeled with fat content, then your expected outcomes will need revision.

The concept of health perception relates to all health disciplines and to the many factors and determinants of health. For this reason, a plan of action specific to nursing may not be appropriate. The plans developed may need to be broad and multidisciplinary in scope. As a result, the plan will help to develop a perception of health for the individual, family, and community.

Key Principles

- Because we are all citizens of the world, health cannot be viewed from only an individual or a local perspective.
- Health is more than the absence of disease.
- Health exists on a continuum.
- Wellness includes positive physiological function and a sense of well-being.
- Population health considers health problems encountered by being a part of a group and focuses intervention on the population rather than on the individual.
- An individual's health is affected by many personal, family, and community factors.
- Families are the primary unit of health.
- Community health studies have revealed that health is also affected by changing conditions in communities.
- Influences from internal and genetic factors and from external sources affect health.

- Assessment of individual health includes physical, social, emotional, intellectual, and spiritual dimensions.
- Family health assessment requires gathering health data on each member of the family and on the function of the family as a whole.
- Community assessment uses statistics on population data, statistics on the use of services, and data that compare community needs with available services.
- The nursing diagnosis *Health-seeking behaviors* addresses the desire or need for positive health action by individuals.
- Primary health care consists of all care necessary to people's lives and health, including health education, nutrition, sanitation, maternal and child health care, immunizations, prevention, and control of endemic disease.
- Nurses carry out preventive health care and health promotion in a multitude of ways each day of nursing practice.

Bibliography

*Airhihenbuwa, C. (1989). Health education for African Americans: A neglected task. *Health Education, 20*(5), 9-14.

*Dunn, H. L. (1959). High-level wellness for man and society. *American Journal of Public Health, 49*(6), 786-792.

Gordon, M. (2002). *Manual of Nursing Diagnosis* (10th ed.). St Louis, MO: Mosby.

Maiese, D. R., & Fox, C. E. (1998). Laying the foundation for Healthy People 2010: The first year of consultation. *Public Health Reports, 113,* 92-95. Access at http://web.health.gov/healthypeople/2010article.htm.

North American Nursing Diagnosis Association. (2001). *NANDA nursing diagnoses: Definitions and classification, 2001-2002.* Philadelphia: Author.

Papenfus, H., & Bryan, A. A. (1998). Nurses' involvement in interdisciplinary team evaluations: Incorporating the family perspective into child assessment. *Journal of School Health, 68*(5), 184-189.

"Putting health in the patient's hands." (1998). *The Globe and Mail,* p. A2, January 21.

Ryan, R. S., & Travis, J. W. (1988). *Wellness workbook.* Berkeley, CA: Ten Speed Press.

Savoi, I., & Pastore, M. T. (1997). *Personal communication,* January 27, 1997.

Stewart, M. J. (Ed.). (1995). *Community nursing: Promoting Canadians' health.* Toronto, Saunders Canada.

Sutherland, R. (1996). *Will nurses call the shots? A look at the delivery of health care twenty years from now.* Ottawa, Tri-Graphic.

U.S. Department of Health and Human Services. (2000). With understanding and improving health and objectives for improving health. In *Healthy People 2010* (2nd ed.). Washington, DC: U.S. Government Printing Office. Retrieved from http://www.health.gov/healthypeople/Document/html/uih/uih_bw/uih_4.htm.

*World Health Organization. (1978). *Primary health care: Report on the international conference on primary health care.* Alma Ata, USSR, 6-12 September, 1978. Geneva: Author.

*World Health Organization. (1981). Global strategy for health for all by the year 2000. In *Health for All Series,* 3, p. 15.

*Asterisk indicates a classic or definitive work on this subject.

19

Health Maintenance: Lifestyle Management

Key Terms

action stage

contemplation stage

counseling

emic dimension

etic dimension

lifestyle

maintenance stage

perceived barriers

perceived benefits

perceived severity

perceived susceptibility

precontemplation stage

preparation stage

referral

self-efficacy

social support

termination stage

Learning Objectives

After studying this chapter, you should be able to do the following:

- Describe world views of health and health care and models of behavioral change that underlie decision making about lifestyle changes to manage a therapeutic regimen
- Describe factors affecting behavioral change
- Assess the client who is experiencing problems in maintaining health when a therapeutic regimen requires alterations in lifestyle
- Write diagnoses for clients who need to manage a therapeutic regimen to maintain health
- Plan nursing interventions that assist the client to effectively manage lifestyle changes needed to implement a therapeutic regimen
- Evaluate the behavioral outcomes of lifestyle changes made to maintain health through a therapeutic regimen

Mr. Oscar Kitchen is a 69-year-old African-American man who keeps house for himself. He is a widower. His only living relatives are distant cousins living in another state. He receives a monthly Social Security check and a small retirement check from his former employment as a janitor in a public school.

Six weeks ago, Mr. Kitchen became short of breath and reluctantly went to a primary health care clinic. The nurse assessed Mr. Kitchen and determined that he had an irregular pulse and pitting edema of the lower extremities. The doctor prescribed medication for his heart and a diuretic. After the first week of medication, Mr. Kitchen felt better and decided to stop the medication. He missed his follow-up clinic appointment.

Two weeks ago, Mr. Kitchen once again became short of breath. He awakened soon after going to bed and was unable to breathe when lying in the supine position. He slept very little during the night. Mr. Kitchen returned to the clinic the next morning.

The nurse discovered that Mr. Kitchen had discontinued medications on several occasions, and that he continues to smoke. The nurse makes the diagnosis *Ineffective therapeutic regimen management* (individuals) related to (1) knowledge deficit regarding current diagnosis, medications, and consequences of failure to comply with treatment, and (2) unwillingness to modify or change an unhealthy lifestyle. Other possible nursing diagnoses relating to lifestyle management are listed below.

KEY NURSING DIAGNOSES FOR   Health Behaviors

Ineffective therapeutic regimen management (individuals, family, or community): A pattern in which the individual experiences or is at risk for experiencing difficulty integrating into daily living a program for treatment of illness and the sequelae of illness that meets specific health goals
Noncompliance (specify): The state in which an individual or group desires to comply, but factors are present that deter adherence to health-related advice given by health professionals

Effective therapeutic regimen management (individual): A pattern in which the individual integrates into daily living a program for treatment of illness and its sequelae that is satisfactory for meeting health goals
Decisional conflict (specify): The state in which an individual or group experiences uncertainty about a course of action when the choice of options involves risk, loss, or challenge to personal life values

CONCEPTS OF BEHAVIORAL CHANGE

A person's **lifestyle** is a behavior or group of behaviors, chosen by the person that may have a positive or a negative influence on health. A healthy lifestyle is evident when one avoids poor health habits, such as smoking and overeating, engages in good habits, such as achieving adequate nutrition and rest, and effectively manages a therapeutic regimen prescribed by a physician (Figure 19-1).

Lifestyle choices are connected to the incidence of heart disease, diabetes, and other chronic illnesses. Pender and others (2002) believe that healthy lifestyle choices are the foundation for preventing chronic diseases. Although health promotion and primary and secondary disease prevention activities will not replace sophisticated medical care, these methods offer hope for achieving improvement in life expectancy and maintenance of health into old age.

The experience of an acute or chronic disease may demand changes in a person's lifestyle and behavioral patterns as part of management of the disease. For an acute illness, these changes are only temporary. For a chronic illness, permanent lifestyle changes are the only avenue to successful living with the illness.

However, helping a client change well-established health and lifestyle habits is challenging. The development of health habits begins in early childhood, and once developed, they become patterns of behavior that are difficult to change. To understand some of the complexities involved in changing lifestyle behaviors, you will need to reconsider the definitions of health in conjunction with theories about behavioral changes.

In Chapter 18, you learned that health may be defined from the multiple perspectives of the individual, the family, and the community. Furthermore, a person's definition of health stems in part from a personal worldview. This is true for the health care provider's definition as well. When client and provider have different worldviews, the result may be misunderstandings and differences in the selection of expected outcomes for health promotion and prevention (Spector, 2000).

Tripp-Reimer (1984) conceptualized health as two-dimensional, having an etic dimension and an emic dimension. **Etic dimension** refers to the objective interpretation of health by a scientifically trained practitioner. **Emic dimension** refers to an individual's or a social group's subjective perception and experiences related to health. Understanding health from the perspective of the client is critical to the development of health services (Jones, Zhang, Jaceldo-Siegl, & Meleis, 2002).

To effectively help others, health care professionals must first understand the health and quality-of-life perspective of the client. A person's identity, role assignment, health, and opportunities in life are greatly influenced by such factors as sex, skin color, age, income, and place of origin. Additionally, health-related quality of life is defined not only by the signs and symptoms of disease or its effects on survival but also by functional status, opportunity, and one's perception of relative well-being (Woolf, Jonas, & Lawrence, 1996).

Worldviews of Health and Health Care

Culture refers to the learned, shared, and transmitted values, beliefs, norms, and lifeways of a particular group that guides their thinking, decisions, and actions in patterned ways

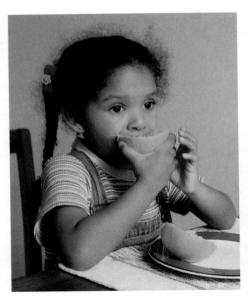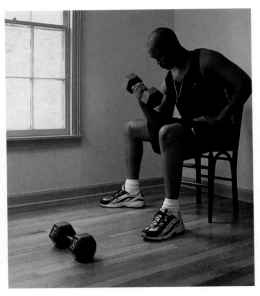

Figure 19-1. Lifestyle patterns associated with health include good nutrition and exercise.

(Leininger, 2001, p. 43). These ways of living, or lifestyles, reflect a person's understanding of health and health practices, as well as the person's view of illness. The experience of illness is determined in part by how illness is defined by one's culture, as well as by the individual or sick person (Spector, 2000).

All cultures have concepts of health and illness. They also have theories of disease causation, which may differ widely from group to group (Clark, 1999). These concepts and theories define the nature of illness, its treatment, and the type of relationships that should occur between client and health care provider. Additionally, ethnic groups with different cultural histories have different approaches to reality, socialization, and health practices. Ideas and beliefs related to health and illness are integral parts of a culture's worldview (Table 19-1).

A client's worldview is important because ideas related to health and illness originate from everyday experiences, family, social network, and the community. Families provide 70% to 90% of health care. Most people seek advice from family, friends, or lay sources before seeking professional advice. Clark (1999) suggests that there are two domains of health care: the folk or generic form and the scientific or professional form (Table 19-2).

The folk medicine system classifies illnesses into two parts: natural and unnatural. "This division of illnesses or diseases into natural and unnatural phenomena is common among persons from Haiti, Trinidad, and Mexico and among Mexican Americans, African Americans, and some southern white Americans" (Giger & Davidhizar, 1999, p. 120). Illnesses treated by folk medicine tend to be described as chronic, nonincapacitating maladies, and those believed to be caused by supernatural agents (Clark, 1999). Natural illnesses in the folk medicine system relate to events that have to do with the world as God made it or as God intended it (Giger &

Table 19-1	Comparison of Nonwestern and Western Worldviews	
Nonwestern	**Western**
Emphasizes group cooperation	Emphasizes individual competition
Values achievement as it reflects group	Values achievement for the individual
Values harmony with nature	Values mastery and control of nature
Sees time as relative	Adheres to rigid time schedule
Accepts affective expression	Limits affective expression
Embraces extended family	Prefers nuclear family
Thinks holistically	Thinks dualistically
Religion permeates culture	Holds religion distinct from other parts of culture
Accepts worldviews of other cultures	Feels own worldview is superior
Emphasizes social orientation	Emphasizes task orientation

Modified from Anderson, A. (1988). Cognitive styles and multicultural populations. *Journal of Teacher Education, 39*(1), 2-9.

Davidhizar, 1999). Unnatural illnesses relate to events that cause disharmony with nature. Therefore unnatural illnesses may be viewed as forces of evil or as events that interrupt the plan intended by God (Giger & Davidhizar, 1999).

Western medicine focuses a biopsychosociocultural (spiritual) approach to explain illness, with an emphasis on cure. Folk medicine focuses on personal data and experiences rather than on scientific persuasion (Giger & Davidhizar, 1999). Health care is provided in dyads (nurse–client or physician–client relationships), whereas in the folk medicine system, people tend to seek health care from multiperson health care networks, including relatives and nonrelatives (Giger & Davidhizar, 1999).

Clark (1999) suggests that many similarities exist between folk and scientific health care systems. One such similarity is

Table 19-2	Similarities and Differences Between Folk and Scientific Health Care Systems	
	Differences	
Similarities	*Folk Health System*	*Scientific Health System*
• Employ similar diagnostic techniques including observation and listening • Use verbal and nonverbal communication • Engage in naming of illnesses and creation of positive expectations • Employ suggestion, interpretation, emotional support, and manipulation of the environment as therapeutic modalities • Use medicinal substances and employ some form of laying on of hands in the care of the sick • Based on asymmetric relationships between experts and laypersons • Provide an explanation of disease, a rationale for treatment, and a rationale for social and moral norms	• Takes into account the religious and social aspects of health • Makes no definite distinction between mental and physical illness • Oriented to the community • Takes place in familiar surroundings • Emphasizes humanistic care • Emphasizes familiar, practical, and concrete behavior • Provides holistic care • Emphasizes caring • Stresses prevention • Emphasizes cultural support • Is of moderate cost	• Focuses primarily on the personal implications of disease • Makes a definite distinction between mental and physical illness • Oriented to the individual • Takes place in unfamiliar surroundings • Emphasizes impersonal care • Emphasizes abstract concepts • Provides fragmented care • Emphasizes curing • Stresses diagnosis and treatment • Does not emphasize cultural support • Is of high cost

From Clark M. J. (1999). *Nursing in the community: Dimensions of community health nursing* (3rd ed.). Reprinted by permission of Pearson Education, Inc., Upper Saddle River, NJ.

the way people initially approach a health problem. According to Kavanagh and Kennedy (1992), "Virtually no one runs for professional help at the first hint of a symptom. Traditional and folk remedies, most of them as benign as herbal tea, might be used and a homemade diagnosis and etiology tentatively constructed. The next resort may be to popular or over-the-counter resources, which may or may not be associated with allopathic medicine. Finally, if relief is not in sight, professional consult is likely to be undertaken" (pp. 19-20).

A person's culturally acquired worldview of health and illness can be modified by social and economic conditions, with the economically disadvantaged forced to adopt lifeways that may be more a product of poverty than of culture.

Models of Behavioral Change

In addition to using culturally specific lifestyle knowledge to promote health, you need to understand theories of behavioral change to explain and predict health-related behaviors. However, these models were not developed as culturally specific models, so no one model is likely to explain the behaviors and belief systems of all specific cultural groups.

Theory of Reasoned Action.

The theory of reasoned action is a human behavior framework designed to explain a person's intention to perform a behavior. The theory is based on the assumption that people are reasonable and, in deciding which actions to take, systematically process and use the information available to them (Poss, 2001). The theory further assumes that behavior is totally under voluntary control and that barriers to performance of the intended behavior do not exist (Pender, et al., 2002).

The theory of reasoned action does not rely solely on facts and logic. It also considers the relations between beliefs, attitudes, and intention in determining behavior. To change or re-

inforce a given intention, the person must change or strengthen the attitude toward performing that behavior.

The theory further holds that a behavioral intention is determined both by attitudes toward the specific behavior and by subjective norms (what others think) regarding the behavior. Thus people intend to perform a behavior when they evaluate that behavior positively and when they believe significant others think they should perform it. Compelling as it is, the theory of reasoned action is, by itself, not sufficient to explain health behaviors.

Remember Mr. Kitchen? A reasonable person might be expected to associate shortness of breath with smoking, to see that the medication caused a decrease in leg swelling, and to take the actions necessary to improve health. Why do you think Mr. Kitchen stopped taking his medication and continued to smoke?

Transtheoretical Model for Behavioral Change.

The transtheoretical model for behavioral change provides stages of change in behavior. People must change their behavior to make major reductions in risks for chronic disease. Prochaska et al. (1994) describe six stages of behavioral change: precontemplation, contemplation, preparation, action, maintenance, and termination. People move through these stages as they consider, and then act on, reducing risky behaviors. Assessing a client's stage of behavioral change can help you determine appropriate interventions to assist the person in reducing risky behavior.

In the **precontemplation stage,** the person does not intend to change a high-risk behavior in the foreseeable future (the next 6 months), primarily because he is unaware of the long-term consequences of the behavior. Furthermore, the person may feel demoralized about his inability to change and defensive because of social pressures to change (Prochaska et al.,

1994). Although unconvinced of the need for change, the person may agree to make changes under pressure from family and friends. These changes are usually minimal and last only as long as pressure continues to be applied.

In the **contemplation stage,** the person intends to change within the next 6 months. However, despite this good intention, the person usually stays in this stage for at least 2 years. He tells himself that he is going to change, but he keeps putting it off. The person is ambivalent about changing and usually substitutes thinking for acting (Prochaska et al., 1994).

In the **preparation stage,** the person intends to take action in the very near future, usually within the next month. This stage has both intention and action. The person usually develops a plan of action and may take small steps toward behavioral change. Furthermore, the person evaluates the advantages and the disadvantages of the risky behavior and decides that the disadvantages outweigh the advantages (Prochaska et al., 1994).

In the **action stage,** the person changes risky behaviors and the context of the behavior (environment, experience) and makes significant efforts to reach goals. This is the busiest but most risky stage because of the chance for relapse. The person is considered to be in the action stage if the behavior is changed for 1 day to 6 months. This stage offers the most external recognition because others become aware of the effort that the person is making toward the change.

The **maintenance stage** takes place during the 6 months after the person changes the high-risk behavior. This stage is characterized by a period of continuing change, with fewer mechanisms needed to prevent relapse. However, the time frame for continuous maintenance is 5 years. Prochaska et al. (1994) discovered that people must continuously abstain from the high-risk behavior for 5 years to prevent the fear of relapse. For example, they found that, even after 12 months of continuous abstinence from smoking, 37% of people will return to regular smoking. After 5 years of continuous abstinence, only 7% will return to regular smoking.

In the **termination stage,** the person is no longer tempted to engage in old behavior. He has confidence in no longer being tempted by previous situations.

Most people go through some or all of these stages several times before conquering an addiction, despite professional help. Movement through the stages occurs in a spiral pattern as the person moves backward into previous stages and forward through later stages. The upward and forward spiral movement toward elimination of the behavior occurs as the person learns from previous experience. The greater the number of successes the person has over time in this spiral movement, the greater the possibility of sustained change.

When the nurse expresses her concern to Mr. Kitchen, he pats her on the hand and says, "Don't you worry none, the good Lord will take care of me." Which of these stages describe Mr. Kitchen's frame of mind concerning his health behaviors? Are any of these stages relevant?

Health Belief Model. The health belief model is a health protection model that provides a framework to explain why some people take specific actions to avoid or treat illness, whereas others fail to protect themselves (Lancaster, Onega, & Forness, 2000; Pender et al., 2002). The model has been used to predict and explain health behavior on the basis of the value-expectancy theory and Kurt Lewin's cognitive theory.

Lewin is a cognitive theorist who conceptualized that certain aspects of a person's life space have negative, positive, or neutral values. He believed that disease has a negative value and, as a result, exerts a force to move the person toward health behaviors. He also believed that behavior is a function of the subjective value of an outcome and of the subjective expectation that a particular action will achieve that outcome (Rosenstock, 1974).

The health belief model states that the probability that a person will take appropriate health care actions depends on the person's value of health, perceptions about disease, and perceived threat of disease. Additionally, action is motivated by perception about the medical team and therapy plans, past experience, contact with risk factors, level of participation in regular health care, life aspirations, and factors in the environment.

Four components of the health belief model have been identified: perceived susceptibility, perceived severity, perceived benefits, and perceived barriers (Rosenstock, 1974). People will take action to ward off, to screen for, or to control ill health if they regard themselves as susceptible to the condition, if they believe it to have potentially serious consequences, or if they believe that actions available to them would reduce either their susceptibility to or the severity of the condition. Action is more likely if they also believe that the anticipated barriers to (or costs of) taking the action are outweighed by its benefits.

Perceived susceptibility refers to a person's subjective perception of the risk of contracting a health condition. For example, with cigarette smoking, the person might not perceive the risk of getting lung cancer. **Perceived severity** refers to the perceived seriousness of contracting an illness or leaving it untreated. In cigarette smoking, the person might not perceive that serious personal harm will occur as a result of smoking. **Perceived benefits** refers to the person's perceptions and beliefs about the effectiveness of the recommended actions in preventing the health threat. **Perceived barriers** refers to perceived negative aspects of a health action or the perceived impediments to undertaking the recommended behaviors (Rosenstock, 1974). Key components of the health belief model can be found in Box 19-1.

Self-efficacy is a central concept in the health belief model. **Self-efficacy** is defined as the conviction that one can successfully execute the behavior required to produce the outcomes (Rosenstock, 1974, p. 40). Bandura (1977) believes that efficacy expectancies differ from outcome expectancies in that efficacy expectancies refer to one's capacity to perform the behavior, whereas outcome expectancies refer to beliefs about what will happen as a result of engaging in the behavior. For example, for a person to quit smoking, he must believe that cessation will benefit his health (outcome expectation) and

Box 19-1 **Key Components of the Health Belief Model**

THREAT

- Perceived susceptibility to an illness (or acceptance of a diagnosis)
- Perceived seriousness of the condition

OUTCOME EXPECTATIONS

- Perceived benefits of specified action
- Perceived barriers to taking that action

EFFICACY EXPECTATIONS

- Conviction about one's ability to carry out a recommended action (self-efficacy)
- Sociodemographic factors (such as education, age, sex, race, ethnicity, and income) are believed to influence behavior indirectly by affecting perceived threat, outcome expectations, and efficacy expectations

From Rosenstock, J. (1974). Historical origins of the health belief model. *Health Education Monograph, 2*(4), 328-335.

also that he is capable of quitting (efficacy expectation). According to Bandura, self-efficacy judgments are based on four major sources of information: the individual's own performance accomplishments, vicarious observation of the performance of others, the influence of external persuasion and social influence, and states of emotional arousal. A person's success with coping in a variety of high-risk situations increases his sense of self-efficacy and decreases the probability of relapse.

Health Promotion Model. The health promotion model, developed by Pender et al. (2002), describes the multidimensional nature of a person's interactions with the environment in the pursuit of health. This model combines nursing and behavioral science perspectives with factors that impact health behaviors. Unlike the health belief model, the health promotion model does not rely on "personal threats." The model uses constructs from the value-expectancy theory and the social cognitive theory.

The value-expectancy theory suggests that behavior is rational and economical. This means that people will not waste their time and resources on behavior changes that have little value to them (Pender et al., 2002). Furthermore, people will not invest in a goal if they perceive that the goal is impossible to achieve. The motivational significance of successfully changing behavior is based on the person having some past experiences with success. In other words, the person must have some confidence in the achievement of the goal. This is why, for some people, achieving small steps is more successful than attempting major change (e.g., cutting down on the number of cigarettes rather than quitting).

Social cognitive theory focuses on the person's beliefs interacting with environmental influences (Pender et al., 2002). Behavior is not solely driven by inner forces or automatically shaped by external stimuli. Rather, there is an interaction between cognitive factors, personal factors, and environmental events.

Beliefs about oneself formed through self-observation and self-reflective thought have the greatest potential for influencing behavior. These beliefs, according to Pender, et al., include self-attribution, self-evaluation, and self-efficacy. Perceived self-efficacy "is a judgment of one's ability to carry out a particular course of action. The greater the perceived self-efficacy, the more persistent individuals will be in achieving the behavior outcome" (Pender, et al., 2002).

FACTORS AFFECTING BEHAVIORAL CHANGE

In helping a client make behavioral changes to manage health, you need to understand the possible areas that can influence the relationship with the client. Some areas are under the control of the nurse and the client; others are not.

Communication

Impaired verbal skills or language differences prevent a client from expressing health needs or communicating effectively with health care professionals. Comprehension and meaning vary among cultures. Words and their meanings carry different nuances and significances, depending on a person's culture, values, and beliefs. Language barriers, whether from foreign languages or varying dialects of the same language, can result in anxiety, fear, and frustration for people who need to communicate, especially when health care is required. Because communication involves body language along with verbal language, the meaning of body position and expression can further facilitate or impede communication. A person's values regarding what personal thoughts and feelings are appropriate to share with others also affect communication.

A client's inability to provide a nurse or physician with accurate assessment data may result in erroneous or ineffective treatment of illness or disease. Likewise, a client's ability to communicate with health care providers can improve the treatment of illness—and the client's satisfaction with treatment.

Cognition and Perception

Cognition is the systematic way in which a person thinks, reasons, and uses language. Perception of information includes the sensing and interpretation of stimuli from the external and internal environments. The person's cognitive–perceptual functioning provides information on the ability to understand and follow directions, retain information, make decisions, solve problems, and use language appropriately. Cognitive–perceptual impairments include limitations of the senses (such as blindness or deafness) or brain dysfunction (such as memory loss or confusion). These impairments may reduce the level of knowledge a person acquires about a health condition or prescribed treatment.

Inability to make deliberate and thoughtful judgments can create a delay in seeking professional assistance. Signs and symptoms may not be understood by the client as being relevant to the disease. Health education or discharge instructions may be misinterpreted instead of being assimilated and remembered, which results in a failure to implement them, with a consequence of inadequate health maintenance or an exacerbation of disease.

Age and Developmental Level

The age and developmental level of the client influence health beliefs and practices. A person's health status can be significantly altered by unachieved developmental tasks. Lack of education about nutrition, safety, fitness, or health-protecting practices during childhood or adolescence can have a significant impact on adult health. An inability to meet basic human needs at various developmental stages may result in the development of a distorted value system or a lack of motivation for self-care.

Age and developmental level may also have a significant impact on the person's ability to manage and maintain health. Although infants and children rely on parents and guardians for the management of health, school-aged children can be taught to manage some self-care activities to promote and maintain health. Common problems may affect the ability for health maintenance. For example, loss of teeth may impede proper nutrition, arthritis may decrease the ability to exercise, and slowed cognitive processes may affect safety practices.

Developmental level plays a significant role in cognitive and perceptual abilities, and the ability to solve problems and conceptualize. As an adult ages, a decline in visual acuity, hearing, touch, and taste occurs.

Advancing age increases susceptibility to certain health risks. For example, the risk of cardiovascular disease increases with age for both sexes. The risks of birth defects and complications of pregnancy increase among pregnant women over age 35. Age risk factors increase in association with other risk factors, such as family history and personal habits. For example, a man at age 60 who has smoked for 40 or more years is at greater risk of developing lung cancer than a man at age 30 who has smoked for 10 years.

Lifestyle and Habits

Lifestyle and health are closely related. Changes in one usually create changes in the other. The family plays a critical role in the development of health-promoting and health-protective behaviors.

Health-related decisions regarding diet and leisure activities affect all family members, with health practices of children and adolescents influenced by actions of adults. Those behaviors that are most satisfying are retained and reinforced and largely determine their pattern for health maintenance. Inappropriate health habits, such as overeating, lack of exercise, use of alcohol and tobacco, and ineffective coping patterns may also be established in early childhood and adolescence and carried through adulthood.

Health practices and behaviors can have positive or negative effects on health. Practices with potential negative effects are labeled risk factors. Overeating or poor nutrition, insufficient rest and sleep, poor personal hygiene, smoking, alcohol or drug abuse, and activities involving a threat of injury, such as skydiving, mountain climbing, or bungee-jumping, are all examples of risk factors. Some habits are risk factors for specific diseases—for example, skin tanning increases the risk of skin cancer and being overweight increases the risk of cardiovascular disease. Ayurvedic medicine is an example of a system of medicine that encompasses the whole lifestyle (see Box 19-2).

Economic Resources

Economic factors can affect a client's level of health by influencing how or at what point the client enters the health care system, or by limiting the ability to comply with a prescribed treatment plan.

People who have health insurance are more likely to seek health care at the onset of symptoms, and they seek health care more frequently than people who have no insurance. People who have no health insurance may feel forced to obtain basic needs, such as food, rather than obtaining health care. Plus, access to health care facilities frequently requires transportation, which may be unaffordable or unavailable to low-income people, who also may not be able to afford the loss of daily wages that results from going to appointments.

Even when good health care is available, the poor cannot generally avail themselves of this important resource to the extent that white-collar, middle-class people can. The poor and the working class cannot put a high priority on minor conditions. Low-income people tend to seek medical treatment only at a relatively late stage in an illness (Box 19-3, p. 374). A person's compliance with a treatment plan designed to maintain or improve health is also affected by economic status. A person who has a high utility bill, a large family, and a low income must give higher priority to the greater good of food and shelter for everyone rather than to costly drugs, treatments, or special diets for one family member.

Crowded living conditions contribute to an increased incidence of illness and disease because of the close proximity of people, the sharing of utensils and belongings, and poor sanitation. Isolation, language or communication difficulties, seasonal work occupations, and migration patterns also affect a person's health status.

Compared with the poor population, middle-class people work in more protected jobs, are better educated, and are more able to seek treatment for minor illnesses. Members of the upper income group face fewer health risks and are able to obtain assistance in promoting and maintaining health more easily.

Cultural Values and Beliefs

Cultural background influences individual beliefs, values, and customs, including entry into the health care system and personal health practices (Box 19-4, p. 374). The range of health definitions, practices, and beliefs about prevention manifested by various ethnic groups is infinite. There are variations in health definitions, beliefs, and practices even within a given ethnic group.

Action Alert! Treat the basic needs of all human beings, regardless of cultural background, the same. How people seek to meet these needs is influenced by their culture and their personal beliefs. Each person is the best source of how he or she would like to be treated.

Box 19-2 *Considering the Alternatives*
Traditional Systems of Healing: Ayurvedic Medicine

Description and History: Ayurvedic medicine, the traditional system of natural medicine in India, has a history of over 5000 years. *Ayurveda* means science of life, and it is a comprehensive approach to health combining mind, body, and spirit and reflecting the values of Indian culture. This is fundamentally a health system, as the goal is to keep the person balanced in all dimensions and in harmony with the environment.

Important Concepts: An individual is a microcosm of the entire cosmos, which is made up of five elements: *earth, ether, air, fire,* and *water.* All of these elements are represented in the human body as well as in the environment. Health reflects a balance of these elements. One's constitution consists of three *doshas: vata*—air and ether, *pitta*—fire and water, and *kapha*—earth and water. Although all people have all three *doshas,* one or more *doshas* are dominant in an individual, and slightly different health practices are required to maximize health depending on the dominant *dosha.* Seven centers, or *chakras* (the Sanskrit word for wheel), represent energy vortices that reflect the essence of a life of health. These are often described by color or energetic properties; they start with the root *chakra* at the sacrococcygeal area and proceed to the crown *chakra* at the top of the head.

Practice of Ayurveda and Therapeutic Techniques: Many of the treatments are classified according to the *doshas,* such as *vata*-stimulating or *vata*-reducing treatments. Examination and diagnosis focus on determining the individual's constitution and balancing the *doshas.* An extensive history is usually followed by examination of pulses and the tongue. Specific healing practices include hygiene, cleansing, purification rituals, diet, use of herbs, and the practice of yoga. Emphasis is placed on purification of the body, mind, and spirit through discipline in daily life. Healing techniques include forms of massage with herbalized oil, enemas, colonics, and physical exercises to cleanse the body of toxins. Mental and spiritual cleansing practices, disciplines, and rituals are incorporated. In India, yoga, which means to yoke or bind the powers of body, mind, and soul to God, is a holistic spiritual discipline that is incorporated into daily life. In the West, various aspects of yoga are extracted and may be practiced as exercise or relaxation. *Hatha yoga* is the most widely known practice of yoga in the West and is closely aligned with Ayurvedic medicine. It includes three practices: *yoga asanas*—physical postures and exercises, often practiced alone; *yoga pranayama*—breathing exercises to balance the life force; and *meditation*—the induction of a relaxed state in the autonomic nervous system.

Practitioners: Ayurvedic practitioners are not licensed to practice in the United States, but some health care providers have integrated principles and techniques of Ayurveda into their practice. Non–health care professionals often act as health consultants or educators of Ayurvedic medicine or the practice of yoga. As Ayurveda is a philosophy of life, several teachers conduct classes or meetings. Yoga classes are available in many cities and health clubs as well as through videotapes. Often these focus mainly on physical positions and breathing.

Potential Benefits in the Use of Ayurvedic Treatments or Yoga: Research on herbal treatments has been conducted, primarily in India, for neurological, cardiovascular, musculoskeletal, respiratory, gastrointestinal, and mental disorders; cancer; and endocrine disorders such as diabetes. As the practice generally uses herbs in conjunction with a holistic approach, it is difficult to demonstrate the efficacy of only one aspect of the treatment. A number of studies have shown some efficacy in the use of yoga to reduce blood pressure and the pain of arthritis, and to treat asthma, multiple sclerosis, epilepsy, and substance abuse.

Concerns Related to the Use of Ayurveda: Some of the cleansing and purification practices are harsh; in particular, the use of colonics is generally not regarded as a healthy practice in Western medicine. Many herbal preparations are imported and not subject to quality control in purity and sanitation or labeling. They may be contaminated with biological materials as well as heavy metals, which can be toxic. It is important to keep in mind that this healing approach is rooted in a holistic cultural belief system, and when parts are taken out of context, the efficacy may be affected. Many of the ideas, such as chakras, energy medicines, and constitutional techniques are being imported to Western culture and are very popular with users of complementary therapies.

Resources
Books

Lad, V. (1984). *Ayurveda: The science of self-healing.* Santa Fe, NM: Lotus Press.

Sheikh, A. A., & Sheikh, K. S. (1989). *Eastern and Western approaches to healing: Ancient wisdom and modern knowledge.* New York: Wiley.

Zysk, K., & Tetlow, G. (2001). Traditional Ayurveda. In M. Micozzi (ed.), *Fundamentals of complementary and alternative medicine* (2nd ed.). New York: Churchill Livingstone.

Journals
Yoga Journal

Websites
National Institute of Ayurvedic Medicine, http://niam.com.
Yoga Research and Education Center, www.yrec.org.
Yoga Paths, www.spiritweb.org.

Spiritual values and beliefs are integrated into all the other dimensions of human beings—physical, mental, psychological, and social. The spiritual dimension helps a person find meaning in all aspect of life, including suffering, pain, illness, and death. Religious beliefs can influence lifestyle choices, attitudes, and feelings about illness that may conflict with interventions to promote, maintain, or restore health. These conflicts are often revealed when clients enumerate the course of an illness, refuse recommended medical intervention, or refuse to comply with treatment modalities for spiritual reasons.

Roles and Relationships

Social relationships within the family, social group, work setting, and the community are significant to one's well-being. The inability to engage in satisfying relationships or to feel comfortable in social interactions may lead to social isolation. Social isolation may prevent the seeking of preventive health services. Conflicting role expectations within the family, social group, and work setting produce stress. Communication patterns, decision-making skills, feelings of self-worth and autonomy, and perceived support will influence patterns of health maintenance.

THE·COST·OF·CARE
Colon Cancer Screening

Box 19-3

In the United States alone, about 109,000 new cases of colon cancer are diagnosed each year. Of these, about 64,000 will be fatal, a number that accounts for about 10% of all cancer deaths each year. Encouraging clients to participate in screening programs for early detection of colon cancer can help to reduce such deaths—and the costs associated with treating colon cancer. However, the screening program itself incurs considerable costs. At least according to one study, it may be possible to lower even these costs safely (Getzen, 1997).

The test used most often to screen for colon cancer is the guaiac test. It uses guaiac as a reagent to detect occult blood in the client's stool. If the results are positive, they raise the suspicion of colon cancer. However, blood in the stool does not always result from colon cancer, which means that, in a certain percentage of people, positive results can stem from a bleeding ulcer, consumption of certain foods, even random error. Nevertheless, each person who has a positive result from a stool guaiac test must have a follow-up barium enema to check for colon cancer. Plus, the American Cancer Society recommends six guaiac tests as a complete screening for colon cancer, with any one positive test raising suspicion of cancer.

In a group of 100,000 people, about 720 will have asymptomatic colon cancer. If the entire group has a stool guaiac test, the initial test will show positive results for about 90% of those who have colon cancer (648 people) and about another 20% of the group for unrelated reasons. So the initial test (at $4 per person) would return positive results in about 20,648 people. Each person must then have a follow-up barium enema, at about $100 each. Thus, following up on false-positive results accounts for more than 80% of the $2,464,800 cost of the initial screening test. Overall, the program has so far cost $3803 per case of colon cancer found.

The second stool guaiac test would cost $1 per person and would detect 90% of the remaining undiagnosed cancers (64.8 cases) and another group of people with false-positive result. At $1.7 million, the total cost for the second test is less than that of the initial test. However, the number of colon cancer cases detected is far lower. Considering the cumulative cost of the first two tests, the average cost per case detected has grown to $5852. More importantly, the marginal cost of cancer detection with the second test is much higher, at $26,335 per additional case found ($1.7 million in additional costs divided by 64.8 additional cases). The marginal cost is "the increase in total costs caused by the production of one more unit of output" (Getzen, 1997, p. 453).

The third, fourth, fifth, and sixth tests would cost $1 per person and would each pick up 90% of the cancers not yet diagnosed. These additional tests are finding very few new cases of colon cancer but are still generating substantial numbers of false-positive results. According to Getzen, "Since 5 tests will have uncovered almost all (719.9928 out of 720) of the cancer, the additional cases of cancer detected by the sixth stool guaiac will account for 100,000 tests and another 6,554 false positives, so that the marginal cost per case detected for the sixth stool guaiac is $755,400 divided by .0065, an almost astronomical $16,574,074 per additional case found" (Getzen, 1997, p. 33).

DISCUSSION

This study demonstrates the obvious benefits of screening tests for colon cancer. It also suggests that undergoing fewer than six tests may produce equal, or nearly equal, benefits at a considerably lower cost. The study also illustrates that the marginal cost can differ from the actual cost. And the study points out that the direct cost (screening tests) may be much less than the indirect cost (barium enemas to rule out cancer among false-positive tests) of the screening program.

REFERENCE

Getzen, T. E. (1997), *Health economics: Fundamentals and flow of funds.* New York: Wiley.

Cross-Cultural Care CARING FOR AN AFRICAN-AMERICAN CLIENT

Box 19-4

Oscar Kitchen is an African-American man who ascribes to the traditional definition of health held by many African Americans. Like people of many other cultures, African Americans have a unique way of classifying illness that aids in diagnosis and treatment. Likewise, many beliefs and values held by African Americans can influence health behaviors and lifestyle. Some of these beliefs include the following:

- Health as harmony with nature, feeling good (no pain), ability to engage in activities of daily living and go to work
- Illness as feeling bad, inability to work or engage in activities of daily living, and disharmony of mind, body, and spirit
- Prayer and a well-balanced diet as helpful in avoiding illness and recovering from illness
- Group orientation
- Spirituality as an influence on perception of health and illness

- Close personal space
- Strong family and kinship ties
- Family resources as a source of support rather than outside assistance
- Health values and beliefs that vary with age, socioeconomic status, and location (rural/urban)
- Dietary pattern that reflects many cultures
- Home remedies accepted for their effectiveness, decreased cost, and lack of segregation and racism that can be found in formal health care
- Distrust of "the system"

During a focused assessment, Ms. Emanuel, the nurse, engaged Mr. Kitchen in a conversation about his health during the past few weeks. He informed Ms. Emanuel he had been fine, "just a little short of breath," which had begun the day before. He revealed that he had stopped taking his medications because he was "feeling fine and no longer needed it."

Coping and Stress Tolerance

Stress can affect health and well-being in any of the adaptive modes: physiological, psychological, spiritual, developmental, and social. In the physical dimension, stress can have a negative affect on homeostasis. In the emotional dimension, stress can threaten the way a person normally perceives information and solves problems. In the social dimension, stress can threaten interpersonal relationships, the support received from others, and a sense of belonging. In the spiritual dimension, stress can threaten a person's view of life and attitude toward a supreme being. In essence, stress can affect a person in all areas of basic human needs.

Workplace and Environmental Conditions

The environment has many influences on health and illness. The physical environment in which a person works or lives can increase the likelihood that certain illnesses will occur. Industrial workers exposed to certain chemicals are more likely to develop some kinds of cancer and other diseases. In some environments, high noise levels, increased emotional stress, environmental pollution, violence, or overcrowding are risk factors.

ASSESSMENT

A thorough assessment of health, attitudes, cultural beliefs, and health practices is critical to developing an effective health promotion plan for your clients (Pender, 2001). Collect information about nutrition, elimination, rest and sleep, activity and exercise, and hygiene. Patterns of psychological health can be determined by assessing coping, interactions, and self-concept. Sociocultural health can be assessed through cultural practices, recreation, and significant relationships. Religious beliefs and values are determinants of spiritual health.

General Assessment of Health Promotion

The health history may be the most important part of the database. Cues from the nursing history can alert you to traits that increase the client's vulnerability to a certain condition or disease. In addition to the health history, you can identify the client's risk factors by using health-risk appraisal tools.

Health Practices. Pender (2001) describes several components of health assessment that focus on wellness including physical fitness evaluation, health risk appraisal, social support systems, and lifestyle assessment.

Physical fitness evaluation is divided into skill-related physical fitness and health-related physical fitness. "Skill-related fitness is defined by those qualities that contribute to successful athletic performance: agility, speed, power, and reaction time. Health-related fitness includes qualities found to contribute to one's general health, including cardiorespiratory endurance, muscular strength and endurance, body composition, and flexibility" (Pender, 2001). Health-related fitness also includes qualities that contribute to a person's general well-being.

Health-risk appraisal includes assessment data that provide clients with essential information about health threats from hereditary factors, lifestyle, and family history (Pender, 2001). Risk factors include genetics, age, biological characteristics, personal health habits, lifestyle, and environment.

The health-risk appraisal provides an average indication of risk. Clients can provide information regarding their own health experience and what improvements they could make in their mortality profile if they adopted more positive behaviors (Pender, 2001).

Social support systems are important in enhancing successful coping and promoting comfortable and effective living. These factors reduce stress and improve health and well-being. **Social support** can be defined as the subjective feeling of belonging, or being accepted, loved, esteemed, valued, and

needed for oneself, not for what one can do for others (Pender, 2001). All people need some type of social support, but the amount and type vary on the basis of the person's age, situation, and personal desires. Types of social support that have been clearly documented in the literature include emotional support, informational support, family support, and instrumental support, which includes assistance with specific tasks (Pender, 2001).

When obtaining assessment data related to cultural beliefs and attitudes, follow these four basic principles (Clark, 1999, p. 324):

- View all cultures in the context in which they developed.
- Examine underlying premises for culturally determined beliefs and behaviors.
- Interpret the meaning and purpose of behavior in the context of the specific culture.
- Recognize the potential for intercultural variation.

Lifestyle assessment is closely related to assessment of cultural beliefs and attitudes (see Box 19-2). Assess life events, dietary patterns, and health habits. "The desired outcomes of health assessment are to (1) identify health assets, (2) identify health-related lifestyle strengths, (3) determine key health-related beliefs, (4) identify health beliefs and health behaviors that put the client at risk, and (5) determine how the client wants to change to improve the quality of life" (Pender, 2001).

> *Action Alert!* Base risk appraisal on current referent group (personal risk age) and the predicted improvement in mortality profile if they were to adopt more positive health-promoting behaviors. A total risk for developing any disease increases on the basis of the number of risk factors present and the intensity of each risk factor.

Illness Practices. A person experiencing a health problem may be told to make adjustments in many aspects of day-to-day living. These changes may be for treatments to restore optimal health, for prevention of additional health problems, or for early detection of other health concerns. Your assessment should include identifying factors and cues that would indicate ineffective management.

Factors to be considered in a therapeutic regimen include the following:

- The client's knowledge of the disease, including severity and prognosis
- Disease history and previous treatment patterns (including the number of previous admissions for acute care)
- Previous history of accessing health care resources
- Treatment and preventive measures
- Pattern of adhering to prescribed therapeutic regimen
- Factors that prevent full implementation or adherence to recommended therapeutic regimen
- Missing knowledge or information that prevents comprehension of the recommended treatment program and its subsequent implementation
- The extent to which adherence to the treatment program has altered the person's life and relationships

Additionally, attention should focus on financial resources, health care resources, presence of sensory deficit, and expressed feelings regarding illnesses or disease process.

KNOWLEDGE OF DISEASE. Knowledge of the disease process includes the client's understanding of the onset of symptoms, causes and consequences of the current condition, and level of overall health knowledge. Solicit the following information from the client: the effects of this illness on present health, personal ideas about the cause of the symptoms, factors that aggravate or alleviate the symptoms, how the present illness affects the performance of role expectations and activities of daily living, and the health promotion and illness prevention activities engaged in since onset.

DISEASE HISTORY. The length of time of the disease process and the frequency of exacerbation of symptoms are cues to the extent to which the client has been able to manage the therapeutic regimen. Soliciting and recording this information in the client's own words will give vital clues when clustered with data collected during the assessment of cognitive-perceptual abilities.

HISTORY OF ACCESSING HEALTH CARE RESOURCES. A person's perception of health and illness, culture and spiritual beliefs, roles, relationships, and support systems are among the many factors that influence his use of health care resources. Each person has a personal definition of health. It may be defined as "good" even though the person has hypertension or symptoms of a respiratory infection. The extent to which a condition has a negative impact will influence the decision to seek health care or engage in health maintenance practices.

The attitudes and behaviors of significant others in the family, social groups, place of employment, or community have an impact on the person's beliefs and actions. When significant others express apathy or distrust in a particular treatment regimen or health promotion practices, the client may have difficulty adhering to the regimen. The family's sociocultural beliefs influence not only how a client perceives illness but also from whom assistance is sought and what types of treatment will be considered most advantageous.

Focused Assessment for *Ineffective Therapeutic Regimen Management*

Defining Characteristics. Several subjective factors may emerge from the health history that suggest that the client is having difficulty managing a therapeutic regimen. The initial defining characteristic is the person's or family member's verbal expression of a desire to adhere to the therapeutic program. Subsequently, the client may report difficulty in carrying out proposed activities or in making choices to incorporate the activities of the regimen into daily living, or the client may report making no attempt to incorporate these activities into patterns of daily living. The difficulty may reflect the person's lifestyle, work patterns, or roles and relationships.

An exacerbation of symptoms is an objective characteristic in making this diagnosis. Failure to seek out health care and related support, to make needed appointments, or to keep appointments would be additional defining characteristics.

Related Factors. Related factors contributing to the diagnosis of *Ineffective therapeutic regimen management (individuals)* include those related to aspects of the treatment regimen, to the health care system, and to personal factors. Factors related to treatment include the complexity of the therapeutic regimen, negative side effects, the financial cost, and the complexity of maneuvering through the health care delivery system. Therapeutic regimens may be complex technological advancements that, although they are useful devices for managing health problems, can create confusion for the clients who must use them. Many electronic devices are used in the home to assist the client in monitoring blood sugar level, blood pressure, urinalysis, and so on. The client's cognitive-perceptual level must be assessed to detect cognitive or sensory deficits that may contribute to the inability to incorporate a complex therapeutic regimen.

Access to care is a factor in the health care system. Some clients enter the system easily through physician's offices, clinics, or hospital emergency rooms. Other clients experience difficulties in entering the system because of confusion or unfamiliarity with the various agencies or because of low income status. Some geographical locations lack adequate health care resources.

Fragmentation of services is a second factor within the system. Specialization and technological advancement throughout the health care system has led to fragmentation in the provision of care. During the course of an illness, a person may be seen by several health care providers that treat, prescribe, and initiate separate health maintenance programs, each of which requires a follow-up visit. This process may overwhelm the client and family and lead to failure to initiate any or all health maintenance activities.

Personal factors also affect a client's adherence to a therapeutic regimen. Individual decisional conflict, family conflict, or excessive demands on the client or family can lead to failure to incorporate the planned program into activities of daily living. A client's unrealistic expectations of care by family members can produce conflict or role strain, which can lead to a breakdown in communication as well as anger.

You must give attention to the premise that a person's health beliefs, locus of control, and self-efficacy influence motivation, learning, and the capacity for behavioral changes needed to manage a therapeutic regimen and maintain health. By assessing the client's health beliefs, you can determine the extent to which the client's ineffective management of a therapeutic regimen relates to mistrust of the regimen, a feeling that the health problem is not serious, or a belief that he is not susceptible to disease. Assess the client's level of self-efficacy by investigating the level of personal confidence the client has about initiating proposed activities and reaching desired outcomes. Remember that the perceived value of the proposed therapeutic program will influence the client's willingness to follow it. If the client believes an activity will be very effective in preventing the development of a health problem, compliance is more likely. Additionally, the perceived benefits of the activities, when weighed against the adverse reactions and the cost, should be assessed as a causative factor.

What questions would you ask Mr. Kitchen to determine his problems with adhering to his therapeutic regimen? Do you think knowledge is a factor? Cost? The need to change his usual pattern of living? His beliefs about health?

DIAGNOSIS

When the objective of care is primarily that the client learns behaviors to improve health maintenance, cluster data (Table 19-3) to help select a diagnosis from the list of related health maintenance diagnoses. The list includes *Health-seeking behaviors, Ineffective health maintenance, Noncompliance, Knowledge deficit, Decisional conflict,* and *Ineffective management of therapeutic regimen.* Related or contributing factors that influence the health status change are listed in Box 19-5 (p. 378).

The diagnosis *Health-seeking behaviors* is appropriate when a person is in a state of wellness but is seeking ways to achieve a higher level of wellness. A person of normal weight, for example, may wish to improve his physical fitness and stamina and may verbalize his unfamiliarity with community resources or a lack of knowledge about how to achieve this goal. The defining characteristics in making this diagnosis include an expressed or observed desire to seek information for health promotion (Carpenito, 2002).

Ineffective health maintenance is appropriate for a person who expresses a desire to change an unhealthy lifestyle. Examples of an unhealthy lifestyle are excessive dissatisfaction with occupation; lack of exercise; failure to be refreshed after rest; diet high in fat, salt, simple carbohydrates;

tobacco use; obesity; excessive alcohol use; and insufficient social support. Because individuals are responsible for their own health, *Ineffective health maintenance* represents a diagnosis that the individual is motivated to treat. This nursing diagnosis is applicable to both well and ill populations. The assessment for *Ineffective health maintenance* includes the collection of both subjective and objective data defining general health status, and data on related factors including familial and environmental risk factors and preventive health activities (Carpenito, 2002). This diagnosis can also be used for a client who must alter health maintenance activities to manage an illness.

The diagnosis *Noncompliance* is used for a state in which an individual or group desires to comply but factors are present that deter adherence to health-related advice given by health professionals. Compliance depends on a variety of factors, including the person's motivation, perception of vulnerability, and beliefs about controlling or preventing illness; environmental variables; quality of health instruction; and the ability to access resources. Because each individual has the freedom to make choices, the nurse is cautioned against using *Noncompliance* to describe a person who has made an informed autonomous decision not to comply. In this situation, the nurse must assess for and validate that all required elements for an informed consent are present (Carpenito, 2002).

Deficient knowledge is best used when the client lacks knowledge about the relationship between an unhealthy behavior or habit and the use of community resources to assist in changing it. Use this diagnosis when the knowledge deficiency is the direct cause or a potential cause of a problem. Defining characteristics of this diagnosis that may be exhibited by the

Table 19-3	*Clustering Data to Make a Nursing Diagnosis*
HEALTH BEHAVIORS	
Data Cluster	**Diagnosis**
An 83-year-old diabetic man lives by himself and prepares his own food when he is feeling well. He feels that family members have abandoned him because they are busy with their own families and jobs. He self-administers insulin when he thinks about it or is feeling "bad."	*Ineffective therapeutic regimen management* related to feelings of abandonment and isolation
A 20-year-old woman has a history of obesity since childhood. She desperately wants to be thin to please her boyfriend. She smokes two packs of cigarettes per day to decrease appetite. She eats a lot of fried and spicy foods and goes on "crash" diets to lose weight quickly. She frequently states, "I can't ever seem to lose weight."	*Ineffective health maintenance* related to poor self-esteem interfering with health care regimen
A 42-year-old woman has four children and works part time outside the home. She feels no need for exercise because she is always chasing the kids around. She loves to bake desserts for her family. She would like to regain her pre-pregnancy figure but states that she "isn't ready to diet or exercise."	*Ineffective therapeutic regimen management* related to altered self-concept and resistance to adopting healthy behaviors at this time
A 50-year-old man is head of a household that includes his spouse, two children, and his aging mother. He has just been informed that he will be let go from his job because the company must show a profit. He immediately made plans to change the family's lifestyle and health care standards because there will be no health insurance. He feels particularly bad because his mother and children will suffer from the lack of money to purchase food and medicines.	*Ineffective health maintenance* related to unexpected change in financial status

Box 19-5   Contributing or Related Factors for Nursing Diagnoses

INEFFECTIVE HEALTH MAINTENANCE

- Information misinterpretation
- Lack of motivation
- Lack of education
- Lack of access to adequate health care services
- Inadequate health teaching

HEALTH-SEEKING BEHAVIORS

- Anticipated role changes, such as marriage, parenthood, retirement
- Lack of knowledge

DEFICIENT KNOWLEDGE

- Lack of exposure
- Lack of recall
- Cognitive limitation
- Misinterpretation

NONCOMPLIANCE

- Impaired ability to perform, for example, because of poor memory or motor or sensory deficits
- Side effect of therapy
- Financial issues
- Nonsupportive family
- Lack of access to health care

DECISIONAL CONFLICT

- Risk versus benefits of therapeutic regimen
- Lack of relevant information, or information is confusing
- Conflict with personal values or beliefs

INEFFECTIVE THERAPEUTIC REGIMEN MANAGEMENT

- Complexity of the therapeutic regimen
- Financial cost of regimen
- Complexity of health care system
- Side effect of therapy
- Insufficient knowledge
- Cognitive deficit
- Mistrust of health care system or therapeutic regimen

client include verbalizing a deficiency of knowledge or skill (e.g., a request for information), expressing inaccurate perception of health status, or failure to correctly perform a desired or prescribed health behavior (Carpenito, 2002).

Decisional conflict is the state in which an individual or group experiences uncertainty about a course of action when the choice of options involves risk, loss, or challenge to personal life values. Many situations can contribute to decisional conflict, particularly those that involve complex medical interventions of great risk. Defining characteristics for making this diagnosis include verbalized uncertainty about choices, verbalization of undesired consequences of alternative actions being considered, vacillation between alternative choices, and delayed decision making (Carpenito, 2002).

The diagnosis *Ineffective therapeutic regimen management* describes individuals or families who are experiencing difficulty in achieving positive outcomes. Individuals or families experiencing a variety of health problems, acute or chronic, are usually faced with a treatment program that require changes in previous functioning or lifestyles. When an individual is faced with a complex regimen to follow or has compromised functioning that impedes successful management, the diagnosis *Risk for ineffective therapeutic regimen management* would be appropriate (Carpenito, 2002)

Use care to differentiate between *Ineffective management of therapeutic regimen*, *Noncompliance*, and *Ineffective health maintenance* (Figure 19-2).

Which of the diagnoses just described would you use for Mr. Kitchen? Consider whether he lacks knowledge, is unsuccessful in his efforts, or has chosen not to comply with the therapeutic regimen. Do you believe Mr. Kitchen has made an informed decision not to follow the therapeutic regimen?

PLANNING

The overall expected outcome for intervention to help the client manage a therapeutic regimen is that the client achieve the desired goals of the treatment plan. Outcomes related to successful movement toward achievement of treatment goals are the following:

- The client makes effective choices in integrating the treatment plan into activities of daily living and actively participates in the regimen as prescribed.
- The client seeks help as needed from family members, support groups, and/or health care providers.
- The client expresses positive ways of dealing with stress and conflict.

INTERVENTION

A person must manage a therapeutic regimen in the context of lifestyle choices. It can require changing patterns of living or incorporating therapeutic management into present patterns of living. It also involves overcoming physical and psychological barriers to the therapeutic regimen. Nursing interventions for clients who are having difficulty managing a therapeutic regimen include assistance with lifestyle changes and with specific aspects of the therapeutic regimen. Nursing care uses the principles of motivation and supportive care while providing the client with education, behavior modification, motivation, and therapeutic relationships.

Interventions to Motivate Health Behaviors

Motivating clients toward more effective management of the therapeutic regimen is based on increasing the client's self-efficacy and beliefs in the value of the therapeutic regimen. Consequently, work with the client to design activities that produce minimal conflict with the client's lifestyle and value system.

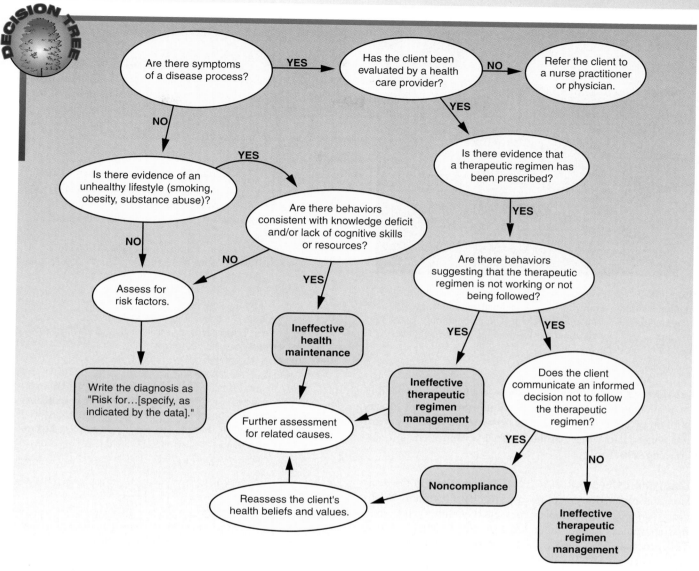

Figure 19-2. Decision tree for health maintenance/lifestyle management nursing diagnoses. Diagnoses are shown in rectangles. Within these rectangles, diagnoses shown in **bold** type are NANDA-approved nursing diagnoses; diagnoses shown in regular type are not NANDA-approved nursing diagnoses.

Increasing Knowledge Level. Although knowledge is not sufficient to produce motivation, it remains a key issue in increasing self-efficacy. The goal is to provide knowledge that will be essential in making informed decisions regarding lifestyles and health promotion practices (Figure 19-3, p. 380). The purpose of health education is to facilitate client decision making regarding personal health behaviors, use of health resources, and general health issues. Teaching a client to plan meals is one example of educating the client. However, appropriate education must be based on the reality of the foods a client may obtain and on cultural desires.

Knowledge helps the client recognize susceptibility to an illness, or the consequences of an illness along with the potential severity of the consequences. The individualized educational plan must focus on increasing awareness of the relationships between the client's specific unhealthy lifestyles (such as tobacco use, poor nutritional habits, excessive alcohol use, drug misuse or abuse, lack of exercise, stress, irresponsible sexual activities, and environmental hazards) and the development of health problems. Box 19-6 (p. 380) offers an example of a way to increase a client's knowledge—in this case about how to lose weight.

Knowledge helps the client weigh benefits against risks. Possible risks involved with health care regimens are side effects, inconveniences, changes in lifestyle, and possibly criticism from family, friends, or co-workers. Benefits can include prolonged life, better quality of life, reduced symptoms, and a return to former activities.

Knowledge contributes to feelings of control. For clients with an internal locus of control, participation in the decision-making process is important. Even when the physician serves as the primary decision maker, understanding how health care

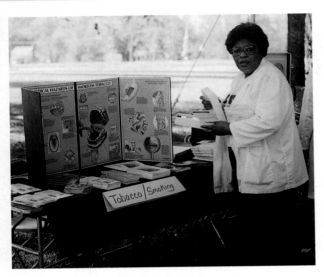

Figure 19-3. Health education is the primary intervention for promoting and maintaining health in individuals, families, groups, and communities. This nurse is participating in a community health fair to educate participants about the far-reaching physical changes caused by cigarette smoking.

providers arrived at their suggestions contributes to a feeling of participating in the decision-making process. For clients with an external locus of control, knowledge may help them recognize factors that can be internally controlled, thus increasing self-efficacy.

Clarifying Values. Values and beliefs play a role in the decision and motivation to follow a health care regimen. *Values clarification* is a self-discovery process that allows a person to find answers to situations or arrive at freely chosen values. This process allows the person to determine what choices to make when faced with alternatives. Your primary goal is to help the client sort out feelings and clarify meanings by listening to the client's comments and appreciating the reason for them.

Lifestyle management involves helping the client develop self-awareness related to attitudes and beliefs regarding smoking, overeating, or other unhealthy lifestyle habits. Help the client identify and examine all available alternatives when faced with choices regarding an unhealthy lifestyle. Guide the client through an examination of consequences associated with each choice to help promote informed decision making. The goal is to get the client to recognize and assume primary responsibility for making healthy lifestyle choices.

Action Alert! Accept the client's choice or point of view, even if it appears to be self-destructive, such as a decision to continue smoking. Confrontation is not beneficial and may actually be detrimental to further cooperation and goal achievement.

Recall that Mr. Kitchen continues to smoke despite his problems with edema and shortness of breath. Although Mr. Kitchen would benefit from a smoking cessation class, the

---

Teaching for Wellness Box 19-6
Helping a Client Lose Weight

Purpose: To support the client's motivation to lose weight through recognition of risk factors and a simple regimen. Teaching supports the client's maintenance of a healthy diet and exercise program.

Expected Outcome: The client will develop a plan to lose weight.

Client Instructions

- In planning for weight loss, make nutritional adequacy your top priority. Most people cannot maintain nutritional adequacy on less than 1200 calories a day, so plan to consume no less than that. To maintain weight, most adults need 2200 to 2500 calories per day, although older adults need less.
- Keep in mind that you will experience a healthier, more successful weight loss with a small energy deficit that provides an adequate intake than with a large energy deficit that creates feelings of starvation and deprivation. These feelings can lead to an irresistible urge to binge. Note the following suggestions:
  - Keep meals small and avoid long periods without food.
  - Choose a diet with plenty of vegetables, fruits, and grain products.
  - Drink plenty of fluids between meals.
  - Avoid foods that are greasy, fried, or highly spiced.
  - Weight loss alone can lower your cholesterol level, decrease your blood pressure, increase your energy level, and lessen joint pain. However, a regular exercise program will enhance these benefits as well as promote self-esteem, reduce the risk of heart disease, and encourage the loss of extra pounds. Note the following suggestions:
  - If you are over 35, have heart trouble, or are taking medicine for high blood pressure, see a doctor before you start a physical exercise program.
  - Initiate your exercise program slowly and build up your activity level gradually.
  - Exercise at least for 20 minutes, four times a week.
  - Listen to your body. Pay attention to warning signals, such as sudden dizziness, cold sweats, fainting, or pressure in the chest.

---

nurse should also recognize that he may be depressed and lonely. Because his wife managed his health care, he may also lack the knowledge to follow through on his care. If he is depressed, he may lack the ability to act. It may be difficult for him to relate to the clinic staff, and he may believe it is acceptable to stop medications if he feels better.

The clinic staff might try a follow-up telephone call a week before Mr. Kitchen's scheduled appointment to determine how the therapeutic regimen is progressing. Can you think of other ways to help Mr. Kitchen?

Engaging Participation. Active participation in learning typically increases learning and motivation. **Counseling** is a method of communication that actively involves the client in the recognition of personal risk factors and management of necessary behavioral changes (Figure 19-4). Counseling is different from education in that it involves guiding the client through decision making rather than merely ensuring that he has the knowledge to make a decision.

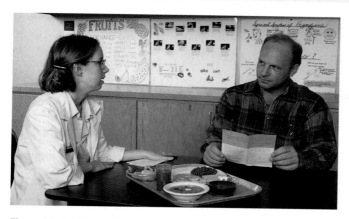

Figure 19-4. Counseling is a method of communication that helps clients recognize personal risk factors and manage necessary behavioral changes.

During counseling, the client plays the major role in identifying and clarifying the problem to be solved. Engage the client in a dialogue to identify the problem and examine the factors that contribute to the problem and those that may enhance or block its resolution. Do not tell the client what to do to solve the problem but instead assist and guide the problem-solving or decision-making process.

Because many people lack the knowledge or skills to approach a problem systematically, teaching and counseling can be combined to help the client solve the dilemma successfully. If the health history reveals that the client is at risk for a sexually transmitted disease, health education would involve providing didactic information to help the person avoid infection. Counseling would involve greater interaction and would entail helping the person identify risky behaviors and developing a plan to reduce the risk. Counseling should be tailored to the individual risk factors, needs, and abilities of each client.

Anticipating Problems. Anticipate problems the client may have in managing the therapeutic regimen. If the client is illiterate, has poor eyesight, has decreased mobility, or has decreased manual dexterity, you can help plan for alternative methods of managing the therapeutic regimen. Also, anticipate side effects of medication and help plan ways to manage them.

Providing Reinforcing Factors. Help the client find motivation from life goals or desirable activities. Playing with grandchildren, traveling to Europe, attending a child's graduation from college, or caring for an elderly parent are among the important activities of life that can motivate a person to work toward better health. If the client does not have motivating factors, you may be able to suggest personal goals that will serve as a reward for effective management of the therapeutic regimen. Rewards can be achieving a major long-term goal or engaging in small daily or weekly pleasures.

Interventions to Provide Supportive Care

Changing lifestyle behaviors to manage a therapeutic regimen can be a complex problem. Although the client may initially have strong motivation and expect to be able to make the

changes, continued support from family and health care providers is often necessary to sustain the changes.

Establishing a Therapeutic Relationship. The most influential factor in increasing the client's participation in effective management of a therapeutic regimen is the relationship with the health care provider. Give the client individual attention by providing information in a face-to-face, two-way communication process.

Probe for the client's level of understanding of and perspective on the problem. A common and sometimes mistaken practice is to wait for the client to ask questions. The assumption is that the client may not want to know everything and will ask the questions that are of the most concern. However, the client may not know what to ask and may not have enough information even to form the questions. Only after you have learned how the client perceives the problem can you offer information that deals with the client's often unspoken concerns (Box 19-7).

Guiding the Client Through the Health System. A major focus of nursing care is to promote and assist the client in receiving the health care necessary to achieve and maintain health. Lifestyle behavioral changes may require the client to seek services from several health care agencies. Getting to and through these systems can prove difficult for many clients.

Helping the client identify services to assist in achieving desired goals should be the initial step. Determine the client's eligibility, as well as the fees involved and methods of payment, to ensure that services are available and affordable. Identify constraints, such as lack of transportation, cultural beliefs, and the ability to communicate. Preparing the client for what will be encountered will help to make the best use of the services available.

The initial step is to help the client recognize the need for these services. A client who is in denial will not see the need for or benefit of services. After the client has acknowledged the problem, discuss the services that are available.

Planning for Discharge. As defined in Chapter 10, *Discharge planning* is the preparation for moving a client from one level of care to another within or outside the current health care agency. It is a systematic process of preparing clients and family members to manage therapeutic regimens and to engage in health maintenance activities once they leave the hospital or other health care delivery system. The objectives of discharge planning are to do the following:

- Make sure that there will be no interruption in the implementation of the therapeutic regimen.
- Provide adequate teaching and instruction or additional demonstrations of procedures to manage the therapeutic regimen.
- Identify or familiarize the client and family with appropriate resources to ensure continuity of care.
- The client and the family should be actively involved in the planning process, goal setting, and all decision making.

Although discharge planning should begin at the time of admission to allow for adequate teaching and preparation, an assessment of the needs of the client and family is ongoing, and final plans are made immediately before discharge. Because most clients stay fewer days in the hospital than they once did, the scope and complexity of the discharge planning has increased. Different clients have different complexities of need, as well. For example, a client being discharged from a substance abuse treatment center would require a more complex discharge plan than a middle-aged client being discharged from an emergency department with a fractured wrist. The substance abuser will require additional community resources, such as substance abuse counselors, a support group, and family members, to assist in managing the treatment plan and the related lifestyle changes needed to remain free of drugs.

During your predischarge assessment, pay attention to any statements that could indicate a potential for ineffective management of health or the health plan, such as an unwillingness or inability to modify personal habits and integrate necessary treatments into the lifestyle. Failure to adhere to a treatment plan while hospitalized (such as refusal to take medication, walk, or follow dietary modification) would suggest a potential for the diagnosis *Ineffective management of therapeutic regimen* after discharge.

Referring to Health Services. **Referral** is a process designed to provide the client with access to health care and supportive services that are not available from the sending institution. The referral process begins after assessment data reveal a need for additional services. A client with chronic obstructive pulmonary disorder who continues to smoke, for example, may be referred to a smoking cessation class. When altered nutritional intake appears to be a family problem, the family may be referred to a nutritionist. An adolescent who shows evidence of anorexia nervosa may be referred to a clinical psychologist or physician. If the assessment data indicate that the client has not completed immunizations for the age group, the client should be referred to the local health department.

As in discharge planning, the client and family should be involved in the decision for referral. This is important to facilitate the client's follow-through. If the referral is recognized by the client as being insignificant, the client probably will not follow through.

Several factors must be taken into consideration when planning for referral. The referred source must be acceptable to the client and it must be specific to the needs of the client. Some clients will not use services that are perceived as "charity" or "demoralizing." For example, a client who is overweight may perceive different implications if referred to Overeaters Anonymous instead of Weight Watchers. Also, the client must be eligible for the services. Services that are designed for Medicare or Medicaid clients will not provide services to people who do not meet the appropriate criteria.

To be effective in making referrals, you will need to know about resources in the client's community, including the location of services, name and telephone number of a contact person, types of services provided, eligibility criteria, operating hours, and a general overview of fees required. When making a referral, give the client all the necessary information. If the client agrees, call ahead to make the appointment.

Promoting Social Support. An assessment of social support involves an analysis of the client's social network to ascertain actual and potential sources of support, the client's perception of need for social support, and the specific helping behaviors that would be of assistance to the client. Help the client make this assessment and develop the social support structure to facilitate the expected lifestyle behavioral changes or to incorporate the therapeutic regimen into daily life. Help the client clarify expectations of support persons and the type of support needed. Encourage open communication of needs among family members, goal setting, and identification of strategies to be implemented to achieve goals.

Action Alert! Assess current actions of significant others and how they are received by the client. When significant others try to be helpful, does the client perceive them as being helpful? Also assess whether significant others are withdrawn or overly protective.

In addition to family and friends, a support group may be helpful with smoking cessation, adjusting dietary habits, or participating in an exercise program. Social support can be provided through groups that provide an opportunity for clients to share the experiences of others in changing behaviors.

EVALUATION

Evaluation involves reassessing the client to determine whether all outcomes were achieved. The outcomes will have been achieved if the client reports participation in activities to increase knowledge of health promotion. Participation in these activities could entail attending classes at the local health center or health department; seeking health information through the media, such as newspaper or television; and building knowledge of preventable diseases and related risk factors.

Additionally, the client may express a desire to achieve better health by participating in health screening clinics or learning to perform self-examinations (Figure 19-5). Reducing the number of risk factors or being successful in integrating the treatment plan into daily life indicates that the client has achieved the outcomes for effective management of the therapeutic regimen. The client should be reassessed for the establishment of new goals.

If no noticeable change occurs in unhealthy behaviors within a reasonable period, or if the client returns with an exacerbation of symptoms, reassess the client to determine what prevented the progress. For example, a client who has successfully followed a reduced-calorie nutritional program may not show a weight loss during the first week because of med-

ications that have fluid-retention properties or other physiological alterations. Mr. Kitchen is an example. Box 19-8 illustrates how the clinic nurse worked with him to improve his management of the therapeutic regimen. Before he left the clinic the nurse wrote the note below.

SAMPLE DOCUMENTATION NOTE FOR MR. KITCHEN
Demonstrates concern for his health and intention to comply with medication schedule. However, he relies on a neighbor for cooking and feels he has no means to control his diet. Instructed to avoid highly salty foods like bacon, and not to add salt at the table. Given a written schedule of his medications. Will do telephone follow-up to reinforce need for compliance.

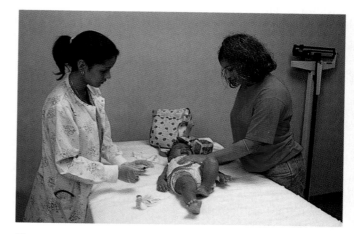

Figure 19-5. Health screening is a primary strategy used to promote health. The young mother *(at right)* understands the importance of health screening in achieving optimal health for her child. During a routine screening visit, the nurse has identified the need to update the child's immunizations.

Nursing Care Plan A CLIENT WITH HEART FAILURE

Box 19-8

ADMISSION DATA

Mr. Oscar Kitchen is a 69-year-old black man who is being seen in a primary health care center. This is the second time he has come in with shortness of breath and edema of the lower limbs. The doctor has told him to stay on the same medication for his heart and on diuretics. With proper instructions, he believes Mr. Kitchen can manage the therapeutic regimen at home.

PHYSICIAN'S ORDERS

Admitting diagnosis: Chronic heart failure
Lasix 20 mg PO daily every morning
Digoxin 0.125 mg PO daily every morning

Low Na diet
Hygroton 25 mg PO daily every morning
Return to clinic in 2 weeks

NURSING ASSESSMENT

BP 160/98, pulse 98, respiration 32 and labored. Height 5 feet 11.5 inches, weight 220 lb, 3+ pitting edema of lower extremities. Widower of 3 months. Wife previously assisted in management of health care regimen. No close relative living near. Very little interaction with neighbors. Smokes two packs of cigarettes each day. He smoked for 55 years.

Continued

Nursing Care Plan A CLIENT WITH HEART FAILURE—CONT'D

Box 19-8

NANDA Nursing Diagnosis	NOC Expected Outcomes With Indicators	NIC Interventions With Selected Activities	Evaluation Data
INEFFECTIVE THERAPEUTIC REGIMEN MANAGEMENT **Related Factors:** • Shortness of breath • 3+ pitting edema • Pulse 98 and irregular • BP 160/98	**COMPLIANCE BEHAVIOR** • Takes medications daily as prescribed.	**MEDICATION MANAGEMENT** • Assists in making a schedule to take medications at planned times that work best for him.	**AT 1-MONTH FOLLOW-UP VISIT** • States medication is taken daily as prescribed. • Pitting edema decreased to < +1 or eliminated. • Pulse regular and within normal range for client.
DEFICIENT KNOWLEDGE RELATED TO TREATMENT REGIMEN **Related Factor:** Made a decision to stop taking medications after the first week because he "feels better."	**KNOWLEDGE:** • Treatment regimen. • Asks questions to clarify understanding of treatment regimen. • Statements reflect an understanding of the implication of not following the prescribed treatment. • Statements reflect an understanding of the effect of sodium on his conditions.	**TEACHING:** • Prescribed medication. • Determine client's understanding of illness. • Explain the disease process of chronic congestive heart failure in very simple terms. • Explain purpose of medications and consequences if medications are not taken. • Explain low-sodium diet and assist in developing a list of low-sodium foods that he likes.	• Voices no misconception about illness. • Answers questions correctly about the disease process. • Reports he takes his medication every day. • Gives a 3-day recall of food eaten, and foods are determined (by the nurse) to be appropriate for a low-sodium diet.

CRITICAL THINKING QUESTIONS

1. Which is the priority nursing intervention? What is the rationale for your choice?
2. Can you think of other ways the nurse could have incorporated Mr. Kitchen's culture into his care? How would you change your approach if the client was of Hispanic or Vietnamese origin?
3. How could the client be motivated to change behavior and accept responsibility for a healthier lifestyle?

Nursing outcome and intervention labels from Johnson, M., Bulechek, G., McCloskey Dochterman, J. M., Maas, M., & Moorhead, S, et al. (2001). *Nursing diagnoses, outcomes, and interventions: NANDA, NOC, and NIC linkages.* St Louis, MO: Mosby.

Key Principles

- Understanding health from the perspectives of the client and the provider is critical to the development of health services and nursing interventions.
- Concepts that differ across cultures include an explanatory model of illness that defines the nature of illness, its treatment, and the type of relationships that should occur between client and health care provider.
- There are two domains of health care: the folk, or generic, form and the scientific form.
- The theory of reasoned action is based on the assumption that people are reasonable and, in deciding what action to take, systematically process and use the information available to them.

- The transtheoretical model of behavioral change is useful across all theories to plan interventions that are appropriate to the stage of change: precontemplation, contemplation, preparation, action, maintenance, and termination.
- In the health belief model, behavior is a function of the subjective value of an outcome and of the subjective expectation that a particular action will achieve that outcome.
- The health promotion model uses concepts from the health belief model but decreases the focus on threats as an avenue to behavioral change.
- Factors affecting behavioral change affect the relationship with the health care provider. They include communication, cognition and perception, age and developmental level, lifestyle and habits, economic resources, cultural values and beliefs, roles

and relationships, coping and stress tolerance, and workplace and environmental conditions.

- Lack of education about nutrition, safety, fitness, or health-protecting practices during early childhood or adolescence can have a significant impact on adult health.
- Wellness assessment focuses on physical fitness evaluation, health risk appraisal, social support systems, and lifestyle assessment.
- Assessment for behavioral change requires assessing the client's level of knowledge.
- Assessment for *Ineffective therapeutic regimen management* often relies on indirect cues suggesting that the client needs to improve the management of the therapeutic regimen.
- The health care system can be a related factor for *Ineffective therapeutic regimen management.*
- Educational interventions aimed at improving behavior can reduce at-risk behaviors.
- Motivation, locus of control, health perception, and a sense of self-efficacy affect participation in activities to promote or maintain health.
- Nursing interventions for *Ineffective health maintenance* would include activities to help the client promote and maintain health through education, health screening, and counseling.
- Nursing interventions for *Ineffective therapeutic regimen management* include teaching the client about the current illness and treatment regimen, supporting the client's well-being through stress-management skills, and promoting health management choices through values clarification.
- Although knowledge is not sufficient to produce motivation, it remains a key issue in increasing self-efficacy.
- Knowledge helps the client recognize susceptibility to an illness or the consequences of an illness, along with the potential severity of the consequences.
- Values clarification is a self-discovery process that allows the person to make choices when faced with alternatives.
- Active participation in learning is expected to increase learning and motivation.
- Anticipation of problems is an effective teaching tool for complex health care regimens.
- The most influential factor in increasing the client's participation in effective management of a therapeutic regimen is the relationship with the health care provider.
- The objectives of discharge planning are to ensure that there will be no interruption in implementation, to provide adequate teaching, and to familiarize the client with appropriate resources.
- Social support is a key element in health promotion activities.

Bibliography

*Bandura, A. (1977). Self-efficacy: Toward a unifying theory of behavioral change. *Psychological Review, 84,* 191-215.

Bernaix, L. W. (2000). Nurses' attitudes, subjective norms, and behavioral intentions toward support of breastfeeding mothers. *Journal of Human Lactation, 16*(3), 201-209.

Carpenito, L. J. (2002). *Nursing diagnosis: Application to clinical practice* (9th ed.). Philadelphia: Lippincott.

Centers for Disease Control (Division of Health Education). (1984). *CDC health risk appraisal user manual* (Publication No. 746-011/15233). Washington, DC: U.S. Government Printing Office.

Clark, M. J. (1999). *Nursing in the community: Dimensions of community health nursing* (3rd ed.). Stamford, CT: Appleton & Lange.

Clarke, K. E., & Aish, A. (2002). An exploration of health beliefs and attitudes of smokers with vascular disease who participate in or decline a smoking cessation program. *Journal of Vascular Nursing, 20*(3), 96-105.

Esser-Stuart, J. E., & Lyons, M. A. (2002). Barriers and influences in seeking health care among lower income minority women. *Social Work and Health Care, 35*(3), 85-99.

Faucher, M. A., & Carter, S. (2001). Why girls smoke: A proposed community-based prevention program. *Journal Obstetrical Gynecologic and Neonatal Nursing, 30*(5), 463-471.

Giger, J. N., & Davidhizar, R. E. (1999). *Transcultural nursing: Assessment and intervention* (3rd ed.). St Louis, MO: Mosby.

Gorek, B., Martin, J., White, N., Peters, D., & Hummel, F. (2002). Culturally competent care for Latino elders in long-term care settings. *Geriatric Nursing, 23*(5), 272-275.

Henderson, J. W. (2002). *Health Economics and policy* (2nd ed.). Cincinnati, OH: South-Western/Thomson Learning.

Johnson, M., Bulechek, G., McCloskey Dochterman, J. M., Maas, M., & Moorhead, S. (2001). *Nursing diagnoses, outcomes, and interventions: NANDA, NOC, and NIC linkages.* St Louis, MO: Mosby.

Jones, P. S., Zhang, X. E., Jaceldo-Siegl, K., & Meleis, A. I. (2002). Caregiving between two cultures: An integrative experience. *Journal of Transcultural Nursing, 13*(3), 202-209.

*Kavanagh, K. H., & Kennedy, P. H. (1992). *Promoting cultural diversity: Strategies for health care professionals.* Newbury Park, CA: Sage.

*Klienman, A., Eisenberg, L., & Good, B. (1978). Culture, illness, and care. *Annals of Internal Medicine, 88,*(2), 251-258.

Kulbok, P. A., Laffrey, S. C., & Goeppinger, J. (2000). Community health promotion: An integrative model for practice. In M. Stanhope & J. Lancaster (Eds.), *Community and public health nursing* (5th ed.). St Louis, MO: Mosby.

Lancaster, J., Onega, L., & Forness, D. (2000). Using NP to Promote Health. In M. Stanhope & J. Lancaster (Eds.), *Community and public health nursing* (5th ed.). St Louis, MO: Mosby.

*Leininger, M. M. (1970). *Nursing and anthropology: Two worlds to blend.* New York: John Wiley.

*Leininger, M. M. (1991). *Culture care diversity & universality: A theory of nursing.* New York: National League for Nursing Press.

Leininger, M. M. (2001). *Culture care diversity & universality: A theory of nursing.* Boston: Jones and Bartlett.

McGahee, T. W., Kemp, V., Tingen, M. (2000). A theoretical model for smoking prevention studies in preteen children. *Pediatric Nursing, 26*(2), 135-138, 141.

McKinlay, A., Couston, M., & Cowan, S. (2001). Nurses' behavioural intentions towards self-poisoning patients: A theory of reasoned action, comparison of attitudes and subjective norms as predictive variables. *Journal of Advanced Nursing, 34*(1), 107-116.

Morgan, D. G., Semchuk, K. M., Stewart, N. J., & D'Arcy, C. (2002). Rural families caring for a relative with dementia: Barriers to use of formal services. *Social Science and Medicine, 55*(7), 1129-1142.

North American Nursing Diagnosis Association. (2000). *NANDA nursing diagnoses: Definitions and classification, 2000-2002.* Philadelphia: Author.

---

*Asterisk indicates a classic or definitive work on this subject.

Pender, N. J., Murdaugh, C. L. , & Parsons, M. A. (2001) *Health promotion in nursing practice.* (4th ed.). Upper Saddle River, N. J. : Prentice Hall.

Pierce, L. L. (2001). Caring and expressions of stability by urban family caregivers of persons with stroke within African American family systems. *Rehabilitation Nursing, 26*(3), 100-107, 116.

Poss, J. E. (2000). Factors associated with participation by Mexican migrant farmworkers in a tuberculosis screening program. *Nursing Research, 49*(1), 20-28.

Poss, J. E. (2001). Developing a new model for cross-cultural research: Synthesizing the health belief model and the theory of reasoned action [Review]. *Advances in Nursing Science, 23*(4), 1-15.

*Prochaska, J. O., Velicer, W. F., Rossi, J. S., Goldstein, M. G., Marcus, B. H., Rakowski, W., et al. (1994). Stages of change and decisional balance for 12 problem behaviors. *Health Psychology, 13*(1), 39-46.

*Rosenstock, J. (1974). Historical origins of the health belief model. *Health Education Monograph, 2*(4), 328-335.

Spector, R. (2000). *Cultural diversity in health and illness* (5th ed.). Upper Saddle River, NJ: Prentice Hall.

Stanhope, M., & Lancaster, J. (2000). *Community and public health nursing* (5th ed.). St Louis, MO: Mosby.

Sumner, J. (2001). Caring in nursing: A different interpretation. *Journal of Advanced Nursing, 35*(6), 926-932.

Swanson, E. A., Tripp-Reimer, T., & Buckwalter, K. (2001). *Health promotion and disease prevention in the older adult: Interventions and recommendations.* New York: Springer.

*Thomas, S. (1992). The health of the black community in the twenty-first century: A futuristic perspective. In R. L. Braithwaite & S. E. Taylor (Eds.), *Health issues in the Black community.* San Francisco: Jossey-Bass.

Toseland, R. W., McCallion, P., Gerber, T., & Banks, S. (2002). Predictors of health and human services use by persons with dementia and their family caregivers. *Social Science and Medicine, 55*(7), 1255-1266.

*Tripp-Reimer, T. (1984). Reconceptualizing the concept of health: Integrating emic and etic perspectives. *Research, Nursing & Health, 7,* 101-109.

*Walker, S. N., Sechrist, K. R., & Pender, N. J. (1987). The health-promoting lifestyle profile: Development and psychometric characteristics. *Nursing Research, 36*(2), 76-81.

Werner, P., Mendelsson, G. (2001). Nursing staff members' intentions to use physical restraints with older people: Testing the theory of reasoned action. *Journal of Advanced Nursing, 35*(5), 784-791.

Wesley, Y., Smeltzer, S. C., Redeker, N. S., Walker, S., Palumbo, P., & Whipple, B. (2000). Reproductive decision making in mothers with HIV-1. *Health Care Women International, 21*(4), 291-304.

Williams, A. M. (2000). Distress and hardiness: A comparison of African-American and white caregivers. *Journal of National Black Nurses Association, 11*(1), 21-26.

Woolf, S., Jonas, S., & Lawrence, R. (1996). *Health promotion and disease prevention in clinical practice.* Baltimore: Williams & Wilkins.

20

Health Maintenance: Medication Management

Key Terms

adverse effect

anaphylaxis

antagonistic effect

bioavailability

biotransformation

chemical name

controlled substance

generic name

hypersensitivity reaction

idiosyncratic response

intradermal route

intramuscular route

intravenous route

loading dose

official name

parenteral route

pharmacokinetics

prescription

side effect

subcutaneous route

synergistic effect

target organ

teratogenic potential

therapeutic effect

topical route

toxic effect

trade name

Learning Objectives

After studying this chapter, you should be able to do the following:

- Discuss important concepts related to safe and effective medication management

- Describe a variety of factors that influence drug actions in individual clients

- Explain how to assess a client who is receiving medication therapy

- Formulate appropriate nursing diagnostic statements for a client receiving medications

- Plan appropriate expected outcomes for a client taking medications

- Incorporate safe and effective nursing interventions in the care of a client receiving medications

- Evaluate the effectiveness of medication therapy in helping to achieve health-related expected outcomes

Daniel Connell is a married 62-year-old Irish American. He came to the emergency department (ED) after experiencing chest pain while carrying an air conditioner up two flights of stairs to the attic. Upon arrival at the ED, vital signs were pulse 96, blood pressure 166/96, respirations 22, and oral temperature 98.8° F. Mr. Connell described the chest pain as a "pressure," and he rated it as 6 on a 0-10 pain scale. The pain did not worsen with inspiration and was relieved with nitroglycerin.

Results of serum laboratory studies and electrocardiogram showed that Mr. Connell did not have a myocardial infarction (heart attack). By taking a more thorough history, the ED nurse learns that Mr. Connell has hypertension but has not been taking prescribed medications. His dietary intake is high in sodium, and he does not exercise regularly. Knowing that Mr. Connell is not doing what is necessary to control his health problems, the nurse considers the diagnosis of *Ineffective health maintenance*. The nurse also considers other nursing diagnoses that may apply to Mr. Connell's situation, such as *Ineffective therapeutic regimen management* and *Noncompliance,* as shown below.

KEY NURSING DIAGNOSES FOR   Medication Administration

Ineffective health maintenance: Inability to identify, manage, and/or seek out help to maintain health

Ineffective therapeutic regimen management: A pattern of regulating and integrating into daily living a program for treatment of illness and the sequelae of illness that is unsatisfactory for meeting specific health goals

CONCEPTS OF MEDICATION MANAGEMENT

Medication administration is a critically important part of the nurse's role. Many clients take medication as part of a therapeutic regimen for health problems. This chapter examines concepts, clinical judgments, and practices needed for safe, effective medication therapy.

Drug Names and Forms

The terms *drug* and *medication* are often used interchangeably, although technically they differ. A *drug* is a chemical substance that alters an organism's function and may or may not have a therapeutic effect. A *medication* is a drug being used for an intended therapeutic effect. Most drugs or medications can be called by several different names. The **chemical name,** often long and complex, is of interest to pharmacists and precisely describes the chemical and molecular structure of a medication. For example, the chemical name for acetaminophen (Tylenol) is *N*-acetyl-*para*-aminophenol.

The **generic name,** or *nonproprietary name,* is the name assigned to a drug by the United States Adopted Names Council when it is first manufactured. Subsequent manufacturers of the drug then use the same generic name. The **official name** is the name assigned by the Food and Drug Administration (FDA) after approval of a drug and is often the same as the generic name. The official name of a drug is how it is listed in the *United States Pharmacopeia* (USP) and *National Formulary* (NF), two publications officially approved by the FDA.

The **trade name,** also known as the brand name or *proprietary name,* is a copyrighted name given by a specific manufacturer to a medication. Because several manufacturers may produce the same medication, a medication may have several trade names in addition to the generic name. It is important to be familiar with both the generic and the trade names of medications. This may be difficult because of the sheer number of trade names on the market and because generic names are often complex or foreign. For example, acetylsalicylic acid is the generic name for Bayer Aspirin, which has other trade names, including Ecotrin and Empirin.

Prescription and Nonprescription Medications. Medications are commonly grouped into two categories, prescription medications or nonprescription (also called over-the-counter, or OTC). A **prescription** is an order for a medication that contains the client's name, medication name, dose, route, frequency, amount of medication to be dispensed, number of refills allowed (if any), and the physician's signature. The physician must sign the prescription and indicate whether a generic interchange may be substituted. Prescription drugs should be used under the supervision of a health care provider. Taking a prescription drug without supervision could lead to harm or result in abuse.

In some states, revised nurse practice acts allow selected groups of advanced practice nurses to write prescriptions. Prescriptive privileges are limited to certified nurse practitioners, nurse anesthetists, nurse midwives, and clinical nurse specialists who work in collaboration with a physician.

Action Alert! Know which groups of health care providers have legal authority to write prescriptions in the state in which you are practicing nursing.

A *nonprescription* or *OTC medication* can be purchased without a prescription and can be used to enhance personal health (e.g., vitamins) or treat common health problems (e.g., constipation or diarrhea). Nurses and pharmacists have an important role in teaching clients about possible interactive effects between medications.

Classification. Medications with similar characteristics may be classified together according to therapeutic effect (bronchodilators), symptoms relieved (antianxiety agents), or clinical actions and composition (opioid analgesics). Classifications have characteristics in common that can help you understand medications. Some medications have more than one classification, so it is important to understand the drug's purpose for each client.

Drug Forms. Medications are manufactured in a variety of forms to make them more useful or easy to administer. Some examples of drug forms include tablets, suspensions, suppositories, and ointments (Table 20-1). The form of a drug guides its route of administration. One form should not be interchanged with another without a specific physician order because the rate of absorption or **bioavailability** (amount available for use by target tissues) may differ among forms or even among brand names (McKenry & Salerno, 2001).

Legislation and Standards

Because medications have a great impact on the health and well-being of clients, their manufacture and use is highly regulated. This protects clients from harm and provides a common set of guidelines for personnel in the pharmaceutical and health care industries. All drugs produced in the United States and Canada must meet legal standards for quality control. Health care personnel rely on these standards to provide safe, effective medication therapy.

Pure Food and Drug Act of 1906. In the United States, the Pure Food and Drug Act of 1906 set the first standards for the quality and purity of drugs. This Act empowered the FDA to monitor drug standards, such as chemical composition, quality, purity, strength, and form. The standards further required that drugs be adequately packaged and labeled. The U.S. standards have been updated over time with various pieces of legislation. Current standards have been broadened to include drug safety and effectiveness. State laws may be even stricter than federal standards. Refer to a pharmacology textbook for detailed information about key drug legislation.

Food and Drug Administration. The FDA is the official government agency responsible for determining that drug manufacturers maintain the standards set by law. Its scope of authority spans several areas, including drug testing, approval of drugs for use, and control of drug sale and distribution. It also specifies whether an individual medication is classified as prescription or nonprescription.

If a pharmaceutical company wishes to produce a new drug, it submits a written proposal to the FDA. Controlled studies, known as clinical trials, are then undertaken in four phases to test the drug. If it meets required standards, it may be approved for use. This rigorous process explains why drugs that are available in some countries may not be authorized for use in the United States.

Controlled Substances. Control of opioid analgesics and other select drugs is an important element of drug legislation. **Controlled substances** are drugs that affect the mind or behavior, may be habit forming, and have a high potential for abuse. They include opioids (also called narcotics), barbiturates, and illegal drugs. Controlled drugs are assigned to a specific category ranging from Schedule I to Schedule V. Their distribution and use is either highly regulated or prohibited (Table 20-2, p. 390).

The Drug Enforcement Agency (DEA) is empowered to enforce narcotics laws. Violations may result in fines, imprisonment, or loss of your nursing license. Health care facilities have detailed policies and procedures for storage, distribution,

Table 20-1	Common Forms for Drug Preparations
Preparation	**General Description**
Caplet	Tablet coated with gelatin that dissolves in the stomach
Capsule	Powder or gel form of drug encased in a hard or soft outer casing that dissolves in the stomach
Elixir	Drug dissolved in a clear liquid containing water, varying amounts of alcohol, and a sweetening agent or flavor
Emulsion	Drug in which one liquid is spread by means of small droplets through another liquid
Enteric-coated tablet	Tablet coated with a substance that blocks drug absorption until the tablet reaches the small intestine
Extract	Highly concentrated form of drug made when the active portion is removed from the other drug components
Liniment	Drug combined with alcohol, soap, or oil that is applied to the skin
Lotion	Drug that is dissolved in liquid and applied to the skin
Lozenge or troche	Drug in a flavored or sweet base that is released as the base dissolves in the mouth
Ointment	Semisolid form of a drug that is applied to and absorbed by the skin
Paste	Semisolid form of a drug that is applied to and absorbed by the skin, thicker than an ointment
Patch (transdermal)	Drug encased in a manufactured material that allows continuous drug absorption through the skin at a steady rate
Pill	Drug in powder form mixed in a cohesive material
Powder or granules	Finely ground form of a drug
Solution	Drug that has been dissolved in a liquid, commonly water
Suppository	Drug mixed in a firm base that melts easily when inserted into the rectum, vagina, or urethra
Suspension	Undissolved particles or powder placed in a liquid that must be shaken vigorously before use
Syrup	Drug dissolved in a solution containing water and sugar
Tablet	Solid drug that is compressed or molded into a particular shape and may be swallowed whole, chewed, or placed in the cheek or under the tongue, depending on its purpose
Tincture	Type of solution in which a drug is dissolved in alcohol or a water–alcohol base

Table 20-2	Controlled Substance Schedule	
Schedule	Explanation	Examples
I	Not accepted for medical use because of their high potential for abuse	• Heroin • LSD • Marijuana
II	Have acceptable medical uses but also have a high potential for abuse or physical or psychological dependency	• Amphetamines • Codeine • Meperidine (Demerol) • Methadone • Morphine
III	Have acceptable medical uses and a potential for abuse or dependence that is less than Schedule II drugs	• Oxycodone • Propoxyphene • Some codeine preparations
IV	Have acceptable medical uses with limited risk of abuse or dependence	• Benzodiazepines • Nonnarcotic analgesics • Phenobarbital
V	Have medically acceptable uses with minimal risk for abuse or dependence	• Opioid-containing antidiarrheals • Opioid-containing cough remedies

and record-keeping of controlled substances. Sample guidelines for controlled substance administration by nurses are outlined in Box 20-1. Adhere to these guidelines to ensure that your behavior is within the law.

Institutional Policies. Hospitals, extended-care facilities, home health agencies, and other health care facilities have policies and procedures for medication administration that are unique to that facility. You have an obligation to be aware of and comply with them.

Institutional policies must be congruent with the nurse practice act for the state in which the facility is located. The nurse practice act for that state includes specific regulations about the nurse's role in medication administration. It is your legal and professional responsibility to understand the legal foundations of your nursing practice.

Sources of Information

Printed Materials. General information about many medications and their classifications is found in pharmacology texts (Lehne, Moore, Crosby, & Hamilton, 2001) and other printed references. Several textbooks have been written with nurses as the primary audience; also published are several drug reference handbooks for easy use.

Detailed information about medications can be found in sources such as the *American Hospital Formulary Service Drug Information* (AHFS DI), *Physician's Desk Reference* (PDR), and the *United States Pharmacopeia: Drug Information for the Health Care Professional* (USP DI). Most health care institutions use one of these as the facility's official drug reference book.

People. Certain key people are good sources of drug information. Other experienced nurses and advanced practice nurses are knowledgeable and available to answer questions during everyday nursing practice. The physician who prescribes a medication can explain its expected action or benefit and why it was ordered for a particular client.

Box 20-1	Controlled Substance Administration and Control Guidelines

- Place all controlled substances in the facility-approved, double-locked storage area.
- Count controlled substances according to facility policy at the beginning and end of each work shift. Have an off-going and an on-coming nurse sign that the count is correct.
- Follow facility protocols for reporting discrepancies in the count.
- Obtain a key from the designated RN or LPN to gain entry to the storage cabinet, or use your assigned code if you have a computerized storage system.
- Make an entry in the controlled substance inventory when removing a medication, unless your computerized system does so automatically. This ensures an ongoing record of the number of drugs used and remaining.
- When you sign out a controlled substance, record the client's name, the date, the time of administration, the drug name, and the dose needed. Make sure to sign the record. If you have a computerized system, your entry code will serve as your signature.
- Have a second nurse witness the disposal of a partial dose of a controlled substance. Both of you should sign the record or use your entry codes as your signatures.

Pharmacists are a primary source of medication information. Larger institutions, such as hospitals, commonly employ pharmacists who are readily available on-site. Smaller facilities, such as extended-care facilities, usually have a contract with a specific pharmacy; these pharmacists are generally available by telephone. Pharmacists employed in local pharmacies are yet another source of information and are the resource most often tapped by consumers.

Pharmaceutical sales representatives often have detailed information about medications produced by a specific company. Keep in mind that their primary objective is sales, not education. Thus they may readily identify the positive aspects of a product while being less vocal about negative ones. They are best used for information about a product's benefits and how to use it for maximum effect.

Purpose: To help the client remain free of the most common side effects of a variety of medications by encouraging health-promoting behaviors.

Expected Outcome: The client will remain free of common medication side effects or will have less severe side effects if they occur.

Client Instructions

Constipation. Many groups of medications, such as opioid analgesics, antispasmodics, and iron supplements, slow the action of the gastrointestinal tract. The following are helpful hints about actions you can take to decrease the risk of getting constipated while taking these medications:

- Drink increased fluids unless contraindicated by another health problem. Because foods also contain fluid, you will probably obtain a sufficient fluid intake by drinking 6 to 8 glasses of water each day in addition to the normal diet, to total 2 to 3 quarts of fluid per day.
- Walk or do some other activity that moves and stretches the abdominal muscles each day. This movement "massages" the intestines and increases peristaltic activity.
- Increase the amount of fiber in your diet. Eat plenty of fruits and vegetables, and include whole grains whenever possible instead of refined carbohydrates.

Sedation. Many medications, such as decongestants, some cough preparations, narcotics, and antianxiety agents, cause drowsiness. Although you may not be able to prevent this side effect, you can modify your activities to reduce the risk of injury while taking these medications. Some suggestions include the following:

- Do not drive or do any other activity that requires concentration for approximately 2 to 3 hours after taking the medication. Resume these activities only after the drowsiness has worn off.
- Make sure travel paths, such as the hallway leading to the bathroom, are sufficiently lighted at night to prevent falls caused by sedation or reduced vision. Remove scatter rugs or other objects that increase the risk of falls.
- If you take the medication once a day, do so at bedtime if possible, to minimize the risks associated with sedation.
- Do not drink alcohol or take any other OTC drugs with a sedative effect while taking this medication. Consult with your physician about specific questions to obtain individualized advice.

Dizziness. Because of their effects on blood vessels, many medications taken for cardiovascular problems cause dizziness (vertigo) when you sit up or stand up. The most common ones are antihypertensives and diuretics. If you are taking one of these medications, try to do the following (especially within the first few hours after taking a dose):

- Sit or stand up slowly when rising from the bed or chair.
- Avoid extremely warm environments or hot baths because they can aggravate the problem by dilating the blood vessels.
- Do not drink alcohol while taking the medication because alcohol dilates blood vessels and causes excessive lowering of blood pressure.
- If you take an antihypertensive medication once a day, do so at night to reduce your dizziness or lightheadedness. If you are taking a diuretic, however, continue to take it in the morning. Taking it at night would interfere with sleep by making you have to get up to urinate.

Computer-Based Resources. Computer-based resources are available for drug reference. Use caution when selecting internet sites, however, because there is no guarantee about the accuracy of information posted on a website. Some facilities have computer-based resources for medication information available within the facility. An example of this type of resource is *Micromedex,* which provides health care professionals with information about drugs, their dosing, drug interactions, and aftercare instructions that can be given to clients.

Drug Actions

Mechanism of Action. The mechanism of action is the physiological change caused by a medication that results in the body's response to that medication. This change alters either the chemistry of the cell environment or the cell itself to either increase or decrease the function of the cell.

Many medications exert a therapeutic effect by interacting with cell receptor sites that have a similar chemical shape. When a medication is linked to the receptor site, similar to a lock and key, a chain of physiological events occurs that ends with the intended therapeutic effect. Because the "shape" of some cell receptor sites may be unique to a certain type of tissue, some medications exert an effect only on that tissue. Others have more systemic or widespread effects. When a medication has a specific effect on one type of body tissue, the tissue is said to be the **target organ** for that medication. An example is a diuretic, which targets the kidneys. The route of administration aids in determining whether a medication exerts a local or systemic effect. For example, a topical medication is more likely to exert a local effect on skin, whereas an intravenous (IV) medication rapidly exerts a systemic effect.

Therapeutic Effect. The **therapeutic effect** is the intended effect or action of the medication. It is accomplished when a drug interacts with cell mechanisms, producing a change in cellular function. Effective drug therapy helps to cure or control disease (antibiotics), relieve pain or other aggravating symptoms (analgesics or decongestants), prevent disease (immunizations), or promote health (vitamin or mineral supplements). Every drug has at least one therapeutic effect and some drugs have several. For example, acetaminophen is an analgesic, but it also reduces fever (antipyretic).

Side Effects. Side effects are effects of a medication that are not intended or planned but may occur as a result of use. Side effects can range from mildly unpleasant to harmful. Although all side effects cannot be avoided, teaching methods to reduce common side effects may help the client tolerate the medication (Box 20-2).

Adverse Effects. An **adverse effect** is a medication side effect that is potentially harmful to a client. Adverse effects can occur even when taking normal drug doses.

Toxic effects are serious adverse effects of medications that may even threaten life. Some examples are a low heart rate with a cardiac glycoside or wheezing or rash with an antibiotic. Be sure to inform clients about important adverse effects and which ones should prompt a call to the primary care provider.

A toxic effect occasionally results from a single ingestion of a large amount of a drug (an overdose). When this occurs, the drug must be inactivated or removed from the body to prevent organ damage or death. This is done using activated charcoal in the gastrointestinal (GI) tract (to bind the incompletely absorbed drug) or hemodialysis (for drugs that are already absorbed or cannot be cleared via the GI tract). Other drugs known as *antidotes* may be used to reverse the toxic effect.

Action Alert! If a client is exhibiting toxic effects of a medication, do not administer the next scheduled dose. Immediately report signs and symptoms of toxicity to the physician.

ALLERGIC RESPONSES. An allergic response is an antigen-antibody response to a medication. Although this can occur with the first administration, the body requires previous exposure to the antigen to develop antibodies. The allergic response could be triggered by the drug itself, a preservative, or a metabolite.

A **hypersensitivity reaction** is a mild allergic reaction to a drug. Symptoms vary according to the drug and the client, but they typically include skin manifestations, such as rash, urticaria, and pruritus. Headache, rhinitis, or nausea and vomiting may also occur.

Anaphylaxis is a life-threatening allergic reaction that requires immediate intervention to prevent possible death. It is a medical emergency. Symptoms are typically cardiorespiratory in nature and include dyspnea, wheezing, stridor, tachycardia, and hypotension. They are caused by bronchoconstriction, laryngeal edema, and widespread vasodilation. Treatment includes supportive care and administration of epinephrine, bronchodilators, antihistamines, and corticosteroids to reduce the allergic response.

Action Alert! If a client begins to exhibit signs of anaphylaxis after receiving a medication, maintain the client's airway and call for help immediately.

Because allergic responses can be serious, carefully question clients about a history of drug allergy. For drugs that are commonly known to be antigenic, such as penicillin, also inquire about a family history of drug allergy. Inquire not only about the drug but also about the specific symptoms of the allergic response. This information helps determine whether the client could safely receive the drug if given with another drug (such as an antihistamine) or whether it must not be used at all. All clients with a history of drug allergy should wear or carry identification that notes the drug allergy. They should also be taught to inform all future caregivers about the allergy.

IDIOSYNCRATIC RESPONSES. An **idiosyncratic response** is an unexplained and unpredictable response to a medication. It may be a suboptimal response, an exaggerated response, or an abnormal type of response. For example, some medications that normally produce drowsiness may cause excitability in children. Idiosyncratic responses may be listed in the drug literature as rare types of adverse effects. Because these are so unpredictable, skilled and conscientious nursing assessment is warranted.

DRUG TOLERANCE. Drug tolerance refers to the diminishing therapeutic effect of the same drug dosage over time, a trend that requires increasing the drug dosage to achieve the same therapeutic effect. Tolerance occurs as the body becomes accustomed to a drug from prolonged use. A classic example involves pain medication. Over time, a client taking an opioid analgesic for chronic pain may require larger doses to control the pain, even if there is no drug addiction. Carefully monitor the degree of symptom relief from a specific dose of a medication, especially if it will be used on a long-term basis.

Drug Interactions. Drug interactions can be either synergistic or antagonistic. A **synergistic effect** occurs when one drug enhances or increases the effect of another drug. This may be either accidental or planned purposefully by the prescriber. An **antagonistic effect** occurs when one drug reduces or negates the effect of another. Antagonistic effects can also be accidental or purposeful. A client who takes multiple medications (called polypharmacy) is more likely to experience accidental drug interactions; thus the medication regimen must be reviewed carefully.

Other substances, such as alcohol or sodium, can also enhance or interfere with drug action. Teach clients about the effects of these substances on prescribed medications. The resurgence of interest in "natural" or "herbal" remedies provides yet another area for assessment. Interactions between medications and these alternative remedies are increasingly of concern and are becoming a more popular area of research.

Pharmacokinetics. The term **pharmacokinetics** refers to a drug's activity from the time it enters the body until it leaves. This process has four parts: absorption, distribution, metabolism, and excretion. All health care professionals responsible for managing client medications should understand these processes.

ABSORPTION. Absorption refers to the transference of drug molecules from the point of entry in the body into the bloodstream. Most medications are absorbed systemically to exert their effects. Drug absorption is influenced by many factors, including route of administration, drug dosage and form, and conditions at the absorption site.

The route of administration has a direct impact on the extent and speed of medication absorption and is related to the physical structure of the tissues. The IV route is fastest because the medication is injected directly into the bloodstream. Medications are also absorbed rapidly through mucous membranes of the mouth, nose, and respiratory tract because these tissues are highly vascular. Injected medications are absorbed fairly rapidly, but their action also depends on conditions at the injection site. Absorption from the oral route can be affected by dose form and conditions in the GI tract. The topical route has the slowest absorption rate because the skin is a natural barrier.

The dosage and form of a medication commonly affect its absorption. Higher-than-average doses may be purposefully ordered when giving a **loading dose,** which is an initial medication dose that exceeds the maintenance or therapeutic dose. A loading dose may be ordered when the client has not recently received the medication and must rapidly achieve a therapeutic serum level. Examples of drugs commonly initiated with loading doses are digitalis and aminophylline. The loading dose is followed by therapeutic doses, and drug levels in the serum may be periodically monitored.

The form of the medication and conditions in the GI tract greatly affect absorption. Liquid forms, such as solutions or suspensions, are absorbed more quickly than solid forms, such as capsules or tablets. Extended-release products gradually release medication for absorption over a period of time. They can usually be recognized by letters at the end of the medication name, such as ER (extended release), SR (sustained release), SA (sustained action), or XL (extended length). Enteric-coated drugs are coated to prevent them from dissolving until they reach the alkaline environment of the small intestine; usually a drug is enteric coated if it would otherwise irritate the stomach lining. Most drugs are absorbed in the small intestine because of the numerous villi there.

Medications are often administered in relationship to meals. Most are better absorbed when taken between meals. Selected medications are given with food to decrease the irritating effect on the stomach. Be sure to read drug reference material to determine whether a medication should be given with food or between meals (1 hour before or 2 hours after a meal).

Medications not given via the GI tract are greatly affected by conditions at the site of absorption, especially the blood supply to the area. Muscles have a rich supply of blood, making the intramuscular (IM) route the second choice after the IV route when rapid absorption is desired. The subcutaneous (SC or SQ) route is slower than the IM route and is a better choice when slower absorption is needed. Local site conditions that interfere with parenteral drug absorption include bruising, scarring, and edema. Local circulatory impairment may also impede absorption.

DISTRIBUTION. The process of drug distribution begins with absorption of a drug into the circulation and ends with its arrival at the site of action. The health and makeup of the client as well as the chemical and physical properties of the medication affect the degree and speed of distribution.

Various circulatory dynamics affect medication distribution. The more blood vessels supplying a tissue, the better the distribution, and vice versa. Blood vessel tone also affects distribution. Vasoconstriction reduces drug distribution, whereas vasodilation enhances it. Thus distribution of a drug to target tissues may be poorer in clients with impaired circulatory status or with edema.

The body also has physiological barriers to certain medications. The blood–brain barrier permits transport of lipid-bound medications while preventing transport of many water-soluble ones. This has important implications when prescribing medications meant to affect the brain. The placental barrier also inhibits transport of some drugs, but it is less selective than the blood-brain barrier. Physicians ordering drug therapy for a pregnant client carefully consider this variable when selecting a medication. This decision is crucial because many medications have a high **teratogenic potential,** which is the possibility that a medication will harm a developing fetus. The FDA, therefore, classifies medications according to a pregnancy category to reflect teratogenicity (Table 20-3).

Most medications are partially bound to proteins such as albumin in the bloodstream, making that portion inactive and unable to be used by the tissues. The active, unbound, or "free" portion exerts the therapeutic effect. Clients with low albumin levels have greater circulation of the "active" drug and require decreased dosages. Low albumin levels are typically found in infants, older adults, and those with poor nutrition or with liver disease.

METABOLISM. Drug metabolism, or **biotransformation,** is the process of inactivating and breaking down a medication. Enzymes chemically alter a drug's structure, converting it to a less potent substance.

Most drug metabolism occurs in the liver by microsomes that trigger the enzymatic breakdown of drugs. The liver can oxidize and transform many substances before they reach the body tissues, called a *first-pass effect.* However, liver function can decrease with age or disease, allowing active drug to accumulate in the body. For this reason, infants, older adults, and those with cirrhosis or other liver diseases experience the same effect even with reduced medication doses. Standard doses would place them at risk for drug toxicity.

Table 20-3	FDA Pregnancy Categories Used to Assess Fetal Risk	
Risk Category	Risk Level	Interpretation
A	No risk	Study results have not shown evidence of fetal harm from use of this medication.
B	Little or no risk	Results of animal studies show no risk, but no well-controlled studies have been performed with pregnant women.
C	Uncertain risk	Results of animal studies indicate that there is risk to the fetus, but no well-controlled studies have been performed with pregnant women. The risks and benefits of using the drug must be assessed.
D	Proven risk	The risks and benefits of using the drug must be assessed and should be considered in the event of life-threatening situations.
X	Proven risk	This drug should be avoided during pregnancy because the risks outweigh any benefits.

Less frequent sites of drug metabolism are the kidneys, lungs, blood, and intestines. Pathology in these areas also requires reduced drug doses to prevent toxicity. Know the sites of metabolism for the medications being given, and monitor the client for intended and adverse drug effects.

EXCRETION. Excretion is the movement of a drug from the site of metabolism back into the circulation and its transport to the site of exit from the body. The route of excretion is determined by the chemical properties of the drug. The kidneys are responsible for excreting most drugs. Other organs of excretion are the lungs, exocrine glands, and GI tract.

The nephrons of the kidneys secrete unwanted substances into the urine in the presence of an adequate glomerular filtration rate. Most medications undergo metabolism before excretion; others are eliminated in their original form. It is important to know how a drug is excreted to anticipate its effectiveness. For example, when a client has a urinary tract infection, the drug of choice is one that is excreted relatively unchanged in the urine. Otherwise, the drug will not effectively treat the infection.

Adequate fluid intake (6 to 8 glasses per day) is generally beneficial to aid excretion, except when the client retains fluid, such as with renal failure or heart failure. A medication dose may be reduced if the client has renal disease that impairs drug excretion.

The lungs, sweat glands, mammary glands, and GI tract excrete drugs to a lesser degree. The lungs excrete volatile gases such as alcohol, nitrous oxide, and ether. The sweat glands help excrete lipid-soluble drugs. Because the mammary glands excrete drugs, women who are breast feeding should use medications only on the advice of a physician. This decision is made after carefully weighing the benefits to the mother and the risks to the infant. The GI tract eliminates medications in bile. The rate of medication excretion by this route can be slowed or accelerated by the same conditions that cause constipation or diarrhea, respectively.

Impaired clearance through any of the routes of excretion could result in drug toxicity. Review the results of periodically drawn laboratory studies, such as liver enzymes or blood urea nitrogen and creatinine (which monitor kidney function).

Blood Level. To be effective, the active component of a medication must be present in the blood within a therapeutic range—that is, the blood level that effectively treats a health problem without creating toxic effects. At its therapeutic range, a medication is in different phases of being absorbed, distributed, metabolized, and excreted.

The blood (or serum) level of a medication is the amount circulating in the bloodstream at a given time. The *peak serum level* of a drug is its highest concentration in the blood, which usually occurs just as the last bit of the most recently administered dose is being absorbed. After this, absorption stops and only distribution, metabolism, and excretion continue. The serum level then falls progressively until the next dose begins to be absorbed. The *trough level* is the term for the lowest circulating level of a drug.

The route of drug administration also influences the blood level. For example, the level of an oral drug typically peaks about 2 hours after ingestion and then tapers steadily (Figure 20-1). Medications given by the IV route reach their peak almost immediately and then taper steadily. In general, therapeutic drug levels are easier to maintain with IV administration, especially when using a continuous pump or drip, because this route avoids the pronounced peaks and valleys of oral administration.

> *Action Alert!* Monitor the results of peak and trough serum drug levels and report values outside the therapeutic range immediately. Assess the client for signs and symptoms of toxicity if results are high, and for symptoms of the original disorder if results are low.

HALF-LIFE. Every drug has a half-life, which is the amount of time the body needs to lower by half the drug's serum concentration by metabolism and excretion. A drug's half-life helps determine how frequently it should be given. Drugs with a long half-life are given less frequently, whereas drugs with a short half-life require more frequent administration.

ONSET, PEAK, AND DURATION. *Onset, peak,* and *duration* are terms frequently used to describe the times of the anticipated effects of a drug. The onset is the amount of time needed after administration of a drug to produce the desired effect. The peak is the amount of time needed for a drug to reach the highest concentration for effectiveness. The duration is the span of time during which the serum drug concentration is high enough to produce the intended effect.

PLATEAU. The term *plateau* refers to the serum concentration or level of a drug that has been reached and sustained with a series of fixed doses. When the plateau is achieved and maintained, the client should receive the optimal therapeutic benefit.

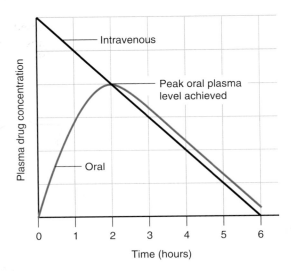

Figure 20-1. The blood level of an oral drug typically peaks about 2 hours after ingestion and then tapers steadily, whereas a drug given by the IV route reaches its peak almost immediately and tapers steadily.

Systems of Delivery

Nurse-Administered Medications. When a client is admitted to a hospital or extended-care facility, the responsibility for medication administration usually shifts from the client to the nurse. Expect to obtain a medication history on admission (including use of OTC drugs), review current medication orders, and consult with the physician about any discrepancies. Anticipate that new medications may be ordered to treat the current health problem. Realize also that medications routinely taken at home are sometimes not reordered in the hospital. This may be intentional, as in the case of digitalis toxicity, because the blood level of the drug must be decreased. Because nurses share the responsibility for ensuring that the client receives medication for ongoing health problems as well as medications ordered for the current problem, consult with the physician whenever discrepancies are noted. Be aware, also, that certain drugs cannot be stopped abruptly, such as steroids or antihypertensives.

Once admitted to a health care facility, most clients receive medications only when the nurse provides them. In other words, you assume responsibility for obtaining the correct medication, dispensing the correct dose and form at the correct time, and recording its administration in the client record. Use extreme caution to avoid errors, which can be harmful to the client, distressing to you, and costly to the institution. The current health care literature contains an increasing number of recommendations to reduce medication errors (Beyers, 2000; Hadaway, 2001; Skuteris, 2000), which have grown in this country at an alarming rate. Increasingly, computerized medication systems (Jech, 2001; Waldo, 1999) are being used to reduce errors in medication order entry and delivery, and to reduce the risk of adverse interactive drug effects.

Prepare medications for administration in an environment that is conducive to safety and accuracy. Plan to work alone to avoid errors that could result from interruptions and distractions. Make sure there is adequate lighting in the work area to promote accuracy.

Maintain the security of medications being dispensed. Do not leave medications unattended after beginning their preparation. If you must leave the area briefly, place medications in a locked drawer, cart, or cabinet until you return. The medication cart or storage area should always be locked when unattended.

> *Action Alert!* Lock the medication cart after use. Do not leave medications unattended on top of a cart during or after preparation.

Client-Administered Medications. Sometimes a client self-administers medications after admission to a health care facility, with a corresponding order from the health care provider. This decision is made after considering the client's reliability, the nature and purpose of the medication, and whether client independence should be promoted. Examples of clients who can benefit from self-administration are alert postpartum women who require analgesics, clients with diabetes who regularly take insulin and know how to administer it, older adult clients who take inhalation medications at home, or clients who take oral contraceptives.

General guidelines should be followed when allowing a client to self-administer medications. First, the client should be alert and reliable. The client should also be able to state when he has self-administered a medication (so you can document it) or reliably record self-medication on a special form placed at the bedside. This form becomes part of the medical record upon discharge. The client should not keep any medications at the bedside other than those permitted for self-administration.

Components and Processing of Medication Orders

Medication orders must be legally entered into the medical record. When a physician or advanced practice nurse enters a medication order, it must include the date and time of the order; medication name, dose, route, and frequency; and the signature of the prescriber (Table 20-4). A complete order not only fulfills the legal standard but also gives sufficient direction to the pharmacist, the nurse, and the client.

Once a drug order has been written, it must be communicated to others. Ideally the pharmacist has direct access to the physician's order entry without transcription. Your legal

Table 20-4	Components of a Drug Order
Component	**Explanation**
Date and time of order	Includes month, day, and year. Also includes time of day on orders for inpatients (written on order sheet instead of prescription pad). Time of day indicates A.M. or P.M. if military time is not used. Time of order is especially important for drugs with automatic stop times.
Name of medication	Should be clearly and precisely written. Most facilities use generic names, but sometimes both generic and trade names are identified. Prescription orders state the trade name if no interchange is permitted.
Dose of medication	Lists exact amount of the drug ordered.
Route of administration	Lists exact route by which to give the drug. This is very important because many medications can be given by more than one route.
Frequency of administration	May specify the number of times per day (such as qid for four times a day) or may state the number of hours between doses (such as q6h for every 6 hours) depending on the drug and its purpose.
Signature of prescriber	Required by law. An unsigned prescription will not be filled in a pharmacy, and you should not implement an unsigned drug order. For a narcotic prescription, the prescriber's DEA number must be provided in addition to the signature.

DEA, Drug Enforcement Agency.

responsibility includes accurate interpretation of the order and administration of the medicine. Note any special conditions or parameters for administration, such as withholding an antihypertensive medication for a systolic blood pressure less than 100 mm Hg. If handwritten orders are illegible or an abbreviation is unclear, clarify the order (Table 20-5). It is not prudent to try to interpret illegible orders (Anonymous, 2000), and nurses could be held accountable for drug administration errors based on faulty interpretation.

Verbal or telephone orders may be given in emergency or unusual situations. Facility policy usually dictates whether and under what conditions these types of orders may be taken. (Nursing students generally cannot take verbal or telephone orders.) When verbal or telephone orders are allowed, record the date and time of the order, as well as the drug, dose, route, and frequency. Write "T.O." or "V.O." to indicate a telephone or verbal order, respectively, and write the name of the ordering physician after the medication order. Record your own signature, followed by title (RN, LPN). Verbal and telephone orders must be co-signed by the physician within a specified time, usually 24 hours or less. To prevent communication errors, repeat back the information to the prescribing physician after taking a verbal or telephone order, including the client's name and room number. These types of orders pose the greatest liability for nurses and physicians. At no time should a medication be administered without an order.

It is an ethical and legal responsibility to clarify a medication order if there are any questions about the order. You could place yourself in legal jeopardy if an error *should* have been noted on the basis of your education and experience. If the physician does not respond appropriately to an inquiry, report the problem following the facility's chain of command to prevent the medication error. If you believe the client could be harmed by the medication as ordered, withhold the medication, document this on the medication administration record, and document the rationale carefully on the nursing progress notes.

Types of Orders

Several types of medication orders exist; it is critically important to understand what type of order is being carried out. The type of order used depends on the goal of the medication therapy.

Standing Orders. A standing order indicates that a medication should be given on a routine basis. It may be written for a specified number of days or it may carry no time limit. If there is no limit, follow the order until another order is specifically written to discontinue it. Facility policy sometimes dictates when standing orders are no longer in effect. For example, opioid analgesics often have a "stop date" that is 3 to 7 days after the original order date. In many institutions, any previously written medication orders are canceled when a client goes to surgery, is transferred to another facility, or is discharged. In these circumstances, new orders must be written because the client's status may have changed and the old orders may no longer be appropriate. Facility policy may also dictate how frequently standing orders must be reviewed.

A special type of standing order may be found in specialty nursing units such as cardiac care or maternity units. In these areas, one or more standardized written medication orders are activated or followed when special circumstances occur (such as cardiac dysrhythmias). These orders are medically safe, time saving for the nurse, and potentially life saving for the client. Once activated, these medications are charted just as any other medication would be.

PRN Orders. A PRN order is an order for a medication that is given as needed. The label derives from the Latin *pro re nata,* meaning "as necessary." It lists the minimum amount of time that must elapse between doses, and it may also specify the symptoms it is used to treat. This type of drug order allows you to use discretion in administering a medication. It also requires that you have good assessment skills, noting both the situation and clinical condition of the client. An example of a

Table 20-5	Abbreviations Commonly Used in Medication Orders
Abbreviation	**Meaning**
ac	Before meals
ad lib	As desired
ASAP	As soon as possible
BID	Twice daily
$\bar{c}$	With
cap	Capsule
d/c	Discontinue
elix	Elixir
gtt	Drop
hs	Hours of sleep, bedtime
ID	Intradermal
IM	Intramuscular
IV	Intravenous
IVP	IV push
IVPB	IV piggyback
KVO	Keep vein open
OD	Right eye
OS	Left eye
OU	Both eyes
pc	After meals
po	By mouth, oral
pr	Per rectum
PRN	When needed, as necessary
q	Every
QD	Every day
qh	Every hour
q3h	Every 3 hours
QID	Four times a day
QOD	Every other day
qs	Quantity sufficient
Rx	Take
$\bar{s}$	Without
SC, SQ	Subcutaneous
SL	Sublingual
stat	Immediately
supp	Suppository
susp	Suspension
TID	Three times a day
tab	Tablet

PRN order is *droperidol (Inapsine) 2.5 mg IV q6h PRN for nausea or vomiting*. This tells you that it may be given for nausea or vomiting, provided the client has not received a dose for at least 6 hours. Another example is *meperidine (Demerol) 75 to 100 mg IM q4h PRN for pain*. This example illustrates that at times you may be allowed to use discretion in determining the dose.

Single Orders. A single order is a medication order carried out one time only. It identifies the drug, dose route, and time for administration. Preoperative and pre-procedure orders are commonly written as one-time orders. An example is *nafcillin (Nafcil) 1 g IVPB on call to OR*. This order states to infuse a specific antibiotic attached to a mainline IV when the client is called to the operating room. (IVPB will be described later.)

Stat Orders. A stat order (from the Latin *stat*) is one that is implemented immediately. These orders are frequently given during emergency or near-emergency situations. An example is impending cardiac or respiratory arrest. Stat orders are more likely to be given as verbal or telephone orders. Most institutions have policies and guidelines stating the time period within which a stat order must be completed.

Medication Distribution Systems

Medication distribution systems are designed to promote safety and accuracy, conserve time and money, and promote client self-care. Within a facility, a single system is used and all personnel and support structures work together to provide streamlined delivery.

Unit-Dose System. The most commonly used system today is the unit-dose system. A unit dose is a single dose of a medication that is prepackaged and labeled by the manufacturer or pharmacist. A new supply of unit doses for each client is delivered to the nursing unit every 24 hours. You then take a single dose of each medication to the bedside at the appropriate time.

Computer-Controlled Dispensing Systems. The most recently developed unit-dose system is the computer-controlled dispensing system. Access to the system is menu driven and resembles (conceptually at least) a small automated teller machine. The unit contains medications stored in specific containers that are labeled and coded in the machine. The computer is programmed with the number of unit doses stocked for each medication. Access the system using a personal identification code. After drug removal, the computer records the transaction in its memory and charges the drug to the client. This system is time saving for you and is cost effective because of better inventory control. It is used most frequently for narcotic and PRN medications, but some facilities use it for all medication dispensing.

Routes of Administration

Oral Routes. Oral or PO (from the Latin *per oris*) means given by mouth. There are three oral routes for medication administration: the oral, sublingual, and buccal routes.

ORAL. A medication given by the oral route is placed in the mouth and swallowed. A client with a nasogastric tube connected to suction cannot receive oral medications. Confused clients or those who are unwilling to swallow should be carefully assessed to determine if this route is appropriate. Clients with an impaired or absent swallow reflex cannot use this route but may have a feeding tube in place. If so, medications may be given by the nasogastric, gastrostomy, or jejunostomy tube and are called enteral medications. A client who is on NPO (nothing by mouth) status may not receive oral medications unless the order specifically states *NPO with/except meds*.

SUBLINGUAL. A medication given by the sublingual route is placed under the tongue and allowed to dissolve. The medication is quickly absorbed through the mucous membranes into the systemic circulation. Tell the client not to swallow a tablet ordered for sublingual use because it will not be effective. The client should avoid eating, swallowing liquids, or smoking while the tablet is dissolving. An example is nitroglycerin, which is used to treat chest pain.

BUCCAL. A tablet or lozenge given by the buccal route is placed against the mucous membranes of the mouth, between the cheek and the gums, near the molars. The drug dissolves and acts either locally on mucosa or systemically after being absorbed from saliva swallowed into the stomach. Teach clients using this route to avoid swallowing liquids while the medication is dissolving and to alternate cheeks with succeeding doses to minimize mucosal irritation.

Parenteral Routes. A **parenteral route** is one that is outside the GI tract. Parenteral medications are given by injection into a body tissue using sterile technique. The four routinely used parenteral routes are intradermal, subcutaneous, intramuscular, and intravenous. These routes provide for faster drug action but are associated with risks of discomfort, infection, and even bleeding in some clients. Other, less frequently used parenteral routes are the epidural and intrathecal routes. These routes are initiated by physicians or advanced practice nurses.

INTRADERMAL. The **intradermal** (ID) **route** involves injection into the dermal layer of the skin. It is commonly used to test for allergic reactions to a substance planted in the dermis. Examples of ID injections are purified protein derivative for tuberculosis and skin testing for mumps and *Candida*.

SUBCUTANEOUS. The **subcutaneous** (SC or SQ) **route** involves injection into subcutaneous tissue just under the dermis. It is commonly used by nurses and by clients self-administering insulin or small amounts of other medications that do not need to be rapidly absorbed.

INTRAMUSCULAR. The **intramuscular** (IM) **route** involves injection into muscle tissue, specifically the body of a muscle. Medications are absorbed quickly, making this a popular route when faster absorption is needed. It is frequently used to administer opioid analgesics, antiemetics, and some antibiotics.

INTRAVENOUS. The **intravenous route** involves injection of a medication into a vein. This route provides the most rapid effect, with distribution throughout the body in a few minutes.

For this reason, smaller drug doses are needed. A disadvantage is that the route is potentially dangerous because drugs given incorrectly cannot be retrieved; this is true for all parenteral medications, but here there is less time to intervene. Antibiotics, histamine-receptor antagonists, and selected pain medications are examples of medications commonly given by the IV route. This route is also used for patient-controlled analgesia (see Chapter 36).

Topical Route. The **topical route** is used to deliver a medication directly to a body site, such as the skin, eyes, ears, nose, throat, vagina, or rectum. A skin preparation may be applied by manually spreading it over a specific area, applying a patch, placing the drug in a medicated dressing, soaking the area in solution, or using a medicated bath.

Topical drugs often have a local effect, although some are absorbed systemically as well. There is a direct correlation between the length of exposure to a topical application and the amount absorbed. Remove a previous dose before the next dose is applied and wash the area to prevent further absorption.

Suppositories are the drug form often used for insertion into the rectum or vagina. Drops may be instilled into the eyes, nose, or ears. Irrigations may be ordered for the eye, ear, bladder, rectum, or vagina. Medications can also be sprayed into the nose or throat, or throat gargles may be used.

Inhalation Route. Inhalation is used to bring medications into the respiratory tract via the nose or throat. Most medications given by this route exert local effects on the bronchial mucosa. They are administered via metered-dose inhaler, nebulizer, or turbo-inhaler (see Chapter 33).

Clients may also receive inhaled medications via an endotracheal tube or a tracheostomy, such as anesthetic gases and some emergency resuscitative drugs. This route allows for rapid systemic absorption because the lungs have a very large and highly vascular surface area.

A nasal inhaler may be used to administer certain medications. The most common example is the use of a decongestant nasal spray to constrict nasal blood vessels and relieve cold symptoms. Another type of nasal medication uses a nasal canister with a thin tube attached. The tube is inserted into the nares and is either squeezed or blown in to deliver a dose of medication. An example is desmopressin (DDAVP), which is used to treat diabetes insipidus.

FACTORS AFFECTING DRUG ACTIONS

A number of client-related factors can influence the action of a medication. These include risk factors that are present across the life span, physiological factors, and cultural/lifestyle factors.

Risk Factors Across the Life Span

Age. A client's age significantly influences medication actions. Infants have immature function of the renal, hepatic, and GI systems. They also lack certain metabolic enzymes needed for proper drug metabolism. Finally, they have relatively more body water and less body mass. These factors cause the infant's system to be highly responsive to medications.

Older adults can also have an altered response to medications because of changes that occur with the aging process (Feinberg & Tobias, 2000; Schafer, 2001; Turkoski, 1999). Absorption, metabolism, and excretion are reduced by slowed or decreased organ function. Drug distribution is altered by decreased size, protein-binding sites, body water, and lean muscle mass. Each of these factors increases the risk for drug toxicity. Older adults also have a higher risk of adverse effects from polypharmacy (Ebersole & Hess, 2001; Hurme & Pourciau, 2001) or from taking medications incorrectly. Nurses play an important role in preventing these occurrences (Ryan & Chambers, 2000).

Psychological Factors. Psychological factors can influence whether a client chooses to take a medication and whether the drug is ultimately effective. These factors include the client's acceptance of medication use, prior experience with medications, fear, motivation, and secondary gain, and the behavior of the nurse administering the medication. Chapter 19 discusses factors affecting compliance with a health care regimen. Box 20-3 discusses research conducted to study compliance with medication regimens.

Physiological Factors
Genetic Differences. Genetic factors can influence the manner in which the body uses, metabolizes, or reacts to a drug. Deficiencies in natural body enzymes used to biotransform drugs may be responsible for these events. Genetics helps to explain why allergies to penicillin, for example, can run in families and why people of one ethnic origin may not obtain the same benefits from a medication dose as those of another origin (Kudzma, 1999).

Gender Differences. Men and women have different amounts of body fat, body water, and muscle mass. They also have different circulating levels of male and female hormones. These factors influence drug actions by affecting one or more of the pharmacokinetic processes. Much clinical drug research is done with male subjects, so drug effects on women may sometimes be unexpected.

Height and Weight. Height and weight are important factors affecting drug actions. Standard drug doses are published for average-size adults, who range in age from 18 to 65 and weigh about 150 pounds. Overweight adults may require an increased dose to achieve therapeutic results. Drug doses for infants and children are calculated according to body weight or body surface area. Record height and weight at the time of hospital admission (or during the intake process in an ambulatory care setting) to provide a ready reference for the physician to determine drug dosages.

Diseases. Diseases that adversely affect any one of the pharmacokinetic processes ultimately affect drug action. For example, impaired GI function may reduce absorption. Heart

---

THE STATE OF NURSING RESEARCH: A Spoonful of Sugar?

Box 20-3

What Are the Issues?

Most chronic illnesses are treated with prescribed medications that people must learn to take at home; however, research indicates that many people do not follow the directions for taking medications. Sometimes people don't understand what they are supposed to do; others can't remember when to take their medications; and still others start to feel better and don't finish the full course of treatment. Researchers are interested in how well clients follow directions as well as how effective various treatments are in improving client outcomes. Both areas of research are important, because even if a medication is shown to be effective in treating a disease its benefits cannot be realized unless the client actually takes the medication.

What Research Has Been Conducted?

Haynes, McDonald, Garg, and Montague (2002) published a comprehensive review of studies on adherence that used a randomized clinical trial as the research design. The interventions studied included such things as "more convenient care, information, reminders, self-monitoring, reinforcement, counseling, family therapy, and other forms of additional supervision or attention by a health care provider (physician, nurse, pharmacist or other)" (p. 1). Many of the studies combined a variety of strategies such as educational sessions about the particular disease as well as the medications, the importance of adherence, and reminder systems. Nurses were actively involved in several of the interventions, with particular emphasis on those involving education for the client and reminder systems such as telephone calls.

What Has the Research Concluded?

The reviewers found studies in which the interventions had a positive effect on improving adherence, including calls to clients to remind them of appointments and more labor-intensive interventions that included education and reminders. The reviewers were quite critical of the small sample sizes in the studies on adherence. They also were not able to determine which components of the complex interventions were the most important.

What Is the Future of Research in This Area?

The reviewers called for more "innovative" strategies for improving adherence, because none of the current interventions have made much of a difference in improving medication administration by clients in their own settings (Haynes, McDonald, Garg, & Montague, 2002). Nurses are in an excellent position to think up creative approaches with the help of clients, because they work so closely with them in hospital settings. Nurses also provide significant amounts of home care and can design interventions that have better real world application.

Reference

Haynes, R. B., McDonald, H., Garg, A. X., & Montague, P. (2002). Interventions for helping patients to follow prescriptions for medications (Cochrane Review). In: *The Cochrane Library*, Issue 2. Oxford: Update Software.

---

failure or other edema-causing conditions may impair drug distribution. Liver or renal disease limits drug metabolism and excretion, putting the client at risk for toxic effects.

Reactions to Environment. Physical agents in the environment can directly affect a client's response to a medication. Heat and cold produce vasodilation and vasoconstriction, which in turn alter drug distribution or even its effects (e.g., antihypertensives). Advise clients to dress appropriately for the weather and to avoid temperature extremes. Ionizing radiation, such as sunlight, can affect enzyme activity in the body, altering drug actions. Many medications have photosensitivity as a side effect, so warn clients to avoid prolonged exposure or to use a strong sunscreen when outdoors.

Cultural and Lifestyle Factors

Dietary Factors. Dietary factors and overall nutritional state can either positively or negatively affect medication actions in the body. Recall that cells manufacture proteins and enzymes. Because most drugs bind with proteins, sufficient protein intake is needed for proper drug distribution. Both proteins and enzymes are also needed for drug metabolism.

Specific foods can trigger drug-food interactions that either increase or decrease the drug's effectiveness. The diet may have to be changed somewhat to manage these nutrients. For example, liver or green leafy vegetables rich in vitamin K should be limited or maintained at a steady level when taking warfarin because they antagonize the drug's action. Clients who take potassium-wasting diuretics should increase intake of high-potassium foods.

Fluid balance also influences drug effects. Sufficient body fluid is necessary to carry drugs to their site of action and to excrete them after use. Thus dehydration can limit the transport of drugs and their metabolites, reducing the effectiveness of drug therapy.

Cultural and Religious Beliefs. Cultural and religious beliefs can influence a client's thoughts about whether a medication will be helpful and whether to comply with therapy. If the client has a cultural heritage in which medication is commonly used to treat health problems, the medication is more likely to be accepted because it is a form of traditional medicine for that client. If the client's cultural heritage does not typically use medication freely, this form of treatment is likely to be viewed instead as an alternative therapy (Spector, 2000) and may not be well accepted. Non-Western healing practices, such as herbal therapy, talismans, and use of spiritual advisors or healers, may complement or interfere with the intended effects of prescribed medications, depending on specific circumstances. Assess the client in a culturally sensitive fashion to build a sufficient database for evaluating drug effectiveness. Become familiar with the basic beliefs and health practices of clients of other cultures to help you to communicate medication information more effectively (Boxes 20-4 [p. 400] and 20-5 [p. 401]).

Socioeconomic Factors. Socioeconomic factors play an indirect role in influencing drug actions. Financially disadvantaged clients may not seek care for a health problem as quickly as those with adequate finances or health insurance. When a disadvantaged client does seek treatment, the medication regimen may be more complex because the health problem was not identified at an early stage. The client may be unable to afford continued medication therapy after the initial episode resolves and may not refill prescriptions or may take partial doses to help the medication last longer.

The Institute for Safe Medication Practices (2001) indicates that more than 40% of clients with a chronic illness are functionally illiterate, that almost one quarter of American adults read at or below the fifth grade level, and that most medical information leaflets are written at or above the tenth grade level. An inability to understand medication instructions will have consequences for the client at some point in the health-illness trajectory.

ASSESSMENT

A client receiving medication therapy deserves a thorough and multifaceted assessment to determine both the need for medication and the likelihood of response. The assessment process is twofold and includes general assessment and focused assessment.

Mr. Connell was diagnosed with hypertension (high blood pressure) 5 years ago. At that time, atenolol (Tenormin, a beta-adrenergic blocking agent) was prescribed. Within a few months, furosemide (Lasix, a diuretic) was also prescribed because his blood pressure was not effectively reduced. This regimen was effective, and he continued with therapy for a little over a year. At that time, he felt quite well and decided that he did not need the medication any longer. He has not seen a physician in more than 3 years. Box 20-6 (p. 402) provides information useful to the nurse working with Mr. Connell and adds to the assessment database gathered thus far.

General Assessment for Medication Administration

Health History. A client's health history provides information about existing health problems being managed with medications, and illnesses or organ dysfunction that may increase the risk of toxicity or other adverse drug effects. Inquire about any significant surgical procedures performed in the past. If a hormone-secreting organ has been removed, such as ovaries or thyroid, the client may take hormone replacement therapy. These medications should be continued during inpatient care.

HISTORY OF ALLERGIES. It is critically important to assess for drug allergies, especially when a client is being treated for the first time. Even if the client has an existing medical record from previous admissions or visits, verify allergies at each encounter. Assess the following factors whenever possible: drug, dose and route, number of times taken before allergy symptoms occurred, and onset and nature of the reaction. Assess for both drug and food allergies because some foods contain ingredients that are also found in medications. For example, clients who are allergic to shellfish cannot receive injectable radiocontrast dye during diagnostic studies because both contain iodine. Some vaccines are made from substances in chick embryos and should not be given to a client allergic to eggs.

Record allergies in large print on the cover of the client's medical record. If handwritten physician order forms are used, place an allergy sticker on each new blank order page as it is inserted into the chart. You may also find allergy notations in nursing admission notes, physician history-and-physical notes, medication administration records, and possibly on or over the bed. On admission, put a bracelet listing all pertinent allergies on the client's wrist and leave it in place until discharge.

Action Alert! Always check for an allergy bracelet before giving medication to a client. If a bracelet falls off or becomes illegible, replace it at once.

MEDICATION HISTORY. On admission, document the name of each drug the client routinely takes, the dose, the route (usually oral), and the time of the last dose. Document whether any medications have been brought to the hospital and their disposition (e.g., sent home or stored on the nursing unit). Question the client about use of prescription, OTC, and herbal or nutritional supplements (Hurme & Pourciau, 2001). Many clients will not mention OTC or herbal drugs unless specifically asked. Assess the dose, frequency, and reason for use.

DIET HISTORY. Because most medications are administered orally, assess the client's usual dietary intake, food preferences, and meal patterns. Several medications are better absorbed when taken either with or without food. Adjust the medication schedule accordingly. This may be more difficult than it seems because most facilities have policies and procedures governing routine medication administration times for standard drug therapy.

CLIENT'S KNOWLEDGE OF DRUG THERAPY. Increased knowledge of drug therapy should positively influence compliance. Assess the client's knowledge of the following:
- What the drug is being taken for
- How and when it should be taken
- If any doses have been skipped and why

Box 20-5 *Considering the Alternatives*
Approaches to Healing From Western Traditions: Homeopathy and Naturopathy

Description and History: A German physician, Samuel Hahnemann, developed *homeopathic medicine* in the nineteenth century. He understood illness symptoms as the body's responses and attempts to self-heal. Remedies then followed that stimulated responses similar to the illness symptoms. This law of similars, *similia similibus curentur* meaning "let likes be cured by likes," is the source of the name homeopathy. This is contrasted with allopathy, which is treating a disorder by counteracting symptoms or providing an action unrelated to symptoms. After the Flexner report in the United States, homeopathic schools were closed; however, homeopathy is still very popular in Europe and around the world.

Naturopathy combines a number of strategies from both Western and non-Western healing systems. Established by Benedict Lust in 1896, it has reemerged and grown in popularity with the more recent focus on the importance of health promotion and disease prevention. Schools developed that incorporated an eclectic array of modalities such as hydrotherapy, nature cures, physical and manipulative treatments, homeopathic remedies, nutrition, and the role of belief and spirituality. Naturopathy uses noninvasive treatments that minimize harmful side effects.

Important Concepts: *Homeopathy* is based on the law of similars, which means treating a disorder with substances that produce the same symptoms as the disease. Hahnemann established a rigorous method of establishing remedies through a process he called *Provings*, in which substances were administered to healthy people and symptoms were carefully monitored and recorded. Sources of these remedies are mostly from the plant kingdom but include substances from mineral and animal kingdoms. The essence of a substance was considered more powerful than the material substance. This *law of infinitesimals* is one of the most difficult for most health care professionals or chemists to understand. The remedies are prepared through a process of dilutions and succussions (shakings) until in many cases the dilutions are beyond the Avogadro limit, where no molecules of the substance can be detected. The more dilute the preparation is, the more potent its healing powers. The *process of healing* from these principles is often a slow process with symptoms getting worse before improvement. The recovery process is believed to progress from the head downward, from inside outward, from vital to less vital organs, and from most recent to earliest symptoms (the reverse order of their appearance).

Naturopathy is based on a holistic framework that views the whole person in relationship to the environment and focuses on wellness and prevention. Practitioners see themselves more as teachers than doctors. Naturopathy is founded on the belief of self-healing, with health and healing within the laws of nature. The principles of naturopathy are based on the principle of "Do no harm": (1) they use the least invasive methods that minimize risk of side effects, (2) they avoid suppressing symptoms that might aid in the natural healing process, and (3) they work within the laws of nature in diagnosis, treatment, and counseling. They use a hierarchy of healing from the least to most invasive forces; for example, the first step would be to reestablish the basis for health and stimulate self-healing. Pharmaceuticals and surgery are at the opposite end.

Practice of Homeopathy: The use of homeopathy is increasing rapidly around the world. The relatively low cost and the philosophy of self-healing are appealing to many people and practitioners. In Europe, 25% to 40% of physicians either use or refer clients for homeopathic remedies. Use of homeopathic remedies in the United States has also increased. A homeopath generally spends more than twice the amount of time with the client than a regular physician.

Practice of Naturopathy: Naturopaths currently use any of the following modalities: clinical nutrition and nutritional and herbal supplements, homeopathic remedies, acupuncture, hydrotherapy, touch, heat, cold, sound, and detoxification. Spirituality and energetic therapies may also be incorporated.

Practitioners: Homeopaths practicing in the United States generally are practicing with another license, such as an MD or a chiropractic or osteopath license. Increasingly, physicians are incorporating these remedies into their practice.

Naturopaths (NDs) are licensed in several states and there are four schools of naturopathy in the United States and one in Canada. These graduate-level schools follow a four-year, formal, standardized, science-based curriculum with clinical practica. There is a standardized licensing exam, and there are professional organizations with standards of practice and peer review.

Potential Benefits From Homeopathy and Naturopathy: Homeopathic remedies may be useful for functional complaints with little or no tissue damage, such as asthma, headaches, and allergies, and some immune and digestive disorders. They may offer relief for some chronic conditions and provide relief for side effects of other biomedical treatments. Naturopathic techniques are often helpful in disease prevention and health promotion and may be very effective in the early stages of disease. They may be used in conjunction with biomedical treatments to offset side effects, facilitate coping, and improve overall health.

Concerns Related to the Practice of Homeopathy and Naturopathy: Because licensed providers generally practice within a defined scope of practice and use referrals to treat conditions that warrant more immediate and invasive treatment, there is little danger if they remain within their scope of practice. There are many conditions that require more immediate and aggressive treatment, such as surgery and pharmaceuticals. Homeopathy as the only line of treatment is contraindicated in advanced stages of diseases, for diseases such as cancer and sexually transmitted diseases, and for diseases where there is irreparable bodily damage. Naturopathy alone is also not appropriate in emergency situations. The practice is best if coordinated with biomedicine. The philosophy underlying naturopathy is very compatible with nursing theory and the nursing role as health counselor.

Resources
Books
Hahnemann, S., & O'Reillly, W. B. (Eds.). (2001). *The organon of the medical art.* Palo Alto, CA: Birdcage Books.

Jacobs, J., & Moskowitz, L. (2001) Homeopathy. In M. Micozzi (Ed.), *Fundamentals of complementary and alternative medicine* (2nd ed.). New York: Churchill Livingstone.

Pizzorno, J. (1998) *Total wellness: Improve your health by understanding the body's healing systems.* Rocklin, CA: Prima.

Pizzorno, J., & Snider, P. (2001). Naturopathic medicine. In M. Micozzi (Ed.), *Fundamentals of complementary and alternative medicine* (2nd ed.). New York: Churchill Livingstone.

Journals
Homeopathy Today

Websites
American Naturopathic Medical Association, www.anma.com.
National Center for Homeopathy, www.homeopathic.org.
Homeopathic Educational Services, www.homeopathic.com.

Cross-Cultural Care CARING FOR AN IRISH-AMERICAN CLIENT

Daniel Connell, the client whose story we've been following through this chapter, is of Irish-American descent. His family came to Boston, Massachusetts, in the late 1800s. Although there are always individual differences among clients, Irish Americans as a group tend to have the following characteristics (Wilson, 1998):

- Believe and expect that life is a difficult process.
- Understate their symptoms when ill and delay seeking health care until symptoms are severe or cannot be ignored.

- Are stoic and resist expressing emotions associated with illness or pain.
- Use facial expressions to communicate nonverbally rather than more expressive gestures, such as hand and arm movements.
- Use traditional home remedies to treat minor illnesses but seek out a traditional health care provider if these fail or if a larger health problem emerges.

- Any side effects experienced
- Other specific information unique to the drug

Inadequate knowledge in any of these areas should guide you to develop an individualized teaching plan (Hayes, 1998; Martens, 1998; Wendt, 1998). If the client cannot learn the necessary information, obtain assistance from others (family or friends), who then become the focus of teaching.

Physical Examination

CURRENT CONDITION. Use knowledge of the client's ongoing condition or health status to assess whether current orders for drug therapy are sufficient and appropriate. Depending on changes in physical assessment data, new medications may be ordered and existing medications may be placed on hold, undergo a change in route, or be discontinued. Assess each client carefully, and report changes in condition to the physician or other person responsible for ordering medication therapy.

Be aware of any specific parameters to assess before giving a medication. For example, you might withhold a dose of digoxin if the client's pulse rate is less than 60. In contrast, you may implement a medication order on the basis of client assessment. For example, you may administer a PRN medication for nausea, pain, or high blood pressure if the client's condition warrants.

PERCEPTION AND COORDINATION. Assess whether the client has any difficulty with perception or coordination. Sensory perceptual deficits usually relate to vision or hearing. Problems with coordination could result from arthritis, muscle weakness or paralysis, or reduced sensation in the hands or fingertips. These clients could have difficulty reaching a medication cabinet, opening medication packages or bottles, splitting scored tablets, or self-administering injections.

Problems with perception or coordination may not seem as important while the client is receiving nurse-administered drugs, but they become significant as the client prepares for discharge. An example is a client newly started on insulin therapy, who has poor vision and cannot see syringe markings. Another is a client with myasthenia gravis who cannot coordinate or control muscle movements. In cases such as these, assess whether family members, friends, or close neighbors can assist. If not, the client may require the services of a home health care agency (Wendt, 1998).

Focused Assessment for *Ineffective Health Maintenance*

Defining Characteristics. Assess the client's knowledge about the need for the medication, the instructions for self-administration, and the need for a temporary or permanent change in lifestyle. Although seemingly simple, for some clients this is complex. For example, an antibiotic prescribed to treat an infection must generally be taken for 5 to 10 days, depending on the antibiotic. Although taking an antibiotic is a temporary change in lifestyle, the client needs to understand that the medication must be taken exactly as prescribed for the full amount of time ordered, even if symptoms disappear. Otherwise, the infection could reoccur and the client's condition could become worse than when originally diagnosed.

Note the client's reported or observed ability to take responsibility for managing medication therapy. Also assess the client's interest in following medication instructions, which may be evidenced by the client's reviewing instructions and asking questions.

Assess whether the client has an adequate support system—that is, one or more other persons to turn to if problems arise in taking or obtaining medications. Clients with no support system are more likely to have difficulty with medication therapy. Remember that this could also involve assistance for follow-up laboratory work needed with some medications (e.g., the International Normalized Ratio, or INR, for anticoagulant therapy). Home health assistance may be required.

Assess the client for inadequate financial and other resources, which can also influence adherence to medication therapy. Assess whether the client can physically obtain the medication and has insurance or other financial resources to pay for it. Some medications are expensive, and the client may stop taking them because of cost. Some clients have no transportation to a pharmacy. Determine whether the client could benefit from referral to a social worker for financial matters or whether resources are available to deliver medication refills to the client.

Related Factors. In general, related factors are those things that increase the likelihood that a nursing diagnosis will apply, although they may not have a cause-and-effect relationship. Examples of assessing and responding to related factors for *Ineffective health maintenance* include the following:

- *Misinterpretation of medication-related information.* A client who inadequately understood previous instructions has *Ineffective health maintenance,* despite prior teaching. Assess the current level of understanding to plan remedial teaching.
- *Inability to take responsibility for medications.* Sometimes clients cannot take their own medications. Two examples are a young child and a client who is not ready to learn because of anxiety. In situations such as these, assess whether other people in the client's support system could be taught about medication therapy.
- *Cognitive impairment.* Assess the client's ability to take in and retain information. A client who has a disorder that impairs cognitive function, such as a cerebrovascular accident (stroke), closed head injury, or dementia, may not be able to respond adequately to medication teaching. For example, a cognitively impaired client may be unable to remember to take a medication at specified times. This client may benefit from a 7-day medication dispenser, which can be prefilled by a family member or home health nurse. If needed, the teaching plan is again directed to others.
- *Physical impairment.* Some clients are physically unable to administer their own medications, open a pill bottle, or manipulate a syringe. They may be paralyzed or have some other limitation that prevents mobility in the environment. Assess whether environmental changes are likely to enable the client to take medications. Determine whether special adaptive devices such as syringe holders or pillboxes could help the client become independent. Some clients with physical impairments must have their medications administered by others.
- *Inadequate communication skills.* A client who cannot comprehend directions will have difficulty taking in and retaining medication information. Examples include clients with a language barrier or receptive aphasia (inability to understand the spoken word). When working with such clients, obtain an interpreter or give the instructions to someone who will be assisting the client after discharge.

If medication therapy is to be effective, the client must be able to obtain the medication, store it properly, take it as directed, watch for expected drug effects, and notice and report important side effects. Difficulty in any of these areas leads you to consider *Ineffective health maintenance* as a nursing diagnosis.

Focused Assessment for *Ineffective Therapeutic Regimen Management*

Defining Characteristics. Clients' beliefs about their ability to regain health or their desire to do so may influence their willingness to take medication. Assess their desire to utilize medication therapy as part of an overall treatment plan. Assess for difficulty in integrating medication therapy into the daily routine. Also, note evidence of compliance with other aspects of the health care regimen and the acceptance of responsibility for self-care as supportive data in determining motivation to comply with medication therapy.

Assess clients' ability to understand and follow the drug regimen. Sometimes clients who are labeled as noncompliant actually have barriers to effective self-administration. These barriers can stem from lack of comprehension, family conflicts, mistrust of the health care team, or the complexity of the medication regimen.

Each of these factors requires a different approach on your part. For example, older adults and those with multiple health problems are most likely to have complex medication schedules. Develop calendars, charts, or other visual reminders for use as needed. Some clients benefit from using prefilled weekly or monthly medication boxes to prevent them from taking the wrong medication or dose. At times, you may enlist the help of family, friends, or a home health agency to ensure that the client receives correct medications.

Related Factors. The related factors for *Ineffective therapeutic regimen management* overlap to some degree with those listed under *Ineffective health maintenance* in relation to perceived barriers, social supports, and economic difficulties. Additional factors include the following:

- *Knowledge deficit.* A client who did not understand or who inadequately understood previous instructions has *Ineffective health maintenance,* despite prior medication instruction. Assess the client's current level of understanding and use a variety of teaching methodologies (oral instruction, written, and audiovisual aids) to improve the client's ability to manage medication therapy.
- *Perceived susceptibility, seriousness, and benefits.* Clients who perceive that they are not susceptible to a worsening of the condition, who believe the condition is not serious, or who do not perceive that there are benefits to medication therapy may not adhere to the medication schedule. They may display no interest in managing medication therapy and may not pay attention to instructions or follow them even if properly understood. Try to assess why the client is not interested so you can include information in the teaching plan that may help counter or change these client beliefs.

DIAGNOSIS

A useful approach for selecting nursing diagnoses may be to think about the goal of care for a particular client. For example, consider an otherwise healthy 68-year-old woman who has been hospitalized with a myocardial infarction. She is concurrently diagnosed with hypertension and shows early signs of heart failure. She is started on daily oral doses of furosemide (a diuretic) and metoprolol (an antihypertensive, antianginal). Nitroglycerin sublingual tablets (antianginal) are prescribed for PRN use. The client is scheduled for discharge within 24 hours and says that she does not understand how these medications will help her. The most logical nursing diagnosis with the information given is *Ineffective health maintenance.* These medications are newly ordered for this client, who was healthy before admission. A sample nursing diagnostic statement could be *Ineffective health maintenance related to insufficient knowledge of newly prescribed medications.*

The goal of care is to return the client to independent living, and the client requires the usual information about medication therapy prior to discharge.

If this client had mild dementia and could not retain information, you might select *Ineffective therapeutic regimen management.* A sample nursing diagnostic statement might be *Ineffective therapeutic regimen management related to cognitive impairment.* The goal of care in this case would be to put safeguards in place to ensure that the client receives both of her daily medications and the PRN nitroglycerin as well.

If an oriented client experienced orthostatic intolerance from the vasodilating effect of metoprolol and fluid loss from furosemide, you might select the nursing diagnostic statement *Risk for injury related to orthostatic hypotension secondary to medication effect.* The goal of care in this instance would be to keep the client from self-injury or experiencing a fall during periods of dizziness and hypotension. The focus of care would be to teach the client to change position slowly, avoid concurrent use of alcohol, and use other standard measures outlined in pharmacology references.

Even if medication use is not the driving force in formulating a nursing diagnosis, administration of medications may be included in the nursing interventions listed for other nursing diagnoses. A client with emphysema may have a nursing diagnosis of *Activity intolerance.* Teaching proper use of bronchodilators may be part of the plan of care for that nursing diagnosis.

The issues and problems that could arise during medication therapy are so broad that several other nursing diagnoses could be relevant. The following is a list of other nursing diagnoses that may apply to individual clients.

- *Constipation* or *Diarrhea related to GI effects of medication therapy.* Opioid analgesics frequently cause constipation, whereas antibiotics may cause diarrhea. Determine any changes in the client's usual pattern of bowel elimination and analyze these changes in relation to the onset and timing of medications. The focus of nursing care is reducing or eliminating the disturbance.
- *Ineffective sexuality patterns related to altered libido secondary to medication therapy.* Common medications that decrease libido are antidepressants, antihistamines, antihypertensives, sedatives, and tranquilizers (chronic use). Medications that increase libido include testosterone, sedatives (low-dose), and tranquilizers. The focus of nursing care is teaching the client about these side effects and about coping mechanisms.
- *Disturbed sleep pattern related to medication side effects.* Some medications cause drowsiness as a side effect (sedatives and hypnotics); others cause excitability (nervous system stimulants). The focus of nursing care is to analyze whether the scheduling of medications could be changed to allow more normal sleep, and to implement these changes whenever possible. Otherwise, take action to reduce interfering stimuli, such as noise, temperature, a full bladder, pain, fear, or stress.
- *Risk for injury related to adverse medication side effects on mobility or sensorium.* Clients with reduced mobility may be at risk for falls from a decreased ability to move pur-

posefully in the environment. Clients with altered sensorium may harm themselves either by falling or by climbing out of bed over the side rails or foot of the bed. Drugs that could cause these effects include sedatives, vasodilators, diuretics, hypoglycemics, antihypertensives, and psychotropics. Assess the client's risk of injury and put precautionary measures in place, such as a call bell, ambulation aids, a night-light, and a clutter-free environment. In general, clients also need to know to avoid drinking alcohol or taking OTC drugs with sedative effects concurrently with many types of medications to avoid adverse interactive effects.

- *Risk for infection related to possible superinfection as a consequence of antibiotic therapy.* Superinfection is an overgrowth of pathogens normally kept in balance by the organisms killed by the antibiotic. Assess for signs of superinfection, such as oral lesions (thrush), diarrhea *(Clostridium difficile),* or vaginal itching (yeast infection). Report these signs and symptoms to the physician so that the new infection(s) may be treated.
- *Risk for infection related to medication-induced immune system depression.* Clients with cancer who receive chemotherapy or radiation therapy and clients taking immunosuppressant drugs after organ transplant are at greatest risk for this diagnosis. Monitor vigilantly these clients' vital signs (especially temperature), white blood cell counts, and other signs and symptoms of infection. Remember that infection may be occurring in immunosuppressed clients when the white blood cell count is too low, not only when it is elevated. Report signs and symptoms of infection immediately.
- *Disturbed sensory perception related to adverse effects of medication therapy (sedatives and tranquilizers).* These medications reduce or change the perception of incoming stimuli. Assess the client for such indicators as disorientation, restlessness, blurred vision, and sometimes auditory or visual hallucinations. Refer back to the nursing diagnosis *Risk for injury.* This diagnosis may also apply when there are toxic drug effects (such as hearing loss from ototoxicity with aminoglycosides). Check the drug literature for adverse neurological effects and report them if noted. Institute a plan to reorient the client as needed, and take measures to maintain client safety.
- *Imbalanced nutrition: less than body requirements related to medication-induced anorexia, GI discomfort, or diarrhea.* Teach clients about the proper timing of medications in relation to meals to reduce the incidence of this problem. Report abdominal discomfort that the client cannot tolerate (such as severe abdominal pain caused by erythromycin). The physician may order a change to a different drug with fewer GI side effects.
- *Impaired swallowing related to cranial nerve impairment.* This diagnosis often applies after cerebrovascular accident (CVA) or other central nervous system problems. Use this nursing diagnosis if the client has an impaired gag reflex, if food remains in the mouth after swallowing, or if the client coughs when swallowing medications, liquids, or food (see Chapter 24). The focus of care is to give medication in a form that the client can manage (crushed medications,

getting an order for a liquid form rather than solid). At times, the physician may need to change the route from oral to enteral (by tube). A client who cannot swallow medications is at risk for aspiration, which could lead to pneumonia.

In summary, clinical diagnostic reasoning is a complex process that becomes easier with time and practice. Assess each client carefully, and cluster the data to form possible alternative nursing diagnoses (Table 20-6). Select the ones that have the best "fit" with the goal or intended outcome of care. *Ineffective health maintenance* is often appropriate to use with a client receiving medication therapy.

PLANNING

During the planning phase of the nursing process, establish the expected outcomes or goals for the selected nursing diagnosis. Next, write the specific nursing interventions that will help the client achieve the identified outcomes.

Expected Outcomes for *Ineffective Health Maintenance*

Sample expected outcomes for the client receiving medication therapy with a nursing diagnosis of *Ineffective health maintenance* are the following:

- Identifies the need to take medication for treatment of health problem
- Verbalizes an understanding of medication purposes, actions, adverse effects, and comfort and safety measures
- Demonstrates initiative in beginning to manage medication therapy
- Utilizes support systems as needed to adhere to medication therapy, such as getting prescriptions from pharmacy or keeping follow-up appointments with health care provider

Expected Outcomes for *Ineffective Therapeutic Regimen Management*

Sample expected outcomes for the client receiving medication therapy with a nursing diagnosis of *Ineffective therapeutic regimen management* are the following:

- Verbalizes an understanding of medication purposes, actions, adverse effects, and comfort and safety measures
- Verbalizes an intention to take medications as prescribed to promote health and limit disease progression

- Correctly self-administers medications
- States proper information about drug procurement, storage, and handling
- States an appropriate plan for medical follow-up for monitoring of medications

These expected outcomes could apply to the client being discharged from nursing care in any setting, including a hospital, an extended-care facility, or a home health agency. The expected outcomes may be modified or made more specific depending on individual client need. For example, the client who is learning to self-inject insulin may need additional intermediate goals to assist in meeting these expected outcomes. The goals developed for a specific client drive the selection of nursing interventions, which are then implemented to provide quality nursing care.

Mr. Connell will be discharged to his home from the ED. His wife has been quietly waiting with him during his evaluation. The diagnosis of myocardial infarction has been ruled out, but he has been diagnosed with hypertension and stable angina. He is being restarted on atenolol and furosemide and is being given a prescription for nitroglycerin for PRN use to relieve chest pain. As the nurse preparing Mr. Connell for discharge, what is your nursing diagnosis? What are your goals? What would you teach him about his medications, and how would it be different knowing he has taken the medications before? What factors should you assess about his home environment and lifestyle? What specific topics would you include in your teaching and why? How would you modify your teaching because Mrs. Connell is present?

INTERVENTION

Interventions to Address *Ineffective Health Maintenance*

The interventions that help a client meet the expected outcomes for *Ineffective health maintenance* are driven by the goals established for the client. They often include the following:

- Explain the medication's purpose, action, dose, and timing in clear and simple terms. Determine the client's prior knowledge and reinforce or reeducate. Provide instruction

Table 20-6	*Clustering Data to Make a Nursing Diagnosis*
MEDICATION THERAPY	
Data Cluster	**Diagnosis**
A client with a newly prescribed medication does not know what effects to expect or how to use the medication properly but has expressed an interest in learning about it.	*Ineffective health maintenance* related to insufficient knowledge of medication use and effects
An older adult client with arthritis in her hands and fingers has been changed from an oral hypoglycemic drug to insulin therapy. Although she expresses interest in managing her insulin therapy, she is unable to draw up the insulin or manipulate the syringe.	*Ineffective therapeutic regimen management* related to poor manual dexterity secondary to inflammation of joints
An older adult client has not refilled a needed prescription because of inability to afford the medication and lack of transportation to a local pharmacy	*Noncompliance* related to medication therapy secondary to financial and physical barriers

Within the apothecary system, use or memorize a conversion table. This enables you to know, for example, that there are 32 ounces in a quart and 64 ounces in a half gallon. Because this system is used so frequently in the United States, you will often make these conversions by memory.

CONVERSION BETWEEN SYSTEMS. In clinical practice, you may occasionally need to convert between the metric and apothecary systems to calculate drug doses. Begin the conversion process by comparing the ordered measurement with what is available. Identify the equivalent needed to make the conversion. For example, an older surgeon has ordered *morphine sulfate gr. ⅙ IM q 3 to 4 h PRN for pain.* The unit dose of morphine is labeled 10 mg/mL. To calculate the dose, you must convert the grains to milligrams. Recall that there are 60 mg in a grain. Set up the conversion as follows:

$$60 \text{ mg/grain} \times \tfrac{1}{6} \text{ grain} = 10 \text{ mg}$$

When you have calculated correctly, you know that one unit dose of the opioid analgesic must be used for the injection. Review a pharmacological math text for ready access to multiple examples and sample problems for converting from one unit of measure to another.

DOSAGE CALCULATIONS. Standard mathematical formulas or calculations are used to compute medication dosages. They may involve dimensional analysis (a variation of ratio and proportion) or other traditional formulas.

TRADITIONAL FORMULAS. Formulas commonly used to solve medication dosage problems are the following:

$$\frac{\text{Dose ordered}}{\text{Dose on hand}} \times \text{Amount on hand} \times \text{Amount to administer}$$

or

$$\frac{\text{Desired}}{\text{have}} \times \text{Quantity} = \text{Dose}$$

The dose that is "ordered" or "desired" is the amount of drug prescribed by the physician that the client should receive. The dose that is on hand (or the "have") is the drug measurement (weight or volume) available from the pharmacy. The dose on hand can be determined by reading the label, which states the amount of drug present in each tablet or capsule or in a certain volume of liquid. The "amount on hand" or "quantity" is the actual unit that contains the dose on hand. This could be "1 tablet" if the medication is a solid, or it could be "5 mL" if the medication is a liquid. For the most part, the "amount on hand" (quantity) is the most confusing part of the equation for nursing students. Some students repeatedly try to put the value of "1" into the equation for "amount on hand" instead of carefully reading the label and inserting the true unit. The following sample problem using a solid medication form illustrates how to calculate a drug dose using this method:

Example: The order states to give *diltiazem (Cardizem) 30 mg PO.* The tablets are labeled 60 mg/tablet. After comparing the order with the medication, you reason that 30 mg is the

dose "desired," whereas 60 mg is the dose available, or the "have." You would then set up the calculation as shown:

$$\frac{30 \text{ mg}}{60 \text{ mg}} \times 1 \text{ tablet} = \text{No. of tablets to administer.}$$

Simplify the fraction by dividing the numerator and denominator by 30 to get

$$\tfrac{1}{2} \times 1 \text{ tablet} = \tfrac{1}{2} \text{ or } 0.5 \text{ tablet to administer.}$$

This example illustrates that a portion of a solid drug may be given. However, this can be done only if the tablet or pill is scored (has an indented line) to allow it to be broken easily into two equal halves. A tablet that is not scored may not be broken into a partial dose because it is highly likely that the dose of the broken pill will be inaccurate. The client could then receive either a high or a low dose of the medication. Both situations are equally dangerous.

DIMENSIONAL ANALYSIS. The use of dimensional analysis by nurses as a method for calculating medication dosages is growing. This method is already popular in the physical sciences as a problem-solving method (Olsen & Giangrasso, 2000). It involves setting up the problem so that all of the units for the entries in the calculation (called factors) cancel each other out except the one being solved for. Use the following steps to solve a problem using dimensional analysis:
- Identify the unit of measure or drug form being calculated (such as mL or tab/cap) to the left of the equation, followed by an equal sign.
- Locate the factor in the problem that contains the unit of measure (such as 500 mg per mL or 325 mg per tab)
- Set up the remainder of the problem so that all units cancel from the numerator and denominator except the one being solved for (again, the mL or tab/cap). Multiply one side of the equation by a conversion factor as needed to help cancel out extra units (this will not change the value of the equation).

The following sample problem illustrates how to calculate a drug dose using this method. Beyond this, you are referred to a pharmacological math text for additional practice.

Example: The order states to give *KCl elixir 20 mEq PO.* The label on the bottle states a drug concentration of 40 mEq/15 mL. After comparing the order with the drug label, you reason that mL is the unit of measure that needs to be calculated. You would set up the problem so that the mL is on the left side of the equation and all other conversion factors are on the right side, until all unnecessary units cancel each other out:

$$\text{mL} = 20 \text{ mEq} \times \frac{15 \text{ mL}}{40 \text{ mEq}}$$

Perform the calculation by multiplying 20 by 15 to get 300, then divide by 40 to obtain the dose of 7.5 mL to administer. Note that the mEq units cancel each other out, leaving only the mL.

When performing drug calculations, make it a habit to perform a "common sense check" at the end of the problem. Compare the answer obtained in relationship to the dose

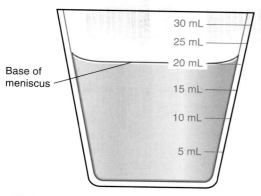

Figure 20-4. When using a calibrated measuring cup, measure the dose at the base of the meniscus.

Interventions Specific to Drug Route

Managing Oral Medications. The oral route is most commonly used for medication administration. Orally administered medications have a slower onset of action and a more prolonged, less potent effect. They are less expensive to manufacture, easy to administer, and do not interrupt the skin and mucous membrane barriers.

Oral medications are most frequently given in solid forms, such as tablets, capsules, and pills. Liquid forms are helpful for clients who have trouble swallowing tablets, and they can be poured using a variety of aids. When pouring a dose into a calibrated measuring cup, hold it at eye level and measure the dose at the base of the meniscus (Figure 20-4).

Remember the following safety points when preparing oral medications for administration:

- If a medication must be removed from a bottle, make sure the label is intact and legible. Return an unlabeled bottle or one that is difficult to read to the pharmacy.
- Pour medications carefully to prevent unnecessary loss. If too much medication is poured, discard the excess. Never return unused medication to a container.
- If pouring a dose from a stock supply, do not return a solid medication to the container if it has been taken out of the cap.
- Do not move medications from one bottle to another, because bottles can be identified by a code number or lot number assigned by the manufacturer. This number may be needed to track medications with quality control problems.

A key concern when giving an oral medication is preventing aspiration. Place clients in an upright position, either on the back or turned to one side. This reduces the risk of medication accumulating at the back of the throat. Provide fluid to drink and give only one pill or tablet at a time. Allow the clients enough time to swallow each medication before giving the next one. If they begin to cough, wait until they have recovered before giving additional medications. Remain with them until all medications have been taken. Do not leave medications at the bedside for clients to take after you leave the room. Make sure that they drink at least 50 or 60 mL of fluid with the last tablet to ensure that the medication reaches the stomach and does not stick in the esophagus. If the clients' intake and output are being measured, record all fluid taken with medications on this record. Specific guidelines for administering medications by the oral route are given in Procedure 20-1.

PROCEDURE 20-1 ADMINISTERING ORAL MEDICATIONS

TIME TO ALLOW
Novice: 10 min.
Expert: 5 min.

Oral medications are administered to provide a pharmacological benefit or effect for a client. They are given carefully, using strict guidelines to prevent error.

DELEGATION GUIDELINES

At no time is it appropriate to delegate medication administration to a nursing assistant. Your knowledge of pharmacological agents, their administration, and ongoing client assessment necessitate that you perform this procedure.

EQUIPMENT NEEDED

- Medication order sheet, computer-generated medication administration record, medication Kardex or cards
- Medication cart or tray
- Disposable medication cups (calibrated plastic or souffle)
- Glass of water, juice, or other preferred fluid
- Drinking straw
- Pill-crushing device (as needed)
- Medications or medication cart (unit-dose system)

---

1. Follow preliminary guidelines for nursing procedures (see inside front cover).

2. Assess the client to verify that the oral route is appropriate. Notify the physician if you find contraindications for giving medications by this route.

3. Confirm the medication order sheet against the original physician orders.
a. Clarify inconsistencies if found.
b. Check the client's record for allergies.
c. Determine any assessments needed (e.g., blood pressure or pulse) before the dose can be given

PROCEDURE 20-1	ADMINISTERING ORAL MEDICATIONS—CONT'D

4. Dispense medications one at a time, for one client at a time.

a. Unlock the drawer of the medication cart or storage area.

b. Select the correct medication and compare its label with the order sheet.

c. Calculate the dose needed.

d. Recheck the dose to be sure it is correct.

e. Place a solid medication into a disposable souffle cup.

f. For a partial dose, use a gloved hand or a cutting device to split a scored medication in half. Discard the unused half of a divided tablet.

g. To remove the dose from a bottle, pour the correct number of tablets into the bottle cap and then transfer them into a clean medicine cup. Do not touch the tablets with fingers; return any untouched extra tablets in the cap to the bottle. Use a new cup for each medication. *This method provides aseptic preparation of medications, avoids allowing medications to touch your hands, and aids in distinguishing one medication from another.*

h. Leave unit-dose medications in their original packaging and place them together in one cup. Do not open the wrappers until you get to the client's bedside. Keep medications that require special assessments in a separate cup. *This approach makes it easier to return refused medications to the pharmacy or to withhold medications as needed on the basis of client assessment.*

i. To give a liquid medication, pour it into a calibrated, disposable medication cup.

  (1) Mix the medication thoroughly, and discard it if it has changed color or become cloudy.

  (2) Remove the lid from the bottle or container and place it upside down. *This position prevents contamination of the container lid.*

  (3) Hold the bottle so that the label is facing up, under the palm of your hand. *This position ensures that the medication label does not become soiled or faded by spilled liquid.*

  (4) Hold the medication cup at eye level and use your thumbnail to mark the level of the correct dose. Pour medication into the cup until the bottom of the meniscus reaches the level of your thumbnail. Do not return any excess medication to the bottle; instead, discard it.

  (5) Wipe the lip of the container with a clean paper towel before recapping.

  (6) Bring a unit dose of a liquid to the bedside without opening it, unless the client needs a partial dose.

5. For medications of all types, recheck the medication and the dose after it is poured but before it is given to the client.

6. Lock the medication cart or storage area and bring the medications to the client.

7. Identify the client.

a. Read the name on client's identification bracelet.

b. Ask the client to tell you his name. *This step requires that client be alert and able to cooperate.*

c. Verify the client's identity with another staff member who knows the client. *Perform this step only if the client does not have an identification bracelet and is confused or unable to communicate.*

8. Perform final assessments (parameters for administration, such as hold Toprol if pulse is <55) and explain the purpose of the medications to client.

9. Give the medications to the client.

a. Allow the client to choose whether to take one or more than one medication at a time and whether to take them in a certain order. *Clients' needs and preferences should be respected if they do not threaten health or safety.*

b. Recheck the accuracy of any medication that the client questions. *Doing so may help to prevent a medication error.*

c. Remove unit-dose medications from their wrappers and give them to the client in a cup or in the hand according to the client's preference. *This method allows the client to see the medication, become familiar with it, and notice any discrepancies from the usual dose.*

d. Offer a full glass of fluid. Have client moisten his mouth with fluid, bow his head slightly to aid swallowing, and follow the medications with an additional 60 to 100 mL. *You may need to use less fluid if the client is on fluid restriction.*

e. Give liquids, chewable medications, lozenges, and sublingual or buccal medications separately from oral tablets, pills, or capsules.

f. Make sure the client has swallowed all medications by questioning him or checking his mouth. Stay with the client until all medications have been taken.

10. Document the medication administration promptly on the client's medication administration record or computerized medication record.

11. Recheck the client when the medication has had time to take effect to assess his response to the medication.

PEDIATRIC CONSIDERATIONS

Children under the age of 5 may need liquid forms of medication because of difficulty in swallowing tablets or capsules. Whenever possible, a child should be allowed to take medication with a beverage of choice. Explanations about medication therapy should be given at an age-appropriate level.

GERIATRIC CONSIDERATIONS

Older adults may need more time than younger individuals to take oral medications. They may also require additional liquid to ensure that all medications are swallowed.

A variation of the oral route used for some clients is an enteral tube, such as a nasogastric tube, gastrostomy tube (G-tube), or jejunostomy tube (J-tube). Important guidelines to follow when administering medications by the enteral route are given in Box 20-9.

Managing Parenteral Medications. Parenteral routes are differentiated by the angle of injection and depth of penetration. To give these medications safely, you must be familiar with the equipment, follow accepted procedures, and have manual dexterity. When preparing medications to be given by this route, keep the equipment and medication sterile.

Medications given by a parenteral route are absorbed more rapidly than those given orally. They cannot be removed or retrieved once given, making safety and accuracy key concerns.

EQUIPMENT. Needles and syringes are used to give parenteral medications. They are available in many sizes and are selected according to the medication dose and site to be injected. All needles have a bevel (an angled end), a shaft, and a hub. All syringes have a tip, a barrel, and a plunger (Figure 20-5, p. 416).

SYRINGES. Syringes must be kept sterile with the exception of the outside barrel and the top edge of the plunger. This means that the syringe tip, barrel interior, and most of the plunger cannot be touched. The plunger moves up and down in the barrel of the syringe so that medication can be withdrawn and injected. The barrel holds the medication and the barrel tip connects to a needle. Barrel tips may be either straight-end or Luer-Lok.

Most syringes used today are disposable and made of plastic. They are individually packaged to ensure sterility. They are clearly labeled with size (1 mL, 2 mL, 3 mL, 5 mL, 10 mL, 20 mL) and may be identified by their use (tuberculin, insulin). Many syringes are prepackaged with a specific-size needle attached, which is also clearly labeled.

The barrel of a syringe is calibrated by volume (Figure 20-6, p. 416). For example, a tuberculin syringe can hold up to 1 mL of volume and is calibrated in units of 0.01 mL. An insulin syringe is calibrated in units (U) of insulin. Most insulin manufactured in the United States and Canada contains 100 units per mL and is therefore called U100 insulin. An insulin syringe may hold up to either 1 mL (most common) or 0.5 mL. Most SC and IM injections do not exceed 2 or 3 mL. A 3-mL syringe is calibrated in units of 0.1 mL. Larger syringes, such as 5 mL, 10 mL, and 20 mL, are calibrated in increments of 0.2 mL. Larger syringes may be used occasionally to draw up IV medications.

NEEDLES. Most needles used today are disposable and made of stainless steel. In selected areas, such as operating rooms, needles may be reused, but they must be resterilized after each use and inspected frequently for wear and tear.

Needles are measured by length and diameter. Lengths range from $\frac{1}{4}$ to 5 inches (with $\frac{5}{8}$ to 1.5 inch most common). A shorter needle is used when the client is smaller in size or when more superficial tissues are being injected (such as insulin and intradermal injections). Longer needles are used to inject deeper tissues (such as IM injections).

The angle at which the needle is inserted also affects the tissue depth reached. In general, IM injections require the use

---

Box 20-9 Guidelines for Administering a Medication Through an Enteral Tube

- Whenever possible, obtain medications in liquid form to lessen the risk of obstructing the tube.
- Crush medications carefully; do not administer large particles or whole medications. Dissolve in warm water first.
- Do not crush enteric-coated, extended-action, sublingual, or buccal medications.
- Administer medications at room temperature rather than chilled. Also, warm the fluids used to flush the tube.
- Put on disposable gloves. Access the tube using standard procedure. Check tube placement before administering a medication. Sit the client upright or semi-upright to reduce risk of aspiration.
- Place a waterproof pad on the bed linens under the area of the tube. Flush the tube with 15 to 60 mL of warm water before and after giving the medication, or as directed by facility policy.
- Administer medications by gravity, pouring them into an irrigation syringe with the plunger removed. Hold the syringe approximately 18 inches high to ensure a slow, steady flow rate. Monitor how the client tolerates the procedure.
- Do not administer a medication through the air vent of a feeding tube.
- After the final flush, clamp the tube that was attached to suction for 20 to 30 minutes. If the client was receiving continuous tube feedings, clamp the tube for a few moments before resuming, if directed by facility policy.
- Help the client to a right-side-lying position with the head elevated for at least 30 minutes after administering the medication.
- Clean up the work area, remove gloves, and perform hand hygiene.
- Document the medication and fluid intake on appropriate charting forms.

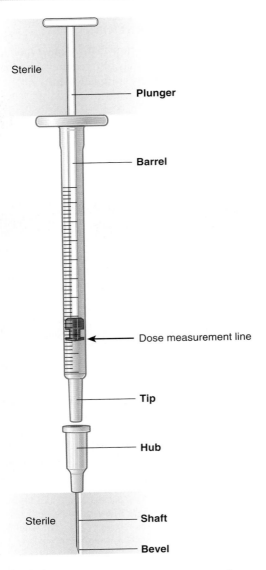

Sterile

Plunger

Barrel

Dose measurement line

Tip

Hub

Sterile

Shaft

Bevel

Figure 20-5. The needle and the syringe each has three parts.

of 1- to 1.5-inch needles, whereas SC injections require use of ⅜- to ⅝-inch needles. Longer needles also have longer bevels, which helps to decrease discomfort at the injection site. Insulin syringes are specially manufactured with a small needle attached to the syringe to meet the needs of clients who must inject themselves regularly.

The diameter of a needle is referred to as its gauge. The diameter size is inversely related to the gauge number. Gauges range from 28 (small) to 14 (large). Smaller-gauge needles are used with smaller drug volumes and produce less tissue trauma. Larger-gauge needles are used when larger volumes are injected, when the medication is viscous, or when the medication must penetrate to deeper tissues.

PREFILLED SYRINGES. Some parenteral medications are manufactured in prefilled, single-dose, disposable syringes (Figure 20-7). These medication systems are available with a preattached needle or in a Luer format (without needle). You simply bring the prefilled syringe to the bedside, remove the needle shield, inject the medication, and dispose of the syringe. However, do not confuse this system with a unit-dose system. You may need to discard excess medication if the ordered dose is smaller than that supplied in the syringe. The purpose of prefilled syringes is to simplify and ease the injection process while decreasing the risk of needlestick injury during medication preparation. Some prefilled syringes may require you to assemble a prefilled cartridge into a holder device and then disassemble the system after use.

SAFE USE OF NEEDLES AND SHARPS. Preventing needlestick injuries is a vital concern in the health care industry. The Occupational Safety and Health Administration (OSHA) mandates the use of standard precautions, which include proper handling and disposal of sharp instruments including needles. After administering an injection, discard the syringe and needle, without recapping the needle, in a rigid container that has been specifically labeled and provided for that purpose (Figure 20-8). The container should be leak-proof and puncture-proof. Rigid containers are kept on medication carts

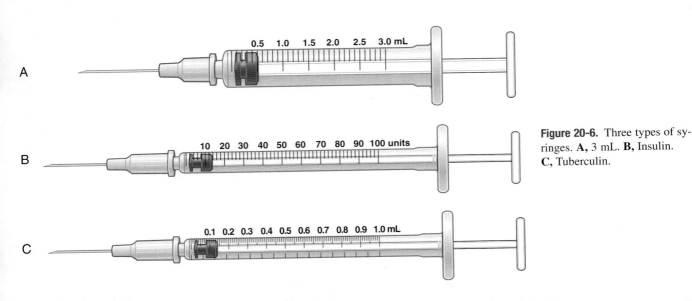

0.5   1.0   1.5   2.0   2.5   3.0 mL

A

10   20   30   40   50   60   70   80   90   100 units

B

0.1   0.2   0.3   0.4   0.5   0.6   0.7   0.8   0.9   1.0 mL

C

Figure 20-6. Three types of syringes. **A,** 3 mL. **B,** Insulin. **C,** Tuberculin.

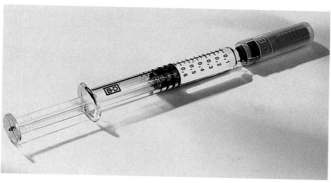

Figure 20-7. The Hypak injection system is an example of a prefilled, single-dose, disposable syringe. It consists of a cartridge holder and a prefilled medication cartridge with a needle. (Courtesy Becton Dickinson Pharmaceutical Systems, Franklin Lakes, NJ.)

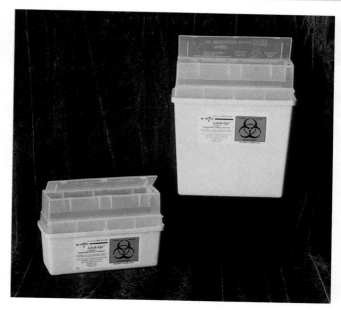

Figure 20-8. Proper use of rigid disposal containers ("sharps" containers) for used needles helps prevent accidental needlesticks. (Courtesy Medline Industries, Mundelein, IL.)

in all client care settings and are wall-mounted in client rooms and treatment areas in many acute care institutions. To prevent the risk of needlestick injury, do not try to place a used syringe into an overfilled container.

If you must recap a needle, do so using the one-handed (or scoop) method. Slide the needle into the needle cover as it lies on a flat surface. Lift the syringe and twist the cover into place near the base of the needle. Never push the cap onto the needle using a finger on the end of the needle cover.

Action Alert! Avoid recapping needles whenever possible. If you must recap, use the one-handed (or scoop) method.

If you cannot discard a syringe immediately, encase it in a protective sheath temporarily. An increasing number of facilities are using safety syringes that cover or encase the needle after use. Follow manufacturer's guidelines and facility procedures if using these devices.

Do not leave needles and syringes (even temporarily) in a pocket, on a client's meal tray, at the bedside, or in the client's bed. Do not discard them in wastebaskets or in a rigid container that is full. Doing so increases the risk of needlestick injury, with possible infection from a number of pathogens, including hepatitis B and human immunodeficiency virus (HIV).

PREPARING AN INJECTION FROM AN AMPULE. An ampule is a glass container that holds a single drug dose and ranges in size from 1 mL to 10 mL or larger. The neck of the ampule is narrow and may have a colored ring indicating where it is prescored for opening. Because bits of glass sometimes found in ampules can be drawn into the syringe, it is prudent to use a filter needle to withdraw the medication (Koschel, 2001). The steps for withdrawing medication from an ampule are given in Procedure 20-2 (p. 418).

PREPARING AN INJECTION FROM A VIAL. A vial is a glass or plastic container with a rubber seal at the top. The seal is sterile before being opened and is protected by a soft metal or plastic cap. A vial may contain either liquid or powder medication. If a powder is used, product literature indicates the type and amount of diluent (such as sterile normal saline solution or sterile water) to use for reconstitution. Read the label carefully to determine the end concentration of the medication to avoid drawing up the wrong dose. Inject the solvent into the vial using the same technique that you would use to inject air. A powdered medication may dissolve easily, or you may have to gently roll or agitate the vial. If needed, the syringe may be removed from the vial before doing this.

Vials are labeled for a single dose or for multiple doses. A single-dose vial must be discarded after one use. A multiple-dose vial may be reused but must be labeled with the date and time opened and your initials. A used vial must be discarded 30 days after being opened, or less according to manufacturer's directions, even if it is not empty. Reconstituted medications in multiple-dose vials often require refrigeration after initial use. The steps for withdrawing medications from a vial are given in Procedure 20-3 (p. 419).

MIXING MEDICATIONS. Two medications may be mixed in one syringe if they are compatible with each other and if their total volume does not exceed the amount that may be given in one parenteral site. Most nursing units and pharmacology texts have charts identifying compatible medications. Consult a pharmacist if the medication is not identified or if you have any questions about compatibility.

MIXING MEDICATIONS FROM AN AMPULE AND A VIAL. When a medication from an ampule must be mixed with one from a vial, first withdraw from the vial and then from the ampule. This prevents the vial from being contaminated with medication from the ampule. It also is easier because the syringe partially filled with medication from the ampule is not used to inject air into the vial. (This recommendation assumes use of a multidose vial.)

WITHDRAWING MEDICATION FROM AN AMPULE

TIME TO ALLOW
Novice: 5 min
Expert: 1 to 2 min.

Liquid medications used for injection may be supplied in ampules. You will need to withdraw the medication properly before you can administer it safely to the client.

DELEGATION GUIDELINES
The withdrawal and preparation of medication is yours alone. You may not delegate this task or any of the component parts of medication preparation to a nursing assistant.

EQUIPMENT NEEDED
- Medication order sheet, computer-generated medication administration record, medication Kardex or cards
- Ampule of medication
- Syringe, filter needle, and needle
- Alcohol swab or gauze pad (2 × 2-inch)
- Container for disposing of sharps and ampule

1. Follow preliminary guidelines for nursing procedures (see inside front cover).

2. Open the ampule.
a. Tap the upper chamber of the ampule quickly but lightly until all the fluid drops into the lower chamber. *This action ensures that all medication is available for use.*
b. Wrap the alcohol swab or gauze pad around the neck of the ampule. *Doing so will protect your fingers from small glass fragments as you open the ampule.*
c. Snap the neck of the ampule so that it opens away from your body (see illustration). *This directs any fragments of glass away from you rather than toward you.*

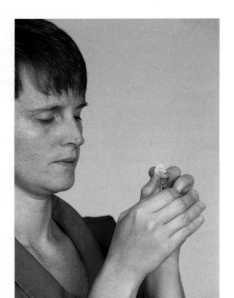

Step 2c. Snapping the neck of the ampule away from your body.

3. Place the ampule upright on a flat surface and withdraw medication into a syringe (see illustration).
a. Attach the filter needle (if used) to the syringe. Hold the ampule while inserting the filter needle into the center of the opening on the ampule. Do not allow the tip or shaft to touch the rim of the ampule. *This prevents contamination of the needle or filter needle, because the rim is considered contaminated.*

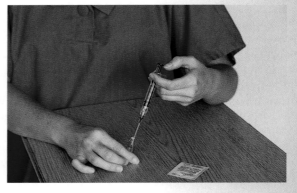

Step 3. Withdrawing medication into the syringe with the ampule upright.

b. Gently pull back on the plunger to aspirate medication into the syringe.
c. Tilt the ampule as needed to keep the needle tip below the level of medication. *This step keeps you from withdrawing air into the syringe.*
d. If air enters the syringe, do not inject it into the ampule. Instead, remove the needle from the ampule, hold the syringe with the needle pointing upward, and eject the air (not the fluid). Then reinsert the needle into the center of the ampule and withdraw fluid again. *These steps provide sufficient room in the syringe to withdraw the full dose*

needed, prevent loss of medication from excess air pressure, and ensure withdrawal of the complete dose.

4. Eject excess air or fluid as needed.

5. Replace the needle or filter needle with a new needle and secure it tightly. Discard the used filter needle properly.

Replacing the needle prevents needle contamination and irritation of the client's tissues caused by tracking of medication through dermal and subcutaneous layers.

6. Compare the volume of fluid in the syringe with the ordered dose.

PROCEDURE 20-3   WITHDRAWING MEDICATION FROM A VIAL

TIME TO ALLOW
Novice: 5 min.
Expert: 1 to 2 min.

Liquid medications used for injection may be supplied in sealed, airtight vials. You will need to add air to the vial to facilitate accurate withdrawal; otherwise you will create a vacuum effect by withdrawing the medication.

DELEGATION GUIDELINES
As in the previous procedures in this chapter, medication preparation is the sole responsibility of you, the RN. You may never delegate this procedure to a nursing assistant.

EQUIPMENT NEEDED
- Medication order sheet, computer-generated medication administration record, medication Kardex or cards
- Vial of medication
- Syringe and needle
- Alcohol swab
- Glass disposal container

1. Follow preliminary guidelines for nursing procedures (see inside front cover).

2. Prepare the vial.
a. Remove the plastic or metal top of a new vial to expose the rubber seal.
b. Cleanse the rubber seal with an alcohol swab.
c. Check the expiration date of a previously opened vial. Do not use the medication if the vial has been opened longer than manufacturer's directions. Check the medication for appropriate color and clarity.

3. Prepare the syringe.
a. Check for a tight connection between the needle hub and syringe barrel. *This action ensures a tight seal and a closed system.*
b. Remove the needle cover.
c. Draw back on the plunger to fill the syringe with a volume of air equal to the dose of medication you will be giving.

4. Withdraw the medication.
a. Insert the needle into the center of the vial's rubber seal using gentle but firm pressure. *The center of the seal is thinner and designed for penetration.*
b. Inject air from the syringe into the vial. *This step creates positive pressure inside the vial to ease medication withdrawal and prevent creation of a vacuum after removing the medication.*

c. Invert the vial while holding it with the first two fingers of your nondominant hand. Use your thumb and last two fingers to brace the barrel of the syringe. Use the thumb of your dominant hand to hold the end of the syringe barrel steady. Use the fingers of your dominant hand to withdraw the plunger. *Proper hand position allows easier medication withdrawal and prevents movement of the plunger or bending of the needle.*
d. Withdraw the medication slowly and steadily while holding the vial at eye level. Keep the tip of the needle in the solution at all times. Touch only the syringe barrel and plunger tip. *This method prevents air bubbles from entering the syringe and prevents contamination of the syringe.*
e. Remove excess air in the syringe by tapping the side of the syringe with a finger and pushing air back into the vial. Remove additional fluid as needed to ensure the full dose.
f. Return the vial to an upright position and remove the needle by pulling back on the syringe barrel, not the plunger. Remove any excess air if present. *This ensures that the correct amount of medication remains in the syringe.*

5. Replace the needle with a new one. Secure the new needle tightly and discard the used needle properly. *Replacing needle prevents needle contamination and irritation of client tissues from medication tracking through dermal and SC tissue layers.*

6. Compare the volume of fluid in the syringe with the ordered dose.

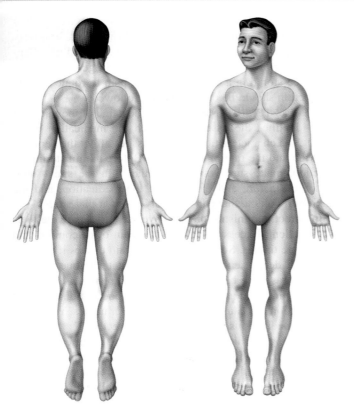

Figure 20-10. Frequently used sites for intradermal injection.

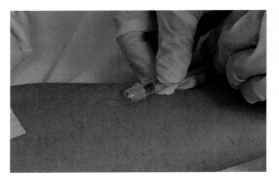

Figure 20-11. Intradermal injection. Insert the needle bevel up, with the syringe almost parallel to the skin at a 10- to 15-degree angle. As the medication is injected, a small wheal should form under the skin.

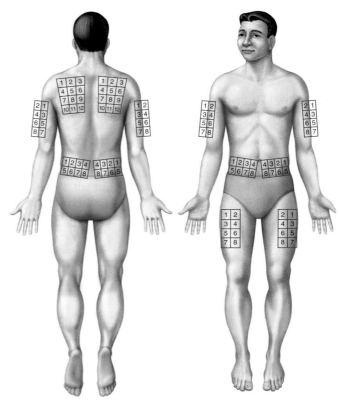

Figure 20-12. Common subcutaneous injection sites.

clearly marked. If there is a reaction (a positive test result), record and report it quickly.

ID injections are administered using a tuberculin syringe, which holds up to 1 mL of medication and is calibrated in 0.1 mL and 0.01 mL. Use a small needle (25 to 27 gauge) with a short bevel that is ¼ to ½ inch long. The usual medication dose is small (0.01 to 0.1 mL) (0.15 maximum). Angle the needle at 10 to 15 degrees from the skin to deposit the medication below the epidermis (Figure 20-11). A wheal forms under the skin with proper administration. The procedure for administering ID injections is given in Procedure 20-5.

SUBCUTANEOUS INJECTIONS. Subcutaneous (SC or SQ) tissue is not as vascular as muscle tissue, so medication is absorbed more slowly with SC injection than with IM injection. The slower absorption rate allows for a more prolonged drug effect.

The body is well supplied with subcutaneous tissue. Common injection sites include the anterolateral upper arms, anterior thighs, and lower abdominal wall between the costal margins and the iliac crests (Figure 20-12). Other acceptable sites are the scapular area of the back and the upper ventral or dorsal gluteal areas. Drugs commonly given by this route include heparin, insulin, and selected immunizations and analgesics.

As with any other injection, the site should be anatomically correct and free of infection, lesions, scars, or bruises. When giving injections frequently, rotate the sites to prevent

local complications, such as sterile abscesses (painful lumps), lipohypertrophy (thickening of the skin), and lipodystrophy (atrophy or dimpling of the skin). This is especially important for diabetic clients who self-inject insulin daily. Identify the site rotation plan on the client's care plan and note the sites of previously administered injections on the medication administration record. Use an injection diagram to help the client remember the site rotation pattern. Individual injection sites may be systematically rotated from

PROCEDURE 20-5 ADMINISTERING AN INTRADERMAL INJECTION

TIME TO ALLOW
Novice: 10 min.
Expert: 5 min.

Intradermal injections are done most often to test for allergies or for diagnostic purposes. The site is evaluated within a specific time period after the injection is given.

DELEGATION GUIDELINES
You may not delegate the administration of an intradermal injection to a nursing assistant.

EQUIPMENT NEEDED
- Medication order, medication administration record, computerized medication order sheet, or medication Kardex or cards
- Medication vial or ampule
- Tuberculin syringe and needle
- Alcohol swab
- 2 × 2-inch sterile gauze pad
- Acetone swab if needed for oily skin
- Disposable gloves

1. Follow preliminary guidelines for nursing procedures (see inside front cover).

2. Check the medication order and note any client allergies.

3. Withdraw medication from the vial as described in Procedure 20-3 (p. 419). Take the syringe and other supplies to the client's room and place them on a clean, flat surface.

4. Prepare the client for the intradermal injection.
   a. Identify the client using an identification bracelet or other accepted means.
   b. Explain the procedure to the client in a calm and confident manner.
   c. Put on disposable gloves and open the swab(s) and gauze package using aseptic technique.
   d. Provide privacy and position the client comfortably. Select and expose the injection site. *These steps reduce client tension and provide a view of the area to be used.*

5. Prepare the injection site and the syringe.
   a. Make sure area is free of bruises, redness, or lesions.
   b. Clean the site with an alcohol swab, wiping skin gently from top to bottom. Allow the alcohol to air dry. Use an acetone swab as well if the client's skin is oily. *Avoids circular motion that could stimulate capillary blood flow. Alcohol reduces the number of pathogens on the skin that could be pushed into the tissues by the needle. Allowing the alcohol to dry prevents tissue irritation.*
   c. Remove the needle-guard or cap with your nondominant hand by pulling it straight off. *This action helps prevent a needlestick injury.*
   d. Check the syringe to make sure that the volume of medication is correct and that it contains no air bubbles.

6. Inject the medication.
   a. Hold the syringe in your dominant hand and spread the skin taut with your nondominant hand. *The dominant hand has better fine motor control. It is easier to inject into taut skin.*
   b. Insert the needle bevel-up at a 10- to 15-degree angle into skin for ⅛ inch or until the bevel disappears from view. The needle should be visible below the skin surface and you should feel resistance. *This step places the needle under the epidermal layer of skin but not into subcutaneous tissue.*
   c. Inject the medication slowly while watching for formation of a small bleb, wheal, or blister (see Figure 20-11). If none is visible, withdraw the needle slightly and continue injecting. *This procedure deposits medication into the dermis.*
   d. Withdraw the needle at the same angle used for insertion. *Doing so will reduce tissue trauma and client discomfort.*
   e. Pat the area dry using the gauze pad. Do not massage the area. *Avoiding massage prevents the medication from spreading beyond the intended injection site.*

7. Dispose of used equipment properly and clean the area.
   a. Discard the needle and syringe in a rigid container without recapping the needle. Dispose of the alcohol swab, gauze, wrappers, and other used materials in a trash receptacle.
   b. Position the client comfortably.
   c. Remove gloves and discard them in a proper receptacle. Perform hand hygiene.

8. Document the procedure carefully.
   a. Observe the site and the client for any immediate allergic reaction. *Anaphylaxis could occur suddenly if the client has a severe allergy to the substance you injected.*

PROCEDURE 20-5 **ADMINISTERING AN INTRADERMAL INJECTION—CONT'D**

b. Use a skin pencil or a ball point pen (according to facility policy) to circle area of the wheal. *Doing so will provide an easy way to identify the site when performing follow-up readings.*

c. Document the date, time, substance, and site of the injection on the client's medication administration record. Document the date and time of follow-up observations, and inform the client and caregivers about their roles. *This will provide clear direction for caregivers responsible for interpreting test results.*

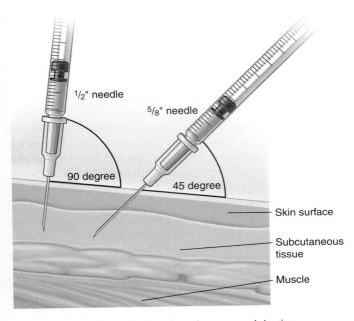

Figure 20-13. Technique for subcutaneous injection.

one area of the body to another (site 1 in one location to site 1 in another location, for example), or the client may rotate among all sites in a given body location. Sites should be separated from each other by 1 inch. Hospitalized diabetic clients often receive insulin in the arms because this site is harder to use at home. Give heparin in the abdomen (unless contraindicated by the client's condition).

Action Alert! Do not aspirate heparin or insulin injection sites. Do not massage heparin or insulin sites, which could lead to bleeding after heparin injection or increased speed of absorption after insulin injection.

The equipment used for SC injection depends on the medication to be given and the client's body size and weight. The amount of medication injected into one site is commonly 0.5 to 1.0 mL but should not exceed 1.5 mL. Insulin syringes are used to administer insulin, whereas tuberculin syringes are commonly used to administer heparin. For other medications, up to a 3-mL syringe may be used.

The needle should be 25 to 29 gauge with a ⅜- to ⅝-inch needle. Within this range, use shorter needles for smaller clients and longer needles for larger clients. In most cases, you may adjust the angle of insertion according to needle length. Shorter needles (½ inch and smaller) are usually inserted at a 90-degree angle, whereas ⅝-inch needles may be inserted at a 45-degree angle or a 90-degree angle, depending on body size (Figure 20-13). Further adjustments may be made for very small or pediatric clients according to need and facility policy. Administration techniques for SC injection are described in Procedure 20-6.

INTRAMUSCULAR INJECTIONS. The IM route may be chosen when rapid absorption is desired or when the medication is irritating to subcutaneous tissue (Procedure 20-7, p. 426). There are fewer nerve endings in muscle tissue, making this area more comfortable when irritating substances are injected. Nonetheless, clients can experience discomfort with IM injections. For this reason, do not inject into muscles that are tender to the client or that are contracted, hard, or tense. Complications of inappropriate site selection or improper technique include abscess formation, skin sloughing and necrosis, continued site pain, nerve injury, and periostitis (inflammation of the membrane over bone).

The volume that can be safely given by the IM route varies with the client's age and the site selected. An adult can receive a maximum of 4 mL in a large muscle, such as the gluteus. Children and older adults should not receive more than 1 or 2 mL because their muscles are less developed. The deltoid should be limited to 0.5 or 1 mL, depending on client size.

The appropriate needle size greatly depends on client size and drug viscosity. The average needle used for IM injection is 21 to 23 gauge and 1 to 1.5 inches long. A 2-inch needle may be used for very large clients so the medication reaches the muscle. Give all IM injections at a 90-degree angle.

There are four common sites for giving IM injections: ventrogluteal, dorsogluteal, vastus lateralis, and deltoid. These sites are safe because they do not lie near blood vessels, nerves, or bones. The gluteus muscles are particularly large and accept medication easily (Figure 20-14, p. 428). As with SC injections, rotate sites if giving repeated injections. Identify the site rotation plan on the care plan, and chart sites used on the medication administration record.

Text continued on p. 428

PROCEDURE 20-6 ADMINISTERING A SUBCUTANEOUS INJECTION

TIME TO ALLOW
Novice: 10 min.
Expert: 5 min.

Subcutaneous injections are given to administer medication into subcutaneous tissue with a written physician's order. This route provides faster medication action than the oral route.

DELEGATION GUIDELINES
You may not delegate the performance or administration of subcutaneous injections to a nursing assistant.

EQUIPMENT NEEDED
- Medication order, medication administration record, computerized medication order sheet, or medication Kardex or cards
- Medication vial or ampule
- Sterile, 3-mL insulin or tuberculin syringe and needle (⅝ inch or smaller)
- Two alcohol swabs
- Disposable gloves

1. Follow preliminary guidelines for nursing procedures (see inside front cover).

2. Check the medication order and note any client allergies.

3. Check the medication for appropriate color and clarity and withdraw the medication from the ampule or vial as described in previous procedures.

4. Take the syringe and other supplies to the client's room and place them on a clean, flat surface.

5. Prepare the client for the injection.
a. Identify the client using an identification bracelet or other accepted means.
b. Explain the procedure to client in a calm and confident manner.
c. Put on disposable gloves and open an alcohol swab wrapper using aseptic technique.
d. Provide privacy and position the client comfortably. Select and expose the injection site. If you select the upper outer arm, place the client's arm at his side in a relaxed position. If you choose the anterior thigh, have the client sit or lie down with the leg muscle relaxed. If you choose the abdomen, have the client lie in a recumbent or semirecumbent position. If you choose the scapula, have the client sit or lie prone or on his side. *These positions give you a clear view of the area to be used.*

6. Prepare the injection site and syringe.
a. Make sure the area is free of bruises, redness, or lesions.
b. Identify the exact site of the injection. Clean the site with an alcohol swab using a circular motion, moving outward from injection site. Allow the alcohol to air dry. Leave the swab in a clean area so you can reuse it when withdrawing the needle.

c. Remove the needle-guard or cap with your nondominant hand by pulling it straight off.
d. Check the syringe to make sure that the volume of medication is correct and contains no air bubbles.

7. Inject the medication.
a. Hold the syringe in your dominant hand between your thumb and forefinger, as if holding a dart. *The dominant hand has better fine motor control.*
b. Pinch or bunch up subcutaneous tissue between the thumb and forefinger of your nondominant hand. If the client has ample subcutaneous tissue or if you are injecting an anticoagulant drug, spread the skin taut. *Bunching the tissue aids needle insertion into SC tissue. Use needle length, the amount of tissue, and tissue turgor as a guide.*
c. Quickly insert the needle up to the hub at a 45- to 90-degree angle, depending on the length of the needle. *This action positions the needle in subcutaneous tissue.*
d. Release the bunched tissue and grasp the distal end of the syringe with your nondominant hand. *Holding the syringe with your nondominant hand steadies it in the tissue, reducing movement and client discomfort.*
e. Unless injecting insulin or heparin, aspirate for a blood return by pulling back gently on the tip of plunger with the thumb and forefinger of your dominant hand. *A blood return indicates that the needle has entered a blood vessel. Avoid aspiration with insulin or heparin because aspiration could cause local trauma.*
f. If a blood return is noted, pull the needle from the injection site, discard the syringe and needle, and begin the procedure again. *This prevents administering the medication intravenously and prevents hematoma formation from blood being introduced into the tissue.*
g. If no blood return is noted, inject the medication slowly and steadily. *Slow, steady injection disperses the medication evenly in the tissues to enhance absorption.*

PROCEDURE 20-6   ADMINISTERING A SUBCUTANEOUS INJECTION—CONT'D

h. Withdraw the needle quickly at the same angle used for insertion. Massage the area gently with the alcohol swab. Do not massage after injecting insulin or heparin. *Massage reduces tissue trauma and client discomfort, but it could increase the rate of insulin absorption or cause bleeding from heparin.*

8. Dispose of used equipment properly.

a. Discard the needle and syringe in a rigid container without recapping the needle. Dispose of the alcohol swab, wrapper, and other used materials in a trash receptacle.

b. Position the client comfortably.

c. Remove your gloves and discard them in the proper receptacle. Perform hand hygiene.

9. Document the procedure carefully.

a. Record the date, time, substance, and site of injection on the client's medication administration record.

b. Check on the client within 30 minutes to assess the effects of the medication.

PEDIATRIC CONSIDERATIONS

Children are often fearful of injections. Use strategies outlined in Box 20-8 (p. 412).

GERIATRIC CONSIDERATIONS

Older adults may have reduced amounts of subcutaneous tissue. Select equipment and injection sites carefully.

HOME CARE CONSIDERATIONS

Subcutaneous injections commonly administered in the home include insulin, heparin, and allergy injections. Subcutaneous injections are easier for the client or family to administer than are intramuscular injections. Teach about the medication, injection technique, site rotation, and management of adverse effects.

PROCEDURE 20-7   ADMINISTERING AN INTRAMUSCULAR INJECTION

TIME TO ALLOW
Novice: 10 min.
Expert: 5 min.

Intramuscular injections are used to administer medication into muscle tissue with a written physician's order. This route provides faster action than the oral or subcutaneous route.

DELEGATION GUIDELINES

You may not delegate the administration of an intramuscular injection to a nursing assistant.

EQUIPMENT NEEDED

- Medication order, medication administration record, computerized medication order sheet, or medication Kardex or cards
- Medication vial or ampule
- Sterile, 3-mL syringe and needle (1 to 2 inches, 20- to 22-gauge, long bevel)
- Two alcohol swabs
- Disposable gloves

1. Follow preliminary guidelines for nursing procedures (see inside front cover).

2. Check the medication order and note any client allergies.

3. Check the medication for color and clarity and withdraw the medication from the ampule or vial as described in previous procedures. Take the syringe and other supplies to the client's room and place them on a clean, flat surface.

4. Prepare the client for the injection.

a. Identify the client using an identification bracelet or other accepted means.

b. Explain the procedure to client in a calm and confident manner.

c. Put on disposable gloves and open the alcohol swab wrapper using aseptic technique.

d. Provide privacy and position the client comfortably. Select and expose the injection site. If you choose the upper arm (deltoid), place the client in a sitting or lying position with the arm relaxed at the side of the body. If you choose the anterolateral thigh (vastus lateralis), place the client in a sitting or lying position with the leg muscle relaxed. If you choose the dorsogluteal location (gluteus maximus), select a side-lying position with the upper leg flexed and in front of the lower leg. You can also use a prone position with the client's toes pointed inward. If you choose the ventrogluteal location (gluteus medius), place the client in a supine position with legs relaxed or a side-lying position with hip and knee flexed. *These positions reduce muscle tension and allow you to clearly see the area to be used.*

5. Prepare the injection site and the syringe.

a. Make sure the area is free of bruises, redness, or lesions.

b. Identify the exact site of the injection. Clean the site with an alcohol swab using a circular motion, moving outward from injection site. Allow the alcohol to air dry. Leave the swab in a clean area so you can reuse it when withdrawing the needle.

c. Remove needle-guard or cap with your nondominant hand by pulling it straight off.

d. Check the syringe to make sure that the volume of medication is correct.

6. Inject the medication.

a. Hold the syringe in your dominant hand between your thumb and forefinger as if holding a dart (see illustration).

b. Spread the skin taut between the thumb and forefinger of your nondominant hand or displace the skin using a Z-track technique (see Figure 20-20, p. 431). *Making the skin taut aids insertion of the needle into the muscle tissue.*

c. Insert the needle quickly at a 90-degree angle up to the hub. *This action positions the needle in the muscle tissue.*

d. Release the skin and grasp the distal end of the syringe with your nondominant hand. *Grasping the syringe steadies it in the tissue, thus reducing movement and client discomfort.*

e. Aspirate for a blood return by pulling back gently on tip of the plunger with the thumb and forefinger of your dominant hand. *Blood return indicates that the needle has entered a blood vessel.*

f. If blood return is noted, remove the needle, discard the syringe, and begin the procedure again. *Beginning again*

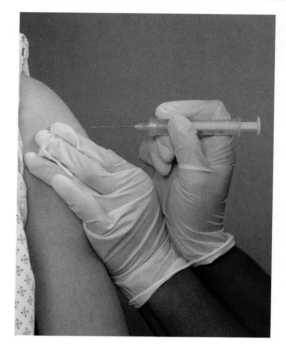

Step 6a. Holding the syringe like a dart and spreading the skin taut (here, over the deltoid).

prevents the medication from being injected intravenously and prevents the reinjection of aspirated blood.

g. If no blood return is noted, inject the medication slowly and steadily, taking about 10 seconds to inject each 1 mL. *Slow, steady injection disperses the medication evenly in the tissue to enhance absorption.*

h. Wait a few seconds, then withdraw the needle quickly at the same angle used to insert it. Apply gentle pressure to the site with an alcohol swab or 2 × 2-inch gauze. *These steps allow the medication to diffuse into the muscle while reducing tissue trauma and discomfort.*

7. Dispose of the used equipment.

a. Discard the needle and syringe in a rigid container without recapping the needle. Dispose of the alcohol swab, wrapper, and other used materials in an appropriate trash receptacle.

b. Position the client comfortably. If medication was injected into a leg muscle, encourage the client to flex and extend leg muscles. *These actions promote client comfort and enhance absorption of medication from sites in the leg.*

c. Remove gloves and discard them in the proper receptacle. Perform hand hygiene.

8. Document the procedure carefully.

a. Record the date, time, substance, and site of injection on the client's medication administration record.

b. Check on the client at an appropriate time after giving the injection (2 to 4 hours for many medications) to assess the client's response to the medication.

Continued

PROCEDURE 20-7 **ADMINISTERING AN INTRAMUSCULAR INJECTION—CONT'D**

PEDIATRIC CONSIDERATIONS

Children are often fearful of injections. Use strategies outlined in Box 20-8 (p. 412).

GERIATRIC CONSIDERATIONS

Older adults may have reduced amounts of subcutaneous tissue. Select equipment and injection sites carefully.

HOME CARE CONSIDERATIONS

The need for intramuscular injections in a homebound client is justification for a home care nurse. Intramuscular injections given in the home include iron, vitamins, antibiotics, and ketorolac tromethamine (Toradol) and other pain medications. The home care nurse must plan for the management of side effects and adverse effects. If a family caregiver is taught to administer intramuscular injections, client teaching should include recognizing and managing emergency reactions such as anaphylaxis. Consider whether the client needs to have injectable epinephrine (Adrenalin) at home for possible emergency use. Teach about the medication, injection technique, site rotation, and the management of adverse effects.

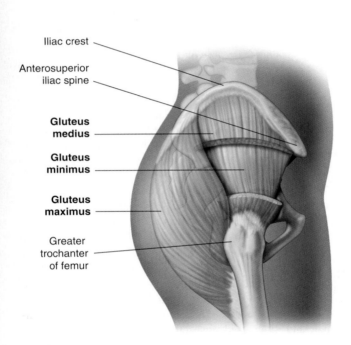

Figure 20-14. The three gluteus muscles are particularly large and accept intramuscular medication easily.

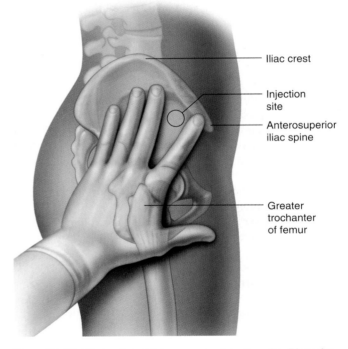

Figure 20-15. Ventrogluteal intramuscular injection site. Place the palm of your hand over the greater trochanter, with your middle finger pointed toward the iliac crest and your index finger toward the anterosuperior iliac spine. Administer the injection in the center of the triangle formed by your fingers.

Ventrogluteal Site. The ventrogluteal site uses the gluteus medius and minimus muscles in the area of the hip. This is a preferred site for adults and for children and infants over 7 months old. It is particularly useful because it does not lie near major bones, blood vessels, or nerves; is relatively free of microorganisms from fecal contamination; and allows the client to lie on the back, side, or abdomen during injection.

Locate the site by placing the palm of your hand over the greater trochanter with your fingers pointed in the direction of the client's head (Figure 20-15). Use your left hand to identify landmarks when the client is receiving the injection in the right hip, and vice versa. Place your index finger on the anterior superior iliac spine at the midaxillary line and extend your middle finger dorsally to the iliac crest. Give the injection in the center of the triangle created by these fingers.

Dorsogluteal Site. The dorsogluteal site uses the gluteus maximus muscles in the buttocks and is another commonly used site for IM injection. This site is recommended for adults

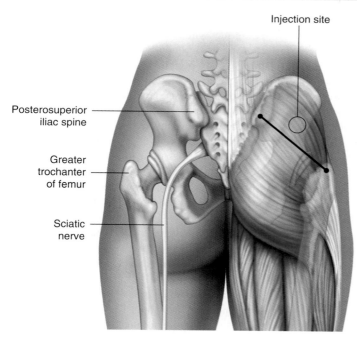

Figure 20-16. Dorsogluteal intramuscular injection site. Identify an imaginary line between the greater trochanter and the posterosuperior iliac spine. Give the injection superior and lateral to that line.

and children over age 3 because these muscles are developed by walking. It is not recommended for infants and children under age 3 because the gluteal muscles are small and underdeveloped. This site is not the preferred site for administering IM injections—there is a potential for injury because of the proximity of the sciatic nerve, major blood vessels, and bone.

To expose the site, the client may lie on the side with the top leg flexed and in front of the lower leg. The client may also lie prone with the toes pointed inward. These positions reduce muscle tension and promote relaxation. Do not allow the client to stand when injection is done in the dorsogluteal site. Make sure you can see the area well. Have the client lower the undergarment, or move aside the hospital gown. Locate the site by drawing an imaginary line between the anatomic landmarks of the posterior superior iliac spine and the greater trochanter. Administer the injection lateral and slightly superior to the midpoint of this line (Figure 20-16).

Vastus Lateralis Site. The vastus lateralis muscle is a thick, well-developed muscle located on the anterolateral aspect of the thigh. In the adult, it extends from a handbreadth above the knee to a handbreadth below the greater trochanter. It measures in width from the midline of the top of the thigh to the midline of the lateral thigh. It is easiest to use this site by injecting the outer middle third of the thigh (Figure 20-17). This is a preferred injection site for adults, children, and infants. It is especially useful in children whose gluteal muscles are poorly developed. There are no large nerves or blood vessels in the area, and the muscle does not lie over a joint. The client may lie supine or be in a sitting position during injection as long as the leg muscles are relaxed.

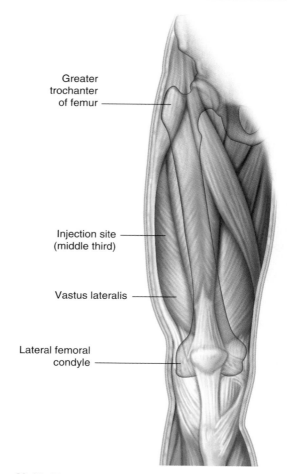

Figure 20-17. Vastus lateralis intramuscular injection site on the right thigh. Divide the thigh into thirds; give the injection in the middle third.

The rectus femoris muscle is located on the midanterior thigh and is another well-developed muscle that lies away from blood vessels and nerves (Figure 20-18, p. 430). It can safely be used in adults, children, and infants. This site is not as popular, however, because it can cause discomfort. In general, it is only used if other sites are contraindicated.

Deltoid Site. The deltoid muscle is found on the lateral aspect of the upper arm. It is not used as often as other sites because it is a small muscle, incapable of absorbing large medication volumes. The deltoid muscle should not be used in infants and children because of its size. In adults, injected volumes should not exceed 1 mL. The client may sit or lie down during injection as long as the arm is relaxed against the body to minimize muscle tension and resistance.

Locate the site by palpating the lower edge of the acromion process. Inject the area that lies two to three fingerbreadths below the acromion process in adults. An alternative method is to locate the triangular muscle area that extends from 2.5 to 5 fingerbreadths below the acromion process (Figure 20-19, p. 430). In a child, locate the site one fingerbreadth below the acromion process.

Air-Lock Technique. Some clinicians use an air lock when giving IM injections. A 0.2-mL air bubble may be drawn into

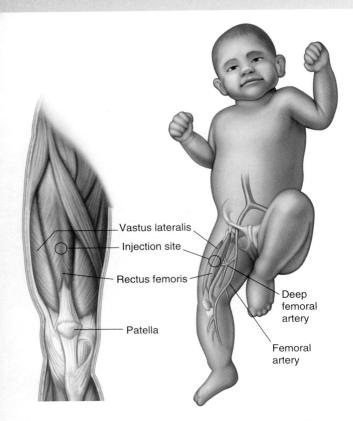

Vastus lateralis

Injection site

Rectus femoris

Patella

Deep femoral artery

Femoral artery

Figure 20-18. Rectus femoris intramuscular injection site on the anterior part of the thigh (used in adults only if other sites are contraindicated). In children, the site is located one third the distance from the patella to the greater trochanter in the center of the anterior thigh.

a syringe and injected to prevent tracking of irritating medication through SC tissue when the needle is withdrawn. Because this procedure is less frequently used than in the past, determine and follow agency policies and procedures about use of air locks. When giving a Z-track medication, use an air lock according to agency policy (see next paragraphs).

Z-Track Method. The Z-track method for giving IM injections seals the medication within muscle tissue. It minimizes tissue irritation by preventing tracking of medication through subcutaneous tissue with needle removal after injection. Although previously used only when giving irritating or tissue-staining medications such as iron dextran (Imferon), Z-track is now being used more frequently to minimize pain and discomfort at any IM injection site.

Use the Z-track technique when giving injections in the ventrogluteal or dorsogluteal areas (Figure 20-20). After drawing up the medication and adding a 0.2-mL air lock, change the needle to ensure that medication is not tracked into SC tissue during needle insertion. The needle should be at least 1.5 inches long. Pull the skin and subcutaneous tissue about 1 to 1.5 inches (2.5 to 3.5 cm) to one side using your nondominant hand. Inject the medication as usual, count to 10 to allow for distribution of medication, withdraw the needle, and release the tissue. The tissue glides back into normal position, eliminating the needle track. Apply gentle pressure over the area, but do not massage (to avoid forcing medication back into the needle track).

INTRAVENOUS MEDICATIONS. The IV route is chosen when medication effect is needed within 1 to 2 minutes or when the medication is irritating to subcutaneous or muscle tissue. Use extreme caution and follow the six "rights" of

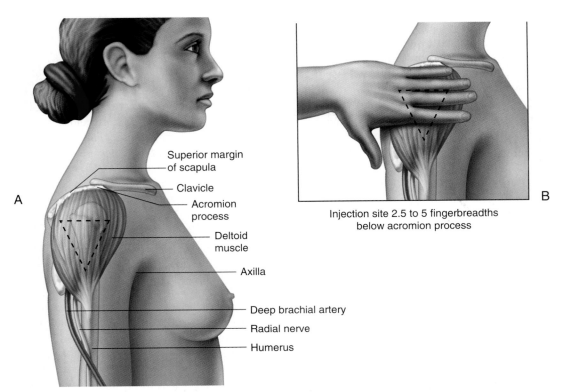

A

Superior margin of scapula

Clavicle

Acromion process

Deltoid muscle

Axilla

Deep brachial artery

Radial nerve

Humerus

B

Injection site 2.5 to 5 fingerbreadths below acromion process

Figure 20-19. **A,** Deltoid muscle injection site in the upper arm. **B,** Locate the site in the triangular area 2.5 to 5 fingerbreadths below the acromion process.

medication administration when using the IV route. If there is an antidote to an IV medication, it should be readily available for emergency use.

Generally, there are three possible methods for giving an IV medication: added to an IV solution, IV piggyback, and IV push. When medication is added directly to a bag or bottle of IV solution, it infuses slowly but continuously into the client. When available, special transfer devices simplify the transfer of medication to an IV solution. See Procedure 20-8 for the correct method for adding medication to an IV solution.

A second method of IV medication administration is the intermittent IV piggyback (IVPB) setup (most common) or an

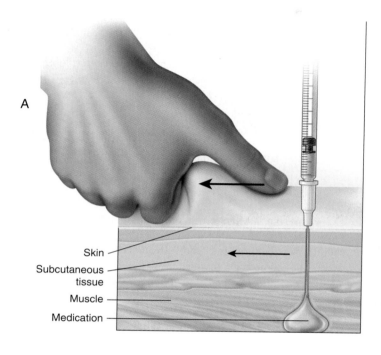
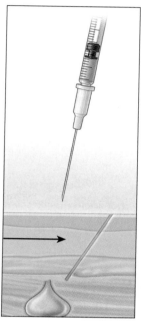

Skin
Subcutaneous tissue
Muscle
Medication

Figure 20-20. Intramuscular injection using the Z-track technique. **A,** pull the skin and subcutaneous tissue 1 to 1.5 inches (2.5 to 3.5 cm) to the side with the thumb or the side of the hand, and inject the medication. **B,** Withdraw the needle, and release the tissue to seal the medication in the muscle.

PROCEDURE 20-8 ADDING MEDICATION TO AN IV BAG

TIME TO ALLOW
Novice: 8 min.
Expert: 3 min.

Some medications are given to clients as part of an intravenous (IV) infusion. The pharmacy may add the medication to the IV infusion bag, or you may need to do it.

DELEGATION GUIDELINES
You may not delegate the addition of medication to an IV bag to a nursing assistant.

EQUIPMENT NEEDED
- Medication order, medication administration record, computerized medication order sheet, or medication Kardex or cards
- Medication vial or ampule

- IV solution
- Medication label
- Sterile syringe and needle of appropriate size (3 to 20 mL and 1 to 1.5-inch, 19 to 21 gauge)
- Needle filter, if appropriate
- Two alcohol swabs
- Disposable gloves

1. Follow preliminary guidelines for nursing procedures (see inside front cover).

2. Check the medication order.

3. Withdraw the medication from the ampule or vial as described in Procedures 20-2 (p. 418) and 20-3 (p. 419).

4. Inject the medication into the bag of IV solution.

PROCEDURE 20-8   ADDING MEDICATION TO AN IV BAG—CONT'D

a. Close the roller clamp on the tubing attached to the IV solution. *This step prevents fluid loss from the IV bag.*

b. Wipe the medication port of the bag containing the IV solution. *Doing so prevents contamination of the needle by microorganisms on the outside of the port.*

c. Insert the needle into the center of the medication port and inject medication from syringe into the solution bag (see illustration). *Using the center of the port prevents accidental puncture of the sides of the port or the IV container.*

d. Withdraw the needle and discard the needle and syringe, without recapping the needle, in an approved receptacle.

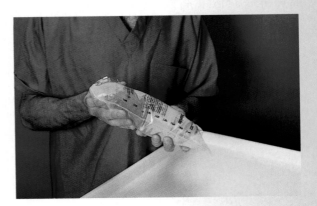

Step 4e. Rotating the solution bag.

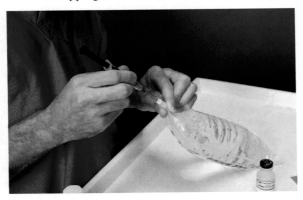

Step 4c. Inserting the needle into the center of the medication port.

e. Rotate the solution bag gently but thoroughly (see illustration). *Rotation distributes the medication evenly throughout the IV solution.*

f. Write the name and dose of the medication, the date, the time, and your initials on a medication label. Affix the label to the IV bag without obstructing the name of the solution or the IV time-tape. *The label clearly identifies what you added to the IV solution without hampering your ability to identify the solution or determine whether the IV is infusing on time.*

g. Dispose of the medication container, alcohol swab, wrapper, and any other used materials in an appropriate receptacle.

5. Prime the tubing, bring the container to the client's room, and hang the solution bag according to standard procedure. Set the drip rate carefully. Follow all procedures needed to monitor IV therapy properly. *This step prevents medication error and possible fluid overload.*

6. Document the date, time, IV solution used, and additive used on the client's medication administration record or other IV charting form.

HOME CARE CONSIDERATIONS

The administration of IV medications is a growing trend in home care. Clients include people with AIDS, cancer, and other serious illnesses. In home care settings today, you may administer chemotherapy, acyclovir, total parenteral nutrition, blood, and medications that were at one time administered only in a hospital setting. You will need to assess for the effects and side effects of medications, recognize serious or life-threatening reactions, and know how to respond. Clients receiving IV medications at home may have prefilled epinephrine (Adrenalin) syringes in the event of an anaphylactic reaction.

IV tandem setup (Figure 20-21). The IVPB method uses gravity to determine flow rate. A roller clamp is used to adjust the flow rate of these infusions as well. The secondary solution (Table 20-8) is plugged into an intermittent IV infusion device using long tubing, or it is added to a primary IV line using either a needle or a needleless system. Preparation and administration of an intermittent IV medication are described in Procedure 20-9 (p. 435).

Use an infusion control pump to control the infusion rate of an intermittent IV medication. Make sure the alarm is always turned on to alert you if the line infiltrates or other problems arise. Remember that these devices are adjuncts to nursing care, not substitutes for careful nursing assessment.

The third method for administering an IV medication is IV push. As with an intermittent IV infusion, you may give IV push medications through a mainline IV or an intermittent infusion device. Medications are usually injected over 1 minute or longer, according to drug literature. If an intermittent infusion device is used, flush the line with normal saline (or, occasionally, heparin) according to facility policy

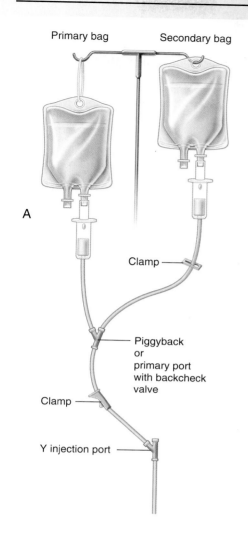

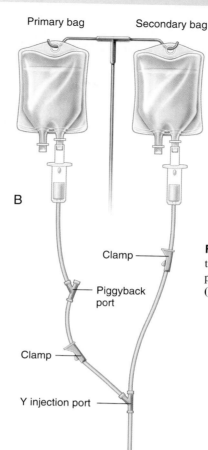

Figure 20-21. Intermittent IV medication administration can be accomplished with the use of IV piggyback (**A**) or tandem (**B**) setups.

to verify that the line is patent. Procedure 20-10 (p. 437) describes how to administer an IV push medication.

Regardless of the specific method used, universal principles apply to the preparation and administration of IV medications. Be especially careful to select the correct medication and draw up the correct dose. Use proper technique when withdrawing medication from a vial or ampule, and wipe the IV port with an alcohol swab before adding the medication or entering the IV line. Label the syringe or bag according to facility policy with the medication name, dose, date, time, and your name or initials. Do not apply a label until you have actually added a medication.

Before giving an IV medication, assess the IV line for patency, and the site for signs of phlebitis (local tenderness, redness, and warmth) or infiltration (local coolness, firmness, pain, and swelling). Refer to Chapter 25 for further discussion of IV site assessment. If signs of phlebitis or infiltration are found, do not use the line; start a new IV line before proceeding. Severe tissue damage could result if irritating medications are injected into an infiltrated IV line. A vein with signs of phlebitis could be damaged further by injection of an IV medication, or the line may be resistant to flushing. Periodically assess the status of the client and the line during the infusion to detect early signs of complications or untoward reactions.

Clients who have veins of poor quality or who require IV medication therapy for prolonged periods may undergo percutaneous insertion of a central venous catheter. Such a catheter may have multiple lumens or a single lumen. Other central venous lines are implanted surgically and are accessed using specific techniques. Such lines may be implanted in clients who need chemotherapy. Adhere to facility policies and procedures when giving IV medications through these catheters. Use strict surgical aseptic technique when accessing these lines, because organisms introduced into a central line could lead rapidly to sepsis.

Managing Topical Medications. Topical medications are often used to produce an anesthetic effect, create a systemic effect, or relieve local irritation or infection. Most are given two to three times a day.

SKIN APPLICATIONS. A medication applied to the skin is manufactured in the form of a cream, lotion, ointment, powder, paste, or patch (also called a disk). Before giving a topical medication, assess the client's skin for breakdown, lesions, rashes, or erythema. The medication may be ordered to treat one of these conditions, or the condition may indicate that the medication should not be applied to that surface,

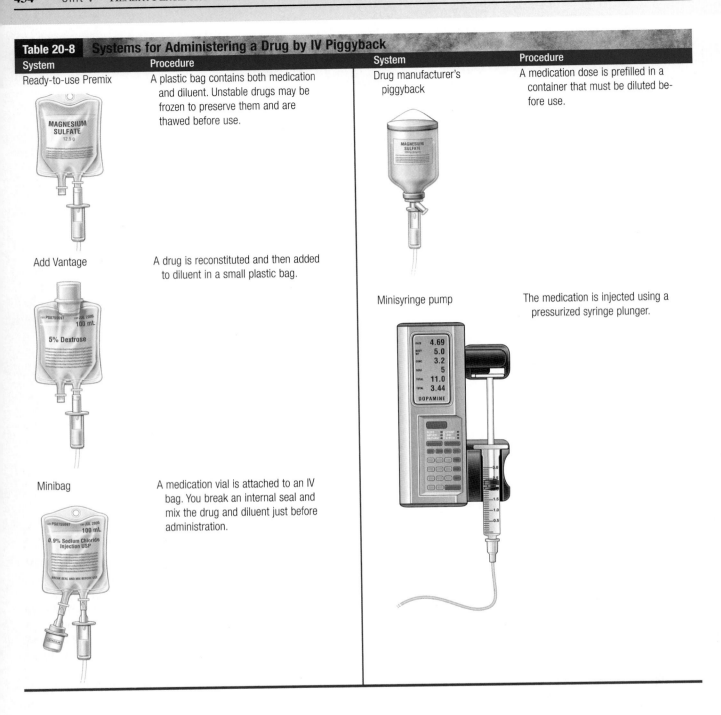

Table 20-8	**Systems for Administering a Drug by IV Piggyback**		
System	**Procedure**	**System**	**Procedure**
Ready-to-use Premix	A plastic bag contains both medication and diluent. Unstable drugs may be frozen to preserve them and are thawed before use.	Drug manufacturer's piggyback	A medication dose is prefilled in a container that must be diluted before use.
Add Vantage	A drug is reconstituted and then added to diluent in a small plastic bag.	Minisyringe pump	The medication is injected using a pressurized syringe plunger.
Minibag	A medication vial is attached to an IV bag. You break an internal seal and mix the drug and diluent just before administration.		

depending on the medication and client circumstances. Use standard precautions when administering a topical drug to protect yourself from contact with the medication and the client's secretions. These precautions also protect the client from microorganisms on your hands.

Before giving a topical medication, cleanse the area with soap and water unless contraindicated. Use sterile procedure as indicated for cleansing an open wound. Medication does not absorb as readily if the skin has accumulated oils, dead cells, or encrustations from lesions. Body oil also reduces the adhesive properties of patches, disks, or tape. Unless there is an open wound or lesion, apply topical medications to dry skin.

Use principles of asepsis when handling topical medications. Use a tongue depressor or swab to remove creams, pastes, or ointments from the original container, such as a jar. Use a new swab or depressor to remove additional medication from the container. If the medication comes in a tube, squeeze the medication onto an applicator before use. Do not squeeze it directly onto the skin. Apply medication evenly using long, smooth strokes, moving in the direction of hair growth to prevent the medication from accumulating in hair follicles. Assess the skin within 2 to 4 hours of the application to assess the medication's effects and possible allergic reaction.

PROCEDURE 20-9 | ADMINISTERING AN IV MEDICATION BY INTERMITTENT INFUSION

TIME TO ALLOW
Novice: 10 min.
Expert: 5 min.

An intermittent intravenous (IV) infusion is administered when a medication to be given by the IV route requires a longer infusion time (typically 30 to 90 minutes) than IV push provides. It is connected into a primary IV line by IVPB or tandem setup or connected to an intermittent infusion device (saline lock).

DELEGATION GUIDELINES
You may not delegate the administration of IV medication by intermittent infusion to a nursing assistant.

EQUIPMENT NEEDED
- Medication order, medication administration record, computerized medication order sheet, or medication Kardex or cards
- Medication premixed in a 50-mL to 250-mL infusion bag (usually 50 to 150 mL), clearly labeled
- Macrodrip or microdrip tubing of appropriate length (primary tubing if attaching to a heparin lock, secondary tubing if attaching to a primary IV line)
- Needleless IV connector or 21- to 23-gauge needle
- Metal or plastic hook (if adding to a primary IV line) or a vial of sterile normal saline and two 3-mL syringes with attached needles (if giving medication through a heparin lock)
- Alcohol swab
- Disposable gloves
- Tape (optional)

1. Follow preliminary guidelines for nursing procedures (see inside front cover).

2. Check the medication order and assess the client's allergies.

3. Prepare the medication at the medication cart or another designated area. Label the IV medication bag/bottle if the pharmacy has not done so already.

4. Administer the medication.

ADMINISTRATION THROUGH AN EXISTING IV LINE (IVPB OR TANDEM SETUP)
a. Attach secondary tubing to the IV bag or bottle that contains the medication according to standard IV therapy protocol. *Tubing may be used for 48 to 96 hours from the time of initial use in most facilities.*
b. Make sure to use nonvented tubing for an IV bag and vented tubing for an IV bottle. Also make sure that the roller clamp on the tubing is closed before attaching the tubing.
c. Prime the tubing and label the secondary IV bag and the tubing with the date, time, and your initials.
d. Bring the medication administration record, IV bag with medication, needle or needleless device, alcohol swab, metal hook, gloves, and tape to client's room.
e. Identify the client using an identification bracelet or other acceptable means.
f. Assess the IV site and put on gloves if the facility requires it.
g. Remove the cap from the distal end of the IV tubing and attach the needle or needleless device.

h. Wipe the IV additive port on the primary line with an alcohol swab and attach the needle or needleless device. Make sure to attach the medication above the flow regulator clamp on the primary line. Although needleless systems are typically manufactured to secure tightly to the IV port, tape the connection if needed for stability. *Cleaning with alcohol prevents the IV line from contamination with microorganisms from the exterior IV port. Attaching above the regulator clamp allows you to regulate the flow rate.*
i. Lower the primary IV solution below the level of the IV medication bag using the metal or plastic hook provided with the secondary tubing set. *The IV medication flows and the primary bag stops flowing because of the effects of gravity.*
j. Regulate the drip rate of the IV medications as ordered, or set the infusion pump rate and volume. Check to be sure that it is running and monitor to determine that the client is tolerating the medication. *If you use a regulator clamp below the site where the IVPB is connected, the primary bag will start flowing when the IVPB is empty.*
k. Come back when the medication has infused and reset the drip rate on the primary line. *Unless readjusted, the primary line will continue to infuse at the rate set for the secondary infusion. If you use an infusion pump, the primary rate should resume once secondary medication is infused.*
l. Reassess the IV site and the client's tolerance of the medication.

Administering an IV Medication by Intermittent Infusion—Cont'd

Administration Through an Intermittent Infusion Device (Saline Lock)

a. Close the roller clamp and attach tubing of adequate length (70″ or longer) to the IV medication bag or bottle according to standard IV therapy protocol. Use nonvented tubing for an IV bag and vented tubing for an IV bottle. Prime the tubing. *Closing the clamp prevents loss of the medication through the tubing. Choosing correctly vented tubing ensures that solution will flow through the tubing. Priming the tubing removes air from the system.*

b. Using standard procedure, draw 3 mL of sterile normal saline solution into a 3-mL syringe (or another solution or amount according to facility policy). *An intermittent infusion device is flushed both before and after use to ensure patency.*

c. Bring the medication administration record, IV medication bag, needle or needleless device, syringe with flush, alcohol swab, gloves, and tape to client's room.

d. Identify client using an identification bracelet or other acceptable means.

e. Assess the IV site and put on gloves if required by your facility.

f. Remove the cap from the distal end of the IV tubing. Attach the needle or needleless device and prime. *Priming removes air from the system.*

g. Wipe the port of the intermittent infusion device with an alcohol swab.

h. Assess the site and flush the infusion device port with sterile saline solution or other ordered solution.

i. Attach the IV medication bag to the infusion device port using the needle or needleless device (see illustration). Tape the connection if needed.

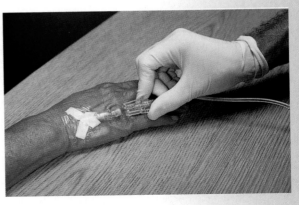

Step 4i. Using a needleless device, attach the IV medication bag to the infusion device port.

j. Regulate the drip rate of the IV medication as ordered. Monitor the client to ensure the client is tolerating the medication.

k. Once the medication has infused, close the roller clamp, and remove the tubing from the port. Recap or attach a clean needle or needleless device to the tubing according to facility policy. *Most facilities allow IV tubing to be reused for 48 to 96 hours after the initial use, if sterility has been maintained.*

l. Reassess the IV site and flush the infusion port with a second syringe filled with the ordered flush solution (often normal saline). Evaluate client response to the medication.

5. Document the date, time, and IV medication given on the client's medication administration record or computerized medication record.

Depending on the type of application, special techniques may be used to enhance medication effectiveness or to protect the client or nurse. Powders are usually applied to prevent friction on the skin and to promote drying. When using powder, apply it lightly and evenly, being careful not to inhale the particles.

Ointments remain in contact with skin for a long time and tend to soften the skin. Massage ointments into skin that is intact. Creams or oils are often used to treat dry or cracked skin. When applying these products to large areas, warm them in your hands before use to keep the client from becoming chilled. Lotions protect and soothe irritated skin. Shake lotions well before use and apply them with gauze or cotton

Pastes (such as nitroglycerin) may be applied for the purpose of systemic absorption. Remove the old dose before applying a new one and rotate sites to avoid skin irritation. Measure these doses carefully using paper supplied by the manufacturer to avoid under- or overdosing.

The newest form of topical administration is the transdermal patch or disk, which allows for time-release medication absorption through the skin. This limits the number of applications needed to maintain the therapeutic effect and reduces fluctuations in circulating drug levels. A transdermal patch may be applied daily or may be left in place as long as 7 days. Examples of drugs administered by this route include nitroglycerin, estrogen, fentanyl, and scopolamine. Box 20-11 (p. 439) outlines important guidelines for using a transdermal patch.

PROCEDURE 20-10	ADMINISTERING AN IV PUSH MEDICATION

TIME TO ALLOW
Novice: 10 min.
Expert: 5 min.

Push means the medication is mixed in a small amount of fluid (usually 1 to 10 mL) and administered directly into the vein (not mixed with IV fluid) over a short time (usually 1 to 5 minutes). The bolus of medication is given by the intravenous (IV) push method when the client needs an immediate effect or the medication cannot be mixed with the fluid. Product literature indicates whether a specific medication can be given using this method.

DELEGATION GUIDELINES
You may not delegate the administration of IV push medication to a nursing assistant.

EQUIPMENT NEEDED
- Medication order, medication administration record, computerized medication order sheet, or medication Kardex or cards
- Medication vial or ampule
- Syringe of appropriate size for the medication dose ordered, with a 21- to 23-gauge needle attached
- Vial of sterile normal saline and two 3-mL syringes with attached needles (if using an intermittent infusion device)
- If a needleless system is used, one needleless device if injecting through a mainline IV and three devices if injecting via an intermittent infusion device
- Alcohol swabs
- Disposable gloves

1. Follow preliminary guidelines for nursing procedures (see inside front cover).

2. Check the medication order and assess the client's allergies.

3. Prepare the medication at the medication cart or other designated area. *Preparing the medication before going to the bedside helps to reduce the client's anxiety.*

4. Administer the medication.

ADMINISTRATION THROUGH AN EXISTING IV LINE
a. Draw up the medication from an ampule or a vial as described in previous procedures. Be certain it reads "for IV use." Recap the needle using one-handed technique. Label the syringe with the medication and dose.

b. Remove the capped needle and attach a needleless device if a needleless system is in use.
c. Bring the medication administration record, IV medication, alcohol swab, and gloves to the client's room.
d. Identify the client using an identification bracelet or other acceptable means.
e. Assess the IV site and put on gloves if the facility requires it.
f. Wipe the IV additive port of the primary line with an alcohol swab. Make sure that the port being used is the port nearest to the client. *Using the closest port ensures the least resistance to flow of medication and helps to control the rate at which the medication reaches client's bloodstream.*
g. Be sure the medication is compatible with the solution in the tubing, then insert the needle into the port and pinch off the tubing above the injection port (see illustrations).

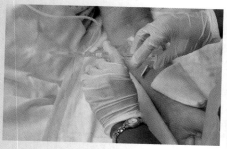
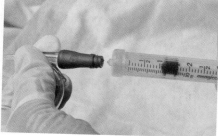
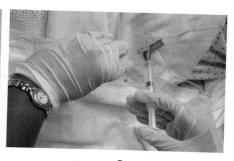

A   B   C

Step 4g. A, Blunt tip plastic access device inserted into needleless port. **B,** Using a syringe to access a needleless access container. **C,** Clamping the tubing to ensure forward injection of medication.

PROCEDURE 20-10 ADMINISTERING AN IV PUSH MEDICATION—CONT'D

Pinching ensures that the medication flows into the client's vein and not upward into the IV tubing. If it is not compatible, remove the IV tubing from the infusion device port; flush the port with a compatible solution, give the medication, then flush the port again and reconnect the IV tubing.

h. Inject the medication slowly and steadily at the rate recommended by the manufacturer. Use a watch to ensure accurate timing. Assess the IV site during injection. *Overly rapid injection could be harmful to the client or cause IV infiltration. Injection that is too slow is not useful and could produce anxiety.*

i. Release the tubing, remove the syringe, and assess the client's tolerance of the medication.

ADMINISTRATION THROUGH AN INTERMITTENT INFUSION DEVICE (HEPARIN LOCK)

a. Draw up sterile normal saline (or another ordered flush solution) into 2 syringes of 3 mL each (or another ordered volume) according to facility policy using Procedure 20-3 for drawing medication out of a vial. Label the syringes. *An intermittent infusion device is flushed with normal saline both before and after use to ensure patency.*

b. Draw up the ordered medication into a syringe from an ampule or a vial (see Procedures 20-2 or 20-3). Recap the needle using one-handed technique. Label the syringe.

c. Bring the IV medication, needle or needleless devices, syringes with flush solution, alcohol swabs, and gloves to the client's room.

d. Identify the client using an identification bracelet or other acceptable means.

e. Assess the IV site and put on gloves if the facility requires it.

f. Wipe the port of the intermittent infusion device with an alcohol swab.

g. Insert one syringe filled with flush solution and inject it slowly into the client. Remove the syringe. *If the line does not flush, evaluate it for patency and placement.*

h. Wipe the port again with an alcohol swab.

i. Insert the syringe containing the medication and inject it slowly and steadily at the rate recommended by the manufacturer. Use a watch with a second-hand to ensure accurate timing. Assess the IV site during the injection. Remove the syringe. *Overly rapid injection could be harmful to the client or cause IV infiltration. Injection that is too slow is not useful and could produce anxiety.*

j. Wipe the port again with another alcohol swab.

k. Insert the second syringe containing flush solution and inject it slowly into the client. Remove syringe and continue to assess the client's tolerance of the medication.

l. Dispose of supplies properly and discard syringe in rigid needle disposal container.

5. Document the date, the time, and the IV medication given on the medication administration record or computerized medication record.

EYE APPLICATIONS AND IRRIGATIONS. Ophthalmic (eye) medications are available as drops, ointments, and disks. They are commonly used for diagnostic reasons or to treat problems such as glaucoma or eye infection. Although the eye is not a sterile area, conjunctival secretions protect the eye against many pathogens, and eye medications are administered as a sterile procedure. Eyedrops have a water base and are easily instilled. Ointments have an oily base and stay in place longer. Because of their composition, eye ointments can cause blurred vision for a period of time after application. If both an eyedrop and an eye ointment are scheduled to be given at the same time, give the eyedrop first.

Disks, which may resemble a contact lens, are the newest form of ocular medication. Disks have prolonged action and can stay in place for up to a week. They are best inserted at bedtime because they may cause temporary blurred vision after insertion.

Because the cornea is sensitive and easily damaged, eye medications are placed in the lower conjunctival sac, not directly on the eyeball. Methods for instilling eyedrops, ointments, and disks are described in Procedure 20-11 (p. 440).

Cross-contamination is a major concern with the use of ocular medications. Follow these guidelines and teach them to clients as appropriate to decrease the risk of infection:

- Do not use eyedrops prescribed for one client on another client. Teach the client not to share them with family or friends.
- Apply ointments from the inner canthus to the outer canthus.
- Apply drops into the lower conjunctival sac.
- Apply medication only to the affected eye.
- Avoid touching the eye with the dropper or tube. Discard and replace contaminated items.

Purpose: To maintain optimal medication effect by using a transdermal patch correctly.

Expected Outcome: The client verbalizes and demonstrates correct application and removal of a transdermal patch.

Client Instructions

- Clean the skin prior to application. Apply the patch to a hairless site on your body. Avoid sites at the ends of your arms and legs. Also avoid areas with cuts or calluses that could interfere with absorption of the medication.
- Use firm pressure when applying the patch, especially around the edges, to ensure good contact with the skin.
- If the patch loosens or falls off, apply a new one. The medication is time-released through the special backing on the patch, so you cannot overdose by replacing a loose patch.
- Do not cut or trim the patch, because doing so would interfere with the time-release absorption of the medication through the special backing.
- Because transdermal patches are waterproof, you may shower or bathe as usual.
- Do not change brands of a transdermal patch without checking first with your physician. The dosage may or may not be equivalent.
- Apply and remove the patch as directed. Some patches remain in place for 12 to 14 hours and then are removed for 10 to 12 hours to prevent tolerance from developing (such as with nitroglycerin). Others can be left in place for 3 days (scopolamine) to 7 days (clonidine). Ask your physician, nurse, or pharmacist if you have questions about how to use your patch.

- Discard unused solution that remains in the dropper after instillation.
- Once opened, try to keep the drug at the bedside rather than replacing it on medication cart.

At times, an eye irrigation is needed to remove secretions from an eye before giving an ophthalmic medication. Irrigation can also be done in an emergency if the eye sustains chemical injury by caustic chemicals. In most emergency situations, the eye should be irrigated for at least 15 minutes with sterile eyewash, if available, or with copious amounts of tap water. The client should obtain professional follow-up after an emergency irrigation. Never irrigate an eye if there is a penetrating eye injury. Procedure 20-12 (p. 442) describes how to perform a routine eye irrigation.

EAR INSTILLATIONS AND IRRIGATIONS. The external ear is not sterile and consists of the external auditory canal and the pinna. The middle and inner ear lie behind the tympanic membrane and are sterile areas. Because a rupture of the tympanic membrane would create an opening between these areas, sterile solutions should be used prophylactically for instillation or irrigation of the ear.

Ear instillations require special care. Warm the solution to body temperature before use if possible, but at least give it at room temperature to prevent vertigo and nausea. Avoid using excessive force when instilling medication or irrigating an ear, to avoid rupturing the tympanic membrane. Do not occlude the auditory meatus during these procedures for the same reason. Assess ear drainage carefully to detect possible infection (Chapter 37).

Otic (ear) medications exert a local effect and are commonly used to soften earwax, fight infection, relieve pain, or destroy an insect trapped in the canal. Different approaches are used when administering otic medications to adults and to children because of differences in the shape of the ear canal. Pull the pinna of an adult's ear up and back to straighten the canal before administering eardrops or ear irrigation. In contrast, pull the pinna of an infant or young child down and back. The recommended methods for administering an ear medication are given in Procedure 20-13 (p. 443).

NASAL INSTILLATIONS. Medications are given by the nasal route to relieve the symptoms of sinus colds and congestion, shrink swollen mucous membranes, loosen nasal secretions, and treat nasal or sinus infection. Occasionally, medications are used for a systemic effect (such as vasopressin). Nasal medications are generally available in the form of sprays (decongestants, vasopressin) or drops (antiinfectives).

Clients have ready access to a number of OTC nasal medications, so teach them carefully about their use. Decongestants, in particular, cause rebound nasal congestion when used to excess. Teach clients how to properly administer them for maximum effect. Warn clients about other active ingredients in these products. For example, many nasal decongestants contain sympathomimetics that exert a systemic effect and are not suitable for use with children or others who could be adversely affected. In these instances, suggest saline drops.

Use clean technique to administer a nasal medication unless the client has undergone nasal or sinus surgery; then use sterile technique. Properly position the client by tilting or hyperextending the head. Procedure 20-14 (p. 444) describes how to give an intranasal medication.

VAGINAL INSTILLATIONS. Vaginal medications are commonly used for contraception or to treat itching, pain, or discomfort from inflammation or infection. They are supplied as gels, creams, foams, or suppositories. Keep suppositories refrigerated to prevent them from melting. Depending on the product, you will administer the medication using a gloved hand and possibly an applicator. Allow the client to self-administer the medication if appropriate.

Before administering the medication, offer the client an opportunity to void. Administer it using standard precautions and aseptic technique as outlined in Procedure 20-15 (p. 445). Once the medication is in the body, it will melt and may produce drainage. For this reason, administer it at bedtime if possible. Offer the client a perineal pad to help absorb drainage. Especially when treating infection, provide meticulous perineal hygiene and carefully assess the characteristics of any drainage.

Text continued on p. 447

PROCEDURE 20-11	ADMINISTERING AN EYE MEDICATION

TIME TO ALLOW
Novice: 10 min.
Expert: 5 min.

A client with glaucoma, an eye infection, or a number of other ocular disorders will need ophthalmic (eye) medications instilled directly into the eye. Following this procedure will allow you to administer the medication without injuring sensitive eye tissue.

DELEGATION GUIDELINES

The administration of eye medications may not be delegated to a nursing assistant.

EQUIPMENT NEEDED

- Medication order, medication administration record, computerized medication order sheet, or medication Kardex or cards
- Medication bottle, tube, or disk
- Tissue or cotton ball
- Warm water and facecloth, as needed
- Disposable gloves

1. Follow preliminary guidelines for nursing procedures (see inside front cover).

2. Check the medication order, noting especially the eye to be treated. Note any client allergies.

3. Prepare the client for instillation of the medication.
   a. Identify the client using an identification bracelet or other accepted means.
   b. Explain the procedure to the client in a calm and confident manner. Help the client to sit or lie down with the head slightly hyperextended. Put on gloves. *This head position assists in correct medication placement and minimizes drainage through the tear duct.*
   c. Assess the condition of the client's eye. Wash away any exudate using the facecloth and warm water, wiping from the inner canthus to the outer canthus. *This observation provides baseline assessment data to evaluate the medication's effect. Removing exudate also removes microorganisms and provides a clean surface to apply the medication.*

4. Administer the medication.

EYEDROPS
   a. Remove the cap from the bottle and place it on its side. Fill the medication dropper (if used) to the prescribed amount. *This position prevents contamination of the cap.*
   b. Place your nondominant hand on the client's cheekbone just under the eyelid and pull downward against the bony orbit to expose the lower conjunctival sac. Hold tissue or a cotton ball under the eyelid and apply slight pressure to the inner canthus. *This action exposes the lower conjunctival sac while preventing pressure and trauma to the eye. Pressing on the inner canthus blocks*

the tear duct temporarily and prevents the medication from leaving the eye through the duct and possibly causing systemic effects.
   c. Rest your dominant hand against the client's forehead for stability and hold the medication bottle or dropper ½ to ¾ inch above the conjunctival sac. *Resting on the client's forehead stabilizes your hand and reduces the risk of contact between eye structures and the medication bottle, preventing trauma, infection, or both.*
   d. Ask the client to look up at the ceiling and then instill the prescribed number of drops into the lower conjunctival sac (see illustration). If the client closes the eye or blinks, or if a drop lands on the eyelid, repeat the missed drop. *Looking up reduces stimulation of the blink reflex and thus promotes accurate delivery of the dose into the conjunctival sac.*
   e. Ask the client to gently close the eye and move it around. Apply gentle pressure over the lacrimal duct for 1 minute or ask the client to do so if possible. *Moving the eye behind the closed lid helps to distribute the medication over the conjunctiva and eyeball. Gently closing it (not squinting or squeezing) prevents loss of medication from conjunctival sac. Pressing the lacrimal duct helps to prevent systemic absorption of the medication.*

EYE OINTMENT
   a. Remove the cap from the tube and place it on its side. Squeeze and discard a small bead of medication. *Placing the cap on its side helps to prevent contamination. The first bead of an ointment is considered contaminated.*
   b. For instillation in the lower lid, separate client's eyelids with the thumb and forefinger of your nondominant hand, pulling lower lid downward over the bony prominence of the cheek. (For instillation in the upper lid, draw upper lid up and away from eyeball.)

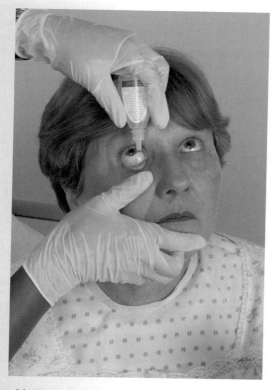

Step 4d. Eyedrops. Administering the prescribed number of drops into the lower conjunctival sac.

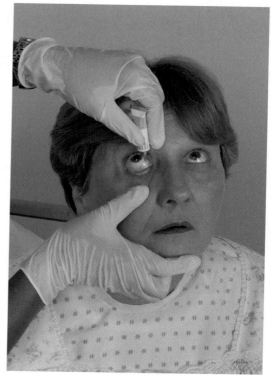

Step 4d. Eye ointment. Applying a thin line of ointment along the inside edge of the eyelid.

c. Ask the client to look up for instillation in the lower lid or down for instillation in the upper lid. *Looking up or down reduces stimulation of the blink reflex and rotates the sensitive cornea away from the medication.*

d. Apply a thin line of ointment along the inside edge of the lower or upper lid as ordered (see illustration), moving from the inner canthus to the outer canthus. *This method ensures aseptic and even distribution of medication as well as the proper dosage.*

e. Ask the client to gently close the eye and move it around. *Moving the eye behind closed lids helps to distribute medication over the conjunctiva and eyeball. Gently closing it (not squinting or squeezing) prevents loss of medication from conjunctival sac.*

MEDICATED EYE DISK

a. Open the package and press the tip of the index finger of your dominant hand against the convex part of disk. Doing so helps the disk adhere to your fingertip.

b. Pull the client's lower eyelid away from the eye with your nondominant hand and ask the client to look up. *This exposes the conjunctival sac and reduces the blink reflex.*

c. Place the disk horizontally in the conjunctival sac between the iris and the lower eyelid.

d. Pull the lower eyelid out, up, and over the disk. Ask the client to blink a few times. If the disk is visible, repeat this step. Otherwise, have the client press her fingers against the closed lids, without rubbing the eyes or moving the disk. *This action ensures proper disk position.*

e. If the disk falls out, rinse it with cool water and reinsert it. *Rinsing the disk reduces the risk of infection.*

f. To remove a disk, pull or invert the client's lower eyelid so you can see the disk, then use the thumb and index finger of your dominant hand to pinch the disk and lift it from the conjunctival sac. If it is in the upper eye, stroke the client's closed eyelid with your fingertip, gently and in long circular motions. Ask the client to open the eye, and look for the disk in the corner of the eye. Slide the disk to the lower lid and remove it as noted earlier. *This minimizes risk of trauma or infection while aiding removal of the disk.*

5. Remove gloves and perform hand hygiene.

6. Document the medication administration promptly on the medication administration record or computerized medication record.

PROCEDURE 20-12	IRRIGATING AN EYE

TIME TO ALLOW
Novice: 15 min.
Expert: 8 min.

Eye irrigation is used to remove infection or other foreign matter from the eye. It should not be done when the client has a penetrating eye injury because it could cause further injury. It can be done on a short-term intermittent basis or as a one-time order based on client need.

DELEGATION GUIDELINES
The performance of this procedure requires your expertise and skill and may not be delegated to a nursing assistant.

EQUIPMENT NEEDED
- Sterile irrigating solution warmed to body temperature
- Sterile irrigation set with irrigating or bulb syringe and a sterile container
- Emesis or curved irrigation basin
- Waterproof pad if not supplied with irrigation set
- Towel
- Cotton balls
- Disposable gloves

1. Follow preliminary guidelines for nursing procedures (see inside front cover).

2. Prepare the client for the irrigation.
a. Identify the client using an identification bracelet or other accepted means.
b. Explain the procedure to the client in a calm and confident manner.
c. Help the client to sit or lie with the head tilted toward the eye that will be irrigated. Place the waterproof pad under the affected side. Put on gloves. *This head position enlists the aid of gravity so solution flows from inner canthus to the outer canthus without flowing through the unaffected eye.*
d. Pour irrigant into the container and draw it into the syringe using aseptic technique.
e. Clean the client's eyelids and eyelashes with a cotton ball moistened with irrigant or normal saline solution. Wipe from the inner canthus to the outer canthus using a new cotton ball with each pass. *This step removes material on the lids and lashes that could be washed into the eye with irrigation.*
f. Place the curved basin under the affected cheek to catch the irrigating solution as it flows from the client's eye. Ask the client to hold the basin if possible.

3. Irrigate the eye.
a. Use your nondominant hand to hold the client's upper lid open and expose the lower conjunctival sac. *Using the conjunctival sac reduces stimulation of the blink reflex and prevents irrigant from injuring the cornea.*
b. Hold the irrigation syringe about 1 inch above the eye. Do not touch the eye with the syringe. Push fluid gently into the conjunctival sac, directing the flow from the inner canthus to the outer canthus. If agency policy allows, you may use approved IV solution (normal saline) with IV tubing, allowing the fluid to gently flow from the medial to the lateral side. *This process uses the least amount of pressure necessary to cleanse the eye while reducing the risk of injury to the eye or contamination of the eye.*
c. Repeat the irrigation until the secretions are gone or the irrigant is used up. Allow the client to close the eyes intermittently during procedure as needed. *Closed eye movements help to move secretions from the upper to the lower conjunctival area.*
d. Dry the area with cotton balls and offer the client a towel to dry the face and neck.

4. Remove gloves and perform hand hygiene.

5. Document the irrigation promptly in the client's medical record. Also record the appearance of the eye, characteristics of drainage, and the client's response to treatment.

PROCEDURE 20-13   ADMINISTERING AN EAR MEDICATION

TIME TO ALLOW
Novice: 8 min.
Expert: 3 min.

Ear infections are relatively common among children and are one of the most common reasons for administering a medication into the ear canal.

DELEGATION GUIDELINES

As with all medication administration procedures, you may not delegate the administration of ear medications to a nursing assistant.

EQUIPMENT NEEDED
- Medication administration record, computerized medication order sheet, or medication Kardex or cards
- Medication (eardrops)
- Tissue or cotton ball
- Cotton-tipped applicator
- Disposable gloves

1. Follow preliminary guidelines for nursing procedures (see inside front cover).

2. Check the medication order, and note any client allergies.

3. Prepare the client for instillation of the medication.
a. Identify the client using an identification bracelet or other accepted means.
b. Explain the procedure to the client in a calm and confident manner. Help the client to a side-lying position with the affected ear upward. Put on gloves. *This position assists in correct placement of medication and minimizes its drainage from the ear canal.*
c. Assess the condition of the ear. Gently wash away any cerumen or exudate using cotton-tipped applicators. Do not force wax or drainage into the ear canal. *This step provides baseline assessment data and cleans the area before application of the medication.*

4. Administer the medication.
a. Remove the cap from the bottle and place it on its side. Fill the medication dropper (if applicable) to prescribed amount. *Placing cap on its side prevents its contamination.*
b. Pull the pinna up and back in an adult client or down and back in a child (see illustration). *This step straightens the ear canal.*
c. Hold the dropper or bottle ½ inch above the ear canal and instill as many eardrops as ordered. *Holding the bottle above the ear canal avoids excess pressure in the canal.*
d. Ask the client to maintain the side-lying position for 2 to 3 minutes. Apply gentle pressure with your finger to the tragus of the ear or ask the client to do so. *Staying in the side-lying position helps to distribute the medication. Because ear infections are painful, the client may prefer to apply the pressure.*

e. Place a cotton ball into the outermost portion of the ear canal. *This helps to prevent medication loss when the client changes position.*
f. Remove your gloves and perform hand hygiene.

5. Document the medication administration promptly in the medication administration record or computerized medication record.

6. Check on the client in 15 minutes to remove the cotton ball from the ear, assess the client's condition, and help her to a comfortable position.

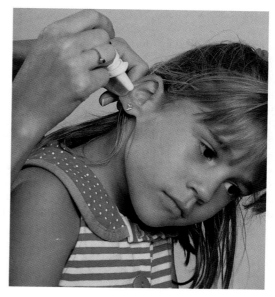

Step 4b. Pulling the pinna down and back.

PROCEDURE 20-14	ADMINISTERING AN INTRANASAL MEDICATION

TIME TO ALLOW
Novice: 8 min.
Expert: 3 min.

Intranasal medications may be ordered to produce local vasoconstriction of blood vessels or for administration of medications for rapid absorption through nasal mucous membranes.

DELEGATION GUIDELINES
You may not delegate the administration of intranasal medication to a nursing assistant.

EQUIPMENT NEEDED
- Medication order, medication administration record, computerized medication order sheet, or medication Kardex or cards
- Nasal spray or drops
- Facial tissue
- Disposable gloves

1. Follow preliminary guidelines for nursing procedures (see inside front cover).

2. Check the medication order and note any client allergies.

3. Prepare the client for instillation of the medication.
   a. Identify the client using an identification bracelet or other accepted means.
   b. Explain the procedure to the client. Mention that the solution may cause choking, stinging, or burning as it drips into the throat. Put on gloves.
   c. Ask the client to the blow the nose unless contraindicated because of risk of nosebleed or increased intracranial pressure. Assess the resulting discharge. *Blowing the nose removes secretions that could interfere with the effectiveness of the medication.*

4. Administer the medication.

ADMINISTRATION OF A NASAL SPRAY
a. Remove the cap from the bottle and place it on its side. *This position prevents contamination of the medication's cap.*
b. Ask an adult client to tilt the head backward and support the head with your nondominant hand. Keep a child's head in an upright position. *This position allows the medication to reach nasal passages without causing the client to swallow it. Supporting the client's head reduces neck strain.*
c. Hold the medication container just inside the tip of the nostril without touching nasal tissue (see illustration). Ask the client to occlude the opposite nostril and inhale while you administer the spray. *Avoiding contact between the container and the nasal tissue prevents contamination of container. Occluding the opposite nostril while inhaling through the target nostril provides maximum effectiveness of the medication.*

d. Assist the client to a comfortable position.

ADMINISTRATION OF NASAL DROPS
a. Remove cap from bottle and place on its side.
b. Position the client to accommodate the intended site of action and support her head with your nondominant hand. For the posterior pharynx, tilt the client's head backward. For the ethmoid or sphenoid sinus, either tilt the client's head back and place a pillow under one shoulder or tilt the head back over the edge of the mattress while supporting the back of the head with your nondominant hand. For the frontal or maxillary sinus, assume the position just described and turn the client's head toward the affected side.

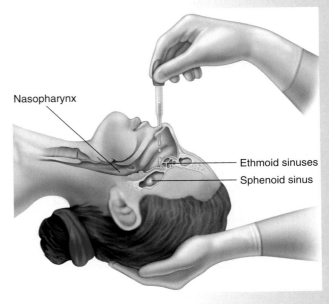

Nasopharynx

Ethmoid sinuses

Sphenoid sinus

Step 4c. Proper position for instillation of nasal medication.

c. Hold the tip of the dropper just above the intended nostril and pointed toward the midline of the ethmoid bone (see illustration). Do not touch the client's nasal tissue with the dropper. Ask client to mouth-breathe, and instill the ordered number of drops. *This process provides the greatest medication effectiveness and prevents contamination of the container.*

d. Ask the client to maintain this position for 5 minutes and then assist to a comfortable position. Maintaining position prevents leakage of medication from the nose and promotes medication absorption.

5. Remove gloves and perform hand hygiene.

6. Document the medication administration promptly on the medication administration record or computerized medication record.

7. Wash nasal spray devices daily in lukewarm water. If used for infection, the remainder should be discarded when no longer needed.

PROCEDURE 20-15   ADMINISTERING A VAGINAL MEDICATION

TIME TO ALLOW
Novice: 15 min.
Expert: 7 min.

Vaginal instillations are usually performed to treat infection. They may also be used by the client as part of a contraceptive method.

DELEGATION GUIDELINES
You may not delegate the administration of vaginal medication to a nursing assistant.

EQUIPMENT NEEDED
- Medication administration record, computerized medication order sheet, or medication Kardex or cards
- Vaginal medication and applicator, if needed
- Water-soluble lubricant
- Perineal pad, if needed
- Cotton balls or facecloth and towel for cleansing, if needed
- Disposable tissue
- Disposable gloves

---

1. Follow preliminary guidelines for nursing procedures (see inside front cover).

2. Check the medication order.

3. Prepare the client for instillation of the medication.

a. Identify client using an identification bracelet or another accepted means.

b. Explain the procedure to the client. Offer her an opportunity to void. Close the curtain or door and help her to a supine position with the abdomen and legs draped. *Maintaining privacy is an important step in this type of medication administration.*

c. Put on gloves.

d. Inspect the client's external genitalia and provide perineal hygiene as needed.

4. Administer the medication using clean technique.

ADMINISTRATION OF A SUPPOSITORY

a. Remove the suppository from its wrapper and insert into the applicator, if used. *Use of either a gloved finger or an applicator is acceptable.*

b. Lubricate the rounded end of the suppository with water-soluble lubricant. If you will not be using an applicator, also lubricate the index finger of your gloved, dominant hand. *Lubrication allows easier insertion by reducing friction.*

c. Separate the client's labia with your nondominant hand and insert the rounded end of the suppository along the posterior vaginal wall for an entire fingerlength (see illustration, p. 446). *This distance ensures complete insertion of the medication and distribution through the entire vagina.*

d. Withdraw your finger or the applicator and wipe away excess lubricant from the genitals.

Continued

PROCEDURE 20-15	ADMINISTERING A VAGINAL MEDICATION—Cont'd

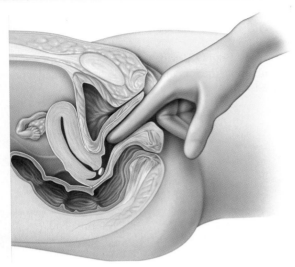

Step 4c. Inserting the vaginal suppository.

ADMINISTRATION OF A FOAM, JELLY, OR CREAM

a. Fill applicator with medication according to the package directions.

b. Separate the client's labia with your nondominant hand, point the applicator toward her sacrum, and use your dominant hand to insert it 2 or 3 inches into the vagina.

c. Depress the plunger on the applicator to push the medication out of the applicator.

d. Withdraw the applicator and place it on a tissue or paper towel. Wipe away excess medication from the genitals. *The applicator may contain microorganisms from the client's vagina.*

5. Help the client to a comfortable position and ask her to remain supine for 5 to 10 minutes or for time frame recommended by medication directions. If needed, offer her a perineal pad. *Lying supine prevents loss of the medication from melting and gravity. The perineal pad absorbs excess drainage.*

6. Wash the applicator with soap and water and store for future use.

7. Remove your gloves and perform hand hygiene.

8. Document the medication administration promptly on the medication administration record or computerized medication record.

PROCEDURE 20-16	ADMINISTERING A RECTAL MEDICATION

TIME TO ALLOW
Novice: 15 min.
Expert: 7 min.

Rectal medications can be used to stimulate a bowel movement or to administer medications when the client cannot take them orally.

DELEGATION GUIDELINES
You may not delegate the administration of rectal medication to a nursing assistant.

EQUIPMENT NEEDED
- Medication administration record, computerized medication order sheet, or medication Kardex or cards
- Rectal medication
- Water-soluble lubricant
- Facecloth and towel for cleansing, if needed
- Disposable tissue
- Disposable gloves

1. Follow preliminary guidelines for nursing procedures (see inside front cover).

2. Check the medication order.

3. Prepare the client for instillation of the medication.

a. Identify the client using an identification bracelet or another accepted means.

b. Explain the procedure to client. Offer an opportunity to void. Close the curtain or door.

c. Put on gloves. Help the client to a left lateral (Sims') position with the upper leg flexed. Drape the client to expose only the anal area. *This position helps to retain the suppository and promotes relaxation of the external anal sphincter.*

d. Inspect the anal area and provide perineal hygiene as needed.

4. Administer the medication using clean aseptic technique.

a. Remove the suppository from the packaging and lubricate the rounded end. Also lubricate the index finger of your gloved dominant hand. *Lubrication eases insertion by reducing friction.*

b. Instruct the client to breathe slowly and deeply through the mouth. *This promotes relaxation of the client's rectal area and anal sphincter to prevent pain.*

c. Separate the buttocks with your gloved nondominant hand. Use your dominant hand to insert the rounded end of the suppository about 4 inches (10 cm) into the rectal canal along the rectal wall (see illustration). Insert the suppository 2 inches (5 cm) for a child. *This distance ensures insertion of the suppository past the external and internal anal sphincters.*

d. Withdraw finger and wipe away fecal material or excess lubricant at the client's anus.

e. Ask the client to remain side-lying for 5 minutes (up to 30 minutes for a laxative). Give an immobile client the call bell and ask her to call you when she feels the need for a bowel movement. *Remaining in position prevents the medication from being expelled.*

5. Remove gloves and perform hand hygiene.

6. Return after 5 minutes to see if the suppository has been expelled. *If so, reinsert it.*

7. Document the medication administration on the medication administration record or computerized medication record.

8. Return 30 minutes after administration to assess effectiveness. Assist the client as needed.

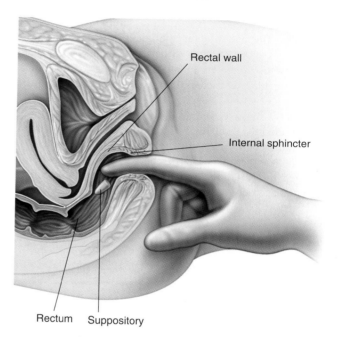

Step 4c. Inserting the rectal suppository.

RECTAL INSTILLATIONS. Rectal instillations are usually used to produce a local effect, such as stimulation of a bowel movement. Less often, they are used for systemic effects, such as relief of fever or nausea when the client cannot tolerate oral medication. Rectal medications typically come as suppositories, but they are often thinner and longer than vaginal suppositories for easier insertion. Many rectal suppositories are kept refrigerated until use.

Use standard precautions when administering a rectal suppository and place it properly for adequate results. Do not place the suppository into a fecal mass because it will not be effective. Administer a small cleansing enema beforehand if needed. The proper method for administering a rectal suppository is described in Procedure 20-16.

Administering Inhalation Medications. Medications administered by inhalation are absorbed into the bloodstream via the alveolar epithelium in the lower respiratory tract. To be effective, a medication must be dispersed in very small droplets, such as a mist, and must be inhaled deeply. Common types of medications administered by inhalation are bronchodilators and mucolytics.

Inhalation agents are delivered either by nebulizer (or atomizer) or by metered-dose inhaler (MDI). A nebulizer uses a forceful flow of oxygen or compressed air to break up liquid medication into tiny particles that can be inhaled. Teach the client to form a tight seal around the mouthpiece and to breathe through the device until the medication has been completely inhaled (often 15 to 20 minutes). Clean the mouthpiece or teach the client to wash it after each use.

An MDI delivers a preset dose of medication when the client discharges the canister. Teach the client the proper method for positioning the mouthpiece. Make sure that the client has manual dexterity and enough strength to push with 5 to 10 pounds of pressure, the amount of pressure needed to depress the medication canister into the device to release a dose. This is an important consideration when working with older or debilitated clients. A turbo-inhaler is a variation of an MDI that must be assembled for use. A spacer may be ordered when a client has difficulty in coordinating the acts of depressing the canister and inhaling at the same time; it attaches to the mouthpiece of the inhaler and holds the medication dose until the client inhales. Important teaching points for using an MDI are found in Chapter 23

EVALUATION

Evaluation of a client's response to medication therapy is just as important as other aspects of administration. Reassess the client to determine whether the original symptoms have been relieved and gather objective data to further evaluate the effects of medication. For example, evaluate urine output, breath sounds, and peripheral edema to determine the effectiveness of diuretic therapy. Document and report medication effects as appropriate.

Use data from laboratory studies as an adjunct in evaluating medication effectiveness. For example, serum drug levels provide useful information about the client's status. Report abnormal values at once so that further adjustments can be made to the medication regimen. Finally, assess for adverse medication effects and report them promptly so corrective action may be taken.

Box 20-12 suggests an initial plan of care that would help meet this client's need for information. Below is a sample documentation note pertaining to Mr. Connell's medication management at the time of his discharge. When Mr. Connell is discharged, the part of the discharge note that pertains to medication management reads as shown below:

> **SAMPLE DOCUMENTATION NOTE FOR MR. CONNELL**
> "Instructions given to client and wife about atenolol, furosemide, and nitroglycerin; they are able to repeat back indications, key actions, adverse effects of medications, and when to call for emergency cardiac care. Client states an intention to follow up with primary care physician. First appointment made by telephone for client before discharge."

 Mr. Connell was ultimately discharged to home with his wife. One month later, he still takes his medications regularly and has started to exercise. His job is still stressful, but he verbalizes satisfaction with his lifestyle and his health. As the nurse working in the physician's office where he is receiving follow-up care, consider the following questions:

- What measures will you use to determine the continued effectiveness of therapy?
- What suggestions can you make to further reduce his risk factors for heart disease?
- What should you teach Mr. Connell, specifically considering his Irish-American cultural beliefs and practices, concerning health?

Nursing Care Plan A CLIENT BEGINNING MEDICATION THERAPY

Box 20-12

ADMISSION DATA

Mr. Connell was admitted to the emergency department following an episode of chest pain. His condition has stabilized and he will be discharged within an hour.

PHYSICIAN'S ORDERS

Atenolol 50 mg PO daily
Furosemide 20 mg PO daily
Nitroglycerin 1/150 gr. SL PRN for chest pain, may repeat × 2

NURSING ASSESSMENT

Before Mr. Connell goes home, he should receive initial instructions to address learning needs he has demonstrated in a variety of areas. He requires information about each of the medications ordered. He would benefit from information about exercise to slow progression of his cardiovascular disease. He could also benefit from initial information on stress management. His understanding and his wife's understanding of sodium restriction should be evaluated and reinforced. He has a definite identified need to understand the importance of continued medical supervision.

NANDA Nursing Diagnosis	NOC Expected Outcomes With Indicators	NIC Interventions With Selected Activities	Evaluation Data
INEFFECTIVE HEALTH MAINTENANCE **Related Factor:** • Insufficient knowledge of treatment regimen	**KNOWLEDGE: TREATMENT REGIMEN** **Medications:** • Verbalizes purpose, actions, and directions for use of all ordered medications.	**TEACHING: PROCEDURE/TREATMENT** • Provide information about atenolol, furosemide, and nitroglycerin. Describe purpose and actions using clear and simple terms. • Review directions for use of each medication (atenolol at night, furosemide in the morning, nitroglycerin at the first sign of chest pain). • Describe handling and storage, especially for nitroglycerin out of light and away from heat). • Outline common side effects of each medication. • Give instructions about when to call physician.	• States he knows "all about atenolol and furosemide" but has never taken nitroglycerin. Reviews the printed material and asks several questions.

Nursing Care Plan A CLIENT BEGINNING MEDICATION THERAPY—CONT'D

Box 20-12

NANDA Nursing Diagnosis	NOC Expected Outcomes With Indicators	NIC Interventions With Selected Activities	Evaluation Data
INEFFECTIVE HEALTH MAINTENANCE—CONT'D	KNOWLEDGE: TREATMENT REGIMEN—CONT'D **Exercise** • Verbalizes the benefits of aerobic exercise to diminish the risk of cardiovascular disease and states intention to begin exercise with physician approval.	TEACHING: PROCEDURE/ TREATMENT—CONT'D • Discuss the benefits of aerobic exercise on the heart, and develop a tentative plan for exercise subject to physician approval.	• States he and his wife will start walking after the evening meal.
	Diet • Client and spouse list foods to be avoided that are high in sodium.	• Review foods to avoid those that are naturally high in sodium. Discuss that foods from animal sources (meats, dairy products) are naturally high in sodium because of physiological saline.	• Is able to list foods high in sodium but expects compliance to be difficult.
	KNOWLEDGE: HEALTH BEHAVIOR **Stress Management** • Verbalizes the importance of stress management as an adjunct to blood pressure control.	TEACHING: INDIVIDUAL • Begin initial teaching about the effects of stress on blood pressure. Develop an initial plan to manage stress effectively to aid in blood pressure reduction. • Stress the importance of continued medical supervision, and develop a specific plan for medical follow-up.	• Has his own business and cannot reduce working hours. • Will visit doctor in 1 week.

CRITICAL THINKING QUESTIONS

1. How would you proceed as a follow-up to Mr. Connell's statement that he knows "all about atenolol and furosemide"?

2. Do you have suggestions to help with planning for diet and exercise?

Nursing outcome and intervention labels from Johnson, M., Bulechek, G., McCloskey Dochterman, J. M., Maas, M., & Moorhead, S. (2001). *Nursing diagnoses, outcomes, and interventions: NANDA, NIC, and NOC linkages.* St Louis, MO: Mosby.

Key Principles

- Drugs have a variety of names, including the official name, chemical name, generic name, and trade name or names. Become familiar with the generic and trade names of medications.
- A client's knowledge base for successful self-administration of medication should include information about therapeutic effect, dose, side effects, adverse effects, directions for use, drug interactions, and storage and expiration.
- Drug manufacture and use is highly regulated in the United States and Canada. There are stringent controls over the distribution and use of highly addictive substances, such as opioids.
- The nurse functions within legal guidelines when administering medications. The nurse practice act in each state specifies the responsibility a nurse has in administering medications.
- Pharmacokinetics refers to the processes of absorption, distribution, metabolism, and excretion. A variety of client-related factors influence a drug's effectiveness.
- Drugs can elicit a variety of responses. Each drug may have a therapeutic effect, adverse effects, and toxic effects. Drugs can

also elicit an allergic response or an idiosyncratic response in some clients. Be aware of potential responses to adequately assess the client.
- Some drugs can cause physiological or psychological dependence in the client. These drugs are labeled as controlled substances and require special precautions.
- Each drug has a specific onset, peak, and duration of action. Each drug also has a specific half-life, which determines how often it must be given to maintain a therapeutic blood level.
- There are various types of drug orders. A standing order is given routinely at prescribed times. A PRN order is given as needed but cannot be given more often than specified. A single or one-time order is carried out once only. A stat order is completed immediately.
- Numerous client-related factors affect drug actions, including life span considerations and various physiological, cultural, and lifestyle factors.
- Medication may be given by the oral, parenteral, topical, or inhalation route. The route has a significant effect on the timing and duration of action. Specific procedures are followed when each of these routes is used.

- All six steps of the nursing process are used when administering medications to clients.
- Many client factors should be considered to safely administer medications: health history, allergies, medication and diet histories, current condition, problems with perception and coordination, knowledge about drug therapy, and individual learning needs.
- *Ineffective health maintenance* is a useful nursing diagnosis for clients receiving medication therapy. Other nursing diagnoses, such as *Ineffective therapeutic regimen management,* may also apply. Assess each client individually to determine whether defining characteristics of one or more nursing diagnoses are exhibited.
- Drug doses are measured using one of three systems: metric, apothecary, and household. Familiarity with all three systems is needed to administer drugs safely.
- It is imperative to give medications correctly to protect the client's safety. Adhere to the "six rights" when giving medications: right client, right drug, right dose, right route, right time, and right documentation.
- The nurse is responsible for safely and accurately administering all medications and documenting administration using established policies and procedures.
- If a medication error does occur, it is your legal and ethical responsibility to report it promptly. Health care facilities have specific policies and procedures to follow if an error occurs. Client safety is the paramount concern.
- Special populations, such as children and older adults, have unique needs with regard to drug therapy. Incorporate your knowledge of these needs when giving medications to these groups.
- Standard precautions are used when administering medications. Use extreme caution when handling needles and other sharps, which can transmit pathogens (such as HIV or hepatitis) from an infected client if a needlestick injury occurs.

Bibliography

American Hospital Formulary Service. *AHFS drug information 2000 (Annual).* Bethesda, MD: American Society of Hospital Pharmacists.

Anonymous. (2000). Transcribing medication abbreviations. *Nursing, 30*(3), 60-61.

Aschenbrenner, D., Cleveland, L., & Venable, S. (2002). *Drug therapy in nursing.* Philadelphia: Lippincott Williams & Wilkins.

Beyers, M. (2000). Ask AONE's experts: About a four-point plan to reduce medication errors. *Nursing Management, 31*(2), 56.

Blazys, D. (2000). Clinical nurses forum: Giving bitter-tasting medicine to children. *Journal of Emergency Nursing, 26*(4), 345, 394-398.

Ebersole, P., & Hess, P. (2001). *Geriatric nursing & healthy aging.* St Louis, MO: Mosby.

Feinberg, J. L., & Tobias, D. E. (2000). MDS-MED GUIDE: Assessing medication effects using resident assessment data. *Geriatric Nursing, 21*(6), 291-299.

Hadaway, L. C. (2001). How to safeguard delivery of high-alert IV drugs. *Nursing, 31*(2), 36-41.

Hayes, K. S. (1998). Randomized trial of geragogy-based medication instruction in the emergency department. *Nursing Research, 47*(4), 211-218.

Hurme, E., & Pourciau, C. (2001). Preventing medication errors in the home. *Geriatric Nursing, 22*(6), 338-339.

Institute for Safe Medication Practices (2001). *To promote understanding, assume every patient has a health literacy problem.* Retrieved April 14, 2002, from http://www.ismp.org/msaarticles/promote.html.

Jech, A. Q. (2001). The next step in preventing med errors. *RN, 64*(4), 46-49.

Johnson, M., Bulecheck, G., McCloskey Dochtermann, J., Mass, M., & Moorehead, S. (2001). *Nursing diagnoses, outcomes, and interventions: NANDA, NOC, and NIC linkages.* St Louis, MO: Mosby.

Johnson, M., Maas, M., & Moorehead, S. (2000). *Nursing outcomes classification (NOC)* (2nd ed.). St Louis, MO: Mosby.

Karch, A. M., & Karch, F. E. (2000). Practice errors: A spoonful of medicine. *American Journal of Nursing, 100*(11), 24.

Koschel, M. J. (2001). Question of practice: Filter needles. *American Journal of Nursing, 101*(1), 75.

Kudzma, E. C. (1999). Culturally competent drug administration: Are one-size-fits-all drugs becoming a thing of the past? *American Journal of Nursing, 99*(8), 46-52.

Lehne, R., Moore, L., Crosby, L., & Hamilton, D. (2001). *Pharmacology for nursing care* (4th ed.). Philadelphia: Saunders.

Martens, K. H. (1998). An ethnographic study of the process of medication discharge education (MDE). *Journal of Advanced Nursing, 27,* 341-348.

McCloskey, J., & Bulecheck, G. (2000). *Nursing interventions classification* (3rd ed.). St Louis, MO: Mosby.

McKenry, L., & Salerno, E. (2001). *Mosby's pharmacology in nursing* (21st ed.). St Louis, MO: Mosby.

Medical Economics Staff, Micromedex. (2000). *Drug information for the health care professional, Volume I: USP DI 2000.* Rockville, MD: USP Convention.

Miller, D., & Miller, H. (2000). To crush or not to crush? *Nursing, 30*(2), 50-52.

National Coordinating Council for Medication Error Reporting and Prevention. *About medication errors.* Retrieved July 1, 2002 from http://www.nccmerp.org.

North American Nursing Diagnosis Association. (2001). *Nursing diagnoses: Definitions and classification, 2001-2002.* Philadelphia: Author.

Olsen, J., & Giangrasso, A. (2000). *Medication dosage calculations* (7th ed.). Upper Saddle River, NJ: Prentice Hall.

Pope, B. (2002). How to administer subcutaneous and intramuscular injections. *Nursing 2002, 32*(1), 50-51.

Ryan, A. A., & Chambers, M. (2000). Medication management and older patients: An individualized and systematic approach. *Journal of Clinical Nursing, 12*(5), 732-741.

Schafer, S. L. (2001). Prescribing for seniors: It's a balancing act. *Journal of the American Academy of Nurse Practitioners, 13*(3), 108-112.

Skuteris, L. R. (2000). Master five common medication administration questions. *Nursing Management, 31*(8), 16-17.

Smetzer, J. (2002). Take 10 giant steps to medication safety. *Nursing 2001, 31*(11), 49-53.

Spector, R. (2000). *Cultural diversity in health & illness* (5th ed.). Upper Saddle River, NJ: Prentice Hall.

Turkoski, B. B. (1999). Pharmacology: Meeting the challenge of medication reactions in the elderly. *Orthopaedic Nursing, 18*(5), 85-95.

Waldo, B. H. (1999). Information systems & technology: Preventing adverse drug reactions through automation. *Nursing Economics, 17*(4), 276-279.

Wendt, D. A. (1998). Evaluation of medication management interventions for the elderly. *Home Healthcare Nurse, 16*(9), 613-617.

Wilson, S. (1998). Irish Americans. In L. Purnell & B. Paulanka (Eds.), *Transcultural health care: A culturally competent approach,* pp. 353-370. Philadelphia: Davis.

Health Protection: Risk for Infection

Learning Objectives

After studying this chapter, you should be able to do the following:

- Discuss the course of an infection, physiological defenses against infection, and chain of infection in relationship to infection control
- Describe the assessment of a client who is at risk for infection, an actual infection, and responses to infection
- Identify appropriate nursing diagnoses for a client with either an active infection or an increased risk for infection
- Plan for goal-directed interventions to prevent infection or control the spread of infection
- Identify specific interventions needed to prevent transmission of infection, manage a client with a compromised immune system, and reduce the personal risk for infection
- Evaluate the outcomes that describe progress toward the goals of health protection nursing care

Six-month-old Luisa Martez lives at home with her parents and two siblings: Rosa, 5 years old, and Jose, 2 years old. The Martez family came to the United States from Mexico. Luisa has been developing normally for her age. She has had a runny nose for the last few days but until last night had not seemed ill.

During the night, she began vomiting. This morning, Luisa's mother noticed that Luisa seemed very sleepy and did not wake up at the usual time. Despite repeated attempts, she would not breastfeed. Also, her skin felt warm. When her mother took her axillary temperature, the thermometer registered 102° F. Mr. and Mrs. Martez took Luisa to the emergency room of the hospital where she had been born. She was admitted to the children's unit with a diagnosis of dehydration secondary to infection. In addition to be-

ing frightened, Luisa's parents were confused about the admission process. Her father speaks and understands English, but her mother speaks no English and does not appear to understand any. The nurse therefore makes plans to obtain a translator to facilitate the management of Luisa's illness, recovery, and follow-up after discharge. Because of Luisa's age, health status, and the risk for hospital acquired infection, the nurse considers the nursing diagnoses *Risk for infection* and *Ineffective protection* from the list of possible nursing diagnoses that relate to infection (see below). Luisa will continue to have *Risk for infection* on discharge because she lives with two older siblings and has altered immunity related to her infancy and possible lack of immunizations.

KEY NURSING DIAGNOSES FOR   Infection

Risk for infection: At increased risk for being invaded by pathogenic organisms.

Ineffective protection: Decreased ability to guard self from internal or external threats such as illness or injury.

CONCEPTS OF INFECTION CONTROL

Nurses have played a major role in preventing infectious diseases since Florence Nightingale demonstrated the effectiveness of nursing care in reducing the infection rate in military hospitals during the Crimean War. Nursing management of infectious diseases encompasses three levels of prevention. In primary prevention, nurses teach health-promotion strategies to stay well. Primary prevention includes practices in the home and in health care institutions that prevent the spread of infection. In secondary prevention, nurses monitor clients both as individuals and in groups to detect infection early, obtain prompt treatment for infection, and prevent the spread to other members of a group. In tertiary prevention, a nurse helps the client manage the medical interventions (commonly with an **antibiotic,** a medication that kills bacteria) to ensure complete recovery from the infection.

An **infection** is a clinical syndrome caused by the invasion and multiplication of a **pathogen,** a disease-producing microorganism, in body tissues. Pathogens cause local cellular injury through their metabolism, toxin production, intracellular replication, or antigen–antibody response. The body responds to the invasion of causative organisms by the formation of antibodies and by a series of physiological changes known as inflammation.

Infections can be either localized or systemic. A localized infection is restricted to a well-defined or limited area of tissue. A systemic infection is one that affects the body as a whole.

Course of Infection

To control the spread of infection, the nurse must have knowledge of the clinical course of the infection, especially the period when the infection can be transmitted to others. The clinical course of an infection varies with the causative organism, the site of infection, and the overall health status of the in-

fected person. In general, however, the course of an infection can be described in four phases that are important to infection control in many cases.

Phases of an Infection. The *incubation period* extends from the time of a client's exposure to the organism to the appearance of the first symptoms. The length of the incubation period is sometimes helpful in diagnosing the specific causative organism. Childhood illnesses, cold viruses, and flu viruses have predictable incubation periods.

The *prodromal phase* is a period of vague, nonspecific symptoms preceding the full manifestation of the infection. The symptoms may include general malaise, low-grade fever, nausea, weakness, and general aches.

The period of *clinical illness* is the time when the symptoms are fully manifested and most clearly recognized as representing a specific infectious process. The diagnosis is made from a specific cluster of symptoms and sometimes after obtaining cultures to identify the specific organism.

The period of *convalescence* is the time following the height of the acute symptoms to the time the person experiences a return to normal health. It is common for a person recovering from an infection to complain of decreased energy or feeling tired before full recovery from an illness.

Infectious diseases can be spread from one person to another during any phase of the illness. Clients are considered to be in a contagious or communicable phase of infection whenever they are able to spread the infection to another person. However, the phases during which illnesses are communicable are variable and depend on the specific infection. With some infections, the disease may be contagious from the prodromal phase through the convalescent phase.

Socioeconomic Factors Affecting Infection. With the development of antibiotics and immunizations since the middle of the twentieth century, health practitioners had hoped that the risk for infectious diseases would become a problem of historic interest. However, infectious diseases are an ongoing health concern.

It is important to develop awareness of clients' susceptibility to infection and to be vigilant in developing plans to minimize clients' risk. It is also necessary to understand the bases for *Ineffective protection*. Public health or community-based nurses, especially, should develop a heightened consciousness of manifestations of infection as they work to prevent infection and decrease its spread.

Infectious diseases were once thought to be all but conquered, at least in developed countries such as the United States and Canada. Since the 1970s, however, there has been reemergence of infectious diseases with the threat of increased incidence in the near future. The most well known of these diseases are acquired immunodeficiency syndrome (AIDS), Ebola virus, drug-resistant tuberculosis, *Cyclospora,* and cholera. A number of factors are thought to contribute to the emergence of new and resistant diseases.

Factors within the social structure can contribute to the spread of disease. One factor is the increasing number of persons who are steadily becoming more economically disadvantaged. The growth of large inner-city ghettos, where public and private services are inadequate or lacking, creates conditions for the spread of infection. As the population grows, crowded living conditions become more common. Although it is easy to assume that the risk for infection could be contained in areas where risk is the greatest, a highly mobile population means that the risk can spread rapidly.

Luisa's family is large and shares a relatively small living area with the extended family. What impact would these living conditions have on her risk for infection?

The desire for a world market for goods and services has created a global economy in which individual nations are less isolated from each other. High-speed travel and migration of the world's population have increased the transmission of disease worldwide. Infectious diseases remain the leading cause of death worldwide. As populations intermingle, both evolving and new pathogens spread to produce infectious diseases where they have previously been unknown.

The potential for infectious disease to spread through the food supply is perhaps greater than it was in the recent past. Large agricultural corporations that have not paid enough attention to controls to ensure a safe food supply have come under scrutiny for the methods of mass production of food. The high demand for fresh fruits and vegetables year-round has resulted in an increase in the importation of these food items, often requiring transportation over great distances and handling at multiple points in the distribution system.

At the same time, health policy in the United States has been treatment driven, with diminishing resources going to public health. The surveillance systems for infectious diseases need to be examined to ensure that the spread of disease can be tracked. Successful early warning procedures can be implemented if reporting procedures and a national system to track infectious diseases is in place.

Infection and Health Care Institutions. The health care system itself is yet another factor in emergent infections. How health care providers prescribe antibiotics is one factor in the development of resistant strains of organisms. New procedures and equipment have led to an increasing variety of methods to perform invasive procedures that in turn create new problems in cleaning and sterilizing equipment. Increases in the number of organ and tissue transplants have further increased the possibility for transmission of disease. **Immunosuppression** therapy (i.e., medications to suppress the body's immune system) has increased because these medications are used with transplants and as new treatments for cancer. Immunosuppressive agents prevent the transplanted organ from being rejected by the body as foreign, but they also limit the ability of the body to fight infection.

The public has a right to expect that the risk for acquiring an infection during hospitalization be minimal; however, controlling infection rates in hospitals is a major problem. Even if infection is not the admitting diagnosis, hospitalized clients are at an increased risk for **nosocomial infection,** an infection acquired in the hospital and more likely to be resistant to several antibiotics.

A nosocomial infection is any infection that was not present or incubating at the time of admission. **Iatrogenic infections** are the direct result of treatments such as invasive procedures. It has been estimated that 5% of clients experience nosocomial infections and, of these, multiple resistant organisms infect 25%. An average of 4 days is added to the hospital stay for persons with nosocomial infections, costing the health care system over $2 billion annually (Box 21-1, p. 454). As many as 20,000 to 40,000 persons die each year from nosocomial infections. Up to 33% of hospital-acquired infections may be preventable.

Defenses Against Infection

Primary Defenses. The human body has a number of refined defenses against infection. The primary defenses include skin and mucous membranes, the respiratory tract, the gastrointestinal (GI) tract, and the circulatory system.

SKIN AND MUCOUS MEMBRANES. The skin and mucous membranes act as a physical barrier to prevent organisms from entering the body through the intact dermis and epidermis. Although the skin harbors many different kinds of microorganisms, we rarely become infected from these organisms if the skin remains intact. The surface of the skin also offers **antimicrobial** properties, which give it the ability to limit the spread of microorganisms. Dryness of the skin promotes desiccation of microorganisms, and the ongoing desquamation of skin cells rids the skin surface of remaining organisms. The skin surface has a low pH that provides additional protection. The low pH is due to fatty acids that occur as a byproduct of lipid conversion of normal skin flora. The mucous membranes of the urinary system, the vagina, the airways, and the GI tract produce mucus that traps and removes organisms. Mucous membranes also destroy bacteria through the action of macrophages and lysozymes.

Clostridium difficile is a spore-forming, gram-positive, anaerobic rod that causes colitis in elderly persons and in hospitalized persons, especially those who are taking antibiotics. It causes diarrhea, ranging from mild to profuse, with watery and mucoid stools. The diagnosis is confirmed by testing a stool sample for the toxin produced by *C. difficile* rather than culturing the stool for this organism.

Patients who acquire *C. difficile* in the hospital often have an increased length of stay and additional cost of treatment. Kyne, Hamel, Polavaram, and Kelly (2002) studied the cost of treating and caring for these clients.

A total of 271 clients were selected who had risk factors for developing *C. difficile,* and they were followed during their hospital stay. The purpose of the study was to determine whether clients whose hospital stay is complicated by diarrhea due to *C. difficile* experience differences in cost, length of stay, and survival rates when compared with clients whose stay is not complicated by *C. difficile*–associated diarrhea.

RESULTS

Forty (15%) of the 271 clients developed diarrhea associated with *C. difficile*. These clients incurred adjusted hospital costs of $3669—that is, 54% (95% confidence interval [CI], 17%-103%) higher than clients whose course was not complicated by *C. difficile*–associated diarrhea. The extra length of stay attributable to *C. difficile*–associated diarrhea was 3.6 days (95% CI, 1.5%-6.2%). However, *C. difficile*–associated diarrhea was not associated with excess 3-month or 1-year mortality after adjustment for age, comorbidity, and disease severity. Using these results, these authors estimated that the cost of this disease in the United States exceeds $1.1 billion per year.

Kyne, L., Hamel, M. B., Polavaram, R., & Kelly, C. P. (2002). Health care costs and mortality associated with nosocomial diarrhea due to *Clostridium difficile. Clinical Infectious Diseases, 34*(3), 346-353.

RESPIRATORY SYSTEM. The respiratory tract filters and warms the air that we breathe. Hairlike structures called cilia that line the respiratory tract continuously sweep debris up and out of the respiratory tract. Cells lining the respiratory tract secrete lysozymes that can destroy certain bacteria. Macrophages engulf and destroy bacteria found in the alveoli.

GASTROINTESTINAL SYSTEM. The GI tract is a hostile environment for many microorganisms because of the pH extremes of the highly acid stomach and the highly alkaline small intestine. Nonetheless, bacterial colonies found normally in the colon aid digestion and provide needed vitamins. They can also provide resistance to colonization by pathogenic organisms by competing for nutrients and by producing inhibitors in the form of proteins that limit the growth of other, possibly pathogenic, bacteria. Cells lining the digestive tract called goblet cells produce secretions that form barriers, preventing penetration by bacteria. These cells also produce enzymes that lyse, or break apart, bacterial cell walls.

CIRCULATORY SYSTEM. The circulatory system is essential to the inflammatory and immune response. Blood carries the components of cellular and humoral immunity and removes waste products of tissue destruction from sites of injury.

Secondary Defenses. The immune and inflammatory responses are the second line of defense against infection. The

inflammatory response is a localized reaction to injury and is activated when there is tissue damage. The immune response is activated in the presence of foreign substances. It has various specific and nonspecific mechanisms to handle invasions of microorganisms. The very complexity of the immune response gives it enormous flexibility and effectiveness.

INFLAMMATORY RESPONSE. The inflammatory response should not be confused with infection. Many physical, chemical, and biological agents that cause damage to tissues can cause inflammation. The inflammatory response is the body's way of protecting and healing itself. Its purpose is to remove or destroy the invasive substance, to localize the invading organism, and to repair damage. Any type of traumatic injury, including surgery, initiates the inflammatory response. Redness, heat, swelling, and pain are the classic signs of an inflammatory response. Many times, loss of function is included as an indicator of inflammation. The inflammatory response results from the increased permeability of blood vessels that allows release of fluid, blood components, and blood cells into the tissue where an injury or infection has occurred.

Local tissue injury releases substances from the damaged cells that cause capillary dilatation and increased capillary permeability. Fluid that contains infection-fighting proteins from the blood then escapes through the walls of the capillaries. These proteins include nonspecific components that fight all infections. Proteins from the complement system can be activated in a series, even in the absence of antibodies. They release factors that attract phagocytic cells that engulf and lyse or destroy the invading microorganism or its toxins. Interferon is another protein released at the site of an infection that is active in fighting viral infections.

Other cells that are present in this fluid-filled space include red blood cells and white blood cells. White blood cells are of various types and have specific roles in fighting infections. Those involved in the nonspecific or innate system include polymorphonuclear leukocytes, macrophages, granulocytes, and null cells.

When the infectious organism or toxin is known to the body's immune system, additional white blood cells, the *B* and *T lymphocytes,* can be found at the site of infection. The B lymphocytes (B cells) are the cells responsible for production of specific antibodies or immunoglobulins. The T lymphocytes (T cells) are the cells that carry the memory of a specific infectious organism, and they are the cells that kill the invading organisms. The B and T cells work together to fight infections that they recognize and, thus, require previous contact with the invading organism.

IMMUNE RESPONSE. Although inflammation is a general protective response, the immune response is specific to the antigen or foreign substance that has invaded the body. The activation of the immune response, therefore, requires that there has been a previous contact with the invading organism or antigen. Immunity (see Box 21-2 for terminology) is a measure of a person's ability to resist disease by forming immunoglobulins (antibody cells that destroy antigens), developing immunologically competent cells, or, in viral infections, producing interferon. The immune system has two

- **Active immunity:** A form of long-term acquired immunity that protects the body against a new infection as a result of antibodies that develop naturally after an initial infection or artificially after a vaccination.
- **Passive immunity:** A form of acquired immunity resulting from antibodies that are transmitted naturally through the placenta to a fetus, through the colostrum to an infant, or artificially by injection of antiserum for treatment or prophylaxis. Passive immunity is not permanent and does not last as long as active immunity.
- **Natural immunity:** The immunity achieved when an animal or human is infected with an organism; the antigenic response occurs naturally within the body.
- **Artificial immunity:** Immunity induced by man-made vaccines or immunoglobulins.
- **Acquired immunity:** A form of immunity that is not innate but is obtained during life. It may be natural or artificial, and actively or passively induced.

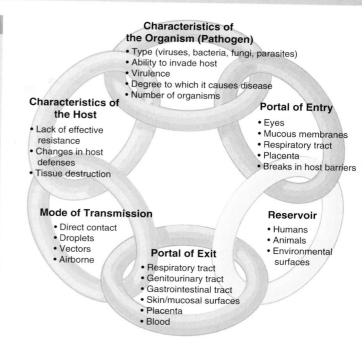

Figure 21-1. Chain of infection.

Table 21-1	Common Pathogens in Nosocomial Infections and Usual Mode of Transmission	
Pathogen	**Mode of Transmission**
Staphylococcus	Contact
Antibiotic-resistant *Staphylococcus aureus*	Contact
Pseudomonas	Contact
Escherichia coli	Contact

closely interrelated components: the humoral and cellular immune responses.

HUMORAL IMMUNITY. The humoral immune response is the antigen–antibody response that takes place in the body fluids (or humors). An **antibody** (immunoglobulin) is a circulating protein that recognizes and destroys foreign invaders. Antibodies are derived from B cells in response to a substance recognized as "not self" (the antigen). Three days after B cells contact an antigen, they divide into immunoglobulins (antibody cells that destroy antigens) and memory cells that can recognize a repeated invasion by the antigen. There are five types of immunoglobulins: IgM, IgG, IgA, IgD, and IgE. IgM is the precursor for the other immunoglobulins and is the initial response to a current infection. IgG is the delayed or secondary response and is present if the person has had an infection in the past.

CELLULAR IMMUNITY. The cellular components of immunity are derived from T and B cells. About 60% to 70% of the lymphocytes in the circulating blood are T cells. T cells have antigen-specific receptors that bind antigens to their surface. The binding of antigens causes the production of sensitized T cells, which travel to the site of inflammation and bind with antigens to release chemicals (lymphokines) that attract macrophages. Because these cells help the B cell recognize an antigen, they are called helper T cells. Suppressor T cells also exist that prevent the reaction to the antigen from becoming an overreaction or hypersensitivity. A third type of T cell actually kills cells and is most effective against viruses and protozoa.

The cellular immune response and its components provide the bases for medications to provide protection against a specific disease or disease agent. An **immunization** is a medication administered to activate an immune response before exposure to the disease agent. One inherent risk of immunization therapy is that any alteration in the immune response also escalates the possibility of infection.

Chain of Infection

The body's ability to internally protect against infection is limited; therefore, preventing infection requires an understanding of how infectious diseases are transmitted or spread.

Thinking of the elements of transmission as links in a chain is a useful figurative way to understand the interlinking nature of these elements (Figure 21-1). Breaking any link in the chain can prevent infection. The elements are the characteristics of the organism (pathogen), portal of entry, reservoir, portal of exit, mode of transmission, and characteristics of the host (the client).

Characteristics of the Organism (Pathogen). Most microorganisms that populate the internal and external surfaces of healthy people normally do not produce disease. The ability of an organism to cause disease is affected by the type of organism and its level of **virulence**—the power of an organism to cause disease.

The number of organisms also affects their ability to cause infection, as does the susceptibility of the host. Table 21-1 lists common pathogens responsible for nosocomial infections and the usual mode of transmission for each.

TYPE. The types of microorganisms that can cause disease include viruses, bacteria, fungi, and parasites, including protozoans, helminths, and arthropods. A brief discussion of each follows.

VIRUSES. A **virus** is a tiny microorganism, much smaller than a bacterium, that can only replicate inside the cell of a host, such as a human. The virus takes over the metabolism of the cell to make more copies of itself. The cell can then no longer function normally because of the infection. The new viral particles are released slowly through the membrane of the cell. They then continue to infect other cells but do not necessarily kill these cells. The cell remains alive but cannot carry out its normal cellular functions. Some viruses do kill the cell and release large numbers of viral particles with cell lysis. Other viruses have the characteristic of latency, which allows the cell to function normally, or with some of its normal functions, while the virus has integrated itself into the genetic material of the cell. At this stage of infection, the individual may not appear to be infected. It is only later, after the virus takes over the cell's machinery and begins to replicate, causing cell death, that it is apparent that the organism is infected.

Because the viruses use the host cell to reproduce, any medications used to kill them must be specific for the viruses' and not the host's metabolism. Few antiviral drugs exist. One antiviral drug is ribavirin, used against respiratory syncytial virus and some herpes viral infections. Many viral infections are eliminated because of the immune system's specific and nonspecific reactions to infection. Because the immune system "remembers" viral infections, it plays an important role in fighting specific viruses. Thus, immunization against specific viral diseases is an important factor in controlling viral infection.

BACTERIA. A **bacterium** is a small, single-celled organism that can reproduce outside of cells. Bacteria cause disease by releasing deadly molecules or toxins, which can kill cells or incapacitate some cellular functions. Some bacteria cause disease by overgrowing and damaging tissues as they grow. Some very small bacteria can only grow inside of cells. They cause diseases in much the same way that viruses do, by taking over the cell's metabolism for their own functions. Again, the body's defense system for specific and nonspecific immune reactions is important in fighting these infections and can be used against specific bacterial toxins. Many antibiotics are developed to kill specific types or strains of bacteria.

FUNGI. Fungi can grow as budding yeasts or as filaments when infecting individuals. Like bacteria, they can replicate very rapidly given the right growing conditions. They can also cause disease by overgrowing and damaging tissues as they grow. Unlike bacteria, their cell walls contain the substance chitin, which makes them very resistant to destruction by the body's resistant mechanisms. Because their cellular metabolism is similar to ours, antibiotics successful in fighting bacteria do not harm fungi, and antibiotics that can harm fungi can also harm our cells.

PARASITES. Multicellular parasites can cause disease by interfering with the nutrition of an organism. They feed off cells and tissues, depriving them of nutrition and causing tissue destruction. This can be life threatening, depending on where the parasite is lodged and which tissues are destroyed.

VIRULENCE. Virulence is a measure of the aggressiveness of an organism in causing a disease. Virulence includes *invasiveness* and *toxigenicity*. Invasiveness has three components: (1) the organism must be able to adhere to the skin or mucous membrane, (2) it must be able to then penetrate that skin or mucosal surface, and (3) once it has invaded the body, it must be able to multiply and evade the body's natural defenses. Toxigenicity is the ability to produce toxic substances, which can damage the host. Much of an organism's disease-causing capability and its ability to cause tissue damage results from the production of enzymes and toxins. Toxins are proteins, or complexes of proteins, polysaccharides, and lipids, that microorganisms release, causing tissue damage or destruction.

Portal of Entry. Organisms can enter a host through the eyes, mucosal membranes (including those of the GI and genitourinary [GU] tracts), respiratory tract, placenta, and any breaks in the host's mechanical or chemical barriers. Controlling the *portal of entry* involves maintaining the integrity of the protective tissues in the host.

Reservoir. A *reservoir* is a place where the infectious agent can survive and, possibly, multiply until it can invade a susceptible host. Three common reservoirs include humans, animals, and environmental surfaces. Reservoirs inside the hospital include clients, health care personnel and equipment, and the hospital environment. When an individual acquires a nosocomial infection, it is acquired from a reservoir in the hospital.

To grow and multiply, an organism needs a food supply and optimal conditions for growth. Many organisms grow best in a warm, moist, dark environment at some optimal pH. Some organisms are aerobic (requiring oxygen); others are anaerobic (not requiring oxygen). Common reservoirs in the home are improperly stored food, improperly cleaned counter surfaces where food has been prepared, and wet surfaces in bathrooms. In hospitals, the same general reservoirs are present. Additionally, the materials used to contain wound drainage create reservoirs. Hence, a bandage removed from a draining wound and discarded in a wastebasket is a good medium for the growth of organisms.

Portal of Exit. Organisms can exit a host through the respiratory tract, GU tract, GI tract, skin or mucosal surfaces, placenta (mother to infant), and blood. Controlling the portal of exit involves management of body fluids and wastes.

Mode of Transmission. Modes of transmission are the mechanisms in which pathogens are transferred from an agent to the host. They include direct contact, droplet, vector, and airborne spread.

DIRECT CONTACT. Contact is a major mode of transmission. Direct contact results in person-to-person spread. Indirect contact also contributes to infection and may involve an intermediate surface or object between the reservoir and the host, such as a dirty instrument.

DROPLET. Droplet transmission occurs when large particles produced by talking, sneezing, or coughing pass through the air from the reservoir to the host. Droplet transmission occurs only through small distances (3 feet or less).

VECTOR. A vector is a vehicle to transmit infection from a reservoir to a host. One example of a common vector is food. Organisms, such as *Salmonella,* can multiply in food before infecting the host. Other organisms do not multiply in the food but are carried on the food, such as the hepatitis A virus.

An important mode of transmission is via a living vector, such as an insect or arthropod. Organisms can be transmitted externally on the vector, such as on the legs of flies. Some vectors carry the organism internally, such as the malarial parasites or yellow fever virus in a mosquito.

AIRBORNE. Airborne spread of infections such as measles occurs when the causative organism can remain suspended in air for extended periods of time. The infection is acquired by breathing in the air that contains the organisms.

Characteristics of the Host.

Once an organism has exited a reservoir, infection can occur in a susceptible host—a person who lacks effective resistance to the pathogen. Any changes in the natural defenses of the host increase the likelihood of infection by a pathogenic agent. Tissue destruction, either accidental or through medical or surgical intervention, accentuates the possibility of infection. Factors affecting susceptibility to infection are discussed later in this chapter.

ASSESSMENT

General Assessment

Prevention of infection in vulnerable clients is a primary nursing concern. All clients entering a health agency, either as an inpatient or outpatient, should be assessed for *Risk for infection.*

Health History.

The health history is a good tool for detecting *Risk for infection.* It should include questions about immunization, possible exposure to communicable disease, and the general health status of the client. The client's history of infections will give you clues about behaviors that may be associated with the incidence of infections and health teaching that should be done. Include assessment of the client's knowledge level and factors in the environment that increase the risk for infection.

Physical Examination.

Follow up findings from the health history during your physical examination. The physical examination may help you tie information from the health history to the physical status of the client. For example, if the client is on immunosuppressants such as cortisone, you will look for the physical effects of the long-term use of cortisone.

Diagnostic Tests

BLOOD CELL COUNT. Because blood cells are important components of the immune system, a blood sample can be useful in determining whether your client has an infection or is at increased risk for infection. The hemoglobin and hematocrit are red blood cell measurements that reflect cell nutrition and repair, whereas the white blood cell count reflects the ability to fight actual infections.

Table 21-2	Interpreting a Differential White Blood Cell (WBC) Count	
Cell Type	Percentage of 100 Counted WBCs	Usual Reason for Increase
Neutrophil	32 to 62	Acute infections, especially localized infections, such as tonsillitis or otitis media
Lymphocyte	31	Certain acute viral infections with early increase; chronic infections
Basophil	0.6	Infrequently increased; when elevated, most often associated with myeloproliferative disorders
Eosinophil	2.2	Allergic reactions and drug reactions
Monocyte	0 to 4	Certain bacteria, such as brucellosis; tuberculosis; protozoa; rickettsiae

HEMOGLOBIN AND HEMATOCRIT. The hemoglobin and hematocrit are measurements of the size and number of red blood cells. A decreased number or size of red blood cells would indicate anemia or blood loss. As a reflection of nutritional status and thus overall health, anemia helps define the risk for infection. Certain genetic diseases or infections can alter the numbers or form of red blood cells, indicating increased risk for infection.

WHITE BLOOD CELL COUNT. The total white blood cell count reflects the body's response to infections. An increase in the number of white blood cells may mean active infection. A decrease from normal in the number of white blood cells indicates a reduction in infection-fighting ability. An individual's risk for infection increases with the decrease in the number of white blood cells. The cause of a decreased cell count is sometimes an active infection. Some viral infections, such as human immunodeficiency virus (HIV), and some cancers cause decreases in the white blood cell count.

When evaluating a white blood cell count, look at what is called the "differential" of the white cells. The **differential cell count** shows the numbers of the different types of white cells. These include neutrophils, eosinophils, basophils, lymphocytes, and monocytes (Table 21-2). The largest group contains the mature or segmented neutrophils. Immature or nonfilamented neutrophils are called bands. A left shift, which is an increased number of immature neutrophils, is a possible indication of infection.

Other diagnostic tests can measure the function of the immune system. Immunoglobulin levels can be used to evaluate the integrity of the humoral immune system or B-cell function. Delayed hypersensitivity tests (skin tests) are used to test T-cell function. It is also possible to quantitatively analyze B cells and T cells, but these tests are not routinely available.

CULTURE AND SENSITIVITY. By determining the actual organism causing an infection, the treatment plan can be specific to the infecting organism. For this reason, cultures are an important diagnostic test. A culture of microorganisms can be grown from samples taken from a site of obvious infection, such as pus draining from a wound. They can also be performed on bodily fluids that may or may not have obvious signs of infection. For example, lung secretions of an intubated client exhibiting signs of infection can be sent for culture, even if there is no obvious change in the secretions. If the site of infection is not apparent in a hospitalized client, samples from various sites can be sent for culture. These can include pulmonary secretions, spinal fluid, and blood cultures. If the client has a surgical incision, a swab of the surgical site might be done even if no change in drainage is noted. Because urinary tract infections are common in the hospitalized client, urine might also be sent for culture.

Culturing of bacteria requires growing the bacteria on a medium that supports the growth. Usually within 3 to 5 days, and often sooner, there will be enough organisms to identify the specific species of bacteria that is causing the infection. The growing bacteria can then be exposed to different antibiotics to determine which one will be most effective in fighting the infection. This is called a *sensitivity test,* and it is needed to determine the organism's resistance to a medication. Resistance is the ability of a microorganism to make genetic changes in response to environmental pressures, such as medications. Because microorganisms reproduce rapidly, they have the ability when resistant to cause new diseases, remain alive during drug treatment, or cause disease in atypical locations of the body. The sensitivity test, then, is a very important tool for telling us which medications will kill the microorganism being cultured.

Various terms are used to describe drug treatment for microorganisms. The term *antimicrobial* is a broad term and generally refers to the ability to limit the spread of microorganisms. This term, then, can also apply to soaps and other chemicals as well as medications. The term *antibiotic* typically refers to a drug that is able to kill a bacterial pathogen. Antiviral drugs are used to treat viral infections. Antifungal agents are used to treat fungal infections.

GRAM STAIN. The **Gram stain** is a specific microscopic test used to obtain rapid results on a culture sent to the laboratory. Although the Gram stain specifically tests the nature of the bacterial cell walls, it can also indicate the presence of cell types, such as epithelial cells or polymorphonuclear leukocytes. The Gram stain divides bacteria into two basic groups on the basis of whether the cell walls take up the stain (gram-positive) or whether they do not (gram-negative). The shape and arrangement of the bacteria are also indicated by this test. Shapes can be round (cocci), rodlike (bacilli), or spiral (spirochetes). Furthermore, the arrangement can be single, in pairs (diplococci), in chains *(Streptococcus),* clusters *(Staphylococcus),* or tetrads *(Sarcina).* This test can quickly give direction for treatment with antibiotics and determine whether any isolation procedures are recommended.

Although the Gram stain can indicate whether the infection is bacterial and narrows the number of causative organisms, culture and sensitivity testing will give a clearer indication of the most effective antimicrobial therapy. Gram stain and sensitivity tests are useful for bacterial infections. Viral cultures are more difficult because viruses must be grown inside cells, not just on culture media. Many times, if a virus is suspected to be the cause of an infection, the culture is sent for antibody testing and not for culturing. The presence of the viral antibody can be determined relatively rapidly, and therapy can then be started. Advances in capabilities for growing and identifying viruses may make viral culturing more commonplace in the future.

The presence of fungi can often be determined from the Gram stain if the laboratory is specifically looking for it; however, fungi grow under much different conditions in the laboratory. If a fungal infection is suspected, the sample for culture should be collected and placed in a special growth medium at the time the specimen is obtained.

In clients with an intact immune system, the inflammatory response and a complete white blood cell count are effective indicators of infection. In immunocompromised clients, however, the culture is a key element in determining whether an infection is present and in determining treatment.

Focused Assessment for *Risk for Infection* and *Ineffective Protection*

Several risk factors make a client more susceptible to infection. These include invasive procedures, trauma, some medications, malnutrition, inadequate primary or secondary defenses, and certain chronic diseases. Assess your clients carefully for these and other factors to better anticipate if they have *Increased risk for infection.* Assess the environment as well; it too can raise a client's risk.

Characteristics of the Host

PRIMARY DEFENSES. Assess the condition of the skin, respiratory tract, and GI and GU systems as the primary defenses against infection. Assess also for tissue damage and circulatory status. Assess the skin for lesions or breaks in the skin and trauma.

Any breaks in the protective barriers of the skin or membranes surrounding tissues will impair an individual's protection again infection. Trauma can break the skin barrier and may break blood vessels and tear other tissues in the area. This has several immediate results. Any infective organisms that were on the surface of the skin or membranes are now closer to the exposed tissue. The ability for the circulation to provide oxygen and remove debris is disrupted. Any immune response is also altered as a result of interrupted circulation. Finally, tissue functioning may be hampered or destroyed.

The rupture of the amniotic membranes of a pregnant woman often signals the beginning of a welcomed end of pregnancy; however, the fetus now loses this defense against invasion of microorganisms in the immediate environment, including the nonsterile environment of the vagina. Thus a prolonged break of these membranes before the birth of the child can put the infant at increased risk for infection.

Assess the amount of trauma caused by invasive procedures. The amount of ineffective protection depends on the amount and location of the trauma. The risk for infection due to a hangnail is considerably less than that due to a gunshot wound to the abdomen. Invasive medical procedures performed by a health care worker can also alter protection. Intravenous lines, especially central venous lines, allow exposure of the circulatory system and tissues surrounding the placement site to infection. Similarly, providing pulmonary support by endotracheal intubation alters a client's risk for infection. The procedure itself can cause trauma to the airway, but there is also ineffective protection from blockage of the natural mechanisms that clear the airway. Artificial suctioning further increases risk for infection by providing a vehicle for introducing pathogens into the airway. Other procedures that alter protection against infection include insertion of nasogastric tubes, other GI tubes, and urinary catheters; spinal taps; and invasive radiographic examinations. Any surgical procedure alters an individual's protection against infection.

Review the client's history for problems in the GI, respiratory, circulatory, and GU systems that can contribute to infection. Some examples are given in Box 21-3.

Assess the person's nutritional status. Malnutrition resulting from malabsorption of nutrients or poor nutrition reduces the body's ability to protect against infection as well as to repair itself after infection.

Luisa was unwilling or unable to breastfeed. What was the impact on her hydration and nutrition?

ALTERED IMMUNITY. Review the client's history for problems that are known to alter immunity. Any alteration in the immune response can increase the risk for infection. Immunosuppression can result from any disease process that removes the secondary defenses against infection. *Leukemia*

Box 21-3   How Selected Diseases Affect Infection Risk

CROHN'S DISEASE

Crohn's disease is a genetic disease that causes chronic inflammation of the gastrointestinal (GI) tract, putting those with the disease at increased risk for infections of the GI tract. They may require hospitalization and antibiotic treatment for food poisoning, although someone with a normally functioning GI tract who ate the same food would not become ill. Other examples of chronic illnesses that increase the risk for GI infections are HIV infection and cystic fibrosis.

CARDIOVASCULAR DISEASE

People with cardiovascular disease may have reduced circulation and thus a poor inflammatory response in the extremities. An ingrown toenail can become severely infected, possibly leading to amputation. Diabetes, sickle cell disease, and multiple sclerosis are other chronic diseases that can result in reduced circulation and thus increase the risk for infection.

ASTHMA

Clients with asthma can have chronic inflammation of their bronchial passages. Because of this alteration in the airways, what would ordinarily be a minor cold and inconvenience can lead to severe pulmonary pneumonia, requiring hospitalization. Other chronic conditions that can alter the airway and increase the risk for infection include cystic fibrosis, emphysema, smoking, and residual lung disease in premature infants.

---

is a term for a group of infections that alter the populations of the infection-fighting white blood cells. *Lymphoma* is a cancer that can affect the lymph system, an important component of the immune response. Chronic diseases that alter the numbers of white blood cells put these people at increased risk for infection. HIV infection reduces the number of T4 cells that can function normally. Diabetes mellitus, especially of the insulin-dependent type, has also been associated with abnormal functioning of the immune system. Cirrhosis of the liver or removal of the spleen can also result in reduced functioning of the immune system.

Take a medication history. Pharmaceutical agents can alter the immune system. A common example is corticosteroid administration, which affects the functioning of white blood cells in the immune response and reduces the inflammatory response. This can be a positive effect. For example, these medications can be life saving by reducing swelling from trauma or from allergic reactions in the airway. At the same time, however, these medications also have some negative consequences. For example, persons on corticosteroid therapy for chronic diseases such as arthritis, asthma, inflammatory bowel disease, or multiple sclerosis may experience alleviation of disease symptoms but also do not have an inflammatory response to infection. Corticosteroids also decrease the delayed hypersensitivity response of the immune system that involves T-cell activity. Furthermore, any antibiotics used to fight infection can themselves increase the risk for infection through their effects on white blood cells and the bone marrow.

Chemotherapeutic drugs used successfully to treat some forms of cancer can attack the white cells or the bone marrow, the site of production for many of the cells in the immune system. Many chemotherapeutic drugs inhibit bone marrow activity, impairing proliferation of cells involved in the immune response. As a result, the client receiving chemotherapy will have reduced protective mechanisms and increased risk for infection because of a decrease in the number of cells that can respond to infection.

An immunosuppressed person is not only at increased risk for infection but, because of the immunosuppression, may not present with the typical signs and symptoms of infection. Increased vigilance is needed to reduce the risk for infection and to observe for signs of infection in these persons.

Finally, review the client's recent history of medical therapies. Radiation therapy, another successful treatment for cancer, can alter primary defense systems against infection, causing immunosuppression.

HEALTH PRACTICES. Assess a client's health practices for factors that contribute to the risk for infection. Contributing factors for clients with the diagnosis *Risk for infection* include contacts with infectious organisms, the environment, and personal health practices. Health practices that increase risk for infection include personal hygienic practices. Young children may not take the time or know the importance of performing hand hygiene. Persons with impaired mental capabilities or physical limitations may not have optimal personal hygiene because of their knowledge base or because of a physical inability to bathe, wash hands, and maintain a clean environment that does not promote growth of microorganisms.

> What are the implications of the presence of other young children in Luisa's family on her risk for infection?

AGE. The client's age should be considered a factor in assessing the client as a susceptible host. An individual's level of immunity is related to age. A newborn infant has no antibodies of its own at the time of birth. Maternal antibodies that have crossed the placenta are the only defenses against infection at the time of birth. The infant, if breastfeeding, continues to receive antibodies from its mother in breast milk. The protective antibodies received from the mother before birth drop rapidly in the newborn period and are almost gone by 4 months of age. The infant begins to make its own antibodies but does not begin to approach adult levels until about age 2. These levels continue to rise gradually over the first 10 years of life.

The unborn fetus has multiple means to guard against infection. Although the immune response is not well developed until after birth, the mother's immunoglobulins cross the placenta and provide protection for the fetus. The placenta and the amniotic sac that contains the fetus are physical barriers that prevent the passage of infective organisms to the fetus. It is normal for the amniotic membrane to rupture at the time of delivery; however, once rupture occurs, the fetus is at increased risk for infection. If the amniotic membranes rupture more the 24 hours before delivery, there is ineffective protection and the fetus is at risk for infection.

After the age of 65, clients lose some of their infection-fighting abilities. Normal age-related changes can alter the protection of those over 65 years of age. The skin becomes more friable, losing some connective tissue layers, and there are changes in the protective oils and layers of outer skin cells. Some older adults also have reduced mobility that can make minor infections more severe. For example, an upper respiratory infection can rapidly lead to pneumonia. These persons may be at increased risk for trauma because of decreased stimulus response times or to changes in the musculoskeletal system. Older persons are at higher risk for falls. Failing eyesight can also be a contributing factor. Mental changes can further contribute to ineffective protection. The ability to provide for personal hygiene and maintain a clean environment can become impaired, altering their protection and leading to an increased risk for infection.

HEREDITY. Heredity can play a role in *Ineffective protection.* Hereditary diseases may be part of the medical history, and sometimes it is pertinent to ask about family history. Clients who lack critical components of the immune response are unable to destroy invading organisms that do not cause disease in those with normally functioning immune systems. For example, hypogammaglobulinemia is a genetic disorder that results in absent B cells, causing loss of protection against invasion by bacteria, viruses, and parasites. Clients with thymic hypoplasia (DiGeorge syndrome) lack T cells, the main line of defense against tumors and reinfection by mi-

croorganisms. People with combined B- and T-cell deficiencies have no defense against any type of infection or tumors.

IMMUNIZATIONS. Ask clients about immunizations that are appropriate to their situation. Much of modern success in fighting infections has resulted from the development of immunizations that protect against a specific agent or toxin. Some common examples of immunizations include measles, mumps, rubella, polio, pertussis, hepatitis B, influenza, diphtheria, tetanus, pneumonia, and meningococcal vaccines. Individuals, particularly young children or older adults, who have not acquired protection with these vaccines have less resistance to infection than those who have received them. According to the American Academy of Pediatrics, immunizations should begin in the newborn period, with a second round occurring at 2 months of age.

> If Luisa has not begun her immunizations, she would be at risk compared with infants her age who have started their immunizations.

Certain cancers can alter protection for their hosts. Persons with myeloma have defects in humoral immunity, resulting in deficiencies of antibodies. Other malignancies have an impact on cell-mediated immunity. Hodgkin's disease is an example of a malignancy that alters the ability to fight intracellular infections (including viruses and those bacteria that invade cells).

IMMUNE STATUS. Clients who are immunocompromised are more likely to experience opportunistic infections, which are those that result from overgrowth of organisms that do not normally cause disease. An example is disease from organisms that are normally present on the skin or mucosal membranes of the body. Although they generally do not cause disease and may even have protective capabilities, they *can* cause disease if they can reproduce in large numbers or establish colonies in tissues where they are not normally found. A reduced immune response can alter the client's protective system so that these normally nonpathogenic organisms can reproduce and cause disease.

PRESENCE OF CONGENITALLY ACQUIRED CONDITIONS. Review the history for congenitally acquired conditions. Any disease that alters the nutritional status increases the risk for infection. Physical defects present at birth can alter many of the defenses against infection. Lung disease in premature infants puts them at risk for pneumonia. Infants with cardiac defects have circulatory changes that impair their ability to deliver oxygen to tissues and remove debris and waste products, altering the tissue's ability to prevent infection. Anomalies such as spinal defects that expose internal tissues alter the protection of these tissues from possible infection.

PRESENCE OF ACQUIRED CONDITIONS. Acquired infections can alter the immune system's response to infection. These infections alter the cell-mediated immune response. Viral infections associated with decreased cell-mediated immunity include measles, mumps, varicella, influenza, Epstein-Barr virus, and rubella. Bacterial and fungal infections include tuberculosis, leprosy, syphilis, coccidioidomycosis, histoplasmosis, and blastomycosis. HIV destroys the cells active in fighting infections and tumors of the immune system.

PRESENCE OF MENTAL ILLNESS. People with mental health problems may have increased risk for infection if they lack the ability or judgment to protect themselves from infection. Decreased ability to recognize or respond to illness alters their protection. Persons with dementia may be unable to protect themselves from infection. Their inability to maintain nutrition, good hygiene, or a safe environment puts them at increased risk.

Characteristics of the Environment

Characteristics of the environment can raise the risk for infection as well and deserve careful assessment.

COMMUNITY. For clients in the community, assess the home and community environment for risk factors. Some clients are at increased risk because of contacts with infectious organisms. Visitors to foreign countries come into contact with microorganisms that are not a significant health concern in the United States. Persons living in milder climates of the United States are more at risk for mosquito vector–borne diseases. Lifestyles can put people at increased risk for some infections. IV drug abusers are at increased risk for the blood-borne infections of HIV and hepatitis B and C. People with multiple sexual contacts are at risk for sexually transmitted diseases. Homeless persons are at increased risks for airborne infections such as tuberculosis because of crowded conditions in shelters.

Environmental factors that contribute to increased risk for infection can include overcrowded living conditions, which can lead to increased contact with individuals who may have an infection. Environments that harbor pests, such as rats or roaches, raise the risk for infection because the pests harbor infectious agents. Lack of screens in mild weather can lead to increased infections caused by mosquitoes or flies.

HEALTH CARE INSTITUTIONS. Assess the health care institution's environment for risk factors. More stringent rules of cleanliness and sanitation are needed in a hospital environment because the clients as a group are at high risk for infection. Hospitalized clients may have weakened defenses to infection because of illness. They also are in close proximity to other persons who harbor infectious agents. In addition to multiple individual risk factors, hospitalized clients come into contact with antibiotic-resistant organisms not present in other places, and they may undergo multiple invasive procedures.

Assessing the hospital environment includes being aware of the infections that are currently present in the hospital. When a hospital has an increased incidence of nosocomial infections, especially those caused by resistant organisms, efforts at infection control should be reviewed and refined to eliminate the spread of these organisms. An example would be an outbreak of *Clostridium difficile* on a nursing unit. The department responsible for infection control may be consulted to review individual client cases and make recommendations for control on that specific nursing unit.

Focused Assessment for Infection

Localized Infection. The clinical appearance of a localized or contained infection has four basic components: *redness* (erythema), *swelling* (edema), *pain,* and *heat.* Often a fifth component, *loss of function,* also is present. This response occurs whether or not the body has experienced this type of infection previously. After an initial decrease of circulation to an infected area, increased permeability of blood vessel (vascular) walls allows a flow of fluid and cells into the affected tissue to aid in fighting the infection. The presence of fluid and red blood cells causes the redness, edema, and increased temperature common at the site of infection. White blood cells result in the formation of pus, a familiar sign of infection found on the surface of the skin.

Systemic Infection. Systemic infections, those that progress to involve more than one organ system, are more difficult to treat and generally result in poorer outcomes. These infections can result from lack of treatment of a localized infection. Clients who are at increased risk for infection with decreased primary defenses or inadequate secondary defenses may experience a systemic infection.

Systemic infections are manifested by signs and symptoms that affect the entire body. These signs and symptoms define a clinical syndrome that determines the diagnosis of infection. Clients with these infections frequently present with a general malaise, fever, myalgia, arthralgia, and nonspecific GI symptoms. Fever, although common with infections, may not always be present. If unrecognized, systemic infections can lead to dehydration, acidosis, septic shock, and possibly death within a short period.

What symptoms did Luisa exhibit that might indicate the presence of systemic infection?

Note pain of any kind: head, chest, abdominal, or in the extremities. Frequently, infants with acute otitis media pull or rub the affected ear. Increased secretions from the nose or abnormal breath sounds indicate the possibility of respiratory infection.

The GI signs and symptoms of general nausea, vomiting, abdominal cramping, and diarrhea could be additional signs of systemic infection. **Septicemia,** or infection in the bloodstream, may be accompanied by nonspecific client complaints, such as tiredness and fever, but can also include chills, sweats, myalgia, and arthralgia. Central nervous system infections can present with general malaise and fever but can also include headache and stiff neck. Urinary frequency, urgency, and dysuria can be presenting symptoms of a urinary tract infection, but there may also be no symptoms at all. Fever is not usually a symptom in such an infection and, if present, along with flank pain, chills, and sweats, probably indicates that pyelonephritis has developed.

Vaginal or other genital organ infections frequently cause symptoms and can result in severe infections involving the uterus and ovaries. Abnormal discharge (changes in color, consistency, odor), itching, and pain with intercourse can be signs of vaginal infection. These infections sometimes lead to pelvic inflammatory disease, which can result in problems with fertility and childbearing.

Symptoms in Immunocompromised Clients.

A client who is immunocompromised may present with a modified clinical picture of infection. The easy-to-recognize initial symptoms of infection such as redness, swelling, heat, pain, and decreased movement can be absent in the immunocompromised client. This lack of response can delay the client's recognition of infection and, in turn, timeliness in seeking treatment. This may lead to more serious infection as well as a spread of infection from the initial site to other tissues.

Assess all clients for *Risk for infection,* and include three major areas in your assessment. First, obtain a history and physical examination, including questions about the characteristics of the host (client) that contribute to the person's vulnerability to infection. Second, obtain information about exposure to infection, the type of organisms to which the individual is exposed, or the characteristics of the agent of infection. This could involve ascertaining the signs of infection in other family members. Finally, examine the environment for factors that contribute to the spread of infection. This might involve questions related to the type of housing a family has.

 To assess Luisa's risk for infection prior to the present illness, what questions would you ask her parents?

DIAGNOSIS

When a client presents with an infection, with increased risk for infection, or with ineffective protection against infection, evaluate the client on the basis of a health history and physical examination that includes any sign of inflammatory response. If the risk factors are present without signs of infection, write the diagnosis as *Risk for infection related to. . . .* If the client has ineffective protection due to physical causes of tissue damage or to altered immune response, write the diagnosis as *Ineffective protection for infection related to. . . .* An active infection puts the client at increased risk for further infection. Some infections that alter the immune system of the client, such as HIV, actually result in ineffective protection. As another example, infants in a day-care center are at increased risk for infection because of the frequent exposure to many children. If those infants have not been immunized as recommended by the American Academy of Pediatrics, they have ineffective protection compared with the infants with proper immunization history. Table 21-3 gives examples of client data with appropriate nursing diagnoses.

Write nursing diagnoses appropriate to the stage of the client's illness and the focus of care. Persons in whom HIV infection is initially diagnosed may need counseling about how to effectively communicate with their partners, and they may not need interventions based on ineffective health protection at this time. The focus of care for persons with HIV admitted to the hospital for *Pneumocystis carinii* pneumonia would initially be improved oxygenation. With recovery, though, the focus of care could shift to that of *Ineffective protection.* Be aware, however, that although the focus of care differs, some of the specific interventions may be similar.

Individuals can and often do respond differently to the same medical diagnosis. The type of response can determine the outcomes for the client in terms of both a willingness to undergo treatment and the actual response to that treatment. It is important to assess the client's and family's responses to the diagnosis. Their responses will form the

Table 21-3	*Clustering Data to Make a Nursing Diagnosis*
INJURIES	
Data Cluster	**Diagnosis**
Client presents with pain, redness, swelling on leg injured during previous week. He is 86 years old and has diabetes.	*Risk for infection* secondary to poor wound healing
This 60-year-old client, living by himself, is readmitted for antibiotic treatment for infected surgical incision. He lacks knowledge of wound care.	*Ineffective health maintenance* related to need to manage wound care
This 2-year-old admitted for dehydration is refusing PO foods, fluids on day 2 of hospitalization. Parents not visiting.	*Ineffective health maintenance* related to fear and lack of social support
Infant at first well-baby visit 6 weeks after delivery. Has normal axillary temperature, respirations 40, and heart rate 100. Appears fussy in mother's arms. Mother expresses concern about the infant receiving immunization.	*Risk for infection* related to age and mother's lack of knowledge regarding immunizations
A 40-year-old woman receiving chemotherapy for cancer of the uterus. White blood cell count 500. Complaining of vaginal dryness and itching.	*Risk for infection* related to decreased WBC and altered vaginal mucous membranes
A 25-year-old man with AIDS. Critically low T-cell count. Rents a room with no cooking facilities. Weight loss 30 pounds.	*Ineffective protection* related to decreased immunity and inadequate nutrition

basis for formulating nursing diagnoses and planning appropriate interventions. A client's culture can significantly influence the response to diagnosis and treatment as well, as suggested in Box 21-4.

Ineffective Health Maintenance.
Determine whether a client's health practices are helpful in preventing the recurrence of a previous illness. Previous experience helps shape one's attitude toward health maintenance. If a previous illness did little to interfere with life or caused minimal discomfort, the client may be unwilling to undertake health maintenance practices to prevent a recurrence. If, however, the previous illness was perceived to cause extreme distress or was life threatening, the client might take major steps to maintain health and prevent a recurrence.

Luisa's siblings had upper-respiratory infections in infancy, but they never experienced ear infections or other secondary infections. How might this family history have had an impact on the parents' response to Luisa's initial cold symptoms?

Anxiety.
Assess for concerns about the risk for infection that may produce anxiety. Concerns about emerging infections and hospital-acquired infection have been publicized and may result in undue alarm. Clients whose immunity is suppressed from an illness or from medical therapy need information about commonsense ways to protect themselves. Although a state of unease can accompany the diagnosis of *Risk for infection*, the knowledge of having a condition that can increase the risk for infection can add to the state of unease. The increased state of anxiety itself can reduce one's protection against infection.

Fear.
Fear of a diagnosis can be reality based but also can be greater than is warranted in a particular situation. Evaluate the fears and provide a climate in which the client feels comfortable in verbalizing them. Knowledge of a particular diagnosis and usual outcomes are helpful in allaying fear of the unknown. At times, you must simply acknowledge your client's fears as being true and feel comfortable in assisting them and their families to access coping mechanisms to assist them through the illness. Your ability to assess the level of fear and help the client cope can help determine the client's outcome. Again, the mind–body connection can be very significant in the healing process.

What factors might put the Martez family at risk for fear?

Impaired Social Interaction.
Many times the diagnoses of *Risk for infection* and *Ineffective protection* for infection require a support system in order for clients to carry out activities of daily living. Without support of friends or family, an infection may develop needlessly into a life-threatening situation. Homeless persons in whom active tuberculosis has been diagnosed and who are unable or unwilling to seek therapy not only endanger their own health but also that of those with whom they come in contact. Clients living alone who are unable to seek medical attention and have no one they can call for help lack a system of support not only for seeking care but also for treatment.

Cross-Cultural Care CARING FOR A MEXICAN-AMERICAN CLIENT

Box 21-4

Luisa's father came to the United States 6 years ago to find employment and lived with his brother's family for 6 months until he could send for his wife in Mexico. He is employed in a local factory, and his entire family continues to live with his brother and his family. In Mr. Martez's culture, it is not unusual for extended families to continue to live together, and this arrangement is not based on financial need.

The family's confusion with the admission process was the result of (1) a lack of understanding about the infant's medical diagnosis and (2) the different health practices of many Mexican Americans, who believe that illness results from imbalance or disharmony that could be caused by natural or supernatural powers. They are accustomed to using folk treatments. They may have some belief that Luisa's illness is caused by the "evil eye," which would require the person who gave the evil eye to touch Luisa to remove it. Luisa's extreme dehydration at the time of admission was probably the result of delay while the parents attempted home remedies and consulted with other family members and possibly a folk practitioner before seeking medical assistance.

Luisa's mother and father stay with Luisa throughout her hospitalization. Other family members care for their other children. Her mother is devoted to her care and follows the agreed-upon plan. The father blames the mother for Luisa's illness but supports the mother because she cares for Luisa. He is not directly involved with Luisa's care but is playful and affectionate when Luisa improves.

Luisa improves dramatically with intravenous hydration and antibiotic therapy. Her mother seems content to be able to breastfeed again. Because of their sense of not having control over their environment, adherence to an immunization schedule begun during this hospitalization will require family- and community-based support. Although every client is unique, Mexican-American clients, like those in Luisa's family, tend to have the following characteristics (Lassiter, 1995):

- They are tactile, communicating with touch and preferring a close personal space during interview.
- They believe in the evil eye, and in the ability of touch to dispel the devil.
- They accept pain as an expected and necessary part of life.
- They use the family as the major support system, and view the family as more important than the individual.
- They view relationships with children as being more important than the marital relationship.
- They exhibit male dominance and demand allegiance from wife and children.
- They exhibit female submissiveness to husbands and devotion to children.
- They are honest and dignified.
- They are focused on relationships rather than tasks.
- They have a present-time orientation.
- They seek a harmonious relationship between social and spiritual realms.

Situational Low Self-Esteem. Self-esteem is another component of a client's mental health that plays a role in determining outcomes for the individual. Low self-esteem can be influenced by society's response to a particular illness. A diagnosis of HIV infection can carry judgment from many in society, despite public campaigns designed to eliminate these prejudices. The client, as a part of society, requires support from you to maintain a positive sense of self-worth. The infection may not even be one that is sexually transmitted (e.g., HIV can also be acquired by other means). An adult may contract chicken pox and be ridiculed by others for having a childhood disease. Even though these examples differ in many respects, the client can have situational low self-esteem in both cases. Because this could hinder the healing process and interfere with client outcomes, it is important to assess for low self-esteem and work with the client to alleviate or eliminate it.

PLANNING

Expected Outcomes for the Client With *Risk for Infection*

The goal of care for the client at risk for infection is to prevent that client from getting an infection. To achieve this goal you must work to reduce risk factors. The expected outcomes are based on primary and secondary prevention strategies (i.e., elimination of those risk factors and early recognition and treatment). Sample client outcomes for the nursing diagnosis *Risk for infection* include the following. The client will do the following:

- Have intact skin and mucous membranes
- Have containment of any infection after the initial diagnosis
- Verbalize knowledge of measures to avoid infection
- Avoid exposure to organisms causing nosocomial infection
- Verbalize early signs of infection and seek appropriate treatment
- Demonstrate no signs or symptoms of infection secondary to medical or nursing procedures

Expected Outcomes for the Client With *Ineffective Protection*

The goal of care for the client with the nursing diagnosis *Ineffective protection* is that the client will have increased ability to safeguard from internal or external threats such as illness or injury. The expected outcomes depend on the specific threat, but the things the client will do may include the following:

- Verbalize knowledge of how to self-protect from infection (if immunocompromised)
- Verbalize knowledge to self-protect from damage to tissue (if anticoagulated)
- Remain free of infection or injury
- Verbalize knowledge of wound management (open wounds due to trauma or surgery)
- Show evidence of wound healing without experiencing an infection
- Reduce the risk factors to minimize the risk for infection

- Be able to identify an infection in its early stages when it can be treated minimally before the infection may become life threatening

Other goals may be formulated, knowing that it is more desirable to treat an infection with oral antibiotics (when able) than with IV antibiotics, and to treat clients at home rather than in the hospital. At times, however, clients with infections cannot be treated in the home setting. A plan of care is then developed to meet the client's needs during hospitalization.

INTERVENTION

Interventions to Prevent Transmission of Infection

Interventions to prevent the transmission of infection are discussed in two categories: hospital infection control and infection control in the home. Infection control measures used in the hospital include medical asepsis, standard precautions, and isolation precautions. The basis of infection control includes maximizing the client's primary defenses against infection by minimizing damage to the skin, respiratory tract, and GI tract. Reducing the number of pathogenic organisms in the environment provides a more sanitary environment. Proper hand hygiene is considered the most effective way to stop the spread of microorganisms between individuals. To prevent the spread of airborne organisms, a well-ventilated environment is essential.

Implementing Medical Asepsis. **Medical asepsis** consists of practices designed to reduce the numbers of pathogenic microorganisms in the client's environment. The desired result is to prevent or reduce the transmission of the microorganisms from one person to another. On the other hand, **surgical asepsis** is the protection of the client against infection before, during, and after surgery using sterile technique. *Sterile* means free of all microorganisms, whereas medical asepsis is free of pathogenic organisms.

HAND HYGIENE. The first line of defense in medical asepsis is good hand hygiene. Hand hygiene refers to any method approved by the Centers for Disease Control and Prevention for decontaminating the hands. Handwashing refers to using soap and water to clean the hands. Friction or rubbing increases the amount of soil and microorganisms removed. When performing hand hygiene, wash from areas of clean to less clean. Procedure 21-1 describes the correct method for hand hygiene using principles of medical asepsis. Box 21-5 (p. 466) provides guidelines from the Centers for Disease Control and Prevention (CDC) for frequency of performing hand hygiene.

> *Action Alert!* Perform hand hygiene before every contact with a client. Hand hygiene is the first line of defense to prevent infection.

ENVIRONMENTAL CONTROLS. Minimizing the spread of infection requires the use of appropriate environmental precautions. Routine cleaning of the environment should be done daily. Any spills, especially those involving infectious

PROCEDURE 21-1   HANDWASHING

TIME TO ALLOW
Novice: 30 seconds
Expert: 30 seconds

Performing hand hygiene is one of the most important ways to prevent transmission of infectious organisms. Make sure you perform hand hygiene properly before and after contact with each client. Perform handwashing when your hands are visibly soiled and when you first come on duty.

DELEGATION GUIDELINES

All staff members are expected to comply with proper hand hygiene technique and adherence to standard precautions. Nursing assistants should follow this hand hygiene procedure before and after any client contact.

EQUIPMENT NEEDED

- Sink with running water
- Soap
- Paper towels
- Prepackaged cleansing sponge with cuticle stick, if needed

1. Follow preliminary guidelines for nursing procedures (see inside front cover).

2. Turn on the faucet so that warm water is running. A sink operated by knee or foot pedal is preferable because your hands do not have to contact the sink surface. *Warm water leaves more protective skin oils in place than hot water and is less chafing to the skin over time, when frequent hand hygiene is done.*

3. Wet your hands and lower arms under running water while holding your hands lower than your elbows (see illustration). *This position helps microbes run off your hands rather than up your arms.*

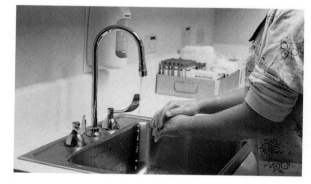

Step 4. Thoroughly rubbing all surfaces of the hand with soap.

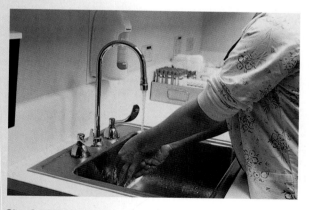

Step 3. Wetting the hands while holding them lower than the elbows.

4. Using soap, thoroughly rub all surfaces of your hands, including your palms, backs of your hands, and wrists (see illustration). Work the soap into a foamy lather while rubbing both hands together using circular movements. *Because bar soap can provide an environment for bacterial growth if continually wet, liquid soap from a dispenser is recommended. Mechanical movements loosen and remove dirt and microorganisms.*

5. Pay special attention to cleansing the following areas that can concentrate microorganisms: between the fingers, at creases and breaks in the skin, at the nail beds, and under the nails (see illustration). Spend 15 to 30 seconds performing hand hygiene. *A cuticle or orangewood stick can be used to assist in properly cleansing under the nails. The washing time may vary depending on the amount of contamination, the type of contamination, and the client's risk for infection.*

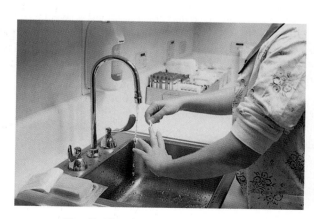

Step 5. Cleaning under the fingernails.

Continued

PROCEDURE 21-1 | HANDWASHING—CONT'D

6. Rinse your hands with warm running water under the faucet, allowing the water to wash down your hands and over your fingertips.

7. Dry hands thoroughly with a towel (see illustration). *In some care situations, paper towels are used for drying the hands.*

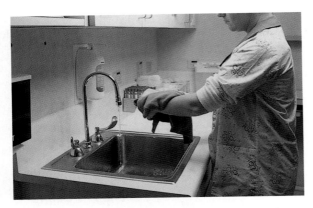

Step 7. Drying the hands thoroughly with a towel.

8. If the sink is not foot-operated, turn off the faucet with the used towel, then discard the towel in the appropriate designated receptacle. *The towel acts as a barrier between your clean hand and the faucet.*

9. Wash hands a second time if indicated by excessive contamination or when you are first entering a nursing unit.

HOME CARE CONSIDERATIONS

If you work in home health care, bring bactericidal soap and paper towels with you to the client's home.

If no running water is available in the home, you may use disposable wipes or alcohol. Be aware, however, that these can be drying to the skin if used frequently.

Box 21-5 | Hand Hygiene Guidelines From the Centers for Disease Control and Prevention

CATEGORIES

These recommendations are designed to improve the hand-hygiene practices of health care workers and to reduce transmission of pathogenic microorganisms to clients and personnel in health care settings. As in previous Centers for Disease Control/Healthcare Infection Control Practices Advisory Committee (CDC/HICPAC) guidelines, each recommendation is categorized on the basis of existing scientific data, theoretical rationale, applicability, and economic impact. The CDC/HICPAC system for categorizing recommendations is as follows:

Category IA. Strongly recommended for implementation and strongly supported by well-designed experimental, clinical, or epidemiological studies.

Category IB. Strongly recommended for implementation and supported by certain experimental, clinical, or epidemiological studies and a strong theoretical rationale.

Category IC. Required for implementation, as mandated by federal or state regulation or standard.

Category II. Suggested for implementation and supported by suggestive clinical or epidemiological studies or a theoretical rationale.

No Recommendation. Unresolved issue. Practices for which insufficient evidence or no consensus regarding efficacy exist.

DEFINITION OF TERMS

Handwashing: Washing hands with plain (i.e., nonantimicrobial) soap and water.

Decontaminate hands: To reduce bacterial counts on hands by performing antiseptic hand rub or antiseptic handwash.

Antiseptic handwash: Washing hands with water and soap or other detergents containing an antiseptic agent.

Antiseptic hand rub: Applying an antiseptic hand-rub product to all surfaces of the hands to reduce the number of microorganisms present.

Alcohol-based hand rub: An alcohol-containing preparation designed for application to the hands for reducing the number of viable microorganisms on the hands. In the United States, such preparations usually contain 60% to 95% ethanol or isopropanol.

RECOMMENDATIONS

1. Indications for Handwashing and Hand Antisepsis

A. When hands are visibly dirty or contaminated with proteinaceous material or are visibly soiled with blood or other body fluids, wash hands with either a nonantimicrobial soap and water or an antimicrobial soap and water (IA).

B. If hands are not visibly soiled, use an alcohol-based hand rub for routinely decontaminating hands in all other clinical situations described in items 1C-1J (IA). Alternatively, perform hand hygiene with an antimicrobial soap and water in all clinical situations described in items 1C–1J (IB).

Box 21-5 Hand Hygiene Guidelines From the Centers for Disease Control and Prevention—cont'd

1. Indications for Handwashing and Hand Antisepsis—cont'd

C. Decontaminate hands before having direct contact with clients (IB).

D. Decontaminate hands before donning sterile gloves when inserting a central intravascular catheter (IB).

E. Decontaminate hands before inserting indwelling urinary catheters, peripheral vascular catheters, or other invasive devices that do not require a surgical procedure (IB).

F. Decontaminate hands after contact with a client's intact skin (e.g., when taking a pulse or blood pressure, and lifting a client) (IB).

G. Decontaminate hands after contact with body fluids or excretions, mucous membranes, nonintact skin, and wound dressings if hands are not visibly soiled (IA).

H. Decontaminate hands if moving from a contaminated body site to a clean body site during client care (II).

I. Decontaminate hands after contact with inanimate objects (including medical equipment) in the immediate vicinity of the client (II).

J. Decontaminate hands after removing gloves (IB).

K. Before eating and after using a restroom, perform hand hygiene with a nonantimicrobial soap and water or with an antimicrobial soap and water (IB).

L. Antimicrobial-impregnated wipes (i.e., towelettes) may be considered as an alternative to washing hands with nonantimicrobial soap and water. Because they are not as effective as alcohol-based hand rubs or washing hands with an antimicrobial soap and water for reducing bacterial counts on the hands of health care workers, they are not a substitute for using an alcohol-based hand rub or antimicrobial soap (IB).

M. Wash hands with nonantimicrobial soap and water or with antimicrobial soap and water if exposure to *Bacillus anthracis* is suspected or proven. The physical action of washing and rinsing hands under such circumstances is recommended because alcohols, chlorhexidine, iodophors, and other antiseptic agents have poor activity against spores (II).

N. No recommendation can be made regarding the routine use of nonalcohol-based hand rubs for hand hygiene in health care settings. Unresolved issue.

2. Hand-Hygiene Technique

A. When decontaminating hands with an alcohol-based hand rub, apply product to palm of one hand and rub hands together, covering all surfaces of hands and fingers, until hands are dry (IB). Follow the manufacturer's recommendations regarding the volume of product to use.

B. When washing hands with soap and water, wet hands first with water, apply an amount of product recommended by the manufacturer to hands, and rub hands together vigorously for at least 15 seconds, covering all surfaces of the hands and fingers. Rinse hands with water and dry thoroughly with a disposable towel. Use towel to turn off the faucet (IB). Avoid using hot water, because repeated exposure to hot water may increase the risk of dermatitis (IB).

C. Liquid, bar, leaflet, or powdered forms of plain soap are acceptable when washing hands with a nonantimicrobial soap and water. When bar soap is used, soap racks that facilitate drainage and small bars of soap should be used (II).

D. Multiple-use cloth towels of the hanging or roll type are not recommended for use in health care settings (II).

OTHER ASPECTS OF HAND HYGIENE

A. Use hand lotions to minimize the occurrence of contact dermatitis associated with hand antisepsis or handwashing.

B. Do not wear artificial fingernails or extenders when having direct contact with clients at high risk (e.g., those in intensive care units or operating rooms) (IA).

C. Keep natural nail tips less than 1/4-inch long (II).

D. Wear gloves when contact with blood or other potentially infectious materials, mucous membranes, and nonintact skin could occur (IC).

E. Remove gloves after caring for a client. Do not wear the same pair of gloves for the care of more than one client, and do not wash gloves between uses with different clients (IB).

F. Change gloves during client care if moving from a contaminated body site to a clean body site (II).

G. No recommendation can be made regarding wearing rings in health care settings. Unresolved issue.

Modified from Guidelines for Hand Hygiene in Health-Care Settings: Recommendations of the Healthcare Infection Control Practices Advisory Committee and the HICPA/SHEA/APIC/IDSA Hand Hygiene Task Force, Centers for Disease Control and Prevention. *MMWR Morbidity and Mortality Weekly Report, 51*(RR-16). Retrieved October 25, 2002 from http://www.cdc.gov/handhygiene.

---

materials, should be cleaned immediately to avoid spreading the infectious organisms. The use of clean materials and antimicrobial soaps for daily cleaning and cleaning between clients is important to reduce the spread of infection.

The housekeeping or environmental services department is responsible for cleaning client rooms, bathrooms, halls, waiting rooms, utility rooms, and the nurse's station. Daily cleaning of the client's room includes removing trash, wiping sinks and countertop with disinfectants, using disinfectants in the bathroom, and sweeping or vacuuming the floor. Disinfectants remove most microorganisms from surfaces, which are then considered clean. They do not prevent microorganisms from returning to these surfaces.

Nursing personnel help the client keep the room clean. The sink and bathroom are generally considered to be dirty areas. When using the sink, consider that it has been used for washing dirty hands and disposing of dirty bathwater. Clean objects that come in contact with the client should not touch dirty surfaces. The bedside table and over-bed table should be clean areas. It is inappropriate to place urinals, bedpans, and even potted plants on a surface that will be used for eating or storing eyeglasses, hearing aids, and dentures.

For even more stringent control of microorganisms, various disinfection and sterilization methods can be used. Disinfection removes microorganisms sensitive to the disinfectant used. It does not limit reintroduction of microorganisms to the surface. Sterilization means to remove all microorganisms. The surface can be easily contaminated, however, by contact with an unsterile surface, equipment, or air currents. Table 21-4 (p. 468) outlines the use and limitations of various methods used to control or eliminate the growth of microbes.

Table 21-4	Disinfection and Sterilization Methods	
Method	**Use**	**Limitations**
Steam	Kills microorganisms sensitive to heat and moisture	• Some bacterial spores seem resistant to this treatment. • Some equipment cannot withstand the high temperatures and moisture.
Gas (ethylene oxide)	Kills microorganisms on products that cannot be steam-sterilized	• Articles must be allowed to release gas by aeration before use. • Cannot use to sterilize liquids, which would absorb gas. • Is expensive and time consuming (2 to 5 hours).
Radiation	Kills microorganisms	• Many spores are resistant, although equipment is not damaged.
Ultraviolet light	Sensitizes microorganisms to other treatments	• May have to be used with other methods to kill additional microorganisms but does not damage equipment.

DISPOSING OF BODILY WASTES. Feces and urine are of course flushed through the bathroom toilet into the sewage system. If the client uses a bedpan, urinal, or bedside commode, use care to prevent spills, and clean the container after disposing of urine or feces. Change any soiled linen as necessary.

PROMOTING AIR QUALITY. Designated hospital personnel monitor the institution's ventilation system to ensure that the quality of air is healthy. Maintenance of the system prevents the growth of molds that could be circulated throughout the hospital, causing disease.

EMPLOYING BARRIERS. Another component of medical asepsis is the use of barriers that can reduce the transmission of organisms from the client to the caregiver. Gloves can be used to avoid direct contact with infectious material. Gloves should never be used as a substitute for good hand hygiene. A clean gown or apron can be used to protect clothing from contamination. To be effective, the gown or apron should be impermeable to water to prevent the soiling of clothing under the covering gown or apron.

Another technique used as part of medical asepsis is cohorting, a process in which clients with similar diagnoses are placed together to minimize the spread of their infections to clients not infected by that organism. In intensive care units and other departments that have more than one bed unit per room, the beds for these clients may be grouped together.

Implementing Standard Precautions. The concept of standard precautions was developed a number of years ago with the developing awareness that any client has the potential for carrying an unknown and possibly incurable infection. Standard precautions include the use of hand hygiene and barrier precautions to prevent the caregiver from exposure to pathogens. Any bodily substance has the potential for harboring infectious organisms, which can be transmitted from client to caretaker and then possibly to another client.

Standard precautions are a set of actions, including hand hygiene and the use of barrier precautions, designed to reduce transmission of infectious organisms; they are applied to every client regardless of whether an infection has been identified. Barrier precautions include gloves, water-impermeable gowns, and eye protection if splashes are possible. Standard precautions are tailored to fit the area, the care delivered, and the client population served. They should be implemented whenever contact with potentially infectious material is anticipated. These precautions are used to protect the caregiver, but keeping the client in mind. Remember that gloves do not re-

Box 21-6	Common Infections Managed With Standard Precautions

- Abscess with minor or limited drainage contained by a sterile dressing
- Acquired immunodeficiency syndrome (AIDS)
- Most pneumonias, including those caused by gram-negative bacteria
- Acute bacterial conjunctivitis, including gonococcal and chlamydial
- Salmonella (use contact precautions if client diapered, incontinent, <6 years of age)
- Hepatitis A, B, C, E (for hepatitis A, use contact precautions if client diapered or incontinent)
- Herpes zoster (localized lesions in immunocompetent client)

place proper hand hygiene. When a task is completed, remove gloves and perform hand hygiene using soap and friction. Change barriers between clients.

Action Alert! **Always** use standard precautions, not just with clients whose infections are known.

The government agency responsible for developing guidelines for standard precautions is the CDC. Box 21-6 lists common infections that are managed using standard precautions. Specific guidelines are part of standard precautions, including hand hygiene; the use of gloves, masks, eyewear, face shields, and gowns; linen; client care equipment; environmental controls; and handling of sharps. Box 21-7 provides specific information about each of these components.

Implementing Isolation Precautions. Historically, health care agencies developed procedures for **isolation**—that is, identification of a client who has an infection and implementation of precautions to prevent the spread of that infection. After an infecting organism was identified, guidelines were implemented specific to the organism. These guidelines were called disease-specific guidelines. The system was cumbersome, however, because the guidelines were listed according to each known organism, and it required extensive education about the mode of transmission of the infecting organism.

Because many infections have similar modes of transmission, similar recommendations could really be used to prevent their spread. For this reason, category-specific isolation precautions were later developed. The number of different kinds of isolation was then reduced to seven, and the mechanisms for prevention were more easily implemented. Category-specific isolation procedures include the following:

Box 21-7 Components of Standard Precautions

HAND HYGIENE

Perform hand hygiene before having any contact with clients and before preparing any items that will be used in client care. Perform hand hygiene again after any contact with a client, especially after touching any blood, body fluids, secretions, excretions, and contaminated items. Even if you wore gloves, you must still perform hand hygiene. When needed, perform hand hygiene during the care of a client to prevent cross-contamination of body sites.

GLOVES

Wear gloves to handle blood, body fluids, secretions, excretions, and contaminated items. Although blood-borne pathogens are the basis for wearing gloves, the blood does not have to be visible in the body fluids for gloves to be required. Remove the gloves immediately and perform hand hygiene before proceeding with the next task or touching noncontaminated items, even on the same client. Change your gloves between tasks on the same client if different body sites are involved.

MASK, EYE PROTECTION, FACE SHIELD, GOWN

Use as needed if you could be exposed to splashes or sprays of blood, body fluids, secretions, and excretions. The risk for splashes or sprays is higher in emergency departments and operating rooms; however, the risk exists with some clients in general care areas as well.

CLIENT-CARE EQUIPMENT

Handle equipment in a manner that prevents personal skin and mucous membrane exposure and cross-contamination to other clients. Ensure that reusable equipment is cleaned and reprocessed before using it in the care of another client.

ENVIRONMENT

Review hospital procedures for routine care, cleaning, and disinfection of environmental surfaces. Spills of blood and body fluid may need to be handled with special procedures.

LINEN

Linen should be handled in a way that keeps it from contaminating skin, mucous membranes, and clothing. Fold soiled linen with the contamination to the inside. Hold it away from your body, place it directly in a plastic bag, tie the bag, and take it directly to the soiled-linen area.

SHARP OBJECTS

Take all possible precautions to prevent needlesticks or cuts with sharp objects (called *sharps* for short). Needles are the primary concern on a general client unit; however, scalpels and other sharp objects are sometimes used. Do not recap used needles in any manner that involves pointing the needle toward any part of your body or another person. If you must recap a needle, place the cap on a flat surface and scoop it onto the needle. After using a needle, immediately discard it in a puncture-proof container. Do not attempt to bend or break a needle before discarding it. Throw the syringe and needle away without removing the needle from the syringe.

- *Blood–body fluid precautions:* To prevent disease transmission by infected blood, saliva, tears, semen, vaginal secretions, urine, or fluid aspirated from body cavities
- *Drainage-secretion precautions:* To prevent disease transmission by direct or indirect contact with drainage from body cavities or with purulent secretions
- *Enteric precautions:* To prevent disease transmission through direct or indirect contact with feces

- *Contact isolation:* To prevent disease transmission by close proximity or direct contact with a client. Private room is required.
- *Strict isolation:* To prevent disease transmission by air and contact with highly contagious or virulent organisms. All barriers are used when entering a private room.
- *Respiratory isolation:* To prevent disease transmission by air through droplets
- *Tuberculosis isolation:* To prevent disease transmission of the airborne organism *Mycobacterium tuberculosis*

Once standard precautions were implemented for all clients, the categories for isolation could be further reduced. Isolation for blood-borne pathogens is no longer necessary because standard precautions, when correctly implemented, already incorporate any precautions necessary for blood-borne pathogens. The CDC now recommends three categories of transmission-based precautions in addition to standard precautions. These three categories are *airborne, droplet,* and *contact.*

AIRBORNE PRECAUTIONS. Airborne precautions are used to prevent infection when the infectious organism is capable of remaining in the air for prolonged periods of time and of being transported in the air for distances greater than 3 feet. The most recognized organism in this group is the tuberculosis bacterium, although the chicken pox and measles viruses are also included in this category. Besides standard precautions, clients with these infections should be placed in a private room with negative pressure, if possible. The room should vent directly to the outside and have a designated minimum number of air exchanges per hour. Anyone entering the room must wear a special particulate filter mask. The CDC also recommends limiting visitors and, in the cases of chicken pox and measles, limiting caretakers to those already immune.

DROPLET PRECAUTIONS. Droplet precautions refer to precautions used for organisms that can be spread through the air but are unable to remain in the air farther than 3 feet. Thus a standard mask (without a special filter) must be worn when standing within 3 feet of the client, in addition to standard precautions. Many respiratory viral infections, including influenza, require droplet precautions.

Figure 21-2 (p. 470) compares three different types of masks. The first is the individually fitted particulate filter mask required as part of airborne precautions. The second is a standard mask that also contains a face shield to guard against exposure to splashes (it is often used in operating rooms). The third is a standard mask that is routinely used as part of droplet precautions.

CONTACT PRECAUTIONS. Contact precautions include standard precautions and the use of barrier precautions such as gloves and impermeable gowns. They are used for clients with diarrhea, when coming into contact with draining wounds not contained by the sterile dressing, or with clients who have acquired antibiotic-resistant infections. An example of this type of infection is methicillin- (or sometimes multidrug-) resistant *Staphylococcus aureus* (commonly called MRSA). The goal of these precautions is to eliminate disease transmission resulting from either direct contact with the client or indirect contact through an intermediary infected object or surface that has been in contact with the client, such as instruments, linen, or dressing materials.

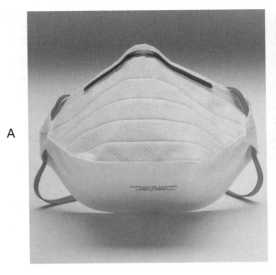

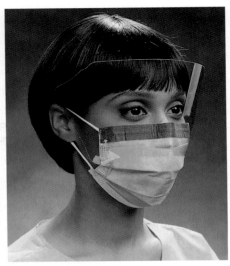

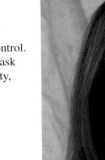

Figure 21-2. Masks used as barrier methods of infection control. **A,** Individually fitted particulate filter mask. **B,** Standard mask with face shield. **C,** Standard mask. (**A** courtesy Uvex Safety, Smithfield, RI; **B** courtesy Kimberly-Clark, Roswell, GA; **C** courtesy Medline Industries, Mundelein, IL.)

The CDC discusses a fourth type of isolation, known as protective isolation. This would be used for immunocompromised clients, who would have a nursing diagnosis of *Ineffective protection*. This type of isolation is discussed further when we look at interventions for clients with this nursing diagnosis.

Table 21-5 (p. 474) outlines common clinical conditions that would require some form of isolation and identifies the potential pathogens for these disorders and the precautions that are warranted. Procedure 21-2 describes how to appropriately don and remove gown, gloves, and mask when working with a client in isolation.

Action Alert! Protective isolation should be used for clients with compromised immune systems.

Isolation rooms can be used to isolate clients with poor hygiene or those with airborne infections. They can also be used for those clients with *Ineffective protection*. When available, rooms with negative pressure are useful for airborne infections such as tuberculosis, measles, or chicken pox. Negative-pressure rooms vent directly to the outside and must have air exchanges with outside air, not with air circulated from the rest of the ventilation system. Positive-pressure rooms are those rooms that prevent the air from the rest of the agency from entering the room, thereby minimizing the possibility of introducing infectious agents to the client. To be effective, doors to both negative- and positive-pressure rooms should be kept closed.

Before the advent of standard precautions, many health care facilities used a special cart with isolation equipment stored on it. Now, as standard precautions are the governmentally mandated standard of care, isolation carts have no particular advantage in most circumstances. Gloves, impermeable gowns, and protective eyewear are stored to be available to all staff. Whenever droplet, airborne, or protective precautions are implemented, these items must be available to all of the client's visitors. In these instances, special carts may be placed at the entrance to the client's room to facilitate the availability of these items to visitors.

Because standard precautions require that all bodily fluids be treated as potentially infectious, laboratory specimens are now all treated as if they are infectious. This usually requires

Text continued on p. 474

| PROCEDURE 21-2 | CARING FOR A CLIENT IN ISOLATION |

TIME TO ALLOW
Novice: Variable
Expert: Variable

Appropriate protective equipment should be used whenever you face a risk for exposure to infectious substances. Likewise, in the case of isolation, appropriate protective equipment should be worn to protect the client from exposure to possibly infectious substances.

DELEGATION GUIDELINES

You may delegate aspects of your client's care to a nursing assistant who has received training in the performance of isolation procedures, consistent with your institution's policies and procedures.

EQUIPMENT NEEDED
- Gown
- Gloves
- Mask
- Goggles (if risk of splash is present)
- Trash receptacle
- Laundry receptacle (if gown is nondisposable)

APPLICATION OF BARRIERS

1. Follow preliminary guidelines for nursing procedures (see inside front cover).

2. Put on gown.
a. Pick up the gown by its collar and allow it to unfold without touching the floor.
b. Put your arms through the sleeves and pull the gown up over your shoulders.
c. Fasten the neck ties.
d. Make sure the gown laps over itself at the back and fasten the waist ties (see illustration). *Overlapping the back reduces the chance of contaminating the back of your clothing underneath the gown, especially when you are removing the gown.*

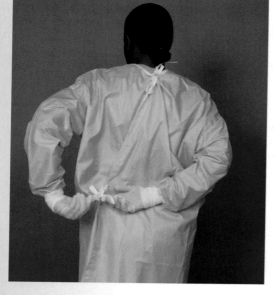

Step 2d. Lapping the gown over itself and fastening the waist ties.

3. Put on disposable gloves.
a. Pull the cuff of each glove over the edge of the gown sleeve (see illustration). *Prevents transmission of microorganisms to you from the client.*

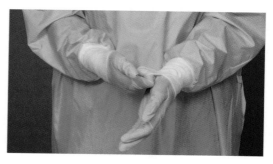

Step 3a. Pulling the cuff of each glove over the edge of the gown sleeve.

b. Interlace your fingers, if needed, to adjust the fit of the gloves.

4. Put on a mask.
a. Position the mask over your nose and mouth (see illustration).

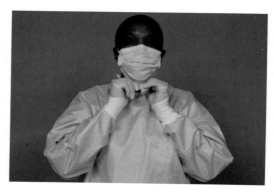

Step 4a. Mask positioned over the nose and mouth.

Continued

PROCEDURE 21-2 CARING FOR A CLIENT IN ISOLATION—CONT'D

b. Bend the nose bar over the bridge of your nose for a snug fit. *Eliminates air entering around the mask rather than through the mask.*
c. Fasten the elastic bands or tie the mask securely in place if it has strings. *A mask reduces potential exposure to airborne droplet nuclei. Plan to change your mask every 30 minutes because its effectiveness dramatically drops after that time period.*
d. Put on goggles, if indicated, after your mask is in place. *Goggles are indicated for situations where splattering of blood or secretions is possible.*

5. Administer care to client. After disposing of soiled items used in client care, tie the bag securely (see illustration). If special disposal methods are used, and the bag is not prelabeled, mark the bag appropriately.

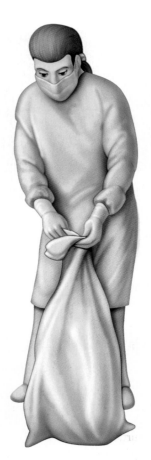

Step 5. Tying the bag securely.

REMOVAL OF BARRIERS

1. At the door to the client's room and next to a trash container, untie your gown at the waist but do not remove it yet (see illustration).

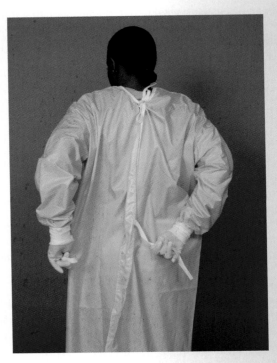

Step 1. Untying the gown at the waist.

2. Remove your gloves.
a. Grasp the outside of the cuff of one glove and pull the glove inside out over your hand (see illustrations). Hold the removed glove in the second hand.
b. Tuck an ungloved finger inside the cuff of the remaining glove.
c. Pull the second glove off inside out (see illustration), and discard both gloves. *This method prevents contamination of your hands by microorganisms.*

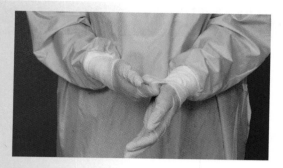

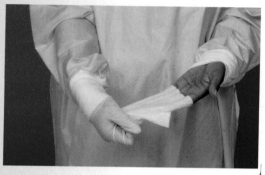

Step 2a. (1) Grasping the cuff. (2) Pulling the first glove inside out.

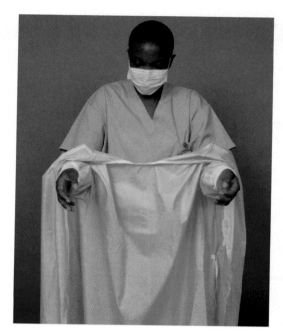

Step 3a. Allowing the gown to fall forward from the shoulders.

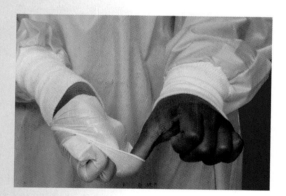

Step 2c. Pulling the second glove inside out.

3. Remove your gown.
a. Untie your gown at the neck and allow it to fall forward from your shoulders (see illustration).
b. Slide your hands through the sleeves and remove them without touching the outside of the gown.
c. Hold the gown at the inside shoulder seams and away from your body, allowing it to turn inside out. Fold the contaminated side of the gown to the inside (see illustration).
d. Discard the gown in an appropriate receptacle.

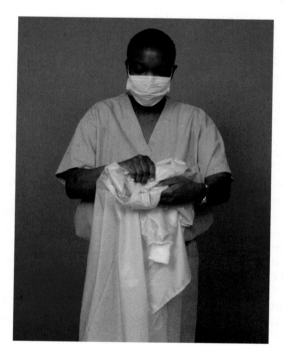

Step 3c. Folding the contaminated side of the gown to the inside.

4. Remove your mask and goggles (if used).
a. Pull the elastic or untie the strings without touching the mask's outer surface.
b. Discard the mask in an appropriate receptacle. *These steps prevent contamination of your hands by microorganisms.*

5. Perform hand hygiene.

Table 21-5	Precautions for Specific Clinical Syndromes or Conditions	
Clinical Syndrome or Condition	**Potential Pathogens**	**Precautions**
DIARRHEA		
Acute diarrhea with a likely infectious cause in an incontinent or diapered client.	Enteric pathogens	Contact
Diarrhea in an adult with a history of recent antibiotic use.	*Clostridium difficile*	Contact
RESPIRATORY INFECTIONS		
Cough, fever, upper-lobe pulmonary infiltrate in an HIV-negative client or a client at low risk for HIV infection.	*Mycobacterium tuberculosis*	Airborne
Cough, fever, pulmonary infiltrate in any lung location in an HIV-infected client or a client at high risk for HIV infection.	*Mycobacterium tuberculosis*	Airborne
Respiratory infections, particularly bronchiolitis and croup, in infants and young children.	Respiratory syncytial or parainfluenza virus	Contact
RISK OF MULTIDRUG-RESISTANT MICROORGANISMS		
History of infection or colonization with multidrug-resistant organisms.	Resistant bacteria	Contact
Skin, wound, or urinary tract infection in a client with a recent hospital or nursing home stay in a facility where multidrug-resistant organisms are prevalent.	Resistant bacteria	Contact

placing the specimen container in another container, such as a bag, that is clean on the outside and has not come into contact with the laboratory specimen. The bag is labeled with a biohazard alert symbol, which tells everyone that the specimen is potentially infectious (Figure 21-3). Health care personnel should wear gloves when handling the actual specimen containers. Laboratory personnel should use gloves and barrier precautions when actually handling the material.

The infection control methods used when transporting clients on isolation depend on the diagnosis or infection. For clients requiring just standard precautions, there are no special precautions. Those with additional precautions should have limited movement and be transported as infrequently as possible out of their room. If it becomes necessary to transport these clients from their room, it is essential to maintain precautions to minimize the risk of transmitting the infecting organism to other clients or to the environment. Additionally, clients with droplet precautions or airborne precautions should wear masks when outside their room.

Controlling Infection in the Home. Whenever a nurse delivers care in the home, interventions must include the input of the client and any other residents into the plan of care. Because the nurse has less control over interventions to minimize the risk for infection, it is critical to have participation of both the client and others living in the household to develop needed interventions to reach the agreed-upon client outcomes. Without the participation of the entire group, outcomes will certainly be less than optimal. Many of the nursing interventions in the home revolve around education and the understanding of the residents. Because the nurse is usually there for only a prescribed period of time, the main caregivers must understand and agree to the plan. These caregivers may consist of family members or family plus home health care workers, depending on the client's situation and ability to provide self-care.

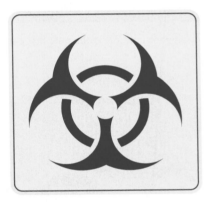

Figure 21-3. Biohazard alert symbol.

MANAGING RISK FOR INFECTION. The basic element of infection control to prevent the spread of infection in the home is the same as in the hospital: good hand hygiene. It is also important for the home caregiver to know how the infection is transmitted to reduce the potential for infecting others. Basic hygiene and pest control might also be issues that may require attention. Principles of good nutrition and signs and symptoms of infection are other educational issues for the nurse working in home care (Box 21-8).

Action Alert! Teach the home care client about the importance of hand hygiene as a basic infection control measure.

The client who is discharged to home after a surgical procedure is often responsible for daily self-monitoring of wound status and self-care for the wound until a follow-up appointment has been scheduled with the surgeon. Because an incision is a break in the skin, a first line of defense, surgical clients are at increased risk for infection by virtue of the surgery. Box 21-9 provides information for clients on how to manage a wound to prevent postoperative infection. The principles of medical asepsis also apply.

Box 21-8 **Teaching Tips for Preventing Infection in the Home**

FOOD HANDLING

- Good hand hygiene is the best defense against infection.
- Perform hand hygiene after using the bathroom and before preparing or eating food.
- When cleaning and cutting chicken, perform hand hygiene before preparing other foods.
- Wash all fresh fruits and vegetables before eating them.
- Store leftover food in the refrigerator.
- Do not refreeze uncooked meat that has been thawed.
- Cook ground meat, chicken, and pork thoroughly.

MANAGING COLDS AND FLU

- Keep tissues handy to catch sneezes and coughs.
- Keep a wastebasket close to the sick person.
- Perform hand hygiene often to help reduce the chance of spreading a cold or the flu.

CARING FOR MINOR SCRAPES AND CUTS

- Clean the wound with mild soap and water, and pat it dry.
- Cover it with a bandage if it is bleeding or likely to become contaminated.

Teaching for Self-Care
Wound Care   **Box 21-9**

Purpose: To keep a wound from getting infected.

Expected Outcome: The client will clean the wound and experience complete healing without incurring an infection.

Client Instructions

- Assemble the supplies you'll need, such as fresh sterile gauze, peroxide, antibiotic cream, tape, and a trash can.
- Perform hand hygiene.
- Remove your old dressing and place it in the trash.
- Look to see if the wound has any new redness, tenderness, or drainage. If it does, tell your doctor or nurse about it.
- Using some sterile gauze moistened with peroxide, wipe your incision from the center out to an edge one time. Then throw the gauze in the trash.
- Using a new piece of moistened sterile gauze, wipe your wound one more time from the center to the edge. Go in a different direction this time.
- Repeat the preceding step until you have cleaned the entire wound.
- Allow the wound to air dry.
- Apply antibiotic cream if your doctor told you to.
- Cover the incision with sterile gauze and tape it in place.

Teaching for Self-Care
Preventing Infection in Immunosuppressed Clients   **Box 21-10**

Purpose: To prevent the client from acquiring an infection at home.

Expected Outcome: The client will continue to function at home without acquiring an infection.

Client Instructions

- Gather as many of your friends and family as possible to learn about keeping you free from infection.
- Perform hand hygiene often with soap and water. This is the best means to prevent infection.
- If you have pets, consider giving them to someone else who can care for them.
- Have any dusting or vacuuming done when you are not in the room.
- If you have living plants in the house, have someone else water them.
- You may need to alter what you eat. For example, all meats should be cooked thoroughly until well done. Also, eat no thin-skinned fresh fruits or vegetables unless they are canned. This includes grapes, peaches, and apples. (Ask clients for their own examples to ensure understanding of this point.)
- Ask your friends to visit you at another time if they feel ill.

MANAGING INEFFECTIVE PROTECTION. Good hand hygiene is an educational issue that can never be addressed too many times and should be reviewed periodically when caring for immunocompromised clients in the home setting. A clear understanding of why their protection for infection is ineffective is essential to minimize their risk. Assess for situations or practices that should be changed because of the ineffective protection, and address these issues with the client and caregivers. Box 21-10 provides instructions for methods to minimize the risk of an immunocompromised client's acquiring an infection in the home.

A health care worker in the home must use the same precautions to prevent the spread of infection from the client to others. Good hand hygiene is still required, but unfortunately some homes may not have running water and soap as readily available resources. In these instances, although not the most desirable, you must use disposable wipes saturated with an antiseptic solution as a stopgap measure. Use barrier precautions as you would in the health care setting if contact with potentially infectious material is possible. The barrier precautions used in the home are the same: gloves, water-impermeable gown, masks, and eye protection. If occupants of the home, other than the client, are at increased risk, they may also need to use barrier precautions. You should ensure that the necessary items are available to them and give instructions on their correct use.

Implementing Sterile Technique. Sterile technique refers to those practices used to prevent the introduction of microorganisms that could cause infection. This is sometimes called *surgical aseptic technique.* Sterile technique is used when there is a break in the first line of defense (i.e., the skin and mucous membranes) and may be indicated for selected procedures performed by the nurse or other health care personnel

at the bedside, or during surgical procedures. Sterile technique as used during surgery requires extensive procedures for preventing microorganisms from entering surgical wounds. There are three areas of application of this technique: the skin, physical barriers (sterile field), and the environment.

SKIN. The skin of the client is thoroughly cleansed before any invasive procedure. This may involve washing first with soap to remove soil. The remainder of the an antimicrobial agent that is left on the skin as an antimicrobial barrier. Hair is sometimes removed by shaving or with depilatory preparations; however, this is a less common practice than in the past because of risk of nicks or scrapes to the skin. If hair is removed, it is done prior to cleansing.

Aside from surgery, sterile technique is used whenever host defenses are interrupted, such as during catheter insertion (e.g., intravenous and urinary), dressing changes of surgical wounds, or endotracheal suctioning. It should also be used during IV fluid or medication administration. Box 21-11 outlines the principles of sterile technique.

STERILE FIELD. Using sterile technique for limited procedures outside the operating room involves setting up a small sterile field with a few pieces of equipment and using sterile gloves to handle sterile equipment. Procedure 21-3 describes how to apply and remove sterile gloves.

When setting up a sterile field, you may open a tray that already contains sterile materials wrapped in a drape. At other times, you may be required to use a drape to set up the sterile field and then place sterile supplies onto that sterile drape. Procedures 21-4 (p. 478) and 21-5 (p. 479) review how to prepare a sterile field using a tray wrapped in a sterile drape and how to set up a sterile field using a sterile drape.

A member of the surgical team who will work within a sterile field scrubs the hands and arms before entering the operating room to put on sterile attire. The hands and arms are first washed with soap and water to remove gross soil. Hands and arms are then washed with an antimicrobial soap using a sponge and/or scrub brush to remove as many microorganisms as possible. The soap leaves an antimicrobial residual that continues to prevent the presence of microorganisms after the washing. Note, however, that the friction from using a sponge or brush is the most effective component of reducing the organisms on the skin. The objective is to remove microorganisms without destroying tissue. Procedure 21-6 (p. 481) describes how to perform a surgical hand scrub.

To maintain the area free of microorganisms, sterile gloves, gowns, and drapes are used to create a barrier between the environment (including the members of the team) and the client. To achieve an outer surface that is sterile, a gown and gloves are put on to cover the body. The technique for putting on a gown and gloves requires not touching the outer surface of the attire. After the procedure, careful removal of the gown and gloves is important to prevent contamination of the clothing under the gown. Procedure 21-7 (p. 483) describes the process for donning a sterile gown and using closed gloving technique. The basics of setting up a sterile field in the operating room include covering the client with sterile drapes, covering work surfaces with sterile drapes, and laying out sterile instruments on the sterile field.

ENVIRONMENT. Environmental controls contribute to reducing the presence of microbes. Special areas may be set aside for special use, such as operating or procedure rooms. These rooms, when not in use, are cleaned using germicidal detergents. The area may have positive-pressure airflow to minimize the introduction of microorganisms into the air, and

Box 21-11	**Principles of Sterile Technique**

- Sterile means the absence of all microorganisms.
- The skin cannot be sterilized, but thorough cleaning can significantly reduce the number of microorganisms present.
- Sterile objects that come in contact with unsterile objects are no longer sterile.
- When a sterile field is wet, capillary action will draw microorganisms from the surface underneath a permeable drape. This is called *strikethrough*. A wet drape is not a sterile drape.
- Consider anything below the waist to be unsterile.
- Consider any part of the sterile field that falls or hangs below the top of the table to be unsterile. Waist level is the limit of a good visual field.
- Consider the edge of a sterile field and 2 inches inward as unsterile.
- Do not cough, sneeze, or talk excessively over a sterile field.
- Do not reach across a sterile field.
- Always face a sterile field. If you turn your back on a sterile field, you cannot guarantee its sterility.
- Use a sterile package immediately once it has been opened. Otherwise, it cannot be considered sterile.
- Consider a bottle of sterile liquid no longer sterile once it has been opened. If you save it to repeat a procedure, you may be performing a clean procedure, but you will not be performing a sterile procedure.
- Sterile packages have expiration dates determined by the manufacturer or the method of sterilization. Do not use packages that have passed their expiration date.
- Sterile packages are labeled as sterile. If a package is not so labeled, consider it unsterile.
- If there is any doubt about the sterility of an object, consider it unsterile.
- If a sterile package is wet or damaged, or if there is evidence that moisture has dried on it, consider it unsterile.

the ventilation system may have more frequent air exchanges to remove any introduced microbes. Any unnecessary visitors and personnel are excluded.

If a special room is not available, the designated area for a procedure can be cleaned ahead of time using a germicidal detergent. Then traffic or other activity in the area can be curtailed during the procedure to minimize the number of microbes deposited on the procedural area by air currents. Screens can be used to designate the area and remind personnel to avoid the area. After a sterile procedure is completed, the area is cleaned using standard precautions, followed by cleaning according to agency policy (which in turn depends on whether the area is specially designated).

Cleaning of equipment used in sterile procedures involves removing any visible soil and then disinfecting with a germicidal cleaner. Any materials used in invasive procedures that are not disposable must be sterilized after cleaning. Items are generally sterilized in autoclaves that utilize steam at high heat and pressure over a period of time. Items that could be destroyed by moisture or high heat and pressures can be sterilized by gas. Many disposable items are bought presterilized. The sterility of these items is guaranteed over a specified time period, assuming no breakage in the packaging has occurred. As a nurse, you are responsible for ensuring that sterilized equipment is properly stored to maintain sterility for use in future procedures.

Text continued on p. 485

PROCEDURE 21-3   DONNING AND REMOVING STERILE GLOVES

TIME TO ALLOW
Novice: 2 min.
Expert: 15 seconds

Sterile gloves should be used when performing procedures requiring surgical asepsis. This will eliminate the risk of introducing microorganisms from the caregiver to a sterile object or to the client.

DELEGATION GUIDELINES
Some of the tasks that you will delegate to your nursing assistant may require the use of sterile gloves. Nursing assistants should receive appropriate training in this skill prior to the delegation of such tasks.

EQUIPMENT NEEDED
- One package sterile gloves of appropriate hand size
- Flat work surface
- Other supplies as needed according to procedure being performed

DONNING STERILE GLOVES

1. Follow preliminary guidelines for nursing procedures (see inside front cover). *Remove rings with stones or irregular surfaces. Reduces microorganisms and the risk of puncturing the gloves with the rings.*

2. Grasp the package at the tabs above the upper sealed edge. Peel down to open the outer wrapper. Discard the outer wrapper.

3. Place the inner package on a flat surface. Open the inner package at the first fold, touching the outside of the folded edge and pulling outward. Then open the next fold, pulling that edge outward without touching the inside of the package. The package is usually labeled "up" and "down," or "left" and "right." Opening in this manner creates a sterile field. The outside of the wrapper is now contaminated. Gloves are now laid out with the left glove on the left and the right glove on the right.

4. Put on the first glove.
a. Grasp the folded edge of the cuff of one glove (see illustration). Usually, the dominant hand is gloved first.

b. Lift the glove above the wrapper and away from your body. *Lift the glove straight up (perpendicular to the wrapper) to avoid dragging the gloves over the contaminated edge of the wrapper. Step back if necessary to give yourself room to glove without touching a contaminated surface.*
c. Slide the opposite hand into the glove. Do not adjust the cuff or fingers now or let your ungloved hand touch the outside of the glove. *This technique maintains sterility by preventing contact of the gloves with unsterile objects, such as the hand, uniform, or other surfaces.*

5. Put on the second glove.
a. Pick up the second glove by sliding your sterile gloved fingers under the edge of the cuff (see illustration). Avoid the tendency to let your gloved thumb touch the (to become) unsterile surface of the cuff of the second glove. *Prevents*

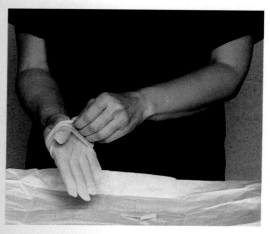

Step 4a. Grasping the folded edge of the cuff of one glove.

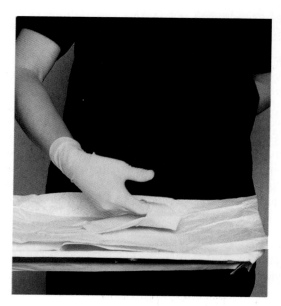

Step 5a. Picking up the second glove.

Continued

PROCEDURE 21-3 DONNING AND REMOVING STERILE GLOVES—CONT'D

the gloved thumb from coming in contact with a surface that will also be touching the ungloved hand.

b. Slide the fingers of your opposite hand into the glove (see illustration). Let go of the edge when your hand is in the glove. As you slide your hand into the glove, the hand that

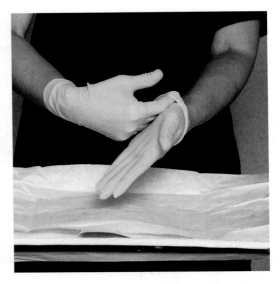

Step 5b. Sliding the fingers of the opposite hand into the glove.

is holding the glove should stretch the edge of the glove out to avoid touching the unsterile wrist.

c. Adjust the gloves for comfort and fit. Your fingers are touching the outside of the glove that will remain sterile. Keep sterile surface to sterile surface. The edges of the glove touching your wrist are not sterile.

REMOVING STERILE GLOVES

1. Grasp the outside of one glove near the base of the thumb and remove it by pulling it inside out. Prevents the used and contaminated glove from coming in contact with the skin of your wrist.

2. Discard the glove or hold it in the palm of the gloved hand. Either method is correct and depends on personal preference.

3. Slide your ungloved thumb or fingers inside the second glove and remove it by pulling it inside out also. If you held the first glove in your hand, they are now wrapped together.

4. Discard into appropriate receptacle.

5. Perform hand hygiene.

PROCEDURE 21-4 PREPARING A STERILE FIELD BY OPENING A TRAY WRAPPED IN A STERILE DRAPE

TIME TO ALLOW
Novice: 1 min.
Expert: 15 seconds

This procedure would be used when a microorganism-free surface is needed to hold materials for dressing changes, insertion of catheters, and other procedures requiring that sterility of objects on the field be maintained.

DELEGATION GUIDELINES
You may delegate the preparation of a sterile field to a nursing assistant who has been appropriately trained in the performance of this task. You would generally not delegate the actual performance of a sterile procedure to a nursing assistant.

EQUIPMENT NEEDED
- Wrapped sterile package
- Flat work surface
- Sterile gloves and other items required to perform the intended procedure on an actual client

1. Follow preliminary guidelines for nursing procedures (see inside front cover).

2. Remove a commercially packaged kit from the outer wrapper.

3. Position the inner package in the center of the work surface so that the outer flap of the wrapper is facing away from you.

4. Reach around (but not over) the package to open the flap away from yourself (see illustration). Touch the outside of the flap only. *Maintains sterility of the package.*

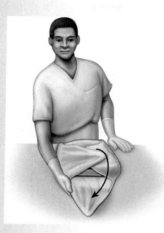

Step 4. Opening the first flap away from yourself.

5. Open the side flaps one at a time, in the same manner as the first, with the uppermost side flap being opened first (see illustration). Remember not to let your hands cross over the sterile field.

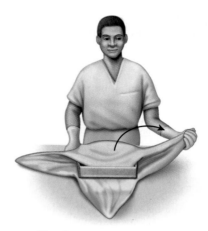

Step 5. Opening the side flaps.

6. Open the innermost flap that faces you last (see illustration). Be sure to stand back sufficiently so that the flap does not touch you during opening.

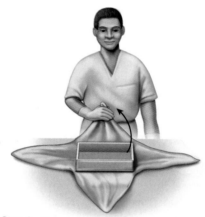

Step 6. Opening the last flap toward yourself.

PROCEDURE 21-5 | **PREPARING A STERILE FIELD**

TIME TO ALLOW
Novice: 6 min.
Expert: 3 min.

This procedure is used when a microorganism-free surface is needed to hold materials for dressing changes, insertion of catheters, and other procedures requiring the sterility of the objects on the field.

DELEGATION GUIDELINES
You may delegate the preparation of a sterile field to a nursing assistant who has been appropriately trained in the performance of this task. You would generally not delegate the actual performance of a sterile procedure to a nursing assistant.

EQUIPMENT NEEDED
- Sterile drape
- Sterile gloves
- Sterile supplies and/or solutions as needed for the planned procedure
- Protective barrier equipment as needed according to the planned procedure

1. Follow preliminary guidelines for nursing procedures (see inside front cover).

2. Arrange your work area. Use a clean, dry, flat, uncluttered surface at waist level. The sterile field should be close to the client. *You should position the field in a manner that allows you to work with the client and keep the field within your line of vision.*

3. Ensure that supplies are sterile by checking the expiration date and for the integrity of the package. *If the package is damaged in any way or shows signs of moisture it cannot be used. This protects the client from being touched by contaminated supplies.*

4. Set up a drape as a sterile field.
a. Prepare a sterile field or surface that is at least 2 inches larger on all sides than the area you need to work with the supplies.
  (1) Open the outer wrapping of a sterile cloth drape, keeping the drape itself sterile.
  (2) Pick up the drape by the loose corner edge and lift the drape into the air and away from your body.
  (3) With your other hand, grasp another corner edge and spread the drape in the air.
  (4) Decide which surface is to remain sterile and spread the drape on the table, with the side that will remain sterile facing up (see illustration). *You can touch the edges of the drape because the edges of a sterile field are not considered sterile.*

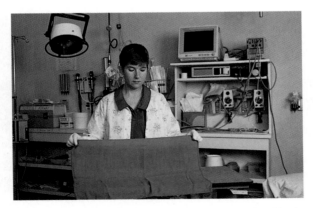

Step 4a(4). Spreading the drape on the table, with the side that will remain sterile facing up.

5. Add sterile supplies
a. **Peel-Apart Packages**
  (1) Use both hands and grasp the edges designed to be peeled open.

(2) Open the package over the sterile field so materials can fall freely from the package onto the field without touching your hands (see illustration).

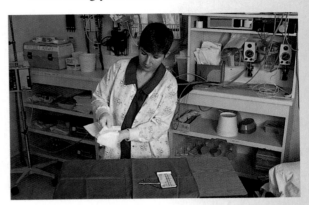

Step 5a(2). Opening the package over the sterile field.

b. **Sterile Liquids**
  (1) Remove or loosen the cap from the bottle of liquid. Do not touch the inside of the cap or the rim of the liquid. Place the cap so the inside is face-up on a flat, unsterile surface to prevent its contamination (see illustration).

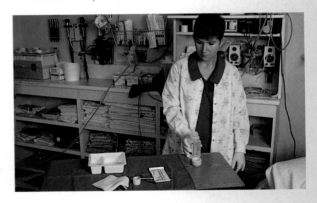

Step 5b(1). Placing the cap with the inside face up on the unsterile surface.

  (2) Label the bottle with the date and time. *Solutions are sometime reused after opening according to agency policy. These solutions that have been opened are considered contaminated 24 hours after opening, or earlier if according to agency policy. When this policy is followed, the procedure is a clean procedure, not a sterile procedure.*
  (3) If the container that will hold the liquid needs to be adjusted, put on one sterile glove.

(4) Use the other ungloved hand to pick up the bottle of liquid so that the label is in the palm of your hand. *This prevents the solution from damaging the label if fluid drips or runs down the side of the bottle. This is only important when the solution is used within 24 hours for a clean procedure.*

(5) Hold the bottle of solution about 10 cm (4 inches) above the container that will receive the liquid. Pour carefully to avoid spills or splashes (see illustration).

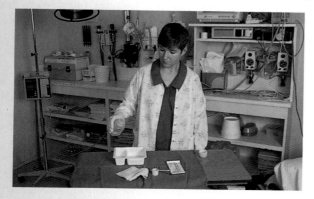

Step 5b(5). Pouring the sterile liquid.

Do not touch the field with the lid of the bottle. *If you get the surface of a permeable sterile field wet, it is no longer sterile. The bottle cannot touch the sterile field for the same reason.*

(6) Replace the lid on the bottle tightly. *Eliminates the risk of spilling the bottle during the procedure.*

(7) Put on the second (or both) sterile glove(s).

c. **Wrapped Packages**

(1) Hold the object in one hand by the bottom or underside of the wrapping.

(2) Unwrap the first corner away from you, then each side, then the last corner toward you.

(3) Stabilize the corners against your wrist. *This prevents the corners from touching the sterile object.*

(4) Turn the object toward the sterile surface and drop it onto the field without touching the field itself.

PROCEDURE 21-6	PERFORMING A SURGICAL HAND SCRUB

TIME TO ALLOW
Novice: Determined by agency policy
Expert: Determined by agency policy

This procedure removes as many microorganisms from your hands as possible before entering a surgical field.

DELEGATION GUIDELINES

The scope of nursing assistant duties in a surgical arena does not generally require the completion of a surgical hand scrub. Nursing assistants may be responsible for the assembly of scrub supplies and should be familiar with this procedure for this purpose alone.

EQUIPMENT NEEDED
- Agency-approved antimicrobial agent
- Surgical scrub brush (with plastic nail-cleaning stick)
- Deep sink with knee or foot controls for water and soap

1. Follow preliminary guidelines for nursing procedures (see inside front cover).

2. Apply surgical attire, including shoe covers, cap or hood, face mask, and protective eyewear (possibly a mask with a face shield).

3. Open a scrub brush so that it is ready for use (see illustration). Turn on the water using the control lever and adjust it to a comfortably warm temperature.

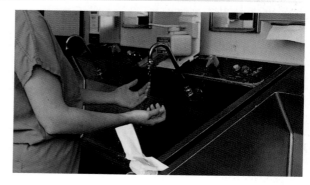

Step 3. Scrub brush ready for use.

PROCEDURE 21-6 PERFORMING A SURGICAL HAND SCRUB—CONT'D

4. Wet your hands and arms, keeping your elbows flexed so that your hands remain higher than your elbows. Water will flow off your arms at the elbows. *Keeps the hands as the cleanest part of the extremities.*

5. Use the plastic nailstick to clean under your nails on both hands (see illustration). *Removes materials under the fingernails that could harbor a variety of microorganisms.*

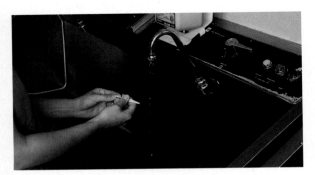

Step 5. Using the plastic nailstick to clean under the fingernails.

6. Remove the scrub brush from its wrapper and wet it. Apply antimicrobial liquid if not already in the brush, or according to agency policy.

7. Scrub the nails of one hand with 15 strokes. Repeat for the other hand. Scrub the palm of one hand (see illustration), each side of the thumbs and fingers, and the back of the hand with 10 strokes each. Repeat for the other hand. *Provides sufficient time for removal of microorganisms by mechanical and chemical means.*

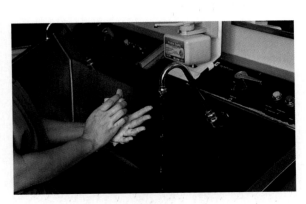

Step 7. Scrubbing the palm.

8. Divide your arms mentally into thirds. Beginning with the section nearest your hands, scrub each third with 10 strokes or by time, according to agency policy. Discard the brush.

9. Flex your arms and rinse from the fingertips to the elbow in a single smooth motion, again letting the water run off at the elbows (see illustration). *Keeps the hands as the cleanest part of the extremities.*

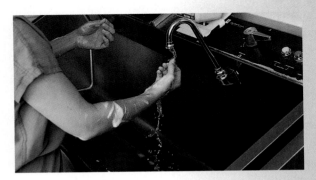

Step 9. Rinsing from the fingertips to the elbow.

10. Release water control and walk backward into the operating room with your hands elevated in front of you and away from your body. *Allows you to keep cleansed hands above waist level and in your line of vision. Reduces the possibility that your hands will become contaminated.*

11. Go to the sterile set up area. Pick up a sterile towel without dripping water onto the sterile field. Using one end of the towel, dry one hand completely using a rotating motion and moving from fingers to elbow. *Dries from cleanest area (fingers) to less clean (elbows).*

12. Using other end of the towel, repeat with other hand and drop the towel into the designated receptacle or an assistant's hand.

PROCEDURE 21-7 · DONNING A STERILE GOWN AND CLOSED GLOVING

TIME TO ALLOW
Novice: Variable
Expert: 7-10 min.

This procedure is done prior to entering a surgical (sterile) field.

DELEGATION GUIDELINES

The scope of nursing assistant duties in a surgical arena does not generally require the donning of a sterile gown and closed gloving. A nursing assistant may be responsible for the assembly of these supplies and should be familiar with this procedure for this purpose alone.

EQUIPMENT NEEDED

- Surgical shoe covers, cap, mask, and protective eyewear
- One package sterile gloves of appropriate size
- One sterile pack containing sterile gown
- Clean, flat, dry surface for opening gown and gloves (such as a Mayo stand)

1. Follow preliminary guidelines for nursing procedures (see inside front cover).

2. Don surgical attire and scrub your arms and hands as described in Procedure 21-6.

3. Have the circulating nurse or other designated person open the sterile gown and gloves.

4. Don the gown.
a. Pick up and unfold the gown.
  (1) Identify the inner surface of the gown and pick up the gown beneath the neckband without touching the sterile field or the outer surface of the gown.
  (2) Make sure you have control of all the folded layers to avoid dangling the gown against unsterile surfaces.

(3) Move away from the table, holding the gown away from your body at arm's length, and allow it to unfold from the top down (see illustration). Do not let the gown touch the floor. *Maintains sterility of the gown.*

(4) Hold the gown just below the neckband near the shoulders and slide both hands into the sleeves until the fingers are at the end of the cuffs but not through the cuffs (see illustration). The fingers remain covered to prepare for closed gloving.

(5) Have someone tie the gown. *The gown should be lapped over itself in the back. The person tying the gown should take care to touch only the ties and not the front or sides of the gown. The front of the gown is sterile.*

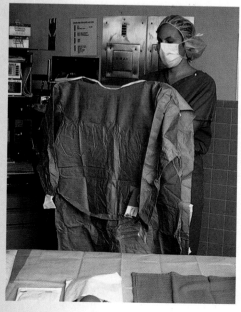

Step 4a(3). Holding the gown at arm's length and allowing it to unfold.

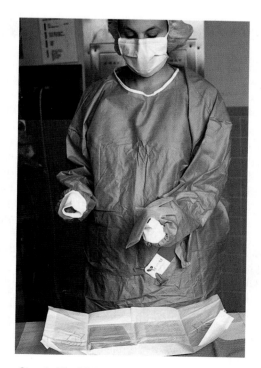

Step 4a(4). Sliding the hands into the sleeves.

PROCEDURE 21-7 **DONNING A STERILE GOWN AND CLOSED GLOVING**—CONT'D

5. Put on the gloves.

a. Apply the first glove.

(1) With your hands covered by the sterile gown cuffs, open the inner sterile glove package and pick up the first glove by the cuff (see illustration). The first glove goes on the dominant hand.

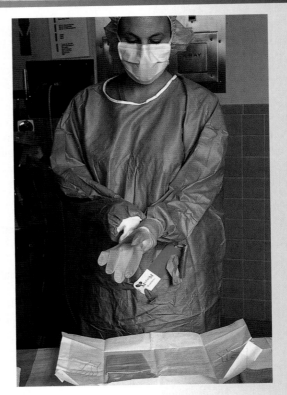

Step 5a(4). Pushing the fingers into the first glove.

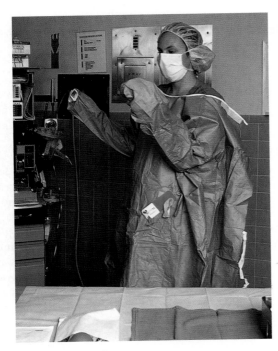

Step 5a(1). Picking up the first glove by the cuff.

(2) Position the glove on the forearm so the cuff faces the hand and the fingers face the elbow.

(3) Begin to put the opposite hand into the glove. Hold the cuff edge of the glove with the sleeve cover of the hand to be gloved. Grasp the back of the glove cuff with the sleeve-covered second hand and turn the cuff over the sleeve. *The fingertips of the hand you are gloving remain inside the sterile sleeve until the sleeve is covered by the sterile glove.*

(4) Push your fingers into the glove (see illustration).

b. Apply the second glove.

(1) Use your sterile hand to pick up the second glove (see illustration). Put the second glove in the same position as the first on the opposite forearm.

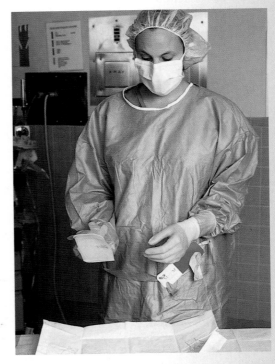

Step 5b(1). Positioning the second glove with the cuff facing the hand and the fingers facing the elbow.

(2) Put on the second glove in the same manner as the first (see illustration).

c. Adjust the gloves for fit and comfort.

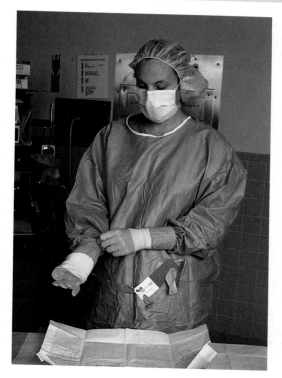

Step 5b(2). Putting on the second glove.

Action Alert! You are responsible for storing sterilized equipment in a manner that maintains its sterility for future use.

Interventions to Protect Clients With Deficient Immunity

Using Environmental Safeguards. Because clients with a compromised immune system have ineffective protection, their entire environment must be altered to minimize their risk for infection. This begins with the type of food that they are able to eat. They must not eat fresh fruits or vegetables except those with thick outer layers that are inedible. They can eat bananas but must handle the skins carefully. Oranges can be eaten, but again, contact with the outer part of the skin must be avoided. They should not eat fresh leafy salads but may have canned or frozen vegetables if well cooked. Fruits, except for those mentioned, must also be cooked before eating. Meats should be eaten only if well done.

The physical environment should be maintained in as clean a state as possible. Not only should these clients avoid dusting and other chores related to cleaning, they should try as much as possible to avoid being in the room when these chores are done. Household pets can be perilous and are not recommended. Living plants are also not recommended, but if there are living plants in the home, they should not be watered by immunocompromised clients.

Preventing Feelings of Isolation. While in the hospital, immunocompromised clients are usually placed in isolation

rooms with the door closed. If available, a room with positive-pressure ventilation to minimize airflow into the room from the rest of the hospital is recommended. Many institutions have special requirements for visitors of these clients. Visitors may be required to perform hand hygiene before entering the room, and to wear gloves, gown, and possibly a mask when inside the room to minimize the spread of normally harmless microbes to the client with ineffective protection. After discharge, because of the extreme risk for infection to those with an altered immune system, these clients should avoid public places, especially those with crowds. Visitors should not be allowed if they think they might have an infection.

Children with up-to-date immunizations and no signs of infection may be allowed to visit in the home. An exception is if they have recently been vaccinated with oral polio vaccine or measles, mumps, rubella, or varicella (chicken pox) inoculations; in this case they should not be allowed to visit. These vaccines are live viral preparations, and although they do not put persons with normal immune systems at risk, those with ineffective protection against infection can become seriously ill from shed viral particles.

To prevent a sense of isolation, encourage clients to have visitors who have no signs of infection. Assess the support systems available to these clients once they go home. Although the number of visitors may be limited at any one time, visiting by friends and relatives is beneficial to the client. Encourage activities that can be done in the home while maintaining relationships with friends and family

Providing Client and Family Teaching. As a starting point for client education, recall that teaching should include any family or friends who will be involved in the client's care. Teach the client about the disease process and its underlying basis. This must include information about the change in ability to fight infections of any kind. Teach the client the basics of infection control and about the importance of keeping the environment as clean as possible, even though all germs cannot be eliminated.

Other important topics for client teaching can then follow. Explain that infections that might be considered a nuisance to some will be life threatening for the client. Teach about the signs and symptoms of infection to watch for, and remind the client that these may be subtle. Tell the client to report any physical changes in general health to the primary health caregiver immediately, so that the client can be evaluated as soon as possible. Subtle signs might include a change in ability to tolerate activity and quite possibly will not include fever or pain. Any rashes or skin breakdown should be reported as well. Changes in bowel habits should be noted as well as any increase in respiratory secretions. Any earache or continuing headache could also be an underlying symptom of infection. The timeliness of reporting these subtle signs is important to reduce the risk for severe infection in the immunocompromised client.

Interventions to Reduce Your Own Risk of Infection

To reduce the risk for infection for the health care worker, strict adherence to guidelines provided by the CDC is necessary. By using hand hygiene and barrier precautions when necessary, health care workers can minimize the risk for infection. Health care workers should use the same precautions to protect themselves that they use for their clients. Use clean technique to prevent the spread of infection to health care personnel when in contact with the client. Perform thorough hand hygiene after client contact to reduce the risk of spreading the infection. If you do have a possible exposure, comply with recommended health service follow-up to minimize the potential risk. Table 21-6 provides an overview of the follow-up treatment recommended after exposure to blood-borne pathogens.

ᐯVALUATION

Evaluation of goal achievement of health protection involves reassessment of the client to determine that the criteria for evaluation have been met.

If the outcomes do not progress as anticipated, a reassessment could provide information as to why. If a client who has received antibiotics for 7 days continues to show signs of inflammation and general malaise, the culture and sensitivity should be reassessed. This may involve reculturing the primary site of infection and looking for additional or new sites of infection.

Evaluation allows continual review of the nursing care. By connecting outcomes to the interventions, nurses can evaluate the effectiveness of those interventions, as suggested in Box 21-12. In most instances, this requires the active participation of the clients and their families. If a client has been instructed to clean a wound twice a day and to re-dress it applying antibiotic ointment and then arrives 2 days later in the emer-

Table 21-6	Follow-Up for Health Care Workers Exposed to Blood-Borne Pathogens
Pathogen	Follow-Up
Unknown	• Contact should be tested for known blood-borne diseases utilizing the fast HIV screening test. • If contact tests positive for HIV, immediate prophylaxis with anti-HIV medications should be begun. • CDC recommends triple-antibiotic treatment at the site of exposure. • If contact does not test positive and health care worker has never undergone hepatitis B immunization, hepatitis B gamma globulin should be administered and immunization should be started per agency protocol. • Health care worker should immediately be screened for the same blood-borne infections and, if negative, return for follow-up screening per agency protocol.
HIV	• If the client was positive for HIV, the health care worker should also be screened and be started on HIV prophylaxis, which could include up to three antiviral drugs. • The health care worker should return for follow-up screening for at least a year or according to the employing agency's recommendations.
Hepatitis B	• If the health care worker is immune, hepatitis B immunoglobulin can be offered. • If the health care worker is nonimmune, hepatitis B immunoglobulin will be offered and immunization begun.
Hepatitis C, D	• Health care worker can be offered immunoglobulin. • Initial and follow-up screening should be done according to agency guidelines.

gency room with odorous, green drainage from the wound, the nurse may question the client's understanding or willingness to participate in the procedure.

A discharge note for Luisa after her treatment for her dehydration secondary to effects of an upper respiratory infection might look like the note below.

SAMPLE DOCUMENTATION NOTE FOR LOUISA MARTEZ
Infant with clear breath sounds and unlabored respirations, and without apparent nasal discharge. Tympanic temperature 98.6° F without receiving acetaminophen during the past 12 hours. Infant appears alert when awake, actively sucking at the breast, voiding freely. Intake has been PO without IV fluids for the last 12 hours. Skin turgor elastic. Infant appears free of pain without any noticeable distress when parents are present. Utilizing the translator, Mr. and Mrs. Martez accurately verbalized the instructions to continue the antibiotic until all of the medication is complete. Additionally, they have stated that they will follow up with the pediatrician at the local clinic within a week. At this appointment they will ask for information on Luisa's immunizations, request that they be updated, and request a record of all their children's immunizations.

Nursing Care Plan **AN INFANT WITH SEPSIS**

Box 21-12

ADMISSION DATA

Luisa is admitted through the emergency department to a general pediatric floor. The emergency room nurse telephones the following report. *"Luisa is a 6-month-old Hispanic infant presenting with dehydration. Intravenous fluids have been started. Blood cultures have been drawn, as well as a CBC. Infant is lethargic. Her parents are at the bedside. She appears to have an upper respiratory infection. A CXR has been done. Her oxygen saturation is 99% on room air. She has mild intercostal and subcostal retractions. Her left ear shows redness and is fluid-filled. Throat swabs were negative for strep."*

PHYSICIAN'S ORDERS

Admitting diagnosis: Dehydration, possible sepsis
IV fluids $D_{10}W$ to infuse at 25 mL/hr
Ampicillin IV q 12 hr
Gentamicin IV q 12 hr

Tylenol PO 50 mg PRN q 3-4 hr for temp > 100.4° F
May breast feed as tolerated, 20 cal/oz formula plus iron on demand when mother not available to breast feed

NURSING ASSESSMENT

Color pale, skin dry, with "tenting" noted, lethargic. Coarse breath sounds with mild retractions noted, rate 40/min. Heart rate regular with no murmur audible, rate = 90/min. Peripheral pulses weak but palpable, equal bilaterally. Bowel sound active. Diaper dry (no urine output since admission). Tympanic temperature 103° F. Mother and father at bedside, quiet, appear frightened.

Luisa recovers with prescribed medical and nursing intervention. When Luisa is ready for discharge the nurse would like to give the parents information about prevention, makes the diagnosis of *Risk for Infection*, and implements the following care plan.

NANDA Nursing Diagnosis	NOC Expected Outcomes With Indicators	NIC Interventions With Selected Activities	Evaluation Data
RISK FOR INFECTION	IMMUNIZATION BEHAVIOR	**INFECTION PROTECTION** • Teach parents about the recommended childhood immunization schedule; use a translator and provide written instructions in Spanish.	• Mr. Martez says they do not have a family physician and do not have health insurance. The nurse makes a referral to a free clinic.
Risk Factor: • Immune status associated with age and presence of siblings in home	KNOWLEDGE: INFECTION CONTROL	**TEACH PARENTS:** • Mode of transmission of disease among siblings and practices to prevent transmission. • Monitor playmates for signs of infectious disease. • Monitor child's general health. • Signs and symptoms of infection. • Diet, rest, and exercise to increase resistance. • Maintain fluid intake during illness. • Follow physician's recommendation about reporting signs of illness.	• Through the interpretor, Mrs. Martez expresses gratitude for the information. She asks questions about how much fluid a child should have when she is ill and what temperature she should report to the physician. She says she does not have a thermometer at home. The nurse provides a thermometer to take home and shows her how to use it. • Spanish instructions are added to the written instructions about fluid needs for all three children and parameters for calling the physician.

CRITICAL THINKING QUESTIONS

1. What other interventions can you think of to make the care delivered to Luisa more culturally specific?
2. What should the nurse be thinking about in order to incorporate cultural considerations in discharge planning?
3. What specific teaching would you provide to Luisa's mother to ensure that another episode such as this does not occur?

Nursing outcome and intervention labels from Johnson, M., Bulechek, G., McCloskey Dochterman, J. M., Maas, M., & Moorhead, S. and others (2001). *Nursing diagnoses, outcomes, and interventions: NANDA, NOC, and NIC linkages.* St Louis, MO:Mosby.

With the sample documentation on page 486, the nurse has documented the data that demonstrates the resolution of the initial diagnosis of *Ineffective protection*. Additionally, the nurse, through a translator, has established new goals for the parents to attain. The nurse can assist the parents in establishing new goals with statements such as "With Luisa more like herself we need to focus on keeping her healthy and at home with her family."

Key Principles

- We are all at risk for infection. There is no environment without organisms having the potential for causing disease.
- We have important physical and physiological mechanisms to protect ourselves from disease-causing organisms.
- Primary defenses against infections include the skin and the membrane barriers of the respiratory, GI, and GU tracts.
- Additional defenses against infection include molecules secreted by skin and membrane cells that provide additional barriers and may break down disease-causing organisms.
- Secondary defenses in the immune system have both nonspecific disease-fighting components and very specific components in the immunoglobulin system.
- Clients with breaks in the primary defenses have the nursing diagnosis *Risk for infection;* those with inadequate secondary defenses have *Ineffective protection.*
- Using the initial assessment of the client, the nurse develops plans of care to provide for the health protection of the client. The assessment includes physical findings and an evaluation of the client's mental status and social support system.
- Interventions may include education, modification of the client's physical environment, administration of antibiotics to eliminate or prevent the spread of infection, and psychosocial support.
- The outcome goals for any client are to minimize the risk for infection and to protect against further spread of infection for both the client and those caring for or associating with the client.

Bibliography

Agut, H. (2001). Prevention and control of viral hospital infections. *American Journal of Infection Control, 29*(4), 244-246.

*Anonymous. (1995). Proposed recommended practices for establishing and maintaining a sterile field. *Association of Operating Room Nurses Journal, 64*(4), 608-610.

Belluck, P., & Drew, C. (1998). Deadly bacteria a new threat to fruit and produce in U.S. *The New York Times,* January 4.

*Centers for Disease Control and Prevention. (1994). *Guidelines for preventing the transmission of* Mycobacterium tuberculosis *in health-care facilities.* Atlanta, GA: Author.

*Centers for Disease Control and Prevention. (1995). *Food and water-borne bacterial diseases.* March [update]. Atlanta, GA: Author.

*Centers for Disease Control and Prevention. (1997). *Guidelines for isolation precautions.* Retrieved from http://www.cdc.gov/ncidod/hip/isolat/isolat.htm.

Chan-Tack, K. M. (2001). Changing antibiotic sensitivity patterns at a university hospital, 1992 through 1999. *Southern Medical Journal, 94*(6), 619-620.

Corrarino, J. E. (1998). Perinatal hepatitis B: Update and recommendations. *American Journal of Maternal/Child Nursing, 23*(5), 246-252.

Engelhart, S., Glasmacher, A., Kaufmann, F., & Exner, M. (2001). Protecting vulnerable groups in the home: The interface between institutions and the domestic setting. *Journal of Infection, 43*(1), 57-59; discussion, 59-60.

Farr, B. M. (2001). Preventing vascular catheter-related infections: Current controversies. *Clinical Infectious Diseases, 33*(10), 1733-1738.

Fleming, C. A., Balaguera, H. U., & Craven, D. E. (2001). Risk factors for nosocomial pneumonia: Focus on prophylaxis [Review]. *Medical Clinics of North America, 85*(6), 1545-1563.

Girouard, S., Levine, G., Goodrich, K., Jones, S., Keyserling, H., Rathore, M., et al. (2001). Infection control programs at children's hospitals: A description of structures and processes. *American Journal of Infection Control, 29*(3), 145-151.

Gross, R., Morgan, A. S., Kinky, D. E., Weiner, M., Gibson, G. A., & Fishman, N. O. (2001). Impact of a hospital-based antimicrobial management program on clinical and economic outcomes. *Clinical Infectious Diseases, 33*(3), 289-295.

Johnson, M., Bulechek, G., McCloskey Dochterman, J. M., Maas, M., & Moorhead, S. and others (2001). *Nursing diagnoses, outcomes, and interventions: NANDA, NOC, and NIC linkages.* St Louis, MO: Mosby.

Kyne, L., Farrell, R. J., & Kelly, C. P. (2001). *Clostridium difficile. Gastroenterology Clinics of North America, 30*(3), ix-x, 753-777.

Kyne, L., Hamel, M. B., Polavaram, R., & Kelly, C. P. (2002). Health care costs and mortality associated with nosocomial diarrhea due to *Clostridium difficile. Clinical Infectious Diseases, 34*(3), 346-353.

*Lassiter, S. M. (1995). *Multicultural clients: A professional handbook for health care providers and social workers.* Westport, CT: Greenwood Press.

Marino, C., & Cohen, M. (2001). Washington State hospital survey 2000: Gloves, handwashing agents, and moisturizers. *American Journal of Infection Control, 29*(6), 422-424.

Oie, S., & Kamiya, A. (2001). Comparison of microbial contamination of enteral feeding solution between repeated use of administration sets after washing with water and after washing followed by disinfection. *Journal of Hospital Infection, 48*(4), 304-307.

Roger, M., St-Antoine, P., & Coutlee, F. (2001). Vancomycin-resistant enterococci in health care facilities. *New England Journal of Medicine, 345*(10), 768-769.

Ruddy, M., Cummins, M., & Drabu, Y. (2001). Hospital hairdresser as a potential source of cross-infection with MRSA. *Journal of Hospital Infections, 49*(3), 225-227.

Sharir, R., Teitler, N., Lavi, I., & Raz, R. (2001). High-level handwashing compliance in a community teaching hospital: A challenge that can be met! *Journal of Hospital Infections, 49*(1), 55-58.

Simor, A. E. (2001). Containing methicillin-resistant *S. aureus:* Surveillance, control, and treatment methods [Review]. *Postgraduate Medicine, 110*(4), 43-48.

Tenover, F. C. (2001). Development and spread of bacterial resistance to antimicrobial agents: An overview. *Clinical Infectious Diseases, 33*(Suppl. 3), S108-S115.

Tokars, J. I., McKinley, G. F., Otten, J., Woodley, C., Sordillo, E. M., Caldwell, J., et al. (2001). Use and efficacy of tuberculosis infection control practices at hospitals with previous outbreaks of multidrug-resistant tuberculosis. *Infection Control and Hospital Epidemiology, 22*(7), 449-455.

Weinstein, R. (1998). Nosocomial infection update. *Emerging Infectious Diseases, 4*(3), 1-7.

Health Protection: Risk for Injury

Key Terms

asphyxiation
aspiration
burn
choking
injury
poisoning
restraint
strangulation
trauma

Learning Objectives

After studying this chapter, you should be able to do the following:

- Discuss the epidemiology of common injuries from falls, asphyxiation, and poisoning
- Discuss the epidemiology of trauma from burns, electricity, motor vehicle accidents, and radiation
- Identify the behavioral, environmental, socioeconomic, developmental, cognitive, and physiological factors that affect safety
- Assess the client's risk for injury
- Distinguish between related nursing diagnoses for the client at risk for injury
- Plan interventions to prevent injury and promote safety in the acute care setting, the client's home, and the community
- Evaluate client outcomes and nursing interventions used to help the client reduce the risk for injury

Juanita Soto is a 75-year-old widow who lives alone in a two-story house. Her sons and daughters live in distant cities and visit her whenever they can. She relies primarily on her neighbors and friends for help. Juanita has been relatively healthy most of her life and has been able to keep up her home despite the fact that 5 years ago she was diagnosed with rheumatoid arthritis. During the last 4 months, however, her condition has worsened. She now uses her wheelchair to get around the house, although she sometimes uses a cane to navigate the flight of stairs that leads downstairs to the washer and dryer. She complains of pain and weakness in her hands and legs. At her last physician visit, she was referred to a local home health agency for evaluation of her condition and her needs.

During the initial assessment visit, the home health nurse notes that, in addition to having limited hand and leg movement, Juanita is partially blind in one eye. The nurse also notes that Juanita's home needs some repairs—especially the stairs, which are old and have no railing for support. Because of the many physical and environmental factors identified, the nurse considers the diagnosis of *Risk for injury*. The nurse also considers related nursing diagnoses for clients with safety needs (see below).

KEY NURSING DIAGNOSES FOR   Health and Safety

Risk for injury: At risk for injury as a result of environmental conditions interacting with the individual's adaptive and defensive resources

Risk for trauma: Accentuated risk for accidental tissue injury (e.g., wound, burn, fracture)

Risk for poisoning: Accentuated risk for accidental exposure to, or ingestion of, drugs or dangerous products in doses sufficient to cause poisoning

Risk for suffocation: Accentuated risk for accidental suffocation (inadequate air available for inhalation)

Risk for aspiration: At risk for entry of gastrointestinal secretions, oropharyngeal secretions, or solids or fluids into tracheobronchial passages

CONCEPTS OF SAFETY

Every person has an inherent need to be and feel safe. Feeling safe allows us to think and act with confidence. Although at birth we depend on someone else for our safety, as we mature we become responsible for our own safety, and eventually we may become responsible for the safety of others. Thus safety is a need that remains with us throughout our lifetime.

Client safety is a major issue in all health care settings. Injuries affect people of all ages, developmental stages, and socioeconomic groups. Injuries can result from behavioral, environmental, or physiological hazards. No matter the cause, they can have devastating effects on both the client and the family when they result in pain, emotional distress, financial hardship, permanent disability, and even death.

As a nurse, you must always be aware of the potential for injury and make it a high priority to promote safety guidelines that help prevent injuries. Prevention can reduce the need for hospitalizations, the risk for complications from medical treatment, the hardship of long-term care, and even the loss of life. Together with your clients, you can develop a plan of action to ensure the safest possible environment.

No matter what type of client you care for—a new mother, toddlers in day care, an older homebound client living alone, a group of clients living in a long-term care facility—safety is a high priority. In fact, you should consider this issue not only with individual clients but also at the community, national, and international levels.

Epidemiology of Injury

An **injury** is trauma or damage to some part of the body. According to the National Center for Health Statistics (Anderson, 1999), accidental injuries are the fourth leading cause of death in the United States. Injury can result from physical, mechanical, biological, or chemical agents. Accidents that result most commonly in death include motor vehicle accidents and falls.

Falls. Older people form the group affected most often by falls, both at home and in institutional settings. Falls are the leading cause of injury-related deaths among people age 65 years and older, with 82% of the deaths occurring in persons age 75 years and older (Centers for Disease Control and Prevention [CDC], 2000a). When a fall occurs, morbidity, immobility, early nursing home placement, or death may result (Fuller, 2000). Because they occur frequently and have serious consequences, falls are one of the most serious problems that acute and long-term care facilities must manage.

Falls occurring in the home are a major concern and account for most reported home accidents in people age 75 and older. The pathophysiological changes that occur with aging—such as an altered gait, decreased mobility, incontinence, and confusion—place many older adults at increased risk for falling (Fuller, 2000).

Action Alert! Assess older clients for unsteady gait, impaired memory or judgment, weakness, and a history of falls.

When older clients fall, the biggest concern is the threat of a hip fracture. Hip fracture is the primary cause of approximately 300,000 hospital admissions each year. In most cases, the affected person is age 65 or older and is more likely to be female (CDC, 2000a).

Falls tend to occur in the home when mobility and coordination are limited, when the person is in a hurry, or when the person is stressed or faced with obstacles. Stairways are commonly involved in falls at home. Factors that contribute to these falls include poor lighting, obstacles on the stairs, and poorly repaired steps. Falls that occur in the bathroom commonly involve a slippery tub or shower.

The risk for falling is significant among hospitalized clients, accounting for up to 10% of all fatal falls (Fuller, 2000). Hospital falls most commonly occur in the client's room when the client is alone and trying to get to the bathroom unassisted. The use of bed side-rails and restraints do not necessarily prevent falls, because clients who fall had either removed the restraints or exited the bed safely, only to fall while walking without assistance. Polypharmacy (the use of several medications at once) is often present in clients who fall.

One day when the home care nurse comes to visit with Mrs. Soto, her daughter is there. The daughter is telling Mrs. Soto that she should sell her home and come to stay with the daughter's family. Can you list the possible concerns that prompted Mrs. Soto's daughter to make this suggestion?

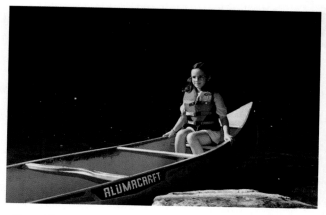

Figure 22-1. The use of a life jacket can promote water safety.

Asphyxiation. **Asphyxiation** refers to an interruption in breathing that results from a severe lack of oxygen (asphyxia) because there is either no source of air, an inadequate supply of oxygen in the air, or a condition where the air cannot be inhaled. Lack of oxygen results specifically from aspiration, choking, or strangulation. **Aspiration** is the inspiration of foreign material into the airway. **Choking** is an internal obstruction of the airway by food or a foreign body. Critical changes in body chemistry caused by choking may quickly become life threatening. If not immediately relieved, they may result in death. Choking can result from aspiration. **Strangulation** is constriction of the airway from an external cause.

Choking on food or objects and aspirating them into the airway, as well as asphyxiation caused by materials that block the external airway, are of special concern in young children and older adults. Death rates from choking are especially high during the first few years of life.

In the older adult or neurologically impaired client, choking and aspiration can result from the loss or absence of protective airway reflexes. Choking and aspiration also can occur in clients who are unconscious from drugs, alcohol, a cerebrovascular accident (stroke), or cardiac arrest, or when a nonfunctioning nasogastric tube allows gastric contents to drain around the tube. Other causes that can lead to choking and aspiration in the older adult or neurologically impaired client include ill-fitting dentures and overzealous feeding. Aspiration of stomach contents is a serious complication that may result in death.

Asphyxiation can result when air is blocked from outside the body, as when a child is caught in an airtight compartment from which the oxygen is gradually depleted by the child's breathing; when airtight material, such as plastic, covers the nose and mouth; or when the chest is compressed so that breathing is impossible, as in some crushing injuries.

Accidental drowning, resulting in asphyxiation, is also of major concern. For children 1 to 3 years old, accidental drowning is a significant cause of injury and death. Drowning is the third most common cause of death among adolescents. For children under 1 year old, drowning occurs most often in bathtubs. Children of ages 1 to 4 years drown most often in residential swimming pools, although bathtubs, toilets, and water buckets are also common. The usual sites of adolescent drownings include lakes and other natural bodies of water. Contributing factors that may increase the risk for drowning include inadequate supervision, lack of safety devices, hazardous swimming conditions, careless boating and water sports, and the use of alcohol and drugs (Figure 22-1).

Strangulation of a child can be caused by unsafe conditions or equipment in the home. Other causes of strangulation include hanging from highchair straps or drapery cords, and wedging of the head between crib slats, in accordion-style safety gates, between a bed and wall, and in electrically operated car windows.

Even in the health care environment, choking, aspiration, strangulation, and asphyxiation can occur. Clients with neurological deficits and impaired mobility are especially vulnerable. You will need to remember that these types of accidents are preventable.

Poisoning. **Poisoning** is clinically defined as an adverse condition or physical state resulting from the administration or ingestion of a toxic substance. Toxic substances can produce injury or death through chemical action. They can enter the body through ingestion, inhalation, injection, application, or absorption of the noxious material. For example, poisoning can result from accidental medication overdose, gases produced when household cleaners are mixed, leaking carbon monoxide, and use of tainted street drugs. There are more than 100,000 chemical entities that the general population could be exposed to and poisoned by. Box 22-1 (p. 492) provides examples. However, despite this multitude of potentially harmful chemicals, only a few have been adequately documented as having caused serious health problems in humans (Loomis & Hayes, 1996).

The reasons for and types of poisonings vary with age. The people most at risk for poisoning include toddlers, young children, and adults with sensory impairment and communication barriers. Lack of adequate supervision and improper storage of toxic household substances are major factors in poisonings in children. Among adolescents and adults, poisoning most often results from snakebites, recreational drugs, or suicide attempts. Poisonings among older adults may result

Box 22-1   Causative Agents in Deaths From Poisoning

The following list presents suspected causative agents in 705 deaths reported to poison control centers in the United States in 1992:

- Antidepressants, such as amitriptyline, desipramine, doxepin, imipramine, and nortriptyline
- Analgesics, such as acetaminophen, aspirin, codeine, morphine, and propoxyphene
- Cardiovascular medications, such as digoxin and verapamil
- Street drugs, such as cocaine, heroin, and methamphetamine
- Sedatives and hypnotics, such as phenobarbital
- Antiasthmatic medications, such as theophylline
- Fumes, gases, and vapors, such as carbon monoxide and hydrogen sulfide
- Chemicals, such as cyanide and strychnine
- Insecticides, such as Diazinon
- Household cleaners, such as sodium hypochlorite (bleach)
- Hydrocarbons, such as butane
- Alcohol, especially the ethanol form
- Automotive products, such as ethylene glycol and methanol

From Loomis, T. A., & Hayes, A. W. (1996). *Loomis' essentials of toxicology,* 4th ed., p. 14, San Diego, CA: Academic Press.

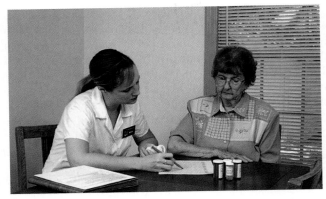

Figure 22-2. Teach a home bound client that the proper labeling and storage of medications can help prevent accidental poisoning.

from medication overdose caused by mental impairment, polypharmacy, or difficulty reading the label due to poor eyesight, illiteracy, or a language barrier (Figure 22-2).

Proper storage, labeling, and use of chemicals and other toxic agents can prevent poisoning, especially in children (Table 22-1).

Action Alert! Teach clients to prevent poisonings through proper storage and labeling of containers. For hospitalized clients, triple-check all medications before administering them.

Epidemiology of Trauma

Clinically, **trauma** is defined as a physical injury or wound caused by a forceful, disruptive, or violent action. The impact from trauma can be profound on all those involved. Trauma is the leading cause of years of potential life lost and the fourth leading cause of death in the United States. Traumatic injury causes morbidity and disability and can create huge problems in lost productivity and medical costs. It has been estimated that each year, 57 million Americans (1 in 4) are injured seriously enough to require medical treatment.

Fires and Burns. Fire hazards can occur in all types of settings. Institutionalized clients are especially at risk for injury from fires because they may be debilitated and unable to escape without assistance. Also, the health care environment contains materials and equipment that may increase the risk of fire. They include flammable gases, such as oxygen combined with anesthetics, and electrical equipment, such as monitors, heating and cooling units, and respiratory equipment. Equipment that is malfunctioning or used improperly may cause sparks that could easily ignite linens, especially in an oxygen-rich environment.

House-fire death rates are highest for children younger than 5 years and for adults older than 65. Older adults are at increased risk for fire death because they are more vulnerable to smoke inhalation and burns and are less likely to recover. Sense impairment (e.g., blindness or hearing loss) may prevent them from noticing a fire or hearing a smoke alarm, and mobility impairment may keep them from escaping a fire (CDC, 2000b). Most house-fire deaths result from the poisoning effects of smoke inhalation rather than from burn injuries.

 Think again about Mrs. Soto. Is she at risk for injury from a fire? What would you assess about her home to determine the level of risk?

The most common cause of house-fire deaths is cigarette smoking. According to one study, alcohol contributed to 40% of deaths in homes (Smith, Branas, & Miller, 1999). The most common causes of house fires are cooking and heating equipment fires (CDC, 2000b).

Action Alert! Urge clients to keep a portable heater at least 36 inches away from anything that might be flammable. Also, recommend that clients install a smoke detector with working batteries on each level of the home. Instruct clients to test the batteries monthly, to change batteries every 6 months, and to keep a multipurpose fire extinguisher on hand in case of fire (Figure 22-3).

A **burn** is clinically defined as any injury caused by excessive exposure to electricity, chemicals, gases, radioactivity, or thermal agents. Besides fire, some of the most common causes of burns in the home or health care institution include exposure to hot bath water, overly hot moist dressings, heat lamps, and other forms of equipment.

People at highest risk for burns include children of age 14 and younger, the handicapped, and older adults with sensory impairments. Children are at risk for burns from misuse of matches and exposure to hot liquids or vapors, and the risk is increased by inadequate parental supervision. Handicapped persons or older adults with sensory impairments risk being

Table 22-1	Preventing Childhood Poisoning
Common Sources of Poisoning	**Client Instructions to Prevent Poisoning**
Medications	• Keep all medications out of the reach of children, preferably in locked cabinets. • Make sure that medication containers have childproof caps. • Store and label medications properly in their original containers. • Read medication labels carefully before administering a medication. • Do not share medications. • Use appropriate measuring devices when administering medications to ensure proper dosing. • Destroy expired medications promptly and appropriately. • Keep emergency numbers—including the local poison control center—near the phone and in plain view. • Never tell a child that a medication is candy. • Keep emergency medications (such as syrup of ipecac) in the home.
Chemicals, cleaning solutions, and other toxic substances	• Keep chemicals, cleaning solutions, and other toxic substances in locked cabinets. • Keep all such substances in their original containers with proper labels. • Maintain adequate ventilation when using chemicals and cleaning solutions. • Do not mix cleaning products, chemicals, and other such substances together.
Houseplants	• Keep out of reach of children. • Provide adequate supervision for young children and infants.

burned from the unsafe use of space heaters, water heaters, stoves, and irons.

Electrical Shock.

Injury from electrical shock can range from trivial burns to charring and destruction of the skin and underlying tissues. Hazards occurring from electrical shock are of concern in both the home and the health care environment. Factors that determine the type and extent of electrical injury include the voltage involved, the type of current, the area and duration of contact, skin resistance, and the path along which the electrical current flows. Other factors include the type of clothing worn and environmental moisture.

The most common type of electrical injuries are low-voltage injuries. They usually are accidental and involve electrical equipment, household appliances, or tools. Electrical shock results when current travels to the ground via the body instead of traveling through the electrical wiring. Fatalities from electrical hazards are relatively uncommon.

Motor Vehicle Accidents.

Motor vehicle accidents are the leading cause of accidental death in the United States (CDC, 2000c). Unsafe driving practices and the use of alcohol and drugs contribute to the occurrences. Depending on the circumstances of the accident, persons at risk for sustaining injuries may include the driver, passengers, pedestrians, bicyclists, and skateboarders. Children on bicycles or skateboards face an increased risk for injury when they fail to use proper safety equipment and precautions, such as wearing safety helmets and padding and following safety guidelines. Guidelines include using signals properly and not riding in traffic or near driveways (Figure 22-4, p. 494). Failure to use safety belts and infant car seats also increases the risk for injury.

Back Injuries.

Back injuries account for nearly 20% of all injuries and illnesses in the workplace and cost the nation an estimated 20 to 50 billion dollars per year. The National

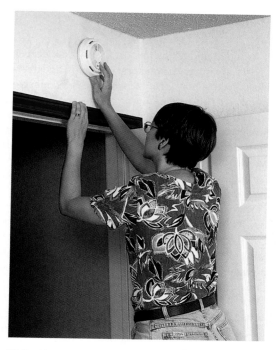

Figure 22-3. All smoke and fire detectors in the home should be installed properly and maintained with fresh batteries.

Institute for Occupational Safety and Health (NIOSH) believes that the most effective way to prevent back injury is to implement an ergonomics program that focuses on redesigning the work environment and work tasks to reduce the hazards of lifting (NIOSH, 1997).

Back injury can often be prevented by following guidelines such as those in Box 22-2 (p. 494). Occupational back injury accounts for a significant number of workers' compensation claims. Back injuries are the main reason for prolonged absence from work; the lost productivity creates substantial costs.

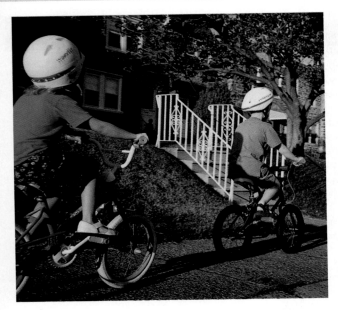

Figure 22-4. Recommend appropriate safety equipment to help prevent head injuries in school-age children.

Back pain and injuries can be caused by disk degeneration, obesity, postural problems, structural problems, and overstretching of the spinal supports. The consequences of injury may include prolonged pain and suffering, decreased quality of life, and a reduced potential for future earnings or job opportunities.

Certain job tasks and personal characteristics increase the probability of back injury. Job tasks include heavy lifting, repetitive lifts (especially while bending or twisting), prolonged sitting, working in a stooped or awkward position, and operating vibrating machinery. Personal characteristics may include lack of job experience, obesity, smoking, alcohol consumption, job dissatisfaction, recent back injury, and lack of strength and overall physical fitness. Most back injuries probably result not from a single, stressful lifting event but rather develop gradually over time. Improper lifting techniques lead to a significant number of back injuries.

Radiation. Exposure to radiation in the form of energy, rays, or waves can lead to a variety of injuries, including radiation burns and radiation dermatitis. Radiation burns result from exposure to radiant energy in the form of sunlight, x-rays, or nuclear emissions or explosion. Exposure to ionizing radiation, as from cancer radiation therapy, can lead to an acute or chronic inflammation of skin known as radiation dermatitis. The signs of redness, blistering, and sloughing of the skin usually appear 3 weeks after exposure.

Exposure to radiation can occur in the community or the health care environment. Community risk increases near nuclear power plants and manufacturing industries that produce radioactive wastes.

In the health care setting, you and other clinicians may be at risk when assisting with diagnostic procedures that use radioactive materials or caring for clients who have radioactive implants. Injury can occur if you fail to use lead shielding or fail to follow the necessary safety procedures involving expo-

---

Teaching for Wellness
Protect Yourself From Job-Related Back Injuries
Box 22-2

Purpose: To prevent back injuries when lifting and moving clients in the acute care setting.

Expected Outcome: The worker will not experience work-related back injuries.

Instructions

- Maintain your health. Eat a well-balanced diet, get a good night's sleep, and reduce stress in your life.
- Maintain your level of physical fitness. Get regular exercise. Exercise for cardiovascular fitness through aerobic exercise and for muscle strength through weight-bearing exercises. Exercise 20 minutes a day to strengthen your back, leg, and abdominal muscles. Include stretching exercises before and after your exercise session.
- Before you lift or move a client, assess the client's ability to help. Can the client move in bed, bear weight when standing, and cooperate with your instructions? How much does the client weigh? Is the range of motion sufficient to accomplish the move?
- Assess your ability to bear the load. How much weight can you lift? Ask for assistance if necessary.
- Arrange the environment to facilitate the move. For example, put the chair close to the bed when you are transferring a client to a chair. Move the furniture to allow you to get close to the client without twisting your back.
- Use assistive devices to lessen your workload. A mechanical lift is suggested when the client is immobile and exceeds the weight you can lift. A gait belt is used to increase leverage and provide a firm grasp. A walker assists the client to balance and bear part of the body's weight.
- Use principles of body mechanics when lifting and moving objects or clients:
  1. Lift using the longest and strongest muscle group; hold your back straight and use your leg muscles rather than your back muscles.
  2. Face the object or person to be lifted; avoid twisting as you lift.
  3. Avoid working against gravity.
  4. Pulling requires less effort than pushing.
  5. Widen your base of support (stance) and avoid working with your center of gravity outside your base of support.

---

sure time and distance from the radioactive source. Radiation can injure the skin, reproductive organs, bone marrow, gastrointestinal tract, and other parts of the body. The international radiation symbol notifies you and other health care workers of the danger of radiation injury (Figure 22-5). The principle of protection from radiation exposure involves three elements: time, distance, and shielding. Reducing the time of exposure, increasing the distance from the source, and using appropriate shielding will reduce the dose of radiation.

FACTORS AFFECTING SAFETY

Lifestyle Factors

A person's lifestyle can raise the risk for injury. Pertinent factors include not taking appropriate safety precautions, choosing a sedentary lifestyle, abusing chemical substances, and being unable or unwilling to provide self-care.

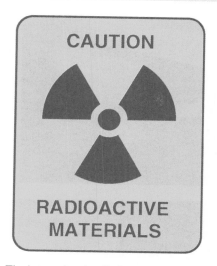

Figure 22-5. The international radiation symbol is commonly used in health care facilities.

Lack of Safety Precautions. Careless behavior occurs when people are in highly stressful situations or have a general disregard for safety. Speeding while driving, smoking in bed, entering high-crime areas at night, riding a bicycle without a helmet, and other risky behaviors invite accidents and injuries. Lack of safety precautions can affect people of all ages and walks of life.

Some people face a greater risk for injury because of their job or high-risk behaviors. They include people who drive or operate machinery under the influence of chemical substances, those who choose not to wear safety belts, those who exceed the posted speed limit when driving, those who work at dangerous jobs, and those who take risks and love the challenge that comes from jumping out of planes, climbing mountains, or racing cars.

Activity and Exercise. A lack of activity and exercise will negatively affect each body system and predispose the person to physiological as well as emotional hazards. Immobility increases the risk for falls and decreases the ability to flee from dangerous situations, including fires and other external hazards.

Despite the fact that activity and exercise are known to be beneficial, many people choose to live relatively inactive lives. A completely inactive lifestyle can limit a person's ability to experience and enjoy life to its fullest, and it will increase the risk for degenerative and chronic diseases, such as hypertension, ischemic heart disease, and diabetes.

Mrs. Soto has gradually become less active. You will need to suggest that she have her arthritis evaluated by a physician before planning a program to increase her activity. How would you approach this situation with her daughter?

Substance Abuse. The use of drugs and alcohol can affect safety in every aspect of a person's life. Substance abuse can reduce judgment and coordination and the ability to complete typical tasks. Operating heavy equipment, driving a car, climbing a ladder, and using a chain saw while under the influence of alcohol are associated with a high risk for injury.

Environmental Factors

Our surroundings, no matter where we live, work, or play, are never completely hazard free. Even when we take all the necessary precautions, there is no guarantee of our safety because we cannot be in total control of our home, community, and workplace environments.

Home. The home environment contains hazards or potential hazards both inside and outside the home. Potential hazards may involve inadequate lighting, steps or handrails missing or in poor repair, cluttered stairways, and the presence of throw rugs, electrical cords, or slippery surfaces. Features that suggest a safe home environment include grab bars in the tub or shower, nonskid rugs, covered electrical plugs, and locked storage cabinets.

Work. The work environment may contain a variety of overt or covert occupational safety hazards. Potential occupational hazards may result from noise, dust, or air pollution; working at heights; working with dangerous machinery; and being exposed to toxic substances. Occupations that raise the risk for injury include those that involve exposure to radiation or high-voltage electricity or the use of heavy equipment. Farm workers, electrical linemen, construction workers, and workers in power plants are a few examples of people at increased risk for injury. Both employers and employees should be aware of potential hazards and the need for precautions, such as wearing appropriate protective apparel.

Community. Hazards that can affect the community environment include crime, landfills, busy intersections, unsafe roads or bridges, dilapidated houses, cliffs, unprotected creeks and swimming pools, toxic waste dumps, air pollution, water pollution, noise from nearby construction, railroad crossings, and airports. Other environmental concerns include a clean water supply, an adequate sewage system, and insect and rodent control. Lack of sanitation in impoverished or less-developed areas increases the risk for disease and infection.

We know that Mrs. Soto's house needs repairs, but we do not know anything about the community in which she lives. How would you assess the community to determine Mrs. Soto's level of safety in her home?

Institution. Potential dangers to health care workers and clients are present within health care institutions. Many appoint safety committees, infection control committees, and hazardous waste committees to address these potential problems. For example, each institution is required to have up-to-date written policies to address such problems as chemical spills, infectious outbreaks, exposure to infectious blood and body fluids, and disposal of hazardous wastes. You must be familiar with your institution's policies and procedures to ensure your own safety and that of your clients.

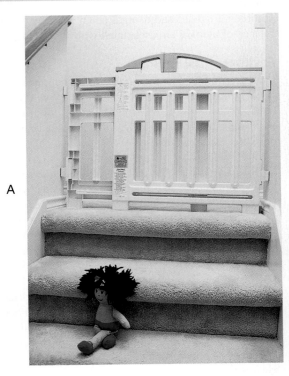

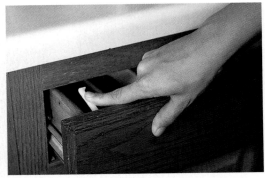

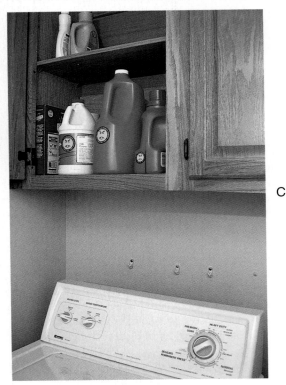

Figure 22-6. Childproofing a home. **A,** Toddler gates on stairs and doors. **B,** Childproof locks for cabinets. **C,** Chemicals labeled with "Mr. Yuk" stickers and placed out of reach.

Socioeconomic Factors

A frequently cited reason for ignoring safety is a lack of financial resources. Buying car seats for children and making repairs to protect the home from a faulty furnace can be expensive. A family may not have the financial means to obtain smoke detectors, fire extinguishers, or carbon monoxide detectors for their home.

However, the cost of *not* preventing accidents can be devastating. When someone is injured or involved in an accident, the costs can be astonishing. They involve lost wages and productivity, medical expenses, administrative expenses, employer costs, vehicle damage, and property losses.

Developmental Factors

Each stage of human development has its own unique risks (Table 22-2). Preventing injury and promoting safety are major concerns and the responsibility of the nurse, client, family, and caregiver. Promoting awareness of potentially haz-

ardous situations is a lifelong process that should begin early (Figure 22-6).

Infants and toddlers are particularly vulnerable to accidents and injuries because of their limited awareness of potential dangers. The type of accident or injury sustained by this age group is closely related to normal growth and development. Because of their oral activity, mobility, and inherent curiosity, toddlers are at increased risk for lead poisoning from ingestion of paint chips, strangulation, drowning, and burns. Box 22-3 (p. 498) is an example of teaching preventive measures.

School-age children face potential dangers as their environment expands from the home to the school. Dangers may exist in transportation to and from school, in after-school and sports activities, and from failure to use safety equipment, such as bike helmets and protective gear. Children should receive specific instructions from parents, teachers, and nurses regarding the safety practices they should follow while at school or play.

Table 22-2   Risk for Injury by Age-Group

Age-Group	Risks	Possible Causes
Developing fetus	• Maternal exposure to smoke. • Maternal use of alcohol or other drugs. • X-rays received during first trimester. • Exposure to certain pesticides.	• Mother cannot or will not assume responsibility for the safety of fetus, or she lacks the knowledge to do so. • Radiograph ordered by physician without inquiry about possible pregnancy. • Mother lives in proximity of fields of crops where the use of pesticides may be common.
Newborn	• Falling. • Suffocating in crib. • Choking or aspiration of formula. • Burns, especially with bath water. • Injuries in automobile accidents. • Injuries in crib or playpen.	• Failure to use approved car seats, cribs, and playpens correctly. • Inappropriate supervision. • Propping bottles while feeding. • Using a microwave oven to warm formula.
Infant or toddler	• Physical trauma from falling. • Banging into objects. • Falling down stairs. • Being cut by sharp objects. • Injuries in automobile accidents. • Burns. • Posioning. • Drowning. • Electric shock from household outlets.	• Environment not childproofed. • No gate at the top of stairs. • Obstructed passageways. • Unsafe window protection. • Improper use of car seats. • Highly flammable toys or clothing. • Pot handles facing front of stove. • Unsupervised bathing. • Unsupervised backyard swimming pool. • Unused electric outlets not blocked.
Preschool and school age	• Injuries in automobile accidents. • Injuries on playground equipment. • Choking. • Suffocation. • Obstruction of airways or ears by foreign objects. • Poisoning. • Drowning. • Electrical shock.	• History of hyperactivity; attention deficit disorder. • Experimenting with chemicals or gasoline. • Playing with matches, cigarettes, candles, or fireworks. • Improper storage of knives, guns, and ammunition. • Improper use of car seats or seat belts. • Unsupervised activities around the pool, electrical outlets, etc.
Adolescents	• Sports injuries. • Automobile accidents. • Drug or alcohol use.	• Lack of proper athletic training. • Lack of experience driving. • Failure to use or misuse of seat belts.
Older adults	• Falls. • Burns. • Pedestrian and automobile accidents.	• *Physical:* Weakness, poor vision, disturbed balance, reduced sensations, poor coordination, impaired eye–hand coordination. • *Environmental:* Slippery floors, snow or ice on walkways, unanchored rugs, no handgrips or rails in shower or bathtub, unsteady ladders or chairs, poor lighting, electrical cords in walkways, clutter or spills, unsteady or absent stair rails, inadequate method to call for assistance, cognitive or emotional disturbance.
All ages	• Fires.	• Gas leaks. • Delayed lighting of gas burners. • Unscreened fires or heaters. • Flowing clothes around open flame. • Inappropriately stored combustibles or corrosives. • Faulty wiring or frayed cords. • Smoking in bed.

Teaching for Wellness
Preventing Lead Poisoning   Box 22-3

Purpose: To educate families about preventive strategies for the prevention of lead poisoning in very young children.

Expected Outcomes: Families will initiate action to detect and prevent ingestion of lead.

Client Instructions

Sources of lead

- Although houses built before 1950 contain the greatest threat, over 80% of houses built before 1978 contain lead-based paint.
- Although all children are at risk, those who live in dilapidated housing face the greatest danger, especially children under age 2.
- Houses in coastal towns may have been painted with paint intended for boats, which has a high lead content.
- Soil near mines, industries that use lead, and smelters can have high lead levels.
- Solder on older plumbing and brass fixtures can contain lead.
- Food grown in soil with a high lead content can contain lead.
- Ceramic tableware from some countries contains lead.
- Ethnic folk remedies, such as the Hispanic remedies *azarcon* and *greta* and the Southeast Asian remedy *pay loo lah,* may contain lead.
- Hobbies that involve working with leaded glass, artist paints, bullets, and jewelry are sources of lead.

Actions

- If you suspect a high level of lead in your home or environment, have your children tested even if they seem healthy.
- Keep your house clean; dust and dirt may contain lead.
- Do not attempt to remove lead-based paint yourself. Improper removal can increase the amount of lead in the environment.
- If you have older plumbing, have your water tested.

Information from (1) National Lead Information Center. U.S. Environmental Protection Agency (EPA 800-b-92, February 1995). (1998). Retrieved from http://www.nsc.org; and (2) Centers for Disease Control and Prevention, National Center for Environmental Health, Childhood Lead Poisoning Prevention. (November 1997). *Screening young children for lead poisoning: Guidance for state and local public health officials.* Retrieved from http://www.cdc.gov/nceh.

The risks for adolescents are motor vehicle accidents, drowning, sexually transmitted diseases, unwanted pregnancy, suicide, homicide, and drug overdose. The need for independence, peer pressure, and the high-risk behaviors common in this age-group greatly increase the risk for accidents and injury.

In adults, the risk for injury tends to result from lifestyle. Excessive use of alcohol raises the risk for motor vehicle accidents. Cigarette smoking raises the risk for cardiovascular and pulmonary diseases. Excessive levels of stress can lead to increased risk for accidents.

The physiological changes normal among older adults can increase the risk for motor vehicle accidents, burns, and falls. Older adults tend to have decreased muscle strength, restricted joint mobility, and postural changes. Nervous system changes include slower reflexes, compromised balance, and a decreased ability to attend to multiple stimuli. Vision and hearing problems are common. Also, older adults are more likely to need to urinate at night, raising the risk for falls. This is especially true if the threat of incontinence requires the person to hurry to the bathroom.

Cognitive Factors

A person's cognitive and perceptual abilities are crucial to promoting safety. The ability to acquire and interpret information is a prerequisite for judgment, orientation, and socially appropriate behaviors. Promoting safety requires a person to think clearly, recall past problems and solutions, and create solutions to current problems. To remain safe, the person must also be able to perceive impending danger. The ability to perceive danger is based primarily on knowledge or learning from past experiences.

Physiological Factors

Impaired neurological function is a major component of risk for injury. To be safe, a person must have the judgment to recognize the presence of danger and the ability to move away. Many physiological factors can raise a person's risk for injury, including poor nutrition, clotting problems, a compromised immune system, a long history of alcohol and drug abuse, a debilitating disease, difficulty swallowing, and a need for tube feedings.

*A*SSESSMENT

General assessment of a client's safety requires gathering subjective data by interviewing the client and family about their safety needs. Gather objective data through physical examination, risk assessment tools, and environmental appraisals.

A home hazard appraisal tool allows you to elicit information objectively about the client's safety (Box 22-4). This tool gathers data contained in the client's nursing history and physical examination, and it may help you obtain specific information regarding the client's behaviors or environment.

Variables used to categorize the client's risk include unsteady gait, dizziness or imbalance, impaired memory or judgment, weakness, and a history of falls. Many health care agencies also use tools that specifically identify a client's risk for falls (Box 22-5).

Health History

To assess the client's safety, you will begin by evaluating the client's lifestyle and health status for factors that affect safety. Take a complete health history, emphasizing areas most likely to reveal issues of safety. They include lifestyle, cardiovascular and respiratory systems, neurological function, mobility, and integument.

Lifestyle. Assess the client's lifestyle for safety risk factors. To elicit a subjective response, ask questions pertaining to the client's awareness of safety practices or plans for management of hazards. Also, ask about the client's occupation, home environment, and habits that may entail a risk for injury. Questions could include the following:

- How often do you use a seat belt in the car?

Box 22-4 **Home Assessment**

To help prevent injuries in the home, assess the client's home and immediate surroundings thoroughly. Make sure your assessment includes the following areas:

- General layout of the home
- Type of access into the home
- Availability of adequate lighting, including night-lights
- Availability of adequate ventilation
- Presence of uneven walkways, stairs, or pathways
- Presence of loose steps on stairways
- Presence or absence of railing on stairways
- Repairs needed to make walkways, stairs, and pathways safe
- Sturdiness and security of all stairs, stepstools, ladders, and handrails
- Potential dangers from cluttered or obstructed hallways, stairways, and walkways
- Presence of unanchored carpet, mats, or throw rugs
- Types of furniture, including sharp or jutting corners, heights in relationship to client, and support provided
- Types of floors, including those in bathrooms, showers, and bathtubs

- Presence or absence of grab bars around tubs, showers, and
- Use of or need for a raised toilet seat or bath chair in tub or sho
- Condition of electrical appliances
- Loose or frayed electrical cords, overloaded outlets or extension cord and proximity of electrical cords to water
- Presence and condition of smoke alarms and carbon monoxide detectors
- Presence and condition of fire extinguishers and plans for an escape route to be used in case of fire
- Appropriate disposal of expired foods and medications
- Proper storage and labeling of medications, cleaning solutions, combustibles (such as paint thinner and gasoline) or corrosives (such as rust remover [phosphoric acid]), and other toxic substances
- Presence of a fence around the pool
- Presence of a reliable heating system
- Accessibility of emergency telephone numbers, such as for the fire department, police department, ambulance, poison control center, and hospital

---

Box 22-5 **Determining an Adult Client's Risk for Falls**

A person may have an increased risk for falling if she has one or more of the following risk factors:

- Age 65 or over
- A history of falling
- Decreased mobility or difficulty walking
- Need for assistance when getting out of bed or transferring to and from a chair
- A history of dizziness or seizures
- Impaired vision, hearing, or speech
- Need for assistive devices, such as a cane, walker, wheelchair, crutches, or braces, for mobility
- Weakness or fatigue caused by a disease process or prescribed therapy
- Confusion, disorientation, impaired memory or judgment, or impaired cognitive function
- Use of certain medications, such as diuretics, laxatives, or those that can alter the client's level of consciousness, including sedatives, hypnotics, tranquilizers, and analgesics

- Are your child's immunizations current?
- How have you childproofed your house?
- Do you have trouble reading warning labels or traffic signs?

Include in your assessment questions about medications the client is currently taking and any side effects that may have been experienced. Cardiovascular medications, sedatives, antidepressants, and other medications that affect the central nervous system are particularly pertinent.

Cardiovascular and Respiratory Systems.
Assessment of the cardiovascular and respiratory systems provides information about the client's activity tolerance. Assess changes in the client's blood pressure, pulse, and respirations with activity. Orthostatic hypotension and dizziness are factors in client safety.

 Mrs. Soto's rheumatoid arthritis has kept her from remaining active, but she is determined to keep trying. How would you assess her cardiovascular status to determine her ability to tolerate an exercise program?

Neurological Function. Assessment of the neurological system can provide information about the client's mental status, sensory function, reflexes, and coordination. Level of consciousness; orientation to time, person, and place; attention span; and decision-making abilities are also included in the neurological assessment. Testing of the senses (vision, hearing, taste, and smell) should be conducted to detect any deficits or alterations. This is important to determine the client's risk for injury during medication administration and while climbing stairs, reading warning labels, and listening for cars, smoke alarms, or other warning sounds.

Mobility. Assessment of the client's mobility is the key element of a safety assessment. Clients who experience impaired mobility because of paralysis, muscle weakness, poor balance, or poor coordination are at increased risk for injury and serious health problems. To be safe, the client needs to be able to move about freely in the environment and avoid hazards.

Integument. Ask the client about any history of accidental injuries while you inspect the skin. During a bath, inspect all areas of the client's skin for bruises, cuts, scratches, and scars. If lesions are present, document their precise location, size, color, and the client's explanation of their cause.

Physical Examination
The collection of objective data allows you to assess the client's safety function and to assess for injuries and risk factors for injuries. Examples of objective data include the client's muscle strength, joint range of motion, gait characteristics,

, results of diagnostic tests, radiographic evidence, , skin turgor, and posture. The physical assessment focus on the neurological system, skin integrity, and lity. Information that can be obtained from assessing se three areas can be of vital importance to the client's erall health and safety.

Focused Assessment for *Risk for Injury*

To assess the general category of *Risk for injury,* you need to observe the client's physical and psychological status and elements of the environment that are unsafe. Often, a combination of factors from the internal and external environments defines the client's risk.

Defining Characteristics. Internal risk factors for injury are classified as biochemical, physical, and psychological (NANDA, 2000). Biochemical factors of the neurological system include sensory, integrative, and motor dysfunction. Additionally, hypoxia affects the ability to form reasoned judgments. Immune/autoimmune dysfunction, malnutrition, and an abnormal blood profile can make even minor injuries serious. Physical factors include altered mobility and the client's developmental status, with the very young and very old being the most vulnerable. Depression and anxiety are psychological factors that affect a person's ability to reason or to be alert to environmental hazards.

External risk factors are characterized as biological, chemical, physical, and people/provider. Biological risk factors include the number and type of microorganisms present in a particular environment, as well as the immunization level of the community. Chemical factors are identified as pollutants, poisons, drugs, alcohol, caffeine, nicotine, preservatives, cosmetics, dyes, nutrients, vitamins, and food types. Physical factors include the design, structure, and arrangement of the community, building, or equipment and the available mode of transportation. People/provider factors include the preventive behaviors of the health care team, staffing patterns, and the knowledge of the health care providers (NANDA, 2000).

Focused Assessment for *Risk for Trauma*

Defining Characteristics. *Risk for trauma* is the nursing diagnosis that indicates the presence of any factor that increases the client's risk for accidental traumatic injury, such as a wound, burn, or fracture. Internal risk factors involve the individual. They include weakness, balancing difficulties, reduced coordination of large or small muscles, lack of safety education or precautions, cognitive or emotional difficulties, poor vision, reduced temperature or tactile sensation, reduced hand–eye coordination, insufficient finances to purchase safety equipment or make repairs, and a history of previous trauma (NANDA, 2000).

External risk factors involve hazards in the client's environment that can result in fires, burns, electrical shock, or accidents, particularly from falls. Falls result from slippery (such as wet or highly waxed) floors, bathtubs without hand grips or traction mats, inappropriate call-for-aid devices for the bedridden client, snow or ice on outside stairs or walkways, unanchored rugs, use of an unsteady ladder or chair for reaching, poor lighting, unanchored electrical wires, clutter or spills on floors or stairs, obstructed passageways, and unsafe window protection in homes with young children.

Burns result from pot handles facing toward the front of the stove, gas leaks, overly hot bath water, experimenting with chemicals or gasoline, and children playing with matches, candles, or cigarettes. Electrical injuries result from faulty electrical plugs, overloaded electrical outlets, and frayed wires or defective appliances. Other types of traumatic injuries can result from knives stored uncovered, unsafe use of dangerous machinery, high-crime neighborhoods, and motor vehicle accidents (NANDA, 2000).

Related Factors. For the client who is at risk for injury or trauma, nursing care may be aimed at reducing the risk or at helping the client compensate for the risk factors. Additionally, care may be aimed at one or more of the following related factors.

LACK OF KNOWLEDGE. Knowledge is an important factor to help prevent accidents. Parents need to be especially aware of the dangers that could cause harm to their children. Assess for high-risk behaviors, such as the use of alcohol or drugs while driving. Referral for an in-depth assessment may be needed to determine the best way to help the client change high-risk behaviors.

LACK OF SELF-CARE ABILITY. The client must have the physical and mental ability to appraise hazardous situations and make the necessary changes to prevent injury. People with physical limitations may be unable to recognize a high-risk situation or take corrective actions. Assess the client's ability to remove risk factors independently. Is there a potential to improve health or make the client more independent by introducing behaviors that reduce risk? For example, could teaching the client how to use a walker prevent falls?

LACK OF ADEQUATE SUPPORT SYSTEM. If your client is cognitively, emotionally, or physically impaired, assess the support systems available. The client may be receiving support from a variety of sources, such as family, friends, volunteer agencies, and professional services. Determine any gaps in service that may leave the client vulnerable to injury.

Focused Assessment for *Risk for Poisoning*

Both internal and external factors are required to produce the *Risk for poisoning.* Internal factors may make clients unable or unwilling to prevent poisoning in the presence of external factors that place them at risk. Assess clients for these factors.

Defining Characteristics. Internal characteristics that increase the *Risk for poisoning* include the use of multiple medications, disability, and reduced vision. Also, assess the client's knowledge of poisonous substances and storage of household chemicals. For young children, the cognitively impaired, and persons with emotional difficulties,

- Verbalize knowledge of the rationale for the use of seat belts, infant and toddler car seats, and bicycle and motorcycle helmets
- Commit to consistent use of seat belts, infant and toddler car seats, and bicycle and motorcycle helmets
- Identify safety measures and practices needed to decrease the risk for fires, electrical hazards, and burns from hot water bottles or heating pads
- Avoid high-risk practices such as diving in unknown places, speeding, and driving while intoxicated
- Describe the safe use of machinery or tools

Expected Outcomes for *Risk for Poisoning*

The client will be able to do the following:
- Recognize potential poisons in the home
- Properly label and store poisonous substances, including medications
- Develop a system for ensuring correct self-administration of medications
- Consult with a physician before combining over-the-counter medications or herbal supplements with prescription medications

Expected Outcomes for *Risk for Suffocation*

The client will be able to do the following:
- Identify risk factors for suffocation
- List preventive measures for suffocation
- Commit to implementation of prevention of suffocation
- Demonstrate correct use of oxygen and other respiratory equipment in the home
- Be protected from hazards associated with oxygen therapy equipment in the health care agency

Expected Outcomes for *Risk for Aspiration*

The client will be able to do the following:
- Sit upright for eating
- Eat small bites of foods of the appropriate consistency
- Select foods that can be easily and safely swallowed
- Be evaluated for factors contributing to aspiration, such as nausea and competency of swallowing mechanisms

INTERVENTION

When a client is at risk for an alteration in safety status, nursing interventions can be instituted to help prevent hazards, trauma, or disease. Nursing interventions should be individualized for each client. They should be holistic in nature and should take into consideration all the factors that are unique to the client, including age, developmental level, health care needs, abilities, support systems, strengths, and weaknesses.

Prevention is a major category of nursing interventions that you should incorporate into the client's plan of care. Preventing hazards, trauma, and illness can be done by focusing on providing or promoting a safe environment, preventing falls, enhancing safety efforts, arranging ongoing surveillance measures to identify risk factors, and providing instruction to increase awareness, knowledge, and a sense of physical and psychological safety and well-being.

Interventions to Promote a Safe Environment

Nursing interventions should focus on promoting a safe environment at home and in the health care institution. Promoting safety at home can be accomplished by creating a safe home environment, especially for infants, children, and older adults. Creating a safe institutional environment, orienting clients to the environment, and monitoring clients carefully can ensure them safety in the hospital.

Promoting Safety at Home. When a client requires care in the home, the environment may need modifications to maintain ongoing safety. The environment may have been safe when the client was well and able to freely move about to manage the activities of daily living and necessary maintenance and repairs. However, when a client becomes physically or mentally compromised, even on a short-term basis, home safety becomes an issue.

CREATING A SAFE HOME ENVIRONMENT. The home should be free of hazards that could result in falls. Measures to promote home safety include using nonskid rugs or tacking down throw rugs to prevent slips and falls, installing and using grab bars in the tub or shower, installing ramps to allow easier access, and keeping rooms, halls, and stairs free of clutter.

Safety practices to prevent burns or electrical shocks should be in place. Potential electrical hazards in the home environment include frayed cords, overloaded outlets and extension cords, use of electrical appliances near water, and lack of supervision of children near uncovered electrical outlets or electrical appliances. Covering electrical outlets when not in use, positioning pans with handles toward the back of the stove while cooking, and avoiding open-flame heaters are examples of prevention strategies.

Proper storage and labeling of bottles containing poisonous substances is essential. Have emergency telephone numbers, including the number for poison control, readily available (Figure 22-7, p. 504). Instruct the client and appropriate family members about proper medication administration. This includes information about the type of medication, dosage, reason for taking, expected effects, and possible side effects.

Encourage the client to call the poison control hotline for immediate access to information about appropriate first aid in a possible poisoning. Emetic agents should be given only after contacting the poison control center and ascertaining the guidelines for the specific poison. Although several emetic agents are available, syrup of ipecac is the most effective one to use in the home setting; administration within 30 minutes is best, but it can be effective for up to 1 hour after ingestion of poison. Syrup of ipecac is contraindicated after ingestion of gasoline, fuel oil, paint thinner, cleaning fluid, or strychnine. Also, children under 6 months old, people with severe heart disease, and pregnant or lactating women should not use syrup of ipecac.

Teaching may also involve instructing the client and family in the use of safe techniques for mobility of the physically impaired client. Provide instructions on the proper use of assistive devices, such as walkers, wheelchairs, or crutches. Teach the client and family ways to prevent back injury, including proper lifting techniques, back exercises to prevent back injury, and proper use of body mechanics.

Teaching may need to address the client's lifestyle as well. For example, the client may need to stop drinking and smoking. The family may need instruction on how to recognize signs and symptoms of choking and carbon monoxide poisoning and how to perform Heimlich's maneuver and cardiopulmonary resuscitation.

Safety precautions are essential for preventing injuries in older adults and in mentally ill or disabled clients. Ways to prevent injury include proper labeling of medications, assessing the home environment for potential hazards, and teaching

appropriate safety measures. Establishing an open line of communication with the client or primary caregiver is of utmost importance in enhancing and promoting the safety of all those involved.

At times you may need to refer a dependent older adult to a home health agency so that a home safety assessment can be performed before the client is discharged from the hospital. If a referral is necessary, it should be done 3 days before discharge to allow appropriate planning and implementation of safety measures. Make every attempt to accommodate the client's cultural needs, as outlined in Box 22-6.

Promoting Safety for Infants and Children. Child safety is taught as part of parenting classes. Nurses may organize parenting classes for populations at risk or as part of a wellness program in a health care facility.

To promote a safe environment for infants and children, teach the family ways to childproof a home. Families can employ a number of important safety measures to prevent accidents. For example, plastic bags should be stored in a cabinet out of the child's reach. Covering an infant's or a child's mattress or pillow with plastic should be avoided. Crib design should follow federal safety regulations, and the mattress should be the appropriate size for the crib frame. Discourage parents from sleeping with their infant or putting the infant down to sleep with a bib, bonnet, or other snug-fitting garment tied around the neck. They should be taught never to tie a pacifier around the infant's neck. To avoid choking accidents, parents should inspect toys for removable parts and avoid feeding the infant such foods as grapes, nuts, and popcorn. When giving medication to a child, parents should avoid trying to entice the child by calling it candy.

Other safety measures that can be taken to ensure a child's safety include keeping doors of large appliances, especially unused refrigerators or freezers, closed at all times. Areas around a swimming pool should be fenced, and children should be supervised and wear protective gear when swimming. Instruct parents to avoid leaving pails of water or cleaning solutions accessible to children. Tell parents to use seat belts or car seats

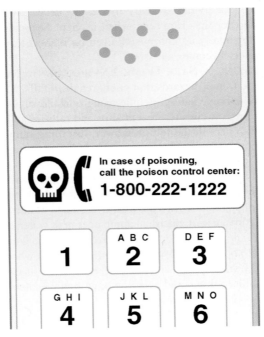

Figure 22-7. An example of a poison control label on a telephone.

Cross-Cultural Care CARING FOR AN OLDER MEXICAN-AMERICAN CLIENT   Box 22-6

Mrs. Soto, the client described in this chapter's case study, lives in a city on the border of Texas and Mexico. She was born in Mexico and maintains close ties with family in Mexico. The following are some key facts to keep in mind when caring for Mexican-American clients:

• Mexican Americans are the most successful of all ethnic groups at retaining their culture and language.
• In southwestern cities, Mexican Americans often live in *barrios* (Hispanic ethnic neighborhoods), where their primary interactions are with members of their own ethnic group.
• More than half (51%) of older Mexican Americans were born in Mexico.
• Older adults constitute less than 4% of the population of Mexican Americans.

• Mexican Americans tend not to retire; they tend to work as long as they are able.
• Mexican-American culture values respectful behavior toward older persons and absolute obedience to their commands.
• Mexican-American women tend to become more outgoing and domineering as they get older.
• Older Mexican Americans tend to function in the role of teacher, delineating proper conduct, relating historic events, and explaining the origin of things.
• Mexican-American grandparents are unlikely to live alone.
• Older Mexican Americans are rarely placed in nursing homes by their families.

Holmes, E. R., & Holmes L. D. (1995). *Other cultures, elder years.* Thousand Oaks, CA: Sage.

appropriate for the child's age and weight. Sharp objects, such as knives and other kitchen utensils, matches, and toxic substances should be kept out of children's reach.

As can be seen from these examples, many safety measures can be emphasized to children's parents, caregivers, or family to help them promote safety and avoid accidents. Community resources are also available and can be accessed through referrals. An important aspect of promoting safety lies in getting clients and their families involved in planning and implementing the safety measures needed to decrease the risk for injury. Solicit involvement of clients and their families through family conferences in which you help them define their mutual goals. This involvement enhances their motivation and increases the likelihood of positive outcomes and the long-term lifestyle changes required.

Most accidents are preventable. By educating yourself, your clients, and their families, you can help reduce the risk for injury, trauma, asphyxiation, poisoning, and aspiration in their homes.

Providing Safety in Institutions

CREATING A SAFE INSTITUTIONAL ENVIRONMENT. In a health care institution, the client, especially one who is incapacitated by illness or disability, depends on the staff to provide a safe environment. This requires a team effort by nursing services, housekeeping, maintenance—indeed, every employee of the institution. Safety issues are similar to those in the home, but a hospital has more equipment, hazardous chemicals, and a large number of people using the facility. Every employee should be trained in electrical safety and fire safety as well as in safe interactions with clients.

Stay aware of the risk for electrical injury, especially in situations that combine moisture with electrical equipment. These situations may involve spills on the floor, a leaking or disconnected intravenous line, or a client with moist skin caused by diaphoresis.

You can help prevent electrical injuries by making sure that electrical equipment stays in good working order and by using devices equipped with three-pronged grounded plugs (Figure 22-8). The third prong of the plug is called the *ground*

because it is specifically designed to carry any stray electrical current into the earth. The two regular prongs carry power to the equipment being used. However, simply having a three-pronged plug does not ensure that the plug is grounded. The maintenance department should check the grounding periodically. Box 22-7 includes additional ideas to reduce the risk for electrical injury. Identifying and correcting potential sources of danger can prevent electrical shock.

> *Action Alert!* Prevent electrical shocks by using grounded equipment. Teach others to avoid the use of faulty equipment and to never overload electrical outlets or extension cords.

Although fires are uncommon in modern buildings when safety precautions are followed, fire safety programs increase the readiness to respond correctly to a fire. Any fire that arises in a health care setting requires quick actions in response. A common response plan incorporates the acronym RACE to help prioritize those actions. It stands for *rescue, alarm, confine,* and *extinguish.*

The first priority in case of fire is to rescue or remove all clients from immediate danger. The second priority is to call for help. Activate the nearest fire alarm, or report the fire to the switchboard operator, whichever is faster. The switchboard operator will page the code for a fire and its location.

Teaching for Self-Care — Box 22-7
Preventing Electrical Shocks

Purpose: To provide information about electrical safety.

Expected Outcome: The client will demonstrate electrical safety practices.

Client Instructions

Equipment
- Make sure that equipment is grounded; the use of a three-prong outlet does not ensure that the outlet is grounded.
- Do not use electrical cords that are frayed or that have visible damage.
- Repair or replace all malfunctioning equipment. If you drop a piece of electrical equipment, have it tested before reusing it.
- Experiencing shocks while using equipment means that it is not safe; have it tested before continuing to use it.
- Learn about all electrical equipment that you intend to use before attempting to use it.

Electrical outlets
- Do not overload.
- Cover outlets not currently in use, especially if small children are present.
- Install outlets with ground fault circuit interrupters near sources of water, such as bathroom and kitchen sinks.
- Never pull a plug from the socket by the cord. Grip the plug firmly and pull it straight out of the socket.

Extension cords
- Avoid using extension cords when possible.
- Anchor extension cords to the floor using specially designed covers to prevent tripping over the cord.

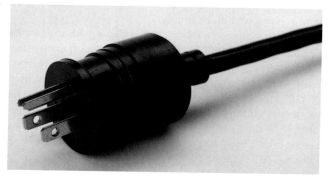

Figure 22-8. A three-pronged grounded plug, used to prevent electrical injuries. (Courtesy Lion Electric, South Norwalk, CT.)

Box 22-8   Fire Extinguishers and Indications for Their Use

WATER PUMP EXTINGUISHER

Use for type A fires, which involve paper, wood, or cloth.

CARBON DIOXIDE (CO_2) EXTINGUISHER/DRY CHEMICAL EXTINGUISHER

Use for type B fires, which involve such flammable liquids as fuel oil, cooking oil, grease, paint, solvents, and anesthetic gases, and for type C fires, which involve electrical sources.

FOAM EXTINGUISHER

Use for type B fires.

MULTIPURPOSE EXTINGUISHER

Use for type A, B, and C fires.

DRY POWDER EXTINGUISHER

Use for type D fires, which involve combustible metals and certain other metals.

The third priority is to confine the fire. Close nearby doors and windows, and turn off oxygen and electrical equipment. Close fire doors to confine the fire to an area of the building. Do not use elevators during a fire. The fourth priority is to extinguish the fire. Be sure to use the proper type of extinguisher for the type of fire involved (Box 22-8).

Also take steps to prevent back injuries—both your back and the client's. Back injuries can lead to lifelong pain, suffering, and disability. Taking care of your back is of vital importance to ensure a healthy, productive life. Many general rules and principles can be applied to home and work environments to reduce the risk for back injuries. Make sure to follow safety guidelines to prevent back injuries from occurring, such as using proper lifting techniques and body mechanics and engaging in appropriate exercise and activity to promote strong bones and muscles.

Action Alert! Prevent back injuries from occurring. Use proper body mechanics and proper lifting and pushing techniques, and always ask for help when needed.

ORIENTING THE CLIENT TO THE ENVIRONMENT. A client newly admitted to a hospital or nursing home needs to be oriented to the new environment. The client and family should know how to operate the bed and any other equipment that the client will be using. One of the most important features of the safety orientation is teaching the client how to call for help using the call light at the bedside and the emergency call light in the bathroom. If the client needs the side rails raised for safety, make a point of saying so; give instructions for calling for help to get out of bed.

Some older clients, very ill clients, and clients under the influence of sedative medications may need ongoing orienta-

tion. A client with borderline dementia may function well at home but become confused in a strange environment. To maintain a client's orientation, provide information about time, person, place, and environment at regular intervals. Use clocks, calendars, even family pictures to help keep the client oriented, especially if there is an impaired awareness of time, place, or person.

PREVENTING INGESTION OF TOXIC SUBSTANCES. To prevent the accidental ingestion of toxic substances in the health care environment, take precautions to not leave medications or toxic solutions in the client's room. Using disposable cups and containers that can be immediately discarded can prevent accidental poisonings.

MONITORING THE CLIENT. While clients are in your care, take every precaution necessary to ensure their safety. By assessing their risk for injury, you can make sound judgments about the type and frequency of monitoring needed to maintain their safety. Clients who need frequent monitoring include those with the following conditions:

- A risk for compromised airway from muscle weakness or sedation
- Impaired mobility, especially when trying to get out of bed on their own
- Unstable (fluctuating) vital signs
- A tendency to be restless in bed, especially if medical therapy includes intravenous lines or nasogastric tubes
- Cognitive impairment, especially if it reduces cooperation with the treatment plan

Monitor totally dependent clients at least once an hour. If they have a high risk for injury, either make sure someone stays with them at all times or place them in a room close to the nurses' station where you can monitor them frequently. A family member or private sitter can be used to provide constant surveillance.

If a client has a high risk for falls, consider using an identification system (colored tape on an arm band, a note in the chart and on the head of bed) to alert other staff members of the client's status. A device called an Ambularm can be attached to the client's leg to warn you when the client tries to get out of bed (Figure 22-9). The device is sensitive to position changes and sounds an alarm when the client's leg goes over the side of the bed. The problem with this device, as with many electronic monitoring systems, is that when multiple false alarms occur, staff members become less sensitive to the sound and respond more slowly.

Frequent monitoring increases the likelihood of detecting risk factors if you form the habit of looking for potential hazards each time you enter the client's room. Assess the client's environment to make sure the bed stays in the low position, side rails are up, bed wheels are locked, and items such as tissues, water, urinal, bedpan, and glasses are within the client's reach. Note the client's level of consciousness, especially if an analgesic, a hypnotic, a sedative, or a tranquilizer has been administered.

The frequent presence of a nurse in the client's room contributes to a sense of security that may prevent the client from

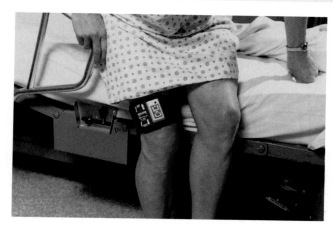

Figure 22-9. An Ambularm is a position-sensitive electronic device that is placed on the client's leg. Because it sounds a warning when the client attempts to get out of bed, it may provide a useful alternative to restraints. (Courtesy Alert Care, Mill Valley, CA.)

trying to get out of bed independently. Inform the client that you are nearby and will respond quickly to a call for help. It may be helpful to inform the client that you will return in a given period of time. However, make sure that you are indeed available when you say you will be.

Think again of Mrs. Soto. Imagine that she is admitted to the hospital. We know she uses a wheelchair and walks with extreme difficulty. She is partially blind. How would you help her be safe in the hospital?

INFANTS AND CHILDREN IN THE HOSPITAL. In the hospital setting, all necessary precautions must be taken to keep children safe. Examples of common safety practices include the following:

- Never leave an infant unattended.
- Keep a bulb syringe readily available in case an infant's oropharynx needs to be suctioned.
- Make sure that periodic safety checks have been performed on emergency response equipment such as suctioning devices.
- Check the infant's or child's armband before giving medications; remember that young children may answer to any name.
- Keep small objects out of reach to help prevent infants and small children from putting them into their mouth, nose, or ears.
- Keep the side rails of the crib up, and inspect all attachments on the crib or bassinet to make sure that they are fastened securely.
- Check the temperature of bath water to prevent scalding or chilling.
- Maintain bodily contact at all times when bathing an infant or toddler; never leave a child unattended during a bath.
- Always check the temperature of food or formula before feeding an infant.
- Never microwave an infant's formula to warm it.

Interventions to Prevent Falls

Interventions to prevent falls, especially in older adults, are of major concern. The environment should be free of potential hazards and equipped with safety devices. Certain basic safety measures should be incorporated into any prevention plan. The use of restraints can be included but only as a last resort and only under a physician's order.

Modifying the Environment. Health care environments are often crowded with equipment and people. Modifying this environment can reduce the risk for falls. For example, make sure that the ambulatory client has a clear path. Remove excess equipment or furniture. Have the client wear rubber-soled shoes or slippers for walking. Make sure that proper transfer precautions are instituted for a heavy or debilitated client in a bed or wheelchair or on a toilet. Teaching safeguards to the family can also minimize the client's risk for falls in the health care environment. Box 22-9 (p. 508) describes measures for preventing falls in the hospital setting.

Using Equipment Safely. Equipment used in the hospital should be in proper working order. Proper training in the use of equipment commonly used in the home or hospital (suctioning machines, monitors, and so on) should be conducted on a regular basis. To ensure proper use of newly acquired equipment, qualified personnel should present training sessions.

Equipment such as wheelchairs, beds, commode chairs, and shower chairs should have brakes that are working properly. Bed wheels should be locked, and the bed should be kept in the low position. Side rails should be kept raised when the client is in bed. Other measures include installing grab bars in the bathroom, applying safety strips in the tub or shower, and not leaving the client unattended while in the bathtub or shower (Figure 22-10, p. 509).

Using Restraints. Restraints are used as a protective measure when clients are in danger of harming themselves or others. The U.S. Food and Drug Administration, which regulates medical devices, defines a **restraint** as a device (usually a wristlet, anklet, or other type of strap) intended for medical purposes that limits movement to the extent necessary for treatment, examination, or protection of the client. Restraints also can be chemical (medications to calm the person's behavior) or environmental (side rails on beds, locked psychiatric units, or quiet rooms).

In the hospital or nursing home setting, the primary use of restraints is to prevent a client from falling and sustaining an injury. The client must be at high risk for falling or injury, be unable to understand that risk, and have no other avenues of prevention available.

The second major reason for restraints is to prevent the client from interrupting therapy, especially when the therapy is life sustaining. When a client is confused or sedated and therefore unable to understand the presence of an intravenous line, nasogastric tube, wound dressing, or other medical

---

Box 22-9   Preventing Falls in the Hospital Setting

On admission, assess each client's risk for falls, and assign one of the following risk levels:

Low Risk: Assign this risk level if the client is alert, ambulates with a steady gait, can perform self-care activities without assistance, has no history of falls, and is cognitively intact and cooperative.

Medium Risk: Assign this risk level if the client may need some assistance or supervision when performing certain daily activities. The person may be alert and cooperative but may have a chronic physical ailment or a barrier (e.g., language) that could prevent calling for help.

High Risk: Assign this risk level if the client experiences periods of confusion or denies obvious problems of ambulation or mobility. This client may refuse to call for assistance and may attempt to perform activities independently. The client may have a history of falls and noncompliance with safety measures.

GENERAL INTERVENTIONS FOR ALL CLIENTS

No matter what your client's risk level, always take the following precautions to help avoid falls:

- When your clients arrive in their room, orient them to their new surroundings.
- Keep the two side rails in the raised position at all times for all clients, regardless of age. Clients at low risk for falls may choose to have the side rails down during the day.

- Keep the call light, bedside table, water, glasses, and so on within the client's easy reach.
- Use a night-light.
- Make sure the client has and wears footwear with nonskid soles when out of bed.
- Use restraints and bed monitors as ordered by the physician.
- Keep the client's bed in the low position at all times except during procedures.
- Teach fall-prevention techniques, such as sitting up for a moment before rising from the bed.

SPECIFIC INTERVENTIONS FOR AT-RISK CLIENTS

- If your clients have a medium risk for falling, allow them to ambulate only with assistance. Make sure their family and other visitors understand this restriction. Anticipate and meet the clients' needs as much as possible. Offer assistance frequently.
- If your clients have a high risk for falling, try to locate them in a room close to the nurses' station. Keep the side rails raised at all times. Answer these clients' call lights as quickly as possible. Assess them more frequently than usual. Maintain their scheduled toileting routine, and provide assistance with all activities of daily living. Encourage family members or other visitors to stay with them.

---

device, it is a natural human instinct to attempt to remove the irritant. Then the client's hands may need to be restrained.

The third major reason for restraints is to prevent the client from self-harm or from harming others. Although violent or self-destructive behavior is more often associated with psychiatric units, it occasionally occurs in general medical or surgical units. Usually, combative behavior results from the confusion and fear that arises in a situation the client cannot understand or control. It sometimes occurs after withdrawal from certain drugs (Procedure 22-1).

The appropriate use of restraints is controversial in the health care setting. Physical restraints are used in health care institutions, especially with confused clients who interfere with medical treatments or devices, demonstrate disruptive behaviors, or face an increased risk for falls. Psychiatric facilities have adopted policies of treating the client in the least restrictive manner possible. In 1987, the Omnibus Reconciliation Act extended this philosophy to nursing home residents, using the following language: "The client has the right to be free from any physical restraints imposed or psychoactive drug administered for purposes of discipline or convenience, and not required to treat, the resident's medical condition."

All health care facilities have well-defined written policies regarding the use of restraints. Unnecessarily restraining a person may be construed as assault or false imprisonment. You must be able to document a clear need for a restraint and that the need is for the client's safety, not for the staff's convenience. The documentation should specify that other avenues of protecting the client have been pursued. Box 22-10 lists alternatives to restraints.

It is important to emphasize that the use of restraints is generally not advocated and should be considered only as a

last resort. Although health care workers usually use restraints with the best of intentions, the complications of restraints can be more devastating than their absence. In spite of the belief that restraints prevent falls, restraints themselves are a source of injury. In fact, the use of restraints in older clients can actually increase the risk for falls because the clients may struggle desperately to free themselves from the perceived bondage (Wilson, 1996). Other potential complications include the following:

- Hypostatic pneumonia from failure to turn and move in bed or from the inability to take a deep breath because of a constricting device
- Skin abrasions, edema, or pressure injuries from the use of improperly padded restraints
- Ischemia and nerve damage if the restraint is applied too tightly
- Strangulation from a vest restraint when the client slides down in bed and is unable to move or call for help
- Contractures from immobility
- Shoulder dislocation from struggling against a restraint
- Aspiration pneumonia

Side rails, stretchers, and other typical types of equipment provide the simplest and least restrictive method of restraint used in the health care environment. If the client needs traditional restraints, several types are available, such as jacket and vest restraints, belt restraints, mitt or hand restraints, and wrist and ankle restraints. Some commonly used restraints must be tied to another object, such as a chair, wheelchair, or bed. They must be tied securely enough to prevent the client from releasing them but precisely enough so that you or another staff member can release them quickly in case of an emergency.

Text continued on p. 513

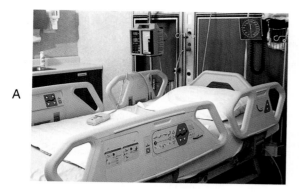

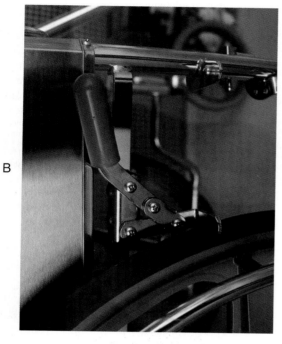

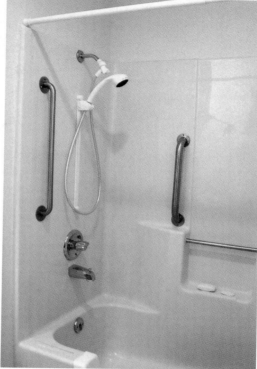

Figure 22-10. Safety devices help prevent falls in health care institutions and in the client's home. **A,** Side rails on beds. **B,** Locking devices on wheeled equipment. **C,** Grab bars in showers.

PROCEDURE 22-1 USING PROTECTIVE RESTRAINTS

TIME TO ALLOW
Novice: 10 min.
Expert: 5 min.

Restraints are any device or method used to restrict or control a client's behavior for the purpose of protecting the client from harm or from causing injury to others. A person can be restrained by confinement to a room or a bed or restrained by the use of drugs that decrease angry or aggressive behavior. The term *restraints* most often refers to restraining devices used to prevent the person from moving the arms or legs.

DELEGATION GUIDELINES

The decision to restrain a client may not be delegated to a nursing assistant. Physical restraint requires a physician's order. As a registered nurse, you will be able to determine whether to restrain a client when the client is deemed to be in immediate danger of causing harm to self or others and no other more appropriate means of managing the behavior exist. However, you must inform the physician and provide di-

rection to continue the restraints. You may delegate observation of the restrained client to a nursing assistant. You may also elect to delegate supervision or assistance with eating, toileting, and repositioning to a nursing assistant, and the reapplication of restraints in these circumstances may be delegated to a nursing assistant. However, you must provide specific criteria for observation and supervision.

Continued

PROCEDURE 22-1	USING PROTECTIVE RESTRAINTS—CONT'D

EQUIPMENT NEEDED

- Restraints: jacket, vest, waist, wrist, or ankle restraint
- Padding as needed

---

1. Follow preliminary guidelines for nursing procedures (see inside front cover).

2. Assess the need for restraints. *The client's behavior could cause self-harm (risk for fall, risk for suicide, risk for wandering into unsafe areas) or injury to others. Alternatively, it could interrupt medical therapy, thus increasing the risk for complications, delaying the healing process, or causing an early death.*

3. Consider alternatives to restraints. *Discuss with the physician and with the client's family.*

4. Choose the least restrictive type of restraint.

a. A *jacket restraint* allows the client to turn from side to side in the bed but prevents getting out of bed or a chair. It secures both the shoulders and the waist (see illustration).

b. A *belt restraint* secures the person at the waist only. Less restrictive than a jacket, it is also not as protective. It also allows the client to turn from side to side in bed (see illustration).

c. A *wrist restraint* secures one or both of the client's hands. By positioning the client's hand or hands away from tubes and dressings, the wrist restraint prevents the client from removing an intravenous line, a nasogastric tube, an indwelling urinary catheter, or a wound dressing. It also can prevent infiltration of an intravenous drug by immobilizing the client's arm. And it can prevent the client from striking people standing nearby (see illustration).

d. An *ankle restraint* secures one or both ankles and prevents injury caused by thrashing about in bed. It also prevents the client from dislodging a femoral arterial line (see illustration).

e. A *mitten restraint* prevents use of the hands while allowing free arm movements. It is useful for a client who is disturbed by wrist restraints but needs to be prevented from dislodging an intravenous line, an indwelling urinary catheter, a nasogastric tube, or a wound dressing (see illustration).

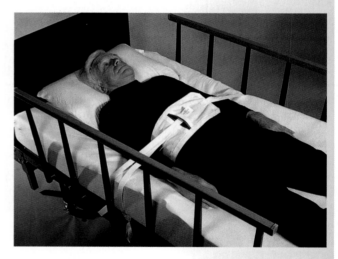

Step 4b. Belt restraint. (Courtesy Medline Industries, Mundelein, IL.)

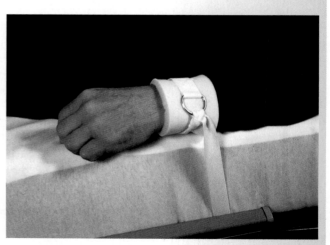

Step 4c. Wrist restraint. (Courtesy Medline Industries, Mundelein, IL.)

Step 4a. Jacket restraint. (Courtesy Medline Industries, Mundelein, IL.)

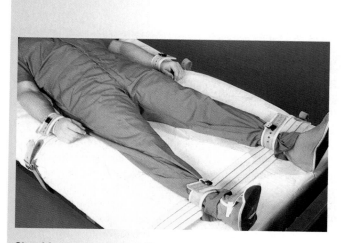

Step 4d. Ankle restraints. (Courtesy Humane Restraint Company, Waunakee, WI.)

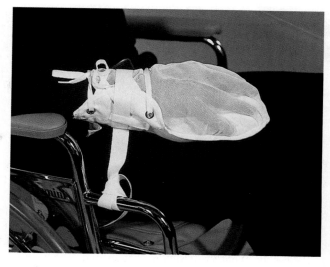

Ste 4e. Mitten restraint. (Courtesy Medline Industries, Mundelein, IL.)

5. Apply the restraint.
 a. Approach the client in a calm, reassuring manner. Avoid sudden or threatening movements.
 b. If the client can understand, explain the need for restraint.
 c. If the client cannot understand the need for restraint, proceed by applying it in a gentle but firm manner.
 d. Pad the skin under the restraint, especially over bony prominences.

 e. Allow room for two fingers to be inserted between the restraint and the client's limb. *Doing so will prevent circulatory constriction.*
 f. Avoid constricting the client's breathing.
 g. Allow the client freedom to turn in bed, if possible.
 h. Tie the restraint to the bed frame rather than a side rail (see illustration). *The side rail can be moved, which may make the restraint too tight (and harmful to the client) or too loose (ineffective).*

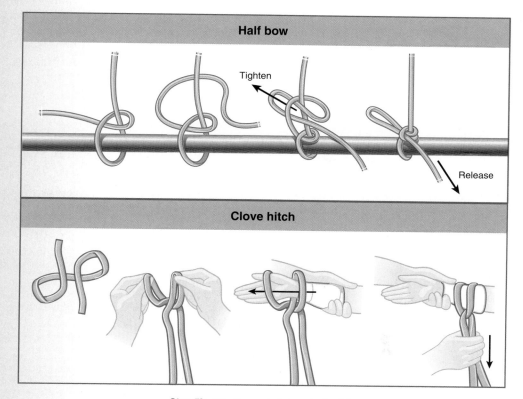

Step 5h. Tie the restraint to the bed frame.

Continued

PROCEDURE 22-1	USING PROTECTIVE RESTRAINTS—CONT'D

i. Tie the restraint in a location where the client cannot reach it but where an attendant can quickly and easily release it in an emergency.
j. Use a slipknot, and never tape a restraint knot.

6. Monitor the client and intervene to prevent complications.
a. Observe the client every 30 minutes.
b. Check the client's skin and circulation every 30 minutes.
c. Provide a regular schedule of toileting.
d. Turn the client at least every 2 hours; position for comfort.
e. Orient the client to the environment every time you check.
f. Assess the client's respirations, cough, and deep breathing every 2 hours.
g. Reassess the need for restraints every 2 hours.
h. Help the client with food and fluid intake as needed.

7. Document the following properly:
a. Rationale or behavior that led to restraint
b. Type of restraint and time it was applied
c. Ongoing assessment and interventions to prevent complications
d. Time restraints are discontinued and client's response

PEDIATRIC CONSIDERATIONS

Restraints for children depend on the age of the child. Provide the least restrictive environment possible, but maintain safety. For some procedures the infant may be held in the mother's arms. For the infant or toddler, a mummy or papoose style of restraint is used for short procedures when it is important that the child be still (e.g., when passing a nasogastric tube, inserting an intravenous catheter, or suturing a laceration).

GERIATRIC CONSIDERATIONS

The older client should receive care in the least restrictive environment possible. Also exercise caution to avoid injury to delicate skin.

HOME CARE CONSIDERATIONS

When the client's behavior in the home requires protection to prevent falls or other self-harm, you should work with the family to provide the protection in the least restrictive manner. If the client needs frequent personal care, a hospital bed may be helpful to family caregivers because of the ease of raising the bed to a working height and of lowering the bed to transfer the client to a chair. If the side rails are sufficient restraint, a hospital bed is a good solution. Otherwise, placing the mattress on the floor may give freedom from restraints and afford protection from falling when trying to get out of bed. Also talk to the family about supervision, and help them work out a schedule to ensure that the client is attended closely.

Box 22-10	Finding Alternatives to Restraints

INCREASE MONITORING FREQUENCY

- Assign the client a room near or within view of the nurses' station.
- Perform hourly safety checks.
- Use an electronic monitoring device, such as an Ambularm, which sounds an alarm when the client's leg reaches a 45-degree angle. An ankle alarm can be used to reveal when an ambulatory client wanders off the nursing unit.
- Have family members or a sitter remain with the client.

PROVIDE A FAMILIAR ENVIRONMENT

- Familiarize the client with the immediate surroundings.
- Provide continuous orientation to person, place, time, and environment. Remind the client to use the call light.
- Use colors as environmental cues.
- Allow the client to use personal belongings, such as a pillow or clothing, when possible.
- Assign familiar personnel, if possible, to help the client feel secure and provide a more accurate needs assessment.
- Encourage the family's participation in the client's care.

PREVENT THE NEED TO GET OUT OF BED UNASSISTED

- Promote a restful environment by minimizing noise, maintaining appropriate lighting, playing relaxing music, and so on.
- Provide comfort measures, such as pain relief and proper positioning.
- Assist with toileting on a regular schedule.

INSTITUTE SAFETY MEASURES

- Use antitip devices, slanted seats, or positioning devices (such as pillows, rolled blankets, and wedge cushions) on wheelchairs to keep the client positioned safely.
- Use bed, chair, or position-sensitive alarms.
- Keep the client's bed in the low position; use half rails or keep the side rails down.
- Increase lighting in the room; use night-lights.

CHANGE THE TREATMENT PLAN

- Consult with the physician to review the need for intravenous catheters, urinary catheters, or nasogastric tubes.

EVALUATION

The effectiveness of nursing interventions used to promote safety and prevent injury is evaluated by comparing the expected outcomes to the goals devised during the planning phase. Nursing interventions are considered effective if the client remains free from injury.

Evaluation of safety is an ongoing process throughout the client's illness or hospital stay. You should continuously reevaluate the client's situation and determine whether new threats to safety have developed or previous ones remain. Additionally, continuous reevaluation will help you make good judgments about discontinuing unnecessary restrictions, especially the use of restraints. The evaluation phase requires frequent assessment of the client's situation to identify specific needs for support services, such as home health care, nursing home placement, or physical and occupational therapy. A care plan for Mrs. Soto can be found in Box 22-11.

It is important to be aware of all the different categories of accidents and hazards that create the potential for risks. Also of importance is an awareness of the people most at risk, such as children and older adults, the handicapped, and the debilitated. You can make a significant difference in the lives of many individuals, especially when safety issues are concerned. Nurses are in a unique position to teach preventive measures, promote safety guidelines, and alleviate alterations in safety.

SAMPLE DOCUMENTATION NOTE FOR MRS. SOTO

Discharge per wheelchair to son's automobile. Alert and oriented, able to walk the length of the hall without dizziness. Son has acquired a walker for his mother's use. Referred to Spring Valley Home Health for evaluation of home setting for safety needs, ability to perform activities of daily living, correct use of walker, need for meals on wheel, and physical therapy services. Will see primary physician on Friday for follow-up.

Key Principles

- To feel safe and to be safe in the home setting or health care facility is a basic human need.
- Nurses are in a prime position to help prevent accidents, promote safety, and alleviate alterations in safety.
- Falls, asphyxiation, choking, and poisoning can be categorized as general injuries.
- Traumatic injuries can result from fires, electrical shock, motor vehicle accidents, and exposure to radiation.
- Falls are the second leading cause of death in people over the age of 74 years.
- The risk for falls is significantly higher in hospitalized older adults.
- Asphyxiation, or suffocation, is a leading cause of mortality during childhood.
- People most at risk for poisoning include toddlers, young children, and adults with sensory impairment.
- Cigarette smoking and the use of alcohol are common factors that can increase the risk for fire injuries.
- Factors that determine the type and extent of an electrical injury include voltage, type of current, area and duration of contact, skin resistance, and path of current flow.
- Motor vehicle accidents are the leading cause of accidental death in the United States.

Nursing Care Plan AN ELDERLY CLIENT WITH A HEAD INJURY   Box 22-11

ADMISSION DATA

Mrs. Juanita Soto is a 75-year-old Hispanic woman who will be discharged from the hospital in a few days and needs reevaluation by her home health nurse. Mrs. Soto had been admitted through the emergency room to the general medical nursing unit after sustaining a head contusion when she fell trying to get out of the shower. Mrs. Soto informed the nurse, "I never have hurt myself this much before. Usually, I catch myself before I fall all the way, but this time I could not. I guess I'm not as strong as I used to be. Since my husband died, I have lived by myself. My sons and daughters live far away, and I don't want to be a burden on anyone." Mrs. Soto lives alone in a two-story woodframe home.

NURSING REPORT TO HOME HEALTH AGENCY

Client was admitted because of a head contusion sustained while trying to get out of the shower. Her son is present and staying with her while she is in the hospital. Client stated that this has happened before but not to this extent. States that she had been feeling weaker. Has limited movement in hands and legs and is partially blind in one eye.

Mrs. Soto is referred back to the home health agency by her physician. Her daughter had expressed concern about her mother living alone safely and being able to manage her arthritis. Because Mrs. Soto refused to leave her home, the physician requested an evaluation by the home health nurse.

PHYSICIAN'S REFERRAL REQUEST

Evaluate client's ability to perform activities of daily living and instrumental activities of daily living. Arrange for home health aide and Meals on Wheels if needed. Monitor compliance with arthritis medication and assess for side effects. Assist client to plan for two 30-minute to 60-minute rest periods during the day. Arrange for physical therapy to teach isometric and range-of-motion exercises. Home paraffin therapy before exercise, BID.

HOME NURSING ASSESSMENT

The home assessment revealed an older, two-story home with no safety equipment in the bathroom, some throw rugs, inadequate lighting at night, cluttered hallways, and broken stairs with no railing.

Nursing Care Plan **AN ELDERLY CLIENT WITH A HEAD INJURY—CONT'D** | Box 22-11

NANDA Nursing Diagnosis	NOC Expected Outcomes With Indicators	NIC Interventions With Selected Activities	Evaluation Data
RISK FOR INJURY: FALL **Related Factors:** • Fall related to limited movement • Partially blind in one eye • Lives alone • Age 75	**SAFETY STATUS: FALL OCCURRENCE** • Number of falls: • While standing • While walking • While sitting • From bed • While transferring • Climbing steps • Descending steps	**FALL PREVENTION SURVELLIANCE: SAFETY** • Identify cognitive or physical deficits that may increase potential of falling at home. • Monitor gait, balance, and fatigue level with ambulation. • Provide assistive devices. • Remove hazards from home (e.g., throw rugs). • Provide grab bars for bathtub, shower chair, nonslip floor. • Increase lighting in home.	**FIRST HOME VISIT** • Mrs. Soto maintains order in her home and is familiar with environment. • Basement stairs are a hazard; son will repair stairs to basement. • Not safe to cook hot meals; will arrange Meals on Wheels with provider who caters to Hispanic food preferences. • Living in her familiar community is an important value to Mrs. Soto. • She has neighbors who are willing to visit frequently and perform small tasks. • She has limited range of motion in lower extremities and sometimes uses a cane to get around; also uses a wheelchair. • She has shoes with nonskid soles. • She stated that the stairs were going to be fixed by her son while he was there. • Her home is about 50 years old; it has four bedrooms and two baths. The bathroom floor has tile, and she usually has throw rugs on the floor because it tends to be cold. She expressed concern over the cost of grab bars.

CRITICAL THINKING QUESTIONS

1. How would you handle the subject of using a copper bracelet rather than the medication the physician has ordered?

2. How would you approach the subject of having a caretaker live with Mrs. Soto?

3. Would adult day care be helpful in this situation?

Nursing outcome and intervention labels from Johnson, M., Bulechek, G., McCloskey Dochterman, J., Maas, M., & Moorhead, S. (2001). *Nursing diagnoses, outcomes, and interventions: NANDA, NOC, and NIC linkages.* St Louis, MO: Mosby.

• Measures to prevent back injuries include using proper lifting techniques and proper body mechanics, and performing proper exercises and activities to promote strong bones and muscles.

• Prevent exposure to radiation by using lead shielding and by observing the increased distance/decreased time rule when caring for a client with radioactive implants.

• Factors affecting a person's risk for injury can be identified in the person's home, work, and community.

• Assessment of clients who are at risk for injury includes the collection of subjective and objective data.

• The nurse's role in home safety includes education appropriate for age and developmental status; it also includes making referrals to help the family attain and maintain safe housing.

• The nurse's role in institutional safety involves the safe use of equipment, appropriate client education, and collaboration with the housekeeping and maintenance departments to ensure a safe environment.

• Clients should be restrained only in the absence of viable alternatives and when there is clear evidence that the failure to restrain could cause harm to the client.

Bibliography

Ahmann, E. (2001). Guns in the home: Nurses' roles. *Pediatric Nursing, 27*(6), 587-590, 605.

Anderson, R. M. (1999). Center for Disease Control and Prevention. *National Vital Statistics Reports, 49*(11), 1-88. Retrieved from http://www. cdc.gov/nchs/data/nvsr/nvsr49/nvsr49_11.pdf.

Benham, S. (2001). Cultural safety values difference. *Nursing New Zealand, 7*(1), 28-29.

Borycki, E. M. (2000). Falls in the elderly: A brief review of some key points. *Perspectives, 24*(3), 20-23.

Casey, A. (2002). Health and safety for parents. *Paediatric Nursing, 14*(2), 3.

CDC (Centers for Disease Control). (2000a). Falls among older adults. *Fact book for the year 2000*. Retrieved from http://www.cdc.gov/ncipc/pub-res/Factsheets/falls.htm.

CDC (Centers for Disease Control). (2000b). Fire related injuries. *Fact book for the year 2000*. Retrieved from http://www.cdc.gov/ncipc/factsheets/fire.htm.

CDC (Centers for Disease Control). (2000c). Motor-vehicle-related injuries. *Fact book for the year 2000*. Retrieved from http://www.cdc.gov/ncipc/pub-res/FactBook/fkmve.htm.

Centers for Disease Control and Prevention, National Center for Environmental Health, Childhood Lead Poisoning Prevention. (1997.) *Screening young children for lead poisoning: Guidance for state and local public health officials*. Retrieved from http://www.cdc.gov/nceh.

Cho, C. Y., Alessi, C. A., Cho, M., Aronow, H. U., Stuck, A. E., Rubenstein, L., et al. (1998). The association between chronic illness and functional change among participants in a comprehensive geriatric assessment program. *Journal of the American Geriatric Society, 46*(6), 677-682.

Cockey, C. D. (2001). New JCAHO patient safety standards. *Association of Women's Health, Obstetrics, and Neonatal Nursing Lifelines, 5*(4), 20-21.

Colgan, J. (2002). Syncope: A fall from grace. *Progress in Cardiovascular Nursing, 17*(2), 66-70.

Cowen, P. S. (1999). Child neglect: Injuries of omission. *Pediatric Nursing, 25*(4), 401-405, 409-418.

Delaney, K. R. (2001). Developing a restraint-reduction program for child/adolescent inpatient treatment. *Journal of Child/Adolescent Psychiatric Nursing, 14*(3), 128-140.

Dunn, K. S. (2001). The effect of physical restraints on fall rates in older adults who are institutionalized. *Journal of Gerontological Nursing, 27*(10), 40-48.

Early, M. R., & Williams, R. A. (2002). Emergency nurses' experience with violence: Does it affect nursing care of battered women? *Journal of Emergency Nursing, 28*(3), 199-204.

Ernst, D. J. (2001). Guide to needle prevention devices. *Home Healthcare Nurse, 19*(6), 348-355.

Forrester, D. A., McCabe-Bender, J., Walsh, N., & Bell-Bowe, J. (2000). Physical restraint management of hospitalized adults and follow-up study. *Journal for Nurses in Staff Development, 16*(6), 267-276.

Fraser, J. (2001). Our children's safety. *The Practising Midwife, 4*(11), 14-15.

Fuller, G. F. (2000). Falls in the elderly. *American Family Physician, 61*, 2159-2168.

Groeneveld, A., McKenzie, M. L., & Williams, D. (2001). Logrolling: Establishing consistent practice. *Orthopedic Nursing, 20*(2), 45-49.

Hall, G. R. (2001). Falls: A more personal look. *Journal of Gerontological Nursing, 27*(10), 5-6.

Hellwig, K. (2000). Alternatives to restraints: What patients and caregivers should know. *Home Healthcare Nurse, 18*(6), 395-402; quiz 402-403.

Hill-Westmoreland, E. E., Soeken, K., & Spellbring, A. M. (2002). A meta-analysis of fall prevention programs for the elderly: How effective are they? *Nursing Research, 51*(1), 1-8.

*Holmes, E. R., & Holmes L. D. (1995). *Other cultures, elder years*. Thousand Oaks, CA: Sage.

Johnson, M., Bulechek, G., McCloskey Dochterman, J. M., Maas, M., & Moorhead, S. (2001). *Nursing diagnoses, outcomes, and interventions: NANDA, NOC, and NIC linkages*. St Louis, MO: Mosby.

Kobs, A. Managing the environment of care. *Nursing Management, 29*(4), 10-13.

Koch, S., Lyon, C., & Lyon, K. S. (2001). Case study approach to removing physical restraint. *International Journal of Nursing Practice, 7*(3), 156-161.

Krumberger, J. M. (2001). Building a culture of safety. *RN, 64*(1), 32ac2-32ac3.

Lassman, J. (2002). Water safety. *Journal of Emergency Nursing, 28*(3), 241-243.

*Loomis, T. A., & Hayes, A. W. (1996). *Loomis' essentials of toxicology* (4th ed.) San Diego, CA: Academic Press.

McConnell, E. A. (1997). Myths and facts about fire safety. *Nursing, 27*(10), 17.

Mion, L. C., Fogel, J., Sandhu, S., Palmer, R. M., Minnick, A. F., & Cranston, T., et al. (2001). Outcomes following physical restraint reduction programs in two acute care hospitals. *The Joint Commission Journal on Quality Improvement, 27*(11), 605-618.

NANDA (North American Nursing Diagnosis Association). (2000). *NANDA nursing diagnoses: Definitions and classification 2001-2002*. Philadelphia: Author.

National Center for Health Statistics. (1999). *Monthly Vital Statistics Report, 46*(1), 1016-1022.

*National Lead Information Center. U.S. Environmental Protection Agency (EPA 800-b-92, February 1995). (1998). Retrieved from http://www.nsc.org.

Nelson, C. M. (2001). Falls prevention in older adults. *Geriatric Nursing, 22*(4), 174-175.

*NIOSH (National Institute for Occupational Safety and Health). (1997). Back belts: Do they prevent injury? Retrieved from http://www.cdc.gov/niosh/backbelt.html.

Owens, M. F. (2000). Patient restraints: Protection for whom? *JONA'S Healthcare Law Ethics, and Regulations, 2*(2), 59-65.

Patrick, L., & Blodgett, A. (2001). Selecting patients for falls-prevention protocols: An evidence-based approach on a geriatric rehabilitation unit. *Journal of Gerontological Nursing, 27*(10), 19-25.

Pennels, C. (2001). Practical ways of putting safety first. *Professional Nurse, 16*(7 Suppl), S7.

Perry, J. (2001). When home is where the risk is. *Home Healthcare Nurse, 19*(6), 338-341.

Sattin, R. W., Rodriguez, J. G., DeVito, C. A., & Wingo, P. A. Study to Assess Falls Among the Elderly (SAFE) Group. (1998). Home environmental hazards and the risk for fall injury events among community-dwelling older persons. *Journal of the American Geriatric Society, 46*(6), 669-676.

Smith, G. S., Branas, C., Miller, T. R. (1999). Fatal nontraffic injuries involving alcohol: A meta-analysis. *Annals of Emergency Medicine, 33*(16), 659-668.

Sullivan-Marx, E. M. (2001). Achieving restraint-free care of acutely confused older adults. *Journal of Gerontological Nursing, 27*(4), 56-61.

Talty, J., Sheese, J., Gunn, S., Stone, J., Chappelow, M., Wyatt, K., et al. (2000). Implementing a comprehensive child restraint program in a pediatric hospital: An effective model. *Pediatric Nursing 26*(6), 619-624.

van Leeuwen, M., Bennett, L., West, S., Wiles, V., & Grasso, J. (2001). Patient falls from bed and the role of bedrails in the acute care setting. *Australian Journal of Advanced Nursing, 19*(2), 8-13.

Walker, B. L. (1998). Preventing falls. *RN, 61*(5), 40-42.

Werner, P., & Mendelsson, G. (2001). Nursing staff members' intentions to use physical restraints with older people: Testing the theory of reasoned action. *Journal of Advanced Nursing, 35*(5), 784-791.

What you must know about new patient safety standards. (2001). *RN, 64*(6), 24hf1-24hf4.

Wilson, E. B. (1996). Physical restraints of elderly patients in critical care. *Critical Care Nursing Clinics of North America, 8*(1), 65.

23

Promoting Healthy Nutrition

Key Terms

amino acids

anthropometric measurements

calorie

carbohydrate

disaccharide

fiber

glycogen

metabolism

minerals

monosaccharide

nutrient

nutrition

nutritional status

polysaccharide

protein

recommended dietary allowance

starch

triglyceride

vitamin

Learning Objectives

After studying this chapter, you should be able to do the following:

- Describe the elements of a nutritious diet and how the body uses nutrients
- Distinguish among various guidelines for normal nutrition
- Discuss the factors that affect nutritional status, such as lifestyle, culture, life span, pregnancy and lactation, and psychological and physiological states
- Describe the assessment of a client's nutritional status
- Identify nursing diagnoses applicable to the client with a normal nutritional balance
- Plan for goal-directed interventions to promote optimal nutrition and reduce nutritional risk factors
- Describe specific interventions and strategies to promote optimal nutrition and reduce nutritional risk factors throughout the life span
- Evaluate the outcomes of nutritional interventions

Joan, a 20-year-old woman, arrives in the nurse practitioner's office for a wellness examination, stating that she feels good and has "no problems." She is of "normal weight" at 115 pounds for her 60-inch (5′0″) frame. Joan says that she has never been hospitalized and has had no serious illnesses. She is an office secretary and participates in many church activities but engages in very little physical activity. Previous medical records reveal that her cholesterol was elevated at an examination 1 year ago.

Joan never eats breakfast but begins a continuous eating pattern beginning about 11:00 A.M. She says that she doesn't really eat a meal at lunch but snacks continually until dinner on cookies, candy, rolls, cheese, potato chips, and other snack foods. For dinner she eats fried foods, potatoes, bread, and dessert, and she admits disliking fruits and vegetables.

The clinical evaluation reveals no abnormalities or specific alterations. The triceps skin-fold measure is within normal limits. Joan's total cholesterol is still elevated, and she wants to know how she can reduce it. In analyzing Joan's status, the nurse considers *Risk for imbalanced nutrition: more than body requirements* from the list of nursing diagnoses that relate to nutrition (see below).

KEY NURSING DIAGNOSES FOR Nutrition

Imbalanced nutrition: more than body requirements: An intake of nutrients that exceeds metabolic needs

Imbalanced nutrition: less than body requirements: An intake of nutrients insufficient to meet metabolic needs

Risk for imbalanced nutrition: more than body requirements: Being at risk for experiencing an intake of nutrients that exceeds metabolic needs

Risk for imbalanced nutrition: less than body requirements: Being at risk for experiencing an intake of nutrients insufficient to meet metabolic needs

CONCEPTS OF NUTRITION

The human body constantly builds, maintains, and heals itself with the molecules it derives from food. For this reason, there is no single factor that influences a person's health more than decisions about the types and amount of food to eat. It is important for optimal health that the daily diet be balanced and high in quality. Health professionals, such as nurses, physicians, and dietitians, are key sources of information about the role of nutrition in promoting health.

Nutrition and Nutrients

Nutrition is the science of food and nutrients and of the processes by which an organism takes them in and uses them for energy to grow, maintain function, and renew itself. To the layperson, the term *nutrition* is synonymous with food or diet. The building block of the diet is a **nutrient,** which is a biochemical substance used by the body for growth, maintenance, and repair. For optimal health, the diet must be sufficient in a variety of nutrients.

Nutritional status is the condition of the body resulting from its use of essential nutrients available to it. A client's nutritional status may be good, fair, or poor, depending on the intake of dietary essentials, on the relative need for them, and on the body's ability to use them. A good nutritional status is essential for normal organ development and function; for normal reproduction, growth, and maintenance; for optimal activity and working efficiency; for resistance to infection; and for the ability to repair bodily damage or injury. Poor nutritional status exists when the body is deprived of adequate amounts of essential nutrients over an extended period.

Nutritional status is relative because the body's stores of some nutrients last longer than others. Additionally, at certain times, demands for particular nutrients may rise. If intake remains constant, stores of these nutrients may be depleted. This may happen, for instance, if a pregnant woman fails to increase her intake of iron, calcium, and certain vitamins.

The Gastrointestinal System

The gastrointestinal (GI) or digestive system converts food into elemental materials that build, maintain, and repair the body's cells. These materials are then absorbed through the intestinal membranes into the bloodstream for use by the body.

Structure. The organs of the GI system include the mouth, pharynx, esophagus, stomach, small intestine, and large intestine (Table 23-1, p. 518). Ancillary organs that play a role in digestion include the liver, gallbladder, and pancreas. Food enters the system through the mouth, passes into the pharynx and is swallowed, and then passes through the esophagus into the stomach.

The stomach is much wider than the rest of the GI tract and has a J-shaped curve at the bottom. It holds food until the food is digested to the right consistency before allowing it to flow into the intestine. The C-shaped duodenum is the first and shortest portion of the small intestine, followed by the jejunum (the longest portion), and the narrow ileum. The ileocecal valve joins the small intestine to the large intestine, which continues to the rectum and anus.

Function. The four main functions of the GI system are digestion, absorption, metabolism, and excretion. This chapter focuses on the first three. Concepts related to excretion are discussed in Chapter 28.

Digestion is a mechanical and chemical process by which the body changes food into elemental nutrients that can be absorbed. The process begins in the mouth, where the food is chewed and mixed with saliva. Ptyalin, the enzyme in saliva,

Table 23-1	Digestive Functions of Gastrointestinal Structures
Structure	**Function**
Mouth	Chews food and mixes it with saliva
Salivary glands	Produce enzymes to begin the breakdown of carbohydrates
Epiglottis	Closes when food is swallowed to prevent aspiration
Esophagus	Transports food bolus from mouth to stomach
Lower esophageal sphincter	Protects the esophagus from regurgitation of hydrochloric acid
Stomach	Mixes food with hydrochloric acid, pepsin, and lipase to form chyme
Pyloric sphincter	Prevents backflow of alkaline intestinal contents into stomach
Liver	Secretes bile for the emulsification of fat
Gallbladder	Stores and releases bile when fat is present in food
Bile duct	Transports bile to duodenum
Pancreas	Produces trypsin, chymotrypsin, amylase, and lipase for digestion of carbohydrates, fats, and proteins
Pancreatic duct	Collects pancreatic enzymes and transports them to duodenum
Duodenum	Mixes chyme with digestive enzymes and begins nutrient absorption across numerous villi
Jejunum	Provides the main area for digestion and absorption across a great number of villi
Ileum	Finishes digestion of chyme and absorption across a smaller number of villi, especially at distal end
Ileocecal sphincter	Slows absorption time and prevents bacteria from entering small intestine
Appendix	Function unknown
Colon	Reabsorbs water and electrolytes and prepares waste for excretion
Rectum	Stores wastes until peristalsis produces urge to defecate
Anus	Controls bowel elimination by means of internal and external sphincters

begins the breakdown of starches into simpler sugars. The powerful peristaltic action of the stomach churns, liquefies, and mixes the food with gastric juices. Pepsin and hydrochloric acid in the stomach break down proteins into proteases, peptones, and polypeptides. Gastric lipase, which is most active in infants for milk digestion, is a weak, fat-splitting enzyme secreted in the stomach.

Food exits the stomach at the pyloric sphincter and enters the small intestine, where most enzymatic digestion and virtually all absorption occur. The pancreatic enzymes—amylase, trypsin, and lipase—are secreted into the small intestine to break down carbohydrates, proteins, and fats into sugars, amino acids, and fatty acids, respectively. Bile from the liver, which is concentrated and stored by the gallbladder, emulsifies fats for the action of the fat-splitting enzymes. Once digested material reaches the large intestine, it contains very few nutrients. Here, water and electrolytes are absorbed from this mass, resulting in semisolid feces.

Absorption is the passage of the end products of carbohydrate, protein, and fat digestion, as well as many vitamin and mineral molecules, through the intestinal wall into the body fluids and tissues. Absorption takes place through diffusion or active transport. The intestinal lining is designed for absorption because it has multiple folds and villi that yield a large surface area.

Metabolism is the process by which energy from nutrients is used by the cells or stored for later use. Individual cells convert chemical energy from molecular bonds into energy for growth, maintenance, and repair as well as for muscle contraction and nerve function. Metabolism can be either anabolic or catabolic. Anabolic processes build up substances and body tissues, whereas catabolic processes break them down. Body reserves are used when a person does not eat sufficient amounts of nutrients or when the body has an increased need for them.

Major Components of Food

The body's main nutrients are carbohydrates, proteins, fats, vitamins, and minerals. An adult's metabolism requires nine amino acids, one fatty acid, 13 vitamins, and 12 minerals. All of the major energy-yielding nutrients are composed of smaller units. Carbohydrates, proteins, and fats must be hydrolyzed into their smaller characteristic units before absorption. Water is another important component of all foods and is also necessary for life. The body's need for water is discussed in Chapter 25.

Energy and Calories. Carbohydrates, proteins, and fats are collectively called the energy nutrients because they contribute the energy value (calories) from food. Their primary physiological function is the production of energy for health and activity. *Energy* is power that can be translated into motion, can overcome resistance, or can effect physical change. Energy production in the body is a chemical process that indirectly involves the use of vitamins, minerals, and water.

The human body may be likened to a machine or engine that must constantly be refueled to enable it to perform work. The fuel needed by the body for both external and internal work is, of course, food. The chemical energy available from food is converted in the body to electrical energy for impulse transmission in the brain and nervous system, to thermal energy for regulation of body temperature, and to other forms of chemical energy for the synthesis of body compounds. Chemical energy from food is also converted into mechanical energy, which allows muscles to contract and for work to be accomplished in the external environment.

Foods are frequently discussed in terms of the calories they contain. **Calorie** is the common term used to refer to the more accurate *kilocalorie* (kcal), a measure of the potential energy of the carbohydrate, protein, and fat content of food. The calorie used in nutrition is defined as the amount of heat needed to raise the temperature of 1 kg of water 1° C. This unit (the kilocalorie) is 1000 times larger than the calorie used in either biology or chemistry.

Three major factors determine a human's daily energy requirement: the *basal metabolic rate* (BMR), the degree of *physical activity,* and the *specific dynamic action* of food. The BMR is the amount of energy needed to maintain essential body functions expressed as calories per hour per square meter of body surface. Essential body functions include respiration, circulation, peristalsis, muscle tone, body temperature, glandular activity, and the other vegetative functions of the body. For infants, children, and pregnant women, growth is an additional factor. Energy requirements are stated in calories.

Carbohydrates. A **carbohydrate** is a simple or complex compound composed of carbon, oxygen, and hydrogen. A **monosaccharide** is a six-carbon sugar (a subunit of carbohydrates). Glucose, fructose, and galactose are examples of monosaccharides. A **disaccharide** is a molecule that forms when two monosaccharides join together to form a double sugar. These include sucrose (glucose and fructose), maltose (two units of glucose), and lactose or milk sugar (glucose and galactose). Notice that glucose is a component of all disaccharides. A **polysaccharide** is a group of monosaccharides joined together in a chain. They can be converted back to monosaccharides through a process called acid hydrolysis.

Carbohydrates are stored differently in plants and animals. **Glycogen** is the form in which carbohydrates are stored in the muscle tissue of humans and animals. When the body needs quick energy, it uses glycogen stores, which can be broken down into glucose by enzymes. **Starch** is the form in which plants store glucose. They use this energy for growth. When a person eats a plant, the plant starch is hydrolyzed by enzymes into glucose, which can then be used for energy or rearranged to form glycogen for storage. Carbohydrate as an energy source provides 4 kcal per gram. The body needs a sufficient daily intake of carbohydrates for energy production to avoid breakdown of proteins and fats. The recommended percentage of dietary carbohydrates is approximately 50% to 60% of total caloric intake.

Fiber. **Fiber** is the structure of which plants are composed, which includes cellulose, hemicellulose, pectins, gums, and mucilages. A diet high in fiber contains foods such as cereals (especially bran), whole wheat bread, and raw fruits and vegetables. Although most fibers begin as polysaccharides, human enzymes cannot further digest or break down the bonds between monosaccharide units of fiber, leading to reduced absorption. Because fiber retains water and increases the rate at which residue moves through the large intestine, people who consume sufficient fiber have fewer problems with constipation.

Other advantages of a high-fiber diet include delayed absorption of glucose and lower blood cholesterol levels. A high-fiber diet also may prevent diverticulosis from developing later in life and may decrease the risk of colon cancer. People who increase fiber in their diet should do so gradually to prevent diarrhea caused by the added bulk and water. They should also drink plenty of fluids to prevent stool impaction.

Protein. **Protein** is a compound containing polymers of *amino acids,* linked together in a chain to form polypeptide bonds. There are over 20 **amino acids,** which are composed of carbon, hydrogen, oxygen, and an amino group. Amino acids can be classified as essential or nonessential depending on whether or not the body can manufacture them from other sources. Essential amino acids are those amino acids that cannot be adequately synthesized by the body to meet metabolic needs and therefore must be supplied by the diet. The body needs a sufficient daily intake of essential amino acids in the diet to meet bodily maintenance and growth needs. Similarly, proteins can be classified as complete or incomplete, depending on whether or not they contain all nine essential amino acids. Some diets, such as a strict vegetarian diet, have a high proportion of incomplete proteins, but incomplete proteins can be successfully combined to form complete proteins (for example, a peanut butter sandwich contains a grain and a legume). See a nutrition text for a more detailed discussion of complete and incomplete proteins in the diet.

Proteins form the structure of the body and regulate body processes. Skin, hair, and eyes are made of protein, as are the enzymes needed for digestion and absorption. The antibodies that defend against disease, hormones that regulate body functions, and red and white blood cells are all made of protein. Even lipoproteins, molecules that carry fat and cholesterol in the blood, have a protein core. Proteins also help to maintain fluid, electrolyte, and acid–base balance.

Enzymes break down dietary proteins or *polypeptides* into individual amino acids or *peptides.* In this form, they can be absorbed through the intestinal wall and into the bloodstream. Some dipeptides (two amino acid chains) and tripeptides (three amino acid chains) are also transported this way. Protein as an energy source provides 4 kcal per gram. When the body is storing protein (anabolism), the person is said to have a positive nitrogen balance. On the other hand, when the body is breaking down protein (catabolism), it is said to be in negative nitrogen balance. Nitrogen that is released during protein catabolism is excreted through the kidneys.

Lipids. Lipids, or fats, are a family of compounds that includes *triglycerides* (fats and oils), phospholipids, and steroids. Like carbohydrates and protein, fat is composed of carbon, oxygen, and hydrogen. A key difference, however, is that there are a greater number of carbon and hydrogen atoms in proportion to oxygen atoms, so lipid molecules yield more energy: 9 kcal per gram. Lipids are a source of fuel for the body, add flavor to food, and assist with satiety.

Triglycerides, each composed of three fatty acids and a glycol unit, are the chief form of fat in the diet and the main form of fat transport in the blood. Ninety-nine percent of body fat is stored in the form of triglycerides. Enzymes and bile salts are needed to break down triglycerides into smaller units (fatty acids, monoglycerides, and glycerol) for use by the body. Small units of digested fat can be absorbed through the cells of the small intestine and into the bloodstream. Larger units are released into the lymph system to enter the bloodstream at the thoracic duct. The body can manufacture many

Table 23-2	Overview of Important Vitamins	
Adult RDA*	**Sources**	**Functions**
Vitamin A (Retinol, retinal, retinoic acid) RDA: 800 to 1000 retinol equivalents	Dark-green and yellow vegetables, broccoli, carrots, winter squash, sweet potatoes, liver, egg yolks, breakfast cereals, dairy products, margarine, fortified milk, peaches, apricots, cantaloupe.	• Better vision in dim light. • Formation and maintenance of skin and mucous membranes. • Normal growth and development of bones and teeth.
Vitamin B$_1$ (Thiamine) RDA: 1.0 to 1.4 mg	Pork, organ meats, liver, enriched and whole-grain grains, eggs, nuts, dried peas, dried beans.	• Energy metabolism, especially of carbohdyrates. • Normal nervous system functioning.
Vitamin B$_2$ (Riboflavin) RDA: 1.2 to 1.7 mg	Dairy products, milk, eggs, organ meats, enriched grains, green leafy vegetables.	• Carbohydrate, protein, and fat metabolism. • Other metabolic functions.
Niacin (Nicotinic acid) RDA: 13 to 19 mg	Lean meat, kidney, poultry, liver, fish, enriched and whole grains, nuts, yeast, peanut butter, and dried peas and beans.	• Carbohydrate, protein, and fat metabolism.
Vitamin B$_4$ RDA: 2.0 to 2.2 mg	Organ meats, pork, egg yolk, potatoes, whole grain cereals, wheat germ, yeast.	• Amino acid metabolism. • Blood formation. • Maintenance of nervous tissue. • Conversion of tryptophan to niacin.
Folic acid RDA: 400 μg	Organ meats, milk, eggs, green leafy vegetables, broccoli, asparagus, wheat germ, yeast.	• RNA and DNA synthesis. • Formation and maturation of red blood cells. • Amino acid metabolism.
Vitamin C (Ascorbic acid) RDA: 60 mg	Citrus fruits and juices, brussels sprouts, broccoli, green peppers, strawberries, tomatoes, cabbage, greens, guava.	• Collagen formation. • Protection of other nutrients from oxidation. • Enhancement of iron absorption. • Conversion of folic acid to its active form. • Metabolism of certain amino acids.
Vitamin D (Cholecalciferol ergosterol) RDA: 5 to 10 μg	Sunlight, liver, egg yolks, fish-liver oils, breakfast cereals, margarine, butter, fortified milk.	• Metabolism of calcium and phosphorus. • Stimulation of calcium absorption. • Mobilization of calcium and phosphorus from bone. • Stimulation of reabsorption of calcium and phosphorus by kidney.
Vitamin E (Tocopherol) RDA: 8 to 10 mg	Vegetable oils, wheat germ, whole-grain products	• Protection of vitamin A and polyunsaturated fatty acids from oxidation. • Maintenance of cell membrane integrity. • Heme synthesis.
Vitamin K RDA: 70 to 140 μg	Dark-green leafy vegetables, vegetables of the cabbage family. Also produced by gut bacteria in the intestines.	• Synthesis of certain proteins needed for blood clotting.

*Others include vitamin B$_{12}$ (cobalamin), 3.0 μg; pantothenic acid, 4 to 7 mg; and biotin, 100 μg to 200 μg.

fatty acids, but the two essential fatty acids (linolenic acid and linoleic acid) need to be obtained from the diet.

Vitamins. A **vitamin** is an organic substance found in food that serves as a coenzyme in enzymatic reactions. Vitamins are essential nutrients required in small amounts by the body for physiological and metabolic functioning (Table 23-2). Vitamins cannot be synthesized by the body and must be obtained from foods. No single food contains all vitamins.

Unlike the carbohydrates, proteins, and fats, vitamins are not linked together in long chains. They are individual units that release energy from food but do not add any energy themselves. Vitamins are measured in very small units, such as milligrams and micrograms.

There are 13 different vitamins, and they are classified as either water soluble or fat soluble. Water-soluble vitamins are the B vitamins and vitamin C; these need to be replenished daily in the diet because they are easily excreted via the kidneys. Fat-soluble vitamins include vitamins A, D, E, and K.

Because the body can store these, it is important to avoid excessive intake, which could lead to toxic levels.

Minerals. **Minerals** are inorganic elements present in small amounts in virtually all body fluids and tissues (Table 23-3). There are 16 minerals essential to human nutrition. Minerals do not yield energy, and they are not metabolized. The major minerals regulate fluid, electrolyte, and acid–base balance and help form the structure of bone. They are also important in the function of muscle and nerve cells.

The major minerals include sodium, chloride, potassium, calcium, phosphorus, magnesium, and sulfur. In addition to major minerals, the body needs trace minerals in smaller amounts. They include iron, zinc, iodine, selenium, copper, manganese, fluoride, chromium, and molybdenum.

A balanced diet composed of a wide variety of foods is the best source of all nutrients needed for good health. Dietary vitamin and mineral supplements, if used, should only supplement nutrients obtained from a balanced diet.

Table 23-3	Overview of Important Minerals	
Mineral and Its Adult RDA*	**Sources**	**Functions**
MACROMINERALS		
Calcium *RDA:* 800 mg	Milk and dairy products, canned fish with bones, green leafy vegetables.	• Bone and tooth formation. • Blood clotting. • Nerve transmission. • Muscle contraction. • Cell membrane permeability. • Activation of certain enzymes.
Phosphorus *RDA:* 800 mg	Milk and milk products, meat, poultry, fish, eggs, dried peas, dried beans, nuts, soft drinks, processed foods.	• Bone and tooth formation. • Acid-base balance. • Energy and metabolism. • Cell membrane structure. • Component of nucleic acids. • Regulation of hormones and coenzymes. • Fat absorption and transport. • Glucose absorption.
Magnesium *RDA:* 350 mg	Green leafy vegetables, nuts, dried peas, dried beans, grains, seafood, cocoa, chocolate.	• Bone and tooth formation. • Smooth muscle relaxation. • Carbohydrate metabolism. • Protein synthesis. • Hormonal activity. • Cell reproduction and growth.
Sodium *RDA:* 1100 to 3300 mg	Salt, sodium-containing preservatives and additives, processed foods, canned meats and vegetables, condiments, pickled foods, ham, soft water, foods prepared in brine solutions, milk, meat, carrots, celery, beets, spinach.	• Fluid balance. • Acid–base balance. • Muscular irritability. • Cell permeability. • Nerve impulse transmission.
Potassium *RDA:* 1875 to 5625 mg	Whole grains, legumens, fruits, leafy vegetables, broccoli, sweet potatoes, potatoes, meat, tomatoes.	• Fluid balance. • Acid–base balance. • Nerve impulse transmission. • Striated skeletal and cardiac muscle activity. • Carbohydrate metabolism. • Protein synthesis. • Catalyst for many metabolic reactions.
MICROMINERALS		
Iron *RDA:* 10 to 18 mg	Liver, lean meats, enriched and whole-grain breads and cereals.	• Oxygen transport via hemoglobin and myoglobin. • Constituent of enzyme systems.
Iodine *RDA:* 150 mg	Iodized salt, seafood, food additives, dough conditioners, dairy disinfectants.	• Component of thyroid hormones.
Zinc *RDA:* 15 mg	Oysters, liver, meats, poultry, dried peas, dried beans, nuts.	• Tissue growth, development, and healing. • Sexual maturation and reproduction. • Enzyme formation. • Immune response.

*Others include copper, 2 to 3 mg; manganese, 2 to 5 mg; fluoride, 1.5 to 4 mg; chromium, 0.05 to 0.2 mg, selenium, 0.05 to 0.2 mg; molybdenum, 0.15 to 0.5 mg.

FACTORS AFFECTING NUTRITIONAL STATUS

Despite an increase in public awareness, good nutrition typically ranks low on the scale of priorities when most people are making food choices. Consequently, you must fully appreciate the meanings and values associated with food because they commonly are more important than the nutrient content and health impact of food in the minds of clients.

A person's dietary pattern is usually slow to change because food habits are deeply rooted in the past. Even among those who want to change, social pressures may make it difficult. Food choices have always been influenced by nonnutritional factors, including religious taboos, ethnicity, gender roles, and social status. Meal preparation, for example, can reflect relatedness, obligation, self-fulfillment, creativity, or love. Mealtimes have historically been viewed as social occasions, bringing together family and friends. Nonetheless, if national nutrition statistics accurately indicate emerging trends, we are experiencing a dietary revolution unprecedented in the history of nutritional science.

Risk Factors Across the Life Span
Infants and Children. Sufficient calorie and protein intake is important in meeting a child's nutritional needs. Growth is especially rapid during infancy, and it is slower but steady during toddlerhood and childhood. Toddlers may also experience physiological anorexia and food jags, in which one or a few foods are preferred to the exclusion of others. Because growth patterns vary at different stages of infancy and childhood, the need for carbohydrates, fats, and other minerals and vitamins is constantly changing. As a health professional, you can support the growth process by supervising the diet and providing dietary teaching to parents.

Adolescents. Adolescents vary in their growth patterns; however, their rapid physical growth requires increased calories to meet their metabolic demands. Specific nutrients also assume added importance, such as calcium (important for the support of long-bone calcification) and iron (critical for maintaining increased red blood cell mass).

Vitamins A and C are necessary at this stage as well, and intake of both vitamins may be inadequate if food intake is erratic. Typically, adolescence is a time when peer group pressure leads to increased snacking and intake of a diet based on a limited number of foods and calories.

Menstrual blood loss in pubescent girls further increases iron needs and put girls at risk for iron deficiency anemia. Young boys may suffer from the same condition if they are growing rapidly.

Middle Adults. Maintaining health for the middle adult includes eating a well-balanced diet. Appropriate calorie intake depends on each person's body type and physical activity. An adequate nutritional program should include balanced nutrients, vitamins, adequate fiber, and sufficient water.

Older Adults. Many nutrition-related changes occur with aging, including decreases in salivation, chewing efficiency, number of taste buds, GI secretions, calcium absorption, renal function, glucose tolerance, and hemopoiesis. The risk of constipation tends to increase. The rate at which these changes occur varies; however, they are common enough to influence general dietary recommendations for older adult clients.

Many older adults have dietary deficiencies in protein, iron, calcium, and zinc. Individual differences may vary and depend on mobility, financial status, and socialization. Other factors that affect nutrient needs and nutritional status include chronic or acute diseases, drug use, and mental health problems.

Drug–nutrient interactions are important in older adults because medications may alter nutrient needs. For example, a client taking a potassium-sparing diuretic should limit or avoid food sources that are high in potassium, because this could lead to excessively high potassium levels. Clients taking warfarin (Coumadin) should avoid ingesting foods high in vitamin K because this vitamin reduces the drug's effect. The timing of food ingestion in relationship to medication administration is another important consideration, particularly among clients who take several drugs. Many older adults take three or more medications daily. Institutionalized older adults may take as many as 10 or more each day.

Pregnant and Lactating Women. Pregnancy and lactation increase a woman's need for calories and fluid. Furthermore, physiological changes occur during pregnancy that can alter body status. For example, increased intravascular volume can cause a pseudo-anemic condition. The overall increase in blood volume and total body fluid can also cause fluid retention and edema, which may be treated in part with diet.

It is especially important during pregnancy that the diet be well balanced, include foods that have high nutrient value, and exclude foods that have low nutrient value. This helps promote optimal fetal growth and development while minimizing excess maternal weight gain. It is also important to take a daily prenatal multivitamin supplement that contains the added vitamins needed during pregnancy. An adequate intake of folic acid, for example, is very important in preventing fetal neural tube defects.

Psychological Factors
People eat for many reasons, only one of which is hunger. Emotional states—such as boredom, anger, depression, or loneliness—can influence the quality and quantity of a person's intake. Emotions can overpower subtle physiological cues that regulate hunger and can result in undereating or overeating, depending on the person. Emotions can also influence poor eating habits.

Food is often used as reward or punishment. We can offer food to express love and approval or withhold it to express disapproval. In the United States, it is acceptable to give children candy, cookies, or ice cream when they are good. Adults may continue this symbolism established in childhood by rewarding themselves with a special food or by going out to dinner if they have been especially good or have worked hard.

Good eating behavior continues when it is positively reinforced. Reinforcement may be physiological, as when hunger is eliminated. Eating may also be situational, such as eating at the same time each day, when arriving at Grandma's house, or when guests come to visit.

Children sometimes rebel against their parents through food. The daughter who develops anorexia nervosa or the son who feels unloved and tends to overeat at mealtime is communicating with us.

Action Alert! Recognize anorexia nervosa or overeating as a possible attempt to cope with frustration, anger, aggression, depression, or unmet needs for affection. Become aware of the behavior exhibited and try to understand the meaning of that behavior in relation to food.

Nutritional Problems in Well Populations. The typical American diet is often abundant in quantity but lacking in quality, containing excess fat and animal proteins and inadequate fresh or unprocessed foods. Even when Americans do consume adequate fresh, unprocessed foods, there are concerns about the health consequences of pesticide residues left on many of those foods. A high-calorie and high-fat diet can lead to obesity over time, especially if coupled with a sedentary lifestyle. It can also lead to high serum cholesterol levels, which increase an individual's risk for atherosclerotic heart disease, stroke, or peripheral vascular disease. A diet high in sodium can lead to hypertension, which increases risk of heart disease, stroke, and renal disease over time. It can also exacerbate existing heart failure by increasing fluid retention.

An important factor when considering diet is the concept of *nutrient density*. Nutrient-dense foods have a high ratio of important nutrients in relation to calories. An increase in these types of foods overall is still needed in the American diet, despite educational initiatives such as *Healthy People 2000* and *Healthy People 2010*.

Physiological Factors

Healthy body functioning promotes optimal digestion and absorption of food. Healthy teeth and gums or well-fitting dentures are important for chewing, which is needed to break down food for digestion. The GI system must function well for optimal use of ingested nutrients. Normal production of insulin and digestive enzymes is also important for food use.

Physical factors can affect a person's ability to buy, transport, cook, and eat food. Physical mobility and energy are needed for shopping, cooking, and eating. When a person physically cannot complete such tasks, assistance may be needed to ensure adequate nutrition.

Cultural, Economic, and Lifestyle Factors

Cultural Factors. Cultural agents of society (those that promote adaptation to a culture and assimilation of its values), such as family, religion, and schools, are all very complex and interrelated. It is difficult to determine the extent to which one agent is more influential than another in determining food habits. Family, particularly parents, usually plays the most significant role in determining foods that are served and eaten.

Certain generalizations can be made about cultural influences on eating habits. The first is that most cultures eat foods in a complex mixture with a staple, such as potatoes, rice, or pasta. These staples, sometimes called cultural superfoods, form the basis of the meal. Second, spices or flavorings are used to make the food more palatable and augment flavor. Third, every cultural group tends to have its unique mixtures of foods, such as the beef bourguignon of the French or the beef Wellington of the English. The continual use of certain foods and their combinations through cultural, technological, and geographical changes shows their value to that cultural group. The use of herbs in the diet may also be culturally influenced, and they can have medicinal effects as well as dietary value (Box 23-1, p. 524).

Characteristic eating habits and patterns of cultures are observed among different nationalities and religious groups. A Jewish client might become ill after eating pork unintentionally, or a Seventh Day Adventist might become upset after drinking punch that has been made with alcohol. To provide or suggest meals that are acceptable as well as promoting good nutrition, it is important to understand the food preferences and taboos of various cultural and religious groups.

Another effect of culture on food preferences is that certain foods have been associated with social class. Refined sugar was once considered a luxury, but today it seems more fashionable to obtain the harder-to-get "natural" sugar. Advertisements today may depict obviously affluent families eating healthful cereals and obviously poorer families eating potato chips.

Economic Factors. Cost is another determinant in food selection, with economics playing a major role in determining food habits. People living in poverty have an increased risk of malnutrition, not because they lack the knowledge to eat nutritious foods (such as fresh fish, organic fruits and vegetables, and fiber-rich breads) but because they lack the money to do so. Some people are unable to purchase what they might "traditionally" choose to eat. For others, a diet reflecting current dietary goals may be completely unaffordable.

An increasing number of people are making changes in what they purchase in supermarkets to save money. They may buy in larger quantities or use generic products rather than brand names. They are also more likely to use food labels both for unit pricing and for counting calories and nutrients, which is a favorable change that over time may result in better nutritional status.

Lifestyle Factors. Lifestyle factors are closely related to food habits. The term *food habits* refers to what people eat and the way they eat. Food habits are derived from total life experience and are very resistant to change. Strong rejections of or desires for foods are learned through either role modeling or compliance (a strong desire to please the caretaker or food distributor, usually the mother). Thus food habits are more closely linked to associations with others and attitudes toward food than to food nutrient value.

A fast-paced lifestyle is consistent with increased consumption of snack foods and fast foods, which are low-nutrient-density foods. The increased dietary fat, decreased complex carbohydrate, and increased simple-sugar components of the fast-food diet are clearly contradictory to nutritional goals. In addition, the typical fast-food meal is high in calories, ranging from 900 to 1300 kcal per meal, which represents a large percent of a typical person's daily calories. The nutritional implications of the trend toward fast and convenient foods are a source of growing concern to many health professionals. Excessive use of these foods is likely to have adverse long-term health effects.

 Remember Joan, who was introduced at the beginning of this chapter? What aspects of her nutritional lifestyle could put her at risk for health problems later in life, even if she is healthy at the present time?

Box 23-1 *Considering the Alternatives*
Complementary Modalities: Ingested and Applied Substances: Herbs or Phytomedicine

Description and History: Plants or plant parts have been used in all cultures throughout history as a major source of medicines. Many pharmaceuticals have come from plants, and individuals have used herbs to self-medicate. Much of herbal use is rooted in cultural practices using local plants. Herbs are used as early primary treatments, to promote good health, and adjunctively with biomedical treatment regimens.

Major Concepts: Herbs can be used as the entire plant or as plant parts, such as the flower, roots, or leaves. The root may have active properties that are different from those of the flower. Herbs can be eaten as food or dried and taken in capsule forms, tinctures, or teas; essential oils may be inhaled. Additionally, herbs may be topically applied as poultices, creams, ointments, or oils. Often herbal preparations use the natural product, which also contains many ingredients other than the one active ingredient. Natural products are not biologically identical, and the active components vary according to soil, growing and harvesting conditions, storage, and preparation. Many people use combinations of herbs.

Practice of Herbal Medicine: The majority of herbs are self-administered and their availability and popularity has greatly increased over recent years. A plethora of lay information about herbs is available to the public. A number of scientific clinical trials have been published in the professional medical literature, and many more studies are currently underway. Herbs are currently categorized by the U.S. Food and Drug Administration (FDA) as food supplements, not drugs. As such, they are subject to standards of good manufacturing and clean preparation. In 1994, federal regulations for labeling required that manufacturers provide the product that is on the label, and to state that it has not been evaluated by the FDA. They cannot make any medical claims or unsubstantiated claims, but they can make structural functional claims. For example, milk thistle carries on its label "supports normal liver function."

Practitioners: Although there are no licensed programs of formal training, many professional herbalists have an academic background in medical herbs (e.g., licensed naturopaths). Some lay herbalists have accumulated much knowledge about herbs but may not have any formal background in medically related fields. Many herbalists are trained in their own cultural traditions and are experts in the use of herbs; for example, traditional Chinese medicine or Ayurvedic practitioners may have an extensive background in the use of herbs. Native American healers and other ethnic groups may also have extensive knowledge and experience in the use of herbs.

Potential Benefits From Herbal Treatments: There is a growing body of knowledge about the benefits of various herbs, but one difficulty encountered in conducting this research is dealing with complex natural products. Most pharmaceutical research involves identifying the active ingredient, isolating it, synthesizing it in a laboratory, and preparing standardized doses. Then it undergoes a rigorous series of tests for safety and efficacy for a particular disease or disorder. Herbs are traditionally natural products, in which one active ingredient often acts in combination with other parts of the plant, which may potentiate, act synergistically, or serve to mitigate side effects. Many herbs are effective in the early development of disease but are not as effective as the disease progresses. For example cran-

berry juice or cranactin capsules, taken with first symptoms of urinary cystitis, may reduce urinary tract infections. Once the infection has advanced, antibiotics may be needed because the infection overwhelms the therapeutic effects of the cranactin. Many other herbs have efficacy for prevention and treatment of mild disorders. Combinations of herbs may also be promising for treatment of many chronic conditions.

Concerns Related to the Practice of Herbal Approaches: Many people have the misperception that since herbs are natural products they are completely safe and can be taken in any amount. Thus people are likely to take excessive quantities and combinations that can be harmful. Any substance that has therapeutic effects can also have dangerous effects when used in the wrong manner. Combinations of herbs, and combinations of herbs and medications, can also have unwanted effects. Many clients do not share information about herbal use with their health care provider, and often providers do not ask clients what herbal preparations they are taking. Nurses should always ask for this information and record it in the chart. Garlic, ginseng, and gingko biloba have an anticoagulant effect and should be stopped prior to surgery or when taking anticoagulants. Echinacea should also be stopped, as it may delay wound healing, and it also should not be used in autoimmune conditions. Kava, St. John's wort, and valerian should also be stopped prior to surgery because they are central nervous system (CNS) depressants and may interact with anesthesia and analgesic medications. They should also not be used with other antidepressants or antianxiety medications. Ma huang or ephedra, a component of many popular diet preparations, is a CNS stimulant and should not be used prior to surgery or by people with hypertension. Most herbs, as well as most over-the-counter medications, should not be used in pregnancy, with the exception of ginger, which is helpful for nausea. With liver or kidney disorders, herbs should be used with caution as they may add to the excretory load. Milk thistle is under study for use in liver disease, as it may have benefits to the liver.

Many medical and nursing journals publish studies on clinical trials of herbal preparations. The following are good sources for reliable data.

Resources
Books
Blumenthal, M., Busse, W. R., Goldberg, A., Gruenwald, J., Hall, T., Rigins, et al. (Eds.). (1998). *The complete German Commission E monographs: Therapeutic guide to herbal medicines.* Austin, TX: American Botanical Council.
Foster, S., & Tyler, V. (1999). *Tyler's honest herbal* (4th ed.). Binghamton, NY: Hawthorn Press.

Journals
Herbalgram

Websites
American Botanical Council, www.herbalgram.org.
Alternative Health News Online, www.altmedicine.com.
NIH Office of Dietary Supplements Databases (IBIDS), http://ods.od.nih.gov./databases/cards.html.
The Illustrated Herbal Encyclopedia, http://www.canoe.ca/HealthHerbal/home.html.
The Longwood Herbal Task Force, http://www.mcp.edu/herbal.

ASSESSMENT

Most people could benefit from an assessment of their nutritional status and dietary patterns. The three purposes of a screening nutritional assessment are to identify clients who need in-depth nutritional assessment, to establish baseline values for evaluating the efficacy of nutritional regimens, and to provide a system for early recognition of increased health risk caused by nutritional factors.

General Assessment of Nutritional Status

Assessment of a client's nutritional status involves measuring both the degree to which the physiological need for nutrients is being met and the degree of balance between nutrient intake and nutrient expenditure. Because nutritional status has an effect on well-being, growth, performance, and resistance to disease, a thorough and accurate nutritional assessment is important. The components of a nutritional assessment include the health history (including diet history), evaluation of food intake, and physical examination and diagnostic tests.

Health History. Refer a client with a severe problem or an unusual eating pattern to a registered dietitian who is trained to evaluate nutritional states and to provide recommendations and sample meal plans. The registered dietitian can be an excellent consultant for you and a resource for your clients, especially if you work in home health care. You would then reinforce the information provided by the dietitian.

To take a diet history, collect and analyze data about the type and amount of food the client eats. It can be difficult and frustrating to accurately record and evaluate dietary intake for several reasons. First, it is difficult to record clients' food intake without influencing it. When people are watched, questioned about what they eat, or asked to write down what they eat, eating patterns tend to change. The extent of change depends on how well clients understand the dietary history and to what extent they are influenced by what they think you want to see or hear.

Second, many people simply cannot remember the types or amounts of food eaten. Third, it can be difficult to accurately evaluate the nutrient composition of food unless the specific ingredients are known. Carefully reading food labels on manufactured foods can be helpful. Food labels are required by law to list, among other things, the calories and specific nutrients in each product. Be aware that methods of cooking can greatly affect nutrient values. Even the area in which a fruit or vegetable is grown can affect its nutrient content.

24-HOUR RECALL. The most popular and easiest method for obtaining data about a client's intake is the *24-hour recall*. The person completes a questionnaire or is interviewed by you, a dietitian, or a nutritionist experienced in dietary interviewing. The client is asked to recall everything eaten the previous day or within the last 24 hours. When performing this test, keep in mind that it has three significant sources of error:

- The client may not be able to recall accurately the amounts of food eaten.

- The previous day's intake may not represent the usual intake.
- The client may not tell the truth for a variety of reasons, including possible embarrassment.

Clients have a tendency to underestimate intake as the portion size increases and overestimate intake as the portion size decreases. Foods that are least likely to be accurately reported are sauces, gravies, fruits, and snack items.

When conducting an interview for a 24-hour recall, compare an actual day (the previous day is best) with a typical day. Be objective, and use open-ended questions, such as *When did you get up? What was the first thing that you ate? What did you drink? What time did you eat next?* This type of questioning may elicit information on snacks and unusual patterns of eating. It is less likely to encourage incorrect information because it avoids giving clients clues about what answers are considered appropriate. To foster accurate reporting, do not react negatively to any response from the client.

FOOD FREQUENCY QUSTIONNAIRE. To help overcome some of the inherent weaknesses in the 24-hour recall method, a *food frequency questionnaire* may also be completed. Using this tool, you can collect information about how many times per day, week, or month a client eats particular foods. This information can help validate the accuracy of the 24-hour recall data and clarify the client's real food consumption pattern. The food frequency questionnaire may be general, containing questions concerning all foods, or selective, containing questions about suspected deficient or excessive foods in the diet.

FOOD DIARY. A *food diary* is a written record of food intake maintained for a specified period of time, usually 3 to 7 days. The time frame depends on the purpose, the nutrients being assessed, and the interest level of the client. This type of assessment may also be used to determine food allergies. Consider carefully the days chosen to observe intake. Food consumption on weekends and holidays is usually different from that on weekdays. A combination of weekday and weekend recordings often reflects a more accurate picture. In the hospital or extended care setting, you may be required to keep track of food intake on a calorie count sheet kept at the bedside or on the chart.

For best results, client teaching must be clear. For each day the food diary is kept, ask the client to record the names of foods eaten, the way the food was prepared, and (if indicated) the time and place the food was eaten. A legitimate concern with the food diary is that the client may change eating patterns on the days of the recording. Encourage clients to eat the foods and amounts that are normal for them on these days. Again, a nonjudgmental manner helps.

When a very accurate record of food consumption is required, the *weighed intake record* is best. Teach the client to weigh all food consumed during the recording and to correct for food waste (food served but not eaten). Disadvantages are that this method is tedious, the client must be well motivated to achieve accurate results, the client may use shortcuts in preparation to make the weighing less time-consuming, and the client's eating patterns may change. The weighed intake method is used in controlled laboratory studies and hospital settings.

HOUSEHOLD FOOD CONSUMPTION. This method involves visiting a household periodically and recording the amounts and types of food purchased for that household and the disappearance of that food. It assumes that the family has eaten any food that is unaccounted for. Household food consumption is most commonly used in large population surveys. It is not a good evaluation of individual intake because it does not record food waste or food consumed by each household member. It is helpful, however, in trying to gain insight into the nutritional situation in a community.

Food in the household can vary with the income of the household, the food available in the marketplace, and other factors. For example, foods available in the market may be limited for some inner-city dwellers, such as frail older adults, who may have to shop at a corner market that does not carry items such as soy milk, salt-free crackers, or fresh fruits and vegetables.

Evaluation of Food Intake. There are two methods by which food intake information is evaluated for adequacy: the food group method and the nutrient composition method. When a client is hospitalized, a calorie count may be done, which evaluates both of these.

FOOD GROUP METHOD. The simplest and fastest way to evaluate food intake data is to determine how many servings from each of the six food groups were consumed during the recorded day. The number of servings from each group is then compared with the number of servings suggested in the food guide pyramid (Figure 23-1). It becomes more difficult to use this method if the diet has many food mixtures or unusual cul-tural foods that do not fit into one of the food groups. For many people, however, gross deficiencies of protein and of a number of vitamins can be detected using this method.

Vitamin deficiencies can often be linked to deficiencies in specific food groups. Intake of folic acid and vitamins A and C is most variable because they are not widely present in foods, except for particular fruits and vegetables. Intake of these nutrients is frequently seasonal, with higher intake in the summer and fall when fresh fruits and vegetables are abundant and cheaper.

Riboflavin, calcium, and vitamin D intake largely depends on the intake of milk and milk products. Daily intake of protein, thiamine, niacin, phosphorus, iron, and vitamins E, B_6, and B_{12} is more consistent because these nutrients are present in a wide variety of foods.

Use the food group method to determine the degree to which Joan, our case study client, is taking in a nutritionally balanced diet.

NUTRIENT COMPOSITION METHOD. Dietary intake can be evaluated more accurately by calculating the amounts of a nutrient in each food consumed. This analysis can be done manually or by computer. The nutrient values for foods can be obtained from several nutrition publications, nutrition labels, and food manufacturers' information on a food's nutrient composition. After recording the nutrient composition for individual foods, you can determine the composition of the total diet.

Once the nutrient composition of the diet is determined, the amount of an individual nutrient can be compared with the **recommended dietary allowance** (RDA). The RDA is the level of a nutrient that is adequate to meet the needs of almost

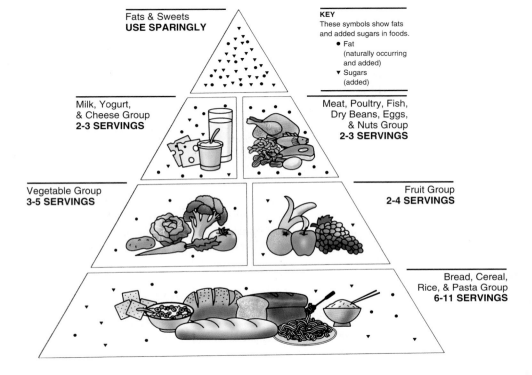

Figure 23-1. Food guide pyramid. (From U.S. Department of Agriculture and U.S. Department of Health and Human Services.)

all healthy people as determined by the Food and Nutrition Board of the National Research Council. Although the RDA is frequently used to evaluate the components of a person's diet, this is theoretically an improper use. RDAs are set at a level slightly above average requirements so they can include everyone in the population who might have an increased need for a particular vitamin or mineral. Because the RDAs include this "safety factor," they are probably higher than a typical person needs. Nutrition textbooks typically contain published tables of RDAs for fat- and water-soluble vitamins and minerals according to age group, height, and weight.

Energy and protein intake should be evaluated on the basis of body weight or, in the case of an underweight or overweight person, on the basis of height. This increases the usefulness of the RDA in individual assessment, especially with children, who at any particular age may differ greatly in size.

RDAs are not meant to be applied to sick people, whose requirements may be very different from those of healthy people. At present, however, there are no established nutrient requirements for various disease states. With these limitations in mind, you can use nutrient RDAs as a general evaluation of the dietary intake of clients who are ill.

CALORIE COUNT. When a client who is hospitalized is nutritionally at risk, dietary intake can be monitored using a calorie count. For each dietary tray that is sent, record the amount of food consumed on a form or on the menu for that meal. Record the client's intake in measurable amounts (such as ounces, teaspoons, tablespoons, or cubic centimeters) or the percentage (%) of the food or beverage portion ingested. Record also any additional foods or fluids consumed during the 24-hour period. Return the forms to the dietitian for analysis, which usually consists of calorie and protein intake. A calorie count is often ordered for a 3-day period. Accurate results depend on your careful assessment of intake and accurate completion of the forms.

Physical Examination
CLINICAL SIGNS OF NUTRITIONAL STATUS. A thorough physical examination will reveal physical signs of nutritional deficiencies. Vitamin and mineral deficiencies can be manifested by clinical signs and symptoms, which are included in Chapter 24.

ANTHROPOMETRIC MEASUREMENTS. Anthropometric measurements are measurements of physical characteristics of the body (such as height and weight) as well as the amount of muscle or fat tissue in the body.

HEIGHT–WEIGHT TABLES. Various tables are available that list average heights and desirable weights for infants, children, men, and women. All suggest approximate weights for healthy adults. Charts listing desirable weights for adults according to frame size are also available. These charts, often produced by insurance companies, list the weight for each inch of height that is associated with the lowest morbidity and mortality. These charts are commonly found in nutrition textbooks.

Another frequently used height–weight figure is the "usual weight." In an older adult, the "usual weight" might be more

indicative of nutritional health than a figure based on the optimal height–weight tables.

Remember that these tables are guides and should be used for screening purposes. To obtain a quick ballpark figure useful for basic screening, use the following:
- A man of 5 feet 0 inch should weigh about 106 pounds. Add 6 pounds for each additional inch.
- A woman of 5 feet 0 inch should weigh about 100 pounds. Add 5 pounds for each additional inch.

Being either underweight or overweight may be associated with increased risk of morbidity and mortality.

A disadvantage of height–weight tables is that they group all adults together without considering age. Insurance tables have also been criticized as underrepresenting lower socioeconomic classes.

BODY MASS INDEX. Because of the disadvantages of height–weight methods, many health professionals prefer to use a mathematical standard called body mass index (BMI). Determine a person's BMI using this formula:

$$BMI = weight (kg) \div height^2 (meters)$$

To do this calculation, recall that 1 kilogram equals 2.2 pounds and 1 meter equals 39.37 inches. The desired BMI for healthy adults is 18.5 to 24.9. A result of 25.0 to 29.9 indicates overweight status, and a BMI of 30 or greater indicates obesity. A BMI of less than 18.5 indicates underweight status and is associated with a health risk such as respiratory or digestive diseases.

BODY COMPOSITION. Various body compartments (fat stores or lean tissue) can be affected by over- or undernutrition. To estimate the degree to which these compartments are affected, use fat-fold measurements and midarm muscle circumference.

About half the body's fat is located directly beneath the skin. Consequently, skin thickness reflects total body fat. The fat-fold measure may be useful when performed by a trained person following a standard procedure and using reliable calipers. The most easily accessible area is the triceps fat fold, making it the most practical in clinical settings (Figure 23-2, A, p. 528).

The midarm muscle circumference is an indicator of lean tissue stores (Figure 23-2, B). It can be derived by measuring the midarm circumference and the triceps fat fold, and then using the following equation:

Midarm muscle circumference = midarm circumference (cm) − [0.314 − triceps fat fold (mm)],

where 0.314 is a conversion factor. The 50th percentile value for midarm muscle circumference is 281 for middle-aged men and 222 for middle-aged women.

Joan's triceps fat-fold measure is within normal limits. Remember also that her clinical evaluation revealed no specific abnormalities. What does this tell you about the impact of her eating habits to this point?

Diagnostic Tests. The most common laboratory indices of nutritional status are serum prealbumin, albumin, transferrin, lymphocyte count, hemoglobin, hematocrit, and urine specific gravity.

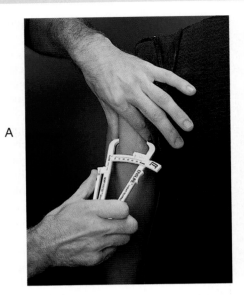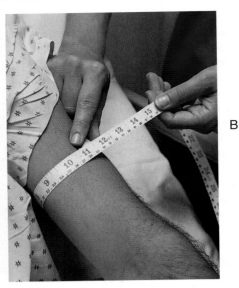

Figure 23-2. Anthropometric measurements. **A,** Using calipers to measure triceps fat fold. **B,** Measuring midarm muscle circumference.

Albumin and *prealbumin* indicate visceral protein status. Albumin is most useful when monitoring long-term nutritional status because normal levels (3.5 to 5.0 g/dL) may be found even in those who are malnourished. Prealbumin (normally 20 to 50 mg/dL) is useful in measuring short-term changes in protein status because of its short half-life of 2 days. The *lymphocyte count* (normally >1500 cells/mm³) is a measure of immune function that is used in conjunction with other nutritional assessments to determine overall nutritional status.

Transferrin and *hematocrit* are measures of iron status. Transferrin is a trace protein needed for iron absorption and transport and is calculated as a percentage (normally 30% to 40%) using the serum iron level and the iron-binding capacity. The *hematocrit* is the percentage of whole blood that is composed of red blood cells (RBCs), and values differ for adult men (37% to 49%) and women (36% to 46%). An increase or decrease in either RBC count or plasma volume affects the hematocrit. Conditions that increase RBC production increase the hematocrit, whereas anemia can lower both hemoglobin and hematocrit. Extracellular fluid volume deficit (e.g., dehydration) may increase the hematocrit, whereas fluid volume excess decreases it.

With normal fluid intake, *urine specific gravity* is usually 1.010 to 1.020. Concentrated urine has a higher specific gravity, and dilute urine has a lower one. These findings correlate with hypovolemia and hypervolemia, respectively.

Focused Assessment for *Imbalanced Nutrition: Less Than Body Requirements*

Some populations at risk for nutritional deficiencies are older adults, adolescents, children, pregnant women, and infants.

Defining Characteristics. Clients with nutritional deficiencies may report any of the following: satiety immediately after eating, food intake less than the RDA for nutrients, lack of interest or aversion to food, altered taste sensations, or inade-

quate or misinformation about diet. Physical signs may include pale conjunctival or mucous membranes; weakness of muscles used for chewing or swallowing; soreness or inflammation of the oral cavity; weight loss despite food intake; body weight 20% or more below ideal for height, frame, and age; abdominal cramping or diarrhea; capillary fragility; and excessive loss of hair.

Because this nursing diagnosis from the North American Nursing Diagnosis Association (NANDA) refers globally to insufficient nutrients to meet metabolic demands, it is often used when the overall diet is inadequate. It could also be useful, however, whenever specific deficiencies arise, such as deficiencies of vitamins, minerals, or proteins. The defining characteristics do not clearly address the healthy client with a poor diet that could be improved.

Related Factors. Related factors for this nursing diagnosis include inability to ingest food, digest food, or absorb nutrients. This inability can result from biological, psychological, or economic factors.

In the well client, nutritional deficiencies may not be severe enough to produce actual signs and symptoms of deficiency; however, general signs may result from a diet that is deficient in one or more nutrients.

> *Action Alert!* Be alert to the presence of fatigue, irritability, frequent colds and flu, and stress-related symptoms as cues to the possibility of mild nutritional deficiency.

Assess the client's lifestyle and dietary pattern for other risk factors, such as overuse of snack foods, using fast foods as a main dietary source, using processed foods, and using cooking methods that destroy nutrients. The nutritional deficiency may be related to lack of knowledge, money, motivation, or time to prepare food.

Focused Assessment for *Imbalanced Nutrition: More Than Body Requirements*

Defining Characteristics. The client may report a sedentary activity level, concentrating food intake at the end of the day, eating in response to external cues (time of day, social situation), internal cues other than hunger (anxiety), or a dysfunctional eating pattern that pairs food with another activity. Anthropometric measurements show a weight that is 10% or more above ideal for height and frame, and a triceps skin fold of more than 25 mm for women or more than 15 mm for men.

Assess the client's intake of nutrients and cluster the data to recognize obesity, high fat intake, and high sodium intake, all of which are linked to negative health consequences, as discussed earlier.

Related Factors. Related factors are any situations in which there is excessive intake in relationship to metabolic need. Lifestyle, knowledge, and motivation could also be related factors for this nursing diagnosis.

Factors that increase the risk of obesity are those that apply to *Risk for imbalanced nutrition: more than body requirements.* They include the following:

- Reported use of solid food as a major food source before 5 months of age
- Concentrated food intake at the end of the day
- Reported or observed obesity in one or both parents
- Reported or observed higher baseline weight at the beginning of each pregnancy
- Rapid transition across growth percentiles in infants or children
- Pairing food with other activities
- Observed use of food as a reward or comfort measure
- Eating in response to internal cues other than hunger, such as anxiety
- Eating in response to external cues, such as time of day or social situation
- Dysfunctional eating patterns

> Although Joan is not overweight, why might the nursing diagnosis *Risk for imbalanced nutrition: more than body requirements* be appropriate? Joan has indicated an interest in reducing her elevated cholesterol level, which should help to motivate her to make healthy changes in her nutritional habits.

DIAGNOSIS

Several options exist in the NANDA nursing diagnosis system for addressing nutritional problems. Diagnostic labels are needed for the well client who seeks a higher level of wellness, the client who has risk factors for nutritional problems, and the client who has an actual deficit or excess in one or more nutrients.

The diagnosis *Health-seeking behaviors: nutrition* can be used for a client who is well but seeks an optimal state of physical and mental well-being. The goals of *Health-seeking behaviors* suggest the need for health promotion activities, one of which is proper nutrition.

The diagnosis *Imbalanced nutrition: less than body requirements* indicates that the client has one or more nutritional deficiencies. The diagnosis *Imbalanced nutrition: more than body requirements* indicates obesity or a diet that is high in nutrients such as fat, carbohydrates, or sodium.

Clients who have related factors for a nursing diagnosis, but do not have the actual defining characteristics, are stated to be at risk for a specific nursing diagnosis. The client may be at risk for imbalanced nutrition that is either more than or less than body requirements.

PLANNING

Planning for clients with a specific imbalance in nutrition involves using assessment data to identify nutritional needs. Goals for nutritional status can then be chosen within the parameters of the specific nursing diagnosis. Guidance, supervision, and education may be incorporated into the plan to help improve the client's nutritional knowledge. Direct nursing care may also be part of the plan.

Expected Outcomes for *Imbalanced Nutrition: Less Than Body Requirements*

Sample expected outcomes for the client with *Imbalanced nutrition: less than body requirements* are the following:

- Discusses the importance of adequate nutrient intake in the daily diet
- Ingests sufficient nutrients to meet daily needs, taking into account activity level and metabolic needs
- Implements shopping and cooking methods for economical food preparation, such as using beans and legumes as a protein source, using powdered milk for cooking, and making soups or stews with leftover food

Expected Outcomes for *Imbalanced Nutrition: More Than Body Requirements*

Sample expected outcomes for the client with *Imbalanced nutrition: more than body requirements* are the following:

- Identifies elements of the daily diet that are not in keeping with nutritional standards
- Plans meals using the food pyramid guide
- Eats the bulk of calories early in the day
- Eats only when seated at the dining table, not in front of the television or while performing other activities
- Increases activity level by using stairs instead of elevators, parking the car in more remote parking spots, and taking a daily walk

INTERVENTION

To succeed in national efforts to promote wellness, prevent disease, and improve quality of life, all nurses must work cooperatively with educators, researchers, industrial and political leaders, and informed consumers to continue to develop positive strategies to improve nutrition. It is also important to be aware of the ever-expanding body of nutritional knowledge generated by research.

Interventions to Promote a Healthy Diet

Knowledge of the nutritional value of foods and their relationship to wellness is essential but is clearly not enough to induce clients to consume appropriate foods. Otherwise, health professionals themselves would be by far the slimmest, best-exercised, optimally nourished group in the nation! What can be done, then, to get clients to change their nutritional patterns?

One key is educating and encouraging the population from infancy. Health professionals too often encounter adolescents and adults who have well-established eating patterns that are far from ideal. As a nurse working with clients at varying points in the life span, you are in a unique position to assess cultural, economic, and environmental factors influencing their food choices. This information is crucial to successful dietary intervention.

Nutrition education is a broad area; however, most nutritional counseling takes place in acute or long-term-care facilities and community-based clinics. Most nutrition education begins with assessment of dietary intake. A broad knowledge of food, nutrition, pathophysiology, and biochemistry is important in analyzing food habits and making recommendations for improved or modified eating behaviors. As in all types of teaching and counseling, you must develop instructional objectives, devise evaluation tools, assess the learner's knowledge, screen for and organize information needs, select education materials, implement the teaching, and critique and revise your instruction. It is also essential to keep the learner's needs in the forefront and work to maintain rapport with the client.

To successfully educate clients, include information about the types and the amounts of foods to eat. To maintain an appropriate body weight and prevent obesity, food intake and physical activity must be balanced. The need for calories can be calculated from the resting energy expenditure (REE), which is calculated as 15.3 times body weight (kg) plus 679 (for men age 18 to 30), and 11.6 times body weight (kg) plus 879 (for men age 30 to 60).

For women age 18 to 30, the formula is 14.7 times body weight (kg) plus 496. For women age 30 to 60, it is 8.7 times body weight (kg) plus 829. Very light physical activity requires 1.5 times the REE, light physical activity uses 2.5 REE, moderate physical activity burns 5.0 REE, and heavy physical activity requires 7.0 REE.

Using Recommended Dietary Allowances. The RDA is the level of intake of essential nutrients considered, on the basis of available scientific knowledge, to be adequate to meet the known nutritional needs of practically all healthy persons. Nutrient requirements during illness may be higher than the RDA, depending on the nature of the illness. Requirements are also known to be higher when the body is under stress or recovering from trauma, infection, or surgery.

To optimize nutrition for relatively healthy clients, teach them to read nutrition labels that appear on manufactured foods, in accordance with the Nutrition Labeling and Education Act of 1990. These labels, titled "nutrition facts," contain information about the percentage of "daily value" that a specific product has for fat, cholesterol, sodium, carbohydrate, protein, vitamins, and minerals. The reference daily intakes (RDIs) are based on the RDA. Another type of labeling is the reference daily values (RDV), which is identified for important nutrients for which an RDA has not yet been established.

Developing Healthy Dietary Patterns. A healthy diet is based on the food guide pyramid, developed in 1992 by the U.S. Department of Agriculture. The design of the pyramid conveys the three essential elements of a healthy diet: proportion, moderation, and variety. Proportion is the relative amount of food to choose from each major food group. Moderation pertains to sparing use of fats, oils, and sugars. And variety emphasizes the importance of eating a selection of foods from each of the major groups every day. Appropriate daily selections of a variety of foods according to the food guide pyramid should provide the RDA of all necessary nutrients.

The base of the pyramid is the foundation of a healthy diet. You and your clients should eat six or more servings of complex carbohydrate foods daily. This group is a source of fiber, vegetable protein, and B vitamins. Whole grains supply more nutrients and fiber than processed grains. A diet high in complex carbohydrates from plant sources is associated with a lower incidence of atherosclerotic disease and some forms of cancer. High-fiber foods, especially cruciferous vegetables (broccoli, cabbage, cauliflower, brussels sprouts), protect against colorectal cancer.

The second level of the pyramid includes fruits and vegetables. These are significant sources of folate, niacin, riboflavin, and vitamins A, C, and K. You and your clients should eat five or more servings of these daily. Fresh fruits and vegetables have a higher vitamin content than when cooked by boiling. To cook vegetables, use a minimum amount of water and cook only until tender. Steaming preserves the vitamin content.

The third level is primarily the animal foods. Protein should be consumed in moderate amounts. The RDA of protein for both sexes is 0.8 g/kg per day; most Americans eat more than this amount. Most protein should come from plant rather than animal sources. Remember, however, that animal proteins are the only source of vitamin B_{12}, the best source of readily absorbable iron, and a good source of zinc.

The small top point of the pyramid suggests that fats, oils, and sweets should make up the smallest part of the diet. To reduce cholesterol and fat intake, limit meat, fish, and poultry to 3 to 6 ounces of cooked weight daily. Ground beef is the largest source of dietary fat in the United States, with half the calories coming from fat even in low-fat ground beef. One egg yolk contains more than two thirds of the RDI of cholesterol. The skin of poultry contains most of its fat. More than 70% of the energy content of cheese comes from fat.

Using General Nutrition Recommendations to Reduce Risk of Disease. Various government agencies and programs in the United States and Canada provide nutritional guidelines for consumers. These include recommendations for nutrient intake, food guides, menu plans, and sample diets. Teaching these recommendations can help clients establish their own goals for improved nutrition; however, knowledge of the recommendations is not usually sufficient to change a dietary pattern.

The importance of dietary habits in preventing disease and maintaining health is becoming more apparent (Box 23-2). A diet high in fat and calories has been associated with heart disease, stroke, and cancer, the three major causes of death in the United States. Fortunately, the incidence of heart disease and stroke has declined in recent years, possibly because of improved dietary habits. As a result of the increased evidence of relationships between diet and chronic diseases, changes in the American diet are being promoted by dietitians, nutritionists, and several organizations, such as the American Heart Association, the American Cancer Society, and the U.S. Department of Agriculture in conjunction with the U.S. Department of Health and Human Services. Nutritional guidelines published in Canada are similar to the U.S. Daily Food Guide.

Fat intake should be 30% or less of caloric intake. Saturated fat intake should be less than 10% of calories, and the intake of cholesterol should be less than 300 mg daily.

Polyunsaturated fats (fats that are liquid at room temperature) have a cholesterol-lowering effect, and vegetable oils containing polyunsaturated fats are the best source of vitamin E. Hydrogenated vegetable oil has a cholesterol-elevating effect. Overall, clients should modify fat intake to keep the cholesterol level below 200 mg/dL, with low-density lipoprotein level (LDL, or "bad" cholesterol) below 130 mg/dL and high-density lipoprotein (HDL, or "good" cholesterol) greater than 60 mg/dL.

Although not all persons are sensitive to salt, limiting the use of salt may help prevent high blood pressure. Total daily salt (sodium chloride) should be limited to 6 g or less. For people who are sensitive to salt, it should be restricted to 4.5 g or less. Most Americans eat more than 6 g of salt (containing 2400 mg of actual sodium) per day. Additionally, eating large quantities of foods pickled or preserved in salt is associated with cancer of the stomach.

> *Action Alert!* Advise salt-sensitive clients to restrict their salt intake to 4.5 g per day or less. Most Americans consume more than 6 g of salt per day.

THE STATE OF NURSING RESEARCH: A Minute on the Lips, A Lifetime on the Hips: Battling Obesity

Box 23-2

What Are the Issues?

More people than ever struggle with obesity and its health consequences. Changing a lifestyle behavior such as eating is a challenging endeavor. Clinicians realize that simply telling people they need to lose weight is not enough. People need more help to lose weight, and to maintain that loss. Interventions that have a theoretical basis may be more likely to succeed than trial and error.

What Research Has Been Conducted?

Keller and Allan (2001) reviewed weight-loss intervention studies that were supposedly based on a theoretical model. The most common models used in the studies were the health belief model, the social learning theory, and the transtheoretical model. All three models have been used in other health behavior studies such as smoking cessation. The health belief model, developed by Rosenstock, Strecher, and Becker, suggests that a person's perceptions will influence the likelihood of behavior change. The model has been used to study a variety of health behaviors. Beliefs about susceptibility, severity, benefits, and barriers are measured and related to the health behavior activity.

The social learning theory developed by Bandura considers the outcome expectations of the individual, "Will what I do have the result I hope for?" and self-efficacy, "How confident am I that I can make the change and do what needs to be done?"

The transtheoretical model describes five stages of behavior change and the processes that individuals use to modify their experience and environment to modify their behavior: precontemplation (not even thinking about changing behavior), contemplation (considering change within 6 months), preparation (getting ready to change within the month), action (trying to change), and maintenance (keeping the behavior change) (Keller & Allan, 2001).

What Has the Research Concluded?

The studies that used the health belief model demonstrated that "individual perception of barriers [was] most consistently associated negatively with health-promoting behaviors" (Keller & Allan, 2001). The studies based on social learning theory usually measured self-efficacy and found it helped explain eating behaviors. For example, one study tried to influence self-efficacy through improving coping and food selection skills. Researchers found a positive effect on food selection for those people who increased their self-efficacy (Shannon, Bagby, Wang, & Trenkner [1990] in Keller & Allan [2001]). Researchers using the transtheoretical model are beginning to develop interventions that target each stage of behavior change. Few of the studies address the contextual factors in the environment that influenced eating behavior, such as culture and public policy. Interventions should be designed to fit the context of the client's lifestyle, beliefs, and values. Nurses need to be sensitive to their clients' readiness to change behaviors such as eating. By identifying people who show signs of readiness and providing them with information and verbal encouragement, you may increase their self-efficacy and improve their efforts to lose weight.

What Is the Future of Research in This Area?

The reviewers recommended that researchers design studies that included interventions more strongly based on theoretical models and that targeted the individual as well as the community.

Reference

Keller, C. S., & Allan, J. D. (2001). Evaluation of selected behavior change theoretical models used in weight management interventions. *Online Journal of Knowledge Synthesis for Nursing,* 8(5), available at http://www.nursingsociety.org.

Shannon, B., Bagby, R., Wang, M. O., & Trenkner, L. L. (1990). Self-efficacy: a contributor to the explanation of eating behavior. *Health Education Research, 5,* 395-407.

Calcium-containing foods (such as dairy products and dark leafy vegetables) promote bone growth just before the onset of puberty and during adolescence. They also protect against osteoporosis later in life. The RDA for calcium is 800 mg for adult men and nonpregnant adult women. The best sources of calcium are milk and milk products. Calcium in dietary supplements is often present in the poorly soluble forms of phosphate or carbonate, which are not well absorbed.

Alcohol consumption should be avoided. Some studies have shown that small amounts of daily alcohol may reduce the risk of coronary disease; however, there are other ways to reduce this risk. If a client must drink, keep the amount to less than one ounce of pure alcohol each day. The "proof" identified on the bottle represents twice the percentage of alcohol it contains; in other words, 80 proof means 40% alcohol.

How would you use the food guide pyramid in teaching Joan how to improve her diet?

Using Dietary Supplements Safely.

Fluoride intake is recommended to prevent tooth decay, particularly when consumed before permanent teeth erupt. This benefit persists throughout life as long as fluoride intake continues. Some communities fluoridate the water supply, making supplements unnecessary.

Controversy exists about the advantages and risks of dietary supplements. Food continues to be the best source of nutrients. Dietary supplements should be unnecessary if a client eats a balanced diet that contains the recommended servings of the basic food groups. Although a single multivitamin with 100% of the RDA is not known to be harmful, it has also not been proven to be decidedly beneficial for the vast majority of people. It may be most useful for those whose diet does not supply the recommended intake of vitamins.

When people take vitamins in megadoses, they are using them as drugs, not as nutrients. Research to date has failed to support the original claims for using megavitamins, for example, curing the common cold, lowering cholesterol levels, and decreasing risk of cancer.

Because fat-soluble vitamins, especially vitamin A, are stored largely in the liver, toxicity from megadoses could possibly lead to liver and brain damage. Most people believe large doses of water-soluble vitamins are not harmful because they are readily excreted, but this is not always true. Prolonged vitamin B_6 therapy at 5 g per day to treat premenstrual syndrome has been shown to cause lack of muscle coordination and occasionally nerve damage, and ascorbic acid (vitamin C) in doses above 2 g per day can cause GI pain, increase the risk of kidney stone formation, and reduce effectiveness of white blood cells against bacteria.

PRINCIPLES OF NUTRIENT SUPPLEMENTATION.

The following principles may be used to guide personal decisions about the use of nutrient supplements:

- Read the labels on dietary supplements as manufacturers of these products supply them, consistent with the Nutrition Labeling and Education Act of 1990.

- Any nutrient can be harmful if taken in excessive amounts; large doses are best used in cases of severe deficiency or problems with absorption or utilization.
- Choose supplements in accordance with personal dietary needs and health care provider recommendations.
- Be aware that excessive intake of one vitamin may lead to deficiency symptoms if that supplement is suddenly discontinued.

PHYTOCHEMICALS. Phytochemicals are recently recognized plant chemicals that are under close scrutiny in nutritional research. Foods containing combinations of phytochemicals are sometimes called healing foods, superfoods, or power foods. Generally, they refer to fruits, vegetables, legumes, grains, nuts, and seeds. Expect to read more about the possible benefits of these chemicals as research results become available:

- *Antioxidants* include selenium, vitamins A, C, and E, carotenoids, and flavonoids. They are found in yellow to red and green leafy vegetables, yellow or orange fruits, citrus fruits, nuts, unrefined grains, and seafood. Potential benefits include preventing cancer.
- *Carotenoids* are plant pigments found in cruciferous vegetables, red and yellow fruits and vegetables, green leafy vegetables, and sea vegetables (kelp). Potential benefits are as antioxidants, precursors to vitamin A, eye protection from excessive light, and reducing risk of prostate cancer.
- *Flavonoids* are plant chemicals that give fruits and vegetables their color. They may help reduce the risk of cancer, act as antioxidants, or have antiallergenic and antiinflammatory properties.
- *Phytoestrogens* are hormonelike substances found in whole grains, legumes, and soy. They may reduce the risk of hormone-related cancers, enhance immunity, inhibit platelet aggregation (blood clotting), and mimic some estrogen effects.
- *Polyphenols* are plant compounds found in red wine, tea, apples, grapes, strawberries, onions, and yams. They may reduce the risk of heart disease and cancer.

Interventions for Special Populations
Promoting Nutrition During Pregnancy and Lactation.

The recommendations for dietary management during pregnancy emphasize an increase in total calories, protein, vitamins, and minerals. Poor nutrition is a factor in excessive maternal weight gain, preeclampsia, postpartum infections, and an increased incidence of premature babies, low-birth-weight babies, anomalies, developmental disabilities, and stillbirths.

Although the mother's preconception nutrition also affects the outcome of pregnancy, most nutritional care begins during the first trimester of pregnancy. Three well-planned meals, plus one or more snacks, provide the RDA for all nutrients with the possible exception of iron and folic acid. Daily supplementation of 30 to 60 mg of ferrous iron and 400 mg of folic acid are recommended. Depending on preferences and tolerance, adequate calcium and zinc may be difficult to achieve in the diet and may require supplementation as well. Prenatal vitamin-plus-mineral supplements are commonly prescribed for pregnant women to minimize the risk of micronutrient (vitamin and mineral) deficiency.

Adequate calories and weight gain are necessary throughout pregnancy. For women entering pregnancy at or near their ideal body weight, a total weight gain of 25 to 35 pounds over the course of the pregnancy is recommended, at a rate of 2 to 4 pounds in the first trimester and 0.75 to 1 pound per week thereafter (roughly an increase of 300 kcal/day). Underweight women should gain the amount they are underweight plus a normal pregnancy gain of 25 pounds. Women whose weight is 120% to 130% of their ideal body weight are encouraged to gain about 20 pounds, whereas those whose weight is more than 135% of the ideal body weight are urged to gain 15 to 16 or 18 to 20 pounds, depending on the source. Most authorities discourage dieting for weight loss during pregnancy. Instead, the emphasis is on high-quality food choices to meet nutrient needs.

Action Alert! Teach pregnant women the importance of appropriate weight gain during pregnancy. Advise them that pregnancy is not the time for dieting to lose weight.

All pregnant women should be counseled about avoiding potentially harmful substances during pregnancy. They should avoid smoking, alcohol, and caffeine. Finally, they should avoid nonprescription drugs, saccharin and other artificial sweeteners, all fad-diet products or regimens, pica (non-nutrient items such as clay or ice), and all recreational drugs.

During lactation, the need for a well-balanced diet continues. Caloric needs are increased by 500 kcal per day from the woman's baseline needs. At least six to eight glasses of water are needed to provide a sufficient volume of milk. Vitamin and mineral supplementation may continue. Harmful substances, such as alcohol, tobacco, and caffeine, should still be avoided to prevent transmission to the infant via breast milk.

Promoting Nutrition in Infants. Breast milk or iron-fortified formula is the only source of nourishment needed for the first 4 to 6 months after birth. The infant who is ready to start solid food has doubled the birth weight and can control head movements and sit up with support.

Vitamin and mineral recommendations are based on the contents of human milk. Daily water requirements are usually met with breast milk or infant formula, except when the weather is hot or the infant has diarrhea or vomiting. Supplemental water is needed at these times to prevent dehydration.

Action Alert! Watch for signs of dehydration (such as decreased urine output, decreased skin turgor, weight loss) in infants with diarrhea or vomiting. With persistent diarrhea or vomiting, severe dehydration can develop quickly in infants.

Promoting Nutrition in Children. Children need adequate calories, protein, water, vitamins, and minerals. Meals should be selected using food from the food guide pyramid for children. Children 1 to 2 years old require smaller servings, more frequent snacks, and 3 cups of whole milk each day (Table 23-4). A good rule of thumb is 1 to 2 tablespoons of a food group with each meal or snack. When planning a child's meals, have the caretaker select from a variety of foods from each food group. Serving sizes increase with age.

A child grows 2 to 3 inches and gains about 5 pounds each year. A standard weight gain–growth chart reflects the child's nutritional health. Weight gain out of proportion to height may reflect overeating or inactivity. If the child's weight-to-height ratio drops below the normal curve, it may indicate malnutrition. By periodically comparing weight to height, you can plot the child's progress on the standard growth curve over time.

Promoting Nutrition in Adolescents. Growth rate increases with the onset of adolescence. In girls, the growth spurt begins at about age 10 and peaks at age 12. Boys begin their growth spurt at about age 12, and it peaks at age 14. Body composition in girls includes a higher percentage of fat tissue. The boys' growth spurt results in a higher proportion of lean body mass, such as muscle and bone.

Table 23-4	Child's Daily Food Plan			
			Average Size of Serving	
Food Group	Servings per Day	*Age 1 to 3*	*Age 4 to 6*	*Age 7 to 10*
Bread and cereals (whole-grain or enriched)[a]	6 or more	1/2 slice	1 slice	1 slice
Vegetables[b]	3 or more	2 to 4 tablespoons or 1/2 cup juice	1/4 to 1/2 cup or 1/2 cup juice	1/2 to 1 cup
Fruits[b]	2 or more	2 to 4 tablespoons or 1/2 cup juice	1/4 to 1/2 cup or 1/2 cup of juice	1/2 to 1 cup
Meat and meat alternatives[c]	2 or more	1/2 ounce	1 to 2 ounces	2 to 3 ounces
Milk and milk products[d]	3 to 4	1/4 to 1/2 cup	3/4 cup	3/4 to 1 cup

Modified from Queen, P. M., & Henry, R. R. (1987). Growth and nutrient requirements of children. In R. J. Grand, L. Sutphen, & W. H. Dietz, Jr. (Eds.), *Pediatric nutrition: Theory and practice* (p. 347). Boston: Butterworths.

[a]1 slice bread = 1/4 cup dry cereal, 1/2 cup cooked cereal, or 1/2 cup potato, rice, or noodles.

[b]Sources of vitamin C (weekly) include citrus fruits, berries, tomatoes, broccoli, cabbage, and cantaloupe. Sources of vitamin A (3 to 4 times weekly) include spinach, carrots, squash, and cantaloupe.

[c]1 ounce of meat, fish, or poultry = 1 egg, 1 frankfurter, 2 tablespoons peanut butter, or 1/2 cup cooked legumes.

[d]1/2 cup milk = 1/2 cup cottage cheese, pudding, or yogurt; 1/4 ounce cheese; or 2 tablespoons dried milk.

Two minerals of special concern include iron in girls from the time they begin menstruation and calcium in both boys and girls for bone growth and optimal bone mass. Adequate calcium remains one of the best protectors against age-related bone loss and fractures.

Promoting Nutrition in Older Adults. Older adults require fewer calories in the diet because of reduced activity levels and because the basal metabolic rate slows as one ages. Caloric intakes for adults over the age of 51 are 1900 kcal for women and 2300 for men. The RDAs for individual nutrients remain the same after age 51, except that increased vitamin D is needed because of reduced bodily synthesis. Proper vitamin and mineral intake is needed to reduce the risk of osteoporosis caused by deficiencies in vitamin D and calcium, and to reduce the risk of anemia due to inadequate iron intake.

Specific dietary recommendations may be made for individual clients if they have disease processes that require dietary management. These commonly include reduced sodium for hypertension, reduced fat intake for those at risk for atherosclerosis, reduced caloric intake to achieve weight reduction for those with type II diabetes mellitus, and other limitations according to the specific health problem.

Nutrition education for older adults requires careful planning because common techniques may not be appropriate. Group discussion, as opposed to lecture, is often more beneficial in teaching normal nutrition. Counseling on strict diet modifications may be less successful because of resistance to changing lifelong eating habits. To simplify instruction, teach the older adult with diabetes that the diet is a normal, healthy diet that restricts concentrated sweets and simple sugars.

Action Alert! Teach older adults with diabetes to eat a normal diet while restricting simple sugars, to establish regular meal times, and to distribute foods consistently among meals.

Improved nutrition at home may also reduce hospitalization rates for older adults and decrease the number hospitalized who have signs of malnutrition. A dietitian can provide you with valuable information about feeding programs for older adults, low-cost nutritious foods, foods that have a longer shelf life and minimal preparation, and programs that provide shopping assistance.

EVALUATION

Education is not complete until learning has been evaluated. Formal and informal tools may be used to measure learning against established nutritional teaching objectives. In general, the client should be able to state the components of the healthy diet and any necessary restrictions added because of disease processes. In addition, the client must have the ability or resources to procure food, store it, cook it properly, and eat it. Inability in any of these areas indicates the need for some type of home health or social service support.

A sample note documenting the outcomes of dietary teaching for Joan, the case study client in this chapter, could be as follows:

SAMPLE DOCUMENTATION NOTE FOR JOAN
Client verbalizes understanding of the food groups in the food guide pyramid and the proper number and sizes of food portions for each group. States she is motivated to change her food intake habits to adopt a healthier lifestyle. Indicates an intention to reduce dietary fat and to return for periodic follow-up monitoring of cholesterol level.

Key Principles

- Good nutritional status is essential for normal organ development and function, for optimal activity and working efficiency, for resistance to infection, and for the ability to repair bodily damage or injury.
- The four functions of the GI system are digestion, absorption, metabolism, and excretion.
- Carbohydrates, proteins, fat, vitamins, minerals, and water are essential nutrients.
- Factors that affect nutrition include life-span considerations, culture and lifestyle, and physiological state.
- General assessment of nutritional status includes a complete health history, diet history, evaluation of food intake, and physical examination.
- The nursing diagnosis *Health-seeking behaviors: nutrition* may be used to promote optimal nutrition for the well client.
- The nursing diagnosis *Ineffective health maintenance* may be used to reduce nutritional risk factors for clients with alterations in health.
- The nursing diagnoses *Imbalanced nutrition: less than body requirements* and *Imbalanced nutrition: more than body requirements* may be used when the diet contains deficient or excess nutrients, respectively.
- Planning for expected outcomes should focus on individual client needs and sound dietary principles.
- The nurse's role in nutritional intervention includes teaching and counseling about appropriate dietary modifications.
- Reading nutrition labels can help relatively healthy clients optimize their nutritional status, and it can improve the nutritional status of those with poor nutrition.
- A healthy diet is based on the food guide pyramid, which includes recommendations for intake of grains (6 to 11 servings), fruits (2 to 4 servings), vegetables (3 to 5 servings), milk and milk products (2 to 3 servings), meats/fish/poultry, eggs, and nuts (2 to 3 servings), and fats and sweets (sparing use).
- Proper diet habits can reduce the risk of heart disease, stroke, and cancer, the three leading causes of death in the United States.
- There may be special dietary needs depending on age, pregnancy status, or disease state.
- Evaluation is necessary to review and improve or change dietary or nutritional plans.

Bibliography

Andrews, M., Angone, K. M., Cray, J. V., Lewis, J. A., & Johnson, P. H. (Eds.). (1999). *Nurse's handbook of alternative & complementary therapies.* Springhouse, PA: Springhouse.

Bernshaw, N. J. (1998). Breastfeeding as the norm. *Journal of Human Lactation, 14*(1), 14.

Center for Medical Consumers. (1998). Dietary fat reconsidered. *HealthFacts, 23*(3), 1-2.

Cerrato, P. L. (2000). Preventing cancer. *RN, 63*(11), 38-40, 43-45.

Dudek, S. G. (2001). *Nutrition essentials for nursing practice* (4th ed.). Philadelphia: Lippincott Williams & Wilkins.

*Food and Nutrition Board, Subcommittee on the Tenth Edition of the RDAs. (1989). *Recommended dietary allowances* (10th ed.). Washington, DC: National Academy Press.

Futterman, L. G., & Lemberg, L. (1999). The use of antioxidants in retarding atherosclerosis: Fact or fiction? *American Journal of Critical Care, 8*(2), 130-133.

Goodwin, J. S., & Tangum, M. R. (1998). Battling quackery: Attitudes about micronutrient supplements in American academic medicine. *Archives of Internal Medicine, 158*(20), 2187-2191.

Grodner, M., Anderson, S. L., & DeYoung, S. (2000). *Foundations and clinical applications of nutrition: A nursing approach* (2nd ed.). St Louis, MO: Mosby.

Holmes, S. (2000). Nutritional screening and older adults. *Nursing Standard, 15*(2), 42-44.

Houston, D. K, Johnson, M. A., Nozza, R. J., Gunter, E. W., Shea, K. J., Cutler, G. M., et al. (1999). Age-related hearing loss, vitamin B_{12}, and folate in elderly women. *American Journal of Clinical Nutrition, 69*(3), 564-571.

McLennan, C. L., & Hartz, D. J. (1998). Use of a pediatric diet history form to create individualized, consistent carbohydrate meal plans. *Diabetes Educator, 24*(4), 459-460, 463-464.

Meydani, M., Lipman, R. D., Han, S. N., Wu, D., Beharka, A., Martin, K. R., et al. (1998). The effect of long-term dietary supplementation with antioxidants. *Annals of the New York Academy of Science, 854,* 352-360.

Murray, M. (1998). Calcium vs. osteoporosis in postmenopausal women. *Natural Medicine Journal, 1*(1), 16-17.

Ottley, C. (2000). Food and mood. *Nursing Standard, 15*(2), 46-52, 54-55.

*U.S. Department of Agriculture (1992). *USDA's food guide pyramid.* USDA human nutritional information service, Publication No. 249. Washington, DC: U.S. Government Printing Office.

U.S. Department of Health and Human Services. (2000). *Healthy People 2010* (2nd ed.). Washington, DC: U.S. Government Printing Office. Available on the internet at http://web.health.gov/healthypeople.

Vitamin E reduces prostate cancer risk. (1998). *Fort Myers News Press,* March 18, p. 1.

Williams, S. W. (2001). *Basic nutrition and diet therapy* (11th ed.). St Louis, MO: Mosby.

Wynn, M., & Wynn, A. (1998). The danger of B_{12} deficiency in the elderly. *Nutritional Health, 12*(4), 215-226.

Yen, P. K. (1998). Stopping heart disease with diet. *Geriatric Nursing, 19*(1), 50-51.

---

*Asterisk indicates a classic or definitive work on this subject.

24

Restoring Nutrition

Key Terms

anorexia
catabolism
deglutition
dysphagia
enteral nutrition
malnutrition
parenteral nutrition

Learning Objectives

After studying this chapter, you should be able to do the following:

- Describe the physiology of malnutrition and starvation
- Discuss factors affecting nutritional deficits
- Assess clients who are experiencing severe nutritional deficits
- Formulate nursing diagnoses for nutritional deficits
- Plan goal-directed interventions for clients with nutritional deficits
- Employ a variety of interventions to facilitate optimal nutrition for clients
- Evaluate the achievement of measurable outcomes for clients with nutritional deficits

Mrs. Rosalie Goldman is a 54-year-old lawyer whose parents came to the United States from Russia in the early 1900s. She has had surgery for cancer of the breast and now is receiving outpatient chemotherapy. Because of her treatments, she experiences early satiety and anorexia and says that food does not have much taste. Mrs. Goldman is 5 feet 4 inches tall and her usual weight is 140 pounds. Currently she weighs 115 pounds. Her serum albumin level is 2.7 g/100 mL.

The clinic nurse is concerned with Mrs. Goldman's weight loss and considers her at risk for malnutrition. She makes the diagnosis of *Imbalanced nutrition: less than body requirements* from the list of nursing diagnoses related to nutrition (see below).

KEY NURSING DIAGNOSES FOR   Imbalanced Nutrition

Imbalanced nutrition: less than body requirements: An intake of nutrients insufficient to meet metabolic needs

Impaired swallowing: Abnormal functioning of the swallowing mechanism associated with deficits in oral, pharyngeal, or esophageal structure or function

Risk for aspiration: Being at risk for entry of GI secretions, oropharyngeal secretions, solids, or fluids into the tracheobronchial passages

---

CONCEPTS OF NUTRITIONAL PROBLEMS

As a nurse, you will observe nutritional problems in clients in all care settings: homes, rehabilitation settings, clinics, and hospitals. Collectively, nutritional problems create a condition known as **malnutrition,** which is any disorder of nutrition caused by imbalanced, insufficient, or excessive diet or by impaired absorption or metabolism of nutrients. To care for clients with malnutrition, you will need a sound understanding of inadequate and excessive nutrition and the many factors that affect nutritional status.

Nutritional deprivation results from inadequate intake, which may be caused by nausea and vomiting, difficulty swallowing, or inability to obtain food. It can also result from problems that raise energy needs, such as infection, trauma, stress, or surgery.

Extreme malnutrition can lead to death through starvation. Starvation is the physiological response to chronic food deprivation. During starvation, the body attempts to reduce its energy use by lowering voluntary activity and the basal metabolic rate (BMR). Next, when nutrient intake fails to meet the body's energy expenditure (energy needs), the body resorts to breaking down muscle and lean body mass (endogenous fuels). This phenomenon, called **catabolism,** yields glucose from protein breakdown in a process called gluconeogenesis. Catabolism results in a negative nitrogen balance. Figure 24-1 summarizes the metabolic changes that occur when the body uses endogenous fuels to meet energy needs. After 10 to 14 days of starvation, the body uses fat rather than glucose for energy. The liver makes ketone bodies for use as fuel by most tissues, including the brain.

If clients have been starving for a period of time, the urine will be positive for ketones and the nitrogen balance will be negative. Because of decreased protein intake, the

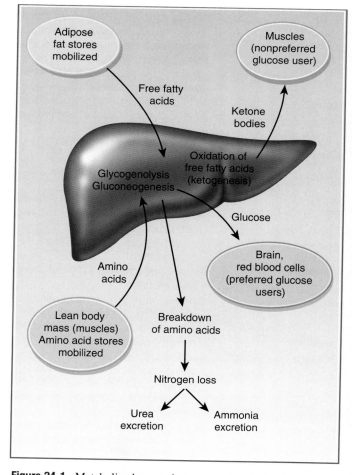

Figure 24-1. Metabolic changes that occur when the body uses endogenous fuels to meet energy needs. (Modified from Lemoyne, M., & Jeejeebhoy, K. N. [1985]. Total parenteral nutrition in the critically ill patient. *Chest, 89* [4], 568.)

blood urea nitrogen (BUN) and creatinine values will fall, reflecting fewer products of protein breakdown. In nonobese adults, fat (the body's main stored fuel) is depleted in about 1 to 2 months. Protein can supply about 2 weeks of calories; however, this protein breakdown affects the body.

The incidence of protein–calorie malnutrition in hospitalized clients ranges from 40% to 70% and results from inadequate assessment and nutritional support. Severe malnourishment may occur in as many as 12% of hospitalized clients (Dudek, 2000). It can be from inadequate calories, inadequate proteins, or both.

Table 24-1 Manifestations of Nutritional Imbalances

Nutrient	Evidence of Deficiency	Evidence of Excess
Vitamin A	Night blindness, dry rough skin, dry eyes (xerosis), dry mucous membranes, decreased saliva secretion leading to difficulty chewing and swallowing, impaired digestion and absorption, diarrhea, increased susceptibility to respiratory, urinary, and vaginal infections, impaired development of bones and teeth	Anorexia, nausea, vomiting, abdominal pain, diarrhea, weight loss, irritability, fatigue, portal hypertension, loss of hair, dry skin, bone pain and fragility, spleen enlargement, extensive liver damage, hydrocephalus (in infants and children)
Vitamin B_1 (thiamine)	Anorexia, edema, enlarged heart, heart failure, mental confusion, peripheral paralysis, fatigue, beriberi, painful calf muscles	None known
Vitamin B_2 (riboflavin)	Reddening of the cornea, dermatitis, cheilosis, glossitis, photophobia, ariboflavinosis	None known
Vitamin B_3 (niacin)	Dermatitis, glossitis, diarrhea, dementia, death	None known
Folic acid	Macrocytic anemia, fatigue, weight loss, pallor, diarrhea, glossitis	None known
Vitamin B_{12} (cobalamin)	Anemia, sore tongue, progressive neuropathy and other neurological changes, such as loss of memory	None known
Vitamin C (ascorbic acid)	Bleeding gums (scurvy), hemorrhage, muscle degeneration, delayed wound healing, softening of bones, soft loose teeth, anemia, increased risk of infection	Kidney stones, scurvy upon withdrawal, nausea, abdominal cramps, diarrhea, false-positive test for urinary glucose
Vitamin D (calciferol)	Infants and children: rickets, retarded bone growth, bone malformation, enlargement of ends of long bones, malformed teeth, tooth decay Adults: osteomalacia, bone deformities, pain, easy fracture, involuntary muscle twitching and spasms	Excessive calcification of bones, kidney stones, nausea, vomiting, headache, weakness, weight loss, constipation, polyuria, polydipsia, mental and physical growth retardation (children), failure to thrive (children), drowsiness, and coma (in severe cases)
Vitamin E (tocopherol)	Possible mild hemolytic anemia in adults, macrocytic anemia in premature infants	With large doses, possible depression, fatigue, diarrhea, cramps, blurred vision, headaches, interference with normal blood clotting and vitamin A metabolism
Vitamin K	Hemorrhagic disease of the newborn, delayed blood clotting	Hemolytic anemia and liver damage with synthetic vitamin K
Calcium	Osteomalacia, osteoporosis, tetany (intermittent, tonic contractions of the extremities, muscular cramps, uncontrolled seizures, possible convulsions)	Nausea, abdominal pain, vomiting, constipation, anorexia, polydipsia, polyuria, calcium kidney stones, excessive calcification of bones and soft tissues, possible coma and death
Phosphorus	Anorexia, weakness, circumoral paresthesia, hyperventilation	Symptoms of hypocalcemic tetany
Magnesium	Increased neuromuscular and central nervous system (CNS) irritability	CNS depression, hypotension, coma
Sodium	Cold and clammy skin, decreased skin turgor, apprehension, confusion, irritability, anxiety, hypotension, tachycardia, headache, tremors, seizures, abdominal cramps, nausea, vomiting, diarrhea	Edema, weight gain, hot flushed dry skin, dry red tongue, intense thirst, restless agitation, oliguria or anuria
Potassium	Muscle cramps and weakness (including cardiac muscle weakness), anorexia, nausea and vomiting, mental depression or confusion, lethargy, abdominal distention, increased urine output, shallow respirations, irregular pulse	Irritability, anxiety, listlessness, mental confusion, nausea, diarrhea, poor respirations, GI hyperactivity, muscle weakness, numbness of the extremities, hypotension, cardiac arrhythmias, heart block, cardiac arrest
Iron	Microcytic anemia, pallor, decreased work capacity, fatigue, weakness, intolerance to cold, pica, spoon-shaped fingernails	Acute iron poisoning from accidental overdose, which leads to GI cramping, nausea, vomiting, possible shock, seizures, coma
Iodine	Goiter	Acne-like skin lesions, "iodine goiter"
Zinc	Impairments of growth, sexual maturation, and immune system functioning; skin lesions; decreased sense of taste and smell	Anorexia, nausea, vomiting, diarrhea, muscle pain, lethargy, drowsiness, bleeding gastric ulcers, decreased serum levels of high-density lipoproteins

Marasmus is a condition of starvation that results from deficient caloric intake. It is a chronic condition that develops over months or years and is characterized by severe fat and muscle loss. Clients appear starved and weigh less than 80% of their ideal body weight (IBW) but have a normal serum albumin level. Fortunately, they respond fairly well to therapy as long as they are not re-fed too quickly.

Kwashiorkor is a condition of starvation, usually in young children after weaning, caused by decreased protein intake; symptoms can develop in a few weeks. A client with kwashiorkor may appear well nourished but is at tremendous risk. The serum albumin level falls below 2.8 g/dL, leading to significant edema. Wounds heal more slowly, and the client risks infection from decreased immunity. The mortality rate is high because of altered immune status and poorer response to refeeding than with marasmus.

Vitamin and mineral deficiencies can also result from decreased intake or increased loss (as with diarrhea or vomiting). Table 24-1 summarizes manifestations of the major imbalances. Vitamin and mineral imbalances commonly affect the skin, peripheral nervous system, hematopoietic system, immunity, calcification of bones, and vision.

FACTORS AFFECTING NUTRITIONAL STATUS

Risk Factors Across the Life Span

Throughout the life cycle, a complex balance exists between the anabolism of growth and the catabolism of aging. Energy expenditure and nutrient requirements are higher early in the life cycle, are stable throughout the middle years, and decline with aging. Specifically, metabolism peaks during the first 5 years and then rises again during puberty. After age 20, the BMR declines steadily. During pregnancy, the BMR increases by about 13%. Uncomplicated stressors (changes in food intake or activity level) or more severe stressors (such as trauma or disease) can increase a client's energy needs significantly (Grodner, Anderson, & Young, 2000).

Infants and Children. Low-birth-weight infants are at risk for undernutrition and need close monitoring. These newborns weigh less than 2500 g (5.5 pounds) and are classified as small for gestational age (restricted intrauterine growth rate) or premature (shortened length of gestation). Premature infants may be given tube feedings in carefully controlled amounts because the suck–swallow reflex does not develop until 32 to 34 weeks of gestation (Wong et al., 1999). These infants also have fewer nutritional reserves because fetal nutrient stores are deposited in the last 3 months of pregnancy.

Infants or children may need extra nourishment if they experience hypermetabolism or decreased growth. Trauma, burns, and failure to thrive are examples of conditions that need special nutritional support.

Adolescents. Eating disorders are common during adolescence, a time of emotional and physical turmoil. Adolescents gain 20% of adult height and 50% of adult weight during this time. They are also developing a sense of self and may feel uncomfortable about their changing bodies. In a society that favors slimness, these factors all encourage the development of eating disorders. About 20 million people in the United States suffer from eating disorders, with a female-to-male ratio that ranges from 6:1 to 10:1. Onset is often between the ages of 13 and 20 years of age. Eating disorders in the United States occur with relatively equal incidence in white and Hispanic females, occur more frequently among Native Americans, and occur less frequently among blacks and Asians (American Psychiatric Association, 2000).

Older Adults. In general, aging causes an increased proportion of connective tissue and a loss of functioning cells. No one knows exactly why this happens, but one theory states that free radicals attack the cells and impair energy production in mitochondria. Antioxidant nutrients (such as vitamin C, vitamin E, and selenium) may reduce free-radical damage to tissues.

Some nutritional deficits may be linked to aging. For example, deficiencies of calcium, iron, zinc, thiamine, vitamin B_{12}, and folate are common in the older adult and may be secondary to problems with chewing, swallowing, and digesting foods. Reduced secretion of gastric hydrochloric acid limits absorption of calcium, iron, and vitamin B_{12}. About half of clients age 65 and older wear dentures, which can create problems with chewing if they do not fit well, limiting intake of nutritious foods. Finally, many older adults take multiple prescription and over-the-counter drugs, increasing the risk of potentially dangerous drug–nutrient interactions. Be especially aware of the possibility of poor nutrition in older adults.

Physiological Factors

Illness can impair the body's ability to maintain normal nutrition by affecting ingestion, digestion, absorption, or metabolism.

Ingestion. Factors that affect the ingestion of food are those that affect the appetite and disorders of the mouth and esophagus that affect swallowing. **Anorexia** is a reduced desire for food, leading to decreased intake and possibly malnutrition if it is prolonged. It is a hallmark of the disorder anorexia nervosa that most frequently affects girls and young women. Anorexia is also caused by liver disease, medications, depression, acquired immunodeficiency syndrome (AIDS), or gastrointestinal (GI) problems. AIDS further inhibits ingestion because of lesions in the mouth and throat (stomatitis). Nausea with vomiting impairs intake and causes loss of certain minerals. This condition may be self-limiting but, if prolonged, may require hydration with intravenous fluids and possible parenteral nutritional support. Even minor disorders such as upper respiratory infection can cause anorexia by reducing the sense of taste and smell.

Swallowing, or **deglutition,** is the reflex passage of food and fluids from the mouth to the stomach (Figure 24-2, p. 540). Swallowing is initiated by voluntary action and is controlled by the central nervous system. The term **dysphagia** refers to difficulty in swallowing.

1.

ORAL PHASE (VOLUNTARY)

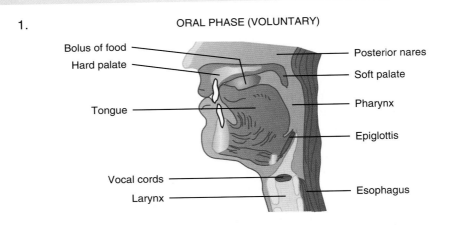

Bolus of food
Hard palate
Tongue
Vocal cords
Larynx
Posterior nares
Soft palate
Pharynx
Epiglottis
Esophagus

2.

PHARYNGEAL PHASE (INVOLUNTARY)

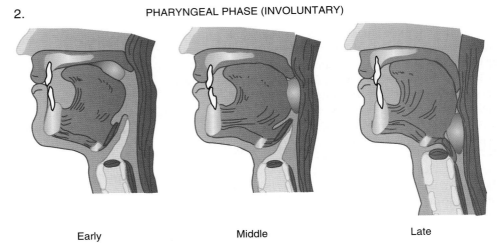

Early   Middle   Late

3.

ESOPHAGEAL PHASE (INVOLUNTARY)

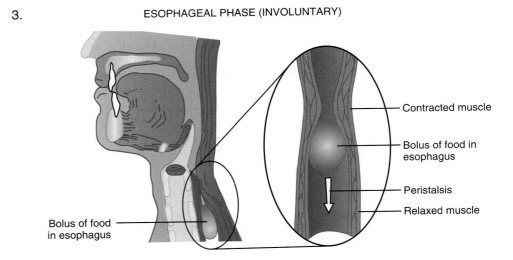

Bolus of food
in esophagus

Contracted muscle
Bolus of food in esophagus
Peristalsis
Relaxed muscle

Figure 24-2. Mechanics of swallowing. Swallowing occurs in three phases: (1) *Voluntary* or *oral* phase. The tongue presses food against the hard palate, forcing it toward the pharynx. (2) *Involuntary, pharyngeal* phase. *Early:* A wave of peristalsis forces the bolus between the tonsillar pillars. *Middle:* The soft palate draws upward to close posterior nares, and respirations cease momentarily. *Late:* The vocal cords approximate and the larynx pulls upward, covering the airway and stretching the esophagus open. (3) *Involuntary, esophageal* phase. Relaxation of the upper esophageal (hypopharyngeal) sphincter allows a peristaltic wave to move the bolus of food down the esophagus. (From Black, J. M., Hawks, J., & Keene, A. (2001). *Medical-surgical nursing: Clinical management for positive outcomes* [6th ed.]. Philadelphia: Saunders.)

Involuntary control of swallowing is coordinated from the swallowing center in the reticular formation of the medulla and the lower pons in the brain. The process uses cranial nerves V, IX, X, and XII. After food is propelled to the back of the throat with the tongue and palate muscles, an involuntary wave of pharyngeal muscle contraction pushes food into the esophagus. Meanwhile, the glottis and epiglottis move to close off the trachea and suspend breathing. When this mechanism malfunctions (such as with a cerebrovascular accident or stroke), food is aspirated into the lungs.

Muscle tension at the upper esophageal (hypopharyngeal) sphincter and the lower esophageal sphincter normally keeps these sphincters tightly closed except during swallowing, when they relax to allow food to move into the stomach by peristalsis. Increased pressure at the lower esophageal sphincter can cause dysphagia. Decreased pressure can cause reflux of acidic stomach contents back into the esophagus. Pressure at the lower esophageal sphincter is increased by parasympathetic drugs and gastrin. It is decreased by anticholinergics, cigarettes, fatty foods, alcohol, and certain digestive substances, such as cholecystokinin and secretin.

Several factors may hinder swallowing. Damage to the cranial nerves that innervate the tongue and pharynx may interfere with initiation of the swallowing reflex, effective chewing, and pushing food back into the pharynx and esophagus. The discomfort of an inflamed throat, obstruction, and decreased muscular contraction of the esophagus also can impede swallowing.

Clients with neurological disease processes or a cerebral vascular accident (CVA) often have problems swallowing because of decreased alertness or partial paralysis of the tongue, mouth, or throat. Examples of difficulties include drooling, inability to form a seal around a cup or a straw, uncoordinated tongue movements, and pocketing of food in the mouth. All of these problems raise the risk of aspiration.

Aspiration occurs when the client cannot protect the airway. This may result from difficulty swallowing, a decreased level of consciousness, seizures, impaired gag or cough reflexes, or a compromised immune system. Weakness of muscles in the soft palate, pharynx, and upper esophagus hinder the cough reflex.

Digestion and Absorption. Certain diseases alter the digestive process and impair food absorption, a condition called malabsorption. Some examples include inflammatory bowel disease (Crohn's disease or ulcerative colitis), diarrhea due to infection, and cystic fibrosis. *Lactose intolerance* is a condition in which the intestinal villi do not produce lactase, the enzyme that breaks down lactose, a carbohydrate found in milk. The lactose remains in the GI tract and draws water into the intestine by osmosis, leading to diarrhea. These disorders require specific management to promote optimal nutrition.

Metabolism. Liver diseases also affect food metabolism. Vitamins normally stored (A, B, C, K) or activated (D) in the liver may be deficient. Liver disease impairs protein metabolism because the liver cannot transform ammonia to urea.

Infection and trauma cause hypermetabolism and catabolism, requiring added calories, protein, vitamins, and minerals. Infection may also cause anorexia and electrolyte imbalances. Anemia is commonly associated with chronic infection; however the mechanism of the association is not fully understood.

When calculating energy needs from predictive equations for clients who have infections, be sure to consider body temperature. Fever increases metabolic needs by 7% for each degree Fahrenheit (13% for each degree centigrade). Clients with massive trauma or burns have very high calorie needs.

Cultural and Lifestyle Factors

Intake of an imbalanced diet, low income status that limits access to affordable nutritious food, and physical problems with obtaining or preparing food place clients at risk for malnutri-

tion. It is important to conduct nutritional assessments with clients to detect any of these factors. Inadequate nutrition over time can impair health, delay recovery from illness or surgery, and decrease overall well-being.

ASSESSMENT

General Assessment for Nutritional Problems

Nutritional assessment and screening can identify cues to nutritional problems (Box 24-1). Chapter 23 discusses general assessment for nutrition status. When the client is identified as having a nutritional problem, assessment focuses on etiology, severity, and factors affecting the problem.

The results of routine and specialized laboratory tests can provide valuable cues to the client's nutritional status (Table 24-2, p. 542). However, no single laboratory test is available to diagnose nutritional problems. A physician will probably order serum studies if the client has unintentionally lost 10% of her weight in the last 6 months or has evidence of a nutritional deficiency.

For example, creatinine and BUN levels rise with kidney disease. If the creatinine level is normal, the BUN level provides useful information on protein status. If the serum creatinine level is high, the BUN alone will not give reliable information about nutrition. In this case, rely on the ratio of BUN to serum creatinine. Serum albumin levels are frequently measured, but albumin has a 21-day half-life. To determine nutritional repletion, look to substances with shorter half-lives, such as prealbumin or transferrin.

Laboratory tests are rarely done to measure vitamin deficiencies. Instead, use the nutritional history, physical examination, and anthropometric measurements. Electrolyte levels are commonly measured, and they can provide information about nutritional problems as well.

Swallowing and aspiration may be evaluated using videofluoroscopy, a procedure also known as a video swallow esophagography, cine-esophagography, a modified barium swallow, or a swallow study. The client swallows barium, which is observed passing through the oropharynx during swallowing. This study is done in the radiology department and exposes the client to a minimal amount of radiation.

Box 24-1	Cues to Possible Nutritional Problems

- Anorexia
- Artificial airway
- Diarrhea
- Increased metabolic need
- Compromised immune system
- Less-than-normal nutrient consumption
- Low socioeconomic status
- Malabsorptive condition
- Polypharmacy
- Greater-than-normal nutrient consumption
- Muscle weaknesses in pharynx, soft palate, or esophagus
- Psychological disturbance (low self-esteem, depression)
- Reduced level of consciousness
- Nausea and vomiting

Table 24-2   Implications of Laboratory Tests for Nutritional Status

Laboratory Test	Normal Range of Values	Possible Nutritional Implications of Abnormal Values
Blood urea nitrogen	8-23 mg/dL	If decreased, low protein intake
Hematocrit	Female: 34%-44% Male: 39%-49%	If decreased, anemia (deficiency of iron, pyridoxine, folate, vitamin B_{12}, protein)
Hemoglobin	Female: 12-15 g/dL Male: 14-17 g/dL	If decreased, anemia (deficiency of iron, pyridoxine, folate, vitamin B_{12}, protein)
Ratio of blood urea nitrogen to serum creatinine	12 or above	If 8 or below, poor protein intake
Serum albumin	3.5-5.5 g/dL	If decreased, compromised protein status (levels under 2.8 are associated with edema and possible kwashiorkor)
Serum creatinine	0.6-1.6 mg/dL	If decreased, muscle wasting
Total lymphocyte count	1500/mm³ or above	If decreased, not specific for any particular nutritional deficiency, but correlates best with protein deficit

Focused Assessment for *Imbalanced Nutrition: Less Than Body Requirements*

While loss of weight is the most commonly identified cue to nutritional deficiency, more subtle cues need to be considered. Cluster various cues to make this diagnosis.

Defining Characteristics. The chief complaints for clients with nutritional problems may include any of the following: weight changes, inability to swallow or eat, fatigue, and skin lesions. Take a detailed history for these clients, making sure to include the following elements:

- Body weight 20% or more under ideal. Assess for weight changes in the last 6 months. Ask clients about their *usual weight* and find out whether they think their current weight differs from their usual weight. Abnormal weight gain can indicate either fluid gain or obesity. Involuntary weight loss can indicate disease or malnutrition and can be a grave sign.
- Changes in appetite: anorexia, early satiety, lack of interest in food, aversion to food, loss of taste
- Symptoms, such as an inability to eat independently
- Nutritional supplements taken
- Medications taken, including prescribed and over-the-counter. Obtain a history of other health problems and use of prescription and over-the-counter medications for them as well
- Difficulty swallowing or chewing; obstructed esophagus or pharynx
- Pale conjunctiva
- GI symptoms, such as abdominal cramping, abdominal pain with or without pathology, hyperactive bowel sounds, diarrhea or steatorrhea, nausea, vomiting, constipation
- A perceived inability to ingest food
- Condition of skin, teeth, and mucous membranes: rashes, scaling, bleeding, poor wound healing, capillary fragility, pale or ulcerated mucous membranes, depapillation of the tongue, bleeding, gum disease, cracks in the mouth, and dental caries; a sore or inflamed mouth or an altered taste sensation
- Hair condition, such as brittleness and how easily it can be plucked

- Fingernail condition, including ridges, clubbing, and brittleness
- Neck characteristics, including enlarged lymph nodes, enlarged thyroid
- Musculoskeletal conditions, such as bone deformities and muscle wasting, muscle weakness, decreased muscle tone
- Central nervous system function, including difficulty walking and peripheral neuritis
- Other medical conditions: liver, specifically any enlargement on palpation; heart condition, such as cardiomegaly; kidney disease; diabetes; cancer; or AIDS

Related Factors. The defining characteristics give cues to the etiology or other related factors. Additional related factors may include the following:

- Economic factors in obtaining food
- Misconceptions, lack of information, or misinformation
- Inadequate caregivers or support systems

Focused Assessment for *Impaired Swallowing*

Defining Characteristics. Defining characteristics for the diagnosis *Impaired swallowing* may arise in any of the three phases of swallowing and include the following:

- Oral phase: lack of tongue action to form a bolus; weak sucking in an infant; incomplete lip closure; food pushed out or falls out of mouth; slow bolus formation; premature entry of bolus; nasal reflux; inability to clear the mouth; coughing, choking, or gagging before swallowing; abnormal results of swallow study; lack of chewing; pooling, drooling, or excessive saliva formation
- Pharyngeal phase: altered head positions, inadequate laryngeal elevation, refusal of food, unexplained fevers, delayed swallowing, recurrent pulmonary infections, a gurgly voice, nasal reflux, choking, coughing, gagging, multiple swallows, abnormal swallow study results
- Esophageal phase: heartburn or epigastric pain, acidic-smelling breath, unexplained irritability at mealtime, vomitus on pillow, repetitive swallowing or ruminating, wet burps, bruxism (teeth-grinding), nighttime coughing or awakening, observed difficulty swallowing, hyperextension of head during or after meals, abnormal swallow study,

Table 24-3 *Clustering Data to Make a Nursing Diagnosis*

NUTRITIONAL PROBLEMS

Data Cluster	Diagnosis
A 27-year-old client presents with a weight 120% of normal; has been overweight since age 10; preoperative for gallbladder surgery and referred for weight loss.	*Imbalanced nutrition: more than body requirements* related to unknown etiology
A 45-year-old client is 120% above his ideal body weight; has been coming to the weight-control clinic for 6 months and continues to gain weight. Refuses to exercise and to keep a food diary.	*Noncompliance* with weight control program related to lack of motivation
A 14-year-old bulimic client comes to the emergency department with a weight of 55 pounds, height of 5'2", blood pressure of 70/20, pulse of 124, respiratory rate of 30, decreased skin turgor, weakness, and thirst.	*Deficient fluid volume* related to frequent vomiting without sufficient fluid replacement
A 76-year-old man has had a stroke and is comatose. He is receiving nasogastric feedings and has developed pneumonia.	*Risk for aspiration* related to esophageal reflux and pharyngeal muscle weakness
A 52-year-old woman receiving chemotherapy for cancer has developed stomatitis, early satiety, anorexia, and decreased taste. Her serum albumin is 2.7 g/dL and she has recent unintentional weight loss.	*Imbalanced nutrition: less than body requirements* related to stomatitis, early satiety, anorexia, and decreased taste
An 81-year-old client with Parkinson's disease is drooling and pocketing food. Recently he has lost 5 lbs unintentionally. His lungs are clear, and he is ambulatory and alert.	*Impaired swallowing* related to muscle rigidity

painful swallowing, limiting or refusing food, complaints of "something stuck," vomiting (including blood)

Related Factors. Factors related to the diagnosis *Impaired swallowing* may include the following:

- Weakness or tiredness
- Decreased or lack of motivation
- Severe anxiety
- Neuromuscular or musculoskeletal impairment
- Perceptual or cognitive impairment
- Pain or discomfort
- Environmental barriers

Focused Assessment for *Risk for Aspiration*

Defining Characteristics. Because this is a risk nursing diagnosis, there are no defining characteristics. Instead, assess the client for related factors.

Related Factors. Factors related to *Risk for aspiration* include the following:

- Conditions that result in decreased GI motility, delayed gastric emptying, increased gastric residual (contents remaining from previous meal or feeding), or increased intragastric pressure
- Presence of tubes such as a feeding tube or other GI tubes
- Presence of an artificial airway, such as a tracheostomy or endotracheal tube
- Reduced level of consciousness, or depressed cough or gag reflexes
- Insufficient elevation of upper body or impaired swallowing
- Trauma or surgery to the face, mouth, or neck
- Medication administration

Diagnosis

It is relatively easy to identify *Imbalanced nutrition: less than body requirements,* but it may be more difficult to distinguish between *Impaired swallowing* and *Risk for aspiration.* If the client has a swallowing disorder but also has reduced intake, use the *Imbalanced nutrition* diagnosis until the nutritional state has stabilized. This allows you to focus your care on improving the client's nutritional state.

Remember that impaired swallowing increases the risk of aspiration. Focus your efforts first on preventing aspiration, since aspiration can be life threatening. Review data from the history and physical examination to find cues to an increased risk for aspiration. If you cannot make a definitive diagnosis of *Risk for aspiration,* then focus on impaired swallowing. Remember that interventions to improve swallowing also help prevent aspiration.

Make the diagnosis that best focuses on nursing care. For example, if a client with anorexia nervosa is acutely ill in the emergency room, use *Imbalanced nutrition: less than body requirements* until the acute episode resolves. If there are life-threatening fluid and electrolyte imbalances, use *Deficient fluid volume.* As treatment continues and the client gets psychological help, focus on *Low self-esteem disturbance* or *Disturbed body image.* Table 24-3 shows how to select nursing diagnoses according to clustered data.

Related Nursing Diagnoses

Noncompliance may be diagnosed if clients do not follow nutritional advice. Obese clients may have trouble following the prescribed dietary regimen. People with eating disorders see themselves in a distorted way and have difficulty thinking about food and weight in the usual way. A related nursing diagnosis to consider would be *Ineffective therapeutic regimen management.*

Clients who are not receiving sufficient fluid may be at risk for dehydration. Consider the diagnosis *Deficient fluid volume.* This is of special concern for older adults or those with swallowing difficulty, anorexia, or eating disorders.

Use the diagnosis *Impaired skin integrity* for a client with nutritional problems that result in skin problems. They may stem from a low serum albumin and decreased protein.

A client with edema may be more prone to skin breakdown. Dehydration causes dry skin and mucous membranes. Another related nursing diagnosis to consider is *Impaired oral mucous membranes.*

Use the diagnosis *Diarrhea* for a client with nutritional problems caused by diarrhea, which leads to a loss of fluids and decreased absorption of nutrients. Diarrhea is a common complication of enteral feedings given to clients with nutritional problems.

The diagnosis *Fatigue* may be appropriate when a client receives insufficient nutrients for metabolism and energy production and, as a consequence, feels fatigue. Fatigue can also be a risk factor for both impaired swallowing and aspiration.

PLANNING

Planning involves setting general goals and specific outcome criteria with the client. Write the outcome criteria so that they are objective and measurable; then you can evaluate whether or not they are achieved. For example, "weight gain of 3 pounds" is objective and easy to measure, whereas "client looks better" is subjective and difficult to measure. Devise a plan for the client to use during the hospital or clinic stay, but also begin discharge planning for the client upon admission.

The clinic nurse sets goals with Mrs. Goldman and her daughter to prevent further nutritional deterioration and to gain 2 pounds per month. The nurse assesses Mrs. Goldman's food preferences and notes that she maintains a kosher diet. What foods would you recommend including in Mrs. Goldman's diet? How would you encourage Mrs. Goldman to monitor her progress toward her nutritional goals?

Expected Outcomes for the Client With *Imbalanced Nutrition: Less Than Body Requirements*

Goals for the diagnosis *Imbalanced nutrition: less than body requirements* focus on an improved nutritional state. Weight gain is a good outcome criterion for this nursing diagnosis.

Generally, if the client gains 2 to 4 pounds a month, the plan is considered successful; however, this rate is individual with each client. In some clients, such as those with eating disorders, the initial plan may be simply to avoid further weight loss. A maximum of 1.5 kg per week can be expected from intensive parenteral nutrition. A weight gain of more than 1 pound per day indicates fluid retention rather than an increase in lean muscle mass.

> *Action Alert!* Report a weight gain of more than 1 pound per day, which indicates fluid retention rather than increased weight from lean body mass.

Laboratory test results may also be used to determine the plan's success. However, make sure to interpret albumin levels cautiously because they take about 3 weeks to reflect results of refeeding. Prealbumin or transferrin levels are better short-term indicators.

If pretreatment physical assessment findings are consistent with nutritional deficiency, then cite improvement in these as outcome criteria. For example, the following might be outcome criteria:

- Wound begins to heal
- Edema resolves
- Petechiae disappear

Expected Outcomes for the Client With *Impaired Swallowing*

The client should be able to maintain a stable weight, show no signs of dehydration, and report no difficulty swallowing. Outcome criteria indicating normal hydration are the following:

- Good skin turgor
- Normal vital signs (no hypotension, tachycardia, or fever)
- Skin and mucous membranes moist, not dry
- No complaints of thirst
- Normal hematocrit (not elevated)

Expected Outcomes for the Client With *Risk for Aspiration*

The client should not experience actual aspiration. The client should also be able to identify and avoid risk factors for aspiration. Examples would include self-positioning upright for eating and drinking, selecting foods according to swallowing ability, and thickening liquids to appropriate consistency.

INTERVENTION

Interventions for nutritional problems in any setting require a team approach. Hospital standards require performance-based interdisciplinary delivery of nutritional support, so you can expect to obtain assistance from nutritional support teams in these institutions. Nurses working in home health agencies may initiate referrals to a dietitian as appropriate. See Figure 24-3 for general guidelines for selecting nutritional interventions.

Interventions to Increase Nutrient Intake

Make sure that the client is comfortable during meals. Clients who are fatigued, immobilized, or paralyzed will need assistance. Until they can eat independently, feed them and teach the family or caregiver about feeding (Figure 24-4). Tell a client who is blind where the food is on the plate in relation to a clock face (e.g., mashed potatoes at 6 o'clock). Consider food preferences and serve food in an attractive manner to improve intake. Young children generally like their food bland, whereas older adults (with diminished taste) prefer food that is seasoned. Fresh herbs are a good choice. Assess the older client's ability to chew, and puree the food as needed if the teeth are in poor condition.

Often, an evaluation team will recommend treatment for complex feeding problems. The team works to improve the client's hand-to-mouth coordination, vision, or ability to suck,

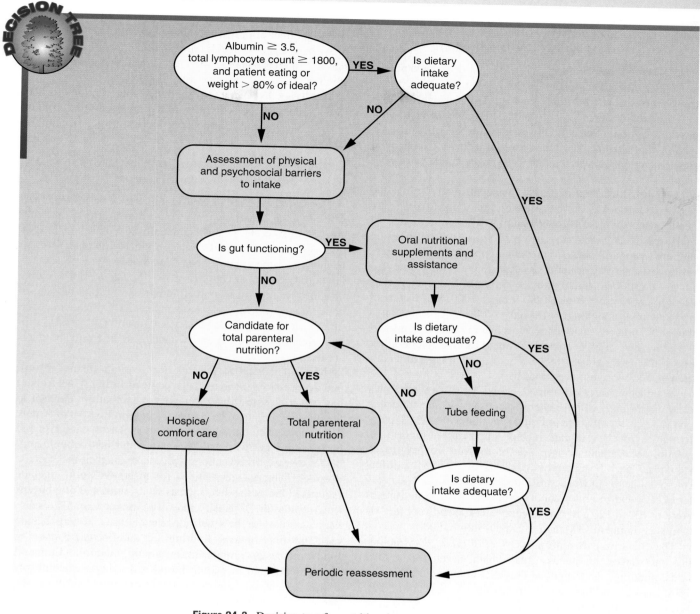

Figure 24-3. Decision tree for nutritional assessment and support.

chew, swallow, or grasp. Special feeding equipment may be used, including weighted utensils, two-handed cups, and unbreakable dishes with suction cups. Battery-powered machines are also available.

Enriching the Insufficient Diet. The diet should be the primary source of good nutrition, but sometimes the diet is insufficient. Pregnant women need extra folic acid, calcium, and iron. Clients with osteoporosis need extra calcium and magnesium, and many chronically ill clients require multiple vitamin or mineral supplements.

Some clients cannot eat enough at mealtime and begin to lose weight. To remedy this, give supplemental feedings to increase calories and nutrients. The extra food should be nutritious and something the client enjoys. Generally, six small meals are preferable to three larger ones.

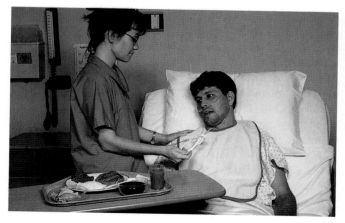

Figure 24-4. Until clients can eat independently, feed them, and teach the family or caregiver about feeding.

Encourage Mrs. Goldman to eat small, supplemental meals. Which types of food would you consider offering her?

Liquid foods are less filling and easier for debilitated people to handle. Milkshakes, puddings, and instant breakfast drinks can be recommended. Adding powdered milk, yogurt, or tofu to foods provides extra protein, and adding sugar or corn syrup provides calories. Sweet additives increase the solution's osmolality but also increase the risk of GI distress. Commercial supplements can add protein, fat, carbohydrate, and calories.

Managing Therapeutic Diets.
In the hospital setting, the physician prescribes the diet. The diet may meet therapeutic needs or be based on the client's ability to tolerate food.

Hospitalized clients may be on *NPO* (*nil per os,* meaning nothing by mouth) status to prevent complications from diagnostic tests, surgery, trauma, or acute illness. Intravenous fluids are prescribed, often with 5% dextrose, to prevent dehydration, not to provide nutrition. It takes 1000 mL (1 liter) of a 5% dextrose solution to yield only *170 kcal.* This amount is thought to prevent catabolism. Most healthy people can tolerate a few days of NPO status but should receive enteral nutrition if the need persists longer than 5 days; infants and children should receive it even sooner.

When a diet order is resumed, clients are often started on a *clear liquid diet,* which generally consists of any fluid that you can see through. These liquids are thin and have no pulp. Examples of clear liquids include apple juice, ginger ale, gelatin, decaffeinated coffee, tea, broth, fruit ices, or frozen ice pops. Check hospital policy because there may be different guidelines as to what constitutes a clear liquid. This diet is temporary and provides about 400 to 500 kcal, 5 to 10 g of protein, 100 to 120 g of carbohydrate, no fat, and very few vitamins and minerals (Mahan & Escott-Stump, 2000).

The client may then progress to a *full liquid diet,* including milkshakes, all juices, gruels, blenderized foods, custards, puddings, and eggnog. This diet contains as much as 1500 calories and has more nutrients than a clear liquid diet. With careful planning and the addition of fiber, it can be used indefinitely.

A *soft diet* is sometimes used as a transition to a general diet or for clients who have difficulty eating. This diet is low in fiber and is devoid of bran, grains, strong vegetables (such as cabbage), and raw fruits or vegetables. However, institutions sometimes differ in their definition of a soft diet, and the trend is to define it more liberally, allowing more whole-grain products, cereals, and vegetables (Mahan & Escott-Stump, 2000).

ANOREXIA. The client with anorexia can benefit from smaller, more frequent meals that include nutritious foods that the client enjoys. The environment should be clean and free from unpleasant odors or other stimuli, to enhance intake. The client with anorexia nervosa needs psychological treatment and medical nutrition therapy using the services of a dietitian with experience in treating this disorder.

NAUSEA AND VOMITING. When nausea and vomiting occur secondary to infection (such as flu), withhold food until nausea and vomiting subside. Encourage sips of fluids (1 to 2 ounces per hour) to prevent dehydration. When nausea occurs as a side effect of drugs, encourage the client to drink liquids between meals or to drink only small amounts of fluids with meals. Cold, carbonated, and clear liquids are easier to tolerate than others.

LACTOSE INTOLERANCE. Dietary interventions for lactose intolerance consist of eliminating foods that contain lactose, such as dairy products or prepared foods containing lactose.

> *Action Alert!* Teach lactose-intolerant clients to read food labels for hidden sources of lactose.

Because the degree of lactose intolerance varies from person to person, small amounts (up to 5 to 8 grams, or 1 to 2 cups of milk per day) may be gradually added back to the diet. Lactose is better tolerated when consumed with other foods or beverages, rather than alone. Dietary supplements such as Lactaid, Lactrase, or Dairy Ease may be taken prior to eating or added to milk 24 hours before use. Restriction of lactose-containing foods may place clients at risk for calcium, vitamin D, and riboflavin deficiency, so mineral and vitamin supplementation is needed unless lactase-treated milk products are used.

MALABSORPTION. Dietary interventions for malabsorption syndromes depend on the specific disorder. When a client has celiac disease (gluten-sensitive enteropathy), damage to the intestine is caused by *gliaden,* a protein fraction of gluten. Thus foods that contain gluten, such as wheat, oats, rye, and barley, must be restricted. When a client has inflammatory bowel disease, interventions vary depending on the specific disorder. Dietary interventions for ulcerative colitis include reducing fiber in the diet, such as seeds, nuts, and dried beans (low-residue diet). Dietary interventions for Crohn's disease vary according to the severity of the disease and may include reducing fiber intake, limiting fat and lactose-containing foods, increasing protein intake, giving vitamin and mineral supplements, and providing bowel rest using elemental formulas for enteral feeding or total parenteral nutrition (see paragraphs that follow).

DIABETES. Clients with diabetes should eat three meals per day, with snacks in the late afternoon and before bedtime as ordered to coincide with peak action times of insulin. The diet should be well balanced, calorie controlled, and avoid concentrated sweets. A dietitian will develop the dietary prescription on the basis of a physician's order.

> *Action Alert!* Urge diabetic clients to immediately report any illness that prevents them from eating.

AIDS AND CANCER. Clients with AIDS and cancer may have cachexia (a syndrome of anorexia, anemia, fatigue, and muscle wasting). They may have a decreased sense of taste (which may respond to zinc supplements). They also tend to eat better in the morning and tolerate small, frequent feedings during the day. Serve foods cool or at room temperature and avoid serving foods with strong odors.

Encourage foods that contain protein, especially milk shakes, poultry, and eggs, but remember that these clients may have an aversion to red meats (Wilkes, 2000). Immuno-suppression may lead to a sore mouth and throat, as well as to xerostomia—mouth dryness caused by insufficient saliva. Encourage fluids, limit spicy or acidic foods, and emphasize good oral hygiene.

HEART DISEASE. Clients with heart disease require a diet low in saturated fat, cholesterol, and salt (Yen, 1998b). Foods to be avoided include butter, whole milk, eggs, red meat, and cheese. Skim milk, poultry, fish, and fresh fruits and vegetables are encouraged, along with foods high in soluble fiber, such as apples, citrus fruits, oats, and barley.

A 2-gram sodium diet (moderate restriction) is common for clients with hypertension. Teach clients on this diet not to add salt while cooking or at the table and to avoid foods high in sodium, such as canned, prepared, and processed foods. Encourage hypertensive clients to increase the amount of calcium and potassium in their diet.

KIDNEY DISEASE. Therapeutic dietary management of kidney disease depends on the type and stage of disease. Protein is generally restricted as the disease advances. Fluid, sodium, potassium, and phosphorus are restricted because the kidneys cannot maintain adequate fluid and electrolyte balance. Vitamin D and calcium levels may be low, causing fractures and bone softening. Administer vitamin D and calcium supplements as ordered. With less erythropoietin to stimulate production of red blood cells, iron supplements are needed to treat anemia.

LIVER DISEASE. Therapeutic nutrition is also important in treating liver disease. Protein intake should be normal to maintain nitrogen balance; however, if the client has impending liver failure, protein is restricted. When the liver fails, ammonia (a byproduct of protein metabolism) is not converted to urea, and ammonia levels rise to toxic levels in the blood. The diet for these clients should provide adequate kilocalories and carbohydrates, as well as vitamins normally stored in the liver (especially vitamins K and B_{12}, thiamine, pyridoxine, folate, and niacin). Sodium and fluid may be restricted because the liver no longer breaks down aldosterone.

Providing Enteral Feedings.
When a client cannot eat sufficient nutrients to sustain life and health, enteral feedings may be initiated. While **enteral nutrition** can refer to any form of nutrition delivered to the GI tract (orally or by tube), it is generally used to mean tube feedings. Feeding a client through a tube inserted into the GI tract can help to keep it functioning normally. Table 24-4 identifies clinical situations in which such artificial nutrition may be necessary.

FEEDING TUBES AND ROUTES OF ACCESS. A feeding tube may be inserted through the nose and placed into the stomach, duodenum, or jejunum. These are known as nasogastric, nasoduodenal, or nasojejunal tubes, respectively. The tube can also be inserted surgically into the esophagus, stomach, or jejunum. These are known as esophagostomy, gastrostomy, and jejunostomy tubes, respectively (Figure 24-5, *A*, p. 548). When endoscopy is used to insert the tube, it is referred to as a percutaneous endoscopic gastrostomy (PEG) or percutaneous endoscopic jejunostomy (PEJ) tube (Figure 24-5, *B*, p. 548). PEG and PEJ often use low-profile tubes because they are comfort-

Table 24-4	Clinical Situations in Which Artificial Nutrition May Be Necessary
Situation	**Possible Cause**
Inability to ingest food	• Cancer of the mouth, tongue, esophagus • Facial trauma • Unconsciousness • Severe stomatitis • Impaired swallowng • Muscle weakness in mouth or esophagus
Inability to digest or absorb food	• Pancreatitis • Cancer of the stomach • Crohn's disease or ulcerative colitis • Biliary disease
Inability to meet nutritional needs	• Increased resting energy expenditure from major trauma or surgery, burns, or severe infection • Anorexia nervosa or bulimia nervosa

able underneath clothing. Figure 24-6 (p. 548) provides some examples of low-profile gastrostomy tubes.

The choice of enteral nutrition support depends on the client's status, the anticipated length of use, the cost, and the availability of a person experienced in placing the feeding tube, as diagrammed in Figure 24-7 (p. 549). The gastric site is preferred to the jejunal site because the stomach has a larger reservoir. However, the jejunal site may be used if the client has significant esophageal reflux, a history or risk of aspiration, or a dysfunctional stomach from gastric surgery or gastritis. Also, function returns to the small intestine faster than to the stomach after stress or trauma.

Endoscopic feeding tube placement is less invasive and less expensive than surgical placement. Surgical placement is done under general or local anesthesia using a laparoscopy or open laparotomy.

Tube feedings are usually initiated with a nasogastric tube. A pliable, small-bore tube is used because it causes less discomfort and less interference with the lower esophageal sphincter than a large-bore tube. To place a feeding tube, follow the relevant procedure in Chapter 25, with the modifications shown in this chapter in Box 24-2 (p. 550).

The definitive way to make sure a tube has reached the stomach is by radiography. The next most reliable indicator is checking the pH of the fluid withdrawn through the tube. If the pH is less than 5.0, the tube is most likely in the stomach, unless the client is receiving medications that alter the gastric pH. With duodenal tube placement, you should note a change of drainage color from green to golden; in addition you should obtain a pH greater than 6.0, and a bilirubin level of greater than 5 in 75% of cases (Metheny, 1998).

The disadvantages of using pH for confirming placement are twofold. First, the flexible, small-bore tubes sometimes collapse during aspiration of gastric contents, preventing removal of the fluid. Second, other factors can affect gastric pH, such as acid-inhibiting agents, aging, pernicious anemia, AIDS, and intestinal bile reflux.

You can also instill 60 mL of air into the tube (in short bursts) and listen with a stethoscope over the left upper quadrant for air

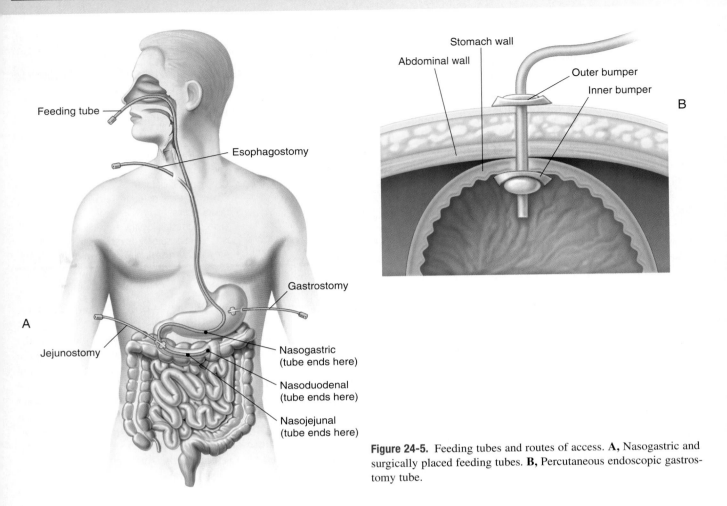

Figure 24-5. Feeding tubes and routes of access. **A,** Nasogastric and surgically placed feeding tubes. **B,** Percutaneous endoscopic gastrostomy tube.

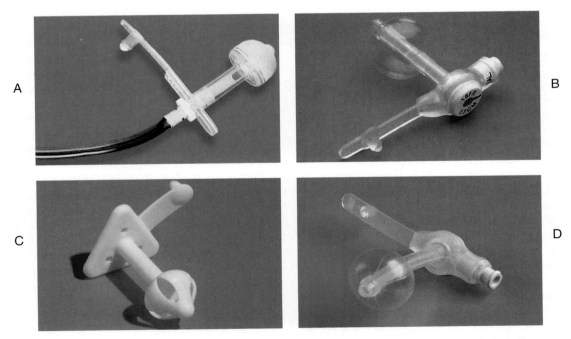

Figure 24-6. Examples of low-profile gastrostomy tubes. **A,** Bard Button. **B,** Ballard Mic-Key. **C,** Ross Stomate. **D,** Ross Hide-a-Port. (**A** courtesy C. R. Bard, Inc., Billerica, MA; **B** courtesy Ballard Medical Products, Draper, UT; **C** and **D** used with permission of Ross Products Division, Abbott Laboratories, Columbus, OH.)

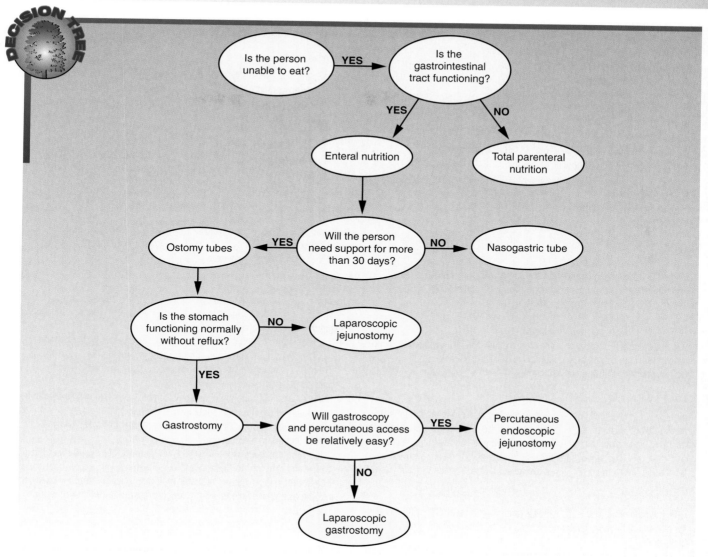

Figure 24-7. Decision tree for route of enteral nutrition support. (Modified from Duh, Q. Y. [1996]. Decision tree for route of enteral nutrition support: Placement techniques. *Current issues in enteral nutrition support: Report of the first Ross Conference on Enteral Devices,* pp. 9-16. Columbus, OH: Ross Products Division, Abbott Laboratories. Used with permission of Ross Products Division, Abbott Laboratories, Columbus, OH. Copyright 1996, Ross Products Division, Abbott Laboratories.)

sounds; however, the "swooshing" sound of air may be heard when the tube has been inadvertently placed in the lungs, making it unreliable as the sole method of determining placement. Aspirating at least 40 mL of the gastric content is also used to verify stomach placement. If more than 10 mL of gastric content cannot be removed, the tube is probably still in the esophagus. Subsequent checks for placement are more reliable if using more than one method.

Action Alert! When placing a feeding tube, be sure that a radiograph is ordered, because it is the definitive method of confirming gastric placement. Determining placement by pH measurement and auscultation do not eliminate the need for an abdominal radiograph.

TYPES OF ENTERAL FORMULAS. Enteral formulas can be made by blenderizing regular foods or using commercially prepared formulas. Blenderized formulas should be refrigerated and the bag hung only long enough to be infused. Baby foods can also be used for clients who will receive tube feedings indefinitely. Polymeric feedings (such as Isocal or Osmolite) are milk based or lactose free and are similar to oral supplements. They contain whole protein, long-chain fatty acids, and complex carbohydrates, and they require an intact intestine for digestion. Elemental or hydrolyzed formulas (such as Vital HN) contain short-chain peptides or amino acids for easy digestion, as well as short-chain fatty acids and simple carbohydrates. These feedings are partially digested and are used for clients with abnormal bowel function. Specialty feedings (Pulmocare, Hepatic-Aid) are designed for

Box 24-2   Modifications for Placement of a Feeding Tube

A feeding tube can be a small-bore tube designed for administration of enteral formula feedings. Feedings can be given through a Levin-type nasogastric tube, but a small-bore flexible feeding tube reduces discomfort and trauma and can thus be safely used for a longer time. To place a feeding tube, follow Procedure 24-1, with the following modifications.

EQUIPMENT

- No. 6-10 French feeding tube with or without guidewire
- 60-mL Luer-Lok or irrigation-tip syringe, as indicated, to fit the specific tube
- Cup of tap water
- Water-soluble lubricant
- pH strips
- Clean gloves

MEASURING

Measuring for gastric placement is the same as for any nasogastric tube. To place the tube in the client's duodenum, you will need at least 75 cm of tube to reach the ligament of Treitz.

LUBRICATION

Use water-soluble lubricant or moisten the surface with water. For some tubes, follow the manufacturer's directions to insert 10 mL of water into tube with a syringe to activate the lubricant.

USING A GUIDEWIRE

A guidewire is provided with small-bore feeding tubes to make the tube rigid during insertion. After you become experienced with tube placement, you may be able to place a tube without a guidewire. If you use a guidewire, insert it into the tube, make sure it fits, and make sure you can remove it easily. The guidewire must be secure to prevent damage to the GI tract.

CHECKING FOR PLACEMENT

Check for placement by x-ray with the guidewire in place. Thereafter, check for placement by determining pH of aspirate, bilirubin content, and using air instillation.

REMOVING THE GUIDEWIRE

Remove the guidewire only after the placement of the tube is confirmed. Never reinsert a guidewire after removing it unless the tube is specifically designed for reinsertion of the guidewire. Reinserting a guidewire could puncture the tube and injure the client.

USING A TOPICAL ANESTHETIC

If you used a topical anesthetic on the client's throat, test for the return of the client's gag reflex with a tongue blade when finished. The use of a topical anesthetic may be contraindicated when a client has dysphagia.

DOCUMENTATION

Document the time you inserted the tube; the type of tube inserted; the amount, color, consistency, and pH of secretions; the amount of water instilled; and the client's response.

HOME CARE

Pediatric tubes should be replaced every 2 to 6 weeks and adult tubes every 6 weeks to 3 months. Health care agencies establish differing protocols. Teach the family as follows:
- The teeth need to be brushed even though the client is taking nothing by mouth. Clean the nostrils daily and inspect for irritation or incrustations. The tape or fixator device on the nose should be changed a minimum of every 5 days. Inspect for any allergic response to the adhesive.
- Some clients can take small amounts of soft foods and swallow around the tube. The tube feeding supplements the diet.
- Maintain tube patency. Flush with water at regular intervals. Always flush before and after medications.
- If the tube becomes clogged, use a 20-mL or larger syringe half filled with water. Attempt to flush in and out. Flushing with a clear diet carbonated beverage instead of water may help unclog the tube. Keep in mind that it is possible to exert enough pressure to puncture the tube. Use caution.

---

use in specific disease situations. The latter two types of formulas are more costly than polymeric ones.

Their components can vary, but formulas usually provide about 1.0 kcal/mL along with recommended amounts of vitamins and minerals. Many formulas now have fiber added to maintain normal GI function. The osmolarity of the formula is another variable. Hyperosmolar (e.g., hydrolyzed) formulas pull water into the GI tract and can cause diarrhea. Standard formulas provide only 80% to 85% of the client's water needs, so tube-fed clients who do not have another source of fluid require additional water to meet their physiological needs.

ADMINISTRATION OF ENTERAL FEEDINGS. Initiate tube feedings slowly, especially if the client has not eaten for a period of time. Monitor the serum phosphorus level for a drop after the metabolism begins to rise. The administration of feedings through various types of tubes at different time intervals is described in Procedure 24-1. Continuous feedings are given over 24 hours. Intermittent feedings deliver no more than 250 mL of feeding over 30 minutes periodically during the day. Bolus feedings of up to 400 mL of formula are given by the nurse or client over approximately 10 to 15 minutes. Because the small intestine tolerates bolus feedings poorly, the duodenum and jejunum require continuous feedings.

The disadvantages of bolus or intermittent feedings include diarrhea and increased resting energy expenditure. The diarrhea results from an osmotic effect and is more common in older adults. The resting energy expenditure increases by 5% to 10% daily because of the fluctuation in fuel reserves with periodic feeding; it does not occur with continuous feedings. Disadvantages of continuous feedings include clogging of the tube and a lower serum protein synthesis. Clogging generally results from a slow feeding rate through a small-bore tube. Decreased protein synthesis occurs because continuous feedings increase insulin and glycogen levels, favoring the use of protein for fuel rather than tissue storage. Bolus and intermittent feeding methods are more natural and allow greater client mobility. Seriously ill clients are often fed continuously, with a goal of intermittent or bolus feedings.

| PROCEDURE 24-1 | ADMINISTERING AN ENTERAL FEEDING |

TIME TO ALLOW
Novice: 15-25 min.
Expert: 10-15 min.

Enteral feedings can be administered into the stomach, duodenum, or jejunum through a tube inserted in the client's nose or a tube implanted in the abdominal wall (gastrostomy or jejunostomy tubes). These feedings are administered on a time schedule specified in the physician's order to provide nutrition to a client who cannot eat or swallow.

DELEGATION GUIDELINES

The assessment of the client and the administration of enteral nutrition via gastric, duodenal, or jejunal tube require the expertise of a licensed nurse. The gathering and assembly of the necessary equipment and the preparation of the tube feeding formula may be delegated to a nursing assistant who has received special training in the performance of this task. You are then responsible for initiating the infusion of the enteral nutrition, and for evaluating the client's response. Institutions vary in their approach to the nursing assistant's role in delivering enteral nutrition; some allow nursing assistants to deliver tube feeding via the bolus method only. It is essential that your actions are in compliance with your institution's policies and procedures regarding delegation of this task.

EQUIPMENT NEEDED

- 60-mL syringe
- Cup of water
- Stethoscope
- Clean gloves
- Feeding pump and IV pole if feeding will be continuous
- pH tape
- Prescribed formula
- Adapter for gastrostomy or jejunostomy tube, if needed
- 4 × 4-inch gauze pads (possibly precut), nonallergenic tape, and soap to clean and dress a gastrostomy or jejunostomy tube site

1. Follow preliminary guidelines for nursing procedures (see inside front cover).

2. Make sure the client is comfortable and the room is private. Raise the head of bed to 30 to 45 degrees. *These steps help the procedure go smoothly and reduce the risk of aspiration.*

3. Assess the client.
a. Listen to bowel sounds.
b. Observe for abdominal distention or distress. *Distention and absence of bowel sounds may indicate paralytic ileus.*
c. Inquire about diarrhea or check with other assigned caregivers if client is nonverbal. *Diarrhea is not always a reaction to the tube feeding; always assess for the cause. If you detect any of these problems, report them and confirm that you should still give the feeding.*

4. Prepare for the feeding.
a. Make sure the formula is at room temperature and within its expiration date. Also check manufacturer's information because some formulas are stable after opening only for a certain time (such as 4 to 8 hours). *Cold formula can cause cramping. Formula left open too long may promote growth of microbes.*
b. Confirm placement and check for residual volume. With the tube clamped, insert a syringe into the end of the tube, unclamp the tube, and aspirate the residual fluid from the client's stomach. For a small-bore tube, use a

10-mL syringe. For a large-bore tube, use a 60-mL syringe. Return the gastric aspirate to the stomach. *If the client has more than 150 mL of fluid or one half of the previous hour's feeding in the stomach, withhold the feeding. Remember that a jejunostomy tube typically has the smallest residual volume.*
c. Test the pH of the gastric fluid.

5. Flush with water. Remove the plunger from the irrigating syringe, and insert the barrel into the end of the tube. The barrel is then used as a funnel to pour the water through. For small-bore tubes, the water is injected slowly with a syringe. *Flushing with water helps keep the tube patent and prevents stomach acid from clumping the formula.*

6. To give a bolus feeding with a syringe, follow these steps:
a. Using the barrel of the syringe as a funnel, add formula until it nearly fills the syringe. *Feedings flow by gravity and may take up to 15 minutes.*
b. When the syringe is almost empty, refill it with formula until the total amount has been instilled. *By refilling the syringe before it empties, you avoid instilling air into the tube. Do not force feedings by using the plunger, because the client will be at increased risk for aspiration, diarrhea, and bloating.*
c. Instill 50 mL water after the feeding is complete (or other amount as ordered by physician). *Instilling water helps to avoid clogging in the tube.*

Continued

PROCEDURE 24-1 ADMINISTERING AN ENTERAL FEEDING—CONT'D

d. Clamp the tube.

e. Remove the syringe, wash it with tap water, and store it for future use.

f. Cover the end of the tube with clean gauze.

7. To give an intermittent feeding with a bag and tubing, follow these steps:

a. After instilling water into the tube in Step 5 clamp the tube and attach the feeding tube.

b. Fill the feeding bag with the prescribed amount of formula and prime the tubing.

c. Hang the feeding bag on an IV stand.

d. Unclamp the feeding tube.

e. Regulate the flow so the formula is instilled over 20 minutes.

f. When formula has finished flowing, clamp the tube and remove the feeding bag. Instill 50 mL water into the feeding tube.

g. Wash out the feeding bag with tap water and store it for future use. *Hints: Change the bag and tubing every 24 hours, or according to agency policy, to avoid bacterial contamination. Fresh formula should be hung after 4 to 8 hours. Consult agency policy.*

h. When hanging a new feeding bag, label it with the time, the date, and your initials.

8. To give a continuous feeding, follow steps 1 through 7 but use an infusion pump (see illustration) to regulate the flow of formula. *The infusion pump ensures a regular rate.*

a. Thread the tubing from the feeding bag through the infusion pump. *Read manufacturer's pump instructions because they vary.*

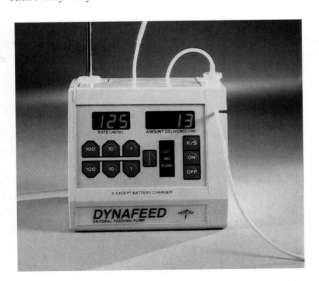

Step 8. Feeding infusion pump. (Courtesy Medline Industries, Mundelein, IL.)

b. Set the infusion pump at the prescribed rate.

9. If you need to give a medication through a nasogastric tube, make sure it is available in liquid form or can be finely crushed. *Medication that is not crushed finely enough could clog the tube.*

10. If necessary, clean and dress the entrance site of a gastrostomy or jejunostomy tube. *Most clients do not require a dressing over the site. If leaking gastric acid is a problem, a hydrocolloid dressing will protect the skin.*

a. Use clean technique to clean the entrance site unless the client is in the immediate postoperative period. Use soap and water to remove all leakage of gastric contents and crusty drainage. Dry the area well. *Using careful cleaning technique and teaching the client thoroughly about cleaning these long-term feeding tubes can help avoid problems and the need for surgical replacement.*

b. Observe for and report any unusual drainage (thick, green, yellow, or foul-smelling), redness, puffiness, or pain at the site.

c. To dress the site, use a precut 4 × 4-inch gauze pad, or make a cut to the middle of a pad. Place the pad around the tube so the tube protrudes from the middle of the pad and use nonallergenic tape to affix the pad in place.

11. Monitor the client.

a. Make sure the tube is taped securely to the client's nose and pinned safely to the gown when you finish with the feeding.

b. Assess the client for gastric distress, distention, cramping, and diarrhea.

12. Tidy the client's environment and discard any used materials. Discard your gloves and perform hand hygiene.

13. Document the amount and type of feeding delivered on an intake and output sheet, the time of the feeding, your assessment findings, residual gastric contents and its pH, and the client's daily weight.

HOME CARE CONSIDERATIONS

Teach family caregivers to administer feedings. Include feeding technique, cleaning and storing equipment, preventing and managing complications, skin care, and monitoring nutritional status.

Regardless of the method used, always ensure correct tube placement and the presence of bowel sounds before giving a feeding. Raise the head of the bed as much as the client can tolerate and keep it elevated for 30 minutes after a bolus or intermittent feeding.

When administering enteral feedings using a feeding bag, perform good hand hygiene to prevent bacterial contamination. Change the bag and tubing as indicated by agency policy, usually every 24 hours. Identify on the bag the date and time it was hung.

COMPLICATIONS OF ENTERAL FEEDINGS. It is very important to monitor any client receiving tube feedings to prevent or minimize complications (Box 24-3). As discussed previously, the most dreaded complication of tube feedings is aspiration. To minimize it, follow the procedures described for confirming tube placement. Check residual volume before giving the feeding, or at least every 4 hours. If the residuals are greater than 150 mL (or 10% to 20% over the hourly flow rate), withhold the feeding. Assess the client's respiratory status at least every shift and note any changes. If a blue dye is added to the feedings and the client's respiratory secretions become blue, stop the feedings immediately because aspiration has occurred.

To prevent clogging of a feeding tube, flush the tube with water before and after giving all feedings and medications. Flush also when adding new formula or at least every 4 hours (even when not in use) to avoid obstruction. Record the amount of water used to flush the tube on the client's intake and output record. If the client is on fluid restriction, consult with the nutrition support team about methods to keep the tube patent. Medications given through the tube should be in liquid form if at all possible. Even finely crushed medications clog small-bore nasoenteric tubes. If the medication is not available in liquid form, dissolve the finely crushed pill in warm water. Enteric-coated tablets should not be given through enteral tubes because crushing the pills circumvents the coating.

If the tube does occlude, various methods can be used to reopen it. Flushing with very warm water is currently the most acceptable method (Brennan, 1998). Pancreatic enzyme or sodium bicarbonate crushed in 5 mL of water may be helpful. Some sources suggest the use of meat tenderizer, cola, or cranberry juice, but others discourage their use. The best treatment is prevention with adequate flushing.

Diarrhea can result from hyperosmolar feedings, medications, or bacterial contamination of the feeding. Assess the cause of diarrhea carefully rather than simply stopping the feeding, decreasing the rate, or diluting the formula. Send a stool specimen and evaluate all medications, especially laxatives and those containing sorbitol elixirs or magnesium.

If the feeding itself is causing the diarrhea, the rate can be lowered, although doing so also lowers calorie intake. Once the problem is resolved, the rate should be gradually increased as tolerated. The formula may also be changed to one that is more elemental or has a lower osmolality. Antidiarrheal medication can be given for symptom management while the cause is treated.

Box 24-3 Monitoring Clients Receiving Tube Feedings

- Measure residual gastric contents every 4 hours. If the amount is greater than half the feeding given in the last 4 hours, stop the feeding, assess the abdomen, and consult the physician.
- Weigh the client daily to detect fluid retention; weekly to detect actual weight gain.
- Assess for signs of edema daily.
- Assess for signs of dehydration daily.
- Obtain fingerstick glucose readings daily.
- Assess intake and output daily.
- Record stool output daily.
- Assess calorie, protein, fat, mineral, and vitamin intake twice weekly.
- Check serum electrolytes, serum phosphorus, blood urea nitrogen, creatinine, and complete blood count two or three times weekly (by physician's order).
- Obtain a chemistry profile weekly (by physician's order).
- Check nitrogen balance weekly (optional).

Other complications that can occur during enteral nutrition include infection at the ostomy site, nausea and vomiting, hyperglycemia, and tube dislodgment. Continually assess the skin around a gastrostomy or jejunostomy site for infection. If the client is nauseated, stop the feeding and report the finding. Nausea and vomiting can stem from contaminated formula or feeding bag or from completely unrelated factors. Perform fingerstick glucose readings daily. If the tube becomes dislodged or clogged beyond repair, it must be replaced.

HOME ENTERAL NUTRITION. Shortening of hospital stays has escalated the number of clients receiving enteral nutrition at home. Adequate home care, professional and family support, and teaching are needed for this to be effective. Box 24-4 (p. 554) describes how to teach a family caregiver to provide home enteral nutrition.

General training for caregivers should include stoma assessment and monitoring of devices. Analysis of associated costs should be ongoing. For example, could the client use syringe feeding rather than an infusion pump and feeding bags? Will the results of future nursing research show that feeding tube bags used in the home can be safely changed less frequently than every 24 hours?

Parenteral Nutrition. **Parenteral nutrition** is the provision of total nutrition through a central or peripheral intravenous catheter. When a central vein (such as the subclavian) is used, this procedure is known as total parenteral nutrition (TPN), hyperalimentation, or central venous nutrition. Sometimes, parenteral nutrition is given in a smaller peripheral vein in an extremity (McConnell, 1998). It is then called peripheral parenteral nutrition (PPN). This peripheral approach is being used more widely for hospitalized clients who need parenteral nutrition for less than 14 days. Parenteral nutrition is indicated for any client who does not have a functional GI tract for an extended period of time.

ADMINISTRATION OF PARENTERAL NUTRITION. Most clients receive continuous parenteral nutrition; however, some clients in the home setting receive cyclic feedings on a

Box 24-4

Teaching for Wellness
Home Enteral Nutrition

Purpose: To teach a client or family member to deliver feedings through a gastrostomy tube and to care for the tube properly.

Expected Outcome: The client or a family member will be able to successfully feed the client through a gastrostomy tube and will prevent infection at the entrance site.

Client Instructions

Giving a Feeding

1. If your feeding formula is refrigerated, allow it to come to room temperature before using it, because cold feeding formula can cause cramping.
2. Perform hand hygiene and put on clean gloves.
3. If your doctor wants you to, check for residual gastric contents before delivering a feeding. To do so, insert a syringe into the tube, unclamp the tube, and use the plunger to remove and measure the volume of gastric secretions. If the amount of residual contents is too great, you may have to withhold the feeding for a while.
4. Measure the prescribed amount of feeding formula.
5. After removing the plunger from a 60-mL syringe, insert the syringe into the end of the tube.
6. Unclamp the tube.
7. Pour enough of the formula into the syringe to nearly fill the syringe. If you unclamp the tube before inserting the syringe, gastric contents may leak out.
8. When the syringe is still about a quarter full, refill it with formula. Refilling before the syringe is empty will prevent air from entering the tube.
9. After instilling all of the formula, flush the syringe and tube with about 60 mL of water.
10. Before removing the syringe from the tube, clamp the tube. Clamping the tube keeps gastric contents from leaking out.
11. Expect this entire process to take about 15 minutes.
12. Wash the syringe after each feeding and change syringes daily.
13. Store the formula according to the package directions.

Caring for the Gastrostomy Site

1. To clean the area where the tube enters your skin, use a washcloth or a 4 × 4-inch gauze pad. Wet it with warm, soapy water and clean around the site. Rinse with clear water and dry thoroughly with a soft towel.
2. Usually, a gastrostomy tube needs no dressing. If your doctor tells you to use one, use a precut 2 × 2-inch gauze pad or use scissors to cut to the middle of the pad. Slide the slit in the pad over the tube so that the tube protrudes from the middle of the pad. Affix the pad in place with nonallergenic tape.
3. Tell your doctor right away if you notice redness, swelling, abnormal drainage (thick, foul smelling, yellow or green), or pain at the tube's entrance site. Also report any abdominal pain, bloating, cramping, or diarrhea.

12- to 18-hour cycle to increase their quality of life. Often, they receive feedings at night so that they can be mobile during the day.

Initiate parenteral nutrition slowly to avoid the refeeding syndrome. A suggested regimen is to start the feedings at 42 mL/hour or 1000 mL/day, and then increase slowly over a 2- to 3-day period. Watch for changes in serum glucose, potassium, magnesium, and calcium levels caused by increased cellular metabolism of these nutrients. Assess for both cellular dehydration and signs of heart failure, because the hyperosmolar serum attracts water from cells. Box 24-5 has recommendations for monitoring a client receiving parenteral nutrition.

Procedure 24-2 describes administering parenteral nutrition through a central line. Ongoing site care is especially important because the client is at risk for infection at the site and in the bloodstream (sepsis). Sepsis is a life-threatening complication with a high mortality rate.

Change the client's central catheter dressing at least every 72 hours—more often if facility policy dictates or if the dressing is wet or no longer occlusive. There is controversy about the correct technique for this dressing change, but generally it includes the use of sterile technique (including sterile gloves and masks) in the hospital setting to avoid nosocomial infection. In the home, clients can use clean technique when changing their own dressing. Most hospitals use transparent polyurethane dressings. The catheter site is scrubbed with an antiseptic, such as povidone-iodine. Some clinicians use an antiseptic ointment at the site as well, but current recommen-

Box 24-5 Monitoring a Client Receiving Parenteral Nutrition

To monitor the nutritional status of a client receiving parenteral nutrition, make sure to complete the following steps. You may need to measure some values more frequently than shown here until the client stabilizes.

GROWTH VARIABLES

- Weigh the client daily.
- Measure an infant's head circumference weekly.
- Measure an infant's length weekly.

METABOLIC VARIABLES

- Assess for signs of edema or dehydration daily.
- Obtain fingerstick glucose levels daily or as ordered.
- Assess intake and output daily.
- Assess calorie, fat, protein, carbohydrate, vitamin, and mineral intake twice weekly.
- Check serum sodium, potassium, chloride, CO_2, phosphorus, blood urea nitrogen, creatinine, and triglycerides twice weekly.
- Assess complete blood count, prothrombin time, albumin, calcium, magnesium, copper, zinc, and liver function tests weekly.
- Obtain a urinalysis weekly.
- Check nitrogen balance weekly (optional).

---

dations from the Centers for Disease Control and Prevention are not to use such an ointment. If used with a transparent dressing, the amount should be small because the dressings are designed to adhere to the skin and promote visualization of the site.

| PROCEDURE 24-2 | ADMINISTERING PARENTERAL NUTRITION THROUGH A CENTRAL LINE |

TIME TO ALLOW
Novice: 20 min.
Expert: 10 min.

Parenteral nutrition is administered to provide fluids and balanced nutrition to a client who cannot eat and who cannot receive such nutrition via the GI tract. Total parenteral nutrition is infused into either a central or a peripheral vein according to a physician's order. This procedure describes using a central line.

DELEGATION GUIDELINES

The assembly of the necessary equipment to perform this procedure may be delegated to a licensed practical or vocational nurse or nursing assistant. The verification of the solution with the physician's order, preparation of the tubing and catheter, and initiation of the infusion are your responsibility and may not be delegated.

EQUIPMENT NEEDED

- Prescribed infusion
- IV tubing with extension tubing
- 0.22-μm filter (or 1.2-μm filter if solution contains lipids or albumin)
- Alcohol sponges
- Infusion pump
- Sterile dressing package
- Labels
- Clean gloves
- Sterile gloves

1. Follow preliminary guidelines for nursing procedures (see inside front cover).

2. Confirm the physician's order and check it against the listed ingredients. *Parenteral nutrition usually requires special physician orders that are written daily, specifying all ingredients and the rate of infusion.*

3. Check the solution.
a. Remove the solution from the refrigerator at least 1 hour before using it.
b. Observe the solution for cloudiness, turbidity, particles, or cracks in the container.
c. If the solution has a brown layer, return it to the pharmacy, because the lipid emulsion has separated from the solution.

4. Assess the client.
a. Know client's potassium, phosphorus, and glucose values. *Glucose and electrolyte values can change dramatically on parenteral nutrition.*
b. Look for any signs of inflammation or swelling at the infusion site.
c. Assess the client's frame of mind and, to ease any fears, reassure that the procedure is not painful. *Clients associate eating with positive feelings and may be upset by not being able to eat.*

5. Prepare the tubing in the infusion pump.
a. Connect tubing, extension tubing, and filter. *Place the filter close to the client.*

b. If the tubing does not have Luer-Lok connections, tape all connections. *Accidental separation of IV tubing could cause air embolism or infection.*
c. Prime the tubing and clamp it.
d. Thread the tubing through the infusion pump.
e. Time and date the IV tubing. *The tubing should be changed every 24 hours or according to your facility's policy.*

6. Prepare the central line catheter.
a. Flush the catheter, according to your facility's policy, with saline.
b. Put on sterile gloves. *Asepsis at the site (see illustration) prevents infection.*

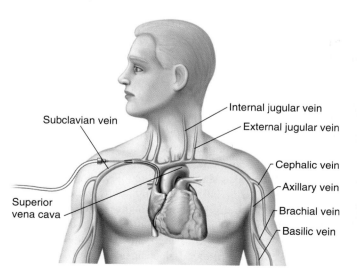

Step 6b. Infusion site for parenteral nutrition through a central line.

PROCEDURE 24-2	ADMINISTERING PARENTERAL NUTRITION THROUGH A CENTRAL LINE—CONT'D

c. Clean the catheter cap with alcohol.

d. Using aseptic technique, insert the needle into the injection cap.

e. Unclamp the tubing.

7. Set the infusion pump at the prescribed rate. Start the flow slowly and monitor the rate carefully.

8. Do not use a single-lumen central line to infuse blood or draw blood. Also, if possible, avoid giving any IV medication during parenteral nutrition. Before adding a piggyback medication to parenteral nutrition, check with the pharmacist to make sure it is compatible. Never add a medication to a parenteral nutrition solution.

9. Monitor and document the client's vital signs, laboratory values (including electrolytes), vital signs, glucose levels, daily weight, urine output, and catheter site. Use sterile technique for dressing changes. *Continued assessment is essential because extravasation of the solution can cause tissue necrosis.*

10. Document the type of solution used, the time and date the bag was hung, the client's response, and the amount of solution added on the intake and output sheet.

HINT

If for any reason you must remove the gummed rubber cap from the central line, *be absolutely sure* the catheter is clamped or the client is performing the Valsalva maneuver. Otherwise, the negative intrathoracic pressure can draw air into the vein, leading to air embolism in a pulmonary artery.

COMPOSITION OF PARENTERAL NUTRITION. Various combinations of protein, fat emulsions, and carbohydrates are used to meet clients' energy needs. The dextrose concentration of parenteral nutrition given through a central vein can vary from 5% to 70%, but it is usually 25%. The dextrose concentration and osmolality of PPN is usually limited to 10% to avoid irritation of vessel walls.

Protein is given in ranges from 3% to 15%. Fat emulsions of 10% or 20% are given to avoid fatty acid deficiency. An all-in-one mixture includes lipids, protein, and carbohydrate and helps to reduce solution osmolarity. Nutrition given through a central vein often includes the carbohydrate and protein in one bag and the fat emulsion in another. Vitamin and mineral contents are slightly lower than the recommended daily amount because they do not undergo digestive processes. The client's fluid needs are calculated and factored into the solution requirements.

COMPLICATIONS OF PARENTERAL NUTRITION. Refeeding syndrome is an important complication of parenteral nutrition. Assess for a drop in serum phosphorus level, which can cause a weakened diaphragm and respiratory failure. Hyperosmolar fluids can cause extracellular fluid overload and pulmonary edema or heart failure. Listen to the client's lungs for crackles and watch the urine output carefully. If the urine output increases significantly, the flow rate may be too fast or erratic. Use an infusion pump to deliver the TPN, and do not try to "catch up" if the infusion has fallen behind.

Obtain fingerstick glucose levels at least daily because hyperglycemia can result from high glucose loads (see Box 24-6 for an overview of blood glucose monitoring). Insulin is sometimes added to the solution or given on a sliding scale as needed. TPN should be discontinued slowly because the client could experience rebound hypoglycemia if it is stopped abruptly.

Infection is a major complication of parenteral nutrition. One of the first signs of sepsis is glucose intolerance. Others include fever or hypothermia, shaking chills, hypotension, and tachycardia. A significant advantage of PPN is that infection, if it occurs, is local rather than systemic. The signs include pain, redness, edema, and warmth at the site.

Some clients react to lipid emulsions. Adverse reactions include fever, chills, vomiting, and pain in the chest or back. A milder symptom is an itchy skin rash. Alert the nutrition support team if these reactions occur. Lipid overload is accompanied by increased triglyceride levels, an enlarged liver, and altered liver function test results. Lipid emulsions are usually discontinued if these reactions occur.

HOME PARENTERAL NUTRITION. Information about home care for clients receiving parenteral nutrition is found in Box 24-7. This therapy is often quite successful with proper professional support to monitor for potential complications and provide information to clients and caregivers (Gorski, 2001).

Interventions to Manage *Impaired Swallowing*

Positioning the Client. The position that best facilitates swallowing is 90-degree flexion at the hips and 45-degree flexion at the neck. Have the client sit as upright as possible and remain there for at least 30 minutes after eating.

If the client has partial paralysis (as from a stroke), rotate the chin toward the weaker side to improve swallowing. Encourage neck flexion to enhance the pharyngeal phase of swallowing and facilitate closure of the glottis. Place food in the unaffected side of the mouth for optimal control.

You can also enhance the swallowing reflex by using an ice collar or by brushing the client's neck with a small brush, such as a small paint brush, just before he eats. Place food behind the client's front teeth and instruct him to tilt his head before swallowing.

Teaching for Self-Care
Blood Glucose Monitoring

Box 24-6

Purpose: Blood glucose monitoring is useful whenever a client is at risk for hyperglycemia or hypoglycemia or to monitor the effects of insulin therapy.

Expected Outcome: The client will demonstrate correctly the ability to measure capillary blood glucose and read and record the results accurately.

Client Instructions

- Assess the skin of the area to be used for puncture (most frequently fingers). Avoid areas with ecchymosis (bruising) or that are broken (open).
- Gather all necessary equipment: glucose meter, reagent strip, sterile lancet or autolet device, alcohol or povidone-iodine swab, and cotton ball. Although health care providers wear clean disposable gloves, it is unnecessary for a client to wear them for self-testing.
- Wash hands with soap and warm water. Assume a comfortable position, such as sitting in a chair.
- Remove the reagent strip from the container, being sure to handle it according to the manufacturer's directions. Place it on a clean, dry surface.
- Select the finger to be punctured, and massage it gently while holding it in a dependent (downward) position to increase circulation to the area.
- Wipe the site with alcohol or povidone iodine swab and allow it to dry completely.

- Remove the cover of the lancet or autolet device; hold the lancet perpendicular to the side of the finger and pierce the skin quickly; if an autolet is used, push the release button to trigger the puncture.
- Use the cotton ball to wipe away the first drop of blood; gently squeeze or massage the skin toward the puncture site to obtain a large drop of blood.
- According to manufacturer's directions, either allow the blood to drop onto the reagent pad or touch the drop of blood onto the pad; in either case, the blood should cover the pad completely. Be sure not to smear the blood.
- If indicated by manufacturer, begin the timer on the meter and wipe the blood from the test strip after the specified amount of time; note that all meters do not require this.
- According to manufacturer's directions, place the reagent strip into the glucose testing meter. Read the results after waiting the specified period of time.
- Remove the reagent strip from the meter, turn off the meter, and dispose of used equipment.
- Record the results per primary care provider directions and store the meter for future use.

Box 24-7 Home Care for Clients Receiving Parenteral Nutrition

ASSESS

- Confirm the physician's order. (Will the parenteral nutrition be given only at night or also during the day? For what length of time will the client need it?)
- Does the client have a support system, such as family?
- What motivation level do the client and family have?
- Can client and family understand the complexities of parenteral nutrition?
- Do the client and family have adequate financial resources to maintain safe, accurate therapy? (Consult a social worker about solving financial problems.)
- Is the client mobile? (If so, consider suggesting that the client wear a lightweight vest with large pockets to hold parenteral nutrition supplies if feedings will occur during the day.)
- What safety problems are present in the client's home?
- Does the client have access to nursing services or a hospital?

TEACH

- Find a quiet space where the client and family can concentrate.
- Include family in all teaching sessions.
- Because the material is complex and important, begin with simple content and use drawings or models as needed. For example, use a teddy bear with a central line site to show procedures.

- Make sure to fully teach the following concepts:
  1. Strict hand-hygiene techniques
  2. How to hang the solution
  3. Setting the feeding rate (operating an infusion pump)
  4. Cleaning the site and changing the dressing
  5. Flushing the catheter
  6. Taking fingerstick glucose readings, if needed
  7. Which problems to report, such as redness, swelling, drainage, or pain at the site; fever; inability to flush the catheter; shortness of breath; increased urinary output; hyperglycemia; chest pain
- When teaching procedures, avoid placing time limits on the client or family members, because manual dexterity can vary from client to client.
- Provide written handouts with specific directions, important adverse responses, and actions to take.
- Provide client with list of phone numbers for reporting problems.

EVALUATE

- Ask the client (and family) to give you a return demonstration of cleaning the site, changing the dressing, and hanging the solution.
- Have the client or a family member keep a record of the amount of parenteral nutrition taken in a 24-hour period and any abnormal responses or symptoms that develop.

Encouraging Appropriate Foods. Certain foods are easier to swallow than others (Box 24-8, p. 558). Thin liquids are the most difficult for clients with dysphagia to handle (Yen, 1998a). Liquids require greater oral coordination and finer motor movements of the swallowing muscles. Dysphagic clients should never "wash food down" with liquids. Fluid requirements for clients with dysphagia must be met with fluids that are thickened with potato flakes, corn starch, fruit, or commercial products.

Box 24-8 Comparing Easy-to-Swallow and Hard-to-Swallow Foods

EASY TO SWALLOW	HARD TO SWALLOW
Warm or cold foods	Lukewarm foods
Flavorful foods (salted or mildly sweetened)	Bland foods
Thickened liquids	Thin liquids and milk
Sauces and gravies	Foods that fall apart (such as peas or rice)
	Pureed foods, which do not stimulate swallowing
Moist pastas, casseroles, egg dishes	Slippery foods, sticky or bulky foods
Blenderized soups	Foods with combination of textures, such as chunky soups

Flavorful foods that are either warm or cold stimulate the swallowing reflex better than bland, lukewarm foods. Flavoring also stimulates the flow of saliva. Sauces and gravies are good choices because they are flavorful and they lubricate food. Fragmented foods, such as corn kernels, peas, rice, and ground meat, are easily aspirated and should be moistened. Moist pastas, casseroles, and egg dishes are good choices for dysphagic clients.

Milk seems to stimulate thick mucus production and should be used cautiously with clients who have excessive phlegm or drooling. The client can drink milk if it is followed by thickened liquids to flush the throat (Mahan & Escott-Stump, 2000).

Pureed foods are not tolerated as well as textured foods because they fail to stimulate swallowing. Sticky foods (such as peanut butter) or bulky foods (such as raw fruits and vegetables) are also more difficult to swallow and should be avoided. Foods with a combination of textures should also be avoided because they are difficult to control. These include chunky soups, although blenderized soups are good.

Interventions to Reduce *Risk for Aspiration*

Many interventions for *Risk for aspiration* have already been discussed, since two major risks for aspiration are impaired swallowing and enteral feedings. Carefully monitor clients because silent aspiration may produce only subtle cues, such as change in

respiratory rate, temperature, breath sounds, or oxygen saturation levels. To check the swallowing reflex, put 3 mL of water on the client's tongue. The swallow reflex should be initiated within 1 second. If it is delayed or absent after three attempts, have the client evaluated (Thelan, Urden, Lough, & Stacy, 1998). Also assess the client's bowel sounds and check for abdominal distention that could indicate increased gastric residual volume. Keep the client's head positioned at a 30-degree angle. If the head cannot be elevated, place the client in a right lateral position to facilitate gastric emptying.

Also, suction oral secretions to keep the oropharynx patent. Treat nausea to prevent vomiting. The physician may order gastric secretion inhibitors to decrease gastric acidity and limit chemical burns to the lungs (Thelan, Urden, Lough, & Stacy, 1998).

EVALUATION

During evaluation, determine if the plan and interventions were successful in achieving the established outcome criteria, as outlined in Box 24-9. Remember, evaluation is an assessment of what actually happened, not what you expected to happen. If goals are not met, revise the plan with new outcome criteria and interventions, and reevaluate the client. Document an evaluation of how well the expected outcomes were met.

A partial documentation note for Mrs. Goldman at a 1-month follow-up visit might look like the one below.

SAMPLE DOCUMENTATION NOTE FOR MRS. GOLDMAN

Weight 116 lb, increased from 115 lb 1 month ago. Serum albumin 2.8 mg/dL, up from 2.7 mg/dL 1 month ago. Goals of 117 lb for weight and 3.0 mg/dL serum albumin level not yet met, although progress has been made.

 How might you revise the interventions? What intervening variables might have interfered with Mrs. Goldman's reaching her goals? What would you add to the documentation note to reflect the changes you would make in the plan of care?

Nursing Care Plan **A CLIENT WITH INADEQUATE NUTRITIONAL INTAKE DURING CHEMOTHERAPY**   Box 24-9

OUTPATIENT CLINIC DATA

Mrs. Goldman is halfway through her 6 months of chemotherapy. She uses prochlorperazine (Compazine) for nausea for 3 days after her treatments, has experienced a 25-pound weight loss, and has signs of depression.

PHYSICIAN'S ORDERS

Assist with diet planning to maintain ideal body weight.

NURSING ASSESSMENT

Client is 54 years old, is 5'4" tall, and weighs 115 pounds. Adheres to a kosher diet. Reports weighing 140 pounds before chemotherapy; weight/IBW = 95%; energy needs from Harris-Benedict equation plus 10% for activity = 2000 calories; serum albumin 3.0 g/dl; hemoglobin 11.5 g/dl and hematocrit 32%; client describes feeling fatigued and has decreased interest in eating. Client is concerned about recent weight loss.

Nursing Care Plan **A Client With Inadequate Nutritional Intake During Chemotherapy—cont'd**   Box 24-9

NANDA Nursing Diagnosis	NOC Expected Outcomes With Indicators	NIC Interventions With Selected Activities	Evaluation Data
IMBALANCED NUTRITION: LESS THAN BODY REQUIREMENTS **Related Factors:** • A 25-lb weight loss • Nausea	**WEIGHT CONTROL** • Weight gain of at least 2 pounds in 1 month. • Eats at least 2000 calories daily.	**WEIGHT GAIN ASSISTANCE** • Offer choices of good-tasting protein supplements to be taken between meals. • Have client keep a calorie diary; consider sugggesting zinc for increasing taste.	**AFTER 1 MONTH OF CARE** • Weight has increased by 1 lb. Reports that supplement is nauseating. • Client reports that she has been eating better and has kept a record of her food intake. Eating 1500 calories.
	NUTRITIONAL STATUS • Increase in hemoglobin and hematocrit by 1 month. • Increase in albumin by 3 weeks. • Decreased fatigue in 1 month.	**NUTRITIONAL MONITORING** • Include a source of iron in diet. Select culturally agreeable foods. • Select high-protein foods that are culturally agreeable. • Establish a contract with client to engage in one pleasurable activity a day. Limit rest periods to one or two per day.	• Hemoglobin and hematocrit show moderate increase after 1 month. • Albumin has begun to slowly increase by 3 weeks. • Has increased number of pleasurable activities. Takes an afternoon nap. Otherwise engages in light activities. Reports that fatigue has improved.

Critical Thinking Questions

1. How frequently does Mrs. Goldman need follow-up once her nutritional status stabilizes?
2. Who is the most desirable member of the health care team to provide this follow-up?
3. What further dietary teaching might be needed if current interventions are not successful?

Nursing outcome and intervention labels from Johnson, M., Bulechek, G., McCloskey Dochterman, J. M., Maas, M., & Moorhead, S. (2001). *Nursing diagnoses, outcomes and interventions: NANDA, NIC and NOC linkages.* St Louis, MO: Mosby.

Key Principles

• Nutrition inadequate to meet the body's needs results from energy needs that exceed the amount taken in and may have many physical and psychological causes.
• Impaired swallowing typically results from neuromuscular problems or a decreased level of consciousness.
• The risk for aspiration is high in clients who receive tube feedings, are intubated, or have decreased consciousness or impaired swallowing.
• There is no single marker for nutritional problems. To detect it, you must review the collected assessment data. Unintentional loss of 10% of body weight within a 6-month period is a red flag for *Imbalanced nutrition: less than body requirements.*
• *Impaired swallowing* can be definitively diagnosed with evidence of aspiration.

• Refeeding of malnourished clients must be done carefully to prevent serious metabolic complications.
• Enteral feeding is a major risk factor for aspiration.
• When making a differential diagnosis for nutritional problems, choose the diagnosis that will best focus care on the client's most immediate needs.
• Interventions for nutritional problems require a team approach, whether carried out in the client's home or in the clinic, hospital, or other health care setting.
• Parenteral and enteral nutritional support includes specialized nursing procedures important for clients with *Imbalanced nutrition: less than body requirements.*
• Interventions for *Impaired swallowing* focus on providing foods and techniques that will encourage the swallow reflex, and on preventing aspiration.

- When evaluating outcome criteria for *Imbalanced nutrition: less than body requirements,* expect a weight gain of at least 2 lb/month; a weight gain of 1 lb/day or more indicates fluid gain.

Bibliography

American Psychiatric Association. (2000). *Diagnostic and statistical manual of mental disorders, ed 4, text Revision.* Washington, DC: Author.

ASPEN Board of Directors & The Clinical Guidelines Taskforce. (2002). Guidelines for the use of parenteral and enteral nutrition in adult and pediatric patients. *Journal of Parenteral and Enteral Nutrition, 26*(1), Supplement.

Ayello, E., Thomas, D., & Litchford, M. (1999). Wound care 1999. Nutritional aspects of wound healing. *Home Healthcare Nurse, 17*(11), 719-730.

Bliss, D., & Lehmann, S. (1999). Tube feeding: Administration tips. *RN 62*(8), 29-32.

Brennan, K. (1998). Going with the flow. *Nursing, 28*(4), 54-55.

Case, K. O., Cuddy, P. G., & McGurk, E. P. (2000). Nutrition support in critically ill patients. *Critical Care Nursing Quarterly, 22*(4), 75-89.

*Clevenger, F., & Rodriguez, D. (1995). Decision-making for enteral feeding administration: The why behind where and how. *Nutrition in Clinical Practice, 10*(3), 104-113.

Cole, L. (1999). Early enteral feeding after surgery. *Critical Care Nursing Clinics of North America, 11*(2), 227-231.

*DeLegge, M. (1996). Continuous vs. intermittent feedings: Slow and steady or fast and furious? *Current issues in enteral nutrition support: Report of the first Ross conference on enteral devices* (pp. 50-53). Columbus, OH: Ross Products Division, Abbott Laboratories.

Dudek, S. G. (2000). Malnutrition in hospitals: Who's assessing what patients eat? *American Journal of Nursing, 100*(4), 36-43.

*Duh, Q. (1996). Decision tree for route of enteral nutrition support: Placement techniques. *Current issues in enteral nutrition support: Report of the first Ross conference on enteral devices* (pp. 9-16). Columbus, OH: Ross Products Division, Abbott Laboratories.

Ellett, M. L., Maahs, J., & Farsee, S. (1998). Prevalence of feeding tube placement errors and associated risk factors in children. *American Journal of Maternal/Child Nursing, 23*(5), 234.

Gorski, L. A. (2001). TPN update: making each visit count. *Home Healthcare Nurse, 19*(1), 15-22.

Grodner, M., Anderson, S., & Young, S. (2000). *Foundations and clinical applications of nutrition: A nursing approach* (2nd ed.). St Louis, MO: Mosby.

Hamilton, S. (2001). Detecting dehydration and malnutrition in the elderly. *Nursing 2001, 31*(12), 56-57.

Johnson, M., Bulechek, G., McCloskey Dochterman, J. M., Maas, M., & Moorhead, S. (2001). *Nursing diagnoses, outcomes, and interventions: NANDA, NIC and NOC linkages.* St Louis, MO: Mosby.

*Kohn, C. (1991). The relationship between enteral formula contamination and length of enteral delivery set usage. *Journal of Parenteral and Enteral Nutrition, 15*(5), 567-571.

Kohn-Keeth, C. (2000). How to keep feeding tubes flowing freely. *Nursing, 30*(3), 58-59.

*Lemoyne, M. & Jeejeebhoy, K. N. (1985). Total parenteral nutrition in the critically ill patient. *Chest, 89*(4), 563-569.

Livingston, A., Seamons, C., & Dalton, T. (2000). If the gut works use it. *Nursing Management, 31*(5, part 1), 39-42.

Loan, T., Magnuson, B., & Williams, S. (1998). Debunking six myths about enteral feeding. *Nursing, 28*(8), 43-48.

Mackin, D. (1997). How to manage PICCs. *American Journal of Nursing, 97*(9), 27.

Mahan, K., & Escott-Stump, S. (2000). *Krause's food, nutrition, & diet therapy* (10th ed.). Philadelphia: Saunders.

*Marian, M. (1993). Pediatric nutrition support. *Nutrition in Clinical Practice, 8*(5), 199-209.

McConnell, M. E. A. (1998). Clinical do's and don'ts: Administering parenteral nutrition. *Nursing, 28*(7), 18.

*Metheny, N. (1993). Minimizing respiratory complications of nasoenteric tube feedings: State of the science. *Heart & Lung, 22,* 213-223.

Metheny, N. (1998). pH, color and feeding tubes. *RN, 61*(1), 25-27.

Metheny, N., & Titler, M. (2001). Assessing placement of feeding tubes. *American Journal of Nursing, 101*(5), 36-46.

Metheny, N., Wehrle, M., Wiersema, L., & Clark, J. (1998). Testing tube placement: Auscultation vs. pH method. *American Journal of Nursing, 98*(5), 37.

Metheny, N., Wehrle, M., Wiersema, L., & Clark, J. (1999). pH and concentration of bilirubin in feeding tube aspirates as predictors of tube placement. *Nursing Research, 48*(4), 189-197.

Metheny, N., et al. (1999). Verification of feeding tube placement. *Current issues in enteral nutrition support: Report of the first Ross conference on enteral devices* (pp. 34-41). Columbus, OH: Ross Products Division, Abbott Laboratories.

Thelan, L., Urden, L., Lough, M., & Stacy, K. (1998). *Textbook of critical care nursing: Diagnosis and management* (3rd ed.). St Louis, MO: Mosby.

Vogelzang, J. L. (1998). Nutrition in home care. Effective use of a registered dietician in home healthcare. *Home Healthcare Nurse, 16*(10), 709-712.

*Welch, S. (1996). Certification of staff nurses to insert enteral feeding tubes using a research-based procedure. *Nutrition in Clinical Practice, 11*(1), 21-27.

Wilkes, G. (2000). Nutrition: The forgotten ingredient in cancer care. *American Journal of Nursing, 100*(4), 46-51.

Williams, S. (2001). *Basic nutrition & diet therapy* (11th ed.). St Louis, MO: Mosby.

Wong, D., Hockenberry-Eaton, M., Wilson, D., Winkelstein, M., Ahmann, E., & DiVito-Thomas, P. (1999). *Nursing care of infants and children.* (6th ed.). St Louis, MO: Mosby.

Yen, P. K. (1998a). Nutrition: Dysphagia diet update. *Geriatric Nursing, 19*(4), 243-245.

Yen, P. K. (1998b). Nutrition: Stopping heart disease with diet. *Geriatric Nursing, 19*(1), 51-52.

*Zaloga, G. P. (1994). *Nutrition in critical care.* St Louis, MO: Mosby.

*Asterisk indicates a classic or definitive work on this subject.

Maintaining Fluid and Electrolyte Balance

Learning Objectives

After studying this chapter, you should be able to do the following:

- Describe the normal physiology of fluid balance, including fluid compartments, functions of body fluids, and types of electrolytes
- Identify mechanisms that contribute to the regulation of fluid and electrolyte balance
- Discuss five common problems related to fluid balance
- Identify the factors affecting fluid balance, including physiological problems and medical and nursing therapies
- Describe the general assessment of a client's fluid balance
- Describe the focused assessment of clients at risk for fluid problems, the manifestations of actual fluid problems, and client responses to fluid problems
- Diagnose the problems of clients with fluid imbalances that are within the domain of nursing
- Plan and carry out goal-directed interventions to prevent or correct fluid and electrolyte imbalances
- Evaluate outcomes in terms of progress or lack of progress toward the goals of fluid balance with revision of the care plan as appropriate

Elli Thompson, an 81-year-old African-American woman, has lived independently in her own home since her husband died 4 years ago. She has one daughter who lives 500 miles away and two sons, one within 10 miles and one within 100 miles. She lately has developed arthritic joint changes and visual changes that interfere with this activity as well as with her ability to drive, cook, and maintain her usual standard of hygiene.

Her physician prescribed a nonsteroidal antiinflammatory (NSAID), an analgesic, and an ophthalmic medication. Mrs. Thompson has found these medications helpful, but she still has problems meeting her everyday needs. She still tries to make three meals for herself, even though cooking has become difficult. The inconvenience has led her to choose foods other than the foods she so dearly loves. In addition, she becomes so full with smaller amounts of food that she has stopped drinking in order to make room for the food. Her fatigue has also resulted in fewer trips to the kitchen for more fluids.

Mrs. Thompson's son Gerald stopped by for a visit and noticed that his mother looked thin and listless. Mrs. Thompson's physician, Dr. Kline, found her to be severely dehydrated. He believed that her lack of energy and change in self-care and social activity were related to the dehydration. Mrs. Thompson also said that the medication "makes me tired."

Dr. Kline recommended a change in her prescription and a home visit from a nurse. The visiting nurse's evaluation supported the diagnosis of *Deficient fluid volume.*

Mrs. Thompson progressed well. To increase Mrs. Thompson's ability to detect problems in the early stages, the nurse reviewed with her a written list of signs and symptoms that should be reported to Dr. Kline.

Mrs. Thompson was on her own again, with support from her family and friends. But she was so concerned about not getting in "this shape" again that she forced herself to drink fluids almost continuously. A week later, Gerald stopped by to check on his mother. This time, she looked puffy and was having trouble breathing. Gerald become alarmed and immediately called Dr. Kline, who admitted Mrs. Thompson to the hospital with a diagnosis of acute congestive heart failure. In analyzing Mrs. Thompson, the nurse considers *Excess fluid volume* from the list of possible nursing diagnoses that relate to fluid imbalance (see below).

KEY NURSING DIAGNOSES FOR Fluid Imbalance

Risk for imbalanced fluid volume: A risk of a decrease, an increase, or a rapid shift from one to another fluid state—intravascular, interstitial, and/or intracellular

Risk for deficient fluid volume: The state in which an individual is at risk for experiencing vascular, cellular, or intracellular dehydration

Deficient fluid volume: The state in which an individual experiences decreased intravascular, interstitial, and/or intracellular fluid; refers to dehydration, water loss alone without change in sodium

Excess fluid volume: The state in which an individual experiences increased isotonic fluid retention

---

Although older adults such as Mrs. Thompson represent the segment most often endangered by fluid imbalance, the risk for fluid imbalances exists at any age and is associated with many conditions. Consider the child who becomes dehydrated from vomiting or diarrhea, the pregnant woman who develops abnormal swelling in her legs and feet, or the alcoholic middle-aged man with an increasingly large abdomen from liver disease.

Fluid and electrolytes are critical to maintain a state of homeostasis. This state must be maintained through a response to continuous changes imposed by both internal physiological processes and by the external environment. As the person takes in fluid and nutrients, the chemical equilibrium of the body is disrupted in the processes of digestion, absorption, and metabolism of nutrients and the excretion of wastes. Additionally, environmental conditions such as temperature and humidity cause changes in physiological functions to maintain a constant body temperature.

In this situation of constant change and adaptation the body maintains precise control over the fluids and electrolytes in the body. Thus the healthy person makes adjustments to a hot day, high humidity, or a temporary delay of a meal. The body responds through chemical reactions and hemodynamic changes to maintain normal physiological processes. Both acute and chronic illness can upset this delicate balance. The client may be too ill to respond to the need for fluid or electrolytes by increasing intake or excreting excess fluid, or there may be abnormal losses that exceed the body's ability to compensate.

The body functions by keeping the total input of water and electrolytes relatively equal to the amount lost. Therefore fluid and electrolyte balance means that total body water and electrolytes are normal, as is their distribution within body compartments. Fluid and electrolytes are interdependent, meaning that an abnormality in one causes an abnormality in the other. Understanding the concepts of fluid balance will help you in planning and administering care appropriately.

In these situations, supportive medical therapy and nursing care is provided to help the body attain and maintain fluid and electrolyte balance. Therapy includes forcing fluids, diuretics, electrolyte administration, and medications that affect hemodynamics (cardiovascular medications).

The nurse's role is to monitor the client for fluid and electrolyte balance, administer the medical therapy, and teach the client health practices to prevent recurrence of the problem. Monitoring is multifaceted because the regulation of fluid and electrolytes is a complex physiological process involving multiple organs and systems.

CONCEPTS OF FLUID BALANCE

Water is not found in its pure state in the body but instead is the medium in which all chemical products of nutrition, metabolism, and excretion are found. The term *fluid* is used to mean water and the components it contains. Chemical compounds are the principal components of most body fluids. An

electrolyte is any compound that, when dissolved in water, separates into electrically charged particles, which are called *ions*. Positively charged ions are called **cations;** negatively charged ions are called **anions.**

The most common compound that becomes an electrolyte in solution is table salt, or sodium chloride (NaCl). Important cations in body metabolism are sodium (Na^+), potassium (K^+), calcium (Ca^{2+}), magnesium (Mg^{2+}), and hydrogen (H^+). Important anions are chloride (Cl^-), bicarbonate (HCO_3^-), sulfate (SO_4^{-2}), and proteinate. **Nonelectrolytes** are substances that do not ionize and thus do not carry an electrical charge. Glucose is an example of a nonelectrolyte compound in body fluids.

Fluid balance is dependent on the chemical and physical properties of electrolytes and plasma proteins. Therefore, from a practical perspective, one cannot address fluid deficit or fluid overload in isolation from electrolytes and proteins because they are so interrelated. In other words, when a client has problems of fluid balance, you will also have to assess the client's electrolyte and protein status. Therefore this chapter presents an overview of major electrolytes as they relate to the person's risk or actual state of fluid imbalance.

There are many fundamental physiological concepts that you must understand to anticipate a fluid imbalance or understand the nature of fluid deficit or fluid excess. These include the functions of body fluids, the storage of fluids in different compartments, the role of electrolytes, the shifting of fluid between compartments, the regulation of fluid balance, and common problems of fluid balance.

Functions of Body Fluids

The body needs at least 1500 mL of water every day in addition to water that comes from the foods we eat (about 700 mL) and the oxidation of food (about 300 mL). Why does the body need so much fluid?

The answer is partly because fluid makes up over half of the normal adult's weight. Fluids transport nutrients and wastes to and from cells and act as a solvent for electrolytes and nonelectrolytes. Fluids also play a role in maintaining body temperature, facilitating digestion and elimination, maintaining acid–base balance, and lubricating joints and other body tissues.

Fluid Compartments

Fluids exist in several compartments in the body. Although fluid is in a continual state of exchange between compartments, the amount of fluid and the relative components in each compartment remain relatively constant.

Body fluid is in a state of balance when the following occurs:

- Its water and electrolyte components are present in the proper proportions.
- Fluids are distributed normally between compartments.
- Lost body water and electrolytes are replaced.
- Excess water and electrolytes are eliminated.

For the body's cells to function normally, the composition of body fluids must remain constant and the distribution among compartments must remain normal. In the average

adult, 50% to 60% of the body weight is from fluid, 70% of which is intracellular and 30% extracellular. Homeostasis depends on the relationship of the components within the intracellular and extracellular fluid compartments (Figure 25-1).

Intracellular Fluid Compartment. Intracellular fluids make up about 70% of the body's fluid and provide cells with the internal aqueous medium necessary for their chemical functions. Therefore anything that affects fluid loss at the cellular level has significant implications for the entire body.

Extracellular Fluid Compartment. Extracellular fluids (30% of the total fluid) are found outside the body cells and serve as the body's transportation system. They carry water, electrolytes, nutrients, and oxygen to the cells and remove the waste products of cellular metabolism. The extracellular compartments are further divided as follows: intravascular (6% of the total), interstitial (22%), and transcellular (2%).

INTRAVASCULAR FLUIDS. The term *intravascular* refers to the spaces within the arteries, veins, and capillaries. As you recall, the major function of these vessels is to carry blood. Blood consists of the fluid known as *plasma* and the cells

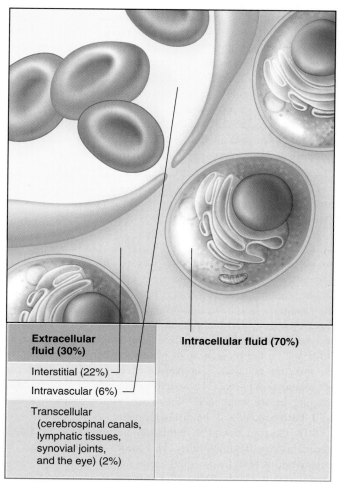

Figure 25-1. Distribution of fluid by compartments in the average adult.

Within the figure:

Extracellular fluid (30%)

Intracellular fluid (70%)

Interstitial (22%)

Intravascular (6%)

Transcellular (cerebrospinal canals, lymphatic tissues, synovial joints, and the eye) (2%)

(white and red blood cells) carried in that plasma. Plasma contains **colloids** (macromolecules that are too large to pass though a cell membrane and that do not readily dissolve into a solution, such as proteins) and byproducts of cellular function and metabolism.

Having too little blood (fluid) in the intravascular space affects the nutrient and oxygen supply to all tissues. Tissues that have a high demand for oxygen and nutrients, such as the brain, heart, and kidneys, are compromised first. A familiar example is the loss of intravascular fluid that occurs with a hemorrhage and results in a drop in blood pressure. Having too much fluid in the intravascular space can damage the intimal lining of the blood vessels and the tissues. Changes in the volume of fluid in the vascular space trigger a series of compensatory neuroendocrine responses (discussed later in the chapter).

INTERSTITIAL FLUIDS. Fluid is everywhere in the body, even between the cells and vascular compartments, in spaces known as the *interstitial spaces.* Interstitial fluid transports nutrients and waste products between the cells and the blood vessels. Too much or too little fluid in this space affects bodily functions.

A sprained ankle is a familiar example of an increase in interstitial fluid. The swelling of the tissue around the ankle bones results from damage to the vessel walls and the release of byproducts of tissue injury. These alter the permeability of the vessel walls, allowing excess fluid to seep into the interstitial spaces. Excess fluid in the interstitial spaces is called *edema.*

TRANSCELLULAR FLUIDS. Transcellular fluids are found in spaces in the cerebrospinal canals in the brain, and in the lymph tissues, synovial joints, and eyes. Although these fluids contribute only about 2% of the total fluid volume in the body, even small changes in fluid volume in these compartments can have a major impact on the health of these organs.

If Mrs. Thompson, from our case study, was eating three meals a day, why didn't the food sustain her? Is drinking water and other fluids really that important?

Electrolytes

As noted earlier, electrolytes are ionized substances that perform their functions within a fluid environment. The electrolytes that are most plentiful inside the cells are potassium, magnesium, phosphate, and protein. Sodium, calcium, chloride, hydrogen, and bicarbonate are the most plentiful electrolytes in the extracellular fluid. Electrolytes exert a major influence on the movement of water between compartments, on enzyme reactions, on neuromuscular activity, and on acid–base regulation. The specific functions of protein, hydrogen, bicarbonate, and other electrolytes as they affect acid–base balance will be discussed later.

It is through complex regulatory systems that the body maintains electrical neutrality. This means that the number of negative ions (anions) is equal to the number of positive ions (cations) in the body. Table 25-1 lists the functions and regulators of ions important in the body.

An example of fluid and electrolyte relationships occurs daily when a person eats. Water, proteins, fats, and carbohydrates are ingested, and minerals, including sodium, potassium, calcium, magnesium, chloride, and phosphate, are consumed. When these minerals are consumed, they ionize and become electrolytes. For example, table salt (NaCl) separates into Na^+ and Cl^- when it dissolves in the body fluid.

Extracellular and intracellular fluids contain the same electrolytes but in different amounts. For example, about 98% of the body's potassium is found in the intracellular compartment, compared with 2% in the extracellular compartment. In contrast, 99% of the sodium is found in the extracellular compartment, and the remaining 1% is in the intracellular compartment.

Sodium. Osmosis is the diffusion of water across membranes, and the osmotic role of sodium is essential to maintaining the proper amount of water in and between compartments. Vascular volume, which affects blood pressure, is a direct response to the level of sodium ions (where sodium goes, water follows). Sodium is also critical to nerve impulse conduction because of its effect on the electrical potential of cells. The sodium–potassium pump is an active transport mechanism that promotes the opening of sodium and potassium channels during different phases of the impulse propagation. In **active transport,** molecules move from an area of lower concentration to an area of higher concentration with an expenditure of energy. These changes in sodium and potassium concentrations are critical to nerve conduction; and without them, cells would die.

Potassium. Potassium plays a key role in maintaining the sodium–potassium pump and thus the transmission of nerve impulses. Potassium balance is critical to the normal function of all cells but especially those of the cardiac and skeletal muscles.

Calcium. Calcium plays a primary role in the formation of healthy bones and teeth. It promotes normal blood coagulation and is critical to nerve conduction. The slow calcium channels open after the more rapid sodium and potassium channels to maintain the electrical potential necessary for the propagation of the nerve impulses across the cell membrane.

Magnesium. Although magnesium is present in low concentration, it also is critical to the function of many body systems through its effect on over 300 enzyme systems. It promotes the release of a phosphate bond (conversion of adenosine triphosphate [ATP] to adenosine diphosphate [ADP]), which provides the energy source for the sodium–potassium pump.

A change in any of these four cations (sodium, potassium, calcium, magnesium) can make the cell more or less responsive to stimuli. The degree and acuteness of the imbalances, as well as the client's adaptive mechanisms, determine the client's responses.

Table 25-1	Electrolyte Functions and Regulators		
Electrolyte	**Normal Plasma Levels (mEq/L)**	**Functions**	**Regulation**
Sodium (Na$^+$)	135-145	• Maintains blood volume • Controls water shifting between compartments • Major cation involved in sodium–potassium pump necessary for nerve impulses • Interacts with calcium to maintain muscle contraction • Major cation in bicarbonate and phosphate acid–base buffer system	**Renin–angiotensin–aldosterone system**
Potassium (K$^+$)	3.5-5.0	• Affects osmolality • Major cation involved in sodium–potassium pump necessary for transmission of nerve impulses • Promotes nerve impulses, especially in heart and skeletal muscles • Assists in conversion of carbohydrates to energy and amino acids into proteins • Promotes glycogen storage in liver • Assists maintenance of acid–base balance through cellular exchange with hydrogen	**Renin–angiotensin–aldosterone system**
Calcium (Ca^{2+})	4.5-5.5	• Nonionized form promotes strong bones and teeth • Promotes blood coagulation • Promotes nerve impulse conduction, decreases neuromuscular irritability • Strengthens and thickens cell membrane • Assists in absorption and utilization of vitamin B$_{12}$ • Activates enzymes for many chemical reactions • Inhibits cell membrane permeability to sodium • Activates actin–myosin muscle contraction	**Parathormone** • Increases calcium resorption from bone • Increases calcium reabsorption by inhibiting phosphate reabsorption from kidney tubules • Increases calcium absorption from gastrointestinal tract
Magnesium (Mg^{2+})	1.5-2.5	• Promotes metabolism of carbohydrates, fats, and proteins • Activates many enzymes (B$_{12}$ metabolism) • Promotes regulation of Ca, PO$_4$, K • Promotes transmission of nerve impulses, muscle contraction, and heart function • Powers sodium–potassium pump • Promotes conversion of adenosine triphosphate (ATP) to adenosine diphosphate (ADP) for energy release	**Parathormone** • Increases or decreases magnesium reabsorption in kidney tubules relative to body need
Chloride (Cl$^-$)	98-106	• Inhibits smooth muscle contraction • Regulates extracellular fluid volume • Promotes acid–base balance through exchange with bicarbonate in red blood cells (chloride shift) • Promotes protein digestion through hydrochloric (HCl) acid; acid pH required for activation of protease	**Renin–angiotensin–aldosterone system**
Phosphate (HPO$_4^-$)	1.2-3.0	• Nonionized form promotes bone and teeth rigidity • Promotes acid–base balance through phosphate buffer system • Necessary for ATP production	**Parathormone** • Increases phosphate resorption from bone • Inhibits phosphate reabsorption in kidney tubules • Increases phosphate absorption in gastrointestinal tract as needed

Chloride. Because chloride is the major anion associated with sodium, its role in osmolality and nerve conduction is also critical. Chloride also plays a key role in the process of digestion because it is the anionic part of hydrochloric acid.

Phosphate. Phosphate works with calcium to promote the integrity of bones and teeth. It is an integral part of ATP and ADP, which maintain our energy sources for all cell functions.

Movement of Fluids and Electrolytes

To maintain homeostasis, fluid shifts constantly between compartments, exchanging nutrients and waste products. For example, nutrients from ingested food are transported from the bloodstream to the cells so that the byproducts of food can be used to build new cells. The waste products from the digestion of these nutrients are then transported from the cells to the bloodstream for removal from the body. Water is the medium that allows the transport of essential particles to the cells and waste products from the cells.

The factors that regulate the shifting of water between compartments are discussed next. Understanding the normal mechanisms of fluid transport will enhance your ability to identify potential or actual fluid and electrolyte problems. Remember that fluid movement depends on the *relationships* between these factors, not on one factor alone.

Osmosis. The cell wall is a semipermeable membrane that selectively allows water and smaller particles to pass through it. Larger particles, such as proteins and glucose, are transported by more complex processes. The movement of fluid between compartments is influenced by osmosis and various pressure forces. **Osmosis** is the movement of water through a semipermeable membrane from an area containing a lesser concentration of particles to an area of greater concentration of particles.

Osmolality and osmolarity are expressions of the osmotic force of a solution. Osmotic force can be illustrated by considering ordinary table salt, sodium chloride (NaCl), as a gargle for a sore throat. The salt particles in the water create an osmotic force that draws fluid from the tissues and reduces swelling (Figure 25-2). The force from the dissolved particles (such as salt) in a solvent (such as water) can be represented as **milliosmoles,** the number of dissolved particles needed to produce one unit of force. **Osmolality** refers to the number of milliosmoles per kilogram of water. The term **osmolarity** is similar but refers to the measurement of milliosmoles per liter of solution. The term *osmolality* is used to describe body fluids, whereas the term *osmolarity* is used more often in reference to solutions measured by volume, such as an intravenous (IV) fluid.

To illustrate osmolality even further, consider two clients, one receiving a hypotonic IV solution and the other receiving an isotonic solution, both solutions given at a fairly rapid rate. An **isotonic** solution has an osmotic pressure equal to that of plasma (solute is evenly distributed within the water). A **hypotonic** solution has an osmotic pressure less than that of

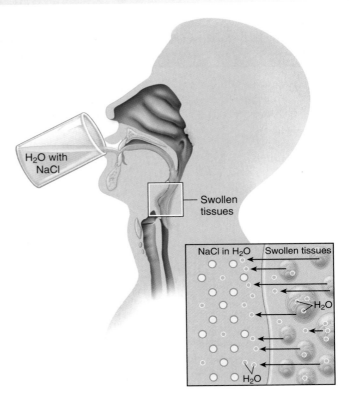

Figure 25-2. Osmosis. When a client uses a saline solution as a gargle for swollen tonsils, the gargle provides a feeling of comfort. This is because of the process of osmosis. The excess water in the swollen tonsils moves from the area of lesser concentration of particles (in the swollen cells) to the extracellular spaces that now have a higher concentration because of the added sodium.

plasma (more water, less solute). A **hypertonic** solution has an osmotic pressure greater than that of plasma (less water, more solute). Whenever there is a difference in osmolality between the cell and the plasma, fluid shifting is likely to occur. For example, when a hypertonic (hyperosmolar) imbalance occurs, cells shrink because they have less water and more solute. In the reverse situation, a hypotonic (hypoosmolar) imbalance results in more water and less solute, causing cells to swell.

Diffusion. **Diffusion** refers to the passive process by which molecules move through a cell membrane from an area of higher concentration to an area of lower concentration without an expenditure of energy (passive transport). For example, gases such as carbon dioxide and oxygen diffuse across the respiratory membrane into the pulmonary capillaries from the area of higher to the area of lower concentration. Electrolytes move passively from an area of higher concentration to an area of lower concentration, such as from the small bowel at the end of digestion into the bloodstream.

Active Transport. In contrast, when an electrolyte moves against a concentration gradient, from an area of lower concentration to an area of higher concentration, energy is required. This active process of molecules moving against a concentration gradient is known as active transport. This is the process necessary to maintain the sodium–potassium pump. This pump is critical to the maintenance of an electrical impulse, such as in the heart. It is the active movement of sodium from inside the cell to the outside of the cell by this pump that results in a negativity on the inside of the cell.

This electrical difference between the outside and the inside of the membrane results in a resting potential, so that the cell can respond to an impulse. When it does so, the response is called an action potential because the cell is no longer in a state of rest but is in a state of action.

Filtration. **Filtration** pressure is the sum of (1) the forces tending to move water and dissolved substances out of the blood vessels and (2) the opposing forces. The balance of fluids within the capillaries depends on both hydrostatic pressure and colloid osmotic pressure. **Hydrostatic pressure** is the pressure exerted by the weight of fluid within a compartment or closed system. Tissue hydrostatic pressure pushes fluid into the capillary. Capillary hydrostatic pressure pushes fluid out of the capillary. **Colloid osmotic pressure** is the osmotic pressure exerted by large molecules, such as proteins. Tissue colloidal osmotic pressure pulls fluid into the interstitial spaces. Capillary colloidal osmotic pressure pulls fluid back into the capillary.

HYDROSTATIC PRESSURE. Arterial hydrostatic pressure is greater than colloid osmotic pressure. On the arterial end of the capillary, the hydrostatic pressure (approximately 32 mm Hg) is greater than the colloid osmotic pressure (approximately 22 mm Hg). This +10 difference is known as filtration pressure and results in the movement of fluid from the arterial end of the capillary into the interstitial compartment in the process known as filtration (Figure 25-3).

In the venous end of the capillary, the pulling force of the colloids draws fluids into the capillaries. The hydrostatic pressure (approximately 12 mm Hg) is less than the colloid osmotic pressure, approximately a −10 difference in filtration pressure. This pulling pressure results in reabsorption of the fluid back into the venous end of the capillary. In other words, a positive filtration pressure at the arterial end leads to fluid being "pushed" into the interstitial compartment, whereas a negative filtration pressure at the venous end leads to fluid being "pulled" back into the capillary.

Any factor that affects blood pressure in the arterial or venous system or the flow of blood through the capillary network can affect hydrostatic pressure. This includes blood volume, size of the vessel lumen, and the opposing forces from all the osmotic molecules. Figure 25-3 shows the approximate pressures found in a healthy adult.

COLLOID OSMOTIC PRESSURE. Colloid osmotic pressure is the osmotic force created by colloids, which are large molecules such as proteins. This pressure draws fluid into the capillary or interstitial space. Colloid osmotic pressure is the major force opposing hydrostatic pressure in the capil-

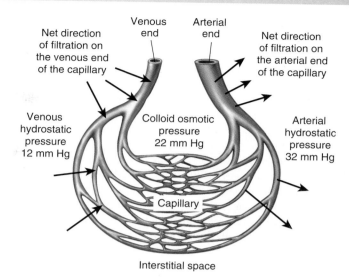

Figure 25-3. Filtration. Complex factors affect the movement of water and nutrients between the plasma, interstitium, and cellular spaces. Two critical factors are hydrostatic pressure and colloid osmotic pressure. Filtration on the arterial end, and reabsorption on the venous end, result in fluid shifting. The lymphatic tissues transport any remaining fluid or proteins to the right atrium.

lary. It maintains a relatively constant value of 22 mm Hg. It is this opposition that affects how much fluid filters from the arterial end of the capillary to the interstitial spaces and the cell itself.

Proteins are the only dissolved substances that do not readily diffuse through the capillary membrane. Thus they exert a greater osmotic force than smaller molecules. The term *oncotic pressure* is used interchangeably with the term *colloid pressure,* and they both refer specifically to the osmotic force of protein and its superior ability to pull in water.

Proteins found in the plasma include albumin, globulin, and fibrinogen. Albumin has the greatest influence on the "pulling" pressure in the capillary. It constitutes 50% of the plasma proteins but is responsible for 80% of the colloid osmotic pressure in plasma. Although proteins play a vital role in fluid shifting, they cannot manage fluid homeostasis by themselves. When a person has a deficiency in protein, more of the fluid stays in the interstitial spaces. This abnormality, called edema, will be discussed later in the chapter.

In a healthy person, the interstitial compartment contains electrolytes and some proteins that have leaked through the capillary membrane; thus it has its own colloid osmotic pressure. However, the concentration of proteins is always greater in the plasma compartment than in the interstitial compartment. Therefore, on the venous end of the capillary, the hydrostatic pressure is less than the colloid osmotic pressure (about 12 mm Hg), and the fluid is "pulled" back into the venous capillary by the osmotic force of protein. This process of fluid being pulled back into the capillary is known as *reabsorption.*

Regulation of Fluid Balance

Thirst. Why do you drink fluids? Is it because of habit or socialization, or are you thirsty? All of these factors probably affect your fluid intake. Western culture emphasizes the provision of beverages at social activities and in the home. Health publications remind us continually to drink plenty of fluids each day. But although habit and culture certainly influence our fluid consumption, our internal thirst mechanism is also a powerful stimulant that encourages us to drink.

The thirst center is located in the hypothalamus. The stimulation or inhibition of the thirst response depends on changes in local plasma osmolality. For example, when the osmolality of the blood flowing around the lateral preoptic cells of the hypothalamus increases, the cells sense the change and trigger the thirst response. Situations that promote increased osmolality include a decrease in fluid intake, excessive fluid loss, or an excessive sodium intake either orally or intravenously. On the other hand, a high intake of fluids, fluid retention, a low sodium intake, and excessive IV infusion of hypotonic solutions inhibit the thirst mechanism.

To return to our case study, why didn't Mrs. Thompson's thirst mechanism stimulate her to drink more? Recall that Mrs. Thompson is 81 years old. Like all older adults, she has a decrease in thirst as a normal consequence of aging. This will be addressed later in the chapter.

Lymphatic System. The lymphatic system performs the essential role of "sponging up" excess fluid that is not reabsorbed into the capillaries. The lymphatic ducts return fluid and some protein to the subclavian veins, which in turn empty into the right atrium of the heart. When the lymphatic system is not functioning properly, fluid excess occurs in the interstitial compartments. Severe lymphatic dysfunction can lead to localized tissue ischemia and cell death. It can also lead to systemic sepsis caused by metabolites from necrotic tissue.

Neuroendocrine System. Another very powerful regulator of fluid intake is the neuroendocrine system. It regulates body fluid volume by producing and secreting hormones that stimulate or inhibit osmotic receptors in the carotid arteries and aortic arch (Figure 25-4). These receptors are very sensitive to blood volume. The neuroendocrine system also uses specialized nerve endings in the walls of the large blood vessels and atria to respond to changes in intravascular fluid volume.

HORMONES. One of the most influential hormones affecting fluid balance is the antidiuretic hormone (ADH). This hormone opposes (i.e., it is "anti") fluid loss (or "diuresis"). ADH is produced by the hypothalamus and stored in the vesicles in the posterior pituitary gland. The osmolality of extracellular fluid as it passes through the hypothalamus is the major stimulant or inhibitor of the secretion of antidiuretic hormone.

The osmolality of Mrs. Thompson's plasma was increased when she was in a state of fluid deficit. It makes sense, then, that her body, in an attempt to compensate, promoted a decrease in water loss. Increased secretion of ADH caused the pores in the distal and collecting tubules of her kidney

nephrons to become larger. This resulted in increased reabsorption of the water back into the capillaries and a decrease in urinary output (oliguria).

Aldosterone is another hormone with a major effect on fluid balance. Although low sodium levels, high potassium levels, and the release of adrenocorticotropic hormone (ACTH) affect the release of aldosterone, the major stimulant for its release is the hormone angiotensin II (the renin–angiotensin–aldosterone [RAA] system). This hormone is produced whenever renin, a proteolytic enzyme synthesized and stored in the juxtaglomerular cells of the kidney, is secreted in response to decreased kidney blood flow. Angiotensin in turn stimulates the release of aldosterone from the adrenal cortex. Unlike antidiuretic hormone, aldosterone has only an indirect effect on water. When it is released, aldosterone promotes the reabsorption of sodium and the excretion of potassium in the distal tubules and collecting ducts of the kidney. Sodium reabsorption results in the passive reabsorption of water.

When fluid excess is present, the opposite occurs: aldosterone secretion is decreased, resulting in sodium and water excretion and potassium retention. Note that when one cation (sodium) is retained, another (potassium) is excreted. This is one of the ways in which the delicate balance of electrical neutrality is maintained. Also recall that cation changes result in changes in the movement of anions. Usually, the chloride ion passively accompanies its leader, the sodium ion, to its destination.

Thyroid hormones (thyroxine [T_4] and triiodothyronine [T_3]) affect fluid volume by influencing cardiac output. An increase in thyroid hormones causes an increase in cardiac output, which in turn increases glomerular filtrate and thus urinary output. A decrease in these hormones has the opposite effect.

The cardiovascular system also plays a role in fluid balance through the release of atrial natriuretic peptides (ANP) whenever the atrial cells are overloaded with fluid. Any condition that causes fluid overload, vasoconstriction, or direct cardiac damage stimulates an increase in the release of ANPs. Their release has an effect opposite to that of the renin–angiotensin–aldosterone system. It causes dilation of the arterioles and venules, sodium excretion (natriuresis), and diuresis.

BARORECEPTORS. Have you ever felt your heart pounding after a stressful event? If someone took your blood pressure at that time, you would see that it was much higher than normal. However, this rise in blood pressure does not cause a problem in a healthy person because of the "minute-to-minute" control of the blood pressure by baroreceptors. These receptors are specialized nerve endings in the walls of the large veins and arteries and in the atria of the heart. They respond to the slightest changes in pressure inside the blood vessels and relay this information to the vasomotor centers in the medulla. Anything that affects the relationship of the size of the blood vessels or the volume inside the blood vessels affects these receptors.

Now that you have an understanding of the major compensatory responses that a person experiences when fluid is lost, you can transfer this knowledge to the opposite scenario, fluid excess. When a person consumes too much fluid, baroreceptors and the hypothalamus sense a decrease

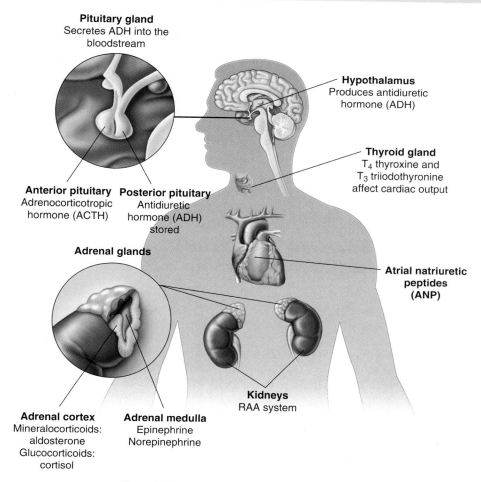

Pituitary gland
Secretes ADH into the
bloodstream

Hypothalamus
Produces antidiuretic
hormone (ADH)

Thyroid gland
T_4 thyroxine and
T_3 triiodothyronine
affect cardiac output

Anterior pituitary
Adrenocorticotropic
hormone (ACTH)

Posterior pituitary
Antidiuretic
hormone (ADH)
stored

Adrenal glands

**Atrial natriuretic
peptides
(ANP)**

Adrenal cortex
Mineralocorticoids:
aldosterone
Glucocorticoids:
cortisol

Adrenal medulla
Epinephrine
Norepinephrine

Kidneys
RAA system

Figure 25-4. Effect of hormones on fluid balance.

in osmolality. This causes a decrease in antidiuretic hormone, an increase in urinary output, and inhibition of the thirst mechanism. The increased volume reaching the kidney will inhibit the release of renin and aldosterone, thus decreasing reabsorption of sodium. This mechanism also promotes diuresis.

Gastrointestinal System. Besides the fluid absorbed from dietary intake, the gastrointestinal (GI) tract produces about 7 to 9 liters (L) of glandular and tissue secretions per day. All but about 100 mL of this fluid is reabsorbed. About every 90 minutes, a volume of blood equivalent to the total body plasma level (about 3000 mL in a person who weighs 70 kg) passes through the intestinal mucosa. The GI fluid contains many nutrients, including electrolytes. Understanding the relationship between fluid balance and normal GI function is essential to anticipating fluid and electrolyte imbalances in a state of altered GI function.

Renal System. The renal system works interdependently with the neuroendocrine system to regulate the volume of extracellular fluid. Recall that the kidney is the target organ for antidiuretic hormone and aldosterone. Antidiuretic hormone

(through the regulation of water) and aldosterone (through the regulation of water, sodium, and potassium) play a major role in fluid and electrolyte homeostasis.

The renin–angiotensin–aldosterone (RAA) system functions to maintain homeostasis between sodium and water as well as regulate the blood pressure. Juxtaglomerular cells secrete renin, an enzyme that converts angiotensinogen to angiotensin I in the liver. Angiotensin I then travels to the lungs, where it is converted to angiotensin II (a potent vasoconstrictor). Angiotensin II has two effects: (1) it raises blood pressure because of its potency, and (2) it stimulates the production of aldosterone from adrenal glands, which also raises the blood pressure. The amount of renin secreted will depend on the volume of blood and the sodium level in the bloodstream. In response to a decreased sodium level or a decrease in plasma volume, the RAA system is triggered.

The kidney also affects many other electrolytes, including calcium, magnesium, phosphate, hydrogen, chloride, and bicarbonate. The renal nephrons regulate electrolyte balance by secreting excess ions into the tubules, where they are later excreted as urine. When a deficit occurs, electrolytes are reabsorbed from the renal tubules back into the capillary network surrounding the tubules of the nephron.

Problems of Fluid Balance

These regulators of fluid balance are important to consider when a client is at risk for or has an actual fluid volume deficit or excess. Compare the following definitions to get a clearer picture of the basic concepts related to fluid imbalance.

Deficient Fluid Volume. *Deficient fluid volume* refers to a state of hypovolemia (low blood volume), or dehydration, in either the extracellular fluid (intravascular or interstitial) compartment or the intracellular fluid compartment. The defining characteristics are a direct or an indirect result of a rapid change in fluid output or a lack of intake without compensation by fluid shifts or other homeostatic mechanisms.

Excess Fluid Volume. *Excess fluid volume* refers to a state of hypervolemia, or water intoxication, in the vascular compartment, the presence of edema in the interstitial compartment, or excess fluid in the intracellular spaces. The defining characteristics are a direct or indirect result of an increase in fluid intake or decrease in excretion without compensation by intercompartmental fluid shifts or other regulatory mechanisms.

Electrolyte Imbalance. *Electrolyte imbalance* means that a person has either a deficit or an excess of one or more electrolytes. Table 25-2 lists the risk factors and manifestations of common imbalances of sodium, potassium, calcium, magnesium, and phosphorus. Note the similarity of some manifestations,

Table 25-2	Common Electrolyte Imbalances: Risk Factors and Manifestations	
Imbalance	**Risk Factors**	**Manifestations**
HYPONATREMIA • Sodium <135 mEq/L • Chloride <98 mEq/L • Plasma osmolality <285 mOsm/kg	• Low-salt diet, especially when taking diuretics at same time • Excess sweating • Athletic events • Vomiting and diarrhea in excess • Dilutional from taking in too much water	*General:* fatigue, weight loss *Musculoskeletal:* weakness *Cardiac:* orthostatic hypotension; rapid, thready, weak pulse; peripheral vein filling takes more than 5 seconds *Respiratory:* tachypnea *Gastrointestinal:* nausea, vomiting, diarrhea *Renal:* oliguria, anuria *Neurological:* hypothermia, decreased thirst, confusion, stupor, seizures
HYPERNATREMIA • Sodium >145 mEq/L	• Increased intake, especially the presence of renal disease • Excessive IV saline solutions • Increased retention from cardiac disease, renal disease, liver disease, Cushing's disease, hyperaldosteronism • Conditions in which water loss exceeds sodium loss, such as diabetes mellitus, diabetes insipidus, hyperventilation, hypertonic feedings, diaphoresis, decreased water intake	*General:* fatigue, pitting edema, puffy eyelids, ascites, weight gain *Musculoskeletal:* weakness *Cardiac:* rapid, bounding pulse; third heart sound; hypertension; peripheral vein emptying takes more than 5 seconds; neck vein distention *Respiratory:* dyspnea, crackles, pulmonary edema, pleural effusion *Gastrointestinal:* anorexia, nausea, vomiting *Renal:* oliguria, anuria *Neurological:* fever, restlessness, confusion
HYPOKALEMIA • Potassium <3.5 mEq/L	• Certain medications, such as diuretics and laxatives • Excess vomiting, diarrhea • GI suctioning • Diet low in potassium • Renal failure	*General:* malaise, fatigue, alkalosis *Musculoskeletal:* weakness *Cardiac:* hypotension; arrhythmias; cardiac arrest; peaked P waves, depressed S–T segments, and flattened T and U waves on ECG *Respiratory:* shallow breathing, apnea, respiratory arrest *Gastrointestinal:* anorexia, nausea, vomiting, distention, paralytic ileus *Neurological:* dysphasia, lethargy, disorientation, irritability, hyporeflexia, paresthesias, tetany, seizures
HYPERKALEMIA • Potassium >5.0 mEq/L	• Increased oral or IV intake, especially in renal disease; stored blood • Decreased output, as from taking angiotensin–converting enzyme inhibitor with potassium-rich salt substitutes or potassium-sparing diuretics, renal failure, postoperative oliguria, Addison's disease	*General:* restlessness, acidosis *Musculoskeletal:* severe weakness *Cardiac:* hypotension, arrhythmias; cardiac arrest; depressed P waves, wide QRS complexes, depressed S–T segments, and tall, tented T waves on ECG *Respiratory:* dyspnea *Gastrointestinal:* nausea, colic, diarrhea *Renal:* oliguria, anuria

ECG, Electrocardiogram.

Table 25-2	Common Electrolyte Imbalances: Risk Factors and Manifestations—cont'd	
Imbalance	**Risk Factors**	**Manifestations**
HYPERKALEMIA—CONT'D		
• Potassium >5.0 mEq/L	• Excessive cellular loss, as from metabolic or respiratory acidosis (except diabetic acidosis) or during the first 3 days after a severe burn or cellular trauma	*Neurological:* restlessness, paresthesias, dysphasia, seizures
HYPOCALCEMIA		
• Calcium <4.5 mEq/L	• Certain medications, such as diuretics and laxatives • Hypoparathyroidism • Renal failure	*General:* bleeding *Musculoskeletal:* muscle cramps, pathological fractures *Cardiac:* hypotension; palpitations; arrhythmias; prolonged QT intervals on ECG *Respiratory:* laryngospasm, stridor *Neurological:* paresthesias, positive Trousseau's and Chvostek's signs, diplopia, tetany, seizures
HYPERCALCEMIA		
• Calcium >5.5 mEq/L • Phosphorus decreased	• Rarely, from excessive intake of milk, calcium–based medications, or vitamin D • Increased loss from bone due to immobilization, cancer (bone, lung, breast, leukemia), multiple fractures, hyperparathyroidism • Decreased opposition, from Addison's disease, hypophosphatemia • Any condition producing acidosis • Decreased loss, from thiazide diuretics	*General:* dehydration, polydipsia *Musculoskeletal:* weak, relaxed muscles; osteoporosis; osteomalacia; bone pain; pathological fractures *Cardiac:* dysrhythmia, cardiac arrest, short QT intervals on ECG *Gastrointestinal:* nausea, vomiting, constipation *Renal:* polyuria, calculi, renal colic, flank pain *Neurological:* confusion, lethargy
HYPOMAGNESEMIA		
• Magnesium <1.5 mEq/L	• Certain medications, such as diuretics • Alcoholism • Malnutrition • Hyperparathyroidism	*General:* refractory hypokalemia, hypocalcemia, or both *Musculoskeletal:* weakness *Cardiac:* tachycardia, arrhythmias *Neurological:* nystagmus, diplopia, disorientation, tremors, hyperactive reflexes, tetany, seizures
HYPERMAGNESEMIA		
• Magnesium >2.5 mEq/L	• Certain medications, such as magnesium antacids • Kidney disease	*General:* flushing *Musculoskeletal:* weakness, dysarthria *Cardiac:* hypotension, arrhythmias, cardiac arrest *Respiratory:* bradypnea, apnea, respiratory arrest *Gastrointestinal:* nausea, vomiting *Neurological:* thirst, hyporeflexia, lethargy, coma
HYPOPHOSPHATEMIA		
• Phosphate <1.2 mEq/L	• Certain medications, such as aluminum antacids and diuretics • Hyperparathyroidism • Malnutrition	*General:* fatigue *Musculoskeletal:* weakness, bone pain, pathological fractures *Cardiac:* decreased cardiac function *Neurological:* confusion, seizures
HYPERPHOSPHATEMIA		
• Phosphate >3.0 mEq/L • Calcium decreased	• Certain medications, such as phosphate antacids and sodium phosphate enemas • Massive trauma, strokes • Renal failure	*Cardiac:* tachycardia *Gastrointestinal:* anorexia, nausea, vomiting *Neurological:* hyperreflexia, tetany

ECG, Electrocardiogram.

as well as the manifestations that are unique to each ion. A client often has more than one electrolyte imbalance as well as an accompanying fluid imbalance.

Acid–Base Balance.
Normal cellular function depends on the maintenance of hydrogen ion concentration within very narrow limits. The normal range of pH (a negative logarithm used to express the H ion concentration) is 7.35 to 7.45. Cellular function is seriously affected when pH drops to 7.20 or lower or rises to 7.50 or higher. Ranges outside of 6.80 and 7.80 are usually incompatible with life. In a healthy state, four systems interactively maintain this narrow margin: cellular buffer systems, the lungs, the kidneys, and three chemical buffer systems. Figure 25-5 illustrates acid–base balance.

Respiratory acidosis is a result of the retention of carbon dioxide (CO_2), which is an acid, and a resultant decrease in pH (Table 25-3). Any pulmonary insufficiency resulting in hypoventilation (which causes the CO_2 level to build up) will result in respiratory acidosis. Conditions that depress the respiratory center (lung diseases, airway obstruction, and situations in which the chest wall and respiratory muscles are hindered) also cause respiratory acidosis. Manifestations include weakness, tremors, confusion, depression of the central nervous system, and even coma. Potassium and bicarbonate are retained, and hydrogen and chloride are lost in order to compensate.

Respiratory alkalosis is a result of rapid or excess elimination of CO_2, resulting in an increase in pH with a decrease in the partial pressure of CO_2 (Pco_2). Any pulmonary insufficiency resulting in hyperventilation will cause the CO_2 to be blown off, leaving an alkalotic state. Manifestations include cardiac dysrhythmias, dizziness, lightheadedness, tetany, and possibly seizures. Hydrogen and chloride are retained, and potassium and bicarbonate are lost in order to compensate.

Metabolic abnormalities are secondary to imbalances in nonvolatile acids or in the amount of alkali and are often more difficult to diagnose. Bicarbonate shifts in the same direction as the pH (hence the memory hint: metabolic equal). Table 25-3 identifies the shifts in pH and HCO_3^- in metabolic abnormalities.

Metabolic acidosis is a pathological condition caused by an increase in noncarbonic acids or a decrease in bicarbonate in the extracellular fluid, or both. Any pathology that results in ineffective tissue perfusion and the accumulation of lactic acid leads to lactic acidosis, a type of metabolic acidosis. Because the kidney is the primary organ responsible for the excretion of acids and the reabsorption of bicarbonate, any state of severe renal insufficiency leads to metabolic acidosis.

The cellular buffering process works as follows. Most dissolved carbon dioxide from tissue cell metabolism diffuses into the red blood cells, combines with water to form carbonic acid, and dissociates into hydrogen and bicarbonate. The bicarbonate shifts across the plasma membrane in exchange for chloride, and the hydrogen combines with hemoglobin and thus is buffered. Any pathology that leads to a deficit of sodium, phosphate, or protein impairs the base component of the chemical buffer systems, resulting in excess hydrogen. A decrease in hemoglobin or chloride can also increase the risk for metabolic acidosis by altering the buffering process.

An increase in potassium ions also increases the risk of metabolic acidosis. Whenever plasma potassium rises, the protective cellular buffer attempts to decrease the risk of hyperkalemia by exchanging potassium for hydrogen across the cell membrane. Thus potassium enters the cell in exchange for hydrogen, which enters the plasma.

The most common manifestations of metabolic acidosis are neurological (headache, lethargy), GI (anorexia, nausea, vomiting, diarrhea), cardiovascular (arrhythmias), and respiratory. The client may develop deep, rapid respirations (Kussmaul's respirations) as the body attempts to blow off carbonic acid. Severe acidosis can lead to coma and death.

In contrast, **metabolic alkalosis** occurs when the pH rises above 7.45. This is a pathological condition caused by an increase in bicarbonate or a decrease in acid in the extracellular fluid, or both. Any pathology or situation that leads to excessive vomiting (and loss of hydrochloric acid) or diarrhea (and excessive loss of the bicarbonate ion) increases the risk for metabolic alkalosis. Potassium deficiency, regardless of the

Figure 25-5. Acid–base balance. In the healthy state, a ratio of 1 part carbonic acid to 20 parts bicarbonate provides a normal plasma pH between 7.35 and 7.45. Any deviation to the left of 7.35 results in an acidotic state. Any deviation to the right of 7.45 results in an alkalotic state.

Table 25-3	Acid–Base Imbalances			
Imbalance	Compensatory State	pH	CO_2	HCO_3^-
Respiratory acidosis	U	↓	↑	N
	PC	↓	↑	↑
	C	N	↑	↑
Respiratory alkalosis	U	↑	↓	N
	PC	↑	↓	↓
	C	N	↓	↓
Metabolic acidosis	U	↓	N	↓
	PC	↓	↓	↓
	C	N	↓	↓
Metabolic alkalosis	U	↑	N	↑
	PC	↑	↑	↑
	C	N	↑	↑

U, Uncompensated; *PC*, partially compensated; *C*, compensated; *N*, normal value.

cause, promotes the shifting of hydrogen into cells and potassium into plasma—thus metabolic alkalosis. An overingestion of bicarbonate (as in antacids), especially in the presence of renal insufficiency, can result in metabolic alkalosis.

Common manifestations of metabolic alkalosis include generalized weakness, muscle cramps, neurological problems (hyperactive reflexes, tetany, confusion, convulsions), cardiac arrhythmias, and respiratory changes. As in metabolic acidosis, the respiratory system attempts to compensate. In this state, however, the respirations become slow and shallow in an attempt to conserve carbonic acid.

FACTORS AFFECTING FLUID BALANCE

Many variables influence a client's risk of fluid, electrolyte, and acid–base imbalance, including lifestyle, developmental stage, physiological state, and clinical factors. Table 25-4 lists the many etiologies of fluid deficit and fluid excess and the contributing factors for each variable.

Lifestyle Factors

Nutrition. An alteration in the intake of fluids increases risk. Although the majority of fluid intake comes from water or other liquids, the importance of the water obtained from foods should not be underestimated (Figure 25-6, p. 575). The water byproduct of food oxidation in the cell also contributes to our fluid balance, but to a lesser degree. The amounts listed in Figure 25-6 are for a healthy, relatively inactive person exposed to a temperate climate. People require at least 1500 mL of fluid daily to maintain essential cellular functions. The usual recommendation for fluid intake is six to eight glasses of fluid daily (about 2000 to 2400 mL).

Now it makes sense that Mrs. Thompson became ill when she stopped drinking an adequate amount of fluid.

In a healthy person, the body compensates for excess fluid, sodium, or both by increasing excretion. However, if the person has cardiac, renal, or liver disease, excess intake only prompts the retention of more fluid. Excess fluid

Table 25-4	Risk Factors for Fluid Volume Imbalance	
Risk Factor	**Contributing Factors**
DEFICIENT FLUID VOLUME	
Life Span	
Children	• Decreased ability to concentrate urine (immature kidneys) • Higher metabolic rate • Greater body surface area relative to weight • Hormonal and growth demands • Compensatory responses less stable • Fevers higher and last longer
Pregnancy	• Increased need for fluid (fetal and supportive tissue changes)
Older adults	• Decreased thirst mechanism, even in healthy older adults • Decreased ability to concentrate urine
Weight Extremes	• Fatty tissue contains less fluid. • Excess fluid may be compartments outside the blood vessels, making it unavailable. • Thirst may be an indicator of plasma deficit. • Women have larger proportion of fat tissue.
Altered Intake	
Decreased thirst	• Older adult population. • Hypoosmolality of the plasma inhibits thirst. • Decreased level of consciousness impairs perception of thirst.
Pain	• Alters desire or perception of thirst.
Dysphagia	• Increases time required for fluid intake. • Makes swallowing more difficult. • Requires thickened fluids.
Decreased access	• Lack of transportation, limited finances, ill health.
Increased Gastrointestinal (GI) Loss	
Diarrhea, vomiting, GI suctioning, ileostomy, fistula	• Rapid movement of fluid through GI tract decreases absorption of water, nutrients, and electrolytes. • Massive amounts of fluid can be lost via these sources regardless of etiology.
Hypertonic feedings (osmolarity >300 mOsm/kg)	• Increased osmolarity of feeding pulls water into bowel, which can cause diarrhea and dehydration.
Lactose-based feedings	• Lactose intolerance is common and may cause diarrhea.
Medications	• Many medications cause GI side effects, including anorexia, nausea, vomiting, and diarrhea. • Many elixirs are made with sorbitol, which can cause osmotic diarrhea.

Table 25-4	Risk Factors for Fluid Volume Imbalance—cont'd	
Risk Factor	**Contributing Factors**	

DEFICIENT FLUID VOLUME

Environmental
- Intolerance to toxins causing vomiting, diarrhea, or both.
- Exposure to high temperature or humidity.

Increased Urinary Loss

Decreased antidiuretic hormone
- May result from hypoosmolality of extracellular fluid, increased blood volume, exposure to cold, acute alcohol ingestion, carbon monoxide poisoning.

Hyperglycemia
Diuretic phase of renal failure
Medications
- Causes osmotic diuresis.
- Excess fluid lost through urine.
- Diuretics are a common cause.

Increased Integumentary Loss

Environmental
Fever
Wounds/burns
- Temperature above 30° C (86° F) and humidity above 50%.
- Insensible water loss, can be large amounts.
- Loss of fluid, protein, electrolytes.
- Damage to capillary membrane with direct fluid loss and secondary fluid loss due to loss of protein.

Increased Respiratory Loss

Hyperventilation
- Increased loss of water through expired air.

Other Losses

Hemorrhage or trauma
Addison's disease
Third spacing
- Increased loss of fluid, nutrients, electrolytes.
- Decreased sodium retention, thus decreased water reabsorption.
- Abnormal amounts of fluid accumulation in compartments that normally have minimal fluid decreases availability of fluids needed to maintain blood volume and cellular function.

EXCESS FLUID VOLUME

Excessive Intake

Excess fluid
- Increased oral or IV volume.
- Electrolyte-free infusion, such as dextrose 5% in water.

Excess sodium
- Increased sodium promotes water reabsorption.

Decreased Excretion

Renal disease
Increased antidiuretic hormone
- Kidney cannot excrete excess fluid.
- More chronic disease in older adults.
- Increase in osmolality of extracellular fluid (water loss, sodium gain), reduced blood volume, pain, stress (emotional and physiological), medications (such as morphine, barbiturates, general anesthetics).
- Excessive stress activates hypothalamic center, causing release of both antidiuretic hormone and adrenocorticotropic hormone.

Increased Capillary Permeability

Sepsis, inflammatory processes, major trauma and burns, acid–base imbalance
- Increased capillary permeability allows more fluid to leak into the interstitial spaces, causing fluid excess or edema.

Hypoproteinemia

Decreased intake or increased loss
- Any state of decreased protein, regardless of etiology, results in a decrease in capillary colloid osmotic pressure that impairs reabsorption. Excess fluid is left in the interstitial spaces, causing edema.

compromises the exchange of nutrients and wastes across the membrane between the cell and the plasma. Fluid output includes both sensible loss and insensible loss. *Sensible fluid loss* is fluid loss that is easily perceived, such as through urination. *Insensible fluid loss* is fluid loss that is not easily perceived, such as through normal respiration (see Figure 25-6).

Hypoproteinemia, or decreased protein in the plasma, either from decreased intake or increased loss, will result in de-

creased intravascular oncotic pressure. This ultimately results in hypotension because of the decrease in reabsorption at the venous end of the capillary.

Exercise. A client who has a risk of fluid deficit does not present with the actual signs and symptoms of an imbalance. However, recognizable risk factors can lead you to believe that the person has a high probability of developing a fluid

Fluid intake		Fluid output	
Ingested water	1200-1500 mL	Kidneys	1500 mL
Ingested food	800-1100 mL	Insensible loss	
Metabolic oxidation	300 mL	through skin	600-800 mL
		Insensible loss	
		through lungs	400-600 mL
		Gastrointestinal tract	100 mL
TOTAL	2600-3000 mL		
		TOTAL	2600-3000 mL

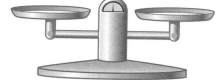

Figure 25-6. Sources of fluid intake and fluid output.

Table 25-5	Proportion of Body Water by Age
Age	Percent of Body Weight
Neonate	77
6 months	72
2-16 years	60
20-39 years	59 (women) to 60 (men)
40-59 years	47 (women) to 55 (men)
65 years and older	45 to 50

deficit. Exercise, especially in a hot, humid environment, is one such risk factor.

In fact, a water loss of only 1.2% has been found to impair thermoregulation. A fluid loss of only 2% can cause increased heart rates, increased body temperature, and decreased plasma volume. It is not just one factor but the relationship of the temperature and humidity that determines a person's response. In an athlete, a low temperature with a high humidity or a high temperature with a low humidity can cause fatal heat strokes.

Stress. Regardless of whether a stressor stems from a physiological, a psychological, an environmental, or another cause, the body's response will vary with the client's perception of the seriousness of the stressor, the actual degree of physical damage, and the body's ability to adapt to the insult. Any stressor activates the general adaptation system, which results in hypothalamic releasing factors that stimulate the anterior pituitary to release adrenocorticotropic hormone which stimulates the adrenal cortex.

Cortisols and aldosterone released from the adrenal cortex play a major role in improving tissue perfusion by increasing blood volume. Cortisols improve vascular volume through healing of the damaged capillary membranes, which decreases capillary leaking, and through increased sodium retention. Aldosterone has an even stronger influence on sodium retention. Both promote the loss of potassium. If the stressor results in marked hypokalemia, metabolic alkalosis may result. To maintain electroneutrality, when the potassium moves out of the cell into the plasma, the hydrogen ion moves from the plasma into the cell, increasing the risk for metabolic alkalosis.

Developmental Factors

Everyone is at risk for fluid and electrolyte imbalance, but older adults and the very young are at greatest risk because of their varying water distribution (Table 25-5).

Infants and Children. The younger the child, the greater the risk for fluid deficit. This is partly because the highest growth rate, or the period of greatest metabolic activity after fetal development, is during infancy. Infants and children also have immature kidneys with a decreased ability to concentrate urine. In addition, an increased body surface area compared with weight leads to increased fluid loss through the skin. Compensatory mechanisms are also less efficient.

Adolescents and Middle-Aged Adults. Adolescents have an increased risk for fluid deficit because of an increase in hormonal activity and increased loss with exercise-related activities. Teenagers who become pregnant further compromise their health because of the increased demands of the fetus during a time when their own bodies have an increased need.

Middle-aged adults are the age group least at risk for fluid imbalance. Developmentally, however, the demands of work-related activities and family rearing can increase the risk for self-care deficit. Pregnancy does increase the need for fluid because of fetal demands and tissue changes.

Older Adults. The older adult is more at risk for fluid imbalances because of the increased incidence of chronic diseases. Fluid deficit, or dehydration, is the most common fluid and electrolyte problem in the older adult population. Even healthy older adults have a decreased thirst mechanism. The aged kidney also has a decreased ability to concentrate urine. Lack of access to food purchasing because of financial, health, or transportation barriers also decreases intake. Older adults usually take more medications, over-the-counter or prescribed, than any other age group. The most common side effects of most of these medications are nausea, vomiting, and diarrhea.

Referring to the case study, Mrs. Thompson was drinking less. She also was losing fluid by four routes. Increased perspiration, diarrhea, vomiting, and, to a lesser extent, rapid respiration each contributed to the dehydration she experienced. Remember that in the early phases of Mrs. Thompson's fluid deficit, her body compensated. Recall that thirst was not a compensatory mechanism for Mrs. Thompson because of her advanced age. Mrs. Thompson's manifestations of oliguria, constipation, and dry skin were expected responses to her body's need to conserve fluid. As her regulatory systems could no longer compensate, she became very ill.

Physiological Factors

The most common physiological factors that increase the risk for fluid, electrolyte, and acid–base problems are pathologies, stressors, or treatments that affect the cardiovascular, respiratory, GI, renal, and integumentary systems. Trauma can affect any one or a combination of these systems.

Uncommon, but just as serious, is the fluid deficit risk raised by conditions that alter the function of the adrenal gland. Hypoaldosteronism can lead to severe sodium deficit and thus fluid loss. Hyperaldosteronism and Cushing's syndrome both increase the risk for fluid retention secondary to sodium retention. Certain cancers (some lymphomas and bronchogenic, pancreatic, and prostatic cancers) also increase the risk for fluid overload secondary to the increased secretion of antidiuretic hormone (also called vasopressin) from the tumor cells.

Cardiovascular Problems. Cardiovascular diseases can lead to a state of weakness or inability to access fluids and food products so that a deficit results. More common, however, is fluid overload caused by heart disease. When the left ventricle cannot contract efficiently, the buildup of fluid pressure has a retrograde effect, causing an increase in left atrial pressure followed by increased pulmonary pressure, which leads to pulmonary congestion.

The most critical consequence of left ventricular failure is pulmonary edema. This can lead to a subsequent increase in right ventricular pressure, followed by systemic fluid overload. Excess fluid or sodium intake in a person who has cardiac or renal dysfunction will only further exacerbate the fluid overload.

Respiratory Problems. Any situation or pathology that increases the respiratory rate also increases the amount of fluid lost in expired air.

Gastrointestinal Problems. Many GI problems, including vomiting, diarrhea, ileostomies, and fistulas, lead to fluid loss. Prescribed therapies such as gastric or bowel suction also increase fluid loss. Decreased fluid intake, as in dysphagia, is a common factor in dehydration. The most common GI pathology that causes fluid overload is liver disease.

Renal Problems. End-stage renal disease is usually characterized by polyuric, oliguric, and anuric phases. During the polyuric phase, a client is at risk for *Deficient fluid volume*. In the oliguric and anuric phases, fluid overload predominates because of the excessive retention of fluid.

Integumentary Problems. Loss of the protective skin barrier results in increased fluid loss. The blisters that accompany partial-thickness burns are filled with fluid that is no longer available to the body. This process by which fluid moves into an area that makes it physiologically unavailable is known as **third spacing.** Other examples of third spacing include the movement of fluid into the peritoneal space (ascites), the pericardial space (pericardial effusion), and the pleural space (pleural effusion).

Protein loss from burn wounds into the interstitial spaces results in decreased plasma colloid osmotic pressure. The etiology of the resulting edema is twofold: impaired reabsorption of water into the capillaries and increased interstitial oncotic pressure. Hypoproteinemia is a common example of how an extracellular fluid deficit (in the plasma) can exist at the same time as an extracellular fluid excess (in the interstitium).

Trauma. As with burns, tissue damage from any type of trauma can lead to fluid loss. Metabolites released by cell damage trigger the inflammatory process, which in turn stimulates the release of byproducts that increase capillary permeability. Increasing permeability allows more fluid to shift from plasma into the interstitial space. This extra interstitial fluid is not available for maintaining body functions, and it alters gas and nutrient exchange in the involved tissues.

Protein loss from traumatized tissues is also a consequence of increased capillary permeability and has the same manifestations as in burn trauma. Sepsis, a possible complication of trauma, promotes increased capillary permeability and more fluid, electrolyte, and protein loss.

A client with head trauma may develop either fluid deficit or fluid excess. Head trauma can result in diabetes insipidus or a syndrome of inappropriate antidiuretic hormone (SIADH). Diabetes insipidus manifests with polyuria (2 to 15 L of urine daily), which can lead to severe fluid deficits. SIADH results in an obligatory increase in antidiuretic hormone, a secondary decrease in urinary output, and thus a risk for fluid overload.

Clinical Factors

Many interventions can increase a client's risk for fluid imbalance. They include surgery, chemotherapy, medications, suctioning, and long-term use of IV therapy.

Surgery. Clients are at risk in both the preoperative and the postoperative phases of surgery. The longer the client has had nothing by mouth or has had a decreased intake or increased loss before surgery, the greater the risk of intraoperative and postoperative complications. For example, the preparation prior to surgery such as cathartics or enemas, as well as excessive blood loss during or after surgery, can also cause a fluid volume deficit. Infection is still one of the most common postoperative complications. The fever, diaphoresis, and tachypnea that accompany infection increase fluid loss.

Chemotherapy. Many chemotherapeutic drugs have a high incidence of GI cell damage, leading to frequent complications of stomatitis, anorexia, taste changes, nausea, and vomiting. These effects promote a fluid deficit through a decreased intake or an increased loss. Fluid volume excess is also a risk with chemotherapeutic drugs that increase the release of antidiuretic hormone, such as vincristine, cyclophosphamide, vinblastine, cisplatin, and oxytocin.

Medications. Medications that cause fluid loss (such as diuretics) and adverse effects that result in fluid loss (such as vomiting and diarrhea) are common causes of fluid deficit. For example, elixirs that contain sorbitol, which are commonly ordered for clients with GI tubes, can cause diarrhea in some people.

Medications such as insulin and oral hypoglycemics are commonly used to control the hyperglycemia of diabetes mellitus. Hyperglycemia, regardless of the cause, increases fluid loss secondary to the osmotic effect of the glucose molecule in the renal tubules.

c. Check for gastric pH by aspirating stomach contents and dipping the pH test strip into the contents. *Contents from the stomach usually have a pH of less than 5. Although usually a good indicator, medications as well as blood can alter the pH.*

d. Use the five-in-one connector to attach the distal end of the tube to the tubing marked "to patient" on the lid of the suction collection device.

e. Finish taping the tube to the client's nose using the method specified by your facility.

f. Attach the tubing to the gown with a rubber band and safety pin. *By leaving some slack in the tube when you affix it to the gown, you can prevent accidental pulling on the tube when the client turns his head.*

g. Set the suction control at the prescribed level. *Usually, you will use low intermittent suction (80 to 120 mm Hg). Only with a double-lumen tube can you safely use high suction (>120 mm Hg). This is because the second lumen allows constant air exchange and thus prevents gastric tissue trauma from the high suction pressure. The second lumen must be kept clear of secretions to decrease this risk. If you notice secretions in the second lumen, instill about 10 to 20 cc of air into it to displace the secretions.*

6. Finish.

a. Document the reason for the nasogastric tube, your collaboration with the physician, the actual procedure, and the client's response. *Documentation is essential to validate care and provide data for future comparison and follow-up.*

b. Provide comfort care for the client's nose and mouth at least every 8 hours and as needed. Use a clean cotton-tipped swab and water-soluble lubricant to clean the client's nostril. Assess the amount and characteristics of the nasogastric drainage as you provide care. Avoid alcohol-based mouth care agents for oral care because they tend to promote dryness.

7. Monitor.

a. Inspect the client's abdomen and auscultate bowel sounds at least every 8 hours. To decrease the possibility of mistaking suction sounds for bowel sounds, pinch the suction tubing as you auscultate the client's abdomen.

b. Monitor and document the amount and characteristics of the client's nasogastric output, manifestations of defi-

cient fluid volume, low electrolyte levels (especially sodium, potassium, calcium, chloride, and magnesium), or plasma levels that suggest deficient fluid volume (elevated sodium, blood urea nitrogen, and hematocrit).

c. Notify the physician if the client's nasogastric output exceeds 100 mL/hour, if total output exceeds total intake, or if there are new or worsening signs of deficient fluid volume. *Signs of deficient fluid volume include hypotension, a pulse of more than 20 beats per minute above the client's baseline when resting, urine production of less than 30 mL/hour for 2 consecutive hours or more, seizures, confusion, sudden behavioral changes, and abnormal electrolyte levels.*

d. If the client's nasogastric tube stops draining well, first assess the equipment for function errors. If this is not the problem, consult a physician for an irrigation order. Irrigate the tube using a 50- or 60-mL cone-shaped syringe with 30 to 60 mL of normal saline. Repeat as necessary. *Normal saline is the only acceptable irrigating solution because its isotonicity will not further compromise the client's fluid and electrolyte balance. Make sure to compute the difference in the amount of irrigant instilled and the amount removed; subtract or add that figure to the client's 8-hour nasogastric drainage total.*

PEDIATRIC CONSIDERATIONS

Measurement of the tube in an infant or young child is from the nose to the tip of the earlobe and then to the point midway between the umbilicus and the xiphoid process. It is often easier for the child to have the tube placed quickly rather than taking pauses. Another nurse or caregiver (even restraints) may be needed to help hold the hands of a child during placement to keep the child from pulling the tube out. The neck of an infant should remain neutral during placement. Taping the tube to the cheek rather than the gown usually works better in a pediatric client.

GERIATRIC CONSIDERATIONS

A geriatric client may need to rest after the tube has been inserted to the posterior part of the nostril (between steps 4c and 4d) before advancing further into the stomach, especially if the procedure is extremely difficult. In very debilitated geriatric clients, another individual may need to hold the head of the client in a forward position while placement is attempted. A geriatric client taking antacids or gastric reflux medicines may have a higher pH because of the medications.

them by mouth (see Chapter 24). Diarrhea resulting in fluid deficit is a common complication of tube feedings. The two most common sources of diarrhea secondary to tube feedings are the use of hypertonic feedings and a rapid delivery rate. The increased osmolality of hypertonic feedings promotes

fluid shifting into the small bowel, which can result in diarrhea and dehydration. Likewise, the client may not tolerate a rapid delivery of a feeding and may develop diarrhea. Giving water boluses with hypertonic feedings and either giving feedings slowly or diluting them will decrease these risks.

PROCEDURE 25-2   REMOVING A NASOGASTRIC TUBE

TIME TO ALLOW
Novice: 10 min.
Expert: 5 min.

This procedure is used to discontinue gastric decompression therapy.

DELEGATION GUIDELINES

The necessity for assessment prior to discontinuation of a nasogastric tube, the risk of aspiration associated with tube removal, and the short nature of this procedure suggest that this procedure not be delegated to a nursing assistant.

EQUIPMENT NEEDED
- Clean gloves
- Towel
- Emesis basin
- Plastic bag
- 50- or 60-mL syringe
- Tissue

1. Follow preliminary guidelines for nursing procedures (see inside front cover).

2. Prepare the client.
a. Before removing the tube, assess for the presence of bowel sounds. *Do not remove the tube if bowel sounds are absent.*
b. Place the emesis basin and opened plastic bag on a nearby table, don clean gloves, and place the towel across the client's upper chest.
c. Turn off the suction machine and disconnect the nasogastric tube from the suction tubing.
d. Unpin the nasogastric tube from the client's gown or untape from the cheek.
e. Instill 20 cc of air into the nasogastric tube to displace secretions back into the client's stomach. *Doing so decreases the client's risk of aspiration.*

f. Loosen the tape on the client's nose while holding the distal end of the nasogastric tube.

3. Remove the tube. Instruct the client to breath-hold, and then pull the tube out in one quick, steady motion. Note the intactness of the tip of the tube.

4. Finish.
a. Assist with or provide skin and mouth care.
b. Document the presence of bowel sounds, the tube removal procedure, and the client's response.
c. Continue to monitor the client for return of bowel dysfunction.

Intravenous Therapy. Many clients receive IV therapy as part of their treatment. If the amount of fluid that the client is receiving is not adequate to meet maintenance and replacement needs, a risk for fluid deficit exists. For example, a client who is receiving IV therapy over several days with no other source of intake is at risk for fluid deficit as well as electrolyte deficit. Fluids, sodium, and potassium are required on a daily basis to maintain homeostasis. When a client has been 3 or more days without food through the oral or gastric route, an IV approach is chosen to provide these nutrients.

When an IV route is used to provide carbohydrates, proteins, fats, and other electrolytes, it is known as total parenteral nutrition. You will need to monitor the client for hyperglycemia and secondary polyuria because of the risk for osmotic diuresis from the high glucose levels in the solution. Frequent monitoring with Chemstrip glucose readings and administration of regular insulin on a sliding scale will prevent this syndrome.

ASSESSMENT

General Assessment of Fluid Balance

Perform a general health history to gather baseline data that will help you screen for specific risk factors. Also, focus your physical assessment on systems that are related to the fluid imbalance.

Health History. Because fluid and electrolyte imbalances affect so many systems, a complete history and a physical examination are necessary. The health history begins with the gathering of more data about the client's chief complaint. When the problem is related to fluid and electrolyte deficit, the client's chief complaint is usually related to one of the following: nausea, vomiting, diarrhea, anorexia, increasing fatigue and weakness, weight loss, fever, blood loss, excess urine output, or a change in mental status. Or the client's chief complaint may be a condition or a traumatic injury, such as a burn, in which manifestations of a fluid and electrolyte imbalance might be hidden by the more obvious problem of the injury itself.

When the problem is related to fluid and electrolyte excess, the client's chief complaint is usually related to one of the following: weight gain, cough, dyspnea, cardiac palpitations, pitting edema, decreased urinary output, or mental status changes.

Whatever the chief complaint, it is important to find out the characteristics of the client's symptoms, including the onset, location and radiation if applicable, frequency, severity, associated signs and symptoms, and aggravating or alleviating factors, and the client's previous history or treatment of this problem.

Also, find out the client's past history of illnesses, hospitalizations, surgeries, trauma, allergies, current or recent medication, and currency of immunizations. Obtain an obstetrical history if applicable. Collect data related to family history and psychosocial history and then complete the review of systems. If the client's condition is acute, collect data pertinent to the immediate problem and intervene quickly. When possible, obtain additional history from family members or old records and complete the history when the client's condition stabilizes.

Physical Examination. A full head-to-toe physical examination may be necessary for an accurate diagnosis. Again, if the client's condition is critical, collect only the data needed for safe and immediate intervention. In addition to the initial physical examination, an accurate diagnosis of fluid and electrolyte imbalances often requires monitoring of the client's intake and output, weight trends, edema levels, diagnostic tests, and ongoing physical assessments.

STANDARD CLINICAL MEASUREMENTS. A basic understanding of standard measurements related to fluid balance is essential to assessing and evaluating a client's fluid status. Volume is commonly measured in liters, milliliters, and cubic centimeters. For all practical purposes, the milliliter and the cubic centimeter are equivalent. Oral fluid measurements are usually expressed as cubic centimeters (cc), whereas IV solutions are expressed as liters (L) or milliliters (mL).

Weight is commonly measured in grams (g) and milligrams (mg). One gram equals 1000 mg. Protein is expressed on a laboratory printout as grams per 100 mL of fluid. The normal plasma protein is 6 g/100 mL.

The **milliequivalent** (mEq), one-thousandth of a chemical equivalent, is the measurement used to express the chemical activity or chemical combining power of an ion. Although electrolytes have variable milligram weights, the weight has no relationship to its chemical combining power. One milliequivalent of any electrolyte is chemically equal to 1 mEq of any other electrolyte. Chemical neutrality, an equal number of milliequivalents of cations and anions, must be present for normal neuromuscular excitability to occur.

WEIGHING THE CLIENT. When the accuracy of intake and output measurements is uncertain, or when the client has generalized body edema, weighing is preferred. A client's weight is a more critical indicator of fluid loss or gain. One kilogram (2.2 lb) is equal to 1 L of fluid loss or gain.

Because interventions are based on the data obtained from weight assessments, standardization is very important. Standardization includes weighing the client at the same time of day, with the same amount of clothing, and on the same scale. When any of these standards are unavoidably changed, the documentation should reflect this change.

MEASURING INTAKE AND OUTPUT. Measurement of intake and output (I&O) is usually advised when a fluid imbalance exists or the client is at risk. This assessment is always used in the acute care setting, where clients are at higher acuity levels and at greater risk for complications.

Most clients in a chronic care setting are older adults. Because dehydration is the most common fluid imbalance in this group, prevention is the key. Giving fluids frequently throughout the day and early evening usually prevents this problem. Monitor I&O for any client at risk for or experiencing an actual fluid volume deficit or excess.

When the problem is fluid overload, assessing the specific systems should be made in addition to measuring I&O. For example, if the client's primary problem is pulmonary congestion, an increase in lung crackles would indicate a worsening condition. In contrast, a decrease in crackles is a positive response to interventions.

Remember to measure I&O from all sources. Intake includes fluids taken orally, by tube, or by IV. Fluid output includes urine, diarrhea, vomitus, suction, wound drainage, diaphoresis, hyperventilation, and other drainage. Insensible fluid loss (through normal breathing and the skin) and sensible fluid loss (through hyperventilation or diaphoresis) should also be considered.

In situations where I&O is critical and normal urinary output cannot be measured, it may be necessary to compare the weight of the clean product that is used (e.g., linens, pads, diapers) with the weight of the soiled product. The difference in grams is equal to the output in milliliters.

To perform an I&O measurement accurately, use the appropriate measurement device for the quantity being measured (e.g., a medicine cup for amounts less than 30 mL, or a graduated cylinder to measure 100 to 1000 mL). Other tools include appropriate documentation forms, such as an I&O form (Figure 25-7, p. 582).

It is essential to document and communicate the amount of IV fluid that is left hanging for the next shift to count. This is known as the "credit" or "claim." For example, if a client receives 1000 mL IV every 8 hours and had 600 mL from the current bag and 350 mL from the previous IV bag, the client received 950 mL. The credit for the next shift, from the current 1000 mL bag, is 400 mL (difference of 1000 − 600). If you use a pump form of delivery, you may just clear the 8-hour intake of feeding or IV fluid and leave the next shift with a starting base of 0 instead of a credit.

Other essential tools include appropriate elimination collection devices (fracture pan or regular bedpan, specimen collection devices for toilet or commode, or urinal) and clean disposable gloves. Some fluid collection devices have

Elkins Park Medical Center

Patient Label

Patient name _____
ID# _____
Physician _____

Intake and Output Record

Date:		0700 – 1900		1700 – 0900	
Intake	Oral				
	Tube feeding				
	Intravenous	Intake	Credit	Intake	Credit
	Primary				
	Secondary				
	Blood products				
	TPN				
	Other				
Output	Urine				
	Gastric				
	Emesis				
	Suction				
	Stool				
	Other				
Total 24° Intake =			**Total 24° Output =**		

Figure 25-7. I&O form. A standard I&O form should include all of the common sources of intake and output to provide cues to the caregiver. Compare the total intake and output over several days with weight changes to identify trends in fluid excess or deficits.

graduations marked on the container. It is acceptable to use these if the measurement can be made accurately.

Adaptation to the home setting includes teaching the client and family how to keep a diary of fluid intake and output. Suggest a simple notebook with a column for the client's sources of intake, a column for measured output, a column for date and time (if appropriate), and a column for other essential data (such as a description of drainage). Graduated measuring cups normally used for cooking purposes will facilitate accuracy. Other supplies—such as a graduated cylinder, specimen pan, bedpan, or urinal—may need to be purchased at a local pharmacy or medical supply outlet.

Tools include more than equipment; knowledge is also essential. For example, you must know which clients should be placed on I&O monitoring. Although collaboration with the physician is vital, measurement of I&O is an independent nursing function. This requires knowledge of who is at risk for fluid imbalance and who has an actual imbalance, as well as appropriate assessment skills.

Your assessment should include the client's and family's willingness and readiness to learn and their level of understanding of the importance of I&O monitoring. It also includes assessing functional abilities, financial resources and barriers, and developmental, cultural, and religious variables. Collaborate closely with the social worker to maximize care,

such as purchasing a bedside commode or other equipment, that is constrained by financial barriers.

Referring to the case study, Mrs. Thompson was very willing to learn but was not capable of cooking or shopping for herself because of extreme fatigue and weakness. Developmentally, her decreased thirst mechanism interfered with her perception of fluid need. Culturally, she didn't like the prepared food items available at the local grocery store. However, because she raised her children with the strong African-American value of family bonding, she had them as a resource. Daily, one of the children assisted her with I&O monitoring, grocery shopping, and the provision of many of her favorite food dishes.

ASSESSING EDEMA. Edema scales vary among different institutions. If your facility has an edema scale, all personnel should use that scale to promote continuity in communication and evaluation of client responses. If no scale is available, measure the level of pitting edema by assessing the residual indentation left by pressing your finger into the area for 5 seconds (+1/5 edema is mild and +5/5 is severe). Document the site, the depth of the tissue indentation in millimeters or centimeters, and the time needed for the tissue to spring back.

Assessment for pitting edema works well with small, localized edematous areas, such as the sacrum, feet, ankles, or tibia. In situations where the edema is more pronounced, however, such as when it involves the entire leg, thigh, or abdomen, you will need a more objective assessment. Because consistency is important, mark the site you are measuring with a marker. Use a centimeter tape to measure the circumference of the leg, thigh, or abdomen. Document the measurement and compare against earlier data for changes. When a client has generalized body edema, called anasarca, weighing is more accurate.

Diagnostic Tests. The plasma levels most commonly used to assist in the diagnosis of dehydration or fluid volume deficit are plasma sodium, plasma and urine osmolality, hematocrit, and blood urea nitrogen (BUN). The sodium ion is used as a direct measure of osmolality because it is the major ion in extracellular fluid. Plasma sodium, osmolality, hematocrit, and BUN levels are elevated in fluid volume deficit. BUN levels may also be elevated in individuals with a high-protein diet. Urine osmolality is also increased secondary to the release of antidiuretic hormone and aldosterone. The kidney still excretes an obligatory amount of urine to rid the body of waste products of metabolism; this is about 30 mL of urine per hour.

Urine osmolality is measured and reported by the laboratory. Less commonly, you may be asked to test specific gravity using a test tube and a floating urinometer. If you test urine specific gravity on the unit, obtain enough urine to half-fill the test tube, spin the urinometer inside the test tube, and read the level of the calibrated mark on the urinometer as it is spinning. Normal specific gravity is 1.005 to 1.026. A specific gravity less than 1.005 indicates excess fluid intake, and greater than 1.026 indicates decreased fluid intake.

Osmolality measurement is often ordered when the concentrating ability of the kidney is being evaluated. This function is significant because, if the kidney cannot concentrate urine, the client loses more fluid and develops a fluid volume deficit. Remember that, in the body, it is the *relationship* of the solute (such as sodium, protein, glucose, or urea) to the solvent (water) that determines the body's response, not the level itself.

Decreased BUN, decreased hematocrit, decreased plasma sodium, and decreased plasma osmolality are classic laboratory findings in fluid volume excess. These diagnostic studies represent the relationship of the solvent (water) to the solute in the plasma. In fluid volume excess, the proportion of water exceeds the normal amount found in the vascular compartment. Therefore the sodium, urea, and red blood cells appear to be decreased when actually they are just diluted.

When plasma levels tend toward the unexpected or the client presents with manifestations that suggest a specific pathology for a fluid volume deficit or excess, the physician will order other plasma studies or diagnostic tests. For example, creatinine levels can help evaluate renal dysfunction, liver function studies can reveal liver pathology, and glucose studies can show glucose intolerance.

Plasma levels are accurate indicators of potassium, sodium, and chloride levels. However, because potassium is primarily an intracellular ion, small deficits in the plasma level are very reflective of a decrease in total body potassium.

Indeed, a level of 3.4 mEq/L, a deficit of only 0.1 mEq/L, requires potassium replacement. On the other hand, the plasma level of sodium, which is predominantly extracellular, gives a much more accurate presentation of total body sodium levels. A client rarely needs replacement if sodium levels exceed 125 mEq/L.

The plasma calcium level helps identify imbalances but can become a false indicator if the client has abnormal albumin levels, an acid–base imbalance, or hypoparathyroidism. Because 99% of the calcium in plasma is bound to albumin and only 0.5% is free (ionized), the amount of albumin has an inverse relationship to the level of functional ionized calcium. For example, when a client has a protein deficit, less calcium is bound, resulting in an increase in free calcium. The plasma level (the bound version) may appear normal when in reality the ionized calcium is higher. The reverse is true when a client has an excess protein intake. The client presents with signs of hypocalcemia because of the excess binding of the calcium to the protein, which leaves less free, ionized calcium.

Alkalosis and acidosis also affect the calcium binding and result in similar manifestations. For example, in alkalosis, more calcium is bound and thus less is ionized, so the client presents with signs of hypocalcemia. In acidosis, less calcium is bound, leaving more free ionized calcium. The client presents with signs of hypercalcemia. In any client with critical calcium regulation, a plasma ionized calcium test should be performed to discover the true functional level of calcium.

Magnesium plasma levels are not commonly ordered because they have not proved accurate as indicators of cellular levels. Assessment of tendon reflexes has been suggested as a more accurate indicator of magnesium imbalance than plasma level.

Because the cardiac conduction system is so sensitive to electrolyte imbalance, an electrocardiogram (ECG) is a helpful diagnostic test. The more serious and acute the imbalance, the more grave the changes are on the ECG.

Arterial blood gases (ABGs) are essential to properly diagnose acid–base imbalances. If only oxygenation data are necessary, an oxygenation saturation level can easily be obtained through pulse oximetry.

Focused Assessment for *Deficient Fluid Volume*

Fluid deficit is a common problem. Many pathologies and situations increase the risk for or result in fluid deficit. Recognizing and intervening in high-risk situations or in early phases of fluid deficit are very important to the client's outcome.

Defining Characteristics. The official definition for *Deficient fluid volume* does not differentiate between vascular, interstitial, and intracellular dehydration. Although all compartments are interactive, the cellular compartments are the last ones to be affected by a fluid deficit. This is because the body's homeostatic mechanisms attempt to correct the deficit. Therefore early recognition and intervention targeted at reversing extracellular fluid deficit will help prevent intracellular dehydration.

Box 25-1 Characteristics of Extracellular Fluid Deficit

GENERALIZED

- Flattened neck veins in supine position
- Sudden weight loss, unless masked by third spacing
- Peripheral vein filling takes more than 5 seconds
- Decreased skin turgor (not accurate in older adults)
- Dry mucous membranes and furrowed tongue
- Speech changes
- Muscle weakness, especially in upper body
- Subnormal temperature if severe loss, fever if moderate loss
- Depressed fontanels in an infant
- Soft and sunken eyeballs

CARDIAC

- Orthostatic hypotension (systolic BP falls more than 25 mm Hg and diastolic BP falls more than 20 mm Hg) with compensatory tachycardia (up to 120 beats/minute)
- Weak, thready pulse
- Narrow pulse pressure

GASTROINTESTINAL

- Constipation or decrease in number and moisture of stools

RENAL

- Urinary output greatly exceeding intake if this is the etiology of the deficit
- Urinary output decreased if compensatory response

EXTRACELLULAR. Box 25-1 provides a list of defining characteristics and age-related manifestations common in a client with extracellular fluid deficit. Muscle weakness results primarily from the altered relationship of fluid to sodium. The decreased plasma volume is responsible for the compensatory increase in pulse rate, orthostatic hypotension, prolonged peripheral vein filling, decreased central venous pressure, flattened neck veins, and compensatory conservation of fluid by the bowel and kidneys.

No one manifestation by itself increases morbidity or mortality as long as compensatory mechanisms or planned interventions reverse the deficit. However, cerebral manifestations indicate cerebral cell involvement that could result in irreversible cerebral tissue damage.

Action Alert! Notify the physician if a client experiences a rapid, unexpected weight loss (more than 3 lb/day); vomiting or diarrhea that lasts more than 24 hours in a child, a pregnant woman, an older adult, or a person with chronic disease; or unexplained tachycardia or other atypical cardiac irregularities.

INTRACELLULAR. Intracellular dehydration is much more serious than extracellular dehydration because of the potential dysfunction of mitochondrial formation of adenosine triphosphate (ATP); ATP is critical to all cell function and transport. Defining characteristics include fever, thirst, and central nervous system changes. Shrinkage of cerebral cells stimulates osmoreceptors in the hypothalamus, which triggers the thirst mechanism. The fluid imbalance also disrupts cortical functioning. Early cerebral manifestations include restlessness, headache, irritability, and a feeling of apprehension. As the fluid deficit progresses, confusion occurs, followed by seizures and, in severe deficit, coma.

Because compensatory mechanisms are so protective, intracellular fluid volume is maintained except in sudden or severe fluid losses or when there is a loss of the body's homeostatic ability to compensate for this loss.

Action Alert! Notify the physician if the client experiences a fever over 38.3° C (101° F) or a change in mental status, such as a headache (new, unrelenting, or increasing in severity), confusion, or behavioral changes such as irritability, seizures, or deterioration in level of consciousness.

Related Factors. Many underlying pathological and situational factors can cause fluid volume deficit. Excessive output from the urinary system, GI tract, skin, or respiratory system can result in extracellular deficit followed by intracellular deficit if not corrected. Decreased intake, whether from lack of access to fluids, financial constraints, pathologies impairing intake, fatigue, weakness, or the decreased thirst mechanism found in older adults, is the other major contributory factor to fluid deficit. If excess output and insufficient intake coexist, the client is at an even higher risk for more serious consequences. The following four major variables determine how critical these manifestations are:

- The acuteness of the loss
- The severity of the loss
- The client's age and state of health
- The degree to which the client's compensatory mechanisms or therapeutic interventions combat the deficit

Focused Assessment for *Excess Fluid Volume*

Defining Characteristics. Again, the official definition of *Excess fluid volume* does not differentiate between extracellular and intracellular excess. Because the cell is the last compartment to undergo shifting (unless the excess is very acute or massive), it is important to be able to differentiate between extracellular and intracellular changes.

EXTRACELLULAR. Box 25-2 provides a list of defining characteristics common in a client with extracellular fluid excess. The excess fluid can be localized to a small area of the body and have little or no effect on overall body function. It can be localized to a specific compartment and cause alterations to specific tissues. Or it can be generalized throughout the body and cause major system dysfunction. An example of extracellular fluid excess at the local level is an ankle sprain. As the fluid accumulates around the joint, joint function is compromised.

If generalized manifestations of extracellular excess are present, they are secondary to fluid accumulation either throughout the body or in large body spaces, such as in the peritoneum. This is called ascites. As excess fluid accumulates, it interferes with the exchange of nutrients and waste

Box 25-2   Characteristics of Extracellular Fluid Excess

GENERALIZED

- Weakness and fatigue
- Body edema (anasarca)
- Pitting or nonpitting edema in dependent areas such as legs, sacrum, and scrotum
- Ascites
- Sudden weight gain of more than 2 lb/week (1 L of fluid = 2.2 lb or 1 kg)
- Peripheral venous distention
- Peripheral vein emptying taking more than 5 seconds
- Jugular venous distention (distended neck veins with client sitting at 45 degrees or higher)
- Bulging fontanels in an infant

PULMONARY

- Progressive worsening of dyspnea, from dyspnea on exertion to orthopnea, and finally to dyspnea at rest
- Increased respiratory rate
- Respiratory rhythm may become irregular or apneic
- Crackles present from fluid congestion in alveoli
- Possible pulmonary edema from severe fluid congestion in alveoli secondary to left ventricular failure

CARDIAC

- Tachycardia
- Bounding pulse
- Hypertension (systolic blood pressure >140 mm Hg or diastolic >90 mm Hg)
- Possible pericardial effusion with audible pericardial rub from fluid congestion in pericardium
- Third heart sound (sometimes called an S_3 gallop) from left ventricular fluid overload

GASTROINTESTINAL

- Anorexia, nausea, and vomiting

RENAL

- Increased output if kidney can compensate
- Decreased output if kidney damage is part of etiology

Possible pleural effusion with audible pleural rub from fluid congestion in pleural spaces

---

products between the cells and plasma spaces. A buildup of waste products leads to feelings of generalized weakness and fatigue, as well as to manifestations of tissue dysfunction.

An example of localized tissue edema that can have systemic effects is pulmonary fluid overload, or pulmonary edema. In pulmonary overload, manifestations are related to fluid in the alveoli of the lungs, which reduces exchange of oxygen and carbon dioxide. The fluid pressure in the lungs may also lead to shifting of fluid into the pleural spaces, a condition called pleural effusion. This complication decreases the ability of the lungs to expand during inhalation and thus can compromise the body's oxygen status even further.

As with any altered health state, the body attempts to compensate. The cardiac signs of bounding pulse, increased blood pressure, and gallop rhythm are all related to the increased volume of fluid in the heart and blood vessels. The bounding pulse and tachycardia are examples of the cardiovascular system's attempt to increase cardiac output by increasing the volume of blood ejected with each heart beat (stroke volume) and by increasing the rate. The same phenomenon of effusion in the lungs can occur in the pericardial spaces when the heart suffers from increased fluid overload. As with pleural effusion, pericardial effusion not only compromises cardiac function further but also affects tissue perfusion to the other body systems.

The renal response to fluid overload varies. The decreased osmolality will result in a decrease in antidiuretic hormone. If the kidneys are healthy, this will lead to an increase in urinary output. However, if the kidneys are part of the etiology of the fluid overload, polyuria followed by oliguria and then anuria will occur as the renal function diminishes.

Action Alert! Notify the physician if the client has a rapid weight gain (more than 2 lb/day); a new onset of severe pulmonary difficulty (respiratory rate greater than 30; irregular or apneic rhythm, marked increase in crackles or bronchial breath sounds, pleural friction rub); new onset or increased severity of cardiac manifestations (pericardial friction rub, arrhythmia, more than 5 premature beats/minute, a rate less than 50 or greater than 120 beats/minute, an S_3 gallop); or a change in urinary output (marked diuresis without taking a diuretic, output less than 30 mL/hour for 2 or more consecutive hours).

INTRACELLULAR. Recall that, in a healthy person, protective mechanisms provide a very delicate balance between intracellular and extracellular fluid compartments. However, many conditions can overpower these protective mechanisms, resulting in abnormal fluid shifting into the intracellular spaces. Because brain cells are very sensitive to minimal changes in fluid balance, the early manifestations of intracellular shifting are cerebral.

Action Alert! Notify the physician if the client shows a change in mental status or cerebral perfusion, such as a new, unrelenting, or worsening headache, confusion, lethargy, irritability, restlessness, or seizures.

The key variable that indicates the need to collaborate with the physician is *change*. This reinforces the importance of thorough and accurate communication and documentation between caregivers. Without this critical communication, client outcomes may be compromised.

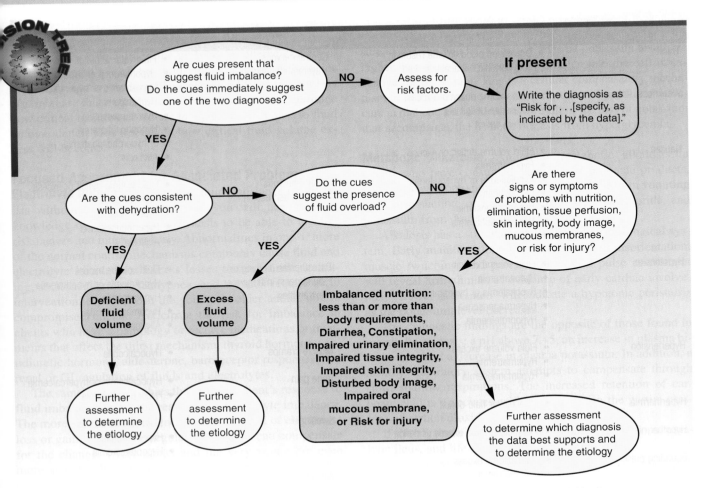

Figure 25-8. Decision tree for fluid balance nursing diagnoses. Diagnoses are shown in rectangles. Within these rectangles, diagnoses shown in **bold** type are NANDA-approved nursing diagnoses; diagnoses shown in regular type are not NANDA-approved nursing diagnoses.

client with a recent myocardial infarction, the diagnosis could be written as *Risk for excess fluid volume related to decreased myocardial contractility secondary to myocardial infarction.* Prevention and early detection of these imbalances influence the level of health alteration in the client. This is especially important in clients with fewer adaptive mechanisms, such as older adults, the young, and those with chronic diseases. Note that in each of the preceding examples, it is the *related to* or etiology component of the diagnostic statement that individualizes the problem. The etiology is derived from the data and explains the pathophysiology behind the problem.

Related Nursing Diagnoses

Clients may have one or many different responses to fluid imbalances. The most common related nursing diagnoses follow. To help make appropriate nursing diagnoses, cluster these and other responses into a data set specific for your client (Table 25-7).

- *Fatigue* related to altered cellular metabolism secondary to deficient (or excess) fluid

- *Anxiety* related to altered stability of the neuroendocrine transmission secondary to deficient (or excess) fluid
- *Ineffective health maintenance* related to inability to care for basic needs secondary to fatigue
- *Imbalanced nutrition: less than body requirements* related to lack of appetite and fatigue
- *Impaired skin integrity* related to lack of transport of nutrients to and waste products from the cells secondary to deficient (or excess) fluid
- *Impaired tissue perfusion* related to impaired cellular function secondary to deficient (or excess) fluid
- *Impaired gas exchange* related to decreased volume of blood available to transport respiratory gases secondary to deficient fluid volume
- *Impaired gas exchange* related to interference with the diffusion of oxygen and carbon dioxide between the capillaries and cells secondary to excess fluid volume
- *Constipation* related to inadequate amount of fluid to provide volume for stool formation
- *Impaired oral mucous membrane* related to cellular dehydration in the mouth secondary to deficient fluid volume

Table 25-7 *Clustering Data to Make a Nursing Diagnosis*

PROBLEMS OF FLUID BALANCE

Data Cluster	Diagnosis
A 9-month-old child has been vomiting for 24 hours. Even a sip of water does not stay down. The mother has noticed a decrease in the number of times his diaper is changed. He has a GI virus.	*Deficient fluid volume* related to gastrointestinal effects of pathogenic organisms
A 25-year-old man has had violent emesis and diarrhea for 2 days after his chemotherapy treatment. He is weak and has dry mucous membranes. He states he is thirsty.	*Deficient fluid volume* related to side effects of medications
An 80-year-old woman arrived in the emergency department struggling for breath with audible gurgling sounds. She has crackles and rhonchi throughout the lung fields. She is in high Fowler's position, appears ashen, and has distended jugular veins. Her blood pressure is 220/110. Her family states that she did not refill her prescriptions last week. She is diagnosed with congestive heart failure.	*Excess fluid volume* related to inability of the heart to pump efficiently secondary to CHF and client's stopping her medication regimen
A 50-year-old man is admitted with +3 pitting edema and decreased urinary output. He was prescribed a short-term treatment of corticosteroids for an episode of bronchitis. He has a history of congestive heart failure.	*Excess fluid volume* related to ineffective pumping action of the heart secondary to CHF and side effect of corticosteroids

- *Impaired oral mucous membrane* related to swollen tissues resulting in a breakdown of cells secondary to excess fluid volume
- *Disturbed sleep pattern* related to anxiety secondary to deficient fluid volume
- *Disturbed sleep pattern* related to inability to find a comfortable position to sleep secondary to excess fluid volume

Action Alert! Notify the physician when the client's fatigue and anxiety interfere with activities of daily living and role functions, when illness persists more than 48 hours or cerebral or cardiac manifestations are present, when an unplanned lack of food intake leads to an unwarranted weight loss greater than 5 lb, when a wound will not heal with basic cleansing and time, when a wound infection develops, or when decreased tissue perfusion becomes progressively worse. In the feet, for example, you might notice that edema continues to increase, the feet are growing cooler, and pulses are barely palpable. Cerebral effects might include atypical confusion. Also notify the physician if the client develops a new productive cough accompanied by increasing dyspnea, especially at rest, constipation that lasts more than 3 days and does not respond to typical remedies, mouth sores that do not heal normally, or sleep pattern disturbances or disturbed thought processes that persist after a few weeks of treatment.

PLANNING

Planning is an essential part of the care delivery. The expected outcomes must be specific to the etiology of the nursing diagnosis. The goal for a client with a fluid imbalance is to improve the existing deficit or excess. If it is not an actual problem but a risk, the goal is to reduce any risk factors that can be controlled. An example of a goal statement is *Client will improve deficient fluid volume as evidenced by . . .* or

Client will improve risk for deficient fluid volume as evidenced by . . . . A listing of expected outcomes that are specific to the etiology follows the goal statement.

Expected Outcomes for the Client With *Deficient Fluid Volume*

Each expected outcome for *Deficient fluid volume* focuses on measurable data that indicate an improvement in the client's fluid deficit. Some examples include the following:
- Increase in fluid intake to at least 1500 mL/24 hr (unless contraindicated)
- Moist mucous membranes
- Absence of tongue furrows
- Absence of tenting when skin turgor assessed
- Neck veins full in a supine position
- Absence of orthostatic hypotension
- Presence of full-volume peripheral pulsations (+2/3 or +3/4 scale)
- Plasma osmolality, hematocrit, sodium, and urine specific gravity values within normal limits
- Client relates the need for, amount of, and type of increased fluid intake during periods of excess loss

Again, the expected outcomes are specific to the etiology. If knowledge deficit is part of the etiology, then *relates the need for . . .* is an example of how to write an outcome criterion focusing on lack of knowledge.

The acuteness and severity of the deficit also influence the focus of the expected outcomes. In very acute states, the expected outcomes address the return to a hemodynamic state in the most critical tissues of the brain, heart, and kidney. Examples of expected outcomes in this situation include the following:
- Absence of confusion, lethargy, hallucinations, seizures
- Decrease in myocardial arrhythmias
- Increase in blood pressure to within normal range
- Increase in pulse volume (+2/3 or +3/4 scale)
- Increase in urinary output with decrease in urine osmolality to within normal limits

convection by using a fan. Administer niacin, if prescribed, to promote a cutaneous flush. Monitor I&O, vital signs, and fluid status hourly.

Remember that thirst is not a reliable indicator of the need for fluid replacement. Up to 3% of body weight can be lost before thirst is stimulated. Administering or consuming fluids only until thirst is relieved can result in only one half to about two thirds of the lost fluid lost being replaced.

Preventing Further Loss. The second major intervention is to provide supportive care to prevent further fluid loss. In addition to fluid replacement, interventions should be individualized to the etiology of the fluid loss. For example, when diarrhea or vomiting is present, antidiarrheal or antiemetic medications are appropriate. When loss is secondary to diaphoresis, choose appropriate interventions such as controlling fevers with medications that fight the etiology of the fever and giving prescribed antipyretics and removing excess bed linens.

Instituting Rehabilitative Care. The third intervention is to provide and recommend rehabilitative care to maximize client and family potential. Teach the client and family the importance of replacing lost fluids, maintaining nutrition, monitoring weight changes, and reporting significant concerns to the physician. Box 25-5 helps clients and families decide when to call a physician. Also, emphasize safety precautions if weakness or orthostatic hypotension is a problem. Safety precautions include changing positions slowly, using assistive devices as appropriate, and removing scatter rugs or other objects that increase the risk of falls.

Administering IV Therapy. Many routes are available for fluid intake: oral, tube (nasogastric, gastric, duodenal, or jejunal tubes), or parenteral (subcutaneous or IV). The oral route is the most preferred, common, and cost efficient. Recall from our earlier discussion that maintaining a balance in body fluid is dependent on the total amount of fluid intake from pure water as well as from other fluids and food products. When fluid homeostasis cannot be maintained through the oral route, alternative methods must be initiated to ensure cellular function. For more information on fluid given via an artificial tube, see Chapter 24.

When a client's homeostatic fluid needs cannot be met through an oral route or tube, or replacement is needed more quickly than either of these two routes can offer, IV therapy is the method of choice. Examples of clients requiring IV therapy include those who receive nothing by mouth, those unable to ingest oral fluids (possibly because of nausea, vomiting, or mental status changes), and those unable to absorb nutrients because of a dysfunctional bowel. Intravenous therapy is also used to deliver medications that would be destroyed by gastric enzymes, when rapid medication response is necessary, or when higher plasma levels are necessary. Clients with life-threatening situations from loss of plasma volume (such as hemorrhage, shock, and severe burns) also require IV therapy.

Teaching for Self-Care Box 25-5
When to Call the Physician for Problems of Fluid Balance

Purpose: To recognize changes in fluid balance that would necessitate a call to the physician

Expected Outcome: The client will seek a physician's advice when a change is recognized in fluid status.

Client Instructions

- Call the physician if the following occur:
- Fluid loss (as from vomiting or diarrhea) lasting more than 24 hours, especially if it involves a child, a pregnant woman, an older adult, or a person with chronic disease
- Rapid weight loss (>3 lb in a day if not an expected outcome of therapy)
- Rapid weight gain (>3 lb in a week or less)
- Increased difficulty breathing or a cough of new onset
- Atypical cardiac irregularity or palpitations
- Confusion or behavioral changes

THE·COST·OF·CARE Box 25-6
Cost-Saving Alternatives in Intravenous Therapy

The cost of health care includes prevention and treatment as well as conservation of resources. Some cost-saving alternatives in IV therapy include the following:

- Promote self-care and family involvement whenever possible, including positive health behaviors, such as fluid maintenance and replacement to decrease the need for IV therapy.
- Use primary prevention strategies to anticipate and prevent complications that could create a need for IV therapy.
- Consider using gravity flow instead of an IV pump if client's baseline health status does not indicate preexisting risk for fluid overload, and if agency policy permits.
- Change IV tubing every 72-96 hours according to agency policy. Label the tubing with the date and time to avoid unnecessary waste resulting from having to replace unlabeled tubing.
- Use retrograde flushing of primary solution through piggyback tubing if solution or medication compatibility is not an issue.
- Collaborate with other caregivers to avoid duplication.

As with any medication, nurses are responsible for the "six rights" (the right client, drug, dose, time, route, and documentation). In addition, nurses must include the proper documentation concerning effects of administration. Table 25-8 lists common IV fluids, their purpose, and specific nursing implications.

Accurate IV administration requires many skills. These include the skills required for the preparatory phase of starting an IV line, the actual starting of an IV infusion, regulating the flow rate, administering IV medications, and discontinuing the IV infusion (Procedures 25-3 [p. 594] and 25-4 [p. 599]). Cost savings is essential component of IV therapy (Box 25-6).

Text continued on p. 599

Table 25-8 Understanding Intravenous Solutions

IV Fluid	Purpose	Nursing Implications
DEXTROSE SOLUTIONS		
Hypotonic <240 mOsm/L, such as dextrose 5% in water (D₅W)	• Provides free water • Dextrose is quickly metabolized, promotes renal excretion of solutes • Without saline in the solution, water may be drawn out of vascular space and cause edema • Adds enough calories to prevent ketosis (170 cal/L) • Never used with blood administration (increases coagulation)	• Risk for hyponatremia and hypokalemia if excess free water given • Not sufficient for nutrition; need other nutrient source if used for long-term therapy • Monitor for hyponatremia (disorientation, headache, lethargy, nausea, weakness)
Hypertonic (>350 mOsm/L), such as dextrose 10% (505 mOsm/L) to 50% (2525 mOsm/L) in water	• Osmotic diuretic • Treats hypoglycemia • Used in total parenteral nutrition • Hypertonic solutions may irritate vein	• Risk for phlebitis and hyperglycemia • Monitor infusion site and glucose levels • Client may need regular insulin administered on a sliding scale (based on blood glucose)
SALINE SOLUTIONS		
Hypotonic, 0.2% or 0.45% normal saline (with or without 5% dextrose)	• Water replacement without increase of osmotic pressure or serum sodium levels • Replaces loss of Na⁺ through normal daily excretion • Adds 170 cal/L if dextrose included	• Risk for hyponatremia and fluid volume excess
Isotonic (310 mEq/L), 0.9% normal saline (with or without 5% dextrose)	• To replace sodium and chloride lost through vomiting • May increase serum sodium level depending on rate of administration and sodium excretion rate • Expands extracellular fluid without changing osmolality (can be used for blood loss to expand volume until blood available) • Used to prime an IV catheter before use and flush it afterward, as indicated • Used as a backup solution to administer blood	• Risk for fluid volume excess (sodium causes the kidneys to retain water)
Hypertonic, such as 3% to 5% normal saline	• Rarely used • Reverses severe sodium deficit	• Risk for hypernatremia, vascular volume overload, pulmonary edema, phlebitis • Give slowly to prevent cellular dehydration
POTASSIUM ADDITIVE		
Usual dose range: 20 to 40 mEq/L × 3L/day to meet an average daily intake of 50 to 150 mEq/day	• Potassium maintenance or potassium replacement; if on a diet, this amount would replace losses • Never administer a concentration >80 mEq/L	• Risk for hyperkalemia, especially if client has oliguria • Agitate IV bag to prevent potassium bolus (could cause cardiac arrest) • Phlebitis is more likely in a small vein • Mix well to prevent potassium bolus (cause of cardiac arrest); may need cardiac monitoring
RINGER'S SOLUTIONS		
Ringer's (isotonic)	• Mimics electrolyte concentration of blood • Replaces fluids, sodium, potassium, calcium, and chloride • Can be used as volume expander in hemorrhage until blood available, or as a volume expander when there is lower GI tract loss	• Risk for fluid volume excess
Lactated Ringer's	• Ringer's plus lactate-precursor bicarbonate; used for metabolic acidosis (except lactic acidosis)	• Risk for fluid volume excess
Total parenteral nutrition—hypertonic	• Provides carbohydrates, amino acids, lipids, vitamins, electrolytes • Provides energy and nutrients for cellular function and repair	• Give via a central IV line • Can give via a peripheral line if tonicity is decreased • Monitor client's glucose levels

Continued

PROCEDURE 25-3	INITIATING PERIPHERAL INTRAVENOUS THERAPY—CONT'D

c. To find a suitable vein, lower the client's arm to below heart level and apply a tourniquet at least 6 inches above the projected site. *If the veins are difficult to see or the client is an older adult, apply a warm, moist pack over the site for 5 to 10 minutes and reassess (see illustration).*

d. Cleanse the site as directed by your facility's procedure manual. *Using alcohol or Betadine, start at the point of needle insertion and wipe in an enlarging spiral until you have cleaned a 3-inch circle around the site. Or, if your facility specifies, use two pledgets. Prepare the site for 30 seconds with the first one by applying friction and multi-directional cleansing around the hair follicles. Then use the second sterile pledget in the same circular method (see illustration).*

e. Remove the needle or catheter from its protective cover and, with your dominant hand, hold it bevel-up at a 30-degree angle to the skin, either directly over or parallel to the vein. *The direct approach usually works better for a larger vein, whereas the indirect approach often works better for a smaller vein. To prevent the vein from wandering, use your nondominant hand to stabilize the vein from above or below the targeted entry site.*

f. Pierce through the skin with one quick motion. As you do, decrease the angle of the needle or catheter to 15 degrees. Continue advancing toward the vein until you see blood return in the catheter or tubing. Then advance the catheter about another ¼ inch to make sure it is well into the vein. If inserting a needle, continue to advance it until the entire needle is within the vein. If you are inserting a catheter, use one hand to advance the catheter and the other to stabilize the needle guidewire. Do not readvance the needle guidewire once you have begun to remove it. When the entire catheter has been threaded, remove the remaining part of the needle guidewire. As you remove the needle from the hub of the catheter, apply pressure over the tip of the catheter to prevent backflow of blood (see illustrations).

g. Attach the IV tubing immediately to prevent blood loss.

h. Attach a saline lock device. Prime the lock with saline before accessing the vein. Then you can immediately attach the lock when you have entered the vein. *Access the IV port with the prefilled syringe. Aspirate to validate blood return, and inject the saline into the vein. If no swelling occurs, proceed to dress the site. If swelling oc-*

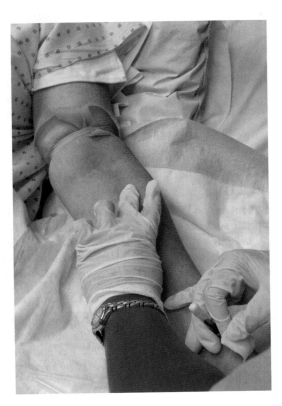

Step 3c. Finding the vein.

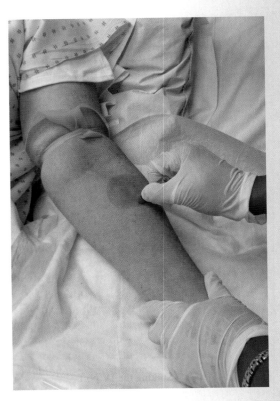

Step 3d. Preparing the site.

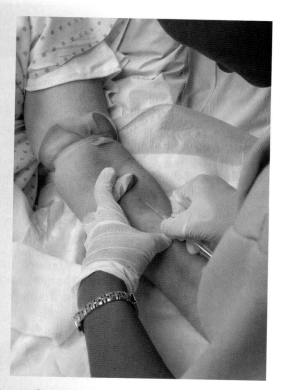

Step 3f(1). Inserting the catheter bevel up.

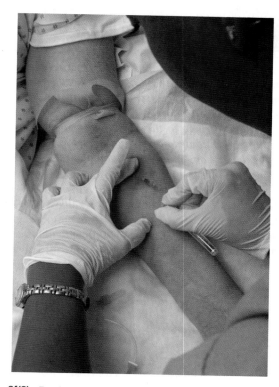

Step 3f(3). Putting pressure on the tip of the cannula to prevent blood flow.

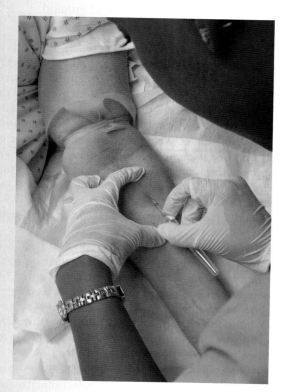

Step 3f(2). Retracting the needle (push white button) after the cannula is threaded into the vein.

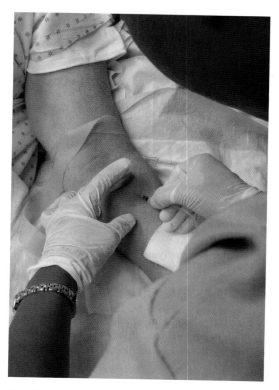

Step 3h. Attaching a primed saline lock to the cannula.

Continued

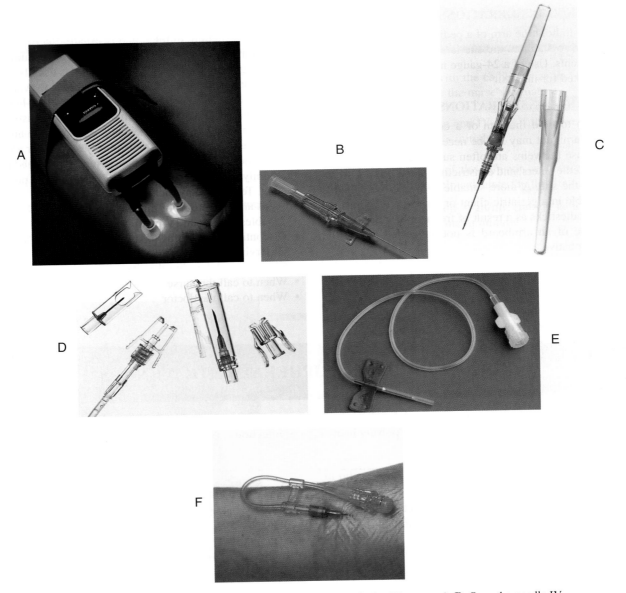

Figure 25-9. Examples of equipment used in IV therapy. **A,** Vein finder (Venoscope). **B,** Over-the-needle IV catheter. **C,** Insyte Autoguard IV cannula. **D,** Two types of protected needles with locking covers and two types of needleless lever locks. **E,** Butterfly infusion set. **F,** Saline lock with transparent dressing. (**A** courtesy Applied Biotech Products, Lafayette, LA; **B** courtesy Becton Dickinson, Sandy, UT; **E** courtesy Medline Industries, Mundelein, IL.)

Continued

(60 drops/mL) and macrodrip (10, 12, or 15 drops/mL). (Sometimes the measurement unit gtt. is used, from the Latin *guttae,* drops.)

Microdrip tubing has less risk of flowing in too rapidly if the IV needle or catheter changes positions in the client's vein. Also, amounts less than 30 mL/hr have to be given by microdrip or on a pump. Use macrodrip tubing when a solution needs to infuse rapidly. Any solution that has potassium chloride in it or any other medication that carries a high risk or needs precise delivery requires an infusion pump. Solutions given through a central vein (subclavian or jugular) also require an infusion pump to decrease the risk of air em-

bolus. Many IV pumps have specialized tubing. Other solutions, such as many blood products and total parenteral nutrition, require an IV pump and filter tubing.

The type of pump also varies. Most pumps are volume specific. The most commonly used pumps deliver 1 mL or more per hour, but there are also micropumps that deliver less than 1 mL/hr. Newer volume pumps can be set for tenths. As an example, if 31.3 gtt./min is needed, the pump can be set at 31.3 and there is no need to round to 31. Specialized tubing is required for some medications, such as nitroglycerin, that can be absorbed by tubing. Specialized tubing with chambers called burretrols is also available and used with children and

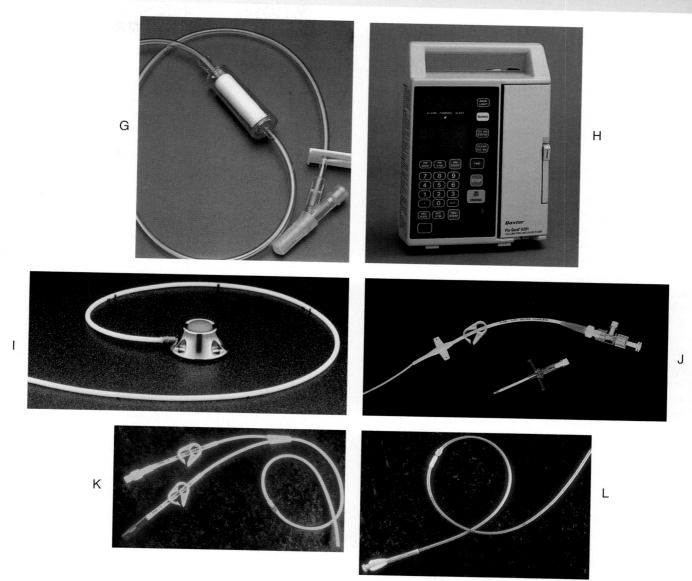

Figure 25-9, cont'd. G, In-line IV filter (Millipore IV Express). **H,** IV pump (Flo-Gard Volumetric). **I,** Implantable vascular access device (Port-a-Cath). **J,** Peripherally inserted central catheter, or PICC (CliniCath). **K,** Hickman catheter. **L,** Groshong catheter. (**G** courtesy Millipore Corporation, Bedford, MA; **H** courtesy Baxter Healthcare Corporation, Deerfield, IL; **I** and **J** courtesy SIMS Deltec, St Paul, MN; **K** and **L** courtesy Bard Access Systems, Salt Lake City, UT.)

critically ill clients to precisely deliver small amounts of fluid or medication. Extension tubing is also available to increase mobility and facilitate position changes. If precise measurement is required, but a pump is not feasible, an in-line flow regulator can be attached to the main IV line. This device adjusts the rate by mL/hr, but it is usually a one-time charge versus a daily charge for a pump.

Often, you will need to "piggyback" a prescribed medication into the client's main IV line. Types of piggyback tubing are specific to the manufacturer. Several manufacturers have created needleless IV equipment to decrease the risk of needlesticks.

In addition to the right solution, tubing, and pump if necessary, you will need more equipment if you are starting an IV line. After assessing the client's veins, choose the correct needle or catheter, and a tourniquet, gloves, dressing, and site preparation agents (alcohol and povidone-iodine [Betadine]) as required by agency policy. The size of the needle or catheter is specific to the type of IV therapy. A 23- to 25-gauge needle and a 20- to 22-gauge catheter are sufficient for most IV therapy. Larger sizes, such as a 16- to 20-gauge catheter, are required if you will be giving blood products or hyperosmotic solutions, or if the client is being prepared for surgery.

SOLUTIONS. Many types of IV solutions are available. Solutions are categorized by the *osmolarity,* or number of milliosmoles per liter of solution, or, more importantly, by their *osmolality*—how they affect the other fluids they are being compared with. Solutions come in three levels of osmolality: isotonic, hypertonic, and hypotonic. To review, an *isotonic* solution is one that has an osmotic pressure very similar to that of the solution or fluid with which it is being compared and thus does not affect fluid shifting. The amount of solute equals the amount of solution. A *hypertonic* solution is one that has a higher osmotic pressure than the one with which it is being compared. An easy way to remember this is that the *hyper* refers to the solute. This type of solution is a high solute concentration with less fluid, thus causing cells to shrink. A *hypotonic* solution is one that has a lower osmotic pressure than the one with which it is being compared. Again, the *hypo* refers to a low solute concentration, and the solution has a low solute concentration and more fluid, thus causing cells to swell.

Both the *hypertonic* and *hypotonic* solutions increase the risk of fluid shifting between compartments. IV solutions that are hypertonic increase the risk for fluid shifting into the plasma and thus for fluid excess because of the increased osmotic pull. *Hypotonic* IV fluids increase the risk of fluid shifting from the plasma to the interstitial compartments and cells because of the decreasing osmolality in the plasma. This concept is discussed later under Potential Complications.

SITES. Sites for IV therapy are categorized as peripheral or central (Figure 25-10). Any IV line that is inserted into the subclavian or jugular vein, or into a peripheral vein and threaded past the axillary line (a peripherally inserted central catheter, also called a PICC line, for peripherally inserted central catheter) is considered a central line. The subclavian veins are accessed more often than the jugular veins, especially for long-term therapy, because of the increased risk of phlebitis, catheter displacement, disconnection, and client discomfort associated with an IV placement in the neck area. All other IV sites are considered peripheral IV sites. The most common site for peripheral IV therapy is the arm. The purpose and duration of the IV therapy, the type of solution, and the age and physical condition of the client are factors that determine the most appropriate IV site.

Avoid starting an IV over a joint to decrease the need for joint immobilization. Avoid the small, thin-walled veins in the hand if possible. This site is more painful and at greater risk for infiltration and limits the client's hand mobility. Also avoid the veins in the legs because their decreased flow rate increases the risk for thrombus or embolus formation. The most recommended site is the most distal site in the forearm above the wrist area. This allows for later venipunctures in more proximal veins. Sites that are compromised by venous or lymphatic flow changes should be avoided. These include veins on the same arm a mastectomy or lymphatic resection has been performed, on arms with fistulas or shunts, or on arms with varicosities or history of phlebitis or thrombosis.

BASELINE ASSESSMENT. To make an accurate evaluation of your client's response to IV therapy, it is important that a baseline head-to-toe assessment be done before the IV therapy is initiated. Repeat the assessment every 8 hours and compare data. Clients with risk factors for overload may need to be assessed more frequently.

A baseline assessment includes vital signs, level of consciousness, mucous membranes for color and moisture, jugular venous distention, heart sounds, lung sounds, abdominal assessment, peripheral pulses, and urinary output. If the client experiences any changes in status, such as changes in level of consciousness, marked changes in vital signs, shortness of breath, chest pain, or feeling that "something is wrong," initiate a thorough assessment immediately. Consult the physician about your findings.

POTENTIAL COMPLICATIONS. Phlebitis is an inflammation of the intimal layer of the vein. The earliest manifestation of phlebitis is the client's report of tenderness when you palpate over the vein. As the inflammation progresses, redness and warmth develop along the vein distal to the end of the IV catheter or needle. The catheter or needle should be removed when tenderness is first present to decrease the risk of clot formation in the vein. If the client still requires IV therapy, an alternative site will need to be selected.

Infiltration means that the IV fluid has leaked through the venous wall into the interstitial tissue surrounding that vein. The area may feel hard or cold and probably will be painful. It is possible to still get blood return when you aspirate via the tubing with a syringe, even though the site is infiltrated. If there is swelling distal to the IV site that was not there when the IV infusion was initiated, you must remove the catheter or needle even if you can get blood return. The longer the infiltration continues, the more the fluid will accumulate and put pressure on the surrounding nerve endings, causing discomfort.

Infiltrated fluid is not functionally useful when it is in the interstitial tissues. Also, if the IV infusion contains medication that is caustic to tissues, it is even more critical that the infusion be discontinued immediately when infiltration is first noted. If this occurs, notify the physician of the infiltration. Depending on the medication, the physician will prescribe an antidote to be given subcutaneously in the infiltrated tissue. Use your procedure manual for further guidance. Table 25-9, p. 604 lists the common data and nursing interventions for other IV complications, including circulatory overload, infection, air embolism, and allergic reactions. The most common risk factors for circulatory overload include the administration of hypertonic solutions, rapid IV administration, and the presence of renal insufficiency.

SITE CARE

PERIPHERAL. Review your facility's procedure manual for specific guidelines for peripheral IV site care. Studies of peripheral IV infection rates have prompted most facilities to require changing of the peripheral IV site every 72 hours. The type of IV dressing will dictate whether the dressing requires changing more frequently. For example, if an occlusive, transparent dressing has been applied at the time of catheter insertion and the dressing remains intact and dry, it does not usually require changing, because it will be

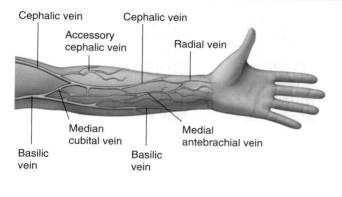

Cephalic vein
Accessory cephalic vein
Cephalic vein
Radial vein
Median cubital vein
Medial antebrachial vein
Basilic vein
Basilic vein

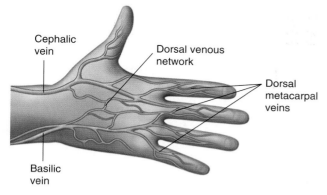

Cephalic vein
Dorsal venous network
Dorsal metacarpal veins
Basilic vein

A

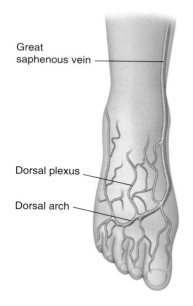

Great saphenous vein
Dorsal plexus
Dorsal arch

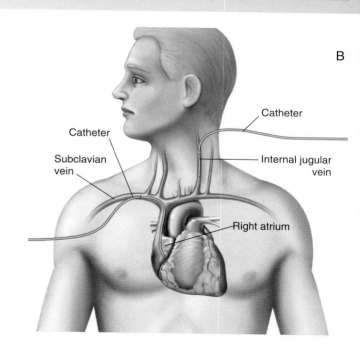

B

Catheter
Catheter
Subclavian vein
Internal jugular vein
Right atrium

Figure 25-10. IV sites. **A,** Peripheral sites. Sites on the inner arm are preferred. Sites on the dorsum of the hand are often used, but the use of these sites increases the risk of vascular trauma and pain. Sites on the dorsum of the foot should be used only as a last resort because they are associated with an increased risk of thrombi. **B,** Central sites: subclavian vein and internal jugular vein.

removed when the IV catheter site is changed. However, if the dressing is not occlusive (gauze, for example), it will need to be changed every 24 hours so that you can perform an accurate site assessment. Many facilities require that a gauze dressing be used if a client is neutropenic, because a neutrophil count below 1000/mm³ increases the risk for bacterial infection and gauze dressings decrease moisture retention.

Whenever you change a dressing or change or start an IV line, you will cleanse the IV site with an antimicrobial sub-

stance. Tincture of iodine (1% to 2%), 70% alcohol, or chlorhexidine (Hibiclens) are the solutions recommended for IV site preparation. Agency policy dictates the type and order of cleansing. All cleansing is done in a circular motion starting at the IV insertion site and moving outward in a 2- to 3-inch circular motion. Let the antimicrobial agent dry before inserting the IV needle or catheter. Place the date and your initials on the IV dressing.

CENTRAL. Many variables influence the physician's choice for the type of IV access device. Among these are cost, ease of

Table 25-9	Managing Complications of Intravenous Therapy		
Complications	**Assessment Findings**	**Interventions**	**Prevention**
Infiltration	• Site is edematous, blanched, painful, cold. • Fluid will not flow by gravity despite confirmed patency of line (blood backflow when bag lowered below site.)	• Discontinue infusion. • Restart in opposite arm. • Elevate arm if edema is severe. • Warm, moist pack may be comforting.	• Tape IV catheter securely in place and protect it from being pulled. • Avoid joints when placing catheter.
Phlebitis	• Heat, pain, redness, and edema develop around the site, or a streak running along the course of the vein may occur.	• Discontinue infusion. • Avoid massage because it might dislodge clots. • Warm, moist pack may be comforting.	• Dilute irritating medications. • Use smallest-gauge catheter appropriate. • Change site every 3 days or as specified.
Infection	• Same as for phlebitis • Possible discharge at site • Possible fever and sepsis • Warmth at site	• Physician will order blood cultures and start antibiotic therapy. • Client may be treated in intensive care unit because sepsis is life threatening.	• Use strict sterile technique for all IV care. • Change dressing every 24 hours.
Air embolism	• Decreased blood pressure • Cyanosis • Tachycardia • Jugular vein distention • Loss of consciousness	• Immediately turn client on left side with head down. • Administer oxygen and monitor vital signs. • Notify physician.	• Remove air from tubing before connecting to catheter (small air bubbles will not be harmful). • Have client perform Valsalva's maneuver or place head below heart level while changing tubing on central line.
Allergic reaction	• Minor reaction produces rash, redness, itching. • Major reaction can cause coughing, dyspnea, swollen tongue, cyanosis, unconsciousness, death.	• Discontinue infusion and notify physician. • Client may need epinephrine, corticosteroids, oxygen, or mechanical ventilation.	• Assess client for history of allergies. • Monitor closely.
Circulatory overload	• In pulmonary edema, findings include dyspnea; cough; cyanosis; frothy, pink sputum; jugular vein distention. • Other findings include ascites, weight gain, edema.	• Slow-infusion and notify physician. • Verify correct fluid and rate of administration. • Diuretics and sodium restriction may be indicated.	• Take precautions to ensure correct fluid and rate of administration. • Monitor client's intake and output.

surgical placement, infection rates, length of therapy, client choice (when possible), quality of vascular tissue, and urgency of placement. Commonly used types include the Swan-Ganz (or introducer) catheter, triple-lumen catheter, tunneled catheter (such as Groshong or Hickman, implanted port (such as a Mediport, Infusaport, or Port-a-Cath), and a PICC line. Figure 25-11 illustrates a tunneled and an implanted central catheter.

Regardless of the type of central line used, you are responsible for following the manufacturer's and the facility's procedural guidelines for care and flushing protocols. For example, a normal saline flush maintains patency in a Groshong (close-ended) catheter and in some implanted ports, whereas heparin is recommended for a PICC line and many other types of central lines. The amount of flushing solution varies with the length and diameter of the catheter and the procedure. For instance, you may need as little as 1

to 3 mL of flush to keep a line open but as much as 10 to 20 mL of saline solution to cleanse the line after blood is drawn. If heparin is recommended, it is always the last solution in the flushing sequence because its only purpose is to prevent coagulation in the catheter system.

Follow your agency's procedure manual for changing a dressing on a central line (Procedure 25-5). The frequency of dressing changes for central lines is similar to that for peripheral dressings. When a client is neutropenic, daily dressing changes with varying types of gauze may be mandated. When a transparent dressing is used without gauze, change the dressing every 72 hours or up to every 7 days, depending on the agency's policy. Sterile technique is required with all IV dressing changes, and a mask is also recommended when changing central line dressings. Sterile technique may be adapted to clean technique in the home setting if the client is not neutropenic.

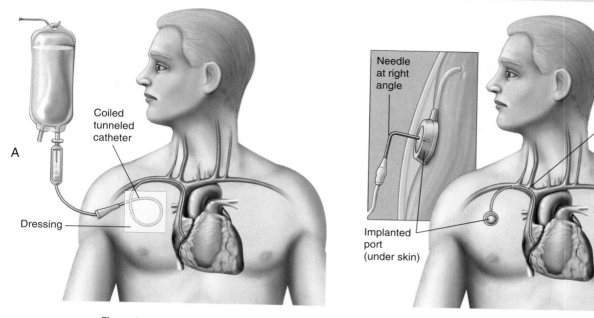

Figure 25-11. A, Placement of a tunneled central venous catheter. **B,** An implanted central port. The distal ends of both the tunneled central catheter and the implanted port are in the subclavian vein.

PROCEDURE 25-5 CHANGING THE DRESSING ON A CENTRAL LINE

TIME TO ALLOW
Novice: 20 min.
Expert: 10 min.

A central venous access line is cleaned and dressed with meticulous care to prevent infection from entering the line. The old dressing is removed, the site cleaned, and the new dressing applied using sterile technique. Infection in the bloodstream (septicemia) is a life-threatening complication.

DELEGATION GUIDELINES
The indications for RN assessment and the potential risks associated with improper care of a central line suggest that this procedure not be delegated to a nursing assistant.

EQUIPMENT NEEDED
- Face mask
- Clean gloves
- Sterile gloves
- Three swabs or sticks of povidone-iodine (Betadine)
- Three swabs or sticks of alcohol
- Sterile, occlusive transparent dressing
- Cap for saline or heparin lock
- Plastic bag
- Black pen or marker
- Bedside table or flat surface for setting up a sterile field

1. Follow preliminary guidelines for nursing procedures (see inside front cover).

2. Remove the soiled dressing. *Remember that a client with a port that is not accessed does not require a dressing.*
a. Don the facemask, wash your hands, and don the clean gloves.
b. Remove the old dressing with your dominant hand while stabilizing the central line device with two fingers of the nondominant hand. The dressing should be removed in the direction toward the insertion of the catheter to prevent the risk of dislodging the catheter. *Be careful not to touch the catheter entry site.*
c. Holding the old dressing in your dominant hand, use your nondominant hand to pull the glove on your dominant hand off over the old dressing. Remove the other glove and discard them both in the plastic bag.
d. Perform hand hygiene.

Continued

3. Clean the site.
a. Set up a sterile field. If a kit is available, open kit to create a sterile field. Don sterile gloves and then tear open the Betadine and alcohol swabs. Check the dressing but do not remove its backing yet. If no kit is available, open the package of sterile gloves but do not don them yet. The inside of the package will become your sterile field. Now, tear open Betadine and alcohol swabs and place them on the corner of the sterile field. Open the outer packaging of the dressing and drop the dressing on the center of the sterile field. Open the plastic bag, make a cuffed edge, and set it to the side of your sterile field. Now, don the sterile gloves. *To do so, grasp the first glove on the top inside of the cuff (so the place you grasped will be against the skin of your arm) and pull the glove over your dominant hand. Now use the sterile gloved hand to grasp the second glove under the cuff and pull it onto your nondominant hand.*
b. Using the elbow of your nondominant arm, hold the packaging of the alcohol swab in place as you grasp the swab with your dominant hand.
c. Starting at the site of IV access, use a circular motion moving outward in a 3-inch circle to cleanse the site. Discard the swab in the plastic bag and cleanse the site in the same manner with the other two alcohol swabs.
d. After the alcohol has evaporated (about 15 seconds), repeat the cleansing motion with the three Betadine swabs. *Allowing the alcohol and Betadine to mix when the alco-*

hol is still wet can cause skin irritation and alter the bacteriostatic properties.

4. Dress the site.
a. If gauze is recommended, apply it over the cleansed site and tape it according to policy. If a transparent dressing is being used, remove the backing and, holding the edges of the dressing taut, place it over the site so the IV access device is in the center of the dressing.
b. Use the fingers of one hand to smooth the dressing from the center outward to make a tight seal. Use a marker or label to show the date and time of the dressing change. Add your initials as well.

PEDIATRIC CONSIDERATIONS

Play therapy is helpful in explaining a procedure to children. If possible, allow the child to participate in handing nonsterile equipment to the nurse.

HOME CARE CONSIDERATIONS

If the client or family members will perform dressing changes at home, teach them how to use clean technique unless the client is neutropenic. In that case, sterile technique is required. If the site has no dressing, teach the client or family member to cleanse the site with soap and water and to place a Band-Aid over the entry site using tape to support the tunneled catheter.

Interventions to Decrease Fluid Volume

There are three primary interventions related to decreasing fluid volume: restoring fluid balance, preventing complications, and instituting rehabilitative care.

Restoring Fluid Balance. Limit the client's fluid and sodium intake. You will need to instruct the client and family about the rationale for fluid and dietary restrictions to ensure compliance.

Administer prescribed medications. Diuretics are often ordered to help rid the body of excess fluid. Another focus of drug therapy is to correct the etiology of the fluid excess. If the overload is from an ineffective myocardial pump, the physician may prescribe an inotropic drug to enhance myocardial contractility, or a medication to decrease myocardial workload, such as a calcium channel blocker or angiotensin-converting enzyme (ACE) inhibitor.

If capillary permeability is the etiology, in addition to treating the underlying sepsis, acid–base imbalance, or other factors, the physician will prescribe corticosteroids to promote healing of the membrane. Careful monitoring of fluid volume should be made if corticosteroids are ordered for a

client with congestive heart failure (CHF). If protein deficit is present, the source of this deficit is investigated and corrected if possible, and additional protein is given if appropriate. The etiologies of fluid volume excess are quite numerous.

Preventing Complications. To prevent complications, provide appropriate supportive care. Monitor and record intake and output (I&O) and weigh the client daily. Compare your findings with previous documentation. Maintain the client's nutritional needs, consulting with a dietitian if necessary. To decrease the client's feeling of mucosal dryness that accompanies the intervention of fluid restriction, you can encourage the family to bring hard candies or lozenges, provide ice chips, and give or assist with oral care frequently (up to hourly if necessary).

Performing a thorough head-to-toe assessment to determine how a client is responding to the interventions is essential to secondary prevention. The frequency of the assessments varies with the acuteness of the fluid overload. Assessments may be needed as often as hourly in a critical care setting, every 8 hours when the condition has stabilized, or weekly or monthly in a chronic-care or home setting.

Fluid retention impairs tissue perfusion. The interventions for impaired tissue perfusion are specific to the organ or system that is involved. Although the goal is to promote optimal perfusion of all body tissues, fluid overload in the heart, lungs, liver, kidneys, and brain must be treated immediately to avoid life-threatening complications.

One of the systems that is often affected by fluid retention is the skin. One of the most common interventions to decrease the risk for impaired skin integrity is pressure relief. Repositioning the client every 2 hours or more as necessary may be enough to decrease the pressure on these tissues. However, if this is not enough, consult the physician about ordering a pressure-reducing mattress or bed. If the edema is localized to an extremity, elevation of that limb will promote venous return and thus decrease swelling. Passive or active range-of-motion exercises five or more times for each joint twice a day will also promote venous return and maintain joint function.

If fluid retention has involved the pulmonary system, elevate the head of the bed to the level necessary for the client's comfort and optimal diaphragmatic excursion. The more pulmonary fluid the client has, the higher the head of the bed will need to be. A client with severe pulmonary fluid overload often needs a 90-degree headrest with arms supported on pillows on a bedside table. Elevating the client's head will also decrease venous return to the right side of the heart and thus decrease cardiac workload. The greater the amount of fluid overload, the more aggressive the interventions need to be. Minimal fluid overload can often be managed with deep breathing, incentive spirometry, repositioning, mild diuretics, inotropic medications, and calcium channel blockers or ACE inhibitors.

Fluid retention is always a risk with a postoperative client who has received a general anesthetic. Administer fluids cautiously in early postoperative or posttraumatic stress periods. Increased antidiuretic hormone during this period can cause fluid overload. The presence of or increase in crackles is an early sign of pulmonary fluid and should alert you that fluids are being given faster than the body can tolerate them. An increase in urinary output is an early sign of the end of this phase.

Instituting Rehabilitative Care.
Self-care is a major component of rehabilitation from fluid volume excess. Promote self-care by teaching the client and family about restricting fluid and table salt, reading food labels, avoiding products high in sodium, keeping a diary of weights, balancing activity and rest, and calling the physician whenever significant health changes occur.

Additional interventions for fluid balance maintenance include the following:

- Control delivery of fluid by using IV and feeding pumps when appropriate.
- Monitor laboratory results specific to fluid and electrolyte homeostasis, such as blood urea nitrogen (BUN), creatinine, hemoglobin, hematocrit, urine or plasma osmolality, and plasma electrolytes.
- Monitor responses to prescribed medications, including expected and unexpected responses.

- Provide referrals to assist with lifestyle changes and financial constraints as appropriate, such as social services, dietitian counseling, home health care nursing services, and home health aide.
- Evaluate fluid balance in relationship to output and compare data with the client's other presenting data.
- Provide client and family teaching.

Interventions to Balance Electrolyte Levels
When caring for a client who has an electrolyte imbalance, your goal is to decrease the risk for serious consequences. With electrolyte deficits, the goals of the interventions include replacing the lost nutrient, decreasing the rate of nutrient loss, or both. With electrolyte excess, the goals of the interventions focus on limiting intake, increasing loss, or both.

General Interventions.
Nutrition is a key intervention in most electrolyte imbalances. Consult with a dietitian for information on specific foods to include or exclude in therapeutic diets specific to each imbalance. Give your client a written handout listing these food items. Keep in mind that dietary changes are among the most difficult for clients to make. Providing resources such as the names of local dietitians or nutrition support groups may help the client with this behavioral change.

Providing practical examples of how to "eat healthier" can also be helpful. For example, you can suggest that the client use fresh lemon on foods and salads instead of prepared sauces. Or, when dining out, the client could request that food be prepared without salt and cooked by grilling, baking, or broiling. The client may also wish to carry along a seasoning that fits the prescribed diet. Also teach the client or food buyer the importance of reading the entire nutritional label for levels of sodium, potassium, and other nutrients. Bold print is often misleading.

When teaching about dietary restrictions, it is very important that the "cook" and other family members be involved. The more support the client has, the more successful the behavioral change will be. Finally, be very clear about whether the dietary restriction is a temporary change or a lifelong change.

In a client at high risk for malnutrition, especially a client unable to consume nutrients orally, the physician may prescribe a nutritional supplement that contains all of the previously mentioned electrolytes as well as some trace electrolytes. This may be delivered by gastric or intestinal tube for a person with long-term nutritional needs or by the IV route in the form of total parenteral nutrition for someone with short-term needs.

Whether the client is experiencing a deficit or an excess, the promptness of the intervention will depend on two key factors: the severity of the imbalance and the presenting manifestations. The following nursing interventions are appropriate to all electrolyte imbalances.

- Monitor the client's liver, kidney, and bowel functions. Normal medication processing and excretion depend on the interactive functioning of these systems. Dysfunction in any of these systems can lead to toxicity, which often includes fluid and electrolyte imbalances.

- Monitor the client's level of plasma electrolytes, especially when giving medications that either affect or are affected by electrolyte levels.
- Assess the client's vital signs. Frequency varies with the severity of the alteration. You may need to assess vital signs as often as every 15 minutes when the electrolyte level is critical, or once a week or month in a more chronic situation.
- Assess an apical pulse for a full minute whenever the peripheral pulse is irregular. Remember that many electrolytes (including sodium, potassium, magnesium, and calcium) affect the rate and rhythm of the cardiac cells.
- A cardiac monitor may be necessary with an irregular pulse. If the client is on a cardiac monitor, watch for arrhythmias and other changes.
- Monitor intake and output (I&O) every hour in an acutely ill client. Teach the client and family to monitor and compare weight trends at least weekly for a stable "at home" client.
- Assess peripheral vein filling and emptying time. Normally, veins take less than 5 seconds to empty or fill.
- Because weakness is a common manifestation of many electrolyte imbalances, remember to initiate fall precautions when appropriate, such as removing obstacles from the environment and providing mobility support.
- Teach clients and families about the importance of consuming foods within the prescribed diet. Encourage intake of a well-rounded diet when possible. Encourage intake of foods that replace nutrients that are lost secondary to an illness or other condition. For a state of electrolyte excess, avoid foods high in that electrolyte.
- Teach clients to follow pharmaceutical recommendations for electrolyte replacement, and to avoid taking more than the recommended daily vitamin–mineral supplement without consultation with a physician. Tell the client to avoid other over-the-counter medications unless approved by a physician, because many of these drugs can alter fluid and electrolyte balance. Implement and teach the client that antacids should be separated from other medications by 1 to 2 hours, as they can alter electrolyte balance or affect the absorption of other medications.
- Irrigate nasogastric tubes with normal saline only; if ice chips are ordered, use sparingly.
- When "enemas till clear" are prescribed, give no more than three in a row. Hypotonic solutions can alter fluid and electrolyte status. Consult the physician before proceeding.

Interventions for Sodium Imbalance.
Hyponatremia is one of the more common electrolyte imbalances. The client's response to hyponatremia varies with the cause, rate of loss, and type of associated fluid imbalance. A client can present with a sodium level of 120 mEq/L and be asymptomatic if the imbalance developed slowly. The same level, if it results from an acute loss, can cause life-threatening manifestations.

The client's amount of body water also affects response. Sodium deficit can occur in the presence of decreased, normal, or increased body water. However, one of the most common types of hyponatremia is caused by fluid overload. When this is the etiology, fluid restriction is the intervention of choice. Fluid restriction is very difficult for any client to abide by. You can help the client understand the importance of this intervention and provide suggestions that will increase compliance. Ice chips, lozenges, frequent mouth care, and small, frequent sips of fluids will provide comfort.

If the hyponatremia is truly due to a sodium deficit, then the physician will prescribe additional sodium either orally, by tube, or in IV form. If the level is 125 mEq/L or greater, diet supplementation and interventions to decrease the loss are the usual treatment. Other common interventions include prescriptions to improve the function of the organs that are causing the problem, such as digitalis and diuretics for cardiac overload.

Interventions for Potassium Imbalance.
Potassium imbalance can be very dangerous. Because potassium is predominantly an intracellular ion, the plasma level is only an indirect reflection of the cellular level. Minor plasma imbalances can indicate serious risk for cellular imbalance. Although many systems are affected by a potassium imbalance, the cardiovascular system is most critically affected. A low serum potassium level increases the risk of dysrhythmia. The risk of digitalis toxicity is also increased. Therefore you should consult the physician before giving digitalis derivatives when potassium is low, when the plasma digitalis level is high, or when the client has bradycardia (pulse less than 60/minute).

Physicians usually prefer to be notified of the bradycardia and often will prescribe the continuance of digitalis as long as the apical pulse is above 50. This is because the client is at a greater risk from the complications of an ineffective myocardial pump without the digitalis.

If dietary replacement is insufficient, oral potassium supplements are usually prescribed. If the level is critical, then the more rapid IV replacement route is chosen.

Oral potassium should be given with food because it is a GI irritant. Intravenous potassium can be given *only* in diluted form; direct IV potassium has been known to cause cardiac arrest. The maintenance dose is 40 to 80 mEq/day. If the potassium level is critically low or the client has serious cardiac arrhythmia, up to 10 mEq/hr can be given in as little as 125 mL of solution, but the client must be on a cardiac monitor during this infusion. An IV pump will ensure a safer delivery of IV potassium. Potassium is a venous irritant; if the client experiences pain at the IV site, the infusion rate may need to be slowed or the potassium diluted further. Potassium is very toxic to interstitial tissues; if infiltration occurs, stop the IV infusion immediately and notify the physician. Because potassium is excreted primarily via the kidneys, it is essential to monitor urinary output. If the output is borderline (about 30 mL/hr), outputs must be monitored hourly. If the urine output drops to less than 30 mL/hr for at least 2 consecutive hours, notify the physician.

Hyperkalemia can be a medical emergency. If the potassium level has caused significant cardiac conduction changes, the physician may order IV glucose and insulin to promote immediate, but temporary, shifting of the potassium from the plasma into the cells. To ensure excretion of potassium from the body, a cation exchange resin (such as sodium KayExalate in oral or rectal form) may be ordered, or, if time permits, peritoneal or hemodialysis may be done to remove excess potassium from the body.

Interventions for Calcium Imbalance.
Calcium imbalance is less common than sodium and potassium imbalances. Therefore, as a cost-conscious effort, the physician tests this level only when a client is at high risk for imbalance or has manifestations that suggest an imbalance. You play an active role in helping the physician identify such clients.

Calcium must be taken with vitamin D to promote absorption. High-phosphate products (such as milk and carbonated beverages) promote calcium loss. Therefore it is important to teach clients to avoid these products if the hypocalcemia is caused by hypoparathyroidism. When a client has normal parathyroid functioning, parathormone is able to manage the high phosphate levels in milk products, and the client is then able to receive the full calcium benefit from the calcium in the milk product.

The bone softening that accompanies calcium deficit or excess can result in a fracture with minimal strain. Teach clients the importance of weight-bearing activities to decrease calcium bone loss. Calcium deficit also increases the client's risk for bleeding; teach clients to report signs of bleeding. If hypercalcemia is present, strain all urine and teach the client to strain urine to identify the presence of renal calculi. Teach the client that forcing fluids will decrease this risk. Also help the client understand the role of prescription medications for hypercalcemia. These include saline IV infusions, diuretics (nonthiazides), etidronate disodium (Didronel), phosphates, and corticosteroids.

Interventions for Magnesium Imbalance.
When a magnesium deficit exists, increasing dietary intake is seldom sufficient. Usually an oral replacement is given unless the situation requires a more aggressive IV approach. The oral magnesium is often given in the form of a magnesium-containing antacid. The parenteral form is usually magnesium sulfate. IV magnesium must be diluted in a nonsaline solution. Monitoring for blood pressure improvement and monitoring the ECG for decreased dysrhythmias are top priorities. Providing safety and seizure precautions for any client who is confused or at risk for seizure is also imperative. Assessing the return of the deep tendon reflexes provides an indication that magnesium balance has been restored.

Interventions for Phosphate Imbalance.
Phosphate imbalances are rare. A deficit is treated by oral or IV replacement. A phosphate excess is treated with calcium or aluminum supplements.

EVALUATION

The time frame for evaluating fluid or electrolyte imbalance, whether deficit or excess, varies with the urgency of the imbalance. For example, if the client is experiencing a life-threatening arrhythmia, cardiac monitoring with narrow alarm parameters will be continuous. Neurological manifestations that indicate a worsening condition also require continuous evaluation. As the client stabilizes, however, the frequency of evaluation decreases. Hourly assessments are followed by assessments every 4 hours, progressing to every 8 hours. In extended-care facilities and in the home, clients may require evaluation of risk or actual imbalances on only a weekly or a monthly basis.

Let us return to Mrs. Thompson. After recovering from her episode of congestive heart failure, she was discharged with home health visits weekly. A nursing progress note for this client might look like the note below.

> **SAMPLE DOCUMENTATION NOTE FOR MRS. THOMPSON**
> Monitoring her fluid intake and the number of voidings every 24 hours. Intake is comparable to output. Compliant with monitoring her weight daily and noting values in her diary. Weight gain of ½ pound in 1 week is noted. No edema or shortness of breath reported. States she feels better and less fatigued since being on her new medications. Skin recoils rapidly, capillary refill less than 3 seconds in nail beds, lungs clear bilaterally. Encouraged to continue monitoring intake and output as well as weight. Reviewed diet and she is compliant with low sodium.

If the client is not improving, collect data to help evaluate the reason that outcomes are not being achieved. There are many possible variables, including barriers such as nausea or lack of access to food or fluids, another etiology or underlying pathology that is not responding to the current treatment, or perhaps a lack of compliance with the prescribed treatments for other reasons.

If a client has an actual fluid and electrolyte imbalance, compare the current manifestations with those present on the last assessment. The desired outcome is an improvement in any of the signs or symptoms discussed in this chapter. Clearly, improvement of manifestations involving life-sustaining tissues is the highest priority. However, even a fluid imbalance at a local level, such as severe edema in an extremity, could pose a threat to the life of that tissue. Naturally, life-threatening signs and symptoms require aggressive intervention. Care plan revision is indicated if the client's responses indicate there is no longer a risk or an actual problem, if improvement is evident, if lack of improvement at the desired or expected rate occurs, or if the condition worsens. See Box 25-7 (p. 610) for more information.

Nursing Care Plan **A CLIENT WITH FLUID VOLUME DEFICIT**  **Box 25-7**

ADMISSION DATA

Mrs. Thompson was examined by her physician's nurse in the out-patient clinic. The nurse reported the following data to Dr. Kline.

NURSING ASSESSMENT

Color pale, skin dry, oral mucous membranes dry with tongue furrows, weight 110 pounds (decrease of 10 pounds in 2 weeks), blood pressure 116/50, pulse 110 and weak, respirations 24 (usually 142/70, 80, 16). Appears restless and is unable to remember when she last ate. Reports extreme fatigue and weakness over the last several weeks; states stools have been hard and infrequent.

Dr. Kline examined Mrs. Thompson and wrote the following on her chart.

PHYSICIAN'S PROGRESS NOTE

Diagnosis: Dehydration secondary to decreased intake, extreme weakness, and fatigue. Early signs of ECF deficit with minimal signs of intracellular affect (confusion). In no acute distress at this time. Believe she can be managed at home because supportive family will assist in monitoring and care delivery. Visiting nurse three times a week for 2 weeks. Hospitalization for IV therapy only if signs worsen.

OFFICE CARE

The office nurse completed teaching with Mrs. Thompson and her son Gerald. While consulting with Mrs. Thompson, especially about her ethnic preferences, a grocery list was compiled. The nurse also reinforced the importance of Gerald's daily visits until his mother becomes stable. She also gave them a list of signs and symptoms about which Dr. Kline's office must be notified. Later, the office nurse contracted the visiting nursing agency and gave Judy Carson, RN, Mrs. Thompson's nurse, a full report with the following orders:

Initial visit today to include the following:
- Home baseline assessment.
- Instruct Mrs. Thompson and her family about schedule for oral fluid replacement.
- Plan to include increasing fluid intake to 1500 mL per day; stopping 3 hours before bedtime.
- Plan to include increasing food intake to 6 small meals per day.
- Validate understanding of teaching.

Additional orders:
- Contact Meals on Wheels about meal supplementation.
- Evaluate progress every 2 days for 2 weeks.

NANDA Nursing Diagnosis	NOC Expected Outcomes With Indicators	NIC Interventions With Selected Activities	Evaluation
DEFICIENT FLUID VOLUME	**HYDRATION**	**FLUID MANAGEMENT**	**HOME VISIT, 48 HOURS LATER**
Related Factors: • Dry skin • Dry mucous membranes • Furrowed tongue	**Fluid balance:** • Maintain moist oral mucous membranes in 48 hours. • No tongue furrows within a week. • Oriented to person, time, and place in 48 hours.	• Assess oral mucous membranes and tongue.	• Tongue furrows absent, but oral mucous membranes remain dry.
• Weight 110 (decrease of 10 pounds in 2 weeks)	**Weight:** • Increased by 1 pound within a week.	• Weigh with approximate amount of clothing had on at initial visit, and at same time of day.	• Weight gain of 1 lb.
• BP 116/50 (usually 142/70) • Pulse 110, R 24 • Restless • Slightly confused	**Vital signs monitoring:** • Improvement seen in BP, systolic <120. • Pulse <100. • Respirations <20 within 48 hours.	• Assess orientation to person, place, and time. • Assess vital signs.	• Able to state name, home address, and month. • BP 118/70, P 96, R 20.
	Constipation management: • Reports softer stools at least once since doctor's visit. **Fluid management:** • Reports taking 60 mL fluids/hour, 6 small meals/day for 1 month.	• Assess stool characteristics since office visit. • Assess fluid and diet history since office visit.	• Stated one stool, moderate amount, still somewhat hard. • Diary of fluid/food intake: • Day 1: 1000 mL, 4 meals. • Day 2: 1200 mL, 4 meals but one bigger; daughter-in-law, Sue, made favorite ethnic dish.
• Fatigue and weakness • Hard, infrequent stools	• Reports more strength. • Improvement in self-care activities.	• Evaluate her ADL since office visit as well as level of fatigue and weakness.	• Able to serve self breakfast, heat up meals from Meals on Wheels; too tired to cook at supper; Gerald fixed supper; Sue helped her with bath each night. Required nap morning and afternoon.

Nursing Care Plan A CLIENT WITH FLUID VOLUME DEFICIT—CONT'D

Box 25-7

CRITICAL THINKING QUESTIONS

1. Mrs. Thompson has made progress toward the expected outcomes but has not achieved them. When the family expresses concern about this and asks you if you think she should come to live with them or be placed in a residential home, how would you answer and why?

2. Referring to the original case study, review the changes that are seen 1 week later. What signs and symptoms is Mrs. Thompson having now? Why? What other signs and symptoms indicate fluid volume excess? Which ones are the most serious, and why?

Nursing outcome and intervention labels from Johnson, M., Bulechek, G., McCloskey Dochterman, J. M., Maas, M., & Moorhead, S. (2001). *Nursing diagnoses, outcomes, and interventions: NANDA, NOC, and NIC linkages.* St Louis, MO: Mosby.

Key Principles

- Fluid and electrolyte imbalances are fairly common and often overlooked.
- Fluid and electrolyte imbalances rarely occur in isolation. It is the relationship of the solute to the solvent that determines the client's response, not the level of the deficit by itself.
- The most common fluid imbalance is dehydration, which occurs most often in the very young and in older adults.
- Fluid overload is common in clients with cardiovascular problems.
- Seventy percent of the body fluid is in the intracellular spaces. Therefore acute or severe loss can have serious consequences for cellular functioning.
- Fluid shifting occurs between the extracellular compartments first, unless the loss or excess is acute or severe. Regardless, cellular fluid shifting occurs last after the extracellular compensatory mechanisms have been exhausted.
- The most common electrolyte imbalance is hyponatremia. It is more common in the older adult population, especially in those on low-salt diets who are taking diuretics.
- Nurses must anticipate imbalances in high-risk clients: the very young; older adults; those experiencing pregnancy, especially teenage pregnancy; and those with acute or chronic illnesses.
- Thorough history and physical assessments including diagnostics are necessary for making an accurate differential diagnosis.
- The outcomes of the imbalance depend on the acuteness and severity of the condition, the age and health state of the client, and the degree to which the client's compensatory mechanisms or therapeutic interventions combat the imbalance.
- The nurse has many roles, including teaching the clients and their families positive health behaviors, promoting nutritional maintenance and replacement, collaborating with the physician for early detection of imbalances and poor responses to treatment, and collaboration with the dietitian in the promotion of positive nutritional outcomes.
- Through individualization of interventions and mutual goal setting with the clients and their families, nurses can facilitate optimal health outcomes.
- Nurses are in a key position to influence cost effectiveness and cost efficiency through utilization of appropriate resources, delegation of appropriate interventions, promotion of primary and secondary prevention, and ongoing care plan evaluation and revision.

Bibliography

*Altura, B. M., Brodsky, M. A., Elin, R. J., Gums, J. G., Resnick, L. M., & Seelig, M. S. (1994). Magnesium therapy: Coming of age. *Patient Care, 28*(2), 79-94.

*Batcheller, J. (1994). Syndrome of inappropriate antidiuretic hormone secretion. *Critical Care Nursing Clinics of North America, 6*(4), 687-692.

Cobbett, S., & LeBlanc, A. (2000). Minimizing IV site infection while saving time and money. *Australian Infection Control, 5*(2), 8-14.

*Constants, T., Delarue, J., Rivol, M., Theret, V., & Lamisse, F. (1994). Effects of nutrition education on calcium intake in the elderly. *Journal of the American Dietetic Association, 94*(4), 447-448.

Cooper, A., & Moore, M. (1999). Clinical update: IV fluid therapy—Water balance and hydration assessment. *Australian Nursing Journal, 7*(5), 26-29.

*Cullin, L. (1992). Interventions related to fluid and electrolyte balance. *Nursing Clinics of North America, 27*(2), 569-597.

*Edes, T., Walk, B. E., & Austin, J. L. (1990). Diarrhea in tube-fed patients: Feeding formula not necessarily the cause. *American Journal of Medicine, 88*(2), 91-93.

Edwards, S. (2001). Regulation of water, sodium and potassium: Implications for practice. *Nursing Standard, 25*(22), 36-44.

Hadaway, L. (1999). Catheter connection: Blood return from a central venous catheter. *Journal of Vascular Access Devices, 4*(2), 41.

*Hall, J. K. (1994). Caring for corpses or killing patients? *Nursing Management, 25*(10), 81-89.

Hand, H. (2001). The use of intravenous therapy. *Nursing Standard, 15*(43), 47-52.

*Hoot-Martin, J., & Larsen, P. D. (1994). Dehydration in the elderly surgical patient. *AORN Journal, 60*(4), 666-671.

Huckleberry, Y. (2001). Intravenous fluids: Which solution and why? *Support-Line 23*(1), 12-13.

Iggulden, H. (1999). Dehydration and electrolyte disturbance. *Nursing Standard, 13*(19), 48-56.

*Incalzi, R. A., Gemma, A., Capparella, O., Terranova, L., Sanguinetti, C., & Carbonin, P. U. (1992). Post-operative electrolyte imbalance: Its incidence and prognostic implications for elderly orthopedic patients. *Age and Ageing, 22,* 325-331.

*Innerarity, S. A. (1992). Hyperkalemic emergencies. *Critical Care Nursing Quarterly, 14*(4), 32-39.

Johnson, M., Bulechek, G. McCloskey-Dochterman, J., Maas, M., & Moorhead, S. (2001). *Nursing diagnoses, outcomes, and interventions: NANDA, NOC, and NIC linkages.* St Louis, MO: Mosby.

*Kaplan, M. (1994). Hypercalcemia of malignancy: A review of advances in pathophysiology. *Oncology Nursing Forum, 21*(6), 1039-1046.

*Kelso, L. A. (1992). Fluid and electrolyte disturbances in hepatic failure. *AACN Clinical Issues, 3*(3), 681-685.

Klein, T. (2001). PICCs and midlines: Fine-tuning your care. *RN, 64*(8), 26-29.

Lipp, J., Lord, L. M., & Scholer, L. H. (1999). Techniques and procedures: Fluid management in enteral nutrition. *Nutrition in Clinical Practice, 14*(5), 232-237.

Macklin, D. (1999). What's physics got to do with it? A review of the physical principles of fluid administration. *Journal of Vascular Access Devices, 4*(2), 7-11.

*Maughan, R. J. (1992). Fluid balance and exercise. *International Journal of Sports Medicine, 13,* S132-S135.

*Mendyka, B. E. (1992). Fluid and electrolyte disorders caused by diuretic therapy. *AACN Clinical Issues, 3*(3), 672-680.

*Newmark, K., & Nugent, P. (1993). Milk-alkali syndrome. *Postgraduate Medicine, 93*(6), 149-156.

*Porth, C., & Erickson, M. (1992). Physiology of thirst and drinking: Implication for nursing practice. *Heart & Lung, 21*(3), 273-282.

*Radke, K. J. (1994). The aging kidney: Structure, function, and nursing practice implications. *ANNA Journal, 21*(4), 181-190.

*Reherer, N. J. (1994). The maintenance of fluid balance during exercise. *International Journal of Sports Medicine, 15*(3), 122-125.

Rigdon, R. O. (2001). Protocols for the prevention of intravascular device-related infections. *Critical Care Nursing Quarterly, 24*(2), 39-47.

*Seshadri, V., & Meyer-Tettambel, O. M. (1993). Electrolyte and drug management in nutritional support. *Critical Care Nursing Clinics of North America, 5*(1), 31-36.

Shirreffs, S. M. (2000). Markers of hydration status. *Journal of Sports Medicine and Physical Fitness, 40*(1), 80-84.

Simmons, J. F., & Assell, C. C. (2001). Acid-base basics. *Support-Line 23*(1), 6-11.

*Sutcliffe, J. (1994). Dehydration: Burden or benefit to the dying patient? *Journal of Advanced Nursing, 19,* 71-76.

*Terry, J. (1994). The major electrolytes: Sodium, potassium, and chloride. *Journal of Intravenous Nursing, 17*(5), 240-247.

Promoting Wound Healing

Key Terms

- abrasion
- débridement
- dehiscence
- eschar
- epithelialization
- evisceration
- exudate
- fistula
- friction injury
- hematoma
- hemorrhage
- laceration
- primary lesion
- pressure ulcer
- secondary lesion
- wound

Learning Objectives

After studying this chapter, you should be able to do the following:

- Describe skin disruptions, wound healing, and problems of wound healing
- Discuss the staging of pressure ulcers
- Explain the effect of lifestyle, age, and illness on skin integrity and wound healing
- Assess the client who is at risk for or has an actual impairment of skin integrity
- Distinguish among the various nursing diagnoses for clients with alterations in skin integrity
- Plan for goal-directed interventions to prevent *Impaired skin integrity* or promote wound healing
- Evaluate the outcomes of interventions for *Impaired skin integrity*

Violetta Jacan is a 72-year-old woman who has been living alone in an apartment since her husband died 3 years ago. Her daughter lives nearby. One morning while getting out of the shower, Mrs. Jacan fell onto the bathroom floor and fractured her right hip. Unable to get to the phone to call for help, she lay on the floor until her daughter checked in on her late the next day. On admission to the emergency department, Mrs. Jacan is diagnosed with a broken hip. She also has reddened areas on her sacrum and heels.

Once Mrs. Jacan arrives on the surgical unit, the nurse prepares her for hip surgery and begins to plan for her postoperative skin care needs. She notes that Mrs. Jacan is over 70 and shows the beginning of pressure ulcer formation. She also considers that the client will have a hip incision and limited mobility during the postoperative period. Because all of these factors put Mrs. Jacan at risk for skin breakdown, the nurse considers the diagnoses of *Risk for impaired skin integrity* and *Impaired skin integrity* (see below).

KEY NURSING DIAGNOSES FOR   Skin Integrity

Risk for impaired skin integrity: A state in which the individual's skin is at risk of being adversely altered

Impaired skin integrity: A state in which an individual has altered epidermis and/or dermis

CONCEPTS OF SKIN INTEGRITY AND WOUND HEALING

Throughout your nursing career and in all practice settings, you will be concerned with your clients' skin care needs and will seek to prevent disruptions in skin integrity. For clients who already have such disruptions, you will seek to promote healing. Some clients will have minor skin disruptions, such as an abrasion or a tape blister. Some disruptions will be major, such as a deep pressure ulcer or a wound from major abdominal surgery. Throughout this range, skin care is an integral part of the overall nursing care plan in virtually all settings.

Skin Disruptions

A primary function of skin is to protect the body from many forms of trauma, including mechanical, thermal, chemical, and radiant. The epidermis serves as a tough mechanical layer that protects against bacteria, foreign material, other organisms, and chemicals. A skin disruption creates a route for the loss of body fluids, and the risk for infection is great.

Skin Lesions. A lesion is any pathological or traumatic discontinuity of tissue or loss of function of a part. This definition includes wounds, sores, ulcers, tumors, cataracts, and any other tissue damage. It is often used to refer to a visible local abnormality in the skin. Skin lesions may or may not relate to the client's medical condition. Lesions can be caused by mechanical injuries, pathological changes, allergies, or bites. To determine the etiology of common skin lesions, you should be able to distinguish between primary and secondary lesions. A **primary lesion** is the first lesion to appear on the skin in response to a causative agent and usually has a recognizable structure. Figure 26-1 identifies and describes 10 types of primary lesions. Changes can occur in a primary lesion and result in a **secondary lesion.** These changes occur in the epidermal layer and are caused by several factors including scratching, rubbing, medications, and the client's medical condition or disease process. Figure 26-2 (p. 616) illustrates secondary lesions.

Wounds. A wound is a type of lesion. A **wound** is a disruption of normal anatomic structure and function that results from bodily injury or from a pathological process that may be internal or external to the involved organ or organs. Wounds can be classified by cause and descriptors of the wound. It is important to be able to identify the cause of the wound and to describe it accurately to the health care team.

The cause of a wound may be intentional or unintentional. Intentional wounds result from a surgical procedure or treatment (such as intravenous therapy). Unintentional wounds result from accidental injury or trauma, animal bites, violence, or adverse effects of health care. The cause of the wound is closely related to the amount of tissue damage that results.

Wounds are classified as open or closed. In an open wound, the skin is broken and a range of soft tissue damage can be present. A surgical wound can be intentionally left open, or it may be open as a complication of healing. A closed wound involves no skin disruption.

Wounds are classified on the basis of the severity and nature of the injury. Superficial wounds involve surface layers of the skin or the body. *Deep* may refer to the deep layers of the skin or mean deep within a body cavity, penetrating internal body organs. Severity also has to do with the amount of tissue damage that results from both the break in the skin and trauma to surrounding tissue. It may also reflect damage to the blood supply to the site of injury.

Wounds are classified on the basis of the risk for infection. A clean wound was created with a clean instrument and contains little or no debris; a dirty wound was created with a grossly contaminated instrument or contains dirt and other debris. The surgical wound is the cleanest of all wounds. Table 26-1 (p. 617) summarizes terms used to classify wounds on the basis of a description of the wound and possible causes.

Most wounds have several characteristics. A surgical incision is created under sterile conditions, tissue damage is minimized, and healthy wound edges are approximated so that new tissue can grow and connect the tissue with minimal scarring. Wounds resulting from trauma are created under "dirty"

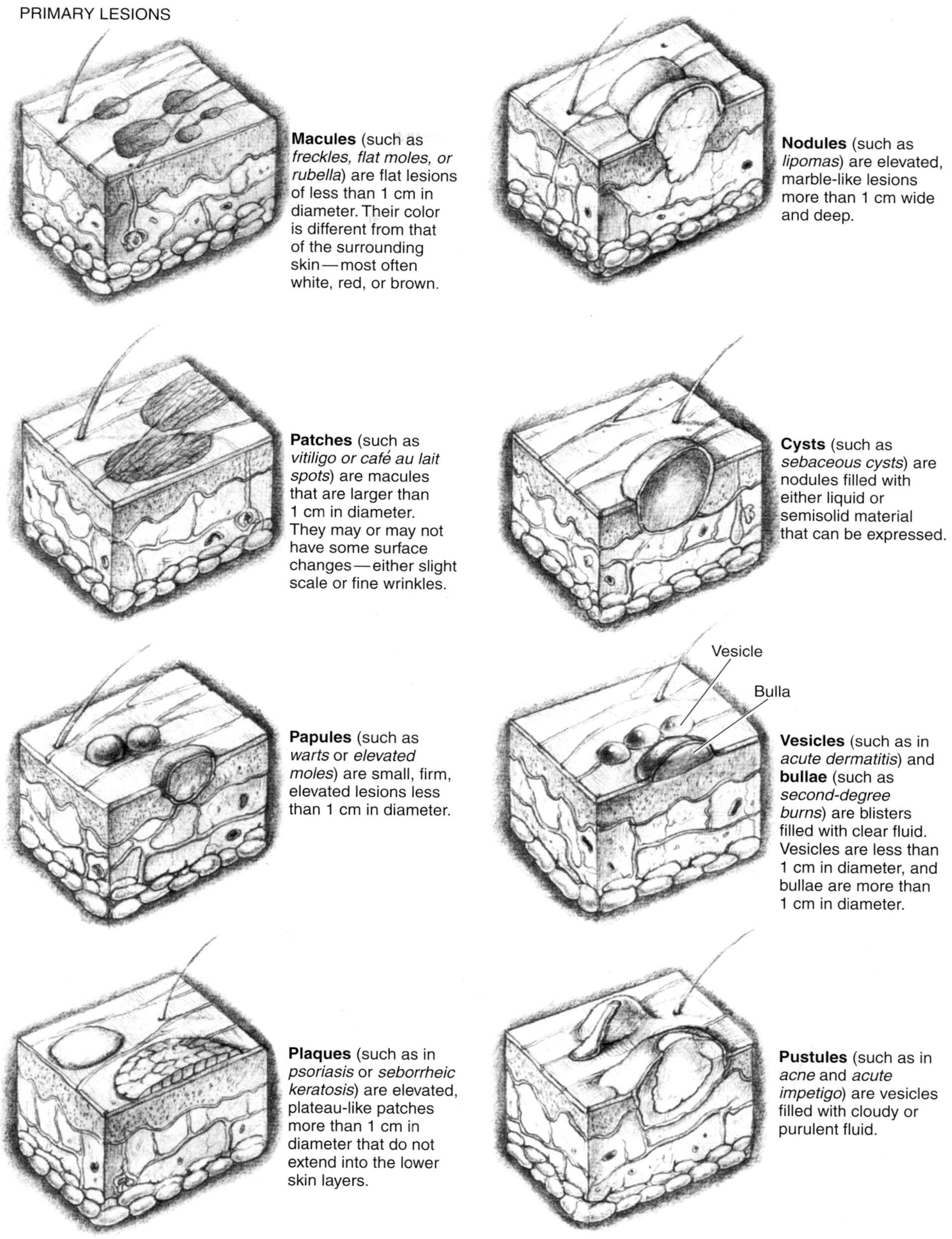

PRIMARY LESIONS

Macules (such as *freckles, flat moles, or rubella*) are flat lesions of less than 1 cm in diameter. Their color is different from that of the surrounding skin—most often white, red, or brown.

Nodules (such as *lipomas*) are elevated, marble-like lesions more than 1 cm wide and deep.

Patches (such as *vitiligo or café au lait spots*) are macules that are larger than 1 cm in diameter. They may or may not have some surface changes—either slight scale or fine wrinkles.

Cysts (such as *sebaceous cysts*) are nodules filled with either liquid or semisolid material that can be expressed.

Papules (such as *warts* or *elevated moles*) are small, firm, elevated lesions less than 1 cm in diameter.

Vesicle

Bulla

Vesicles (such as in *acute dermatitis*) and **bullae** (such as *second-degree burns*) are blisters filled with clear fluid. Vesicles are less than 1 cm in diameter, and bullae are more than 1 cm in diameter.

Plaques (such as in *psoriasis* or *seborrheic keratosis*) are elevated, plateau-like patches more than 1 cm in diameter that do not extend into the lower skin layers.

Pustules (such as in *acne* and *acute impetigo*) are vesicles filled with cloudy or purulent fluid.

Figure 26-1. Primary skin lesions. (From Ignatavicius, D., & Workman, M. L. [2002]. *Medical-surgical nursing: Critical thinking for collaborative care* [4th ed.]. Philadelphia: Saunders).

Continued

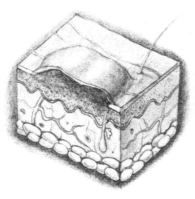

Wheals (such as *urticaria* and *insect bites*) are elevated, irregularly shaped, transient areas of dermal edema.

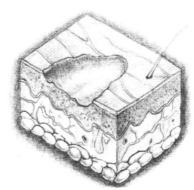

Erosions (such as in *varicella*) are wider than fissures but involve only the epidermis. They are often associated with vesicles, bullae, or pustules.

Figure 26-1, cont'd. Primary skin lesions. (From Ignatavicius, D., & Workman, M. L. [2002]. *Medical-surgical nursing: Critical thinking for collaborative care* [4th ed.]. Philadelphia: Saunders).

SECONDARY LESIONS

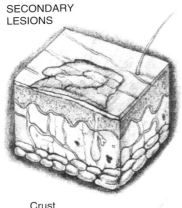

Scales (such as in *exfoliative dermatitis* and *psoriasis*) are visibly thickened stratum corneum. They appear dry and are usually whitish. They are seen most often with papules and plaques.

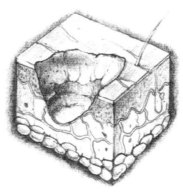

Ulcers (such as *stage III pressure sores*) are deep erosions that extend beneath the epidermis and involve the dermis and sometimes the subcutaneous fat.

Crust

Oozing

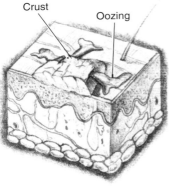

Crusts and oozing (such as in *eczema* and *late-stage impetigo*) are composed of dried serum or pus on the surface of the skin, beneath which liquid debris may accumulate. Crusts frequently result from broken vesicles, bullae, or pustules.

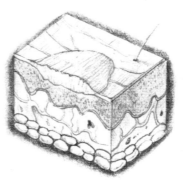

Lichenifications (such as in *chronic dermatitis*) are palpably thickened areas of epidermis with accentuated skin markings. They are caused by chronic rubbing and scratching.

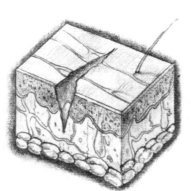

Fissures (such as in *athlete's foot*) are linear cracks in the epidermis, which often extend into the dermis.

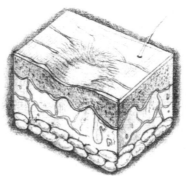

Atrophy (such as *striae* [stretch marks] and *aged skin*) is characterized by thinning of the skin surface with loss of skin markings. The skin is translucent and paper like. Atrophy involving the dermal layer results in skin depression.

Figure 26-2. Secondary skin lesions. (From Ignatavicius, D., & Workman, M. L. [2002]. *Medical-surgical nursing: Critical thinking for collaborative care* [4th ed.]. Philadelphia: Saunders).

Table 26-1	Types of Wounds	
Type	**Description**	**Possible Cause**
Open	Disruption or break in skin	Penetration by sharp object or instrument (such as knife, scalpel, bullet)
Closed	No disruption or break in skin	Trauma caused by blow with blunt object
Clean	Wound free of infectious organisms	Surgical incision not entering or affected by secretions from respiratory, gastrointestinal, or genitourinary tracts
Contaminated	Wound with microorganisms	Penetration of skin by dirt, bacteria
Penetrating	Wound with break through epidermis, dermis, and underlying tissues; may enter organs	Penetration by object or instrument (usually accidental)
Abrasion	Superficial injury caused by rubbing or scraping of skin against another surface	Friction injury resulting from fall or rubbing against bed linens
Laceration	Open wound with jagged edges	Penetration of skin by sharp object
Contusion	Closed wound; may be swollen, discolored, and painful	Blunt trauma, such as being hit by object

conditions, tissue damage is variable, wound edges may not be easily approximated, and scarring is more likely. Healing an open traumatic wound may be impeded by damage to soft tissue surrounding the open wound.

A chronic wound is a wound that has an insidious onset and heals slowly or is resistant to healing. Pressure ulcers are an example of a chronic wound in which the wound is open, increasing the risk for infection; blood flow to the wound bed is impaired, resulting in the presence of necrotic tissue; and a large amount of scar tissue will be needed to fill the wound bed for healing to occur. The etiology of pressure ulcers is discussed in Chapter 32. Chronic wounds are often classified by a description of the wound, including color of the wound bed and characteristics of drainage.

The red-yellow-black (RYB) classification system is based on wound bed color. Use this system in conjunction with other wound classification criteria. Based on the wound healing process, the RYB system identifies the wound on a continuum of wound healing. Generally, red wounds are healing wounds with clean, healthy granulation tissue. A yellow wound bed indicates that the wound is not yet ready to heal because it has fibrous slough or exudate that must be cleansed and removed. A black wound bed indicates the presence of **eschar,** a thick, leathery, necrotic, devitalized tissue (Hess, 2000).

Another important characteristic used to classify and describe a wound is its drainage. Wound drainage, or **exudate,** refers to fluid and cells that have escaped from blood vessels during the inflammatory response and remain in the surrounding tissues. Wound exudate varies with the type of tissue involved, the amount of inflammation, and the presence or absence of bacteria or other microorganisms.

Types of wound exudate include serous, sanguineous, serosanguineous, and purulent. Serous drainage is clear and watery plasma. Sanguineous drainage (from the Latin word for blood) is bright red. Serosanguineous drainage, a mixture of serous and sanguineous drainage, consists of plasma and red blood cells and is pale red and watery. Drainage from a surgical wound is initially sanguineous. Over several days, it changes to serosanguineous and then serous. Purulent drainage is pus, a protein-rich liquid product of the liquefac-

tion of necrotic tissue. It is made up of cells and cellular debris and is usually caused by an infection. It is thick and yellow, green, tan, or brown.

Wound Healing

The human body is able to heal itself and uses complex physiological processes to aid skin and wound healing and promote restoration of function and structure.

Phases of Wound Healing. The inflammatory phase, the first phase of wound healing, begins at the time of tissue injury and lasts 3 to 4 days. The cardinal signs of inflammation are edema, erythema, heat, and pain at the wound site. Hemostasis, the control of bleeding, is the process by which injured blood vessels constrict and platelets accumulate to stop the bleeding. The blood clots that subsequently develop in the wound area form a fibrin matrix, which acts as a structure or framework for further cellular repair. A scab forms on the wound surface, promoting hemostasis and helping to prevent wound contamination. Histamine is secreted by mast cells and damaged tissues, leading to capillary dilation, which increases the supply of blood and nutrients to the wound. Cell migration occurs when leukocytes (neutrophils) move into the wound and begin to ingest bacteria and wound debris. Monocytes change into macrophages and clean the wound bed of cellular debris and dead cells through phagocytosis. This process rids the site of cellular debris and prepares the wound bed for healing.

Monocytes continue cleaning the wound and stimulate the formation of fibroblasts (connective tissue cells). The fibrin network of the clot provides a structure to aid the formation of fibrous bridges as well as epithelial cells that move inward from the wound edges to create an epithelial layer.

The proliferative, or reconstruction, phase of healing lasts 4 to 21 days. During this phase, collagen fills the wound bed, new blood vessels develop (angiogenesis), and granulation tissue is formed by fibroblasts, giving the wound a bright red granular appearance. Also, the wound closes by **epithelialization,** a process in which epithelial cells grow to cover the wound bed. By day 5, the wound has filled with highly vascular fibroblastic connective tissue. By day 7, the surface epithelium has a normal thickness and the subepithelial layers are bridged. Progressive collagen accumulation during the second week results in the basic structure of the scar, which is bright red when new. The scar does not achieve its full tensile strength for a long time.

The final stage of wound healing is the maturation, or remodeling, phase. Although much maturation occurs by 3 to 4 weeks, the scar may not achieve maximum strength for up to 2 years. This phase is characterized by reorganization of the collagen fibers, wound remodeling, and maturation of the tissues to approximate the skin's original strength. Although the wound is considered fully healed, the tissue will always be at risk for breakdown because the wound's tensile strength never exceeds 80% of its preinjury strength.

Types of Wound Healing.

Most acute wounds and surgical wounds close by primary intention (Figure 26-3). The clinician brings together (approximates) wound edges or margins that are without **hematoma** (an accumulation of bloody fluid beneath tissue), debris, or exudate, and secures them using sutures, staples, or tape. The wound bed then fills in with granulation tissue, and the scar is usually thin and flat. Primary intention healing occurs in the first 14 days after injury. Wounds that heal by primary intention have a lower risk of infection, little tissue loss, and minimal scarring. Healing by primary intention takes a predictable course through the stages of inflammation, proliferation, and maturation.

In contrast, healing by secondary intention is prolonged (Figure 26-4). When the skin or wound edges cannot be approximated, as in a pressure ulcer or a wound that is large or infected, all dead (necrotic) and infectious tissue must be removed and the wound must fill with new tissue. The wound bed fills mostly with granulation tissue, but some tissue regeneration (epithelialization) proceeds from the margins. Wound contraction plays a greater role in healing by secondary intention, reducing the size of the final surface scar. Secondary intention healing generally involves greater tissue loss, higher risk for infection, and a prolonged healing time.

Tertiary intention, or delayed primary closure, occurs in wounds that may be contaminated, infected, or draining exudate (Figure 26-5). These wounds may be left open intentionally for 3 to 5 days to let healing begin by allowing the contaminated or infected matter or exudate to drain out. Once the infection clears, the wound is closed with sutures, staples, or tape.

Pressure Ulcers

The Agency for Health Care Policy and Research (AHCPR) (Bergstrom et al., 1994) defines a **pressure ulcer** as any lesion caused by unrelieved pressure that leads to damage of underlying tissues. Pressure ulcers develop when soft tissue is compressed between a bony prominence (such as the hip) and an external surface (such as a mattress). With prolonged pressure, the blood supply to the tissue's capillary network is disrupted, causing impeded blood flow to the surrounding

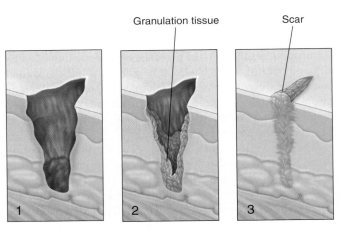

Figure 26-4. Wound healing by secondary intention.

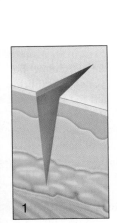
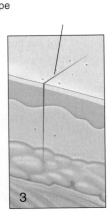
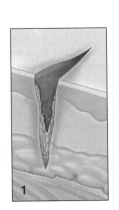

Figure 26-3. Wound healing by primary intention.

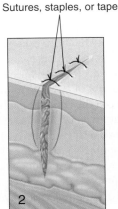
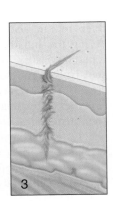

Figure 26-5. Wound healing by tertiary intention.

tissues. This leads to local tissue ischemia and hypoxia, edema, inflammation, and cell death. Pressure ulcers are sometimes called decubitus ulcers, pressure sores, or bed sores. However, the Wound, Ostomy, and Continence Society considers *pressure ulcer* the correct term.

The economic impact of pressure ulcers is significant, both for hospitals and for long-term-care facilities (Box 26-1).

Two clinical practice guidelines developed by the AHCPR address pressure ulcers. The first, *Pressure Ulcers in Adults: Prediction and Prevention Guidelines No. 3* (Bergstrom, Allman, & Carlson, 1992), lists strategies for identifying clients at risk and describes preventive strategies and treatment guidelines. The other guideline, *Treatment of Pressure Ulcers No.15* (Bergstrom et al., 1994), focuses on treating adults with pressure ulcers. Developed after an extensive literature review, these clinical practice guidelines are supported by clinical research and expert opinion. This chapter dis-

cusses pressure ulcers in reference to these practice guidelines as well as other current nursing literature.

The National Pressure Ulcer Advisory Panel (Margolis, 1995; NPUAP, 1998) identifies four stages of pressure ulcers (Figure 26-6, p. 620).

- *Stage I:* An observable, pressure-related alteration of intact skin whose indicators, as compared with the adjacent or opposite area on the body, may include changes in one or more of the following: skin temperature (warmth or coolness), tissue consistency (firm or boggy), and sensation (pain, itching). The ulcer appears as a defined area of persistent redness in lightly pigmented skin, or persistent red, blue, or purple hues in those with darker skin tones.
- *Stage II:* Partial-thickness skin loss involving the epidermis, dermis, or both. The ulcer is superficial and presents clinically as an **abrasion,** blister, or shallow crater.
- *Stage III:* Full-thickness skin loss involving damage to or necrosis of subcutaneous tissue that may extend to, but not through, the underlying fascia. The ulcer presents clinically as a deep crater with or without undermining of adjacent tissues.
- *Stage IV:* Full-thickness skin loss with extensive destruction, tissue necrosis, or damage to muscle, bone, or supporting structures (such as tendon, joint capsule).

Note: If the wound involves necrotic tissue, staging cannot be confirmed until the wound bed is viable.

According to the NPUAP, pressure ulcer staging is appropriate only for defining the maximum depth of tissue involvement. Beware of using reverse staging (also called downstaging) to describe a healing pressure ulcer. For example, if a client has a stage IV pressure ulcer that has healed and now looks like a stage II ulcer, identify it as a healing stage IV ulcer instead of as a stage II ulcer.

What stage pressure ulcer do you think Mrs. Jacan has on her heels and sacrum?

Problems of Wound Healing

Many factors affect wound healing (Box 26-2, p. 622). Local factors can affect the wound site itself, whereas a systemic condition may affect overall healing. Complications—such as infection, hemorrhage, fistulas, dehiscence, and evisceration—can occur during wound healing.

Infection. Wound infections most commonly occur within 36 to 48 hours after surgery, with symptoms of infection arising 5 to 7 days after surgery. Postoperative monitoring must include assessing for signs and symptoms of infection, such as fever, wound drainage, swelling, and tenderness. Increased drainage, drainage of another color, erythema at the wound perimeter, an elevated white blood cell count, and general malaise may indicate wound infection.

An infected wound must be cleansed of the infecting organism and cellular debris so that healing can begin. Factors that can predispose a client to wound infection include obesity, a debilitating condition, advanced age, a long and

---

THE·COST·OF·CARE Wound Care	Box 26-1

The cost of wound care involves much more than simply the cost of dressings. In general, wound care involves direct costs and indirect costs, as listed here.

DIRECT COSTS

- Primary wound dressing
- Secondary dressing
- Other materials needed (normal saline, tape, underpads)
- Caregiver time (assessment, positioning, dressing changes)
- Consultations
- Diagnostics
- Equipment (specialty beds and mattresses)
- Pharmacy

INDIRECT COSTS

- Extra inpatient days
- Client days lost from work
- Treating complications
- Costs of waste of disposal of used wound care materials
- Litigation costs

DISCUSSION

Reducing and preventing infection play a significant role in reducing the cost of wound care (Hermans & Bolton, 1996). Indeed, spending money to prevent pressure ulcers can save much more money by avoiding the need to treat pressure ulcers, which are usually difficult to resolve.

Additionally, research into new products has identified less costly treatments than the traditional methods. For example, research was conducted on the use of moist gauze versus a hydrocolloid dressing in treating pressure ulcers. Results indicated that the hydrocolloid dressing was more cost effective; the dressing was less expensive and saved 29 minutes of nursing time per wound.

RESOURCE

Collwell, J. C., Foreman, M. D., & Trotter, J. P. (1993). A comparison of the efficacy and cost effectiveness of 2 methods of managing pressure ulcers. *Decubitus, 6*(4), 28-35.

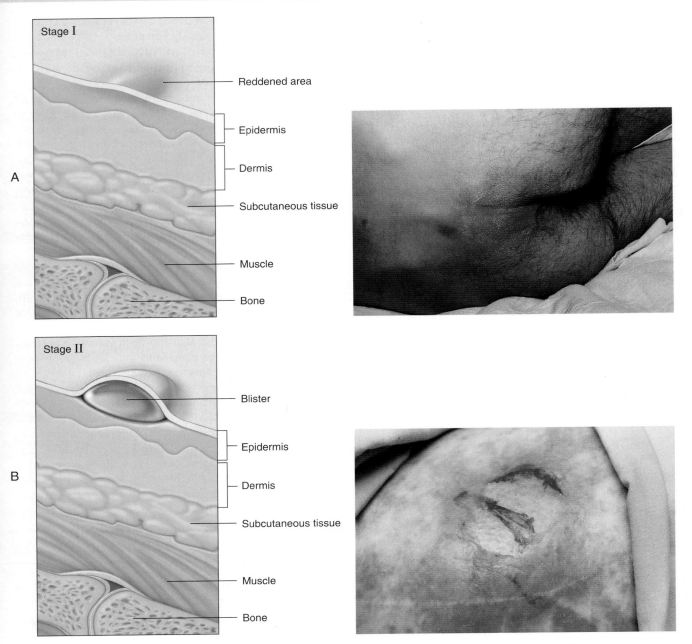

Figure 26-6. Stages of development of pressure ulcers. *A,* Stage I. *B,* Stage II. (From Ignatavicius, D. D., Workman, M. L., & Mishler, M. A. [2002]. *Medical-surgical nursing: Critical thinking for collaborative practice* (4th ed.). Philadelphia: Saunders.)

complicated operative procedure, other medical conditions, corticosteroid use, radiation therapy, and wound dehiscence and evisceration.

Hemorrhage. **Hemorrhage,** or bleeding from the wound bed or site, can occur in the immediate postoperative or initial postinjury period. Normally, hemostasis occurs quickly and clotting begins. However, hemorrhage may occur if a blood vessel continues to bleed or the client has poor clotting function. Causes include a surgical drain, a loose surgical suture, and infection. Internal hemorrhage can occur with no external

evidence of bleeding. To assess for internal hemorrhage, check for distention or swelling of the affected area, a change in the amount or type of drainage from a drain, and signs and symptoms of hypovolemic shock (decreased urine output, elevated heart rate, and decreased blood pressure).

External hemorrhage is easily detected as bloody drainage on the surgical dressing, especially if the dressing becomes saturated rapidly. However, be sure to assess not just the dressing but also the area around the dressing and posterior to the wound site. For instance, if a client has an incision and dressing on the anterior part of the neck, check

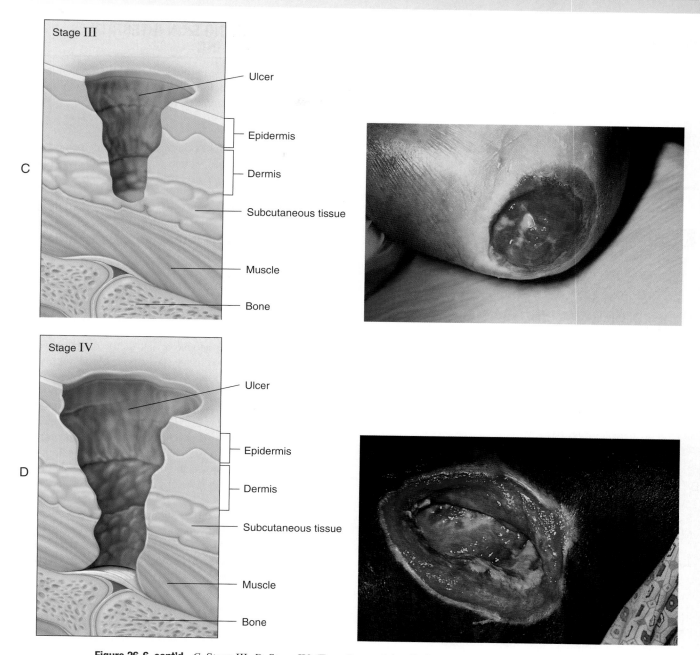

Figure 26-6, cont'd. *C,* Stage III. *D,* Stage IV. (From Ignatavicius, D. D., Workman, M. L., & Mishler, M. A. [2002]. *Medical-surgical nursing: Critical thinking for collaborative practice* (4th ed.). Philadelphia: Saunders.)

the posterior neck region for drainage. A hematoma also may form during the early postoperative period. To detect a hematoma, assess for hard painful swelling around the incision site. Assess all surgical wounds closely during the first 24 to 48 hours postoperatively.

Fistula. A **fistula** is an abnormal passage between two internal organs or between an organ and the external skin surface. A fistula forms because healing tissue layers do not close. A fistula may result from an abscess or infection, traumatic in-

jury, inflammatory process (radiation), or a disease process such as cancer.

Dehiscence and Evisceration. Dehiscence refers to separation of wound edges (Figure 26-7, p. 622). **Evisceration** is the protrusion of an internal organ (such as a bowel loop) through the incision. Wound eviscerations are medical emergencies. If one of these complications occurs, contact the physician immediately. Box 26-3 (p. 622) describes your role in caring for a client with wound evisceration.

Box 26-2 Factors Affecting Wound Healing

LOCAL FACTORS

- Dry environment
- Edema
- Eschar
- Infection
- Pressure
- Sloughing
- Trauma
- Wound stress

SYSTEMIC FACTORS

- Age
- Body build
- Chronic disease
- Poor nutritional status
- Prolonged steroid use
- Smoking
- Vascular problems

Box 26-3 Responding to Wound Evisceration

If a client's wound eviscerates, you will need to respond swiftly and accurately, as outlined here.

1. Stay calm. Projecting a calm and confident manner will help keep the client and family calm as well.
2. Ask a colleague to obtain supplies and to notify a physician while you stay with the client.
3. Help the client into semi-Fowler's position with the knees slightly flexed after gatching the foot of the bed. This position will ease pressure on the wound, prevent further tearing of the wound edges, and reduce the risk of further evisceration.
4. Cover the protruding intestine with a sterile dressing moistened with sterile normal saline solution to help prevent wound contamination and keep the abdominal contents moist. If no sterile dressing is available, use clean towels or dressings.
5. Monitor the client closely and assess vital signs and pulse oximetry readings. Frequent monitoring will help detect impending shock.
6. Establish intravenous access to provide fluids and prepare the client for surgery as ordered. The client will most likely need surgery to repair the wound and will not be permitted oral intake.
7. Continue to provide emotional support to client and family. Wound evisceration can be extremely frightening. A calm, supportive approach can help the client through this emergency.

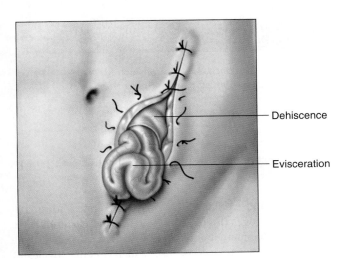

Figure 26-7. Wound dehiscence is the opening of the edges of a surgical wound. Evisceration is the protrusion of internal organs through the incision.

FACTORS AFFECTING SKIN INTEGRITY AND WOUND HEALING

Several factors affect skin integrity and the potential for wound healing. They include lifestyle, developmental, physiological, and environmental factors.

Lifestyle Factors

Lifestyle factors that affect skin integrity include personal hygiene, nutrition and fluid status, activity and exercise level, smoking, and substance abuse.

Personal Hygiene. People with poor hygiene may have increased risk for a wound infection or skin disorder. Routine skin cleansing removes bacteria, sweat, and other substances that may cause skin problems.

Nutrition and Fluid Status. Malnutrition with deficiencies of protein and vitamins A and C can impair wound healing. In a severely underweight or emaciated client, cells cannot transport sufficient oxygen and nutrients to the tissues to aid wound healing. Obesity is also a risk factor for poor wound healing, because adipose tissue has a poor blood supply and less resistance to infection.

Activity and Exercise. Active people who get adequate exercise tend to experience fewer skin problems. On the other hand, immobilization (such as from advanced age or spinal cord injury) increases the risk for skin breakdown and other skin problems. Clients who cannot change position independently for any reason have a greater risk for pressure ulcer formation.

Smoking. Smoking constricts blood vessels and reduces the blood's oxygen-carrying capacity, resulting in decreased tissue oxygenation. Smoking also increases platelet aggregation, which in turn may cause hypercoagulability with decreased perfusion to the skin or wound.

Substance Abuse. People who abuse substances, such as alcohol or illicit drugs, often have poor nutrition, which can lead to poor wound healing and skin condition.

Developmental Factors

Skin problems can occur at any time of life, from infancy to advanced age. However, infants and children heal faster than older adults, who may be less mobile and have more fragile, slowly healing skin than younger adults.

Physiological Factors

Factors such as advanced age, immunosuppression, incontinence, hypoxemia, diabetes, infections, neurological impairments, medical–surgical procedures, and medications can affect wound healing.

Age. Age plays an important role in wound healing. As a person ages, the wound healing phase can be prolonged because of decreased initial inflammatory responses. Changes in the vascular, immune, and respiratory systems can also impair wound healing.

Immunosuppression. Immunosuppressed persons may have a slowed inflammatory response, slowed reepithelialization, and a decrease in leukocyte activity.

Incontinence. Bowel and bladder incontinence can affect and delay wound healing because contact with stool or urine can contaminate a wound, prolonging healing and providing a medium for bacterial growth and subsequent infection.

Hypoxemia. Poor or impaired blood flow to a wound and surrounding tissues impairs wound healing. Decreased tissue oxygenation impairs collagen synthesis and epithelialization.

Diabetes. Diabetic clients may have microvascular disease, which can impair tissue oxygenation and tissue perfusion. Hyperglycemia inhibits leukocyte activity, can delay formation of granulation tissue, and provides an ideal environment for the growth of yeast and fungi.

Infection. Wound infection causes a prolonged inflammatory response and delayed wound healing. Wounds cannot heal when infection is present.

Neurological Impairment. Clients with neurological impairments, such as spinal cord injury, dementia, or diabetic neuropathy, are at greater risk for *Impaired skin integrity.* These people may be unable to care for themselves and, because they may lack sensation, cannot feel pressure or irritation to the skin. Clients with a change in level of consciousness (such as comatose or sedated clients in intensive care) also cannot protect themselves from factors that can lead to skin breakdown.

Procedures. Medical and surgical procedures, such as operative incisions, intravenous therapy, venipuncture, and radia-

tion therapy, can raise the risk of *Impaired skin integrity.* Orthopedic clients who undergo traction or cast application to treat fractures are at increased risk for skin breakdown. Friction and pressure from medical devices, such as cervical collars, oxygen tubing around the nose and ears, and nasogastric tubes can also cause skin breakdown.

Medications. Drugs—such as steroids, antiinflammatory medications, and chemotherapy—can alter protein synthesis and cellular growth, and slow the inflammatory phase of wound healing.

Environmental Factors

Environmental factors that can affect skin integrity include skin dryness, friction from bed linens, and moisture from incontinence, perspiration, emesis, and wound drainage. Skin may become macerated (wet and softened) if exposed to moisture for a prolonged period. Friction and shear from wrinkled bed linens can lead to pressure ulcers unless appropriate preventive strategies are implemented.

Even general environmental factors can affect a client's ability to relax and heal (Box 26-4).

ASSESSMENT

Collecting client data is the first step in the nursing process. You will use that data to develop a plan of care for the client. The two primary skin integrity diagnoses are *Risk for impaired skin integrity* and *Impaired skin integrity.*

General Assessment of Skin Integrity and Wound Healing

A thorough skin assessment is an important part of the physical examination, especially if the client was treated for or has risk factors for *Impaired skin integrity.* Make it a practice to identify risk factors and assess the skin of all clients routinely, especially those who need long-term care.

Health History. When obtaining the health history, use a holistic perspective. Consider the client's medical history, history of present illness, surgical history, current and past medications, nutritional state, mobility level, circulatory status, continence status, and presence of current infection. Perform a psychosocial assessment that includes the client's age, marital status, occupation, living arrangements, financial status, insurance coverage, cultural beliefs, and spirituality. Also assess the client's learning potential to determine learning needs.

Physical Examination. If a client has *Impaired skin integrity* or a *Risk for impaired integrity,* be sure to conduct a thorough physical examination. Assess height, weight, activity level, muscle mass, circulatory function, and respiratory function.

During a physical examination, you may notice a wide variety of lesions on your client's skin. Some are harmless variations; others are evidence of a disease process. If your client has a wound, assess it carefully.

Diagnostic Tests. Several diagnostic studies help identify skin or wound infection, poor oxygenation, and general nutrition status—factors that can affect skin integrity and wound healing. Use these laboratory values to assess the client's hydration status, identify possible infections, and help you formulate nursing diagnoses and develop a plan of nursing care.

COMPLETE BLOOD COUNT. The complete blood count (CBC) reveals the blood's oxygen-carrying capacity and may suggest an infection. For instance, the hemoglobin (Hgb) level indicates the blood's oxygen-carrying capacity, and an elevated white blood cell count may suggest a systemic or local infection.

ERYTHROCYTE SEDIMENTATION RATE. The sedimentation rate can help assess the client's inflammatory, infectious, and necrotic processes.

PREALBUMIN AND ALBUMIN LEVELS. Abnormally low prealbumin and albumin levels indicate poor nutritional status, which slows wound healing.

RADIOLOGICAL STUDIES. If a client has a suspected infection in a wound over a bony prominence (such as the sacrum or heel), a physician will typically order radiological studies to rule out osteomyelitis. Standard radiographs or a bone scan can be used to detect infection.

Focused Assessment for *Impaired Skin Integrity*

Defining Characteristics. Defining characteristics for *Impaired skin integrity* include invasion of body structures, disruption of the epidermis, and destruction of the dermis. When assessing a client's wound, you must document many characteristics of the wound and the surrounding area, including those described here.

LOCATION. Always document the exact anatomic location of a wound. For example, write "client has 4-cm abdominal incision in the right lower quadrant" or "pressure ulcer on left lateral malleolus."

SIZE. When measuring the wound, determine its length, width, and depth, in centimeters (cm) unless directed otherwise. Accurate wound measurement is important to develop an appropriate treatment plan and to aid evaluation of skin and wound healing.

To properly define a pressure ulcer, measure the length, width, and depth of the affected area. Use the concept of the face of a clock to help define landmarks and areas of the wound or impaired skin area. Measure wound length from head to toe (with 12 o'clock representing the client's head and 6 o'clock representing the feet). Measure the width of the wound from side to side (3 o'clock to 9 o'clock). Also assess wound depth by measuring how far the wound extends below the skin surface. Be sure to check for tunneling (a sinus tract or tunnel) or undermining of the wound or pressure ulcer.

Various measuring instruments are available to assess a wound. One of the easiest methods involves using a cotton-tipped applicator and a centimeter ruler (Figure 26-8). Another common method employs a tape measure or ruler. In the client's chart, record the wound length and width in centimeters, the measurement method used, and the client's position at the time of measurement.

Another way to measure a wound is to trace it. Hold a disposable acetate sheet, a measuring guide, or a plastic bag over the wound and trace the edges with a fine-tip permanent marker. Also write the date, the client's name or number, your name, and location markers (such as head or toes) on the tracing. Calculate the wound area, and document the area, the method of obtaining and calculating the measurement, and the client's position at the time of the measurement. Also place the tracing itself in the client's chart.

The advantages of this method, especially for a large wound, are that it is easy, quick, and reliably reproduced by the same person and by other people. Wound tracings can be a valuable addition to the client's medical record, and they allow easy monitoring of changes in the wound. The expense incurred by this method depends on the materials you use. Disadvantages of this method are that it may be difficult to see the margins of the wound while tracing it, and the accuracy of the tracing declines in smaller wounds. If the transparency does not contain a grid, you will need to copy the tracing to grid paper to calculate the size of the wound.

COLOR. Document the color of the wound bed. A red wound bed is ready for healing and consists of viable tissue. A yellow wound bed indicates fibrinous slough, old tissue, or

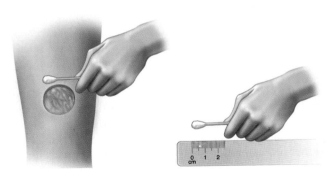

FIGURE 26-8. An easy method for measuring a wound using a cotton swab and a centimeter rule.

exudate that must be removed for healing to occur. Black tissue indicates eschar, a thick, leathery necrotic tissue that is not viable (Bryant, 2000).

SURROUNDING SKIN. Note the condition of the wound edges or margins. Assess the skin around the wound for redness or induration, temperature, moisture, color, and odor. Erythema around the wound edges may indicate underlying infection.

DRAINAGE. Assess any wound drainage for color, amount, consistency, and odor. Describe the drainage as serous, sanguineous, or serosanguineous. Be aware that the wound location, depth, and extent determine the amount of drainage. Noting drainage color can help identify the type of organism that may be infecting the wound. A foul, fecal, musty, or strong odor from a wound may indicate infection.

Action Alert! Be careful when documenting drainage and infection. Yellow drainage from a wound does not always indicate wound infection. Slough from the wound bed can be yellow and consist of wound debris, old white blood cells, and macrophages.

TEMPERATURE. Be sure to assess the temperature of the wound. Increased warmth of the wound bed or surrounding tissues may indicate pressure ulcer formation or an infection. To assess temperature, palpate the wound and surrounding tissues.

PAIN. Always assess for pain at the wound site. Absence of pain may indicate nerve impairment or involvement. Although pain at the wound site indicates intact nerves, severe pain may indicate infection and underlying tissue involvement.

WOUND CLOSURES. Surgical wounds and incisions are usually closed using sutures or stainless steel staples. Suture material may be silk, nylon, cotton, linen, wire, or Dacron (polyester). When suturing, the physician sews the inner tissue layers together, usually with a suture material that is absorbed by the body during healing. Usually, skin sutures are left in place for 7 to 10 days. If sutures are removed in 3 to 4 days, Steri-Strips are used to reinforce the wound.

Several different suturing methods can be used (Figure 26-9). They include intermittent suturing (in which each stitch is knotted) and continuous suturing (in which one thread is used to create several stitches and is tied only at the beginning and the end). Retention sutures (large sutures covered by rubber tubing to prevent further skin disruption) are used for large abdominal incisions in which additional support is needed (such as in obese clients), if swelling is substantial, or when the sutures must be left in place for a prolonged period.

Stainless steel staples are commonly used to approximate incision edges (Figure 26-10). Staples have advantages over sutures because they are stronger and less irritating to the skin, and the final scar is more cosmetically acceptable. Steri-Strips (small, thin strips of tape) can be used for smaller incisions (Figure 26-11). These strips may minimize incisional irritation, swelling, and scar formation. Topical skin adhesives (glues) may be used for wound closure in the place of sutures and staples and form a fast, strong, flexible bond between the wound edges. There are no stitches to remove because the adhesive "sheds" from the skin naturally as the wound heals.

Postoperative assessment of a surgical wound should include inspecting the skin around the incision for redness, irritation, or excessive swelling. These signs may indicate a

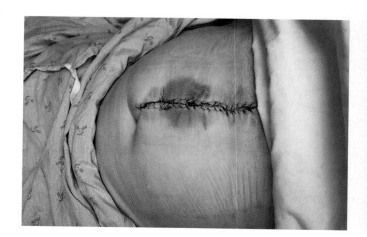

Figure 26-10. Staples in an incision line.

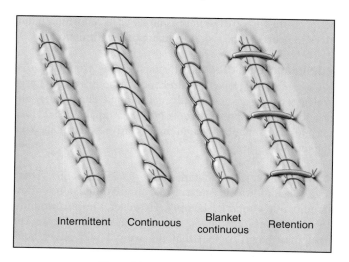

Figure 26-9. Types of sutures.

Intermittent Continuous Blanket continuous Retention

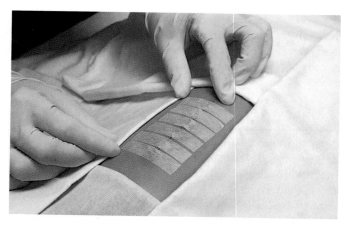

Figure 26-11. Steri-Strips.

wound infection or an overly tight wound closure, which ultimately can lead to wound edge separation.

Related Factors

Factors related to the diagnosis *Impaired skin integrity* may be either internal or external. External factors include the following:

- Extreme heat or cold
- Chemical substances
- Mechanical factors, such as shear, pressure, or restraints
- Physical immobilization
- Moisture and humidity
- Medications
- Radiation
- Diminished circulation

Internal factors include the following:

- Altered metabolism
- Skeletal prominence
- Immunological deficit
- Altered sensation, circulation, turgor, pigmentation, or nutritional state (such as obesity or emaciation)

Keep in mind that proper wound healing requires adequate perfusion. Altered circulation may lead to poor tissue oxygenation and subsequent ulceration. Decreased arterial circulation causes ulcers because the tissues fail to receive enough oxygenated blood. These ulcers most commonly appear on the bony prominences of the ankle and toes. Chronic diminished circulation produces atrophic changes, including hair loss and thin, shiny skin. Also, pulses may be absent or weak. Venous stasis ulcers, caused by poor venous return, are associated with varicose veins and thrombophlebitis. Arterial pulses are present but venous blood is not returning to the heart. The chronic skin changes of dark pigmentation and stasis dermatitis are usually present.

Chemical irritation can result from urinary or fecal incontinence, gastric secretions, and harsh products that can cause skin irritation and breakdown. To help prevent chemical irritation, make sure the client's plan of care includes measures to protect the epidermis from contact with these irritants.

Radiation is the least common mechanism of skin injury. Excluding occupational radiation accidents, the most common type of radiation injury results from radiation therapy. The skin is vulnerable to radiation injury because the cells of the basal layer are continually and rapidly dividing. Signs of injury develop 2 to 3 days after radiation exposure and peak in 2 to 3 weeks. When the skin is severely affected, ulceration may develop.

DIAGNOSIS

Risk for impaired skin integrity applies to a client with a medical, surgical, developmental, or mobility problem that could affect skin health. *Impaired skin integrity* results from skin injury caused by moisture, pressure, friction, shear, and other factors.

Be sure to take a thorough assessment, including a complete health history, physical examination, and evaluation of

has a nursing diagnosis of *Risk for impaired skin integrity* or *Impaired skin integrity*. If the client has risk factors without signs or symptoms of skin impairment, use *Risk for impaired skin integrity*. Typical candidates for this nursing diagnosis include clients who are bed-bound with poor nutrition and those with an altered level of consciousness. In contrast, a client who is being treated for pressure ulcers has a nursing diagnosis of *Impaired skin integrity*. Figure 26-12 illustrates how to choose among these nursing diagnoses.

Assigning an appropriate nursing diagnosis depends on the assessment data you collect. In some cases, another nursing diagnosis may be more suitable. For example, for a client recovering from a total hip replacement, you might choose *Impaired physical mobility* because it addresses skin integrity as well as mobility problems. *Risk for infection* may be appropriate for the postoperative client with an abdominal incision after an appendectomy. Table 26-2 provides examples of ways to formulate appropriate nursing diagnoses.

Related Nursing Diagnoses

Other client conditions and factors may impact selection of a nursing diagnosis, such as the following.

Risk for Infection. Assess the client with a pressure ulcer or postoperative surgical incision for infection. The skin opening creates an entrance site for microorganisms to enter the wound.

Impaired Tissue Integrity. Assess the tissues surrounding the client's wound for further skin breakdown or interruption. A client may have *Impaired tissue integrity* even without skin breakdown on the surface. Palpate the area around the incision or pressure ulcer to assess for bogginess or hardened tissue.

Impaired Physical Mobility. Assess for other conditions, such as visual or neurological impairment. These clients may also be at risk for *Impaired skin integrity*. For example, clients with spinal cord injury or multiple sclerosis may be unable to feel pressure and other skin sensations or to reposition themselves to decrease the risk of pressure ulcer formation.

Body Image Disturbance. Clients suffering from *Impaired skin integrity* may have a disturbance in body image. Large surgical wounds or pressure ulcers can make clients feel self-conscious and apprehensive about their appearance. Take measures to help clients maintain a positive body image (see Chapter 40).

Hopelessness. Clients with *Impaired skin integrity* may feel a sense of hopelessness. Most surgical incisions follow a predictable course of healing. However, chronic wounds, especially pressure ulcers, can take months to heal. The client may begin to feel that the wound will never heal. Encouraging the client to focus on wound healing stages and to participate in wound care may help ease feelings of

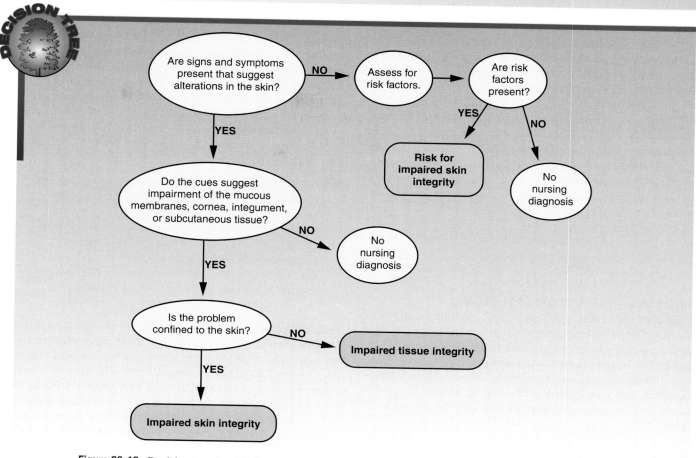

Figure 26-12. Decision tree for skin integrity nursing diagnoses. Diagnoses are shown in rectangles. Within these rectangles, diagnoses shown in **bold** type are NANDA-approved nursing diagnoses; diagnoses shown in regular type are not NANDA-approved nursing diagnoses.

Table 26-2	*Clustering Data to Make a Nursing Diagnosis*
SKIN PROBLEMS	

Data Cluster	Diagnosis
A single, 44-year-old woman on the third postoperative day is very concerned about the large abdominal incision created during her hysterectomy and worries about her future cosmetic appearance.	*Disturbed body image* related to large abdominal incision secondary to hysterectomy
An 18-year-old man injured while body-surfing at the beach sustained a C4 fracture and now is quadriplegic.	*Risk for impaired skin integrity* related to impaired physical mobility
A 72-year-old woman in a motor vehicle accident needs balanced suspended traction for a fracture of her right femur. Has a stage II pressure ulcer measuring 2 × 3 cm on left buttock.	*Impaired skin integrity* related to bed rest and traction

Imbalanced Nutrition: Less Than Body Requirements. The client with *Impaired skin integrity* needs adequate nutrition for wound healing. Assess for poor appetite, actual intake, and the need for nutritional and/or daily multivitamin supplements.

PLANNING

After choosing appropriate nursing diagnoses, you must develop a plan of care on the basis of the diagnoses. When planning care, assign priorities to the nursing diagnoses, select appropriate nursing interventions to achieve expected outcomes (client-centered goals), and document the nursing diagnoses, outcomes, interventions, and evaluations on the plan of care.

For a client who is bed-bound after a motor vehicle accident, the goal is to prevent skin breakdown and pressure ulcer formation. For a client with a pressure ulcer, the goal is to achieve timely healing of the pressure ulcer.

Expected Outcomes for the Client With *Impaired Skin Integrity*

The expected outcome for a client with the nursing diagnosis of *Impaired skin integrity* is to achieve wound healing without complications. Outcomes for the client may include the following:

- Maintains a normal temperature or baseline vital signs
- Maintains nutritional intake to support wound healing

- Maintains adequate fluid intake
- Performs activities of daily living
- Performs wound care and dressing changes as instructed
- States the signs and symptoms of infection
- Verbalizes discharge instructions for wound care

INTERVENTION

Interventions for a client with *Impaired skin integrity* are developed by the multidisciplinary team, including the nurse, physician, physical and occupational therapists, and dietitian, as well as the client and family. A valuable resource to the medical and nursing staff is the certified enterostomal therapist nurse. This nurse, specially trained in wound, ostomy, and incontinence care, can assist in selecting dressings and support surfaces, planning and implementing care, and evaluating the plan of care.

Interventions to Promote Skin Healing

Skin care and wound care have changed dramatically over the past 30 years. Extensive research has led to new wound care treatment protocols and products. However, wound healing cannot be approached solely from a procedural perspective. Instead, the treatment plan must take the client's entire condition into consideration. Physical condition, nutritional status, and treatment methods all affect the healing process (Hess, 2000).

Providing Adequate Nutrition. Adequate nutrition is essential for the client with *Impaired skin integrity* (Hess, 2000). Malnutrition inhibits wound healing and may increase the risk for wound infection (Table 26-3). Commonly, a client with *Impaired skin integrity* needs assistance in meeting daily nutritional requirements. Wound healing depends on the availability of adequate protein, vitamins, and minerals. Postoperative clients and older, debilitated clients with pressure ulcers require particularly close nutritional monitoring.

Improving clients' nutritional status requires a multidisciplinary effort. Assess their intake and help them meet nutritional needs. One way to help clients choose nutritious meals is to assist them in filling out the dietary menu. Also

consult a dietitian, as appropriate, to help determine a client's minimal caloric intake required to promote wound healing. The dietitian may request a calorie count to monitor intake and determine whether nutritional requirements are being met. As previously mentioned, clients may require dietary supplementation, such as multivitamins or liquid supplements. Vitamins C, A, and B complex, and iron, copper, and zinc are especially important for wound healing. A client who cannot take nutrition orally may require enteral or parenteral feedings.

Postoperatively, Mrs. Jacan has little appetite and is not getting adequate nutrition. What effect might Mrs. Jacan's nutrition have on wound healing and development of pressure ulcers? Although Mrs. Jacan tries some nutritional milkshakes, she just cannot eat the solid food on her tray. Keeping in mind Mrs. Jacan's admission history, what foods might the nurse want to include in her diet? How might the nurse involve Mrs. Jacan's daughter in promoting good nutrition for her mother?

Cleansing the Wound. For a wound to heal, the wound bed must be clean and free of infection. Bacteria, devitalized tissue, and exudate must be removed to promote healthy granulation tissue. To cleanse a wound, you will need a wound cleansing solution and a method for applying the solution to the wound. Numerous wound cleansing solutions or antiseptics are available. However, the benefits of a clean wound must be weighed against the potential trauma to the wound bed that could result from cleansing. Use caution when applying these products. Povidone-iodine, acetic acid, sodium

Table 26-3	Nutrients and Their Roles in Wound Healing
Nutrient	**Role in Wound Healing**
Carbohydrates, fats, and calories	Energy for wound regeneration and repair
Copper	Cross-linking of collagen fibers
Iron	Oxygen transport
Protein	Collagen synthesis, epidermal proliferation, and immune reesponse
Vitamin A	Collagen synthesis, epidermal proliferation, and immune response
Vitamin B complex	Protein synthesis and cross-linking of collagen fibers
Vitamin C	Collagen synthesis and capillary wall integrity
Zinc	Collagen synthesis and immune response

Table 26-4	Irrigation Pressures by Device
Device	**Irrigation Pressure (psi)**
Spray Bottle-Ultra Klenz (Carrington Laboratories, Inc., Irving, TX)	1.2
Bulb Syringe (Davol Inc., Cranston, RI)	2.0
Piston Irrigation Syringe (60-mL) with catheter tip (Premium Plastics, Inc., Chicago, IL)	4.2
Saline Squeeze Bottle (250-mL) with irrigation cap (Baxter Healthcare Corp., Deerfield, IL)	4.5
Water Pik at lowest setting (#1) (Teledyne Water Pik, Fort Collins, CO)	6.0
Irrijet DS with tip (Ackrad Laboratories, Inc., Cranford, NJ)	7.6
35-mL syringe with 19-gauge needle or angiocatheter	8.0
Water Pik at middle setting (#3) (Teledyne Water Pik, Fort Collins, CO)	42
Water Pik at highest setting (#5) (Teledyne Water Pik, Fort Collins, CO)	>50
Pressurized Cannister-Dey wash (Dey Laboratories, Inc., Napa, CA)	>50

From Beltram, K. A., Thacker, J. G., & Rodeheaver, G. T. *Impact pressures generated by commercial wound irrigation devices.* Unpublished research report. Charlottesville, VA, University of Virginia Health Sciences Center.

hypochlorite, and hydrogen peroxide are toxic to fibroblasts. Dakin's solution and some commercial wound cleansers have also been found to be cytotoxic.

Normal saline solution is the preferred cleansing agent because it is physiologically compatible, does not harm tissue, and adequately cleanses most tissues. Irrigate wounds with a device that provides 4 to 15 pounds of pressure per square inch (Table 26-4). Using adequate irrigation pressure enhances wound cleansing without damaging the tissues. An easy way to irrigate a wound is to use a 35-mL syringe with an angiocatheter. This method provides enough force to remove eschar, bacteria, and other debris. Procedure 26-1 (p. 630) outlines the steps of wound irrigation.

Commonly, a physician will order that an incision be cleansed. When cleansing around an incision or drain, always wipe from the cleanest area to the dirtiest (Figure 26-13). Remember that, generally, the wound is cleaner than the surrounding skin. To apply the "clean to dirty" rule, clean from the center of the incision and wipe outward. To cleanse around a drain, wipe in a circular direction, changing swabs with each concentric circle.

Maintaining a Moist Wound Bed.
Moisture enhances wound reepithelialization, helping a wound heal faster and with less scar tissue. In contrast, a scab that forms when a wound is kept dry does not allow the movement of epidermal cells in the healing process. Moist wound healing does not promote infection. The infection rate for moisture-retentive dressings is 2.5% compared to 9% for dry dressings (Thompson, 2000).

Dressing the Wound.
Most surgical wounds heal by primary intention and proceed through the three healing phases previously described. Optimal dressings absorb drainage and provide an aseptic environment that provides a barrier against further trauma (Bryant, 2000). To support the "moist wound" concept, numerous wound care products, including transparent films, hydrocolloid dressings, hydrogels, and foams, have been developed (Table 26-5, p. 631). It may be difficult to determine which type of dressing to apply. Table 26-6 (p. 632) suggests specific dressings for each stage of a pressure ulcer.

> *Action Alert!* Always check the physician's dressing orders for the specific site, method, dressing type, frequency of dressing changes, and time frame to evaluate healing.

Dry sterile dressings (DSDs) are most commonly used for closed surgical incisions. These dressings protect the incision and absorb drainage or exudate. The initial postoperative dressing is usually left in place for 24 to 48 hours. Some surgeons prefer to change the first postoperative dressing themselves, so check the physician's order and agency policy on initial postoperative dressing changes. Remove the dressing correctly, as described in Procedure 26-2 (p. 633). Remember that repeatedly applying and removing a dressing can further impair a client's skin integrity. Montgomery straps are a good choice for clients who need frequent dressing changes or have sensitive skin (Figure 26-14, p. 632). They reduce skin irritation caused by repeated dressing changes.

Occasionally, a dressing will stick to the wound bed. To loosen the dressing easily without disturbing new granulation tissue, moisten it with normal saline solution.

Secure dressings in place using tape, other bandages, or binders, as described in Procedure 26-3 (p. 634). To determine the best method for securing a bandage, assess the wound (including its size), the client's activity level, and the frequency of ordered dressing changes.

Generally, open surgical wounds are managed by keeping the wound clean, moist, free of necrotic tissue, and protected with dressings. When caring for an open surgical wound, follow principles for providing pressure ulcer care.

Keep in mind that all pressure ulcers are colonized with bacteria; on occasion, you may need to culture a wound to assess the bacteria growing in it (Procedure 26-4, p. 635). The AHCPR

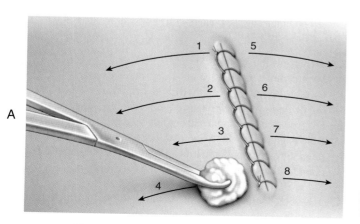
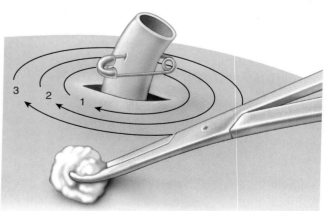

Figure 26-13. Cleaning a surgical wound. **A,** Start at the incision and clean outward. **B,** Start at the drain site, and clean around the drain in a circular fashion. Use a clean, new sterile swab for each stroke to prevent contamination of the wound.

PROCEDURE 26-1 · IRRIGATING A WOUND

TIME TO ALLOW
Novice: 15 min.
Expert: 7 min.

Wound irrigation promotes wound healing by removing exudate, drainage, pus, and slough. Irrigation is a method of cleaning a wound with a gentle flow of a solution. It washes the wound without wiping delicate tissues with a fabric that might cause damage to newly forming granulation tissue. Irrigation also has the advantage of penetrating tunnels or fissures in the wound. The irrigation solution should not be harmful to the tissues and should be injected at a pressure of 4 to 15 psi (pounds per square inch).

DELEGATION GUIDELINES

You may not delegate wound irrigation to a nursing assistant. The complex nature of this type of wound requires your on-going assessment and careful attention to irrigation technique. The nursing assistant may help with assembling the necessary equipment and positioning the client for your performance of wound care.

EQUIPMENT NEEDED
- Irrigation kit or sterile basin
- 18- or 19-gauge needle or angiocatheter
- 35-mL syringe
- Sterile normal saline 150 to 500 mL or other irrigant ordered by physician
- Clean gloves
- Sterile gloves
- Waterproof underpad
- Protective eyewear (if needed)

1. Follow preliminary guidelines for nursing procedures (see inside front cover).

2. Prepare for the procedure.
a. Check the wound care order and the specific order for irrigant. *Wound irrigations are prescribed by a physician or advanced practice nurse.*
b. Premedicate the client for pain if you anticipate discomfort.
c. Perform hand hygiene and apply protective eyewear and a gown if you anticipate splashing during the irrigation procedure. *Following these steps maintains standard precautions.*
d. Place the underpad and/or clean basin to catch the irrigant fluid when it drains from the wound.
e. Decide whether the procedure should be clean or sterile. Set up a clean or sterile field by opening the irrigation tray. Add new sterile dressings to the field or open packages where sterile dressings can be accessed once you have donned your sterile gloves.
f. Pour irrigant into the sterile basin.

3. Remove the old dressing using clean gloves.
a. Remove the outer layer. If the dressing is stuck to delicate granulation tissue, moisten it for easier removal.
b. Remove any packing from the wound. Dispose of the dressing according to hospital policy for standard precautions for blood and body fluids.

4. Irrigate the wound.
a. Apply sterile gloves.

b. Fill the syringe with irrigant. With the tip of the needle about 2 inches from the wound bed, flush with slow continuous pressure (see illustration). Repeat as needed. Irrigate the wound thoroughly.

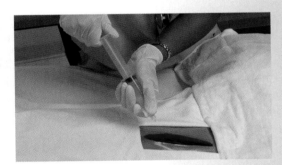

Step 4b. Flushing the wound with slow continuous pressure.

5. Re-dress the wound.
a. Wet-to-moist packing with a dry outer dressing is often used in conjunction with wound irrigations. *Re-dressing the wound with an appropriate dressing promotes healing.*
b. Dispose of used supplies according to standard precautions. If hospital policy dictates that a wound irrigation be a clean procedure, the irrigation kit can be reused for 24 hours. The open bottle of normal saline is good for 24 hours.

6. Document the client's tolerance of the wound irrigation and dressing change, as well as a description of the wound bed. *Documentation of client tolerance and the appearance of the wound bed facilitates communication of the client's condition and allows ongoing assessment of the client plan of care.*

Table 26-5 Common Wound Care Products

Product	Action	Indication	Advantages	Disadvantages
Gauze dressing	Wound débridement	• Prevent trauma and infection • Wick exudate away from wound • Provide a moist environment for healing (when moistened)	• Moderately absorptive • Cost-effective • Universally available • Can be combined with other dressings • Can be packed into wounds	• May require frequent changes • May adhere to wound bed and débride healthy tissue
Transparent film	Provides a moist environment that promotes granulation tissue and autolysis of necrotic tissue, allowing oxygen and water vapor to escape while remaining impermeable to bacteria and contaminants	• Superficial wound • Partial-thickness wound • Wound with sloughing or necrosis • Wound with little or no exudate	• Retains moisture • Impermeable to bacteria and other contaminantion • Promotes autolysis • Allows visualization of wound	• Not recommended for infected wounds or those with heavy exudate • May be difficult to apply • May not stay in place in high-friction area or if exudate is heavy
Hydrocolloid dressing	Provides a moist environment that allows a clean wound to granulate and a necrotic wound to débride autolytically	• Superficial or partial-thickness wound • Wound with necrosis or sloughing • Wound with light-to-moderate exudate	• Impermeable to bacteria and other contaminants • Promotes débridement • Self-adhesive and molds well • May be left in place for 3 to 5 days, minimizing skin trauma and disruption of healing • May be used under compression	• Not recommended for sinus tracts, infection, fragile skin, exposed bone or tendon, or wounds with heavy exudate • May become dislodged if wound produces heavy exudate • May curl at edges
Hydrogel dressing	Water- or glycerin-based amorphous gel, impregnated gauze, or sheet dressing used to maintain a moist wound	• Partial- and full-thickness wounds • Deep wound with light exudate • Wound with necrosis or sloughing	• Soothes and reduces pain • Rehydrates wound • Promotes débridement • Is easily removed	• Not recommended for wounds with heavy exudate • May be difficult to secure • Becomes dehydrated easily
Alginate dressing	Interacts with exudate to form a soft gel that keeps the environment moist	• Partial- or full-thickness wound with moderate to heavy exudate • Wound with tunneling or sinus tracts • Wound with necrotic tissue and exudate • Infected or noninfected	• Can absorb up to 20 times its weight in exudate • Forms a gel over wound • Promotes débridement • Fills in dead space	• Not recommended for wounds with dry eschar or light exudate • May dry out wound bed • Requires secondary dressings
Composite dressing (combination of two or more products)	Combines moisture retention with absorption	• Partial- or full-thickness wound with moderate-to-heavy exudate and with healthy tissue • Necrotic tissue or mixed wounds	• May promote débridement • May be used on infected wounds • Easy to apply and remove	• Not recommended for wounds with minimal or no exudate
Exudate absorber	Conforms to wound surface, eliminates dead space, and absorbs exudate while maintaining a moist environment	• Full-thickness wound with moderate-to-heavy exudate • Wound that requires packing and absorption • Wound with necrotic tissue	• Absorbs at least 5 times its weight in exudate • Fills in dead space • Promotes débridement • Easy to apply	• Not recommended for wounds with light exudate or dry eschar • May rehydrate wound bed • Requires secondary dressings
Foam	Creates a moist environment and can be removed without trauma	• Partial- or full-thickness wound with minimal-to-heavy exudate • To absorb drainage around tubes	• Nonadherent • Will not injure surrounding skin • Easy to apply and remove	• Not recommended for wounds with no exudate • May macerate surrounding unprotected skin

Table 26-6	Choosing the Right Dressing for a Pressure Ulcer*	
Pressure Ulcer Stage	Dressing Options
Stage I pressure ulcers	• Hydrocolloids† • Lubricating sprays • Moisturizing lotions • Skin sealants • Transparent films†
Stage II pressure ulcers with light exudate or drainage	• Collagen • Composites • Foams • Hydrocolloids† • Hydrogel wafers • Moist impregnated gauzes • Specialty absorptives • Transparent films† • Contact layers
Stage II pressure ulcers with moderate exudate or drainage	• Alginates • Collagens • Composites • Foam (covers) • Hydrogel wafers • Moist impregnated gauzes • Specialty absorptives • Gelling fibers
Stage III pressure ulcers with light-to-moderate exudate or drainage; no necrosis	• Collagens • Foam (fillers) • Hydrocolloids (pastes, fillers) • Hydrogels (amorphous, gauze) • Moist impregnated packing gauzes • Wound fillers
Stage III pressure ulcers with moderate-to-heavy exudate or drainage; necrosis present; tunneling or undermining present	• Alginates • Collagens • Débriding agents • Foams (fillers) • Wound fillers • Gelling fibers
Stage IV pressure ulcers with light-to-moderate exudate or drainage; no necrosis present	• Collagens • Foams (fillers) • Hydrocolloids† • Hydrogels (amorphous, gauze) • Moist impregnated packing gauzes • Wound fillers
Stage IV pressure ulcers with moderate-to-heavy exudate or drainage; necrosis present; tunneling or undermining present	• Alginates • Collagens • Débriding agents • Foams (fillers) • Moist impregnated gauzes • Wound fillers • Gelling fibers

Modified from Hess, C. T. (1988). *Nurse's clinical guide to wound care* (2nd ed.). Springhouse, PA: Springhouse.
*It remains the responsibility of the nurse to know the actions, indications, and contraindications of wound care products (see Table 26-5) before selecting a dressing.
†Contraindicated for infected wounds.

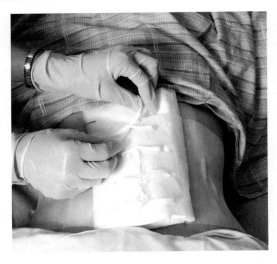

Figure 26-14. Montgomery straps are useful for clients with sensitive skin who cannot tolerate tape, or for those clients who require frequent dressing changes.

recommends effective wound cleansing to minimize wound colonization. When culturing a wound, do not use swab cultures because they detect only surface colonization. The Centers for Disease and Control and Prevention (CDC) recommend obtaining fluid through needle aspiration or through tissue ulcer biopsy.

Topical antibiotics can be used on a clean ulcer that is not healing. Local pressure ulcer infections do not require systemic antibiotics.

> *Action Alert!* A pungent, foul, fecal, or musty odor coming from a wound or pressure ulcer suggests infection. Check with the physician about obtaining a wound culture.

Draining the Wound. Drains are placed in some wounds before the surgical incision is closed to prevent fluid from collecting between the surfaces of the wound, which would separates wound surfaces and prevent them from growing together to heal the wound. Drains are commonly left in place for 3 to 7 days, depending on the type of incision and the surgeon's preference. Common drains include the Penrose, Hemovac, and Jackson-Pratt. A Penrose drain is a small, pliable, flat latex tube placed in the wound to promote drainage (Figure 26-15, *A*, p. 636). Although sometimes sutured in, this drain may simply be placed in the wound. Use caution when changing a dressing with a Penrose drain in place to avoid dislodging it. Hemovac and Jackson-Pratt drains are closed drainage systems that perform self-suction and collection of drainage. Both are opened to air, compressed, and held compressed while closed, thus creating a vacuum. A Jackson-Pratt drain (Figure 26-15, *B*) has a bulb, and a Hemovac drain (Figure 26-15, *C*) has a cartridge, either of which creates its own suction. As the bulb or cartridge fills with drainage, less suction is placed on the wound.

PROCEDURE 26-2 | REMOVING A DRESSING

TIME TO ALLOW
Novice: 10 min.
Expert: 5 min.

Removal of a dressing allows direct observation of the client's wound and replacement of the contaminated dressing with a clean (or sterile) dressing. The physician will order the frequency of dressing changes.

DELEGATION GUIDELINES
A nursing assistant may be helpful in assisting you in the general performance of wound care. The assembly of necessary equipment and removal of a dressing may be delegated to a nursing assistant who has received specific training in this procedure. You are then responsible for directly assessing and dressing the wound.

EQUIPMENT NEEDED
- Clean gloves
- Red trash bag

1. Follow preliminary guidelines for nursing procedures (see inside front cover).

2. Perform hand hygiene and apply gloves. *Performing hand hygiene and applying gloves decreases the risk of spreading infection.*

3. Gently begin to remove old dressing by pulling the tape toward the dressing and parallel to the skin. Simultaneously apply pressure to the client's skin at the edge of the tape to prevent the skin from being pulled with the tape. *Applying pressure to the client's skin while pulling off the dressing can reduce both the chance of causing further skin breakdown and increasing the client's pain. If the tape has been in place for several days, use of an acetone-free adhesive remover may help you remove the tape. Do not use acetone if the skin is irritated or broken.*

4. Observe the removed dressing for drainage, especially noting the amount, color, and odor (if any) of the drainage. *Thorough assessment of the dressing can assist with evaluation of the client's treatment plan.*

5. Dispose of the dressing according to agency policy and government regulations. If the dressing is heavily soiled with body fluids or bloody drainage, dispose of it in a red (biohazard) trash bag.

6. Document the odor, color, amount, and consistency of the drainage. Describe the appearance of the wound.

GERIATRIC CONSIDERATIONS
Be careful when removing tape from the skin of an older adult; the skin is more friable and more easily damaged. If the older adult has an abdominal dressing, put the head of the bed as flat as tolerated for easier dressing removal. Be aware, however, that older adults may have respiratory disorders that do not allow them to breathe easily with the head of the bed flat.

HOME CARE CONSIDERATIONS
For a nondraining surgical wound, before sutures or staples are removed, the client may wish to use a light dressing to protect the wound under clothes. Clothes should fit loosely and comfortably over the wound without binding. A dressing is not essential, however.

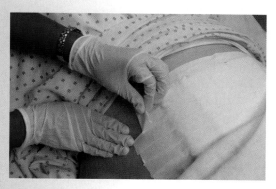

Step 3. Pulling the tape toward the dressing and parallel to the skin.

PROCEDURE 26-3   DRESSING A SIMPLE WOUND

TIME TO ALLOW
Novice: 10 min.
Expert: 5 min.

Wounds are covered with dressings to protect them from contamination and injury, to provide compression, to absorb drainage, to débride necrotic tissue, and to apply medication. A simple nondraining wound is covered for protection and in most cases the dressing is optional.

DELEGATION GUIDELINES

Institutional policies regarding delegation of this procedure vary widely. In many institutions, the performance of simple, clean dressing changes may be delegated to nursing assistants who have received specialized training in this skill. However, application of new postoperative dressings should not be delegated, nor should dressing changes to open wounds that are known to contain fistulas, that contain draining sinus tracts, or that require packing. The ongoing assessment of the wound and the effectiveness of the dressing technique lie with you; you may therefore determine not to delegate this procedure. A nursing assistant may assemble the necessary equipment and assist in positioning the client for the dressing change.

EQUIPMENT NEEDED

- Clean gloves
- Type of dressing ordered by the physician
- Tape, bandages, or binders needed to secure the dressing in place

1. Follow preliminary guidelines for nursing procedures (see inside front cover).

2. Answer any questions client may have. *Allowing the client to ask questions sets the stage for the client to provide self-care at home. If the client or a caregiver will be changing dressings at home, practicing in the hospital will be helpful.*

3. Confirm the dressing change order. *Dressing changes are commonly ordered by a physician, so you will need to verify the specific order.*

4. Assemble the supplies needed for the dressing change.

5. Perform hand hygiene and apply gloves. *Dressing changes should be done in sterile fashion.*

6. Remove the dressing from its package and apply it to the center of the wound (see illustration). The dressing change is sterile as long as the surface of the dressing placed next to the client is sterile. The wound and 1 inch beyond should be covered with the dressing. *A sterile field may be used to hold all dressings, or individual packages may be opened and left in their original packaging.*

7. Secure the edges of the dressing to the client's skin with tape. *Use the least amount of tape necessary to hold the dressing in place.*

8. If the dressing will be changed frequently or the client has sensitive or impaired skin, consider using Montgomery straps rather than tape. *Montgomery straps will allow you to change the dressing repeatedly without having to pull tape from the client's skin each time.*

HOME CARE CONSIDERATIONS

If the client or family will need to change a dressing at home, ensure that they have the necessary clean or sterile supplies. An array of sterile dressing supplies can generally be purchased at a pharmacy. If special dressings are needed, determine whether the hospital can supply the needed items on discharge.

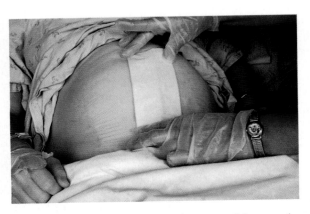

Step 6. Applying the dressing to the center of the wound.

PROCEDURE 26-4   CULTURING A WOUND

TIME TO ALLOW
Novice: 15 min.
Expert: 5 min.

Wounds are cultured to determine the type of bacteria that may be present in them. Swab cultures are used to detect surface colonization.

DELEGATION GUIDELINES

The sterile nature of this procedure generally precludes the delegation of wound culturing. However, nursing assistants in specialized burn and wound care units, having received specialty training, may perform wound cultures under your direct supervision.

EQUIPMENT NEEDED

- 18- or 19-gauge needle or angiocatheter
- 35-mL syringe
- Normal saline solution
- Sterile swab
- Sterile culture tube
- Gloves

1. Follow preliminary guidelines for nursing procedures (see inside front cover).

2. Rinse or irrigate wound thoroughly with sterile normal saline before obtaining a culture. *Cleansing the wound before culturing it will remove any surface bacteria.*

3. Swab the entire wound bed using a zigzag technique starting at the top of the wound and proceeding to the bottom of the wound (see illustration). *Using this technique will cover the entire wound bed.*

4. Place the swab in the culture tube and send it to the laboratory. *Prompt delivery of the swab specimen will facilitate prompt culturing of the swab.* **Note:** Swab cultures generally should not be used because they detect only surface bacteria, and a diagnosis should not be based solely on a swab culture. The Centers for Disease Control and Prevention recommends that you obtain fluid through needle aspiration or tissue ulcer biopsy.

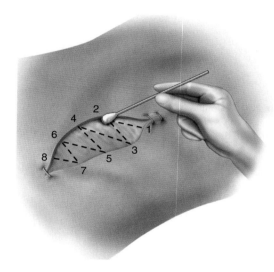

Step 3. Swabbing the wound bed in a zigzag pattern.

Your responsibilities in caring for a drain include the following:

- Maintaining its patency
- Emptying fluid from the drain, usually once a shift when intake and output are measured
- Maintaining accurate measurements of wound drainage and documenting accurately
- Maintaining the dressing around the drain
- Checking the wound for signs that drainage is incomplete
- Describing the drainage
- Securing the drain to prevent tension on the wound

Débriding the Wound. Débridement is the removal of dirt, foreign matter, and dead or devitalized tissue from a wound. Moist, devitalized tissue supports the growth of organisms. Thus removing this tissue promotes wound healing.

Débridement methods include sharp, mechanical, enzymatic, and autolytic. Always use the method most appropriate to the client's condition and care goals.

SHARP DÉBRIDEMENT. Sharp débridement is the removal of necrotic tissue using a scalpel, scissors, or laser. This method is rapid and efficient but should be performed only by persons skilled at and specially trained to perform this technique. Check your state's nurse practice act for details.

MECHANICAL DÉBRIDEMENT. Mechanical débridement removes dead tissue by applying a mechanical force, such as scrubbing, whirlpool therapy, or a wet-to-moist dressing. The latter is a gauze dressing that is applied wet and removed after it has partially dried (Procedure 26-5, p. 637). As the dressing dries in the wound, the gauze adheres to the wound bed. Removing the dressing

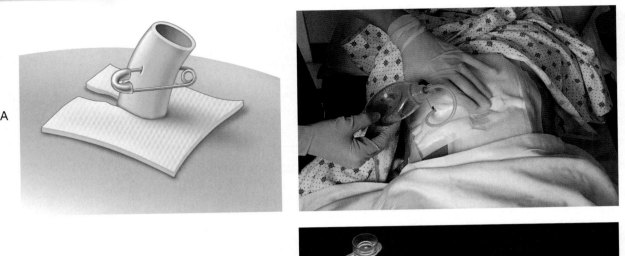

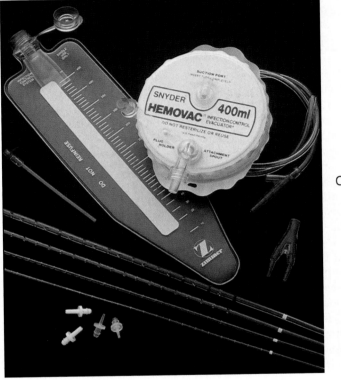

Figure 26-15. Common drainage systems. **A,** Penrose drain. **B,** Jackson-Pratt drain (shown in use on a client). **C,** Hemovac drain. (*C,* courtesy Zimmer, Inc., Warsaw, IN.)

tissue. Be aware that mechanical débridement is nonselective and can lead to removal of healthy as well as dead tissue.

ENZYMATIC DÉBRIDEMENT. Enzymatic débridement is a form of chemical débridement in which enzymes are used to break down necrotic tissue without targeting viable tissue. This method must be monitored closely because it can cause erythema around the wound perimeter.

AUTOLYTIC DÉBRIDEMENT. Autolytic débridement uses the body's ability to digest devitalized tissue. It is most often performed by applying a moisture-retentive dressing (such as a hydrocolloid dressing) to the wound bed (Procedure 26-6, p. 638). The dressing creates an occlusive seal, and then macrophages and neutrophils eliminate the necrotic tissue. Using an occlusive dressing does not promote infection. In fact, such a dressing has many benefits, including less pain at rest, during ambulation, and during dressing changes.

Action Alert! Do not use hydrocolloid dressings for immunocompromised clients.

Figure 26-16 summarizes the treatment of pressure ulcers.

Removing Sutures and Staples. Sutures and staples are typically removed 7 to 10 days after surgery by the physician's order. The physician may order only a certain number of sutures or staples to be removed. For example, removing every other suture may allow continued wound healing. Check agency policy to determine which personnel are permitted to remove sutures.

PROCEDURE 26-5 | APPLYING A WET-TO-MOIST DRESSING

TIME TO ALLOW
Novice: 15 min.
Expert: 5 min.

The purpose of a wet-to-moist dressing is to mechanically débride a wound. This type of gauze dressing is applied wet and removed moist. As the dressing changes from wet to moist in the wound, the gauze adheres to the wound bed. Thus removal of the dressing removes necrotic tissue as well. The dressing should not be allowed to become dry, because this type of débridement is nonselective and can result in the removal of healthy tissue as well as dead tissue.

DELEGATION GUIDELINES

The nature of a wound requiring a wet-to-dry or wet-to-moist dressing change is such that you would not want to delegate it to a nursing assistant. The assessment, sterile procedure, and intervention of mechanical débridement require your expertise. Within a burn or wound care unit, some unlicensed personnel receive specialized training to perform such dressing changes; these are generally the exception. Assembly of the necessary equipment and supplies, along with positioning the client for the dressing change, may be delegated to a nursing assistant.

EQUIPMENT NEEDED

- Sterile gauze dressing or type ordered by physician
- Sterile dressing to cover wet dressing as ordered by physician
- Tape or Montgomery straps
- Sterile normal saline or other solution as ordered by physician
- Sterile gloves
- Sterile cotton swabs

1. Follow preliminary guidelines for nursing procedures (see inside front cover).

2. Confirm the physician's dressing order and assemble the needed supplies.

3. Use sterile normal saline solution (or another ordered solution) to dampen the dressing that will be placed into the wound. *Wetting the dressing will promote a moist healing environment.*

4. Don sterile gloves and twist the wet dressing so it remains wet but is not dripping. Open the dressing fully and fluff it open. *The dressing should be damp to moderately wet.*

5. Gently place the dressing into the wound (see illustration). Do not pack the wound tightly. *Packing the dressing tightly will block air from entering the wound and will keep the dressing from partially drying.*

6. Cover the damp dressing with a dry sterile dressing and secure it with tape. If the client is allergic to tape, has sensitive skin, or needs repeated dressing changes, consider using Montgomery straps to affix the top dressing.

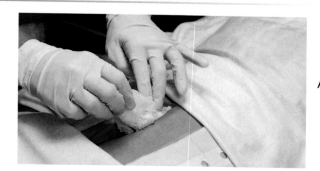
A

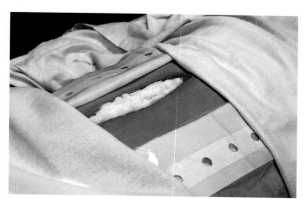
B

Step 5. A, Packing the wound. **B,** Packed wound with the wound edges free.

PROCEDURE 26-6   Applying a Hydrocolloid Dressing

TIME TO ALLOW
Novice: 15 min.
Expert: 5 min.

Hydrocolloid dressing is a type of autolytic débridement. This type of dressing causes an occlusive seal, then uses the body's own macrophages and neutrophils to eliminate necrotic tissue. Instead of drying out a wound, this treatment aims at maintaining the moisture in a wound bed.

DELEGATION GUIDELINES

The application of a hydrocolloid dressing requires your assessment and expertise and should not be delegated to a nursing assistant. However, assembly of the necessary equipment and supplies may be delegated to a nursing assistant. You may also need the help of a nursing assistant in positioning a client for dressing application.

EQUIPMENT NEEDED

- Sterile gauze dressing or other dressing according to physician's order
- Sterile normal saline or other solution as ordered by physician
- Sterile gloves
- Sterile cotton swabs
- Hydrocolloid dressing; size will depend on the size of the wound
- Hypoallergenic tape

1. Follow preliminary guidelines for nursing procedures (see inside front cover).

2. Confirm physician order.

3. Clean the wound by irrigating it or lightly swabbing it with a gauze dressing soaked in sterile normal saline solution. *The wound bed must be cleansed and debris removed before applying the hydrocolloid dressing.*

4. Select a hydrocolloid dressing of an appropriate size. It should extend past the wound margins by at least 1 inch. *If the dressing is too small, it will not adhere to the wound bed and, consequently, will not function properly.*

5. Apply the dressing from one side of the wound to the other side. Use hand pressure to hold the dressing in place for a minimum of 1 minute (see illustration). *Applying pressure and warmth with your hands will make the dressing adhere better to the wound.*

6. Depending on the location of the wound and the hydrocolloid dressing used, you may need to place hypoallergenic tape around the edges of the dressing to secure it. *Applying tape will help prevent the edges of the dressing from rolling back.*

7. Leave the dressing in place for 5 to 7 days. Remove the dressing if it is leaking or peeling off and apply another one. *Leaving the dressing in place will allow moist wound healing to occur.*

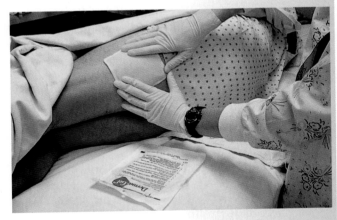

Step 5. Applying a hydrocolloid dressing. Apply pressure with your hands over the dressing for at least 1 minute to ensure good adherence of the dressing.

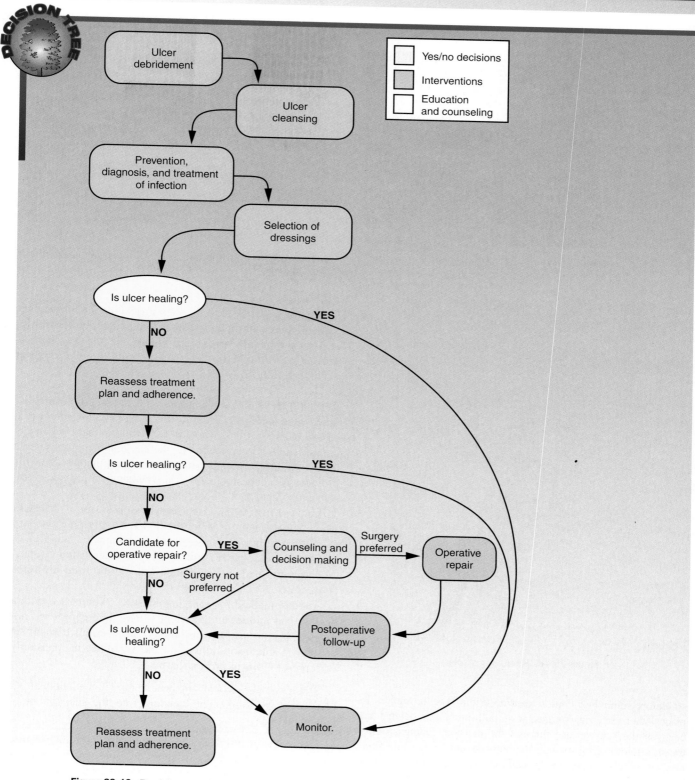

Figure 26-16. Decision tree for ulcer care. (Modified from Bergstrom, N., Bennett, M. A., Carlson, C. E., et al. [1994]. *Treatment of pressure ulcers: Practice guideline No. 15.* [Publication No. 95-0652]. Rockville, MD: U.S. Public Health Service, Agency for Health Care Policy and Research.)

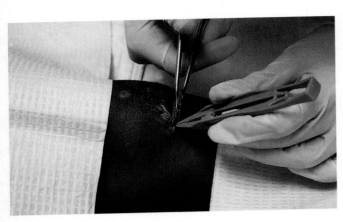

Figure 26-17. Removing sutures.

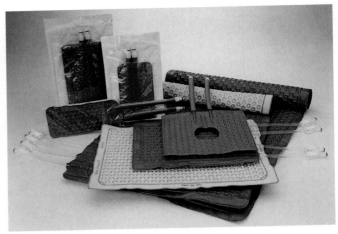

Figure 26-19. Aquathermia pads. (Courtesy Zimmer, Inc., Warsaw, IN.)

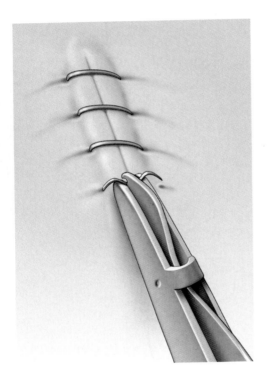

Figure 26-18. Removing staples.

Before removing sutures, determine the type of sutures in place. When removing sutures, never pull suture material that has been on the skin surface through the incision. Doing so may transmit microorganisms into the incision and lead to infection. Use suture scissors designed specifically for suture removal. Cut the suture material as close to the skin as possible and pull the suture material through the other side of the incision (Figure 26-17).

To remove staples, obtain a staple remover and insert the two lower prongs of the staple remover beneath the staple and the middle upper prong on top of the staple. Then squeeze the staple remover closed. The staple should separate from the skin (Figure 26-18). Avoid pulling the skin with the staple as it is removed. Remove the staple with a smooth steady hand and quickly squeeze the staple remover to cause

less dragging of the skin. It is common practice to spray the wound edges with tincture of benzoin and apply Steri-Strips at 1-inch intervals across the wound. Teach the client to shower with Steri-Strips in place and discontinue their use when they fall off.

Applying Heat and Cold. Applying heat and cold can create therapeutic local and systemic effects. For example, cold constricts blood vessels, whereas heat dilates them. Cold decreases capillary permeability, whereas heat increases it. Cold decreases cellular metabolism, whereas heat increases it. Cold provides local anesthetic effects, whereas heat provides local sedative effects. Both therapies relax muscles.

HEAT THERAPIES. Heat can be applied in a variety of dry or moist methods. One method for applying either dry or moist heat is with a disposable Aquathermia pad (Kpad). A small electrical unit heats water-filled tubes. Aquathermia pads are moldable and can be used on limbs (Figure 26-19).

Another method for applying constant, even heat is with a heating pad molded to the client's body. Use care when applying a heating pad because it can cause serious burns if set too high. Some institutions allow the use of heating pads only with preset limits to prevent burns.

Action Alert! Avoid using heat therapy immediately after surgery to prevent bleeding into the incision or wound bed.

COLD THERAPIES. Cold decreases pain and inflammation and can reduce bleeding. To apply cold therapy, use a compress, an ice pack, or an ice bag. Compresses are moist, cool dressings. Cold packs come in a variety of shapes and are activated by striking or twisting the pack (Figure 26-20). To prepare an ice bag, place crushed ice into a small or large plastic bag depending on the size of the area to be covered. For a small area, such as a finger, consider filling a glove with ice. For a larger area, such as a fractured ankle, fill a plastic bag. Always cover an ice bag before placing it on a client's skin to avoid a cold injury.

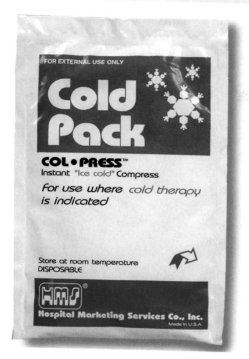

Figure 26-20. Cold pack. (Courtesy Hospital Marketing Services, Naugatuck, CT.)

Action Alert! Do not use heat or cold therapies for a client with neurological impairment, impaired mental status, or impaired circulation.

Bandaging the Wound. Bandages and binders secure dressings in difficult-to-secure areas (such as the elbow) or provide support to a wound. They may also be used for other purposes, such as the following:
- Apply pressure (e.g., after central line removal or postoperative incision)
- Immobilize a body part (e.g., an elastic bandage wrapped around a sprained wrist)
- Maintain splint placement (e.g., in an elastic bandage placed over an ankle splint)

Before applying a bandage or binder, be sure to use the following assessment strategies:
- Inspect the area for swelling, wounds, and wound drainage.
- Assess the client for pain and provide prescribed medication as appropriate.
- Assess the client's ability to apply the bandage.
- Assess the client's ability to perform activities of daily living with the bandage in place.
- Assess circulatory function in the bandaged area.

Several types and sizes of bandages are available. Woven or gauze dressings, the most common type, are considered the gold standard in dressing supplies. These inexpensive bandages provide support to other bandages, allow air circulation to the skin, and can be used on many different body parts, including extremities. Gauze also wicks away moisture and exudate from the skin, preventing maceration, and can assist in débridement. This type of dressing is used in wound packing.

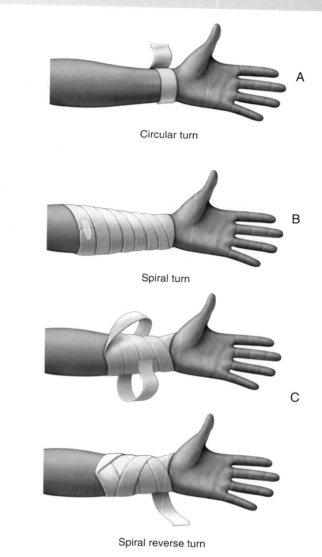

Circular turn

Spiral turn

Spiral reverse turn

Figure 26-21. Methods of bandage application. **A,** Circular turn. **B,** Spiral turn. **C,** Spiral reverse turns.

Continued

Nonwoven dressings are made of synthetic fibers (most often rayon or polyester). These dressings are soft and most often are used for skin preparation and cleansing. They are not ideal for absorbing drainage. Elasticized bandages are used to provide support or pressure to a specific area.

Choose a dressing type and size on the basis of the area to be bandaged. Generally, a narrow bandage is suitable for smaller areas (such as hand or wrist), whereas a larger bandage is more suitable for a leg. Applying a bandage of the wrong width may cause constriction or excessive pressure on the skin.

Five basic methods or turns can be used to start a bandage, wrap it evenly, and secure the dressing (Figure 26-21). Circular turns are used to anchor the beginning and end of the bandage (Figure 26-21, *A*). Spiral turns are used to bandage extremities by ascending up the extremity (Figure 26-21, *B*). Each turn overlaps the previous turn by half or a third. Spiral reverse turns are used to bandage oblong body parts (such as the forearm, thigh, or calf) (Figure 26-21, *C*). Recurrent turns are used to

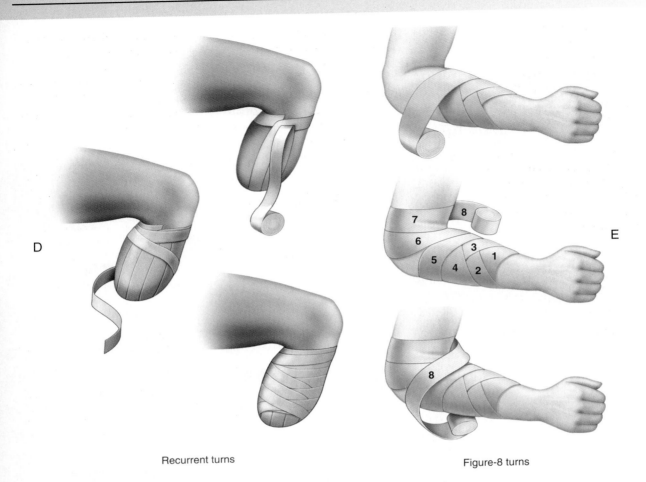

Recurrent turns

Figure-8 turns

D

E

Figure 26-21, cont'd. D, Recurrent turns. **E,** Figure-8 turns.

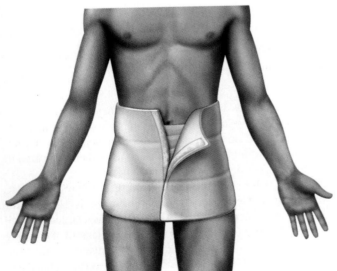

Figure 26-22. Abdominal binder.

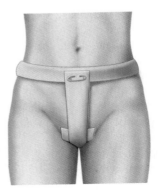

Female

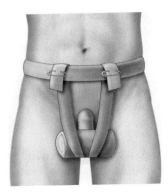

Male

Figure 26-23. Female and male T-binders.

skull, or finger). The bandage is first secured with two circular turns and then folded back on itself and brought to cover
the distal end. Again, each turn covers the affected body part
and overlaps the previous turn by half or a third (Figure
26-21, *D*). The figure-8 turn is most often used to bandage

joints because it allows mobility after application. Apply this
bandage over the joint in a figure-8 motion above and below
the joint (Figure 26-21, *E*).

Binders are used to provide support and protection to
larger areas, such as the abdomen or chest (Figure 26-22).

A Velcro attachment secures the binder around the client. Apply the binder snugly to provide support, but not so snugly that it creates excessive compression. T-binders are used to provide support for dressings in the perineal area. Use a single T-binder for a female client and a double T-binder for a male client (Figure 26-23).

EVALUATION

Evaluation of the plan of care is in an ongoing part of the nursing process (Box 26-5). Outcome measurement in wound management is essential to evaluating the plan of care and wound healing. To measure outcomes, consider questions such as the following:

- By what percentage has a client's wound decreased in size?
- By how much has a wound been reduced in depth?
- By how much has the client's pain been reduced?
- By what percentage has necrotic tissue covering the wound been reduced?
- To what extent has the client returned to normal activities?
- Was the client's wound kept free of infection?

Naturally, in the largest sense, the desired outcome is that the client has an intact integumentary system that serves its normal functions. If the client has *Impaired skin integrity*, the expected outcome is wound healing without infection and prevention of further areas of *Impaired skin integrity*.

Nursing Care Plan A CLIENT WITH A HIP FRACTURE

Box 26-5

ADMISSION DATA

Mrs. Jacan was admitted through the emergency department to an orthopedic unit, where she was prepared for surgery. Phone report from the postanesthesia recovery unit is as follows: "72-year-old woman who fell at home in bathroom 2 days earlier sustained a right femoral neck fracture. She lay on the bathroom floor for 2 days before being discovered by her daughter and had a reddened area to her sacrum and bilateral heels. Underwent pinning of right hip."

PHYSICIAN'S ORDERS

- Turn every 2 hours to unaffected side only
- Keep heels elevated off bed at all times
- Out of bed (OOB) BID with physical therapy starting tomorrow

NURSING ASSESSMENT

Quiet, cooperative older adult woman after hip surgery with stage II pressure ulcer formation on sacrum and bilateral heels. Right hip dressing intact, no drainage on dressing. Slow to progress in physical therapy as well as positioning in bed because of postoperative pain.

NANDA Nursing Diagnosis	NOC Expected Outcomes With Indicators	NIC Interventions With Selected Activities	Evaluation Data
IMPAIRED SKIN INTEGRITY	**PRIMARY HEALING**	**WOUND MANAGEMENT**	**AFTER 24 HOURS OF CARE**
Related factors: • Surgical incision on hip • Stage II pressure ulcer on hip and heels	**Incision:** • Right hip incision will heal by primary intention and be free from infection.	• Change hip dressing per physician order maintaining sterile technique. • Assess for drainage from right hip incision.	• Right hip dressing clean, dry, and intact. • Dressing changed qd by RN using sterile technique.
	Dressing: • Dressing to sacrum and heels will prevent further breakdown and will promote wound healing. **Skin:** • No further skin breakdown	• Apply hydrocolloid dressing to sacrum. • Turn and reposition q2h. • Apply air mattress to bed. • Explain importance of repositioning and need to be OOB.	• Hydrocolloid dressing intact. • No further skin breakdown noted.

CRITICAL THINKING QUESTIONS

1. Before falling at home, Mrs. Jacan was living independently. Her daughter is concerned about her mother's future ability to care for herself and asks you about nursing home placement for her mother. How would you respond?
2. Mrs. Jacan's daughter thinks that she can care for her mother at her home. With which members of the multidisciplinary team would you consult regarding the appropriateness of the plan? What information would you teach the client and her daughter?
3. Mrs. Jacan prefers to lie only on her back while in bed. What rationale would you give her daughter for the need to reposition and turn her mother onto her side?

Nursing outcome and intervention labels from Johnson, M., Bulechek, G., McCloskey Dochterman, J. M., Maas, M., & Moorhead, S. (2001). *Nursing diagnoses, outcomes and interventions: NANDA, NOC, and NIC linkages.* St Louis, MO: Mosby.

After 24 hours of care, documentation for Mrs. Jacan's nursing diagnosis of Impaired skin integrity may include the data shown below.

SAMPLE DOCUMENTATION NOTE FOR MRS. JACAN
Right hip dressing clean, dry, and intact. During dressing change, right hip incision noted to be clean with no areas of redness, swelling, or drainage; sutures intact. Hydrocolloid dressings on sacrum and heels are intact with no drainage. No further areas of skin breakdown noted. Client assists with turning and repositioning every 2 hours.

Key Principles

- The functions of the skin are protection, sensation, thermoregulation, and excretion.
- There are four stages of pressure ulcers.
- Wounds can be classified into different categories. Intentional wounds are those caused by surgical procedures or treatments (operations, intravenous therapy). Unintentional wounds are accidental in cause (abrasion or laceration from a fall).
- Although not all pressure wounds can be prevented, the nurse plays an important role in the care of the client in assessing for risk, providing care to a surgical wound, or participating in the treatment of a pressure ulcer.
- A multidisciplinary effort is required to maintain and facilitate intact skin of clients. Members of the multidisciplinary team include physicians, nurses, rehabilitation therapists, enterostomal therapists, social workers, and home care providers.
- The skin diagnoses are *Risk for impaired skin integrity, Impaired skin integrity*, and *Impaired tissue integrity*.
- The goals of wound healing include keeping the wound and wound bed clean, moist, and free from infection.
- Moisture was once thought to be harmful in the wound healing process. Through research, we now know that moisture facilitates wound healing.
- When the client has an impairment of skin integrity, the expected outcome is wound healing without infection and further prevention of *Impaired skin integrity*.

Bibliography

Beltram, K. A., Thacker, J. G., & Rodeheaver, G. T. *Impact pressures generated by commercial wound irrigation devices.* Unpublished research report, University of Virginia Health Science Center, Charlottesville, VA, University of Virginia Health Science Center.

*Bergstrom, N., Allman, R. M., & Carlson, C. E. (1992). *Pressure ulcers in adults: Prediction and prevention. Clinical practice guideline No. 3* (AHCPR Publication No. 92-0047). Rockville, MD: Agency for Health Care Policy and Research, U.S. Public Health Service.

*Bergstrom, N., Allman, R., Alvarez, O., Bennett, M. A., et al. (1994). *Treatment of pressure ulcers. Practice guideline No. 15* (Publication No. 95-0652). Rockville, MD: U.S. Public Health Service, Agency for Health Care Policy and Research.

*Bolton, L. L., van Rijswijk, L. A., & Shaffer, F. A. (1996). Quality wound care equals cost effective wound care. *Nursing

Bryant, R. A., (2000). Acute and chronic wounds: Nursing management (2nd ed.). St Louis, MO: Mosby.

*Collwell, J. C., Foreman, M. D., & Trotter, J. P. (1993). A comparison of the efficacy and cost effectiveness of 2 methods of managing pressure ulcers. *Decubitus, 6*(4), 28-35.

*Field, C. K., & Kerstein, M. D. (1994). Overview of wound healing in a moist environment. *American Journal of Surgery, 167*(Suppl. 1A), 2S-6S.

Fowler, E. (1998). Wound infection: A nurse's perspective. *Ostomy & Wound Management, 44*(8), 44-52.

Geissler, E. M. (1998). *Pocket guide to cultural assessment* (2nd ed.). St Louis, MO: Mosby.

*Guarlnik, J. M., Harris, T. B., White, L. R., & Cornoni-Huntley, J. C. (1988). Occurrence and predictors of pressure sores in the national health and nutrition exam survey follow-up. *Journal of the American Geriatric Society, 36*(9), 801-812.

*Hermans, M. H., & Bolton, L. L. (1996). The influence of dressings on the costs of wound treatment. *Dermatology Nursing, 8*(2), 93-100.

Hess, C. T. (1998). *Wound care: Nurses' clinical guide* (2nd ed.). Springhouse, PA: Springhouse.

Ignatavicius, D., & Workman, M. L. (2002). *Medical-surgical nursing: Critical thinking for collaborative care* (4th ed.). Philadelphia: Saunders.

*International Committee on Wound Management. (1995). An overview of economic model of cost effective wound care. *Advances in Wound Care, 8*(5), 46.

Johnson, M., Bulechek, G., McCloskey Dochterman, J. M., Maas, M., & Moorhead, S. (2001). *Nursing diagnoses, outcomes, and interventions: NANDA, NOC, and NIC linkages.* St Louis, MO: Mosby.

Kalailieff, D. (1998). Vacuum-assisted closure: Wound care technology for the new millennium. *Perspectives, 22*(3), 28-29.

*Lazarus, G. S., Cooper D. M., & Knighton, D. R. (1994). Definitions and guidelines for assessment of wounds and evaluation of healing. *Archives of Dermatology 130*(4), 489-493.

Leininger, M. M. (2001). *Cultural care diversity and universality: A theory of nursing.* Boston, MA: Jones and Bartlett Publishing.

*Lineaweaver, W., Howard, R., Saucy, D., McMorris, S., Freeman, J., Crain, C., et al. (1985). Topical antimicrobial toxicity. *Archives Surgery, 120*(3), 267-270.

National Pressure Ulcer Advisory Panel. (1998). *Proceedings of the Fifth National NPUAP Conference.* February, 1997. The NPUAP Task Force on Darkly Pigmented Skin and Stage I Pressure Ulcers.

*Miller, H., & Delozier, J. (1994). *Cost implications of the pressure ulcer treatment guidelines* (Contr 282-9-0070, 17). Sponsored by the Agency for Health Care Policy and Research, Center for Health Policy Studies.

Margolis, D. J. (1995). Definition of a pressure ulcer. NPUAP Proceedings. *Advances in Wound Care, 7*(4), 28.

North American Nursing Diagnosis Association. (2001). *Nursing diagnoses: Definitions and classification 1999-2000.* Philadelphia: Author.

Ovington, L. G. (1999). Dressings and adjunctive therapies: AHCPR guidelines revisited, *Ostomy & Wound Management, 45*(Suppl. 1A), 94S-106S.

*Ponder, R. B., & Krasner, D. (1993). Gauzes and related dressings. *Ostomy & Wound Management, 39*(5), 48-60.

Thompson, J. (2000). A practical guide to wound care. *RN, 63*(1), 48-52.

---

*Asterisk indicates a classic or definitive work on this subject.

Managing Body Temperature

Learning Objectives

After studying this chapter, you should be able to do the following:

- Describe fever, hyperthermia, and hypothermia
- Identify characteristics of clients with fever, hyperthermia, or hypothermia
- Describe the assessment of the client with fever, hyperthermia, or hypothermia
- Write a nursing diagnosis for the person with fever, hyperthermia, or hypothermia
- Plan for nursing interventions for clients experiencing fever, hyperthermia, or hypothermia
- Evaluate the effectiveness of interventions for clients with fever, hyperthermia, or hypothermia

Andrew Stephen is a 64-year-old African-American man transferred to the cardiac telemetry unit 36 hours after having coronary artery bypass surgery. His vital signs after transfer include a heart rate of 120 beats per minute, a temperature of 38.9° C (102° F), a blood pressure of 140/82, and a respiratory rate of 16. Mr. Stephen is complaining of feeling cold and has asked for additional blankets. The nurse's physical examination indicates decreased breath sounds on the left posterior side of his chest. The most likely cause of Mr. Stephen's fever is atelectasis. Less likely causes are wound infection, respiratory infection, or urinary tract infection.

Treatment of fever in Mr. Stephen may include administration of an antipyretic to decrease core body temperature. Considerations when treating fever in Mr. Stephen include the facts that an elevated body temperature contributes to host defense and that an elevated body temperature increases metabolic demands. The report regarding Mr. Stephen's cardiac function is important to consider in treating him. If he has diminished cardiac function, his fever should be treated to decrease the demands on his heart. The nurse considers the diagnosis of *Fever* from the list of possible nursing diagnoses related to thermoregulation (see below).

KEY NURSING DIAGNOSES FOR Thermoregulation

Hyperthermia: Body temperature elevated to above normal range
*Fever: A regulated rise in body temperature (hyperthermia) that is mediated by a rise in temperature set-point

Hypothermia: Body temperature reduced to below normal range

*Diagnoses with an asterisk are not NANDA approved.

Fever presents significant problems to the nurse in managing the responses of the client and in providing education to the public about evaluating and making decisions about the meaning of a fever. Fever, resulting from infection or inflammation, is the most common change in body temperature requiring nursing care.

Fever is a host defense response that frequently occurs in hospitalized people either from the primary diagnosis or from complications. Therefore you are likely to encounter this phenomenon while caring for clients in an acute care setting. In outpatient and home settings, you will be responsible for providing information to clients and families to help them evaluate and manage a fever.

Fever can be caused by a wide variety of processes, including infection, inflammation, autoimmune diseases, vascular diseases, neoplasia, and drug reactions. The most frequent causes of fever are infection and inflammation. Nurses who understand fever and its management can (1) assist parents who have fever phobia to make good decisions about seeking health care, (2) prevent complications in the hospitalized client through early detection, and (3) impact health care costs (Box 27-1).

CONCEPTS OF THERMOREGULATION

Understanding fever is enhanced by a brief introduction to problems in thermoregulation. It helps to understand that body temperature is the balance between heat production and heat loss (Figure 27-1).

Physiology of Thermoregulation

The thermoregulatory system consists of a control center, a sensory component, and effector mechanisms. The temperature of the body is regulated almost entirely by nervous feedback mechanisms in the hypothalamus. Temperature sensa-

THE·COST·OF·CARE — Box 27-1
Managing a Fever

The role of the nurse in the management of a client with fever has the potential to reduce the cost of care. The areas where this potential exists include the following:

- *Encouraging routine preventive care.* Routine use of intranasal influenza vaccine among healthy children may be cost effective and may be maximized by using group-based vaccination approaches (Luce et al., 2001).
- *Using correct technique for technical procedures.* During a 4-year period, 9465 specimens for blood culture were obtained from 11,911 highly febrile, otherwise healthy young children. Of these specimens, 87 (0.9%) yielded nonpathogens and were considered to be false-positive blood culture results (Waltzman & Harper, 2001).
- *Educating parents to help them evaluate their child's health condition.* Visits for otitis media, sinusitis, and particularly allergic rhinitis appear to be overrepresented in children with asthma and contribute to the high utilization rate. Once a high-risk cohort is identified, the needs of those children can be addressed through targeted, organized systems of care that may include guidelines or other disease management strategies (Grupp-Phelan, Lozano, & Fishman, 2001).

Data from Grupp-Phelan, J., Lozano, P., & Fishman, P. (2001). Health care utilization and cost in children with asthma and selected comorbidities. *Journal of Asthma, 38*(4), 363-373; Luce, B. R., Zangwill, K. M., Palmer, C.S., et al. (2001). Cost-effectiveness analysis of an intranasal influenza vaccine for the prevention of influenza in healthy children. *Pediatrics 108*(2), E24; Waltzman, M. L., & Harper, M. (2001). Financial and clinical impact of false-positive blood culture results. *Clinics in Infectious Diseases, 33*(3), 296-299.

tion occurs in the skin, with the face and hands having the greatest concentration of thermoreceptors for hot and cold sensation. Deeper structures, especially the spinal cord and abdominal viscera, are also thought to have the ability to sense temperature. A combination of sensory neuron activity from the periphery and the central nervous system provide

Heat production and conservation

Heat production
- Basal metabolism
- Muscle contraction
- Increased metabolic rate

Heat conservation
- Shivering
- Vasoconstriction

Heat loss

- Evaporation (sweating)
- Conduction (contact with cold surfaces)
- Radiation (vasodilation of blood vessels in the skin)
- Convection (contact with air currents)

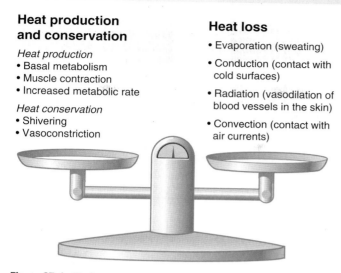

Figure 27-1. Body temperature is the balance between the production of heat and the loss of heat.

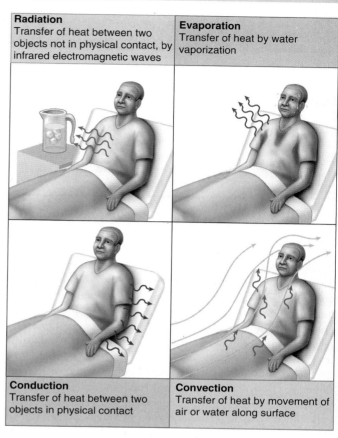

Figure 27-2. Mechanisms of heat loss.

sensory input. The temperature control centers interpret the sensory signals and activate effector mechanisms that raise or lower the body's temperature.

These effector mechanisms are activated when body temperature is above the person's **set-point**—the temperature that thermoregulatory mechanisms attempt to maintain. The resultant actions, such as sweating, dilation of the blood vessels in the skin, and decrease in heat production, promote heat loss into the surrounding environment by the mechanisms of evaporation, conduction, radiation, and convection (Figure 27-2). Effector mechanisms activated when body temperature is below the set-point include shivering (piloerection), constriction of the blood vessels in the skin, and increase in heat production. Shivering generates heat by causing muscle contraction, and it increases heat production up to four to five times normal (Guyton and Hall, 2000). Vasoconstriction of the skin decreases the amount of heat that would have been lost by radiation, convection, and conduction.

Definitions of Thermoregulatory States

Regulated Rise in Temperature. **Fever** is a regulated rise in body temperature that is mediated by a rise in the temperature set-point. Mediators released in response to a pathophysiological process, such as infection or inflammation, facilitate the rise in the temperature set-point in the central nervous system. Physiological effector mechanisms are activated by the central nervous system in an attempt to attain this new elevated temperature set-point.

Nonregulated Changes in Temperature. Although the term *hyperthermia* means elevated temperature, it is generally used to refer to extremes of temperature elevation. Thus, specifically, **hyperthermia** is a nonregulated elevation in body temperature related to an imbalance between heat gain and heat loss. In contrast to during fever, the temperature set-point during hyperthermia is not elevated. Instead, the problem is an imbalance between heat loss and heat gain. The

problem may be neurological damage that prevents the control of body temperature.

The most common example of hyperthermia is **heat stroke,** which is an extreme elevation of body temperature, usually above 40.6° C (105° F), resulting in altered central nervous system function and shock. Heat stroke results from failure of the temperature-regulating capacity of the body, caused by prolonged exposure to sun or high temperature. Heat loss cannot keep up with heat gain; therefore the body temperature increases.

Hypothermia is a state in which body temperature is reduced to below normal. It too is a problem of imbalance between heat gain and heat loss. In this case, heat production cannot keep up with heat loss; therefore body temperature decreases. For example, hypothermia occurs when a person falls through the ice of a lake and loses heat rapidly in the cold water.

Fever

Differentiating between fever and hyperthermia is important in terms of diagnosing and treating a rise in body temperature (Table 27-1, p. 648). Fever is often associated with infection and requires additional diagnostic evaluation based on localizing signs and symptoms. Antipyretic medications reduce the fever by decreasing the elevation in temperature set-point. Other therapies promote heat loss rather than decreasing the set-point.

Table 27-1	Comparison of Fever and Hyperthermia	
Characteristic	Fever	Hyperthermia
Etiology	Infection or inflammation	Elevated environmental temperature, physical activity, impaired heat loss
Temperature range	Usually less than 40.6° C (105° F)	In severe cases, such as heat stroke, 40.6° C (105° F)
Mechanism	Host defense response	Loss of ability to thermoregulate
Manifestations	Increased heart rate, chills, sleepiness, anorexia	Decreased level of consciousness, increased heart rate, decreased blood pressure, tissue injury
Nursing interventions	Monitor temperature frequently, provide fluids, prevent shivering, change linen to keep client dry, administer antipyretics as ordered, obtain blood cultures as ordered	Remove from warm environment and actively cool the client in more severe cases, monitor temperature and other vital signs frequently, prepare for insertion of IV line to provide fluids, monitor urine output

Pyrogens. A **pyrogen** is any agent that causes or stimulates a fever. The initial stimulus for fever is often an exogenous pyrogen. The word *exogenous* indicates an outside stimulus that is introduced into the body. Exogenous pyrogens include bacteria, viruses, fungi, allergens, incompatible blood products, and foreign substances. Exogenous pyrogens stimulate the production of *endogenous* pyrogens, internal stimuli that act directly on the hypothalamus. Some of the endogenous pyrogens that are produced in response to exogenous pyrogens include hormonelike chemical messengers called cytokines. Endogenous pyrogens are produced by monocytes, macrophages, neutrophils, and eosinophils. Endogenous pyrogens may result from inflammatory reactions, such as those that occur in tissue damage, cell necrosis, rejection of transplanted tissues, malignancy, and antigen–antibody reactions.

Phases of a Fever. There are three phases of fever: initiation, plateau, and defervescence (Figure 27-3). Thermoregulation during these phases involves activation of the effector mechanisms discussed earlier, as well as initiation of behavioral and experiential responses.

During the initiation phase of fever, pyrogens act on the hypothalamus to reset the temperature set-point to higher than body temperature. Activation of effector mechanisms, such as shivering and decreased blood flow to the skin, increases body temperature to attempt to reach the set-point. Additionally, the feverish client exhibits behaviors to decrease heat loss, such as putting skin surfaces together in a fetal position and increasing insulation by adding blankets or clothing. The client will feel cold and may have chills.

During the plateau phase of fever, the body temperature has risen and is maintained at this new elevated set-point. The client may feel quite warm because of this elevation in core body temperature.

During the defervescent phase of fever, the body's effector mechanisms are activated to promote heat loss because of the lowering of the temperature set-point. The client will feel warm and may sweat and appear flushed. Behaviors include shedding of clothing and blankets and requests for ice and fluids. Fever may resolve by a rapid return to normal over a period of a few hours (resolution by crisis) or resolve slowly (resolution by lysis).

Fever Patterns. The pattern of the rise and fall of body temperature is occasionally useful for the diagnosis of a particular causative organism. *Continuous* or *sustained fever* is sometimes seen with drug-induced fever. *Remittent fever* is defined as an elevation and fall in temperature each day, with the baseline temperature remaining above normal for the entire day. Malaria is one example of a disorder that causes remittent fever. *Intermittent fever* is defined as an elevation and fall in temperature to baseline each day. Some forms of infection may present with intermittent fever, although this finding is not necessarily helpful in determining the causative organism. With many infections, fever is most likely to be elevated in the late afternoon.

Physiological Responses. Associated physiological responses that occur during fever include increased cardiovascular demands and altered metabolism and immune system function. Cardiovascular responses related to fever include increased heart rate and increased cardiac output. Metabolic rate during fever increases 10% per 1.0° C (1.8° F) of elevation in body temperature; if the client shivers, the rise in metabolic rate is approximately 100% to 200% above baseline. Other changes in metabolism include the production of acute-phase proteins that assist with host defense. Effects of fever on immune system function have not been determined fully. The signs of increased metabolic need do not accompany drug reaction fevers.

Recall Mr. Stephen, the client in the case study. His fever is in the initiation phase. What behaviors would Mr. Stephen display next?

Action Alert! Observe for fever that occurs without associated changes or an increase in heart rate—the cause may be a drug reaction.

Additional behavioral responses that occur as part of fever include malaise, anorexia, drowsiness, and altered

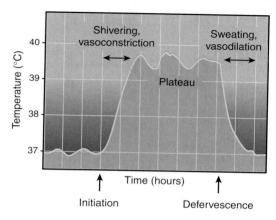

Figure 27-3. The three phases of fever: initiation, plateau, and defervescence.

sleep patterns. **Malaise,** a feeling of indisposition, is thought to be an adaptive response that decreases most daily activities, thereby maintaining energy stores for fever generation.

 Because Mr. Stephen has had cardiac surgery, his caregivers should be concerned about the effect of fever on the workload of his heart. What changes in vital signs might be attributed to his fever?

Hyperthermia

A person who develops hyperthermia does so either by generating too much heat, as during sports activities in hot weather, or by failing to lose heat while in a warm environment (more common in older adults and children).

Sweating is an effective mechanism of heat loss, unless the environment is humid. Increased water saturation in the air prevents evaporation of sweat from the skin, thus decreasing heat loss. Therefore hyperthermia is more likely to occur in humid environments. The amount of fluid loss attributed to sweating varies with the environmental humidity but can be more than a liter per hour with intense exercise. Fluid balance always needs to be monitored in clients at risk for hyperthermia. Maintenance of fluid balance is necessary to maintain perfusion of body systems and perfusion of the skin. Inadequate hydration will reduce blood flow to the skin, thus reducing heat loss.

Increased blood flow to the skin in response to temperature elevation may be impaired in older adults and in some clients with autonomic nervous system dysfunction, such as those with diabetes (Vinik et al., 2001). The autonomic nervous system controls vasoconstriction and vasodilation in the skin. Problems with nervous system control of blood flow to the skin predispose clients to hyperthermia.

Another population at risk for hyperthermia consists of clients with central nervous system injury, such as head injury, cerebrovascular accident (stroke), or subarachnoid hem-

orrhage. Hyperthermia in this group is thought to result from interference with thermoregulation in the hypothalamus.

Heat exhaustion is a rise in body temperature that is usually related to inadequate fluid and electrolyte replacement during physical activity in intense heat, or the inability to acclimatize to intense heat. Physiological responses associated with heat exhaustion from physical exertion include an increase in cardiac output, release of antidiuretic hormone, increased production of aldosterone, and increased release of norepinephrine. Serum sodium levels usually become concentrated because perspiration represents a relatively greater loss of water than sodium.

In heat stroke, in which the body temperature exceeds 40.6° C (105° F), the client develops alterations in central nervous system function, such as confusion, convulsions, or a coma. Physiological responses associated with heat stroke include dry skin, hypotension, tachycardia, vomiting, and diarrhea.

Hypothermia

Accidental hypothermia occurs because of decreased heat production, increased heat loss, or impaired thermoregulation. Hypothermia is often associated with clinical conditions or factors that predispose clients to a decrease in core body temperature.

Circumstances related to hypothermia (temperature 32.2° C [91.9° F] or lower) include drowning, serious illness, systemic infection, trauma, frostbite, and overdose (including drug addicts found sleeping outside). A common finding in hypothermic clients is the incidence of high alcohol or other drug intake. Alcohol ingestion affects thermoregulation in a number of different ways. It provides a false sense of warmth, inhibits shivering, and causes the skin to vasodilate, thus promoting heat loss. Alcohol also impairs judgment and decisions, raising the person's risk of making inappropriate decisions about exposure.

Hypothermia that occurs in hospitalized clients may be related to treatment (intentional) used to decrease the metabolic rate. This might occur in clients with head injuries. Or hypothermia may be associated with therapies implemented in the hospital. Medications, particularly anesthetic agents, inhibit shivering and vasoconstriction, therefore promoting heat loss. In the operating room, not only do anesthetics contribute to heat loss, but surgical incisions contribute significantly to evaporative heat loss. Hypothermia is also associated with rapid infusion of large volumes of fluid, known as fluid resuscitation.

Classification of hypothermia and physiological responses are based on the level of body temperature. Mild hypothermia is a temperature between 35° C and 32° C (95° F and 89.6° F); moderate hypothermia is a temperature between 32° C and 28° C (89.6° F and 82.4° F); and severe hypothermia is a temperature below 28° C (82.4° F). Physiological responses associated with hypothermia affect the cardiovascular, respiratory, renal, nervous, and endocrine systems (Box 27-2, p. 650).

Box 27-2 Physiological Responses to Hypothermia

CENTRAL NERVOUS SYSTEM

- Apathy
- Poor judgment
- Paradoxical undressing
- Dilated pupils

CARDIOVASCULAR SYSTEM

- Decreased heart rate at temperatures <32° C (89.6° F)
- Decreased cardiac output at temperatures <32° C
- Ventricular fibrillation at temperatures <28° C (82.4° F)

RENAL SYSTEM

- Cold diuresis
- Decreased glomerular filtration rate at temperatures <32° C

ENDOCRINE SYSTEM

- Increased aldosterone
- Increased T_4 and T_3

From Granberg, P. (1991). Human physiology under cold exposure. *Arctic Medical Research, 50* (Suppl. 6), 23-27.

FACTORS AFFECTING THERMOREGULATION

Factors That Place Clients at Risk for Fever

Clients most likely to develop acute fever are those at risk for infection or inflammation. Bacterial infection accounts for about 50% of nosocomial fevers in hospitalized clients (Arbo et al., 1993). The most likely site of infection is the respiratory system.

Immunosuppressed people are at particular risk for fever because of their high incidence of infection. An immunosuppressed person is still able to generate a fever. Examples of causes of immunosuppression include neoplasms, infection with human immunodeficiency virus, and medications received after an organ transplant.

Factors That Place Clients at Risk for Hyperthermia

There are two classifications of hyperthermia: classic and exertional. Classic heat stroke is most likely to occur in people who have problems with thermoregulation, such as children, older adults, and people with chronic diseases. Additional risk factors include alcoholism, an urban residence, poverty, the use of major tranquilizers, and living on higher floors of multistory buildings. People with classic heat stroke typically have a limited ability to lose heat.

Exertional heat stroke occurs in people who have been physically active in hot, humid conditions. Examples of people at risk for exertional hyperthermia are marathon runners, football players, and military recruits. Heat gain is typically the problem in people with exertional heat stroke. Heat stroke is more common in the humid southern climates. Heat-related deaths occur in prolonged periods of high temperature and humidity.

Factors That Place Clients at Risk for Hypothermia

People at risk for hypothermia have an altered ability to thermoregulate, or they have experienced excessive exposure to a cold environment. Ineffective thermoregulation occurs in older adults and in people who have diseases that alter autonomic nervous system function, such as diabetes mellitus. Decreased ability to vasoconstrict in response to cold in these people will inappropriately promote heat loss. Children are at increased risk for hypothermia because of their high ratio of body surface to mass, which promotes rapid heat loss.

ASSESSMENT

Temperature is measured as part of the vital signs during a general health screening or when the client presents with evidence suggesting a fever or is at risk for developing a fever.

General Assessment

For the client with altered body temperature, you should perform a complete history and physical examination. As you take the health history, listen for information about the risk for infection and other causes of altered body temperature. You are also looking for signs and symptoms that suggest the presence of an infection. You need to assess the client's general condition and other health problems that might affect the course of the illness. Age and general health status are often important factors in an individual's response to infection.

Diagnostic Tests

TEMPERATURE MEASUREMENT. A thermometer is the instrument used to measure body temperature. Thermometers measure temperatures via many routes: oral, rectal, axillary, and tympanic membrane. The most common type of thermometer used today is an electronic device, although glass thermometers may still be used on occasion. (See Procedure 7-1 in Chapter 7 for measuring body temperature.)

BLOOD CULTURES. One of the frequently ordered diagnostic procedures in a febrile client is a blood culture. Blood cultures can indicate to the clinician the etiology of a fever. Most blood cultures are used to identify bacteria in the blood (bacteremia), but they can also be used to identify viruses in the blood (viremia). It is important to realize that in bacterial pneumonia, urinary tract infection, and wound infection, bacteria may not be present in the blood even though the client has developed an infectious process.

Blood cultures are ordered when body temperature reaches a specific threshold. This threshold varies, depending on characteristics of the client and on practitioner preference. Blood cultures are sometimes drawn at lower temperature levels in immunosuppressed clients because of the likelihood of a life-threatening infection.

When drawing blood cultures from a client, the blood should not be drawn through an intravascular device, such as a central line or intravenous catheter. Blood cultures should be drawn from a peripheral site to prevent contamination of the culture. Drawing blood cultures through the intravascular device may be appropriate, however, if you are trying to determine whether the device itself is the source of the infection.

Action Alert! If a blood culture is ordered at the same time as an antibiotic, draw the blood culture before giving the antibiotic. Administration of an antibiotic will alter the results.

Focused Assessment for Fever

Most hospitalized clients are at risk for an elevated temperature. Inflammation and infection commonly affect the hospitalized client. (See Chapter 21 for a discussion of *Risk for infection.*)

Defining Characteristics. The definition of fever is an elevation of set-point manifested as a rise in body temperature and usually associated with chills. Acute fever is considered a temperature rise to higher than 37.8° C (100° F), but circadian variation must be taken into consideration when assessing fever. A temperature of 37.8° C at 5:00 A.M. is more of a rise above normal than a temperature of 37.8° C at 6:00 P.M. in a client with a normal circadian rhythm.

Chronic fever or fever of unknown origin is defined as fever of 3 weeks' duration with evaluation by a medical team for 1 week. Chronic fever is most likely to occur in people with neoplasia, autoimmune disease, and vascular disease.

Fever is often associated with increased heart rate and cardiac output. In a person with an increased body temperature but not an increased heart rate, fever may be the result of a drug reaction. A person with underlying cardiac problems may not tolerate the additional cardiovascular stress associated with fever.

Another consequence of fever is a change in the metabolic absorption and distribution of medications in the gastrointestinal tract. Acid secretion decreases and transit time decreases, altering the absorption of medications. The increase in cardiac output that occurs with fever also alters the distribution of medications.

In some clients, fever may not be present during infection. Older adults can have bacteremia without a fever. In older adults, fever does not develop as readily and diagnosis of infection may be delayed, leading to serious consequences. Fever is also a poor indicator of infection in clients receiving nonsteroidal antiinflammatory medications for conditions such as rheumatoid arthritis.

Related Factors. Fever is related to a variety of etiologies, including infection, inflammation, neoplasia, autoimmune disease, vascular disease, drug reaction, and miscellaneous causes (Box 27-3).

Assessment of Responses. Responses associated with fever that need to be monitored include increased cardiac demand (such as increased heart rate), increased metabolic rate, altered drug metabolism, and altered comfort. Treatment will be based on the client's ability to tolerate fever and the discomfort associated with the fever. Table 27-2 summarizes decision making in the assessment of temperature for different age groups.

Box 27-3   Etiologies of Fever

INFLAMMATION
- Pancreatitis
- Cholecystitis
- Thrombophlebitis

BURNS

TRAUMA

INFECTION
- Bacterial
- Viral
- Parasitic
- Fungal

DRUG FEVER

NEOPLASTIC DISEASE

VASCULAR OCCLUSION
- Myocardial infarction
- Stroke

Table 27-2   Decision Making in Assessing Temperature for Different Age-Groups

Age	Assessment Data	Decision Considerations
Infant	• Infants have immature thermoregulation. • A temperature of 38° C (>100.4° F) in the first 12 months of life is considered significant. • Convulsions and delirium may occur.	• Protect from environmental changes; keep dry and appropriately clothed. • The parent is often advised to see the primary care provider. • Tympanic or axillary site is preferred. • Risk for febrile convulsions begins at 6 months. Febrile convulsions generally occur as the temperature is elevating.
Child	• Risk for febrile convulsions and delirium lasts up to 6 years. • May experience temperature elevation after exercise.	• Educate parents about the risk for convulsions and appropriate actions. • Tell the child experiencing hallucinations that the image is not real and will go away when the fever is down.
Adult	• 37.1° to 38.2° C (98.8° to 100.6° F) low grade. • >38.2° C (>100.6° F) significant fever. • >40.5° C (>104.9° F) hyperpyrexia.	• Temperature regulation is still labile.
Older adult	• Body temperature drops to an average of 36° C (96.8° F) in the older adult.	• Older adults may have decreased sensitivity to temperature changes. • Confusion may be a sign of impending infection with fever.

Focused Assessment for Hyperthermia

Hyperthermia includes heat exhaustion and heat stroke. Heat exhaustion is defined as a body temperature greater than normal but less than 40.6° C (105° F). Heat stroke is a body temperature greater than 40.6° C. At both of these levels of hyperthermia, heat gain occurs at a greater rate than heat loss.

Defining Characteristics. *Heat exhaustion* is more severe than simple heat-related symptoms that can be relieved by resting in a cool environment and replacing fluids. Symptoms associated with heat exhaustion include weakness, fatigue, headache, giddiness, anorexia, nausea, vomiting, diarrhea, and skeletal muscle cramps. Heat stroke is a severe and sometimes fatal condition. It is characterized by hot, dry skin; the absence of sweating; and neurological manifestations.

A person with exertional *heat stroke* still produces sweat. Manifestations associated with heat stroke include central nervous system alterations, acute renal failure, liver damage, cardiovascular abnormalities, and electrolyte imbalance. Neurological manifestations that occur with heat stroke include confusion, seizures, and coma. Sinus tachycardia and hypotension are common. Electrolyte abnormalities include increased serum sodium and decreased serum potassium levels. Potassium is initially decreased because the person has a metabolic acidosis. Box 27-4 lists teaching points to help parents prevent or manage febrile convulsions in their small children.

Related Factors. Various factors may be involved in heat-related illness.

AGE. Several factors contribute to an increased risk for heat exhaustion or heat stroke in older adults. The size, number, and activity of the sweat glands diminish, making the body less efficient at losing excess heat. Decreased mobility may affect the ability of older adults to get water, and they may also have decreased thirst sensation. Diminished cognitive capacity in an older adult client may also affect decision making related to heat exposure and water intake. Table 27-3 lists other factors that can affect thermoregulation.

SOCIOECONOMIC CONDITIONS. Prevention of heat stroke is a public health issue, particularly in crowded urban areas where it may be difficult to maintain cool, well-ventilated housing. In conditions of prolonged heat and humidity, ventilation and air conditioning become important. The cost of electricity and air conditioning units may be prohibitive for the poor.

OCCUPATION. Heat-related illness, a concern for an occupational health nurse, may occur where a significant number of employees work in conditions of extreme heat. Laborers who do heavy physical work in the hot sun or in metal foundries, mines, or closed shops are vulnerable. Regular breaks, ventilation, lightweight clothing, and plenty of liquids may be helpful in preventing heat-related problems.

MEDICATIONS. Hyperthermia can also occur as a side effect of medications. Malignant hyperthermia can occur in re-

Teaching for Wellness
Managing Febrile Convulsions   Box 27-4

Purpose: To provide parents of small children information about febrile convulsions.

Expected Outcome: Parents will feel confident that febrile convulsions can be prevented or safely managed.

Client Instructions

General information
- Febrile convulsions are associated with a fever of 38.9° C to 40° C (102° F to 104° F).
- They occur as early as 3 months of age and as late as 7 years of age; 95% of febrile convulsions occur before the age of 5 years, and they are most likely to occur before the age of 24 months.
- Febrile convulsions occur in only 3% to 4% of children, but the risk is greater if the child has had a previous febrile convulsion.
- The child's electroencephalogram remains normal during a febrile convulsion; the child will have little of the confusion that occurs after other types of convulsions; and most importantly, febrile convulsions do not cause brain damage.
- The height of the child's fever does not seem to trigger febrile convulsions as much as a sudden spike in body temperature.
- You can treat your child at home with the specific dosage of medication that the physician prescribes.
- Dress the child with a fever in lightweight clothing; infants should be dressed only in diapers.
- Febrile convulsions occur mostly at night, when parents are not aware of temperature elevations until the temperature is quite high.
- If your child has had one episode of a high fever, try to prevent a second high fever to reduce the risk of febrile convulsions.
- Make sure you take the child with a high fever to the doctor.

Treatment of febrile convulsions
- Remain calm, and protect the child from injury.
- Following the convulsion, put a cool cloth to the child's head, and call the physician to determine where the child can be checked (physician's office, emergency department).
- Do not put the child in a tub of cold water; extreme cooling is a shock to the nervous system.
- Do not use alcohol to cool the child; the skin will absorb it, and the fumes are toxic.
- Do not give the child any medications by mouth.
- Do not use an oral thermometer to measure the child's body temperature.

sponse to general anesthetic agents, such as halothane. This increase in body temperature is the result of a genetic abnormality that causes muscle rigidity, leading to a rise in body temperature. Neuroleptic malignant syndrome can occur in clients receiving antipsychotic medications such as clozapine. Neuroleptic malignant syndrome is a potentially fatal complication consisting of hypertonicity, pallor, dyskinesia, hyperthermia, incontinence, unstable blood pressure, and pulmonary congestion. Other medications can make the person vulnerable to heat stroke. Diuretics reduce the amount of total body fluid. Beta-blockers, phenothiazines, and anticholinergics decrease the ability to sweat.

Table 27-3 Factors Affecting Thermoregulation

Factor	Effect
Age	Children have a greater body-surface-to-mass ratio, and children also have a higher metabolic rate. Older adult clients have a lower average body temperature.
Percent body fat	Increased body fat prevents heat loss. This can be beneficial in cold environments or detrimental in warm environments.
Gender	Women have changes in body temperature that are related to the menstrual cycle.
Chronic illness	Some chronic illnesses, such as diabetes mellitus and renal failure, interfere with thermoregulation.
Medications	Neuroleptic medications affect thermoregulation by impairing thirst. Fever may not occur in clients taking nonsteroidal antiinflammatory agents.
Environment	Living areas that have poor ventilation because of windows that cannot be opened or materials that hold heat, such as concrete, may impact thermoregulation in clients.
Occupation	Work that requires exposure to cold environments or physical labor in warm, humid environments affects thermoregulation.
Recreation	Activities such as running, football, etc. generate heat and may be of concern in warm, humid environments.

Assessment of Responses. In addition to treating the manifestations of hyperthermia, you will be involved in assessing and managing complications. Complications associated with hyperthermia include altered perfusion of the central nervous system, altered perfusion of the kidneys, and breakdown of muscle. Clients with a family history of malignant hyperthermia may have anxiety before surgical procedures. Clients with neuroleptic malignant syndrome will often have decreased thirst, which contributes to the development of hyperthermia. Nursing diagnoses that may be appropriate are *Anxiety, Fluid volume deficit, Confusion,* and *Ineffective tissue perfusion.*

Focused Assessment for Hypothermia

In clients with hypothermia, heat gain is at a lower rate than heat loss. Because of the higher heat loss, body temperature decreases.

Defining Characteristics. Hypothermia has been categorized as mild (35° C to 32° C [95° F to 89.6° F]), moderate (32° C to 28° C [89.6° F to 82.4° F]), and severe (less than 28° C [82.4° F]).

Thermometers normally used in clinical practice do not provide a scale low enough to assess hypothermia. A thermometer with a lower range should be available, particularly in emergency departments, for accurate assessment of body temperature in clients with hypothermia.

The levels of hypothermia are associated with pathophysiological responses. Life-threatening sequelae, such as ventricular fibrillation, are associated with severe hypothermia.

Level of consciousness will be diminished in severely hypothermic clients as well.

Manifestations associated with hypothermia depend on temperature level (see Box 27-2). Shivering caused by hypothermia will become progressively more intense to the point at which the hypothermic person will have trouble performing voluntary motor functions. Level of consciousness will also decrease as body temperature decreases. Hyporeflexia occurs with severe hypothermia.

Initially during hypothermia, cold diuresis occurs, possibly because of peripheral vasoconstriction or reduction in antidiuretic hormone. Cold diuresis is increased urine production resulting from a smaller vascular compartment. Subsequently, the hematocrit level will increase because of the fluid loss. As body temperature decreases, cold diuresis slows, renal blood flow decreases, and urine output decreases.

Cardiovascular responses also depend on temperature level. Sinus tachycardia occurs with mild hypothermia. Sinus bradycardia with death resulting from ventricular fibrillation occurs with moderate and severe hypothermia. The major concern with hypothermia is preventing cardiovascular compromise caused by ventricular arrhythmias.

Related Factors. The primary related factors are exposure and medical procedures.

EXPOSURE. People exposed to the cold—for example, hikers, hunters, and others who spend time outdoors—are at risk for hypothermia, particularly if some unforeseen injury occurs and the person is a distance from assistance. Heat loss, and thus death, occurs at a much faster rate in people accidentally submerged in cold water than in those exposed to cold air. In the southern United States, a case of hypothermia is less common than in northern regions.

MEDICAL PROCEDURES. Hypothermia is also a consequence of procedures performed in the hospital. Clients undergoing surgery and clients receiving fluid resuscitation may be hypothermic after these procedures.

DIAGNOSIS

An elevation in body temperature is due to either hyperthermia or fever. To differentiate fever from hyperthermia, it is useful to consider client history and setting, and this is most difficult in clients admitted to the hospital with neurological injury. The elevation in temperature could be due to the underlying injury or to an infectious process. You need to assess for signs of infection to make the final determination. Table 27-4 (p. 654) shows examples of clustering data used to support thermoregulatory nursing diagnoses.

Determining the cause of fever can be difficult because of the many possible etiologies. It requires examining for localizing signs, such as increased sputum production, abdominal pain, or cloudy urine. Without localizing signs, the fever may have to be classified as fever of unknown origin.

The age and other demographic data about the client may be useful in knowing what questions to ask when you are

Table 27-4 *Clustering Data to Make a Nursing Diagnosis*

PROBLEMS OF BODY TEMPERATURE

Data Cluster	Diagnosis
A mother calls the pediatrician's office, concerned that her 4-year-old has a temperature of 37.5° C (99.6° F). The child is active, does not appear ill, and does not have any gastrointestinal symptoms or respiratory symptoms. Further assessment reveals that the child has a sunburn after swimming yesterday.	*Low-grade fever* related to inflammation
A 90-year-old woman is admitted to the hospital with a temperature of 40.6° C (105° F). The city is experiencing a heat wave, and the woman lives in a high-rise apartment without air conditioning or adequate ventilation. She has no signs of infection.	*Hyperthermia* related to environmental conditions
A first-day postsurgical client has a temperature of 39° C (102.2° F). Respirations are 10, breath sounds diminished, and the person is unable to cough.	*Fever* related to postoperative hypoventilation

looking for the cause of an elevated body temperature. As an example, assessment for causes of fever in children is illustrated in Figure 27-4. A pattern of body temperature change during fever in some cases is related to particular diseases.

One of the clues that an elevation in body temperature is a drug-related fever is that there is no change in heart rate with the rise in body temperature. Generally during fever, there is an associated elevation in heart rate; during drug fever, this may not occur.

PLANNING

Expected Outcomes for the Client With Fever

Fever is a component of the host defenses and should be treated only in clients who cannot tolerate the additional physiological or experiential stress caused by the fever. In these clients, body temperature can be brought within normal range using therapies that do not induce shivering. Therefore the goal may be to make the client comfortable rather than to reduce the fever. Sometimes the goal is to teach the client self-care. Possible outcomes are that the client is able to do the following:

- Maintain a body temperature that is normal for the client
- Maintain dry skin, clothes, and linens
- Maintain comfort
- Maintain fluid intake sufficient to prevent dehydration
- Demonstrate the correct method for measuring a temperature
- Identify when a nurse or physician should be consulted for a fever

Expected Outcomes for the Client With Hyperthermia

Body temperature will be brought to within normal limits to prevent complications related to hyperthermia, such as muscle breakdown. Ideally, there will be no neurological deficits present after cooling. Fluid balance as assessed by serum sodium and urine output will be within normal limits. Precipitating causes of hyperthermia will be evaluated to determine etiology and to prevent future episodes of hyperthermia. Box 27-5 (p. 656) is a guide to teaching preventive measures.

When the diagnosis is *Risk for hyperthermia,* the goal is to prevent heat-related problems. Possible outcomes are that the client is able to do the following:

- Modify the environment to prevent hyperthermia, such as by repairing an air-conditioning unit or increasing ventilation with fans or open windows
- Identify appropriate dress for a hot, humid environment
- Identify precautions to take when exercising or working in a hot environment

Expected Outcomes for the Client With Hypothermia

The goal in hypothermia is to bring temperature to a normal level without complications. Therapies should be monitored closely to prevent the afterdrop that may occur during peripheral warming. Possible outcomes include that the client is able to do the following:

- Have minimal or no tissue necrosis
- Return to a normal sinus rhythm
- Have urinary output within normal limits
- Have blood pressure and pulse within normal limits

When the diagnosis is *Risk for hypothermia,* the goal is prevention. Possible outcomes include that the client is able to do the following:

- Recall safety precautions for walking or skating on frozen ponds
- Demonstrate appropriate dress for cold weather
- Modify the environment to maintain heat in the home, such as by repairing the furnace, seeking public assistance for utility bills, or insulating the home
- Implement a plan for checking on the welfare of older adults in the family

INTERVENTION

Interventions to Monitor Temperature

Temperature is monitored as part of routine vital signs. The scheduling of routine vital signs varies for an outpatient clinic, a general nursing unit in a hospital, a long-term care

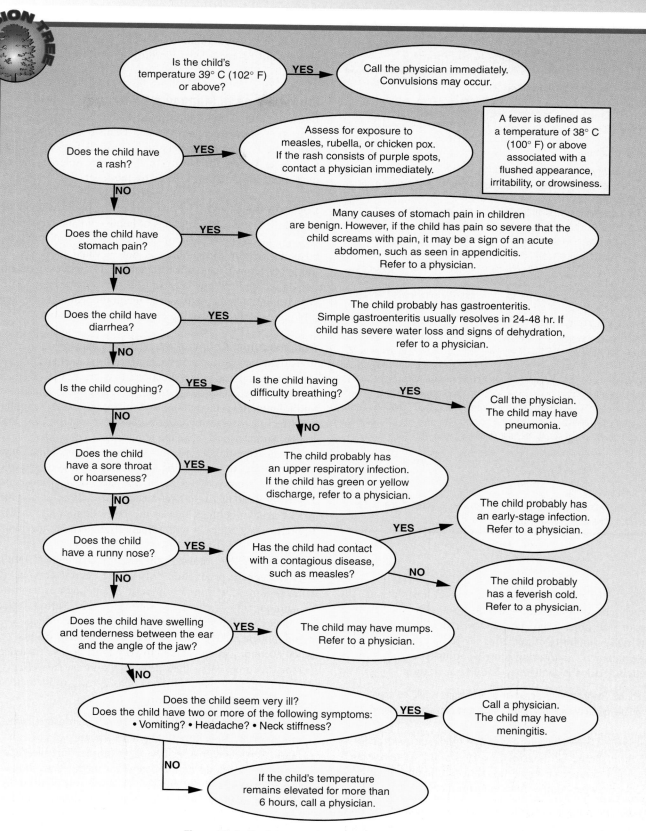

Figure 27-4. Decision tree for screening fever in children.

facility, or the client's home. On a general hospital unit, the routine depends on institution policy; it may specify two, three, or four times a day. For the low-risk client, twice a day has a high probability of detecting a rise in temperature.

Frequency of monitoring must be adjusted on the basis of the client's risk for changes in body temperature.

For Mr. Stephen, what schedule of vital signs would be appropriate, given his postoperative status and present vital signs?

Action Alert! The temperature of clients at risk for infection should be measured every 4 hours. If temperature is monitored every 8 hours, a febrile episode may occur between temperature measurements.

If the client has an elevated temperature, monitoring every 4 hours is usually sufficient. However, you should be aware of signs of possible fever and take the client's temperature more often if needed. Clients with severe alterations in thermoregulation, such as hyperthermia or hypothermia, should be monitored as often as every 15 minutes.

Temperature is reported in either centigrade or Fahrenheit units; both units continue to be used clinically. The temperature should be recorded according to the agency's charting format.

Interventions to Manage a Fever

Because fever is considered a host defense response, treatment is somewhat controversial. Decisions to treat fever should be based on the benefits of host defense associated with fever versus the ability of the host to tolerate the cardiopulmonary demands created by the fever.

Covering the Client. The first sign of the onset of fever may be a chill. The client complains of being cold and requests additional covering. The temperature may be collected as a baseline measurement, but it is not elevated until the chill phase has passed. Chills last from 10 to 30 minutes. Cover the person with a light blanket, but avoid heavy covering. Covers will aid in the body's attempt to maintain heat and may actually increase the impending elevation of temperature.

Administering Antipyretics. The two classes of interventions used for treating fever include antipyretics and physical cooling. Antipyretics (medications that are effective against fever) include acetaminophen, aspirin, and other nonsteroidal antiinflammatory medications. Aspirin and other salicylates are effective for treating fever because they act directly on the hypothalamus to decrease the temperature set-point.

Because treating a fever masks the symptoms of an illness, it is important to know if the absence of fever is a sign of recovery or simply a result of the use of an antipyretic. Knowing the half-life of the medication will help. The half-life of acetaminophen, one of the more commonly used antipyretics, is 2 hours. It will influence temperature for about 4 to 6 hours.

Acetaminophen, unlike other antipyretic agents, inhibits cyclooxygenase production only in the central nervous system. Treatment with an antipyretic agent, such as aspirin or acetaminophen, is relatively safe. However, serious effects can occur in high-risk clients. One of the side effects of acetaminophen is hepatic toxicity. This usually occurs only when acetaminophen is taken in very large doses or when the person has preexisting liver disease. Common side effects of aspirin include bruising of the skin as a result of its anticoagulant effect and tinnitus (ringing in the ears).

Action Alert! Teach clients to avoid overdose of acetaminophen, especially if they have a history of liver disease. Persons with a history of gastrointestinal bleeding or who are taking an anticoagulant medication should avoid aspirin and the ibuprofens. Aspirin is contraindicated in children and teenagers with chicken pox or flu because of the risk of developing Reye's syndrome.

Acetaminophen can be administered either orally as tablets or an elixir, or rectally as a suppository. One of the problems with administration of acetaminophen to acutely ill people is variable absorption when the client has a nasogastric tube or slow gastric emptying. Only the more commonly used antipyretics, such as acetaminophen, are available as preparations that can be administered via the nasogastric tube.

Providing Physical Cooling.
Methods used for cooling include cooling blankets, ice packs, fans, and tepid baths. Physical cooling does not alter the set-point; therefore use of these interventions to decrease temperature is controversial. Physical cooling decreases body temperature by increasing the temperature difference between the skin and the environment. Subsequently, the difference between the skin and the core of the body increases heat loss.

Various physical cooling methods are available. Cooling blankets promote conductive heat loss. Fans promote convective heat loss by moving air closest to the skin away from the client. The body warms air that is close to the skin. When the fan moves this air away, colder air moves next to the skin, increasing the difference between the skin and air temperature. Tepid baths used on febrile clients promote evaporative heat loss. Heat can be lost through evaporation of water on the skin in a manner similar to sweating.

One of the more recent innovations in cooling is the convective cooling blanket. This system blows cool air by the client to increase convective heat loss. This system is very similar to mechanisms of heat loss. Remember, however, that cooling systems that blow air by a client who has a wound infection may promote movement of infectious agents into the air.

Action Alert! The decrease in skin blood flow caused by cooling measures increases vascular resistance and may increase the work of the heart. The decreased skin blood flow may also lead to skin breakdown, particularly if the cooling blanket is placed under the client.

Another consequence of using physical cooling is shivering. Because physical cooling does not affect set-point, the thermoregulatory response to cooling will be to maintain the current body temperature. This increase in metabolic rate may add stress to the client who is already physiologically compromised.

Providing Nutrition and Fluids.
Anorexia (loss of appetite) is often associated with fever. In an otherwise healthy person, not eating for a short time will not change the course of the illness or result in nutritional deficits. If the person is compromised, however, maintaining nutrition is important. Assess the likelihood of the person tolerating food. Decreased bowel sounds, a distended abdomen, or nausea would suggest the person may not tolerate eating. As soon as the person is able, provide a well-balanced diet that includes proteins, minerals, and vitamins. Carbohydrates may be the food of choice because they are easily digested and provide energy.

Action Alert! Maintaining fluid volume is essential for maintaining the balance between heat loss and heat gain. Inadequate circulating blood volume impairs an individual's ability to eliminate heat because there is less blood transferring heat to the skin.

Dehydration often contributes to the development of hyperthermia. Clients with fever often lose fluid because of the sweating that occurs when set-point decreases. They sweat to decrease body temperature to attain this lower set-point. Fluid replacement should take these losses into consideration.

Providing Comfort and Rest.
Treatment of fever often affects client comfort. If fever is treated with antipyretics on a regular schedule, the client will avoid the cycle of chills and defervescence. Treatment with antipyretics on a less frequent schedule leads to defervescence when the antipyretics are administered and chills when the effects of antipyretics end. This may be more uncomfortable than not being treated for fever at all.

Interventions to Manage Hyperthermia
The treatment of hyperthermia is considerably different from treatment of fever because hyperthermia is not a rise in set-point but an alteration in thermoregulation. Appropriate treatment of hyperthermia depends on the etiology, but the goal of therapy in most cases is to promote heat loss. Therefore physical cooling measures that promote heat loss are the standard treatment.

Methods of physical cooling for individuals with hyperthermia include warm air spray, cooling blankets, ice packs, iced gastric lavage, and convective cooling blankets. Warm air spray is an effective means for heat loss because the water sprayed on the client promotes heat loss by evaporation, and the blowing of the air on the client promotes convective heat loss. Although the person is hyperthermic, the warmth of the spray prevents vasoconstriction of the skin, which would impair heat loss. Warm air spray systems can be seen on the sidelines of football games in warm, humid environments. They are being used in an attempt to prevent hyperthermia in football players.

Cooling blankets increase the gradient between core and shell temperature by cooling the skin temperature. However, cold applied to the skin also causes vasoconstriction of the vessels in the skin, decreasing heat loss. Methods that avoid cooling the skin, such as iced saline gastric lavage, do not directly stimulate vasoconstriction in the skin and may be more effective at decreasing body temperature.

Managing Malignant Hyperthermia.
Malignant hyperthermia is an autosomal dominant genetic disorder that affects calcium levels within the skeletal muscle. Treatment of malignant hyperthermia due to general anesthesia focuses on decreasing heat production.

Action Alert! Increased calcium levels in the skeletal muscle in response to general anesthetic agents such as halothane lead to skeletal muscle hyperactivity. The skeletal muscle hyperactivity increases body temperature to life-threatening levels.

Treatment of malignant hyperthermia is based on decreasing heat production by the skeletal muscle. The medication that is most effective in treating malignant hyperthermia is dantrolene.

Dantrolene decreases the calcium available for excitation in the skeletal muscle cells. Physical cooling measures are also applied to promote heat loss and decrease body temperature.

Managing Neuroleptic Malignant Syndrome.

Treatment of neuroleptic malignant syndrome is similar to that for malignant hyperthermia, although the underlying mechanisms causing neuroleptic malignant syndrome are not well understood. Treatment of neuroleptic malignant syndrome includes administration of dantrolene, physical cooling, and hydration. Dehydration is thought to be a contributing factor because many neuroleptic medications inhibit thirst. Decreased fluid volume will impair the person's ability to lose heat because less heat can be transferred to the skin through the blood.

Interventions to Manage Hypothermia

Treatment of hypothermia varies according to the level of body temperature. Passive warming methods—such as blankets and increased ambient temperature—will be used to decrease heat loss if the hypothermia is mild. Active warming methods may be incorporated in more severe cases.

Peripheral methods of active warming, such as warm blankets and radiant warmers, will have more of an effect on the shell of the person. Central methods of warming are more invasive and include administration of warmed intravenous fluid. If hypothermia is severe, active methods such as extracorporeal warming of blood by means of a device similar to a cardiac bypass machine may be utilized to warm the client. Other invasive methods of warming include instillation of warm fluid into the peritoneum.

Action Alert! One of the consequences that may occur during peripheral rewarming is a decrease in body temperature termed afterdrop. As warming of the skin increases skin blood flow, the blood becomes cooler than usual because of the coldness of the peripheral tissues. Blood returning to the core will then decrease core temperature. Therefore, during attempts to warm a client peripherally, one of the consequences may be an even lower core temperature.

Hypothermia occurs not only in outlying settings but also in hospitalized clients after surgery.

EVALUATION

To evaluate the care provided for a client with an altered body temperature, ask yourself the following four questions. First, was the client's comfort maintained? Second, was the body temperature controlled in a timely manner? Third, are there any residual effects? Fourth, are appropriate measures in place to prevent future occurrences?

Fever is uncomfortable and commonly produces a feeling of drowsiness. Appropriate care includes relieving the discomfort and providing a quiet environment to allow the client to rest. Usually, fever is relatively easy to control. Evaluation data include the client's level of satisfaction with the care. Evaluation of prevention measures includes the effectiveness of teaching the client to avoid infections. Box 27-6 demonstrates the nursing process for Mr. Stephen.

🍲 Nursing Care Plan A CLIENT WITH A WOUND INFECTION AND FEVER Box 27-6

ADMISSION DATA

On the 12th postoperative day, Mr. Stephen was visited at home by a friend who is a registered nurse. She took his temperature: 39° C (102.2° F). Further assessment revealed the following about Mr. Stephen: feeling hot for 2 days, with no chills for 24 hours; malaise; lack of appetite; unwilling to drink adequate fluids even though the mucous membranes are dry; lung sounds are clear, blood pressure is 138/84, pulse 130, and respirations 20. The incisions were healing except one suture line that was oozing a foul-smelling butter-yellow discharge that was enough to saturate a 2 × 4-inch gauze in about 2 hours.

The nurse suggested to the family that the physician should be notified. The family asked the nurse to call the physician and report her observations.

Following the report of client status to the physician, the client was transported to the hospital for admission.

PHYSICIAN'S ORDERS

Admitting diagnosis: wound infection
Vital signs every 4 hours

Acetaminophen 650 mg PO or rectally every 4 hours, now and prn
   if temperatures over 39° C (102. 2° F)
Culture and sensitivity of wound
IV of 1000 mL $D_5W/1/2NS$ at 100 mL/hr
Cefoxitin sodium (Mefoxin) 2 g every 8 hours IV
Dressing change as needed
Fluids of choice at 240 mL/hr while awake
Diet as tolerated
Up ad lib
Laxative of choice

NURSING ASSESSMENT

Color pale, diaphoretic, vital signs: BP 136/82, T 39° C (102.2° F), P 126, R 20. Reports feeling weak and tired. Incision draining thick, yellow, foul-smelling drainage, edges are red and not approximated distally for about 1 inch. Mucous membranes dry, lips cracked, skin flushed and warm to touch. Sleeping, easily aroused.

Nursing Care Plan A CLIENT WITH A WOUND INFECTION AND FEVER—CONT'D

Box 27-6

NANDA Nursing Diagnosis	NOC Expected Outcomes With Indicators	NIC Interventions With Selected Activities	Evaluation Data
HYPERTHERMIA: FEVER RELATED TO POSTOPERATIVE WOUND INFECTION	THERMOREGULATION • Body temperature WNL • Hydration adequate • Reports thermal comfort • Skin color changes not present	FEVER TREATMENT (AND WOUND CARE) • Monitor temperature q4h. • Monitor for insensible water loss. • Monitor intake and output. • Monitor WBC, Hgb, and Hct. • Administer acetaminophen as ordered.	• Acetaminophen administered; temperature 99.2° F in 4 hours. • Skin pink, warm, and dry. • WBC 8000, Hgb 13.5, Hct 35. • For 8 hours intake (including IV fluids) 1600 cc and output 800.

CRITICAL THINKING QUESTIONS

1. What factors related to aging might be contributing to the client's impaired immune status?
2. What difference in treatment would there be if the client were a 3-year-old child?
3. What part of the ordered treatment could be carried out in the home?

Nursing outcomes and intervention labels from Johnson, M., Bulechek, G., McCloskey Dochterman, J. M., Maas, M., & Moorhead, S. et al. (2001). *Nursing diagnoses, outcomes and interventions: NANDA, NOC and NIC linkages.* St Louis, MO: Mosby.

In hyperthermia, evaluation includes assessment for residual effects. If a hypothermia blanket was used, the client's skin should be inspected for damage. The client's neurological status should also be assessed to determine that no neurological damage has occurred.

The hypothermic client should be assessed for comfort during the course of treatment. In severe hypothermic states, skin damage and sloughing of tissue can occur. Inspect the skin carefully, especially the toes, finger, and earlobes, for damage from frostbite.

Mr. Stephen's pneumonia resolves and his recovery from heart surgery proceeds as desired. He is discharged on the 7th postoperative day. The nurse includes the following in a discharge note to address the infection.

SAMPLE DOCUMENTATION FOR MR. STEPHEN

Lungs clear, temperature 98.0° F. Instructed to notify physician if he has difficulty breathing, pain with respiration, temperature >101° F. Avoid contact with individuals with respiratory infections. Given a prescription for a 7-day course of antibiotics. Instructed to take all of his prescription as directed even if he is not currently experiencing symptoms. Has an appointment with the cardiologist in 1 week. Instructed to call primary care physician for follow-up appointment.

Key Principles

• Fever is a regulated rise in temperature mediated by a rise in temperature set-point.
• Fever is a host defense response and may have a beneficial effect; therefore treatment of fever is controversial.
• The etiology of a fever can be a wide variety of processes, including infection, inflammation, autoimmune disease, vascular disease, neoplasia, and drug reaction.
• A chill may be the first sign of a fever; the temperature rises after the onset of the chill.
• Hyperthermia is a nonregulated rise in body temperature that occurs when a person is unable to lose sufficient heat or is generating more heat than can be lost.
• Hypothermia is often associated with clinical conditions or factors that predispose clients to a decrease in core body temperature, such as severe illness, trauma, immersion, and frostbite.
• Temperature should be monitored frequently enough to detect elevations in temperature.
• Fever is treated with antipyretics to lower the set-point or with physical cooling to increase the temperature difference between the environment and the skin. Although the most common antipyretics (aspirin and acetaminophen) are relatively safe medications, serious side effects can occur in high-risk clients.
• When a client has a fever, management should include measures aimed at nutrition, fluid and electrolytes, and physical comfort.

Bibliography

Anonymous. (1998). Coming of age. Hyperthermia: A hot-weather hazard for older people. *AARC Times, 22*(6), 15-17.

Anonymous. (2000). Long-term care too quick on the transfer trigger: Fever does not warrant hazardous hospitalization [Healthcare Infection Prevention insert 3-4]. *Hospital Infection Control, 27*(12), 168.

Arbo, M., Fine, M., Hanusa, B., Sefeik, T., & Kapoor, W. (1993). Fever of nosocomial origin: Etiology, risk factors, and outcomes. *American Journal of Medicine, 95*(5), 505-512.

Bailey, J., & Rose, P. (2001). Axillary and tympanic membrane temperature recording in the preterm neonate: A comparative study. *Journal of Advanced Nursing, 34*(4), 465-474.

Blumenthal, I. (2000). Fever and the practice nurse: Measurement and treatment. *Community Practitioner, 73*(3), 519-521.

*Bor, D. H., Makadon, H. J., Friedland, G., Dasse, P., Komaroff, A. L., & Aronon, M. D. (1988). Fever in hospitalized medical clients: Characteristics and significance. *Journal of General Internal Medicine, 3*(2), 119-125.

Bower, J. R., & Powell, K. R. (2001). Unexplained fever in infants and young children: How to manage. *Consultant, 41*(5), 712-715.

Casey, G. (2000). Fever management in children. *Paediatric Nursing, 12*(3), 38-42.

Creechan, T., Vollman, K., & Kravutske, M. E. (2001). Cooling by convection vs cooling by conduction for treatment of fever in critically ill adults. *American Journal of Critical Care, 10*(1), 52-59.

Edwards, I. L. (1998). Update: High temperature. *Professional Nurse, 13*(8), 521-526.

Erickson, R. S., Meyer, L. T., & Moser Woo, T. (1996). Accuracy of chemical dot thermometers in critically ill adults and young children. *Image, 28*(1), 23-28.

*Granberg, P. (1991). Human physiology under cold exposure. *Arctic Medical Research, 50*(Suppl. 6), 23-27.

Gray-Vickrey, P., & Colucci, R. (1999). Taking charge in a geriatric emergency. *Nursing, 29*(1), 41-47.

Grupp-Phelan, J., Lozano, P., & Fishman, P. (2001). Health care utilization and cost in children with asthma and selected comorbidities. *Journal of Asthma, 38*(4), 363-373.

Guyton, A. C., & Hall, J. E. (2000). *Textbook of medical physiology* (10th ed.). Philadelphia: Saunders.

Henker, R. (1999). Evidence-based practice: Fever-related interventions. *American Journal of Critical Care, 8*(1), 481-489.

*Henker, R., Kramer, D., & Rogers, S. (1997). Fever. *AACN Clinical Issues, 8*(3), 351-367

Henker, R., Rogers, S., Kramer, D. J., Kelso, L., Kerr, M., & Sereika, S. (2001). Comparison of fever treatments in the critically ill: A pilot study. *American Journal of Critical Care, 10*(4), 276-280.

Hoffmann, K. J. (2001). Letter to the editor re: Creechan, T., Vollman, K., & Kravutske, M. E. (2001). Cooling by convection vs cooling by conduction for treatment of fever in critically ill adults (in *American Journal of Critical Care, 10*[1], 52-59). *American Journal of Critical Care, 10*(4), 294-295.

Joaquin, A. M. (2000). Hypothermia and hyperthermia. *Clinical Geriatrics, 8*(9), 54, 57, 61-63.

Johnson, M., Bulechek, G., McCloskey Dochterman, J., Maas, M., & Moorhead, S. (2001). *Nursing diagnoses, outcomes, and interventions: NANDA, NOC, and NIC linkages.* St Louis, MO: Mosby.

Jones, S. G., Holloman, F., & Coffin, D. (1998). Research utilization: Body temperature alterations in hospitalized HIV/AIDS patients. *MEDSURG Nursing, 7*(4), 217-222.

Koschel, M. J. (2001). Rewarming a hypothermic patient. *American Journal of Nursing, 101*(5), 85.

Little, D. J. (2000-2001). Factors influencing clinical decision-making for fever management by multi-ethnic acute care nurses. *Interaction, 18*(4), 6.

Luce, B. R., Zangwill, K. M., Palmer, C. S., et al. (2001). Cost-effectiveness analysis of an intranasal influenza vaccine for the prevention of influenza in healthy children. *Pediatrics, 108*(2), E24.

Marks, C. (2001). Reflective practice in thermoregulatory nursing care. *Nursing Standard, 15*(43), 38-41.

McConnell, E. A. (1998). Hospital nursing. What's wrong with Mrs. Nash? *Nursing, 28*(2), 32hn10-1.

McKenzie, N. E. (1998). Fever: Upping the body's thermostat. *Nursing, 28*(10), 41-45.

Nelson, D. S. (1998). Emergency treatment of fever phobia. *Journal of Emergency Nursing, 24*(1), 83-84.

North American Nursing Diagnosis Association. (1999). *Nursing diagnoses: Definitions and classification 1999-2000.* Philadelphia: Author.

Sarwari, A. R., & Mackowiak, P. A. (1996). The pharmacologic consequences of fever. *Infectious Disease Clinics of North America, 10*(1), 21-32.

Sharber, J. (1997). The efficacy of tepid sponge bathing to reduce fever in young children. *American Journal of Emergency Medicine, 15*(2), 188-192.

Sloan, A. (2001). Advice of counsel: Nurse should monitor feverish child despite physician's order. *RN, 64*(5), 86.

Thompson, S. (1999). Nursing care of a patient with fever due to sepsis/SIRS. *Nursing in Critical Care, 4*(2), 63-66.

Vinik, A. I., Erbas, T., Park, T. S., Stansberry, K. B., Scanelli, J. A., & Pittenger, G. L. (2001). Dermal neurovascular dysfunction in type 2 diabetes. *Diabetes Care, 24*(8), 1468.

Waltzman, M. L., & Harper, M. (2001). Financial and clinical impact of false-positive blood culture results. *Clinics in Infectious Diseases, 33*(3), 296-299

Watson, R. (1998). Controlling body temperature in adults. *Nursing Standard, 12*(20), 49-55.

Yarbrough, S. S., Cole, L., & Holtzclaw, B. J. (2001). "Riding it out": Living with uncertainty of HIV-related fever at home. *Southern Online Journal of Nursing Research, 2*(2), 1-23.

*Asterisk indicates a classic or definitive work on this subject.

Managing Bowel Elimination

Key Terms

bowel incontinence

cathartic

colostomy

constipation

diarrhea

fecal impaction

feces

flatus

flatulence

guaiac

ileostomy

laxative

occult blood

ostomy

paralytic ileus

peristalsis

steatorrhea

stoma

Learning Objectives

After studying this chapter, you should be able to do the following:

- Describe the structure and function of the lower gastrointestinal tract

- Discuss problems of bowel elimination, including constipation, diarrhea, and bowel incontinence

- Explain the effect on bowel elimination of the client's diet and exercise, personal habits, cultural background, age, and physiological and psychosocial factors

- Assess the client for manifestations of and responses to problems of bowel elimination

- Distinguish among the variety of nursing diagnoses for problems of bowel elimination

- Plan for goal-directed interventions to prevent or correct problems of bowel elimination

- Evaluate the outcomes that describe progress toward the goals of bowel elimination

Ninety-two-year-old John Daly lives in a private room in a long-term-care facility. He lived alone in his apartment in independent living as long as he could, until bone cancer and declining functional abilities required him to move. Dr. Daly is a retired neurosurgeon. He knows the consequences of immobility and decreased dietary intake and the side effects of pain medications. He called the nurse to report lower abdominal pain and difficulty having a bowel movement that morning. He reported that he had had a small bowel movement the day before, but it was not his usual pattern. Questioning the client further, the nurse ascertained that Dr. Daly's usual pattern of elimination was daily after intake of a high-fiber breakfast. When his routine was regular, the stool was usually formed and soft. The nurse considers the diagnosis of *Constipation* from the list of nursing diagnoses for bowel elimination (see below).

KEY NURSING DIAGNOSES FOR ▸ Bowel Elimination

Constipation: A decrease in normal frequency of defecation accompanied by difficult or incomplete passage of stool and/or passage of excessively hard, dry stool

Perceived constipation: Self-diagnosis of constipation and abuse of laxatives, enemas, and suppositories to ensure a daily bowel movement

Diarrhea: Passage of loose, unformed stool

Bowel incontinence: A change in normal bowel habits characterized by involuntary passage of stool

Risk for constipation: At risk for a decrease in normal frequency of defecation accompanied by difficult or incomplete passage of stool and/or passage of excessively hard, dry stool

*Fecal impaction: Hardened feces in the sigmoid colon and/or rectum that cannot be passed voluntarily

*Flatulence: The presence of an excessive amount of air or gas in the stomach and intestinal tract, causing distention of the organs and in some cases mild to moderate pain

*Diagnoses with an asterisk are not NANDA approved.

CONCEPTS OF BOWEL ELIMINATION

The nurse's role in helping a client with bowel elimination involves both independent and dependent actions. As a nurse, you may be responsible for assessing the client's bowel status, helping him maintain a normal bowel pattern, collecting stool specimens, performing diagnostic tests, and intervening in collaboration with the physician to meet the client's bowel elimination needs.

A number of bowel elimination needs can be met through independent nursing measures that do not require a physician's order. You can initiate them after appropriate assessment and application of relevant scientific principles. Nursing diagnoses relevant to the lower gastrointestinal (GI) system that have been approved by the North American Nursing Diagnosis Association (NANDA) include *Constipation, Perceived constipation, Diarrhea, Bowel incontinence,* and *Risk for constipation.*

Structure and Function of the Lower Gastrointestinal Tract

To understand and successfully treat bowel elimination problems, you will need to understand the structure and function of the GI tract. Naturally, a change in any aspect of the GI tract can affect a client's elimination process.

Organs of Bowel Elimination.
The GI tract, also called the alimentary canal, is a hollow, muscular tube that extends from the mouth to the anus (Figure 28-1). Food is broken down in the stomach into a semiliquid mass called chyme, which is more easily absorbed than solid food. Chyme leaves the stomach and enters the small intestine, which is divided into the duodenum, jejunum, and ileum. The 10-inch-long duodenum plays a role in digestion because it receives bile and pancreatic enzymes from the common bile duct. In the jejunum, chyme mixes with digestive enzymes and most of the nutrients are absorbed. Unabsorbed chyme enters the large intestine through the ileocecal valve in a semiliquid state. The large intestine, or colon, begins at the ileocecal valve and is the primary organ of bowel elimination. The four segments of the colon are the ascending, the transverse, the descending, and the sigmoid.

Formation of Feces.
The colon absorbs water and electrolytes, leaving approximately 150 cc of water per day to be excreted with body waste materials. These processes require a number of ancillary organs and anatomic structures, chemical substances, and physiological processes. As digested, unabsorbed food travels through the colon, it changes from a liquid to a solid as the colon absorbs water from it.

Feces are the body waste discharged from the intestine. This waste is also called stool, excreta, or excrement. It moves through the large intestine propelled by peristaltic waves and segmental contractions (Figure 28-2). **Peristalsis** is the rhythmic smooth-muscle contractions of the intestinal wall that propel the intestinal contents forward. Although the force could propel intestinal contents in either direction, movement in the GI tract is toward the anus. In segmental contractions, circular muscles in a segment of the colon mix the contents of the colon.

In addition to constant peristalsis, periods of mass peristalsis occur two or three times a day, usually following meals, and are facilitated by the gastrocolic reflex. The gastrocolic reflex occurs when the bolus of food enters the stomach

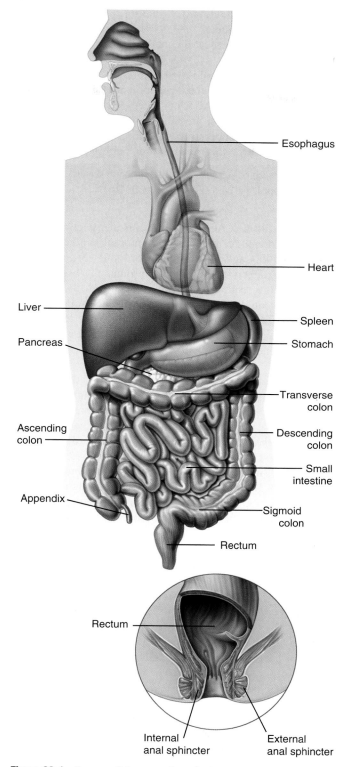

Figure 28-1. Organs of the gastrointestinal tract. (The heart is shown for reference.) **Inset:** Detailed anatomy of the rectum.

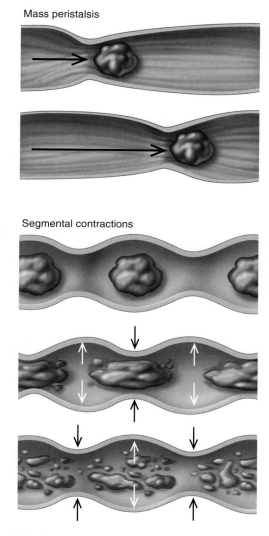

Figure 28-2. Movement of feces through the large intestine by mass peristalsis; segmental contractions break up chyme.

Eventually, fecal material enters the sigmoid colon, where it stays until it passes into the rectum and is eliminated through the anus. The time required for food to move through the entire GI tract, called transit time, is affected by such factors as rate of motility, amount of residue, and the presence or absence of irritating substances in the colon. However, it may take up to 4 hours for gastric emptying and 3 to 10 hours for food to move through the small intestine.

Flatus is swallowed air and gases (especially carbon dioxide, hydrogen, and methane) produced through the digestive process. The GI tract removes this flatus through the anus.

Defecation. To complete passage from the body, feces and flatus move through the rectum, anal canal, and anus. This process is referred to as defecation, or "having a bowel movement," and is under both voluntary and involuntary control. Defecation is initiated by reflexes mediated by local enteric nerves and by the parasympathetic nerve center in the sacral segments of the spinal cord.

and stimulates peristalsis throughout the entire GI tract. The duodenocolic reflex acts in a similar but less forceful manner. The gastrocolic and duodenocolic reflexes are strongest when a person eats after a period of fasting—for example, at breakfast after a night's sleep.

The rectum usually remains empty until just before and during defecation. When the fecal mass or flatus moves from the sigmoid colon into the rectum, the defecation reflex begins. Feces enter the rectum either from an involuntary mass propulsive movement in the colon or from a voluntary increase in intraabdominal pressure caused by contraction of the abdominal muscles and increased intrathoracic pressure against a closed glottis. This straining or bearing-down action is called *Valsalva's maneuver*. It forces the diaphragm downward, thus increasing pressure. Rectal distention then causes increased intrarectal pressure and the urge to evacuate the bowel. Voluntarily forcing feces into the rectum to stimulate the defecation reflex is less efficient than the involuntary mass propulsive movement.

The anal canal has two sphincters, as shown in Figure 28-1. The internal sphincter is made up of smooth muscle and is innervated through the autonomic nervous system. Distention of the rectum by feces causes this sphincter to relax and allow passage of the feces. The external anal sphincter consists of striated muscle and is under voluntary control in most healthy people. When the internal sphincter is being stimulated to relax by descending feces, the external sphincter is stimulated as well. However, the person can voluntarily constrict the external sphincter to delay defecation. In that case, stool remains in the rectum until the defecation reflex is again stimulated.

Problems of Bowel Elimination

Bowel elimination is a basic human need susceptible to a number of problems. Common bowel elimination problems include constipation, fecal impaction, diarrhea, bowel incontinence, and flatulence.

Constipation. **Constipation** is a condition in which feces are abnormally hard and dry and evacuation is abnormally infrequent and may be difficult. Discomfort created by constipation typically interferes with the client's daily activities and sense of well-being. The term *constipation* is used in various ways to include any or all of the following: character of stool, frequency of defecation, time required for passage of the stool through the intestinal tract (intestinal transit time), and difficulty expelling rectal contents through the anal sphincter.

On the basis of the popularity of over-the-counter aids for elimination, constipation appears to be a common worry. In fact, some people feel constipated if they have not had a daily bowel movement. Constipation is a major complaint among older adults; about 30% use laxatives at least once a week.

Besides being uncomfortable, constipation can be hazardous. The hazard exists when the constipated person uses Valsalva's maneuver in an effort to pass feces. This action can cause angina pectoris (chest pain) or even cardiac arrest if the person has underlying cardiac disease. It may also be detrimental to a person with head injuries (by increasing intracranial pressure), respiratory disease (by increasing intrathoracic pressure), or thromboembolic disorders (by

causing thrombi to dislodge). Exhaling through the mouth during straining reduces the chance of increasing intrathoracic pressure. The best precaution, however, is to avoid constipation.

Straining to pass a stool is detrimental in other ways. Over time, it may contribute to the development of hemorrhoids. If the person has had recent bowel surgery, straining might disrupt the suture line. As a precaution, the surgical client may be given enemas preoperatively to eliminate the need for a bowel movement for several days after surgery.

What evidence do you see in this description to suggest that *Constipation* is the correct diagnosis for Dr. Daly?

Fecal Impaction. A **fecal impaction** is a collection of puttylike or hardened feces in the rectum or sigmoid colon that prevents the passage of a normal stool and becomes more and more hardened as the colon continues to absorb water from it. As the fecal mass moves down from the sigmoid colon, additional fecal material may be added to it. Eventually, the mass becomes so hard and large that it cannot pass through the anal canal. It is essentially a lower intestinal obstruction.

Diarrhea. **Diarrhea** is the rapid movement of fecal matter through the intestine, resulting in poor absorption of water, nutrients, and electrolytes and producing abnormally frequent evacuation of watery stools. As with constipation, some people consider the frequency of defecation as part of the definition, but stool consistency is the primary component.

In general, diarrhea indicates increased intestinal motility, which causes GI contents to move rapidly through the tract. Because of the rapid transit time, normal amounts of water are not removed from the feces. In addition, irritation of the mucosal walls may stimulate increased secretions, which add moisture to the fecal mass. Therefore, when the feces reach the rectum and anus, they are still liquid.

Bowel Incontinence. **Bowel incontinence** is the inability to voluntarily control the passage of feces and gas. Bowel evacuation usually occurs voluntarily in response to defecation reflex stimulation. Lack of control is accepted through the first 3 years of life. However, following toilet training, the embarrassment of incontinence causes people to arrange their lives to conceal the problem.

Flatulence. A certain amount of gas occurs normally in the GI tract—usually about 150 cc. Some of it is swallowed, some of it is produced by fermentation in the intestine, and some of it comes from diffusion of gases from the bloodstream. **Flatulence** refers to the presence of abnormal amounts of gas in the GI tract, causing abdominal distention and discomfort. Belching is the expulsion of gas from the upper GI tract and has its origin as swallowed air. Flatulence is expelled from the lower GI tract. Because it may be painful, noisy, and malodorous, flatulence can be distressing to the client.

FACTORS AFFECTING BOWEL ELIMINATION

The bowel elimination process can be affected by many factors, such as a person's lifestyle, culture, and developmental level. Physiological and psychological factors can influence the bowel elimination process as well.

 As you read about the factors affecting bowel elimination, can you relate the information to Dr. Daly? What factors may have influenced his bowel elimination problem?

Lifestyle Factors

The client's lifestyle affects bowel elimination through personal habits of elimination, fluid intake, diet, and exercise. Healthy bowel function is maintained through regular patterns of elimination.

Personal Habits. Personal habits of bowel elimination are important to health. As discussed later, the bowel can be trained to evacuate at a certain time. If this pattern is followed, and all other variables remain constant, the bowel continues to empty regularly. On the other hand, if a person continually ignores the urge to defecate, no rhythmic pattern is established. Travel, which usually disrupts a person's normal schedule, often leads to constipation and sometimes to diarrhea.

Along with timing, many people have other established habits related to bowel elimination, such as drinking warm or cold water, eating prunes, having a cup of coffee, or reading. Continuing these activities may trigger conscious mental stimulation of the defecation reflex.

Nutrition and Fluids. Diet strongly influences bowel habits. Fiber, or indigestible dietary residue, provides bulk in fecal material. Bulk assists peristalsis and increases stimulation of the defecation reflex. A low-fiber, high-carbohydrate diet tends to diminish the reflex. Reduction of overall intake also directly reduces the amount of bulk present. Gas-producing foods may stimulate peristalsis by distending the intestinal walls.

How the GI tract reacts to a particular food depends on the individual (Box 28-1). For instance, chocolate has no effect on many people but causes constipation in some and diarrhea in others. Likewise, milk and milk products constipate some people and cause diarrhea in others. Various foods can also adversely affect defecation patterns and act as irritants. Irritants, such as spicy foods, within the GI tract usually stimulate peristalsis by local reflex stimulation.

The amount of water in the fecal mass affects stool consistency. The lower the water content, the harder the mass, and the more difficult it is to pass the mass through the anus. If the person is fluid depleted, more fluid is absorbed from the GI tract to maintain adequate hydration. Thus dehydration can result in constipation.

Exercise. Muscle tone affects not only the activity of the intestinal musculature itself but also the ability of the supporting skeletal muscles to aid the process of defecation. Weak or atrophied muscles in the abdomen or pelvic floor are ineffective in increasing intraabdominal pressure or assisting the anus to control defecation. This inadequate musculature may result from lack of exercise, immobility, neurological impairment, or multiple pregnancies.

Cultural Factors

Cultural teachings significantly influence a person's defecation habits. In Western society, we are taught strict rules about when and under what conditions defecation can take place. Failure to follow these rules results in social censure and even isolation. Defecation is a private matter and people go to great lengths to ensure this privacy. Many people avoid any discussion of bowel activity. Therefore some people feel highly anxious when forced to seek out a health professional about problems with bowel elimination. Even more dangerous, some people with such problems avoid seeking professional help altogether because they are too embarrassed. Although people in some cultures tend to be very bowel conscious, not all people are embarrassed or reluctant to discuss bowel habits. Assess the client's lifeways for information pertinent to bowel elimination (Box 28-2, p. 666).

Box 28-1	Foods That Alter Gastrointestinal Function		
FOODS THAT MAY CAUSE GAS • Beans • Beer • Cabbage-family vegetables • Carbonated beverages • Cucumbers • Dairy products • Onions • Radishes **FOODS THAT CAUSE ODOR** • Beans • Cabbage family • Cheese	• Eggs • Fish • Garlic • Onions **FOODS THAT THICKEN STOOL** • Applesauce • Bananas • Bread • Cheese • High-fiber foods • Marshmallows • Pasta • Peanut butter	• Rice • Tapioca **FOODS THAT LOOSEN STOOL** • Alcohol • Beans • Beer • Chocolate • Coffee • Fried foods • Prune or grape juice • Raw fruits and vegetables • Spicy foods • Spinach	**FOODS THAT MAY BLOCK AN ILEOSTOMY** • Celery • Coconut • Coleslaw • Mushrooms • Corn • Nuts • Popcorn • Raisins • Raw vegetables and fruits • Seeds • Stringy meats

Developmental Factors

Age plays a role in establishing bowel patterns. Before a child acquires bowel control through toilet training, defecation occurs whenever stool stimulates the rectum. In infancy, the stomach is small and secretes a smaller amount of digestive enzymes. Rapid peristalsis propels food quickly through the GI system, and, because the neuromuscular system is not developed, the infant cannot control defecation.

Bowel elimination usually is not a problem in the adolescent unless the person has a health problem. However, adolescents can experience changes in bowel habits associated with growth and irregular patterns of eating and sleeping. During adolescence, the large intestine grows rapidly. At the same time, adolescents tend to eat more. Adolescent eating habits vary from very good to poor, with the person's self-concept influencing the intake.

Among older adults, vulnerability to GI disturbances rises. Cancer occurs more frequently, and motor and neurological disturbances are more prevalent. Box 28-3 addresses screening for colon cancer. In addition, diverticulosis (an outpouching in the intestinal wall) occurs almost exclusively after age 40.

Nutritional intake commonly changes in older adults as well. Inadequate dentition impairs mastication, allowing food not adequately chewed to enter the GI tract. Furthermore, the amount of digestive enzymes in saliva and gastric acids in the stomach declines, reducing the ability to break down foods. Along with upper-GI changes, the lower GI tract develops deficiencies in proteins, vitamins, and minerals. A muscular decline occurs as well, and the internal and external sphincters may not be controlled normally. In addition, slowing of nerve impulses to the rectum may cause some people to be less conscious of the need to defecate.

Physiological Factors

Bowel elimination problems can be caused by such physiological factors as pregnancy, motor and sensory disturbances, intestinal pathologies, medications, surgical procedures, and diagnostic procedures.

Pregnancy. Pregnancy itself and medications taken during pregnancy can influence a woman's normal bowel elimination pattern. As the fetus grows, pressure may be exerted on the rectum, slowing the passage of feces through the intestine. Exertion for defecation can cause other elimination problems, such as hemorrhoids. Iron and vitamin supplements prescribed for many women during pregnancy are constipating, which can cause additional problems.

Motor and Sensory Disturbances. Motor or sensory disturbances may result from spinal cord injury, head injury, cerebrovascular accident (stroke), neurological disease, or any condition that causes immobility or otherwise interferes with motor or sensory function. Immobility hinders the person's ability to respond to the urge to defecate. For instance, the person who is unable to walk to the bathroom or reach a call bell to summon help may (1) suppress the urge to defecate, which could eventually lead to constipation, or (2) suffer fecal incontinence.

Intestinal Pathology. Pathological conditions in the intestine itself can be heralded by constipation or diarrhea. These conditions can result from obstruction, inflammation, infection, or cancer.

- *Bowel obstruction:* Partial or complete blockage caused by a tumor, inflammation, strangulation, or adhesion that prevents the movement of chyme through the intestine. Bowel obstruction may initially present with constipation or diarrhea associated with abdominal distention, pain, and hyperactive bowel sounds in one quadrant.
- *Crohn's disease:* A chronic inflammatory bowel disease of unknown origin, usually affecting the ileum, the colon, or another part of the gastrointestinal tract. It is characterized by frequent attacks of diarrhea, severe abdominal pain, nausea, fever, chills, weakness, anorexia, and weight loss.
- *Ulcerative colitis:* A chronic, episodic, inflammatory disease of the large intestine and rectum. It is characterized by profuse watery diarrhea containing varying amounts of blood, mucus, and pus.
- *Cancer:* Signs and symptoms that may indicate referral are a change in bowel habits and blood in the stool. Encourage clients to obtain routine screening tests for colon and rectal cancer (see Box 28-4).
- *Infectious diarrhea:* Sudden onset of watery diarrhea that can signal acute viral, bacterial, and protozoal infections. Most bacterial or viral diarrhea will resolve in 1 to 7 days. However, severe fluid and electrolyte disturbances can be life threatening, especially to the very young and very old.

Medications. Common side effects of medications are constipation or diarrhea. Medications administered for bowel regulation, antibiotics, narcotics, sympathomimetics, antidepressants, and anticholinergics are examples. A drug given to prevent constipation may cause diarrhea, and a drug given to prevent diarrhea may cause constipation. The overuse of laxatives can lead to physiological and psychological dependence on them. Additionally, some medications may affect the color and odor of the feces.

Surgical Procedures. Surgical procedures commonly result in constipation for several reasons. For one, direct handling of the bowel during abdominal surgery can temporarily stop peristalsis; when the absence of peristalsis persists beyond 3 days, the condition is called **paralytic ileus.** For another, any procedure involving the pelvis or perineum, such as rectal, hip, or gynecological surgery, can affect defecation patterns through the effects of postoperative edema and discom-

THE·COST·OF·CARE   **Box 28-4**
Screening for Colorectal Cancer

Common wisdom in health care today suggests that preventive health care strategies will result in earlier detection of cancer, and thus will make the cost of treatment less for the overall health care system. However, when you screen more people you not only detect more cases of cancer, you also screen more people who do not have cancer. Thus the cost of screening is high. In fact, it is estimated that the cost, per year of life saved by colorectal screening, is about $15,000 to $20,000.

Nurses are participating in reducing this cost by becoming trained to perform endoscopy. However, the training needs to be sufficient to ensure that these nurses can be effective in the technique of endoscopy, examination of the intestinal mucosa, and biopsy of suspicious lesions. The training at one center includes 3 months of didactic training and performing 50 endoscopies under direct supervision. It was felt that after 250 examinations, the nurse endoscopist has developed the skill and confidence to provide a more comfortable examination for the client. This program includes ongoing periodic monitoring of the nurse endoscopist.

Nurses in a general practice setting can also help in the cost and accuracy of screening by providing client education about the need for periodic screening, risk factors for colorectal cancer, and education to ensure the correct technique in collecting specimens for Hemoccult tests.

Modified from Eslemon, N., Stucky-Marshall, L., & Talamonti, M. S. (2001). Screening for colorectal cancer: Developing a preventive health care program utilizing nurse endoscopists. *Gastroenterology Nursing, 24*(1), 12-19; Frazier, A. L., Colditz, G. A., Fuchs, C. S., & Kuntz, K. M. (2000). Cost-effectiveness of screening for colorectal cancer in the general population. *Journal of the American Medical Association, 284*(15), 1954-1961.

fort. Operative and postoperative medications can contribute to constipation as well.

Additionally, bowel function can be altered permanently by surgical intervention. Fecal diversion involves channeling intestinal contents out of the body at a site other than the anus. The surgical procedure used to create an opening through the abdominal wall and into the intestine is called an **ostomy** procedure. An **ileostomy** is a surgical procedure involving the creation of an opening between the ileum and the abdominal wall. Because water is not reabsorbed until feces reach the colon, the feces from an ileostomy are liquid. A **colostomy** is a surgical procedure involving the creation of an opening between the colon and the abdominal wall. Feces from this area of the colon are semisolid or solid, depending on the segment of the colon that is resected. Each of these surgical procedures establishes a **stoma,** which is an opening between the abdominal wall and the intestine through which fecal material passes.

An ileostomy may be performed because of cancer, a congenital defect, or trauma. However, the most frequent reason stems from ulcerative colitis or regional ileitis (Crohn's disease). Because of the placement of the stoma in the small intestine, the flow of fecal material in most cases is constant and cannot be regulated. Surgical techniques do exist in which a continent ileostomy is formed by creating an internal pouch with a nipple valve that can be emptied with a catheter at the person's convenience.

A colostomy may be performed because of trauma, intestinal obstruction, birth defect, or cancer. It may involve

One-piece drainable pouch
with wire closure

One-piece drainable pouch
with narrow valve

One-piece
nondrainable pouch

Clamp
closure

Two-piece drainable pouch
with stoma wafer

Stoma wafers

Figure 28-3. Examples of ostomy pouches, closures, and stoma wafers.

ascending (rarely), transverse, descending, or sigmoid portion of the colon. The farther down the intestine the stoma is placed, the better are the chances of regulating the bowel. Some people develop such reliable bowel control that they wear no fecal collection bag and only a small dressing to protect the stoma from irritation by clothing. However, most people with ostomies wear a collection pouch or bag that is changed periodically (Figure 28-3).

Psychosocial Factors

Clinical evidence suggests a relationship between bowel elimination patterns and stress, although the relationship is not completely clear. Agitation and nervousness can cause diarrhea, usually in the form of frequent small stools without a large-volume fluid loss. Some disease processes that cause diarrhea, gaseous distention, and ulcer formation may have psychological elements either as cause or effect. On the other hand, mental depression can contribute to constipation by slowing all bodily activities. Indeed, it may be the depressed client's chief complaint.

ASSESSMENT

The need for assessment of bowel elimination problems commonly arises after a client reports a problem. However, it should also be a routine part of any health assessment because bowel elimination is frequently disrupted by illness, surgery, or other treatment.

General Assessment of Bowel Elimination

The general assessment of bowel elimination should include the usual pattern of elimination, a history pertinent to bowel elimination, a physical assessment of the abdomen, observation of feces, and review of diagnostic tests.

Health History. The health history should include questions regarding the client's normal elimination pattern, health habits, and any psychological or physiological alterations pertinent to bowel elimination. The following are pertinent historical questions:

- What is your normal bowel elimination pattern, including time of day and frequency?
- How often do you use laxatives or bowel elimination aids?
- What is your normal dietary intake for a day? Has it changed recently?
- What is your normal fluid intake for a day? Has it changed recently?
- What kind of exercise or physical activity do you get? Has it changed recently?
- Are you unusually anxious or do you have excess stress in you life?
- What medications do you take?
- What do your feces look like, including amount, color, consistency, constituents, frequency, odor, and shape?
- Have you noticed any changes in your bowel elimination pattern?
- Has your use of bowel elimination aids changed recently?
- Have you had any gastrointestinal surgery?
- Do you have a history of stomach or bowel problems?
- How is your current emotional state? Is it different from your normal?
- Have you experienced recent weight gain or loss?

Analyze symptoms (abdominal pain, nausea, vomiting, constipation, diarrhea, incontinence) for onset, duration, frequency, severity, associated symptoms. Elicit a history of other, possibly related, health problems: thyroid disease, diabetes, lactose intolerance, gastroesophageal reflux disease, peptic ulcer, gallbladder disease, pancreatitis, diverticulitis, or ulcerative colitis.

 What questions would you ask Dr. Daly to determine the best course of action to assist with his bowel elimination problem?

Physical Examination. Physical assessment of the bowel system should include inspection, auscultation, percussion, and palpation of the abdomen. It should also include inspection and palpation of the anus. With the client in the supine position, inspect the abdomen for peristalsis, contour, symmetry, scars, distention, and masses. Look for signs of hernia, dehydration, striae, or engorged veins. Auscultate the client's bowel sounds, noting their frequency and character. Use percussion to elicit tympani, which indicate the presence of gas, or dullness (indicating fluid and feces) in the GI tract. Use palpation to assess for areas of tenderness, guarding, rebound tenderness, or palpable masses in the abdomen. Turn the client to the side and inspect and palpate the anus to assess for lumps, ulcers, inflammation, rashes, or excoriations.

Evaluate the client for abdominal distention and "gas pains." Ask about the duration of any problem, abdominal cramps, dietary and medication intake, and anxiety, stress, or systemic disease that might contribute to the problem.

Diagnostic Tests.
Review the results of diagnostic tests. Prepare the client for and assist with additional diagnostic tests that have been ordered to help identify problems with bowel elimination. Common tests include observation of fecal characteristics and laboratory analysis of feces, radiographic examination of the bowel, and direct endoscopic visualization of the bowel.

STOOL ANALYSIS

SPECIMEN COLLECTION. Stool specimens are collected in a clean, dry container. If the client uses a toilet, place a receptacle under the seat. If the specimen is collected at home, the client can drape a piece of plastic wrap over the toilet seat so it droops in the middle to catch the feces. After depositing the specimen, the client then finishes the collection process by bringing the corners and edges of the wrap together and twisting them to form a sealed package.

To perform a test on the specimen, use a tongue blade to transfer a portion of it to a smaller, covered specimen container for transport to a lab. Visible blood or mucus should be included in the sample. Avoid mixing urine, soap, or detergent with the specimen.

If the client cannot produce any feces, gently pass a rectal swab beyond the internal sphincter and rotate it carefully to collect fecal material. Then place the specimen in a suitable container for transport to the laboratory.

When collecting stool specimens, make sure you maintain the conditions needed for accurate test results. For example, collect specimens for culture in a clean, dry container and send them to the laboratory immediately. A specimen to be tested for ova and parasites should be examined immediately because the organisms die if they cool below body temperature. On the other hand, you can refrigerate specimens not needing microscopic examination if you are unable to deliver them to the laboratory right away.

Action Alert! Take care in collecting specimens. Urine, soap, detergent, and drying of the specimen destroy bacteria.

To check for pinworms, you will need to collect a specimen from the perianal area. To do so, press the sticky side of a strip of nonfrosted cellophane tape over and around the client's anus. Remove it immediately, place it on a glass slide (sticky side down), and send it to the laboratory for examination. Because the female worm deposits eggs on the perianal area during the night, you will want to collect the specimen early in the morning, before the person has bathed or had a bowel movement.

CHARACTERISTICS OF FECES. Fecal material is composed of food residues, bacteria, some white blood cells, epithelial cells, intestinal secretions, and water. Assessing frequency, amount, color, consistency, shape, and odor can help to identify GI problems (Table 28-1, p. 670).

Bile pigments produce the normal brown color of stool. Absence of bile causes the stool to be white, gray, or clay-colored and may indicate biliary obstruction or lack of bile production (acholia). Light-colored stools also can result from barium or antacid ingestion. A gray stool mixed with observable fat and mucus is called **steatorrhea** and results from the malabsorption of fat. In infants, the first stools (called meconium) are normally black and tarry from ingested amniotic fluid, epithelial cells, and bile.

The consistency of stool is a reflection of its water content. Stools can be liquid, unformed, soft, or hard. An abnormal consistency indicates constipation or diarrhea.

The shape of the stool normally resembles that of the rectum. An abnormal finding would be that of a consistently narrowed, pencil-shaped stool, which indicates obstruction of the distal portion of the large intestine, as might occur with carcinoma.

The odor of the stool is characteristically pungent and is produced by bacterial flora and by some foods and medications. Blood or infection in the GI tract causes detectable noxious changes in the normal odor.

LABORATORY ANALYSIS OF FECES. In the laboratory, stool specimens can be examined for bile or bilirubin, blood, microorganisms, ova, and parasites. Bacteria are detected through cultures. Microscopic examination may reveal meat fibers and fat, indicating a malabsorption syndrome.

A test used to detect **occult blood** in feces (an amount too small to be seen without a microscope) may be your responsibility. You will perform the test in the clinical setting or teach the client to collect the specimen in the home setting. The instructions in Procedure 28-1 (p. 670) are for the Hemoccult test, which uses **guaiac** as a reagent. Other brands may have slightly different instructions.

Besides supplying information about a current bowel disorder, this test also can be used as a screening procedure for colorectal cancer. The American Cancer Society recommends that people over age 50 have annual tests for occult blood in the stool.

Radiographic Examination of Bowel.
Radiographic examination reveals the location and contour of the bowel and supporting structures as well as the presence and distribution of fecal material and gas in the bowel. A flat plate of the abdomen is taken without contrast material and therefore requires no special preparation. It shows shadows, fluid levels, and gas.

More specific information can be obtained from a barium radiographic study, usually called a "lower GI series." Barium is instilled as an enema to provide a contrast medium to outline the bowel. For maximum visualization, the bowel should be thoroughly cleansed prior to a barium enema. After the study, a laxative is administered to ensure its complete evacuation. Barium left in the colon can cause impaction (a stool mass too large and hard to pass through the anus) and even obstruction. Although a barium enema is relatively safe, it can produce an anaphylactic reaction in about 1 in 750,000 examinations.

Action Alert! Be prepared to manage an anaphylactic reaction in a client who has a barium enema.

Direct Visualization of Bowel. A fiberoptic endoscope inserted through the anus and advanced through the bowel allows direct visualization of the lower GI tract. The physician may perform a proctoscopy, sigmoidoscopy, or colonoscopy, depending on the area of the colon to be examined.

Table 28-1	**Characteristics of Feces**		
Characteristic	**Normal**	**Abnormal**	**Possible Cause**
Amount	150 g (varies with diet)		
Color	Adult: brown	Black or tarry	• Iron ingestion
	Infant: yellow		• Bismuth ingestion
			• Charcoal ingestion
		Black and tarry (melena)	• Upper GI bleeding
		Pale	• Malabsorption of fat
			• Diet high in milk and low in meat
		Red	• Lower GI bleeding
			• Ingestion of beets
			• Ingestion of pyrvinium pamoate, an antiparasite agent
			• Hemorrhoids, if the red is smeared on the surface of feces
		Red orange	• Ingestion of rifampin, an antibiotic
		Green or orange	• Large amounts of ingested chlorophyll
			• Intestinal infection
		White or clay colored	• Absence of bile
Consistency	Formed, soft	Liquid	• Diarrhea
			• Increased intestinal motility
		Hard	• Constipation
Constituents	Cells lining intestinal mucosa,	Blood	• GI bleeding
	dead bacteria, bile pigment,	Fat	• Malabsorption
	fat, protein, undigested	Foreign objects	• Accidental ingestion
	food, water	Mucus	• Inflammatory condition
		Pus	• Bacterial infection
Odor	Pungent (affected by client's	Noxious change	• Blood in feces
	own bacterial flora)		• Infection
Shape	Appearance of diameter of	Narrow, pencil shaped,	• Obstructive condition
	rectum, about 2.5 cm	or stringlike	
	(1 inch) for adults		

PROCEDURE 28-1 TESTING FECES FOR OCCULT BLOOD

TIME TO ALLOW
Novice: 5 min.
Expert: 5 min.

The Hemoccult test is one of many commercial products used as a screening test for blood in the feces that is not visible to the naked eye. The test is used to detect gastrointestinal bleeding and to screen for colorectal cancer. Testing three separate specimens reduces the incidence of false-negative results. Restricting red meat for 2 to 3 days before the test reduces false-positive results.

DELEGATION GUIDELINES
The test for occult blood is a simple test that may be delegated to a nursing assistant. Review of the instructions for collecting the specimen and test performance can ensure uniform test results.

EQUIPMENT NEEDED
- Hemoccult test slide folder
- Clean gloves
- Wooden applicator
- Hemoccult developing solution

1. Follow preliminary guidelines for nursing procedures (see inside front cover).

2. Instruct the client about the purpose of the test and have him defecate into a collection container. Tell him to avoid urinating in the container. Urine may contaminate the stool sample. If the client has to urinate, he can do so before collecting the stool sample. *Hospital policy may require that the specimen be sent to the lab.*

3. Put on clean gloves. Clean gloves help to prevent transmission of microorganisms from the client's feces.

4. With the applicator, obtain a small specimen of feces and smear a thin layer in the first box of the cardboard Hemoccult slide. While obtaining the specimen, observe and document its characteristics. A small specimen is sufficient to perform the test accurately.

5. With the opposite tip of the applicator, obtain a second specimen of feces from another location and smear it thinly in the second box of the cardboard Hemoccult slide. Using the opposite end of the applicator prevents contamination of the second sample with the first.

6. Close the cardboard Hemoccult slide cover and turn it over to the reverse side. Open the cardboard flap on the reverse side and apply two drops of Hemoccult developing solution to the guaiac paper. Apply the exact amount of solution specified (one or two drops) to ensure the accuracy of the test.

7. As soon as you apply the developing solution, start keeping track of the time. If you notice a bluish discoloration on the guaiac paper 30 to 60 seconds after applying the solution, the sample contained occult blood. Consider the result positive if both samples show a positive result (see illustration).

8. Dispose of the Hemoccult slide in a biohazard waste container, discard your gloves, and wash your hands. Standard precautions dictate that human excrement be treated as hazardous waste.

9. Document the characteristics of the client's feces and the results of the guaiac test in the client's chart. Charting both objective findings and test results gives a complete picture of the specimen.

HOME CARE CONSIDERATIONS

Clients are often taught to collect a specimen for screening for occult blood in the home. Supply the person with the Hemoccult slide, a tongue blade, mailing pouch for returning slides, and the Hemoccult product instructions. Some labs may supply the developer or reagent for testing at home.

You may give the client the following instructions:
- Read and carefully follow the instructions included in the package.
- Wait 3 days after the end of a menstrual period; do not collect when you have blood in your urine or from hemorrhoids.
- Collect from a toilet bowl only if it is clean and free of chemicals; flush three times before collecting.
- Collect samples and test (if instructed) from three different bowel movements.
- Protect Hemoccult slides from heat, light, and chemicals.
- Seven days prior to the test, stop taking aspirin or nonsteroidal antiinflammatory drugs. Acetaminophen is allowed.
- Three days prior to the test, stop eating vitamin C, red meat, and raw broccoli, cauliflower, horseradish, parsnips, radishes, turnips, and melons.

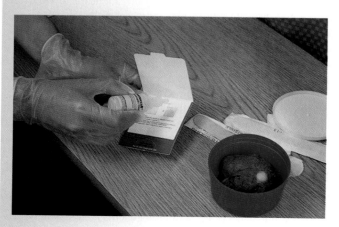

Step 7. Applying Hemoccult developing solution to the guaiac paper.

The endoscopes used to observe the bowel are hollow tubes through which the examiner can see GI structures. They also allow suction and collection of tissue for biopsy.

Before an endoscopic procedure, explain the test to the client to allay any anxiety. Also, make sure that bowel preparation is complete. If the person's bowel has not been thoroughly cleansed, feces can obscure the fiberoptic examination. Typically, preparation begins 24 to 48 hours before the procedure and includes dietary and fluid restrictions, laxatives, enemas, or a combination of laxatives and saline enema.

A common method of emptying the bowel uses a solution called GoLYTELY (pronounced "go-lightly"). GoLYTELY cleanses the bowel without causing the excretion or absorption of fluid and electrolytes by the body that often occurs with traditional purgatives and enemas. This method is safer for people with congestive heart disease, chronic obstructive pulmonary disease, or controlled renal failure. The solution is consumed cold at a rate of 1.2 to 1.8 L per hour. The client soon develops diarrhea and, within 2 to 4 hours, the rectal output is clear. Because the solution works so quickly, make sure the client has ready access to toilet facilities.

Throughout the endoscopic procedure, provide emotional support. Before the procedure, administer a relaxant medication, as prescribed. Then help the client into the position chosen by the physician, often a side-lying position with one knee pulled up to the chest. Assess the client throughout the procedure because of the awkward position and the effects of the medication. Monitor the vital signs regularly during the procedure. Assist the physician with equipment and specimens, as necessary.

After the procedure, continue to monitor the client's vital signs. Inspect often for fresh anal bleeding, which may indicate continued oozing at a biopsy site. Severe abdominal pain could indicate a bowel perforation.

> *Action Alert!* Monitor for circulatory and respiratory problems during endoscopy examination.

Focused Assessment for *Constipation*

Assessment for *Constipation* is initiated from a client complaint or your observation that the client has been 3 days without a bowel movement. Assess for signs and symptoms and the probable cause.

Defining Characteristics. The client usually recognizes or suspects constipation when the frequency of bowel movements is less than usual and the abdomen feels full and distended. Additionally, the client may report a feeling of fullness or pressure in the rectum, straining to evacuate the stool, abdominal pain, appetite impairment, back pain, headache, interference with daily living, and the use of laxatives. Sometimes the fecal mass can be palpated in the abdomen (NANDA, 2001). Hard, dry stool or difficulty passing stool confirms the diagnosis of *Constipation.*

Clients sometimes complain of constipation when digestive signs are absent. The diagnosis of *Perceived constipation* should be made only after ruling out actual constipation. The diagnosis is made when the client expects a daily bowel movement and uses laxatives, enemas, and suppositories to make it happen. The expectation may include passage of stool at the same time every day. Perceived constipation is common among older adults who have health practices ingrained from another era.

Related Factors. To select appropriate nursing actions, you need to identify the cause or causes and determine if the problem is expected to be acute or chronic. An acute problem would need immediate, definitive intervention, whereas a chronic problem would demand long-term lifestyle management. Common causative lifestyle factors include a lack of established bowel pattern; inadequate diet, fluids, and exercise; emotional depression; and weak pelvic floor muscles.

Other, less obvious lifestyle factors may contribute to constipation. Inconvenience is frequently a factor. When the urge to defecate is repeatedly ignored, stool remaining in the rectum continues to lose water and stops stimulating normal reflexes. Overuse of laxatives, suppositories, and enemas contribute to the problem primarily through the resulting loss of intrinsic innervation and atrophy of the smooth muscle necessary for defecation. Constipation frequently accompanies pregnancy, both because of hormonal changes and because of external pressure on the intestine.

Constipation is often associated with an acute illness because of the change in routine, diet, fluid intake, and mobility. Immobility alone is sufficient cause. Constipation may be a symptom of intestinal pathological conditions, including neoplasm, stricture, hernia, megacolon (excessive dilation or stretching of the colon), diverticular disease, and painful anal lesions, in which case the underlying pathology must be considered in developing a plan of intervention.

Constipation may be associated with chronic health problems. Besides the lifestyle changes required to manage a chronic health problem, medications for pain, hypertension, depression, and gastric hyperacidity contribute to constipation. Additional examples include anesthetics, anticholinergics, and iron supplements.

Focused Assessment for *Diarrhea*

Defining Characteristics. To assess the client with *Diarrhea,* analyze the symptom with particular attention to fluid and electrolyte loss. Question the client carefully about the frequency and characteristics of the stool. In diarrhea the stool is described as loose, liquid, or unformed. It may contain blood or mucus. Ask the client to describe the nature of the diarrhea. Diarrhea may involve frequent, small stools, or it may represent the loss of a large volume of water. In the latter case, the person may become dehydrated and deficient in important electrolytes. Estimate the amount of water loss on the basis of the number and volume of stools. Is the person able to replace the fluid loss? Look for signs of dehydration—sluggish skin turgor, sunken eyes, low urine output. In the pediatric client, you may notice an absence of tears.

Ask about associated systemic symptoms such as fever, myalgia, malaise, anorexia, and headache. Also ask about associated abdominal symptoms, such as urgency, flatus, pain, abdominal cramping, nausea, and vomiting. Diarrhea is usually alkaline, because it contains digestive enzymes. Assess for skin breakdown or irritation in the perianal area.

Related Factors. Also ask questions that will help determine the cause of the diarrhea. Ask about the duration of the problem, recent exposure to infected people, recent travel, dietary and medication intake, and the existence of anxiety, stress, or systemic disease that might contribute to a change in elimination patterns.

The causes of diarrhea are numerous and different for acute and chronic diarrhea. *Acute diarrhea* may be caused by emotional states, especially anxiety; infectious organisms, such as bacteria, viruses, and parasites; alterations in diet, such as increased greasy or spicy foods, or food to which the person is allergic; and medications, such as iron supplements, thyroid agents, magnesium-containing antacids, antibiotics, lactulose, cimetidine, antihypertensives, colchicine, digitalis, and laxatives.

Causes of *chronic diarrhea* have been identified as lactose-containing or hyperosmolar nutritional supplements; sorbitol and mannitol (ingredients); such diseases as hyperthyroidism, diabetes mellitus, adrenal insufficiency, hyperparathyroidism, inflammatory bowel diseases, and cancer of the colon; GI surgery; radiation enterocolitis; laxative abuse; alcohol abuse; and chemotherapeutic agents.

Focused Assessment for *Bowel Incontinence*

The risk for *Bowel incontinence* is associated with physical and mental disabilities. An older adult with decreased mobility or cognitive impairment is the most likely to have bowel incontinence. Developmentally disabled people with physical handicaps and mental retardation are the second largest group in whom incontinence is seen.

> *Action Alert!* Investigate any fecal odor that arises near a person or a source of soiled clothes or linens.

Defining Characteristics. Fecal incontinence is almost always involuntary and can occur at any age. A primary question to ask is whether or not the person is aware of the incontinence. Then you need to determine if the client is able to assist in the solution or if the nurse needs to assume responsibility for managing the problem. Determine if the client recognizes the incontinence but cannot control it because of the explosive nature of the diarrhea, an inability to move to the toilet in a timely manner, a loss of rectal sphincter control, or the presence of a colostomy or an ileostomy. On the other hand, the person may not recognize that incontinence has occurred.

The focus of the assessment then becomes to determine if the problem is correctable or manageable. Determine the frequency, the duration of the problem, and the presence of associated symptoms such as abdominal cramps.

Related Factors. Related factors for *Bowel incontinence* are the following:

- Gastrointestinal disorder with explosive diarrhea (urge to defecate too overwhelming to control)

- Neuromuscular disorders in which the person lacks the sensation to recognize the urge to defecate
- Loss of anal sphincter control, ileostomy, colostomy; may be secondary to hemorrhoids, tumors, lacerations, rectal prolapse, fistulas, and loss of sensory innervation
- Impaired cognition

Psychologically, incontinence may be secondary to mental illness, as well as being itself the cause of various emotional problems. *Encopresis* is the socially inappropriate passage of a stool when no physical reason exists to account for the behavior. It is believed to occur because of an emotional disturbance or delay in the maturation process. Sometimes a formerly continent child or adult becomes incontinent as a means to gain attention or to express anger.

Probably the most important consequence of incontinence is the loss of self-respect, which is intensified by the reactions of significant others in the person's environment, including nurses, physicians, friends, and relatives. Also, incontinence causes skin irritation and breakdown, and soiling of clothes and linen.

Focused Assessment for *Flatulence*

Flatulence is recognized from a swollen feeling, abdominal distention, cramping, and eructation from the anus (flatus). Respiratory distress may also occur if the distended abdomen pushes against the diaphragm. Abdominal percussion produces a tympanic sound.

Probably the most common predisposing factor in flatulence is excessive air swallowing, which results from chewing gum, drinking carbonated beverages, eating rapidly, or sucking through straws. Anxiety and postnasal drip can also lead to excessive air swallowing.

Other causes of gaseous distention include constipation; slowed intestinal motility, as may occur after abdominal surgery; bowel obstruction; medications that decrease peristalsis; decreased physical activity; and eating such foods as beans, cabbage, radishes, onions, cauliflower, and cucumbers.

Focused Assessment for *Fecal Impaction*

Impaction consists of hardened feces that a person cannot pass voluntarily or involuntarily. Probably the most common predisposing factor is immobility. Other predisposing factors are nutritional intake, abuse of laxatives, and poor fluid intake.

> *Action Alert!* Assess for fecal impaction when there is a continuous seepage of loose feces.

Suspect a fecal impaction when the client has abdominal distention, small amounts of liquid stool, and the absence of a bowel movement over several days. However, a fecal impaction can be present even if the client has had small regular bowel movements that have not emptied the colon. The impaction is confirmed by abdominal palpation, digital exam for the presence of hardened stool in the rectum, or radiographic confirmation. Inquire about the date of the client's last known bowel movement, any previous impaction problems, dietary and medication intake, and immobility that might contribute to the problem. Previous bowel surgery, decreased bowel sounds, immobility, and chronic use of

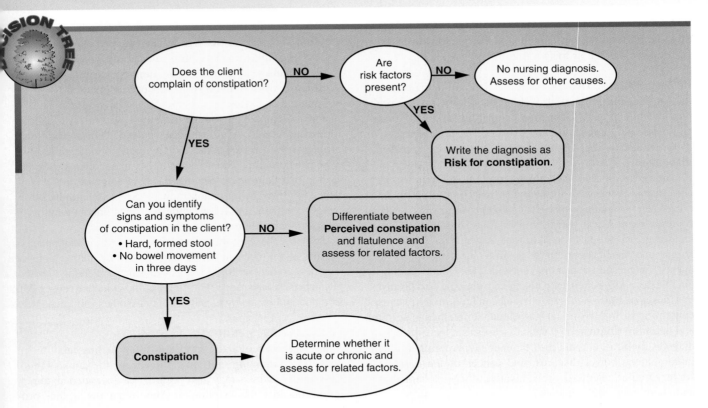

Figure 28-4. Decision tree for constipation. Diagnoses are shown in rectangles. Within these rectangles, diagnoses shown in **bold** type are NANDA-approved nursing diagnoses; diagnoses shown in regular type are not NANDA-approved nursing diagnoses.

suppositories are risk factors. It is usually associated with decreased mental status.

Often the first symptom of a fecal impaction is the inability to pass a normal stool. However, probably the most definitive symptom is the seepage of liquid stool from the anus. Liquefaction provides the only way that fecal material can get around the impaction. Usually the liquid appears in small amounts, which helps to differentiate it from diarrhea. However, bacterial action on the fecal mass sometimes causes the production of copious amounts of liquid stool. Also, the seepage of stool is usually uncontrolled, since the anal sphincters have become less competent, secondary to prolonged stimulation of the defecation reflex by the hardened mass. Other symptoms indicating impaction include an almost continuous urge to defecate, rectal pain, abdominal fullness, nausea and vomiting, shortness of breath, hypertension, and abdominal distention.

Confirm the presence of an impaction by performing a digital rectal examination. With a gloved hand, insert a well-lubricated forefinger through the anus into the rectum. If you feel a hard fecal mass, an impaction probably exists. If you do not feel a mass but symptoms are present, the mass may be higher up in the colon, out of reach.

DIAGNOSIS

The use of a "risk for" diagnosis is based on the philosophy of early detection and prevention of health problems. For example,

a postoperative client is at risk for constipation. Once the diagnosis is actual, it could be written as *Constipation related to immobility and anesthesia.* Figure 28-4 offers more information.

When considering a nursing diagnosis, be sure that the focus of care and interventions are appropriate to the client. Examples of nursing diagnoses that are pertinent to bowel elimination are *Diarrhea related to excessive use of laxatives, Bowel incontinence related to cognitive impairment, Perceived constipation related to impaired thought process,* and *Bowel incontinence related to effects of medication.* Clustering appropriate data can help you arrive at the most appropriate nursing diagnoses (Table 28-2).

Disturbed body image disturbance may be present in the client who has had a fecal diversion procedure, such as an ileostomy or a colostomy. The presence of an ostomy is an actual change in body image and may result in the client being reluctant to learn to manage the ostomy care. Bowel incontinence also can produce a body image disturbance because it represents a socially unacceptable activity. Embarrassment is often a major factor in managing incontinence.

Ineffective health maintenance is present any time a client has to undergo a lifestyle change to manage a bowel elimination problem. The client with an ostomy clearly has to change methods of self-care for bowel elimination. However, any client who is required to change diet, take medications, or alter the usual pattern of activity and exercise will have to manage the effect of those changes on bowel elimination.

Table 28-2 *Clustering Data to Make a Nursing Diagnosis*
BOWEL ELIMINATION PROBLEMS

Data Cluster	Diagnosis
An 84-year-old ambulatory woman with Alzheimer's disease has an incontinent bowel movement every morning after breakfast. She cannot find her room in the nursing home; it is not clear if she feels the urge to defecate.	*Bowel incontinence* related to impaired cognition and sensory perception
The 3rd day after gallbladder surgery, a 50-year-old woman calls the doctor's office complaining of abdominal distention and cramping. She reports that she has not had a bowel movement since the surgery. She has been taking acetaminophen with codeine for pain.	*Constipation* related to decreased physical activity and use of pain medication
A 70-year-old woman has been admitted to the hospital with leukemia. She tells you that she must have milk of magnesia every morning before breakfast. She reports that her stool is unformed and a small amount.	*Perceived constipation* related to possible inaccurate health belief
After returning home from traveling in a foreign country, parents report that their 18-month-old infant has developed loose stools that have occurred about seven times a day for more than 2 days.	*Diarrhea* related to possible infectious processes
A 47-year-old man had abdominal exploratory surgery. On the 2nd postoperative day, he complained of abdominal cramping and gas pains.	*Flatulence* related to slowed peristalsis secondary to surgery and decreased mobility
A resident of a long-term-care facility has been unable to ambulate or move herself for about 2 years. She recently began losing weight, about 2 to 3 pounds per month, because she was refusing her meals. She also began refusing to take her laxatives on a regular basis. A nurse's aide reported to the charge nurse that she was constantly cleaning up loose, seeping stool for this resident.	*Fecal impaction* related to decreased mobility, decreased nutritional intake, and refusal of laxative medications

Many times, older adult clients have the nursing diagnosis *Ineffective health maintenance* because they cannot identify and manage a bowel elimination problem. For example, a client may be homebound with very poor nutritional intake. Mobility has declined over time and, as a result, the usual routine of a daily bowel movement after a high-fiber diet is gone. The visiting nurse becomes involved with the client and identifies the nursing diagnosis *Ineffective health maintenance* not only for bowel elimination but for dietary intake and hygiene needs.

Risk for impaired skin integrity is appropriate when the client has bowel incontinence. The contents of the colon are alkaline compared to the skin and, therefore, highly irritable to the skin. The risk for impaired skin integrity is especially high when other risk factors for *Impaired skin integrity* exist.

Toileting self-care deficit is highly associated with bowel elimination problems. The client may be unable to independently perform toileting activities because of immobility, lack of full range of motion, weakness, or intolerance for activity.

PLANNING

After performing a thorough bowel history and assessment, you will plan care to address the nursing diagnoses. During the planning phase of the nursing process, nursing interventions are identified to assist the client in achieving outcomes for problem resolution.

Expected Outcomes for the Client With *Constipation*

The goal for a diagnosis of *Constipation* is that the client resume a normal bowel elimination pattern. Most of the time, a

positive outcome is inferred from observation of frequency and the client's subjective experience and report that bowel elimination is normal.

If the problem is a direct result of an acute illness, such as a postoperative client who had no bowel elimination for 76 hours after surgery, the outcome of normal bowel elimination by discharge from the hospital is usually sufficient. However, if the problem can be expected to return—that is, the client is at continued risk or the problem is the result of chronic illness—the outcomes need to include evidence that the person is prepared to manage the risk.

The outcomes may include the following:
- Listing foods with high-fiber content
- Explaining the importance of exercise in relationship to the GI system
- Stating types of laxatives available
- Identifying side effects and contraindications of bowel laxatives
- Administering appropriate laxatives to maintain normal bowel elimination

Expected Outcomes for the Client With *Diarrhea*

The expected outcome for the diagnosis *Diarrhea* is also that the client resume a normal bowel elimination pattern. No evidence of diarrhea will be present, as manifested by a soft, medium-size to large bowel movement every day or every few days, as is the client's routine. The client with diarrhea should be evaluated for risk for reoccurrence. The outcomes may include the following:
- The client will be clean and dry.
- The client will avoid foods that contribute to diarrhea.
- The client will note the frequency and amount of diarrhea.

Expected Outcomes for the Client With *Bowel Incontinence*

The expected outcome for a diagnosis of *Bowel incontinence* depends on the illness that has caused the problem. If the bowel incontinence is a permanent problem, the appropriate outcome is that the client's skin integrity remain intact. If the bowel incontinence is not permanent or can be minimized by intervention, then outcomes could be that the client will do the following:

- Have a daily bowel elimination on a commode or bedpan
- Alter diet and fluids to control elimination
- Establish a set routine for elimination
- Decrease episodes of incontinence

Expected Outcomes for the Client With *Fecal Impaction*

Outcomes for the client with *Fecal impaction* could be that the client will do the following:

- Experience manual removal of feces without pain or other side effects
- Initiate or be placed on a preventive bowel program

Expected Outcomes for the Client With *Flatulence*

Outcomes for the client with *Flatulence* could be that the client will do the following:

- Decrease the production of flatus by modifying diet and/or air swallowing
- Expel excess flatus
- Experience a decrease in symptoms of flatulence

INTERVENTION

Interventions to Promote Healthful Elimination

You can help clients meet the goal of healthy defecation habits through learning activities. Support normal bowel habits through adjustments in diet, fluids, exercise, and positioning and by providing relaxation and privacy.

Developing a Plan for Lifestyle Management. Even clients whom you assume to be knowledgeable may have misconceptions about defecation. For example, many people incorrectly believe that it is necessary to defecate every day. If they fail to have a daily bowel movement, they may use laxatives, suppositories, or enemas to induce one. As described later, continued use of such measures begins a cycle that may lead to physical dependence. Because there are many other misunderstandings about defecation, you must give clients accurate information about this normal body function. With appropriate teaching, a client who needs intervention is more likely to be compliant.

TOILET HABITS. Many factors influence the timing of bowel movements, such as availability of a bathroom and the demands of personal and professional responsibilities. Consequently, you will need to assess each client's daily routine before planning a bowel program. However, keep in mind that, although defecation can occur at any time, it is best to encourage bowel movements during stimulation of the gastrocolic reflex. As described earlier, this reflex is usually strongest after breakfast. Therefore attempts to have a bowel movement at this time are likely to be the most successful.

Frequency of bowel movements varies from person to person. The normal range for an adult is from three times per week to three times per day. Infants often have three to five stools per day, but for adults and older children, passing stools more than three times a day or less than once a week may indicate a problem. Because many people worry needlessly about the frequency of their bowel movements, emphasize to your clients that the frequency of bowel movements varies among individuals.

> *Action Alert!* Stress that the frequency of bowel movements is individualized, and that it is not necessary to have a bowel movement every day.

The amount of stool varies according to the amount and type of food ingested, fluid intake, and frequency of bowel evacuation. It is normally about 150 g per day. Because much fecal material is not dietary in origin, the person with no oral intake still passes stool. Also, it may take several days for food to move through the entire GI tract. The colon therefore is not empty even if the person has not eaten for several days. Inform people of these facts to motivate them to take measures to prevent constipation.

Help people select a time during the day when they can take time to attend to bowel needs. As indicated, timing depends on lifestyle and daily activities. Once it is decided, encourage clients to make this habit a daily routine. If the time selected is inappropriate, alter it until a suitable one is found. People who have little routine in their lives are a particular challenge.

In addition, hospitalization often alters established routines. During this time, determine the client's normal routine, and then help him to maintain it.

DIET. Dietary fiber is one of the most important elements in maintaining normal bowel function. Dietary fiber increases the weight and water content of feces. It also speeds the progress of feces through the GI tract. Fiber may be soluble or insoluble. The digestive system cannot break down insoluble fiber from a plant. Likewise, fiber does not break down in water but rather retains water. Water retained by fiber softens the stool and promotes regularity. Thus supplementing diets with bran, whole-grain cereals, nuts, and raw fruits and vegetables is effective in promoting normal bowel elimination.

A high-fiber diet can also prevent diverticular disease. A diverticulum is an outpouching of the colon wall that results from weakened muscles in the intestinal wall. This condition can cause problems if the diverticula fill with feces. Perforation, ulceration, and infection can also develop. Diverticular disease is commonly asymptomatic when the client eats a high-fiber diet.

The National Cancer Institute recommends a daily intake of 25 to 35 g of fiber. To increase a client's consumption of fiber, add high-fiber foods slowly to allow time for the GI tract to adapt. Large amounts of dietary fiber added abruptly can cause abdominal cramps, gaseous distention, and diarrhea. The client's fiber consumption should include both insoluble and soluble fiber. It should come from foods rather than from supplements, which may not contain needed vitamins and minerals.

In addition to adding fiber, help the client identify and avoid foods that disrupt bowel function. If there are several suspect foods, urge the client to eliminate all of them from the diet and then add them back, one at a time. Tell the client to wait for several days, longer if necessary, between introductions, to see which foods cause the problem.

FLUIDS. Hydration helps maintain normal bowel function by keeping stools soft. Although experts recommend different amounts of fluid to maintain adequate hydration, most consider about 1200 to 1500 mL per day to be a reasonable minimum for adults. A client with significant fluid replacement needs (such as from increased sweating caused by activity or fever) should consume more. Immobility also requires increased fluid intake because one of the normal aids to defecation—exercise—is limited. However, before increasing a client's fluid intake, make sure that the person has no contraindications, such as cardiac disease, renal disease, or head injury. Fluid requirements for infants and children are based on kilograms of body weight. Infants and children are more vulnerable to changing fluid needs related to ambient temperature and exercise.

Although the amount of fluid intake is critical, the type of fluids consumed may also be important. For example, milk constipates some people. Prune juice is a natural laxative for most people. Other fruit juices, such as apricot, lemonade, cranberry, and orange, can also stimulate bowel activity.

EXERCISE. Encourage and assist clients, as necessary, to take part in daily physical activity, because exercise improves muscle tone and strengthens the muscles used in defecation. Walking, for example, is an excellent body toner.

Also, teach exercises specifically designed to strengthen the abdominal and pelvic floor muscles. Probably the most effective are isometric exercises in which the client contracts or tightens muscles as strongly as possible for about 10 seconds, and then relaxes them. Instruct the client to repeat each exercise 5 to 10 times, four times a day. Remember that isometric exercises raise blood pressure and may cause coronary ischemia (deficient blood flow to the cardiac muscle) in a client with cardiac disease. Therefore you may need to consult a physician about the client's health status before instituting an exercise program.

USE OF LAXATIVES. Laxatives are short-acting medications that cause defecation. Healthy people should not use them on a routine basis. For clients who cannot defecate because of constipation or fecal impaction, laxatives are used to aid in the bowel elimination process.

Positioning the Client.

Proper positioning for elimination promotes comfort and aids defecation in several ways. For one, it makes use of the force of gravity. For another, good positioning facilitates contraction of the abdominal muscles, thereby increasing intraabdominal pressure. Because squatting is the best position for defecation, position the client as near to this posture as possible. The commode and toilet promote this position. You can increase external pressure on the abdomen by having the client lean forward.

If the person is short, place a footstool or other appropriate device under the feet at the toilet to increase hip flexion. Exercise caution, however, with a client who has had hip surgery, especially total hip replacement. This client must avoid flexing the hips beyond 90 degrees to prevent dislocation of the prosthesis. Some clients can use the toilet only with the aid of a device that raises the seat height to decrease hip flexion. Instruct these clients not to lean forward.

If the client must use a bedpan, raise the head of the bed into a high-Fowler position, if not contraindicated. If head elevation is contraindicated, use a fracture bedpan instead.

Promoting Relaxation and Privacy.

Relaxation is critical to normal bowel function. Probably the most important factor in achieving relaxation is privacy. Clients may become anxious if they feel that the odors and sounds that naturally accompany this body function may be communicated to others. Anxiety causes tension in the voluntary musculature, which in turn can suppress defecation. Provide as private an environment as possible to facilitate normal defecation.

For example, if the client is using the bathroom, make sure that other people know the room is occupied. This is especially important when the bathroom has two doors opening into adjacent rooms. If the client must use a bedpan or commode in the room, pull the bed curtains around the bed, ask all visitors or staff to leave the room, open the window if appropriate, and turn on the television or radio. Use room deodorizers to reduce odors.

Make sure that clients have a way to call you when they are finished or need help. In addition to providing a call light, assure them that there is no hurry. Communicate this fact by your actions as well as your words. For example, avoid interrupting them simply to see if they are finished. On the other hand, do keep careful watch on any client who is at risk for accidents, such as fainting or falling. In fact, fainting in bathrooms is a rather frequent occurrence. Bathrooms are notoriously warm and stuffy and, when a weakened person strains to have a bowel movement, the cardiovascular system may not be able to maintain sufficient blood flow to the brain.

Some clients may need pain relief before trying to defecate. If you must administer a narcotic pain reliever, time its administration carefully because these drugs depress central nervous system function. Time the administration so that the client can attempt defecation when pain has been relieved but before drowsiness and sleep set in.

Interventions to Manage Constipation

The treatment of typical constipation requires all the preventive measures mentioned: learning and teaching activities; changes in diet, fluid intake, and exercise; and development of healthy bowel habits (Box 28-5, p. 678). Sometimes, additional intervention is needed.

𝒯HE STATE OF NURSING RESEARCH: Have You Had a Bowel Movement Today? Box 28-5

What Are the Issues?

Questions about daily routines related to bowel patterns are a routine part of a nursing assessment. Many illnesses and treatments as well as immobility can alter normal bowel patterns and cause mild discomfort to severe complications. Dietary intake, fluid intake, and exercise also influence bowel patterns. Helping clients maintain normal bowel function is an important nursing care issue. What is normal for one person may be considered constipation for another person.

What Research Has Been Conducted?

Fiber is thought to have a laxative effect on bowel function through its water-absorbing properties (Hinrichs & Huseboe, 2001). Increasing the amount of fiber in the diet can be one way to reduce the risk of constipation. Hinrichs and Huseboe (2001) describe a protocol for bowel management that includes 20-35 grams per day as long as the person also has fluid intake of a least 1500 milliliters. The protocol includes a variety of recipes that increase dietary fiber. The protocol recommends exercise in the form of walking or bed exercises. "Toileting is recommended 5-15 minutes after meals and as needed, especially after breakfast" (Hinrichs & Huseboe, 2001). Two other researchers systematically reviewed studies that used dietary fiber as an intervention for constipation (Kenny & Skelly, 2001). In their review, "dietary fiber was defined as a product or mixture including at least one food item high in dietary fiber (bran, whole grain, fruit, or vegetable)" (p. 120). Of the eight studies that met their review criteria, only two used the strongest design, randomized controlled trial.

Dietary fiber has also been tested as a treatment for clients with fecal incontinence by Bliss et al. (2001), who used random assignment to decide the treatment and placebo groups. After obtaining a baseline pattern, people in the treatment groups took dietary supplements of either psyllium or gum arabic mixed in juice twice a day. The control group was given a placebo of pectin. Besides the self-report data recorded by participants, researchers conducted laboratory analysis on stool samples to determine fiber content. Stool incontinence dropped and consistency increased during the study for those in the treatment groups.

What Has the Research Concluded?

Kenny and Skelly (2001) found major design weaknesses in most of the studies on the use of dietary fiber. The two studies that were strong in design reported conflicting results. They noted that other possible factors such as laxative use and fluid intake were not controlled.

What Is the Future of Research in This Area?

Kenny and Skelly (2001) recommended that future studies look at "clinically meaningful outcome measures" (p. 127), such as comfort and incontinence. The use of dietary fiber to control fecal incontinence shows some promise. Studies that look at the long-term effects of such treatment are needed. Certainly, as the population ages, bowel patterns will continue to be an important nursing consideration. Interventions that can keep people comfortable will be valued.

References

Bliss, D. Z., Jung, H., Savik, K., Lowry, A., LeMoine, M., Jensen, L., et al. (2001). Supplementation with dietary fiber improves fecal incontinence. *Nursing Research, 50*(4), 203-213.

Hinrichs, M., & Huseboe, J. (2001). Research-based protocol: Management of constipation. *Journal of Gerontological Nursing, 27*(2), 17.

Kenny, K. A., & Skelly, J. M. (2001). Dietary fiber for constipation in older adults: A systematic review. *Clinical Effectiveness in Nursing, 5,* 120-128.

Administering Medications. **Laxatives** are agents that stimulate defecation and **cathartics** are strong laxatives that produce a watery stool. Laxatives come in four categories: bulk forming, lubricant, saline, and stimulant. Besides these oral medications, laxatives are also available as medicated suppositories. When inserted into the rectum, they stimulate defecation.

Bulk-forming laxatives are the most natural and least irritating laxative preparations and are frequently used to wean laxative-dependent people from medication misuse. They use synthetic or natural polysaccharides and cellulose derivatives to absorb water and add bulk. This increased volume stretches the intestinal wall, thus stimulating peristalsis. Common examples are bran, psyllium, karaya gum, agar, and methylcellulose. Mix bulk-forming agents with water and follow the dose with additional fluid to make sure that it has been cleared from the esophagus. Results usually occur in 12 to 24 hours, but they may take up to 72 hours. Encourage high fluid intake to improve the action of the laxative and to avoid GI tract obstruction.

Lubricant laxatives include mineral oil and the docusates. They coat the outside of the fecal mass, making it slippery and inhibiting fluid absorption from it. Mineral oil is a classic example of a lubricant laxative. It is not very palatable, but you can mask the oily aftertaste by mixing it with orange juice or root beer. Administer mineral oil when the client's stomach is empty to keep it from interfering with the absorption of fat-soluble vitamins. Watch carefully if the client has trouble swallowing, because mineral oil aspiration can cause pneumonia. The docusates act as wetting and dispersing agents. Common examples are Dialose, Colace, Doxidan, and Surfak. Poloxamer 188, a nonionic surfactant, is a stool softener.

Saline laxatives, or osmotic agents, contain poorly absorbed salts and sugars, which, through osmotic activity, draw water into the intestine to increase bulk and lubricate feces. These drugs usually act within 1 to 3 hours. Many are purgatives that empty the bowel completely. Magnesium sulfate (Epsom salts), magnesium hydroxide (milk of magnesia), magnesium citrate, and lactulose are osmotic agents. Lactulose causes a severe osmotic reaction and, unless the dose is calculated carefully, causes intestinal rumbling, colic, and flatulence. Because of the salts used and the severity of their action, osmotic agents are usually contraindicated in people with renal, cardiac, or inflammatory bowel disease.

Stimulants (also called irritants) increase peristalsis by stimulating sensory nerve endings of the colonic epithelium or by directly irritating the GI mucosa. In addition, some (such as bisacodyl) may increase GI secretory activity, thus producing bulkier feces. Examples of stimulants include cascara, castor oil, senna, glycerin, and bisacodyl. Be aware that these medications are transmitted through breast milk, causing diarrhea in the nursing infant.

Laxatives are one of the most widely used and misused over-the-counter drugs. Most laxative abuse results from advertising that supports the public's misconceptions about the need for a daily bowel movement. In addition to teaching clients about the proper use of laxatives, warn them never to take these drugs in the presence of undiagnosed abdominal pain or cramps, nausea, vomiting, or diarrhea. These symptoms may indicate appendicitis, inflammatory bowel disease, or obstruction.

> *Action Alert!* Daily laxative administration is detrimental to normal bowel elimination.

Suppositories are semisolid, cone-shaped, or oval-shaped masses that melt at body temperature. To stimulate defecation, medicated suppositories are inserted into the rectum, where they release their active ingredients as they melt. Many types of suppositories are refrigerated because it is easier to insert a cold, firm suppository than a warm, soft one.

The suppositories used most often are glycerin and bisacodyl. Each acts as a local irritant to stimulate GI mucosal secretion. Fecal softeners may also be given by suppository to moisten and lubricate the fecal mass. After administering the suppository, cleanse the client's anal area to remove excess lubricant. Instruct the client to retain the suppository as long as possible—at least 20 to 30 minutes. If appropriate, teach the client how to self-administer the suppository.

Administering Enemas.

An enema involves the instillation of fluid into the rectum to stimulate defecation. People who have had no formal instruction in the procedure commonly administer this treatment in the home. Indeed, some people use a daily enema to prevent constipation. Consequently, most people consider enemas to be a harmless, necessary treatment for constipation. This is a misconception. To achieve the safest and most effective results, it is necessary to understand and apply the scientific principles underlying enema administration.

PURPOSE. Enemas are given for several purposes. The *cleansing enema* is used to treat constipation or fecal impaction, to clean out the bowel before diagnostic procedures or surgery, and to help establish regular bowel function during a bowel-training program. A *retention enema* is retained in the bowel over a prolonged period. It is usually administered to lubricate or soften a hard fecal mass with oil, thus facilitating its expulsion through the anus. Less frequently, a retention enema is used to administer medications, to protect and soothe the mucous membrane of the intestine, to destroy intestinal parasites (anthelmintic), to relieve distention (carminative), or to administer fluids and nutrition (nutritive). Another kind of enema, the *return flow enema*, relieves gaseous distention. It is sometimes called a Harris flush and is described later, in the discussion of flatulence.

Enemas stimulate peristalsis through bowel distention, irritation of the mucosal wall, or both. Bowel distention results from filling the colon with fluid, either via a large-volume enema, which injects large amounts of fluid into the colon from an external source, or via a small-volume enema, which draws internal fluid into the bowel.

The concepts of osmosis and concentration gradient are important to an understanding of how some enemas work. Briefly, osmosis is the movement of water through a semipermeable membrane to equalize the concentration of particles on both sides of the membrane. Although water continuously flows back and forth across the membrane, the major net flow of water is toward the solution with a higher concentration of molecules.

TYPES OF ENEMAS. A cleansing enema may use a hypotonic, isotonic, or hypertonic solution. Hypotonic solutions (such as tap water) have a lower osmotic pressure than the fluid in the interstitial tissues, so the net flow of water is out of the bowel into the tissues. The net flow occurs slowly, however, and defecation is usually stimulated before any appreciable fluid is absorbed into the body. Significant absorption can occur if the client is fluid depleted or receives multiple enemas. Isotonic solutions (such as normal saline solution) produce equal concentrations on both sides of the semipermeable membrane. Consequently, no net water flow occurs. Hypertonic solutions are of higher concentration than the interstitial fluid. Thus the net water flow is into the colon, leading to distention and stimulating the defecation reflex.

Hypotonic and isotonic enema solutions are used for large-volume enemas (500 to 750 mL) that result in immediate colonic emptying. The large volumes, however, may present a danger to people with weakened colon walls. In addition, these enemas often require special preparation and equipment. On the other hand, hypertonic small-volume enemas (120 to 250 mL) are available commercially and are easier to administer. A commonly used over-the-counter product is the prepackaged enema, such as the Fleet brand (Figure 28-5, p. 680). These commercially packaged enemas are available as normal saline enemas or as mineral oil enemas. People who have problems with sodium retention should avoid using hypertonic solutions.

One common enema additive is Castile soap. Added to either tap water or saline solution, it causes mucosal irritation. Other enema solutions, such as milk and molasses, vegetable oils, hydrogen peroxide, and champagne, are reported in the literature. However, these types are rarely used. Various medicated and nutritive formulas, such as sucralfate enemas, are also used, depending on the person's needs.

Procedure 28-2 (p. 680) describes the techniques for preparing and administering a large-volume enema. Use these methods for enemas of any volume, but make any necessary changes when preparing the solution.

Administration of a hypertonic enema requires several variations in the procedure for an enema, mainly because the solution comes prepackaged and ready to inject. You do not need to warm the solution, but make sure that it is at room temperature to prevent intestinal cramps. The client may be in any position to receive this enema; however, the left lateral position with right leg flexed is recommended to distribute the solution throughout the colon.

To administer a commercially prepared hypertonic enema, remove the cap and insert the prelubricated tip into the

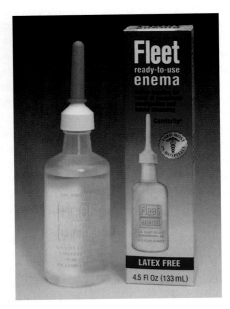

Figure 28-5. A Fleet enema. (Courtesy C. B. Fleet Company, Lynchburg, VA.)

client's rectum. Squeeze the collapsible reservoir steadily until the solution is gone. Have the client retain the solution until the urge to defecate is very strong. Clients can be taught to self-administer a hypertonic enema, and they may be asked to administer one at home before radiographic studies or proctological examinations.

Administration of a retention enema is similar to administration of a hypertonic enema except that the solution must be retained over a prolonged period, usually for at least an hour. Some enemas (such as medicated or nutritive enemas) are never evacuated. The method of solution preparation depends on what type of solution has been ordered. A smaller administration tip is used (usually a No. 14 to No. 20 French catheter for adults) to avoid stretching the sphincter, thereby diminishing stimulation of the defecation reflex. Make sure you elevate the reservoir only high enough to allow the solution to run slowly into the rectum. Administration under higher pressure distends the rectum, causing defecation. Finally, protect the bed linen in case the client cannot retain the fluid.

COMPLICATIONS. Enema administration is not without its hazards. Complications include fluid and electrolyte imbalances, tissue trauma, vagal nerve stimulation, and dependence. Fluid imbalances usually occur because of the tonicity of the enema solution. Remember that the body absorbs water from hypotonic solutions. Use caution when administering enemas to people who are susceptible to fluid imbalance (such as infants or clients with decompensated cardiac or

---

PROCEDURE 28-2 PREPARING AND ADMINISTERING A LARGE-VOLUME ENEMA

TIME TO ALLOW
Novice: 15 min.
Expert: 10 min.

A large-volume enema is defined as 500 to 1000 mL of fluid to stimulate the colon to empty. It is unpleasant at best, may have some hazardous consequences for the client, and is seldom used in the health care environment. A large-volume enema is useful when rapid cleansing or evacuation of the bowel is needed. It may also be useful when the gentler forms of bowel cleansing are not effective.

DELEGATION GUIDELINES

An enema requires a physician's order. Administration of a large-volume enema may be delegated to a nursing assistant. First, however, you must assess the client for risk factors associated with receipt of an enema and instruct the nursing assistant in safety precautions. If the client has diverticular disease or another disorder of the colon, you may instruct the nursing assistant to use a smaller volume of solution or choose to administer the enema yourself.

EQUIPMENT NEEDED

- Enema solution container
- 36 inches of tubing with rectal tip (adult, No. 22 to No. 30 French; child, No. 12 to No. 18 French)

- Solution: tap water or normal saline, with 1 teaspoon mild liquid soap without additives. (Normal saline solution is the safest option for an enema solution, and tap water requires the least preparation. If the client has severe constipation or needs a thorough cleansing of the bowel, soapsuds may be most useful because they irritate the colonic mucosa.)
- Water-soluble lubricating jelly
- Clean gloves
- Waterproof pad
- Bedside commode or bedpan

1. Follow preliminary guidelines for nursing procedures (see inside front cover).

2. Set up the equipment and close the door or draw the curtain. Position the client on his left (or most comfortable) side. Drape him so only his buttocks are exposed. If you expect that the client will be unable to retain the enema solution, position him on a bedpan or commode instead. *Positioning the client on his left side allows gravity to help the enema solution flow into the rectum. Exposing only his buttocks will help to give him a sense of privacy. Allowing him to face the door may help as well.*

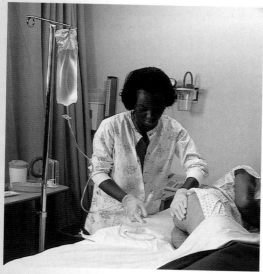

Step 2. Positioning and equipment for administering a large-volume enema.

3. Make sure the enema solution is lukewarm, about 40.5° C (105° F). Coat the tip of the enema tube with water-soluble lubricant and gently insert it 2 to 3 inches into the client's rectum. *If the client has hemorrhoids, consider using extra lubricant. Insert the tip gently, with a twisting motion, to pass the hemorrhoids.*

4. Allow 500 to 750 mL of the enema solution to flow slowly into the client's rectum, over about 10 minutes. The enema bag should be approximately 18 inches above the rectum. *Keep the flow rate slow enough to prevent cramping and an uncontrollable urge to evacuate the bowel. If the client develops an uncontrollable urge, stop the flow until the urge passes.*

5. Encourage the client to retain the solution in the bowel for up to 15 minutes. *With a large-volume enema, most clients will need to expel the solution quickly.*

6. Help the client to the toilet or assist him with the bedpan or commode, as needed. *If the client has mobility problems, you may be able to place him more quickly on a bedpan than on the toilet. However, the best position for bowel evacuation is on the toilet or bedside commode.*

7. After bowel evacuation, cleanse the client's perianal skin, control odors, and make the client comfortable. *Cleanse the skin thoroughly and gently. Controlling odors promptly can help to minimize the client's embarrassment.*

8. If the physician has ordered enemas until clear, you may need to administer up to three large-volume enemas as described here. If three enemas fail to produce clear results, consult the physician. *Remember that a large-volume enema may produce more than one bowel movement. Allow time between enemas for maximum results.*

PEDIATRIC CONSIDERATIONS

Hospitalized children are prone to constipation and should be carefully observed for this problem. Isotonic saline is often the preferred solution for a large-volume enema in a child. The amount of fluid and the position varies with the age of the child:

- Infant, 150 to 250 mL
- Young child, 250 to 300 mL
- Older child, 300 to 350 mL
- Adolescent, 500 to 750 mL

GERIATRIC CONSIDERATIONS

Enemas in older adults with mobility problems can be challenging. An enema can be given on a bedpan for the person who cannot hold the solution or cannot move to the toilet easily. You may be able to insert the catheter and then turn the client onto the bedpan. Large-volume enemas should not be routinely used to manage chronic constipation. Avoid giving an enema more frequently than every 3 days to prevent dependence on enemas and to prevent the excess loss of electrolytes.

HOME CARE CONSIDERATIONS

Enemas should not be used with any frequency in the home setting. Teach the family that cleansing enemas and laxatives should not be used any more often than once every 3 days. Once the bowel is thoroughly cleansed, the client may not need another bowel movement for 3 days. If the client is in the habit of managing constipation with enemas, help family caregivers with an overall bowel management program designed to reduce the need for enemas kidney reserve). Water intoxication can occur. Symptoms of this condition include weakness, dizziness, pallor, sweating, and respiratory difficulties. Signs of congestive heart failure or cerebral edema may also be present. On the other hand, hypertonic solutions draw fluid from the interstitial tissues and can lead to fluid depletion, especially in children and other people susceptible to dehydration.

Electrolyte imbalances also occur. Usually, normal saline is the safest enema solution because of its isotonicity. However, in clients who have problems with sodium retention (such as those with congestive heart failure or cirrhosis of the liver), the body absorbs sodium, which leads to fluid retention. Therefore these clients should not receive saline solutions. Depending on the contents of the enema solution used, other electrolyte imbalances may also occur, such as hypokalemia, hypocalcemia, or hyperphosphatemia.

Action Alert! Avoid giving an enema to a person with inflammatory bowel disease.

Enemas can also cause tissue trauma. The four major sources of trauma are the administration tip, solution delivered under high pressure, a soapsuds solution, and increased peristalsis. If the enema tip has any chips or broken areas, it may lacerate or abrade the rectal mucosa. High fluid pressures can rupture the intestinal wall without causing pain at the time of perforation. In fact, the first indication of rupture may be signs of peritonitis (inflammation of the peritoneum). Do not use a bulb syringe to administer an enema, because you will not be able to control the pressure. Tissue trauma from peristalsis can occur in clients with inflammatory bowel disease. Increased bowel motility enhances cramping and bleeding.

Although the use of soapsuds enemas is questionable, they are still sometimes ordered. As stated, the soapsuds solution chemically irritates the mucosa. This irritation commonly leads to rectal inflammation and colitis, sometimes lasting up to 3 weeks after administration. The higher the concentration of soap in the solution, the greater is the chance of inflammation. Thus the practice of swirling a bar of soap or soap pieces in the enema reservoir is extremely dangerous, since it is impossible to determine the concentration. A soapsuds solution is somewhat safer if you use standardized packages of soap.

As is true of laxatives and suppositories, people can develop physical and psychological dependence on enemas. The underlying mechanism is the same: the enema cleans the bowel so that it takes 2 or more days for enough fecal mass to collect again to stimulate defecation. In the meantime, the person becomes anxious because he has not had a bowel movement. Thus he self-administers another enema. Gradually, the bowel becomes less sensitive to normal defecation reflex stimuli, and the person becomes physically dependent on bowel aids. Table 28-3 summarizes agents used to relieve constipation.

Removing an Impaction. The goal of treatment for a fecal impaction is removal of the mass from the rectum. Oral laxatives or cathartics may be used to moisten and lubricate the fecal mass, although their action may be too slow. A program of enemas may be instituted, starting with the administration of an oil-retention enema and followed by a cleansing enema. These two enemas may need to be repeated.

If the fecal mass is extremely large or the enemas are ineffective in expelling it, you will have to remove the impaction digitally. To do this, insert a gloved, heavily

Table 28-3 Agents Used to Relieve Constipation		
Type	Action	Examples
LAXATIVES		
Bulk-forming	Increases the fluid, gaseous, or solid bulk in the intestines and absorbs water into the intestine	• Methylcellulose • Hydrolose • Psyllium (Metamucil)
Lubricant	Softens and delays the drying of feces	• Mineral oil • Docusate sodium (Colace, Dialose)
Saline	Draws water into the intestine to increase bulk and lubricate feces	• Magnesium sulfate (Epsom salts) • Magnesium hydroxide (milk of magnesia) • Magnesium citrate
Stimulant	Irritates the intestinal mucosa, increasing peristalsis	• Bisacodyl (Dulcolax) • Castor oil • Cascara sagrada
ENEMAS		
Hypertonic	Distends colon and irritates mucosa	• Sodium phosphate • Fleet enema
Hypotonic	Distends colon, stimulates peristalsis, and softens feces	• Tap water
Isotonic	Distends colon, stimulates peristalsis, and softens feces	• Normal saline solution
Soap	Irritates mucosa and distends colon	• Castile soap
Oil	Lubricates the feces and the colonic mucosa	• Mineral oil • Olive oil • Cottonseed oil

lubricated finger into the client's rectum (Figure 28-6). Remove pieces of the mass manually with a bedpan close at hand. Even though you can use a topical anesthetic agent such as lidocaine, this intervention is uncomfortable and embarrassing for the client. Gentleness may help, but prevention is the best treatment. Sometimes, a fecal impaction must be removed surgically.

Interventions to Alleviate Diarrhea

The usual intervention for diarrhea is to inhibit peristalsis. However, because this action may slow the expulsion of pathogenic organisms or irritants, it may actually prolong the problem. Consequently, treatment involves removing the precipitating factors, then stopping the diarrhea itself. For example, a client with a GI infection typically receives antibiotics and possibly antidiarrheals.

Administering Medications. Commonly used antidiarrheal drugs, such as kaolin and pectin, may be used. These medications bind and remove irritants from the GI tract and form a soothing, protective coating on the mucosa. In severe diarrhea, the physician may prescribe opiates (such as paregoric or codeine) or anticholinergic drugs (such as diphenoxylate/atropine sulfate [Lomotil]) to inhibit peristalsis. As stated, antibiotics can be used to eliminate the cause of the diarrhea. Normal intestinal bacterial flora can be reestablished by giving the client yogurt, buttermilk, or bacillus-containing medications such as Bacid or Lactinex.

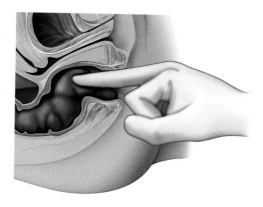

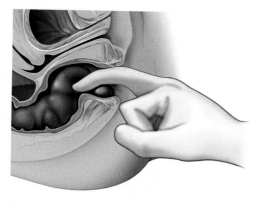

Figure 28-6. Digital removal of a fecal impaction.

Limiting Food Intake. Good nutrition is important during episodes of diarrhea. Diet modification may be necessary to counteract the decreased absorption. For mild to moderate diarrhea, short-term therapy involves decreasing or eliminating food intake to reduce stimulation of peristalsis. For severe diarrhea, dietary modification may include a diet low in residue and high in calories and vitamins. Food may also be withheld or restricted to clear liquids, followed by a soft diet in frequent small amounts. Raw fruits, vegetables, whole grains, and concentrated sweets should be avoided and added to the diet later.

The BRATY diet is recommended for children and adults with nausea and vomiting associated with gastroenteritis. The diet can be used for up to 24 hours. The initials stand for bananas (mashed or whole), rice, apples (or applesauce), toast (or crackers—preferably dry), and yogurt (plain).

Restoring Fluids and Electrolytes. Fluid and electrolyte losses are a common complication of diarrhea. Infants and debilitated clients are especially susceptible to this complication. In fact, age is a significant factor when a person has diarrhea. A young infant can soon have a serious depletion of electrolytes, water, and nutrients unless the disorder is promptly corrected. Fluids and electrolytes must be replaced by either oral or parenteral (intravenous) therapy. Emphasize to the client that decreasing fluid intake will not stop the diarrhea.

Using a Bedpan. Many clients need to use a bedpan for elimination, including those restricted to bed rest because of a fracture, recent surgery, or illness. A client receiving an enema or who has diarrhea may need to use a bedpan as well.

Bedpans come in two styles: a regular bedpan and a fracture bedpan. The regular and fracture bedpans shown in Figure 28-7 (p. 684) are made of metal or plastic. Fracture bedpans were developed for clients with fractures of the lower limbs who could not elevate easily to have a regular bedpan placed. Because of the ease of use of the fracture bedpans, it has become a common practice to use fracture bedpans with all clients. A metal bedpan of any style is cold; if possible, warm it before use by running warm water over its edges. This is not necessary for plastic bedpans.

You can place a bedpan by having the client lift his hips and sliding it under him. Or you can have him roll onto his side, place the bedpan against his buttocks, and have him roll back onto his back. You will need to judge the best method for each client. Either way, the closed-lip end of the bedpan should be placed under the buttocks, making sure that it is positioned to collect the waste (Figure 28-8, p. 684).

Preventing Skin Breakdown. Skin care is especially important for the client with diarrhea. Provide the client with soft material for wiping after each stool to help reduce the irritation. Also, washing the client's perianal area with soap and water after each stool reduces the time that irritating diarrhea stays in contact with the skin.

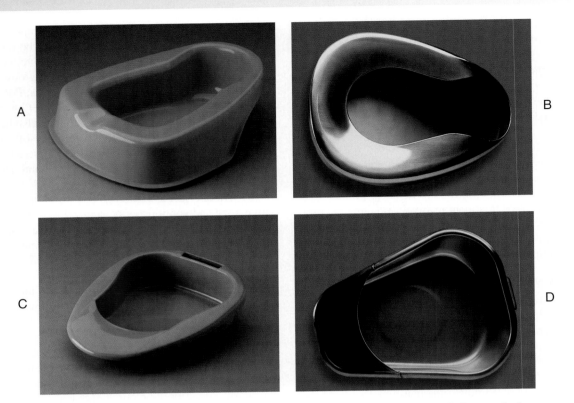

Figure 28-7. Types of bedpans. **A,** Regular bedpan—plastic. **B,** Regular bedpan—metal. **C,** Fracture bedpan—plastic. **D,** Fracture bedpan—metal. (*A* and *C,* courtesy Bemis Health Care, Sheboygan Falls, WI; *B* and *D,* courtesy Vollrath Group, Gallaway, TN.)

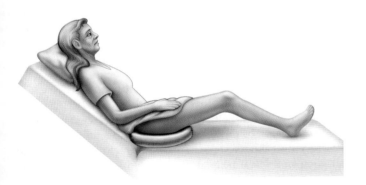

Figure 28-8. Proper client position on a bedpan.

Ensuring Privacy. The frequency and urgency of bowel movements causes fatigue and embarrassment. Therefore make sure that the client has quick and easy access to the bathroom, commode, or bedpan. Place the call bell nearby at all times. Provide privacy and odor control.

Interventions to Restore Bowel Continence

Interventions for bowel incontinence include promoting continence through bowel training and maintenance of skin integrity. Caring for the skin of an incontinent person may be a time-consuming task. The main goal is to prevent prolonged contact between the skin and fecal material, which leads to excoriation and breakdown.

Maintaining Skin Integrity. Washing the perianal area with soap and water and drying it thoroughly after each stool keeps the skin in good condition and controls fecal odor. Nonionic detergent preparations (such as Peri-Wash) are even more effective than regular soap. Use powders and creams with caution because they may contribute to skin breakdown.

Application of a rectal incontinence pouch for a client with bowel incontinence protects the skin and the bed linens (Figure 28-9). The rectal pouch has a circular paper adhesive backing that adheres to the perianal skin. An attached plastic bag collects the feces. The adhesive opening can be altered in size to facilitate individual fitting. Perianal hair should be shaved to allow a tight fit of the adhesive back.

If a rectal pouch is not in use, the bed and clothing of the incontinent person must be kept clean. When using plastic or rubber sheeting to protect bed linens, make sure that it does not contact the skin, thus causing irritation. A client with severe incontinence may need to wear waterproof undergarments to protect clothing. Adult-size disposable briefs are available with cellulose padding to draw fluid away from the skin by capillary action. However, diapers make the person feel infantile and appear to give "permission" to be incontinent. Avoid using them whenever possible. The best way to

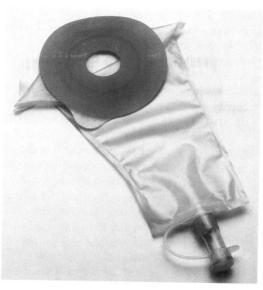

Figure 28-9. A rectal incontinence pouch. (Reproduced with permission of Hollister Inc., Libertyville, IL.)

reduce the physiological and psychological effects of incontinence is to reestablish bowel control.

Providing Bowel Training. Bowel training programs are effective for regaining bowel control. They require time, patience, and commitment from nurses and the client, but the results are well worth the effort.

First, assess and diagnose the factors causing the incontinence. Then, discuss bowel training with the client and significant others. Together, decide on a routine for bowel elimination. Base the routine on the person's previous bowel habits and on alterations in bowel habits that have resulted from illness or trauma. In addition, note when the client is most likely to be incontinent during the day.

All bowel training programs include independent nursing measures used to aid normal defecation: diet, fluids, exercise, and maintenance of defecation patterns. Probably the most crucial element of the program is timing. The schedule for defecation should be carefully determined and then strictly followed. If possible, position the client on the commode or toilet at the designated time to take advantage of gravity.

Bowel programming is individualized, although there are many common factors. Habit training, control of diarrhea, and biofeedback are possible strategies for bowel programming. Most programs include stool softeners to facilitate passage of feces. This intervention is especially important for clients with spinal cord injuries or extreme debilitation, because they frequently cannot bear down. Suppositories may be used every 1 to 3 days to stimulate evacuation. In people with spinal cord injuries, the suppository is usually followed in 20 to 30 minutes by digital stimulation of the anal sphincter to augment stimulation of the defecation reflex. In some programs, enemas are used in place of the sup-

positories. Suppository or enema administration is usually discontinued as soon as bowel elimination can be maintained without them.

Modify the training program as needed until a successful routine is found. Generally, a person is kept on a particular program for at least 3 days before it is changed. This period allows you to be sure that changes are indeed necessary.

Other methods of treating incontinence are available. For example, biofeedback therapy works for some people. This method helps the client modify the incontinence using feedback from instruments. Surgical intervention to create new tissue sphincters has been tried. Electrical stimulation of sphincter control has also been successful in some cases.

Interventions to Reduce Flatulence

The goal of therapy is to remove gas from the GI tract. The most effective and natural way to expel the flatus is by exercise. Exercise stimulates peristalsis, which speeds the transit time of the gas through the colon. Walking is the best method but, if this is not possible, moving around in bed will help. Prevention is also important. Teach clients to avoid situations and substances that cause flatulence.

If simple, natural methods fail, you may need to use a rectal tube to allow gas to escape from the body. To insert a rectal tube into an adult, lubricate a No. 22 to No. 32 French rubber or plastic rectal tube and insert it about 10 cm (4 inches) into the rectum. Place the distal end of the tube into a collecting receptacle to catch any feces that may be expelled. Tape the tube in place and leave it there for 20 minutes or less. Longer periods may cause sphincter damage. Reinsert the tube every 2 or 3 hours if necessary.

A return-flow enema (Harris flush) also relieves flatulence, although this intervention is controversial because it can cause intestinal trauma. In this procedure, the rectum is alternately filled and drained to move flatus by stimulating peristalsis. Prepare the client, the equipment, and the solution (tap water or saline) as shown in Procedure 28-2. After inserting the rectal tube, infuse about 200 to 300 mL of fluid into the colon. Then lower the solution container 45 cm (18 inches) below the level of the anus to allow the solution and flatus to drain back into the reservoir. Expelled gas bubbles up through the solution in the container. When the return flow ceases, raise the reservoir 45 cm above the anus and allow 200 to 300 mL to flow in. Repeat this process until the returned gas is minimal.

Several medications may help to relieve flatulence. Simethicone-containing medications cause gas bubbles to coalesce, making them easier to expel. Some physicians order neostigmine to be given intramuscularly about 20 minutes before a rectal tube or return-flow enema is administered. Neostigmine increases GI motility and facilitates downward movement of the gas. However, this practice is controversial because of the drug's numerous side effects, such as dizziness, severe abdominal cramping, respiratory depression, and nausea and vomiting. If postnasal drip causes excessive air swallowing, a decongestant or antihistamine may eliminate the problem.

Interventions to Manage Fecal Diversions

As with any condition, fecal diversions must be assessed to detect problems and determine appropriate nursing interventions. Physiological problems vary depending on whether the type of ostomy is an ileostomy or colostomy (Figure 28-10).

The major problems with ileostomies are obstruction, diarrhea, and skin irritation. Obstruction is prevented by chewing food thoroughly, and it can usually be relieved by massaging the abdomen around the stoma or by gentle lavage (washing out) of the stoma with a catheter. Diarrhea is treated as described earlier. The client with an ileostomy is particularly susceptible to fluid and electrolyte imbalances. Therefore diarrhea must be quickly controlled.

Skin irritation is best treated by preventive measures, such as proper fitting and fixation of the collection bag. If irritation does occur, the skin must be kept clean and dry, and a protective skin barrier should be used between the pouch faceplate and the skin. Use topical medications to treat severe irritation.

Emptying and Changing the Ostomy Pouch or Bag. Except for continent ileostomies, ostomies continually drain fecal material. After surgery, and after the stoma heals, the client is fitted with a reusable ostomy pouch or bag. (A client with a colostomy usually wears an ostomy pouch rather than an ostomy bag.) Regardless of whether the client has a continent ileostomy or a colostomy, however, the ostomy pouch or bag must be emptied at regular intervals.

The client empties the pouch or bag whenever necessary (typically at the time of urination) through an opening at the bottom. To do so, the client removes the clamp from the end of the pouch or bag, places the end into the toilet, and lets the pouch or bag drain (Figure 28-11). Once the pouch or bag is empty, the client replaces the clamp on the end until it needs emptying again.

In addition to emptying an ostomy pouch or bag, the appliance needs to be changed when it is loose, or about every 3 days (Figure 28-12). When an ostomy bag needs to be changed, the old pouch and stoma wafer are removed. The stoma and skin are washed with warm water and soap and patted dry. To replace the appliance, the stoma is first measured to ensure a proper fit. Once the size of the stoma has been measured, the stoma wafer is cut to the proper size. If the client is very active, a special skin preparation is applied to the skin as a protectant. Next, an adhesive paste is applied. The backing material is removed from the stoma wafer, and the center hole of the stoma wafer is placed over the stoma with light pressure applied to ensure adherence to the skin. The ostomy pouch or bag is then snapped onto the ring of the stoma wafer. The ostomy pouch or bag may be closed or open at the

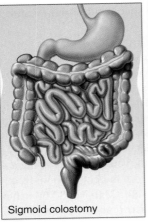
Sigmoid colostomy

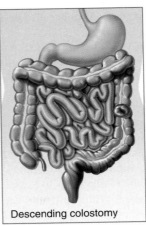
Descending colostomy

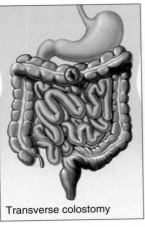
Transverse colostomy

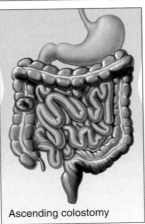
Ascending colostomy

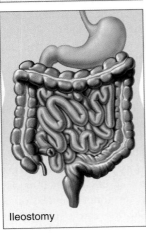
Ileostomy

Figure 28-10. Locations of ileostomies and colostomies.

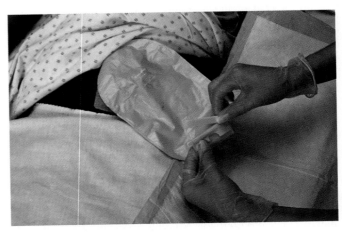

Figure 28-11. Emptying an ostomy pouch or bag.

end, depending on the location of the stoma and the client's preference.

Irrigating the Bowel. A colostomy can function adequately without irrigation, but irrigation helps to avoid fecal spillage during the day. Most clients are taught to care for their stomas and irrigate the bowel if necessary. Clients with a stoma who come into the hospital may prefer to continue their own care, or you may temporarily assume these tasks.

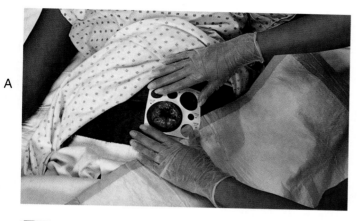

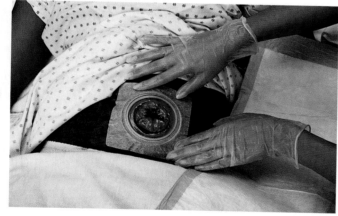

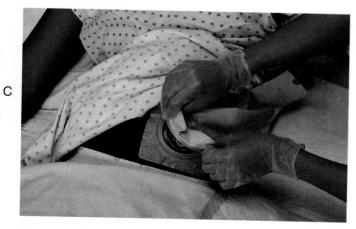

Figure 28-12. Changing an ostomy pouch or bag. **A,** Measure the stoma size to ensure a proper fit. **B,** Place the center hole of the stoma wafer over the stoma. **C,** Snap the ostomy pouch or bag onto the ring of the stoma wafer.

Irrigation of a colostomy is very similar to administration of a normal saline enema. The major differences are the insertion site and the client's inability to control the expulsion of solution and fecal material. Consequently, some variation in equipment and technique is necessary. An irrigation sleeve channels the expelled contents into the toilet or bedpan. This is a plastic tunnel that fits around the stoma and is held in place by a belt around the waist (Figure 28-13). The irrigating solution and enema equipment are prepared as for a volume enema. Cone-shaped irrigation tips are preferred to catheters because they reduce the danger of bowel perforation. The nipple cone also seals off the stoma so that the irrigating fluid cannot leak. Make sure of the location of the stoma before inserting the cone. If using a catheter, gently insert it about 7.5 to 10 cm (3 to 4 inches) and infuse the solution.

When you are ready to remove the administration tip, be sure the irrigating sleeve is well in front of the stoma, because the initial drainage may gush out. Close the top of the sleeve with clips, and allow most of the contents to be expelled. This usually takes about 10 to 15 minutes. Control odor by occasionally rinsing the sleeve with water and flushing the toilet. When the client is sure that the irrigation returns have finished, the irrigation sleeve may be removed, the peristomal skin cleaned, and either a clean pouch or dressing applied.

Teaching the Client Ostomy Self-Care. Clients with ostomies should be taught to live independently and care for their ostomy needs on their own, if possible. Changing the ostomy pouch or bag is the first step in learning and is the same as the procedure just described. If the client will be irrigating the colostomy, the irrigation procedure needs to be taught. Odor control and medication use are other topics of concern (Box 28-6, p. 688).

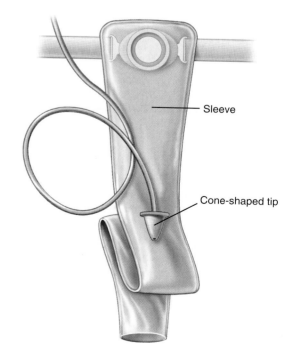

Sleeve

Cone-shaped tip

Figure 28-13. Sleeve and cone-shaped tip for colostomy irrigation.

Teaching for Self-Care
Ostomy Care

Box 28-6

Purpose: To make the client independent in the management of bowel elimination in the presence of an ostomy.

Expected Outcome: The client will demonstrate the ability to manage bowel elimination through an ostomy, prevent complications, and manage lifestyle changes.

Client Instructions

Maintain a regular bowel elimination pattern by following these steps
- Plan for daily elimination at a time most consistent with the urge to defecate.
- Keep in mind that regular patterns of meals and activity may be helpful.

Maintain the necessary supplies
- Skin barriers
- Ostomy pouches
- A pouch belt, if needed
- Clamps or closing devices
- Hypoallergenic tape
- Towel and washcloths
- A mild skin cleanser

Use a pouching system to collect waste from the bowel
- Ensure a proper fit of the pouch to prevent leaks and protect your skin.
- Measure the stoma diameter and prepare a skin barrier/pouch with each pouch change. The opening should be no more than ⅛ inch larger than your stoma. Measure the stoma weekly for at least 8 weeks or until the stoma has stopped shrinking.
- Apply the skin barrier first. Then ensure that there are no wrinkles in the barrier.
- Apply the pouch to the barrier. Center and apply the pouch. Practice applying the pouch while sitting and standing.
- Change the appliance any time it leaks or is not intact.
- To remove the ostomy appliance, support the skin of your abdomen and gently loosen the seal.
- Cleanse the skin around the stoma. Waste from an ileostomy is especially irritating to the skin.
- Use a mild soap and carefully dry the area with a clean cloth or towel.
- Choose an ostomy pouch with an open end or a closed end. An open-ended pouch is best for liquid wastes, and the bag can be emptied without changing it.
- Use a clamp that you can manage easily, given your eyesight and manual dexterity.
- Empty an ileostomy pouch when it is one third full. Empty a colostomy pouch as needed.
- To close the pouch, fold the tail up once around the bar of the clamp and fasten the clamp.

Keep in mind the following lifestyle tips
- Avoid foods that cause odor and gas.
- Do whatever you need to do to avoid constipation.
- Treat diarrhea promptly.
- Check periodically to make sure that your ostomy is not blocked.
- Drink six to eight glasses of water daily, 10 to 12 if you have an ileostomy.
- Exercise regularly, especially to strengthen abdominal muscles.
- You can bathe and shower with or without the pouch.
- You can swim with the pouch, but use waterproof tape around edges of the pouch in a picture-frame fashion.
- You can continue to wear your normal wardrobe after an ostomy. No change in clothing is necessary.

Manage skin irritation
- Assess for irregularities in the skin that might cause leaks.
- Use a skin barrier to protect the skin.
- Use a skin barrier paste, if needed, to fill in any abdominal creases or irregular contours.
- Change pouching systems to maintain or create a well-functioning appliance.
- Add an ostomy belt, if needed.
- Notify your health care provider if you detect the following signs and symptoms of a *Candida* (yeast) infection: itching, burning, pain around the stoma, redness of the skin, or whiteheads (pustules).
- Apply an antifungal powder or spray, such as Mycostatin, to the skin around the stoma.

Follow a dietary plan
- Follow a well-balanced diet.
- Watch for foods that cause gas or changes in the consistency of your stool.
- Avoid foods that tend to block your stoma.

For the ostomate who wears a pouch, odor control can be a problem. Careful washing, pouch deodorizers, and medications are possible solutions. The client should also avoid gas-forming foods. Cabbage, cauliflower, onions, and turnips often increase fecal odor. Yogurt, buttermilk, parsley, and green leafy vegetables may reduce fecal odor. Odor control, which can be very distressing, can be managed by the following:

- Carefully washing the appliance after use
- Placing a deodorizing agent in the pouch
- Using internal medications, such as bismuth subgallate
- Ingesting yogurt, buttermilk, parsley, or orange juice
- Placing a few drops of Dispatch in the collection receptacle to mask the odor while emptying the pouch

Review of the new ostomate's medication regimen can help eliminate contraindicated medications. Diuretics, laxa-tives, enteric-coated medications, and sustained-release oral medications are usually not administered for the ileostomate and some colostomates.

EVALUATION

Evaluation of nursing care for the management of bowel elimination problems involves making decisions about the expected time frame for the intervention to be successful, ongoing monitoring, and measuring the parameters of the outcome criteria. Decision making is centered on whether the problem is acute or chronic. Look for data that suggest the problem is improving, the client is participating in care, and the problem is resolving.

Evaluation of the effectiveness of interventions for constipation is based on ongoing assessment to determine that

Nursing Care Plan A CLIENT WITH CONSTIPATION

Box 28-7

ADMISSION DATA

Dr. Daly reported that, yesterday, he consumed only one fourth of his usual intake of prune juice and bran flakes for breakfast. He consumed only half of his other two meals becaue of severe pain from bone cancer. He reported that he was concerned about increasing his morphine for fear of falling and other side effects.

Because Mr. Daly is having difficulty with his bowel elimination this morning, the nurse realizes that his nursing diagnosis of *Constipation* may lead to impaction.

PHYSICIAN'S ORDERS

Diet as desired
Laxative of choice

NURSING ASSESSMENT

Dr. Daly has not had his usual bowel movement in 3 days, his bowel sounds are hypoactive, and a fecal mass can be palpated in his lower abdomen. Therefore, the nurse considers the possibility of an impaction.

NANDA Nursing Diagnosis	NOC Expected Outcomes With Indicators	NIC Interventions With Selected Activities	Evaluation Data
CONSTIPATION **Related Factors:** • Decreased mobility and morphine use	**BOWEL ELIMINATION** • Elimination pattern in expected range. • Stool soft and formed. • Constipation not present. • Ease of stool passage. • Comfort of stool passage.	**BOWEL MANAGEMENT** • Note date of last bowel movement (BM). • Monitor BM frequency, consistency, shape, volume, and color. • Monitor bowel sounds. • Report diminished bowel sounds. • Monitor for signs and symptoms of constipation and impaction. • Teach about alternative foods that help in promoting bowel regularity. • Instruct in foods that are high in fiber. • Give warm liquids after meals as appropriate. • Evaluate medication profile for GI side effects. • Allow client choices in bowel management.	**AFTER 24 HOURS OF CARE** • Laxative administered at client's request. Large, hard, formed BM today. • Passage was difficult. • Dr. Daly chooses to continue his usual routine.

CRITICAL THINKING QUESTIONS

1. How would you prevent further constipation in Dr. Daly?
2. Is reducing the dose of morphine an acceptable method of preventing constipation in this client?
3. The client prefers to use fiber as a means of managing constipation. What would you say to him about continuing to use this method?

Nursing outcome and intervention labels from Johnson, M., Bulechek, G., McCloskey Dochterman, J., Maas, M., & Moorhead, S. (2001). *Nursing diagnoses, outcomes, and interventions: NANDA, NIC, and NOC linkages.* St Louis, MO: Mosby.

the problem is resolving. When the problem is constipation, the client should have a bowel movement usually within 24 hours of the onset of treatment. Collect data to determine that the signs and symptoms of constipation are not persistent. When the problem is chronic, data are collected over time to determine that the client establishes a regular pattern of elimination without the signs and symptoms of constipation (Box 28-7).

Evaluation of the effectiveness of interventions for diarrhea requires ongoing monitoring to determine that the diarrhea is resolving, usually within the first 24 hours. Monitor for signs of dehydration and electrolyte loss. Intake and output measurements should be taken. The time frame for diarrhea resolution is directly related to the cause of the diarrhea. For example, some viral infections may have a natural course of 24 to 48 hours. On the other hand,

a client with inflammatory bowel disease will have outcome criteria that suggest the problem is controlled rather than cured.

For the problem of fecal impaction, the initial outcome criterion is that the impaction has been removed. Long-term goals are set to prevent the problem from recurring. The client's bowel management program must be modified on an ongoing basis.

For the problem of bowel incontinence, the time frame for evaluation depends on the cause of the problem. If the cause is a medication combined with weakness from an acute illness, the problem can often be resolved quickly. If the problem is a permanent change in mental status combined with immobility, management will be ongoing. It may take several weeks to determine the best schedule of toileting to prevent bowel incontinence.

The nurse enters the following note into the chart about Dr. Daly's constipation.

SAMPLE DOCUMENTATION FOR DR. DALY

Reports relief of constipation. Will resume his usual routine of a high-fiber breakfast and a warm drink with breakfast.

Key Principles

- The lower GI tract is the main organ system responsible for the elimination of the body's solid waste. It consists of the ascending, transverse, descending, and sigmoid portions of the colon, and the rectum.
- Physiological and psychosocial factors have a strong influence on the act of defecation.
- Assessment of bowel elimination needs includes noting the history of psychological and physiological factors affecting elimination; completing a physical assessment of the abdomen and observing fecal characteristics; and noting the outcome of diagnostic tests completed by radiographic examination, direct visualization, and laboratory analysis.
- The current NANDA list of nursing diagnoses relevant to bowel elimination needs includes *Bowel incontinence, Constipation, Perceived constipation,* and *Diarrhea.*
- The nurse does not order diagnostic tests but, along with assessment findings, does use the results in diagnosing nursing problems.
- Interventions to treat acute constipation would meet the goals of rapid relief from the acute problem and reestablishing a regular bowel elimination pattern; for chronic constipation, the goal is to help the client establish a long-term plan of management.
- Interventions to treat diarrhea would meet the goals of no loose stools and a return of regular bowel elimination pattern.
- Interventions to treat bowel incontinence would meet the goals of maintaining skin integrity and promoting normal bowel elimination.
- Evaluation of outcomes should show that the fecal contents and bowel movements are as near to normal as possible for the client, or that the client has adapted successfully to elimination changes.

Bibliography

Campbell, T., Draper, S., Reid, J., & Robinson, L. (2001). The management of constipation in people with advanced cancer. *International Journal of Palliative Nursing, 7*(3):110, 112-119.

Chiarioni, G., Bassotti, G., Monsignori, A., Menegotti, M., Salandini, L., Di Matteo, G., et al. (2000). Anorectal dysfunction in constipated women with anorexia nervosa. *Mayo Clinic Proceedings, 75*(10), 1015-1019.

Eslemon, N., Stucky-Marshall, L., & Talamonti, M. S. (2001). Screening for colorectal cancer: Developing a preventive health-care program utilizing nurse endoscopists. *Gastroenterology Nursing, 24*(1), 12-19.

Fennig, S. (1999). Management of encopresis in early adolescence in a medical-psychiatric unit. *General Hospital Psychiatry, 21*(5), 360-367.

Fish, C. (1995). *In good hands: The keeping of a family farm.* New York: Farrar, Straus & Giroux.

Frazier, A. L., Colditz, G. A., Fuchs, C. S., & Kuntz, K. M. (2000). Cost-effectiveness of screening for colorectal cancer in the general population. *Journal of the American Medical Association, 284*(15), 1954-1961.

Gruver, R. A. (2000). Case study: Antibiotic-induced acute diarrhea. *Physician Assistant, 24*(11), 56-58.

Hinrichs, M. D., & Huseboe, J. (2001). Research-based protocol: Management of constipation. *Journal of Gerontological Nursing, 27*(2), 17-28.

Jarrett, M. E., Lustyk, M. K., Cain, K. C., & Heitkemper, M. M. (2000). Exercise across the health continuum: A paradigm shift—Exercise as a therapeutic for women with constipation-prone IBS. *Communicating Nursing Research, 33,* 113.

Jensen, L. L. (2000). Assessing and treating patients with complex fecal incontinence. *Ostomy Wound Management, 46*(12), 56-61.

Johnson, M., Bulechek, G., McCloskey Dochterman, J., Maas, M., & Moorhead, S. (2001). *Nursing diagnoses, outcomes, and interventions: NANDA, NOC, and NIC linkages.* St Louis, MO: Mosby.

Kachourbos, M. J., & Creasey, G. H. (2000). Health promotion in motion: improving quality of life for persons with neurogenic bladder and bowel using assistive technology [corrected] [published erratum appears in *SCI Nursing, 17*(4), 221 (2000)]. *SCI Nursing, 17*(3), 125-129.

*Leininger, M. M. (1991). *Culture care diversity and universality: A theory of nursing.* New York: National League for Nursing Press.

Moore, K. (2001). Measurement challenges in fecal incontinence. *Journal of Wound, Ostomy, & Continence Nursing, 28*(3), 121.

Mylonakis, E., Ryan, E. T., & Calderwood, S. B. (2001). *Clostridium difficile*–associated diarrhea: A review. *Archives of Internal Medicine, 161*(4), 525-533, 617-618.

North American Nursing Diagnosis Association. (2001). *Nursing diagnoses: Definitions and classification, 2001-2002.* Philadelphia: Author.

Norton, C., & Chelvanayagam, S. (2001). Methodology of biofeedback for adults with fecal incontinence: A program of care, including commentary by Bliss, D. Z. *Journal of Wound, Ostomy & Continence Nursing, 28*(3), 156-170.

Palmer, D., & Barker, P. (2001). Increasing fibre: Why and how. *Nursing Times, 97*(16), 19-25, 54-55.

Rew, L. (2000). Possible outcomes of holistic nursing interventions. *Journal of Holistic Nursing, 18*(4), 307-309.

Rogers, J. (2000). The causes and management of constipation in children. *Community Nurse, 6*(3), 39-40.

Sneddon, D. (2001). Continence in MS [corrected] [published erratum appears in *Professional Nurse, 16*(8), 1268 (2001)]. *Professional Nurse, 16*(7), 1241-1244.

Tanner, C. A., (2000). Critical thinking: Beyond nursing process. *Journal of Nursing Education, 39*(8), 338-339.

---

*Asterisk indicates a classic or definitive work on this subject.

Managing Urinary Elimination

Learning Objectives

After studying this chapter, you should be able to do the following:

- Describe the normal structure and function of the urinary system
- Identify common problems of urinary elimination
- Discuss factors affecting urinary elimination
- Assess urinary function and identify a client experiencing urinary elimination problems
- Diagnose problems of urinary elimination that can be managed with nursing care
- Plan expected outcomes for goal-directed nursing interventions for managing problems in urinary elimination
- Implement basic nursing care for a client experiencing problems with urinary elimination
- Evaluate care for a person experiencing problems with urinary elimination

Urinary Tract Infection. A urinary tract infection can occur in any portion of the urinary tract. The infection is termed cystitis if it affects the bladder, urethritis if it affects the urethra, and ureteritis if it affects the ureters. Pyelonephritis is an infection of the kidney. Urinary tract infections are more common in women than in men.

Urinary Obstruction. Urinary obstruction can occur from stones, strictures, tumors, prostatic hypertrophy, or edema. Stones, or calculi, cause symptoms when the kidneys, ureters, or bladder are blocked or partially blocked or the stone is moving. You may hear the condition called urolithiasis. Most renal calculi are composed of calcium, but they may also contain magnesium, uric acid, and cystine.

Urinary Diversion. Urine can be diverted from its normal pathway, either by congenital malformation or by surgical creation. Hypospadias, in which the urethra opens on the underside of the penis or inside the vagina, is an example of a congenital malformation.

Various types of urinary diversions can be created surgically to treat cancer, a birth defect, an obstruction, or a neurogenic dysfunctional bladder (Figure 29-4). Although the principles of care for urinary diversions are similar, understanding the nature of the following surgical procedures may help you anticipate normal findings in the function of the diversion.

- An *ileal conduit* connects the distal ureters to a resected portion of the terminal ileum, which is used to form a stoma, or opening, onto the surface of the abdomen.

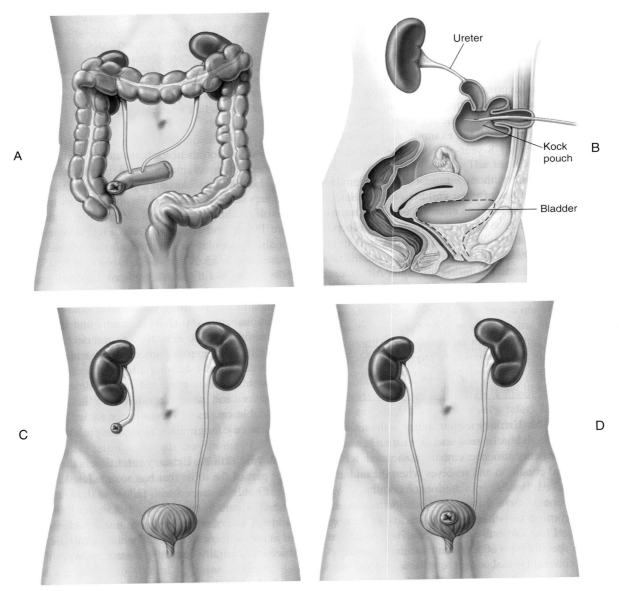

Figure 29-4. Types of urinary diversions. **A,** Ileal conduit. **B,** Kock pouch. **C,** Cutaneous ureterostomy; **D,** Vesicostomy.

- A *Kock pouch* is a special type of ileal conduit in which a surgeon uses a segment of ileum to create a pouch for holding urine. Nipple valves created from intussuscepted portions of the ileal segment help keep the pouch continent. The client drains the pouch by inserting a catheter through the stoma.
- A *ureterosigmoidostomy* procedure connects the ureters to the sigmoid colon, which allows urine to drain through the colon. The procedure (not shown in Figure 29-4) is a variation of the Kock pouch procedure.
- In a *cutaneous ureterostomy,* the distal end of the ureter is brought to the surface of the skin to create a stoma.
- In a *vesicostomy* (also called cystostomy), an opening is made directly into the bladder.

Unless the client has a Kock pouch, attach a bag to the skin around the stoma to collect urine as it drains from the stoma. The client must be taught to manage drainage from the stoma, to care for the skin, to recognize signs and symptoms of abnormal function, and to manage the feelings associated with a change in body image.

FACTORS AFFECTING URINARY ELIMINATION

Most people do not give much thought or planning to maintaining a normal pattern of urinary elimination. Voiding typically occurs five or six times daily, although the actual number may vary widely with the volume of fluid intake, the size of the person's bladder, and the availability of toilet facilities.

Urinary output has diurnal variation. The action of antidiuretic hormone and decreased renal blood flow in the recumbent position decrease the volume of urine produced at night. However, some people need to urinate at night, possibly because of a small bladder capacity, increased fluid intake before bed, habit, or certain health problems. **Nocturia** is the term used for nighttime urination. Many factors can affect urination, both at night and during the day.

Lifestyle Factors
Nutrition and Fluids. The amount of urine produced in a 24-hour period is directly related to the amount of fluid consumed in the same period. The kidneys function to maintain a balance of body water by excreting excess fluids that the body does not need. Six to eight glasses (1200 to 2000 mL) of water daily is the recommended amount to maintain optimal renal function. Because fluid is also lost through perspiration and respiration, any activity that increases these functions also increases the body's need for water. Diarrhea and vomiting may lead to excessive loss of fluids from the gastrointestinal tract.

The water taken in through foods balances the water lost through perspiration and respiration. Foods contain various amounts of water. Fruits, especially watermelon, will add to the fluid intake and increase the production of urine. **Diuresis** is the increased formation and excretion of urine. Watermelon may actually have a diuretic effect. Drinks with caffeine (coffee, tea, some carbonated beverages) and alcoholic beverages (especially beer) cause diuresis and increase the urge to urinate. Artichokes may have some diuretic effect. Foods high in sodium encourage fluid retention.

Psychosocial. Privacy is probably the most important psychosocial issue and may relate to larger cultural issues (Box 29-2). Most people consider urination to be a private matter; some people have difficulty initiating urination in the presence of others. Both men and women may have difficulty voiding in the presence of a person of the opposite sex.

Stressful life events can interfere with complete emptying of the bladder or cause a person to urinate more frequently

---

Cross-Cultural Care CARING FOR A WEST INDIAN HINDU AMERICAN
Box 29-2

Fatami Shireem is a 60-year-old woman who emigrated from India to the United States with her family as an adult. She belongs to the Hindu religion, which evolved over 4000 years, represents no single creed or founder, and has diverse, spiritually based health practices and customs. Formal religious organization is minimal and there is no religious hierarchy. Mrs. Shireem married a West Indian Hindu American whom she chose, but it was important that her parents approved of her choice. She alternates between traditional Indian dress and American-style dress. Although every client is unique, many West Indian Hindu people hold certain unifying beliefs (Giger & Davidhizar, 1996), such as the following:
- Awe, respect, or reverence for life
- Belief in reincarnation (transmigration of the soul at the time of death into another body)
- Belief in dharma, or moral responsibility, as in law, religion, virtue, morality, custom; dharma requires the pursuit of Nirvana as defined by the priests
- A divine mandate to separate people by castes, in which those of a lower caste can advance to a higher caste in the next life by fulfilling moral obligations in the present life

- Use of the Hindi language to maintain cultural unity, especially for older West Indian Hindu people; younger people often adapt to the use of English
- The social status of women being below that of men (with a female client, a greeting should be first addressed to the husband)
- Avoidance of direct eye contact between a man and any woman other than his wife
- Avoidance of handshaking as a greeting between a man and any woman other than his wife
- A family orientation, in which the entire family may gather at a client's bedside, in part to help guard the client's personal space and to increase her feelings of control
- A preference for being stoic rather than praying for recovery because praying for recovery is the lowest form of prayer
- Requirement for a daily bath as a religious duty
- The importance of the mother-in-law in making health care decisions
- Soft-spoken manner
- Vegetarian diet

Expected Outcomes for the Client
With *Urinary Retention*

For a client with a diagnosis of *Urinary retention* as a result of overflow incontinence caused by a neurogenic bladder, expected outcomes could include that the client will be able to do the following:

- Express motivation to perform self-catheterization
- Master self-catheterization
- Maintain clean technique
- Have no urinary tract infections

For other causes of *Urinary retention*, the expected outcomes could include that the client will be able to do the following:

- Establish a normal pattern of voiding without residual urine
- Void within 8 hours of removal of an indwelling (Foley) catheter
- Report no discomfort with voiding
- Recognize the signs of bladder distention
- Have no signs or symptoms of reflux, bladder damage, or renal damage

INTERVENTION

Interventions to Promote Urinary Continence

Many interventions are available to help control urinary incontinence, as summarized here and in Table 29-4.

Establishing Continence

PELVIC MUSCLE EXERCISES. **Kegel exercises** are exercises performed to strengthen the pelvic and vaginal muscles to help control stress incontinence in women (Box 29-5). They are named for Dr. Arnold H. Kegel, the gynecologist who first developed them. Performed correctly, Kegel exercises can reduce or eliminate incontinence in approximately 60% of cognitively intact, cooperative women (AHCPR, 1996). The exercises are described in Box 29-6 (p. 710). Although used primarily for stress incontinence, they sometimes can be beneficial for reducing urge incontinence.

Performing the exercises correctly depends on the woman's ability to selectively contract the muscles of the pelvic floor. The initial tendency is to contract the abdominal muscles or the muscles of the buttocks. The correct muscle can be located by starting the stream of urine, then contracting the muscles to stop the flow. Another method is to place one finger in the vagina and contract the pelvic floor muscles around the finger. Biofeedback training is useful for some women to become familiar with the contraction of the correct muscle. A vaginal or rectal probe may be used to provide visual feedback when the correct muscle has been contracted. Two thirds of women will need some practice to find the correct muscles.

BLADDER RETRAINING. For the person with urge incontinence associated with a small bladder capacity, training is designed to increase the bladder capacity by having the client

Table 29-4	Interventions for Urinary Incontinence
Intervention	**Application**
Basic evaluation	• Obtain history, physical examination, postvoid residual volume, and urinalysis on all clients with urinary incontinence. • After basic evaluation and initial treatment, clients who fail or are not appropriate for treatment based on presumptive diagnosis should undergo further evaluation.
Routine or scheduled toileting	• Offer to incontinent clients on a consistent schedule. • This technique is recommended for clients who cannot participate in independent toileting.
Habit training Prompted voiding	• Use for clients in whom a natural voiding pattern can be determined. • Recommended for clients who can learn to recognize some degree of bladder fullness or the need to void, or who can ask for assistance or respond when prompted to toilet. • Clients who are candidates for prompted voiding may not have sufficient cognitive ability to participate in other, more complex behavioral therapies.
Bladder training	• Use to manage urge incontinence, mixed incontinence, and stress incontinence.
Exercises to strengthen pelvic muscles	• Use to decrease the incidence of urinary incontinence. • Pelvic muscle exercises are strongly recommended for women with stress incontinence, men and women with urge incontinence who also receive bladder training, and men who develop urinary incontinence after prostatectomy. • Pelvic muscle rehabilitation and bladder inhibition using biofeedback therapy are recommended for clients with stress incontinence, urge incontinence, and mixed incontinence.
Vaginal weight training	• Recommended for premenopausal woman who have stress incontinence. • Used to decrease incontinence in women with stress incontinence.
Pelvic floor electrical stimulation	• Used to decrease incontinence in women with stress incontinence. • May be useful for urge and mixed incontinence.
Medications	• Alpha-adrenergic agonists are the first line of therapy when not contraindicated. • Estrogen is recommended as adjunct therapy in conjunction with alpha-adrenergic agonists. • Anticholinergic agents (especially oxybutynin) and tricyclic antidepressants are reportedly useful for detrusor instability. However, tricyclic antidepressants produce adverse effects, especially in older adults.
Surgery	• May be used as first-line treatment for some clients with stress incontinence; used uncommonly for urge incontinence. • Surgery to relieve the obstruction is used for overflow incontinence.

From Urinary Incontinence Guideline Panel (1982). *Urinary incontinence in adults*. AHCPR Publication No. 92-0038 and 92-0041. Rockville, MD: Agency for Health Care Policy and Research.

adopt a gradually lengthening voiding schedule. Strategies to control the urge to urinate are practiced.

For the cognitively competent person, a bladder diary may be useful for selecting the most useful training protocol. A daily record is kept of the time of urination, whether the person was incontinent, whether the incontinence involved a small or large amount, and associated events or the reason for the incontinence. For the cognitively impaired person, training is different, and a scheduled toileting regimen may be successful. The client's voiding pattern should be recorded for several days to determine whether a pattern exists. Electronic devices to monitor for wetness are sometimes useful in establishing the pattern.

People often need to urinate on arising in the morning, after meals, and at bedtime. However, for some older clients, the schedule may need to be as frequent as every 2 hours. Patience is required. Over time, the regimen becomes habitual and incontinence will improve. Success is partially related to a consistent daily schedule of meals and fluid intake.

For clients with some ability to recognize the need to urinate, a schedule of prompted voiding may be successful, as described later in the chapter.

Maintaining Dry and Intact Skin

EXTERNAL CATHETERS. External catheters are devices that can be attached to the skin to collect urine. External collecting devices for women are not widely available and have tended to leak and cause skin abrasions. Condom catheters are used successfully for men, however. The condom is a heavy rubber sheath that fits over the penis and is secured with a soft, flexible band (Procedure 29-2, p. 710). The end of the condom has a drainage tube molded into the condom and connected to a bedside drainage bag or leg bag (Figure 29-8, p. 710).

The risk for urinary tract infection is reduced with an external catheter. The advantages of using a condom catheter are keeping the skin dry and controlling odor. The disadvantages are the difficulty in securing the catheter adequately to control leakage of urine and to keep the catheter in place without causing edema to the penis and excoriation to the skin. The catheter should be removed at least daily to inspect the skin.

Complications include abrasion, dermatitis, ischemia, necrosis, edema, and maceration of the penis. The incidence of urinary tract infection is less than with an indwelling catheter but is still a factor in using condom catheters. An alternative to a condom catheter for men is a retracted penis pouch (Figure 29-9, p. 712). This device is sometimes successful if the man has a retracted penis that cannot support a condom catheter.

> *Action Alert!* Avoid constricting the penis with a condom catheter, because doing so will cause edema. Remove the condom and inspect the skin daily.

⊄HE STATE OF NURSING RESEARCH: It's That Problem No One Wants to Talk About

Box 29-5

What Are the Issues?

Urinary stress incontinence occurs unwanted in susceptible women when they cough or sneeze. Having stress incontinence can cause a woman to limit her activities and to resort to such interventions as wearing pads on a daily basis. Efforts to control urinary incontinence have focused on improving pelvic floor muscles that control urinary outflow.

What Research Has Been Conducted?

One group of researchers randomly assigned older rural women living at home to either treatment (behavioral management) or control group (Dougherty et al., 2002). Women kept a diary of such things as "fluid intake, voids, and incontinent episodes throughout the day and night" (p. 5). Women wore pads to collect urine lost during incontinence episodes. The researchers also measured quality of life with a questionnaire. The intervention included bladder training and pelvic muscle exercises (PME). "The women performed PME (15 repetitions per day increased by 15 repetitions every 3 weeks to 45 contractions per day) three time a week for 12 weeks" (p. 7).

Another researcher (Johnson, 2001, p. 33) randomly assigned women with incontinence to one of two types of exercise protocols, maximum voluntary contractions or submaximal voluntary contractions. Measures of muscle contraction strength and urine leakage were compared for the two groups.

What Has the Research Concluded?

Training women to improve pelvic muscle function appears to decrease urinary incontinence in women living at home. Over the 2 years of the study, the behavioral management group in the first study (Dougherty et al., 2002) showed dramatic decreases in urinary incontinence and increases in quality of life over that of the control group. Researchers were somewhat surprised that women in the control group whose incontinence worsened were not offered other forms of treatment from their health care providers. It may be that incontinence continues to be underassessed and not talked about.

Johnson's (2001) study using two types of exercise instruction found that those women in the group who used submaximal contraction strengthened both their pelvic floor muscles and endurance.

What Is the Future of Research in This Area?

Both studies were limited in the types of women studied. A wider variety of clients could be recruited to see if the results can be repeated. Johnson recommended a study that combined training protocols to see if both pelvic muscle strength and control could be improved.

References

Dougherty, M. C., Dwyer, J. W., Pendergast, J. F., Boyington, A. R., Tomlinson, B. U., Coward, R. T., et al. (2002). A randomized trial of behavioral management for continence with older rural women. *Research in Nursing & Health*, 25(1), 3-13.

Johnson, V. Y. (2001). Effects of a submaximal exercise protocol to recondition the pelvic floor musculature. *Nursing Research*, 50(1), 33-41.

Teaching for Wellness — Box 29-6
Exercises for the Pelvic Floor Muscles

Purpose: To help control stress incontinence in women.

Expected Outcome: The client will experience no urine leakage with an increase in abdominal pressure.

Client Instructions

- To perform Kegel exercises correctly, you must first locate the proper muscles. To do so, sit on the toilet, begin urinating, and try to stop the urine in midstream. The muscles used to stop the urine stream are the ones you need to exercise. Another way to locate the proper muscles is to insert one finger into your vagina and contract the muscles of your pelvic floor around your finger.
- Strengthen your pelvic floor muscles by contracting them for 5 to 10 seconds, relaxing for 5 to 10 seconds, and repeating.
- Perform this exercise three times daily, contracting the muscles 15 times during each exercise period. For example, perform 15 contractions in the morning before rising from bed. Perform 15 more contractions in the afternoon while doing a task that requires you to stand up without moving around. Finally, perform 15 more contractions in the evening while sitting, such as while watching television or reading a book.
- Make these exercises a part of your daily routine. You will begin to see results in about 2 weeks, and you will continue to improve for about 6 weeks.

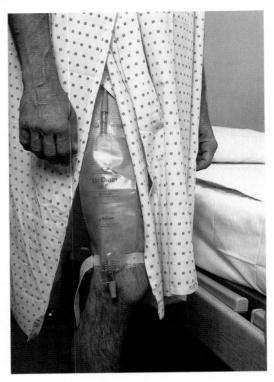

Figure 29-8. For the ambulatory client with an indwelling catheter, a drainage bag can be attached to the leg and hidden by the client's clothes.

PROCEDURE 29-2 APPLYING A CONDOM CATHETER

TIME TO ALLOW
Novice: 10 min.
Expert: 5 min.

The purpose of applying a condom catheter is to control incontinence in a male client without the risk for urinary tract infection and with greater comfort to the client than an indwelling catheter.

DELEGATION GUIDELINES
The application of a condom catheter is a noninvasive procedure that you may delegate to a nursing assistant who has received specific instruction in this skill. Instruction should include safety and skin care considerations.

EQUIPMENT NEEDED
- Commercially packaged condom catheter
- Soap and water
- Disposable clean gloves
- Drainage bag and tubing

1. Follow preliminary guidelines for nursing procedures (see inside front cover).

2. Position the client on his back and drape him to expose only his penis.

3. Clean his genitals with soap and water and dry thoroughly.

4. Apply skin-protecting cream packaged with the catheter to the client's penis. Allow it to dry.

5. Wrap the adhesive spirally around the shaft of the penis (see illustration). *Be careful not to apply the adhesive too tightly. Severe edema can result if the adhesive strip constricts the shaft of the penis, and the client will develop pain and difficulty urinating.*

possible, help a female client sit up in bed on the bedpan to simulate the usual position for urination. It may be helpful to warm the bedpan by filling it with warm water, emptying it, and drying it thoroughly before offering it to the client. Using a small amount of talcum powder on the rim helps prevent the bedpan from sticking to the skin as it slides under the buttocks.

If the client cannot raise the buttocks enough to place the bedpan in the correct position, turn the client to the side, place the bedpan in the correct position, and turn the client back onto the bedpan. As you turn the client, push down on the side of the bedpan to help it stay under the buttocks. As an alternative, use a fracture pan, which was specially designed for clients who have fractured bones and cannot raise their buttocks. The client simply raises one leg and the small end of the pan is placed in the angle between the buttocks and the bed. It is not necessary for the client to raise the hips to slide the pan under the buttocks.

Some clients have difficulty with the initial voiding after an indwelling catheter is removed or after having surgery in the pelvic region. The problem can be the result of edema, irritation, or tenderness. It is exacerbated by feeling tension about being able to urinate or about the possibility of pain when urinating. You can try methods to help the person relax, such as relaxation breathing techniques. Running water in a nearby sink may stimulate urination. Using a spray of warm water over the perineum may relax the perineum and help start the stream of urine. The client's sitting in a warm sitz bath can also be helpful. If the client's urine must be measured, however, you will not be able to use a method that mixes the urine with water.

Remember Mrs. Shireem from the introductory story? On the second day after surgery, she can walk to the bathroom. What methods would you think are the most appropriate to help her urinate for the first time?

Using Catheters. A urinary catheter is a tube inserted into the bladder to drain urine. Urinary catheters can be used to prevent incontinence, to avoid the inconvenience of a bedpan in a client confined to bed, to collect urine specimens, and to drain urine from a person unable to void. The primary purpose of a urinary catheter is to prevent urinary retention.

CATHETERIZATION. Catheterization refers to inserting a tube into the bladder through the urethra for the purpose of draining urine from the bladder. It may have various indications (Box 29-8). For one-time relief of retention, the catheter is passed, urine is drained, and the catheter is removed. Sometimes referred to as straight catheterization or in-and-out catheterization, intermittent catheterization is also used by clients who need self-catheterization.

When a problem is expected to persist, an indwelling (Foley) catheter is used. This type of catheter has two or three lumens. One drains urine, the second allows inflation of a balloon in the client's bladder, and a third can be used to irrigate the bladder with fluids or medications (Figure 29-10, p. 714).

Box 29-8   Indications for Catheterization

SHORT-TERM INDWELLING CATHETERIZATION

- After surgical procedures known to interfere with normal urination, such as bladder surgery, pelvic surgery, some types of hip surgery
- When the client's kidney function must be monitored, as when renal function is compromised or the client has a critical illness and a high risk for shock
- After surgical procedures involving the urinary tract, when a catheter can help prevent obstruction from blood clots
- When an orthopedic client cannot be safely turned and repositioned
- When frequent moving causes pain
- To empty the bladder during childbirth (labor and delivery)

INTERMITTENT CATHETERIZATION

- For relief of discomfort from an overdistended bladder when the client cannot initiate urination
- When obtaining a sterile urine specimen for culture
- When assessing residual urine volume after the client voids
- For long-term management of urination in spinal cord injuries, multiple sclerosis, or other causes of incompetent bladder

LONG-TERM CATHETERIZATION

- For irreversible incontinence, when skin rash, ulcers, or wound management is negatively affected by urine on the skin
- For a terminally ill client (especially one in severe pain) whose comfort is improved by minimizing the amount of turning and cleaning needed
- For irreversible, severe urinary retention, especially when the client develops frequent urinary tract infections

---

Action Alert! Check an indwelling catheter regularly for patency to prevent urinary retention. Crusts formed with long-term use, blood clots when bleeding is present, or kinking and incorrect positioning of the tube can obstruct catheters.

Indwelling catheters are used for short-term problems that will benefit from catheterization to relieve or prevent urinary retention that cannot be corrected medically or surgically, that cannot be managed practically by intermittent catheterization, and, occasionally, to manage the incontinent client. A client with chronic retention may benefit from a catheter if bothered by persistent overflow incontinence, symptomatic urinary tract infections, or an increased risk for renal dysfunction. If an incontinent client has pressure ulcers, skin lesions, or surgical wounds that are being contaminated by urine, an indwelling catheter may be beneficial as well. Indwelling catheters are sometimes used for short-term management of elimination in the severely ill, in clients undergoing major surgery, and in the terminally ill (Procedure 29-3, p. 715).

Action Alert! Maintaining straight, gravity drainage from an indwelling catheter will prevent backflow of possibly contaminated urine into the bladder.

Urinary catheterization carries a high risk for urinary tract infection and should be avoided unless the potential benefits outweigh the potential risks. After a single catheterization

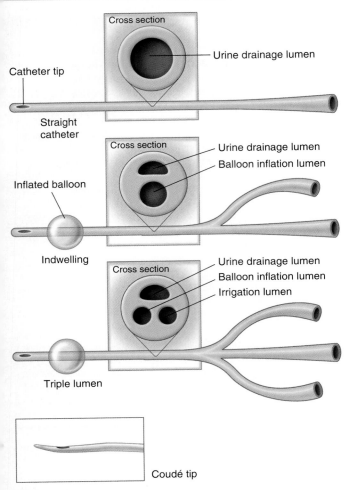

Figure 29-10. Types of catheters. **A,** A straight catheter is inserted to drain the bladder and then immediately removed. **B,** An indwelling (Foley) catheter has a second lumen, used to inflate a balloon that holds the catheter in place in the bladder. **C,** A triple-lumen indwelling catheter has a third lumen for instillation of fluid into the bladder for irrigation. **D,** A Coudé tip.

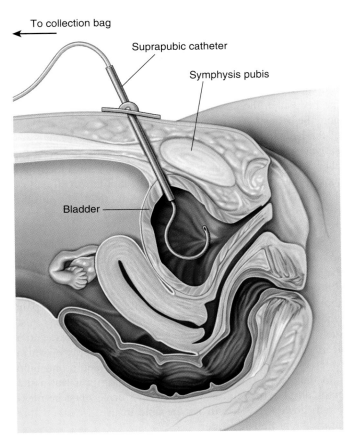

Figure 29-11. A suprapubic catheter is surgically placed through a puncture wound to drain urine until the client can void normally through the urethra.

(not indwelling), 1% of ambulatory clients will develop infection. With an open drainage system, most clients will develop an infection in 4 to 7 days.

Suprapubic catheters are sometimes placed to reduce the incidence of infection. A puncture wound is made through the abdominal wall into the bladder and a catheter is inserted (Figure 29-11). The incidence of infection is less than with a typical indwelling catheter because the abdominal skin has a lower bacterial count than the urethra.

MANAGING URETHRAL CATHETERS

MAINTAINING COMFORT. The client with an indwelling catheter should be physically and mentally comfortable. Probably the greatest discomfort for most people is embarrassment and invasion of privacy.

MAINTAINING A PATENT CATHETER. The catheter should be taped to the leg (women) or abdomen (men) to prevent it from pulling on the urethra and to ensure the free flow of urine. Disposable anchoring devices are available, but nonallergenic tape can be used as well. Keep enough slack in the catheter to

allow the client to move about without having the catheter pull on the urethra. Taping a male catheter laterally to the side or to the abdomen more naturally follows the normal anatomic direction of the male urethra and avoids the possibility of abscess formation at the penoscrotal junction.

When the client is in bed, the connecting tubing can be placed under the leg or over the leg. Under-the-leg placement may use gravity more effectively for drainage, but the tubing is made of hard plastic and may cause discomfort or pressure on the skin. Coil any excess tubing on the bed to prevent stagnation of urine in dangling loops of tubing. Keep the drainage bag below the level of the bladder, even when moving the person in and out of bed or to a stretcher. Urine in the collection tubing is not sterile and, because bacteria growing in the collection bag could travel up the tubing, urine should not be allowed to flow back into the bladder.

RELIEVING BLADDER SPASMS. Bladder spasms are involuntary, sudden, violent contractions of the muscles of the bladder that can be prolonged and painful. Spasms can occur as a side effect of catheterization or secondary to surgery on the bladder or urethra. Even though the client has a catheter, the urge to urinate is often strong.

PROCEDURE 29-3   INSERTING AN INDWELLING CATHETER

TIME TO ALLOW
Novice: 20 min.
Expert: 10 min.

Unlike a straight catheterization, in which you insert a urinary catheter, drain the urine, and remove the catheter right away, an indwelling catheter remains in the client's bladder to provide continuous urine drainage. An inflated balloon holds the catheter in place in the urinary bladder. Besides providing continuous urine drainage, an indwelling catheter can be used to prevent bladder distention, obtain sterile urine specimens, and irrigate the bladder with fluids or medications.

DELEGATION GUIDELINES

The assessment and complexities of sterile technique suggest that the insertion of an indwelling catheter not be delegated to a nursing assistant. This is particularly true in an acute care setting, where the risk for nosocomial infection exists, or in a client in whom difficulty passing a catheter may be anticipated. In a long-term-care setting, it may be appropriate to consider delegation of this procedure after a careful client assessment.

EQUIPMENT NEEDED

- Bottom drape
- Sterile gloves
- Fenestrated drape
- Catheter, connecting tubing, and collection bag
- Syringe prefilled with sterile water
- Antiseptic cleaning solution
- Cotton balls
- Forceps
- Water-soluble lubricant
- Gooseneck lamp or flashlight, especially for a female client

1. Follow preliminary guidelines for nursing procedures (see inside front cover).

2. Select a catheter of appropriate size and material, with a balloon of appropriate size. *Catheters range from No. 6 French (the smallest) to No. 24 French (the largest). For a child, you probably will use a No. 8 to 10 French. Most adult women need a No. 14 to 16 French. Most men need a No. 16 to 18 French. A client who has had an indwelling catheter for a long time will need a larger catheter to prevent urine leakage from the stretched urethra.*

For short-term catheterization, you probably will use a plastic catheter. It can be inserted easily when well lubricated but may be less comfortable because it is stiff and inflexible. For catheterization lasting up to 3 weeks, you may use a latex or rubber catheter, which is softer than plastic. For catheterization lasting 4 to 6 weeks, you may use a polyvinylchloride catheter, which softens at body temperatures. For catheterization lasting 2 to 3 months, you may use a silicone or Teflon catheter, on which secretions are less likely to adhere and form crusts that could irritate the urethra or obstruct the catheter.

Pediatric catheters usually come with a 3-mL balloon; adult catheters have either a 5-mL or a 30-mL balloon. You may need to use the 30-mL balloon if the client has had an indwelling catheter for a long time or if he has had a transurethral resection of the prostate. The larger balloon is thought to provide some hemostasis at the neck of the bladder after prostate resection.

3. Position the client for catheterization.

a. If the client is female, have her lie in a supine position with her knees flexed and separated. *This position allows access to the urinary meatus and typically is comfortable for the client. If the client cannot hold her knees open, ask a colleague to hold them for you; do not spread the client's knees if doing so causes her pain. If the client cannot lie on her back or open her knees, place her in Sims' position with her upper leg flexed at the hip and knee.*

b. If the client is male, have him lie in a supine position.

4. Drape the client for privacy.

a. If the client is female, expose only her labia. To do so, place one corner of a sheet between her legs so that two corners cover her legs and the remaining corner covers her abdomen. Leave the drape fully in place over the client's labia until you are ready to perform the catheterization. You can then lift the corner of the drape that covers her labia and fold it back.

b. If the client is male, use his gown or a bath blanket to cover his upper body down to his penis. Use a bed sheet to cover his lower body up to his penis. *Draping should make the client feel covered and as private as possible but should be simple and not add significantly to the length of the procedure.*

PROCEDURE 29-3 | **INSERTING AN INDWELLING CATHETER**—CONT'D

5. *Establish a sterile field.*
a. Open the prepackaged catheter tray and place it in a convenient location. If your client is female, consider placing the opened tray on the bed near her perineum. If your client is male, consider placing the opened tray on an overbed table.
b. Place the bottom drape adjacent to a female client's buttocks (see illustration). Hold the drape only by a corner, allow it to fall open, and place it under her buttocks, still touching only the corners. Place the drape so it overlaps the outer wrapper of the open catheter tray. This will form a continuous sterile field from the tray to the client's buttocks. *This procedure is not practical for female clients who are likely to move their legs during the catheterization procedure.*

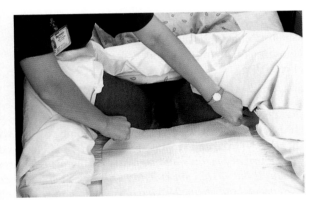

Step 5b. Placing the bottom drape. Touch only the corners to avoid contamination. (The edge of a sterile field is never considered to be sterile.)

c. Put on sterile gloves. If you wish, or according to your facility's policy, use a fenestrated drape (see illustration) to create a sterile field that encircles a female client's labia or a male client's penis.

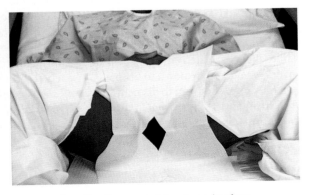

Step 5c. Fenestrated top drape in place.

d. Inflate the catheter balloon to test it for leaks (see illustration).

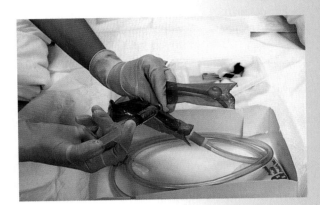

Step 5d. Testing the catheter balloon for leaks.

6. Clean the area around the urinary meatus
a. Pour antiseptic on all three cotton balls.
b. If the client is female, spread her labia with your nondominant hand (see illustration) while using forceps to hold a cotton ball in your dominant hand. *Remember that the hand used to spread the labia is no longer sterile.*

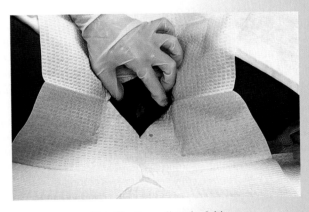

Step 6b. Spreading the labia.

c. With the first cotton ball, clean to the right of the client's urinary meatus. Make one stroke from top to bottom and discard the cotton ball (see illustration). With the second cotton ball, clean to the left of the client's urinary meatus, again making one stroke from top to bottom before discarding the cotton ball. With the third cotton ball, clean down the middle of the client's perineum, directly over the urinary meatus. Then discard the cotton ball. Keep the client's labia spread until the catheter is inserted.

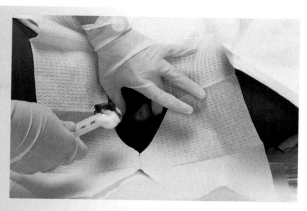

Step 6c. Cleaning the labia and meatus from top to bottom.

d. If the client is male, use at least two cotton balls soaked in antiseptic. Use the first to clean around the glans penis. Use the second to clean over the meatus. Make sure to retract the foreskin if the client has not been circumcised. *Remember to replace the foreskin to avoid edema of the glans penis.*

7. Lubricate and insert the catheter.

a. Holding the catheter 2.5 to 5 cm (1 to 2 inches) from its tip, lubricate it and insert it into the urinary meatus. If the client is male, use your nondominant hand to hold his penis perpendicular to his body, using your fingers to gently encircle and stabilize the shaft. *If you meet resistance when inserting a catheter, do not force it. Instead, have the client take a deep breath as you twist the catheter while trying to pass it. Often this method will allow the catheter to slide in easily. If it does not, try using a catheter with a Coudé tip; it is smaller and curved to help the catheter pass an obstruction, such as prostatic hypertrophy.*

b. Insert the catheter until urine begins to flow (see illustration). *The catheter should enter a female client by 5 to 7.6 cm (2 to 3 inches) or a male client by 15.2 to 20.3 cm (6 to 8 inches).*

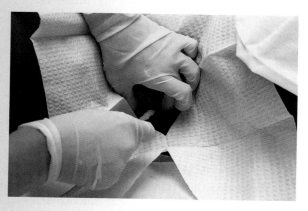

Step 7b. Inserting the catheter.

c. After urine begins to flow, insert the catheter 2.5 cm (1 inch) more. *Doing so will ensure that the balloon is in the bladder, not the urethra.*

8. Inflate the balloon (see illustration). If the syringe has been previously attached to the pigtail, simply inject 8 to 10 mL of water (30 mL +3 if the catheter has a 30-mL balloon). This recommendation is based on most catheters' needing 3 cc more than the amount that fills the balloon, to fill the lumen of the catheter. *You should check the recommendations of the manufacturer.*

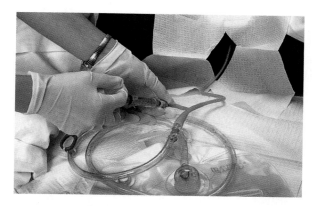

Step 8. Inflating the balloon.

9. Tape catheter to the inner aspect of the thigh (see illustration). *Allow enough slack in the catheter tubing to avoid tugging on the catheter when the client's leg moves.*

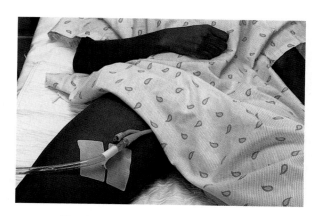

Step 9. Catheter taped to the inner thigh.

10. Establish the drainage system.

a. If the client will use a leg bag to collect urine, attach the catheter to the inner thigh.

b. If the client will use gravity drainage, attach the bag to the bed frame below the level of the client's bladder (see illustration). *In a hospital bed, the bag and tubing should go*

Continued

PROCEDURE 29-3 INSERTING AN INDWELLING CATHETER—CONT'D

under the side rails in a position that allows for straight gravity drainage and does not interfere with the operation of the side rails. Do not attach to moveable side rails.

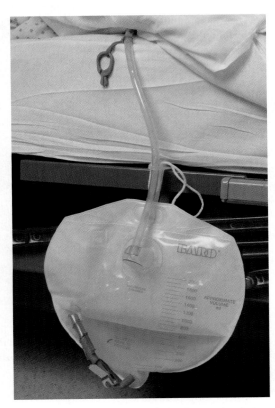

Step 10b. Bag attached to bed frame for gravity drainage.

11. Complete the procedure
a. Discard all trash.
b. Make the client comfortable. Blot or rinse excess solution from the perineum.
c. Document the time the catheter was inserted, the amount and characteristics of the urine that drained from the bladder, and the size of the catheter and balloon.

PEDIATRIC CONSIDERATIONS

When you catheterize a child, you should take time to enlist the child's cooperation. Prepare the child for the sensations associated with cleansing and inserting the catheter. Demonstrating on a doll may be helpful. Encourage the parents to comfort and assist the child to remain still. Praise the child for cooperation.

GERIATRIC CONSIDERATIONS

Assess for the ability to abduct the thighs. It may be helpful to have an assistant help the person to maintain the position for catheterization. Do not attempt to abduct the thighs beyond a comfortable angle. Privacy is sometimes more important for older adult female clients than for younger clients.

HOME CARE CONSIDERATIONS

In the home setting, you will need to be creative in positioning yourself, setting up the sterile field, and establishing adequate lighting to insert the catheter. Provide perineal hygiene before catheterizing. Teach any family caregivers about maintenance of the catheter.

Manipulating the catheter to move the balloon away from the neck of the bladder may alleviate the spasms. Increasing fluid intake may be helpful as well. Anticholinergic medications may be prescribed to reduce bladder tone and relieve the spasms. Narcotics will relieve the pain.

REESTABLISHING URINATION AFTER CATHETERIZATION. Because of the high incidence of infection, an indwelling catheter should be removed as soon as possible. The criterion may be that the person is able to ambulate to the bathroom, the edema has subsided, or the initial inflammatory stage of healing of a surgical wound has passed.

To remove the catheter, select a syringe appropriate to the amount of water in the balloon (usually 5 mL), insert the syringe into the pigtail used to inflate the balloon, aspirate the water from the balloon, and pinch and withdraw the catheter (Figure 29-12). The client may feel a pulling sensation as the catheter is removed. For clients who have urethral irritation, the procedure may be momentarily uncomfortable. Ask the client to take a deep breath and remove the catheter slowly. A small amount of urine may escape, so it is useful to have a towel under the catheter as it comes out. Empty the bag and measure the urine in a graduated container; discard the bag. The marks for measuring on the bag are for estimation only. Removing a catheter is a clean procedure employing standard precautions.

Following removal of the catheter, monitor the client for the return of a normal pattern of urination. The client should drink extra liquid to fill the bladder and relieve irritation. Most people void after 2 to 4 hours. Sometimes, measures to help the person relax and initiate the stream are needed for the first voiding. The time to the first voiding should be 4 to 6 hours (a maximum of 8) depending on the person's bladder capacity and fluid intake. If the bladder becomes overdistended, it may be more difficult to void the first time. If the client has had surgery on the bladder or urethra, the urine should be monitored for diminishing amounts of blood.

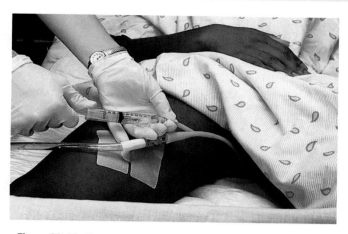

Figure 29-12. To remove an indwelling catheter, attach a 10-mL syringe (without a needle) to the pigtail port, and withdraw the normal saline from the catheter balloon.

For a client who has had an indwelling catheter for a prolonged period of time, training or reconditioning of the bladder before removing the catheter may be helpful. Bladder tone and capacity may have diminished. To do so, clamp the catheter, allow time for the bladder to fill, and then drain the bladder. When the client can tolerate having the catheter clamped for 4 hours, the catheter can be removed.

SINGLE AND INTERMITTENT CATHETERIZATION. Single catheterization refers to the practice of inserting a catheter, draining the bladder, and removing the catheter. If the client is unable to void, the catheter can be inserted again when the bladder needs to be emptied. Intermittent catheterization is performed to check for residual urine, to manage long-term lack of control over urination, and to collect urine specimens.

A physician may prescribe intermittent catheterization after a surgical procedure that produces a high risk for urinary retention. The order is often written as "catheterize PRN" or "in-and-out catheter PRN." You must make judgments about the need for catheterization and the frequency of catheterization. This judgment is based on the client's report of fullness, the interval since the last voiding, and an examination for bladder distention. Before inserting the catheter, have the client attempt to urinate. Then immediately insert the catheter. Because the client has just emptied the bladder, the amount of urine remaining in the bladder represents retention and is referred to as residual urine.

Ultrasonography is sometimes used to detect the presence of residual urine. It is a noninvasive bedside test. Catheterization can be avoided for the client who does not have residual urine in the bladder.

Intermittent self-catheterization is a procedure that can be taught to clients who are unable to spontaneously empty the bladder and have chronic urinary retention with overflow incontinence. These clients are usually relatively young, cognitively intact victims of spinal cord injury with permanent paralysis from the waist down. The procedure may also be used for a client with an underactive or a partially obstructed bladder. It is easier for a male to perform self-catheterization than for a female.

Before teaching self-catheterization, determine the reason that the client needs the procedure. The way the procedure can be performed by a client with a neurogenic bladder is different from the way a client who is paraplegic will perform it. Also assess the client's ability and motivation to learn. The client may need a period of adjustment before deciding to master self-catheterization. Assess the client's usual health practices to determine the likelihood of safe management of the procedure.

If the client's immune system is not impaired, you most likely will teach self-catheterization as a clean procedure (Box 29-9, p. 720). Clean technique has not been shown to result in a higher incidence of urinary tract infection than sterile technique. Long-term use of intermittent catheterization may be preferable to indwelling catheterization from the standpoint of preventing infections and formation of stones.

TEACHING AT-HOME USE OF URINARY CATHETERS. If necessary, the client and family will need to know how to manage a catheter safely at home (Box 29-10, p. 720). The client and family caregivers should understand the functions and purpose of the catheter. Preventing urinary tract infection is probably the most important concept to teach. Clean technique and adequate fluid intake should be included in the teaching. The caregiver should have the knowledge to monitor for the signs and symptoms of urinary tract infections.

Interventions to Irrigate the Bladder

Surgery on the bladder or prostate may result in bleeding into the bladder. Therefore, when a client has had surgery on the bladder or a transurethral resection of the prostate, the indwelling catheter will need to be irrigated to maintain its patency by preventing the formation of blood clots or removing those that do form.

Irrigation can be accomplished using a closed-bladder irrigation system or by opening the system and using an irrigation syringe attached to the indwelling catheter. Because the urine and bladder are normally free of bacteria, either method should be used with sterile technique.

Action Alert! In high-risk populations, such as hospitalized clients, you will need to maintain sterile technique for catheterization or irrigation of a catheter.

A closed irrigation system uses a three-lumen indwelling catheter (Figure 29-13, p. 721). The advantage of this closed irrigation system is a reduced risk for infection. The disadvantage is that the client is attached to multiple tubes and the bag of irrigation fluid. The physician's order usually specifies irrigation of the bladder to maintain patency. The fluid can be run continuously through the bladder or instilled intermittently. You will use a sliding clamp to regulate the flow of irrigant to keep the urine pink. If the urine becomes burgundy or red, you will need to increase the flow rate of the irrigant. If the urine stops flowing, the catheter may need to be irrigated with an irrigation syringe, which applies more force to remove clots. Preventing clots is preferable to irrigating forcefully, because forceful irrigation increases the risk for bleeding.

Box 29-9

Teaching for Self-Care
Self-Catheterization

Purpose: To help the client manage bladder elimination and establish skills for independent living.

Expected Outcome: The client will be able to self-catheterize successfully to minimize incontinence and the risk for urinary tract infection.

Client Instructions

Establishing a schedule for catheterization
- Together with your health care providers, determine an optimal schedule for self-catheterization. It will depend in part on how often you experience incontinence, which may relate directly to your bladder capacity and fluid intake. Consider your work and social schedules as well.
- Seek to maintain a routine catheterization schedule, such as three or four times daily or after a certain number of hours have passed. Some people need self-catheterization every 4 hours.

Performing catheterization
- Plan to drain the urine into a receptacle or directly into the toilet. If you drain it into a receptacle, you may want to have a towel on hand to catch any spills.
- Assume a position that allows access to your urinary meatus. If you are female and find it helpful, you can use a mirror to locate the meatus. Many women locate it by feel.

- Clean your urinary meatus with warm, soapy water and rinse.
- If you are male, retract your foreskin, if necessary, and hold your penis erect or at a right angle to your body. If you are female, spread your labia.
- Holding the catheter about ½ inch from the tip, insert it into your urinary meatus. This should not hurt, and you should feel no resistance. The first time you perform self-catheterization, you may feel some pressure as your urethra stretches.
- Advance the catheter until urine begins to flow (about 2 to 3 inches for a woman and 6 to 8 inches for a man). Then advance the catheter 1 to 2 inches farther to make sure it is in your bladder.
- When the urine has stopped flowing, lean forward and use your abdominal muscles to remove any residual urine.

Maintaining safety measures
- Wash your hands vigorously before and after self-catheterization.
- Clean the catheter with warm, soapy water and rinse it thoroughly after each use.
- Once the catheter is clean and dry, store it in a clean plastic bag or towel.
- Immediately report any signs and symptoms of urinary tract infection to your doctor, such as burning or pain on urination, increased incontinence, malodorous or cloudy urine, or swelling or redness at your urinary meatus.

Box 29-10

Teaching for Self-Care
Maintaining an Indwelling (Foley) Catheter at Home

Purpose: To maintain the function of the catheter, maximize comfort, and prevent complications from the use of an indwelling catheter.

Expected Outcome: The client will not experience a urinary tract infection as a result of the use of an indwelling catheter.

Client Instructions

Care of the catheter
- Cleanse the area around the catheter's exit site with mild soap and water. Some people prefer to clean the area around the catheter while showering. Afterward, rinse thoroughly. If you are not bathing in the shower, use a squeeze bottle filled with warm water to rinse the area while sitting on the toilet. Do not soak in the bathtub.
- Use nonallergenic tape to secure the catheter to your thigh. Allow enough slack in the tube to avoid pulling on the catheter when you move in bed or walk.
- Keep the drainage bag below your bladder at all times.
- Avoid using powders and sprays on your perineal area.
- Call your doctor if your temperature goes above 38.3° C (101° F).

Care of the drainage bag
- Empty the drainage bag often.
- To drain urine, open the port at the bottom of the bag and allow the urine to drain into the toilet or into a receptacle that you can easily empty into the toilet. When urine stops flowing, reclamp the drainage tube.
- If you use a receptacle, rinse it after emptying it to prevent odor and bacterial growth.

Removing the catheter
- If your physician prescribes it, schedule an appointment to check for residual urine in your bladder.
- Before you leave the hospital, review the instructions for removing the catheter.
- As instructed, remove the catheter 2 hours before your office visit. To do so, first perform thorough hand hygiene with soap and warm water.
- Sit on the toilet. Insert a 10-mL syringe (without a needle) into the pigtail on the catheter and withdraw all the water from the pigtail. It should be about 5 mL.
- Gently pull the catheter out of your urinary meatus. It should slide out easily.
- Drink 32 ounces of water, and urinate when you feel the urge. If you have trouble starting your urine stream, try running water or rinsing your perineum with warm water from a squeeze bottle. Do not panic if you are unable to urinate.
- At the doctor's office, you will be asked to urinate and your urine will be measured. You will then have a catheter inserted to check for residual urine. If you have more than 3 ounces of residual urine, the indwelling catheter will need to remain in place.
- If you are not ready to have the catheter out, you will be given another appointment and will repeat the same procedure. It is not uncommon to need the catheter for an additional period of time. It does not mean that anything is wrong.
- If you have any questions, always feel free to ask a doctor or nurse.

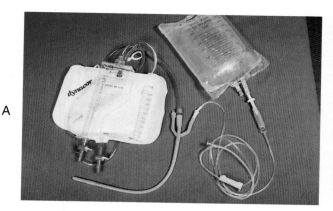

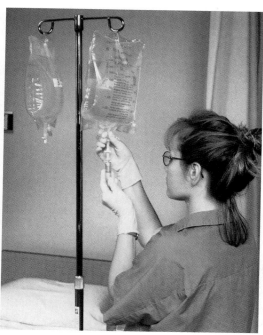

Figure 29-13. Closed bladder irrigation. **A,** The setup for closed bladder irrigation consists of a three-way indwelling catheter, a bag of irrigant with tubing, and a gravity drainage system. **B,** The irrigant is hung on an IV pole and is regulated with a sliding clamp on the tubing.

The catheter also may be irrigated to remove sediment, to reduce the number of microorganisms in the bladder, and to instill medications. When catheters are used for the long-term management of urinary incontinence, sediment is formed from minerals excreted in the urine, and it may solidify in and around the catheter. Keep in mind that irrigation for the purpose of removing sediment is controversial because it increases the chance of urinary tract infection.

Interventions to Manage a Urinary Diversion

In the initial postoperative period, you will monitor the client for postoperative complications. This involves tracking the flow of urine and watching for signs of peritonitis, hemorrhage, and a decrease in vital signs. The newly created stoma may have a stent to maintain its patency. If urine leaks from the operative site into the peritoneum, the client will report pain and you will note abdominal distention, guarding, and tenderness.

The goal for the client is to learn to manage life with a urinary diversion. If the person does not have a continent stoma, an appliance will be attached to the skin around the stoma and urine will drain into a bag either at the site or attached to the client's leg. The person with a continent stoma must learn self-catheterization.

Because of the absence of the normal protective mechanisms of the urinary tract, a urinary diversion is prone to infection. So the client must learn to maintain clean technique and must know the signs and symptoms of infection. The skin around the stoma must remain dry and must be monitored for irritation.

Interventions to Manage Urinary Tract Infections

Urinary tract infections usually are treated with specific or nonspecific antibiotics. When a client has a urinary tract in-fection, increased fluid intake keeps urine dilute and promotes rapid reduction of the bacterial count in the urinary tract. On the other hand, it can hinder therapy by producing increased urine output, thus lowering urinary concentrations of antimicrobial agents. Therefore the client should drink six to eight glasses of fluid per day but should not force fluids when taking most urinary antibiotics. Encourage clients to void when they feel the urge.

Changing the pH of urine has been recommended as an adjunct to therapy. Lowering the pH enhances the antibacterial activity of urine by increasing the concentration of organic acids normally found in urine. The pH of urine also affects the activity of some chemotherapeutic agents. The activity of methenamine mandelate, methenamine hippurate, and nitrofurantoin (all urinary antibacterials) is increased at a low urinary pH, whereas aminoglycoside antibiotics are more effective at an alkaline pH.

Acidification can be achieved by the use of ascorbic acid or methionine, by a modification of the diet, and by restricting milk, sodium bicarbonate, and fruit juices (except for cranberry juice). However, urinary acidification can be difficult to achieve and can cause precipitation of urate stones. Lowering the pH of the urine with a special diet or with ordered medications is advised. For the client with frequent urinary tract infections, preventive measures should be taught.

EVALUATION

Evaluation of urinary tract problems should be specific to the nature of the problem. Ask yourself if the problem is resolvable or expected to be ongoing. Examine the outcomes, the methods to achieve the outcomes, and the client's level of satisfaction with care (Box 29-11, p. 722).

Nursing Care Plan A POSTOPERATIVE CLIENT AT RISK FOR URINARY TRACT INFECTION   Box 29-11

NURSING HISTORY

Mrs. Shireem is in the 2nd postoperative day following a vaginal hysterectomy. She has no history of difficulty with urination.

PHYSICIAN'S ORDERS

Clear liquids; advance diet as tolerated
Activity as tolerated
Demerol 50-100 mg q4h PRN for pain
Vicodin i or ii PRN for pain
Tylenol 650 mg PRN for temperature over 38.8° C (102° F)
$D_5/^{1}/_2$ NS @ 100 mL/hr
Discontinue IV fluid when able to take fluids by mouth
Discontinue Foley catheter
Laxative of choice

NURSING ASSESSMENT

(Morning change-of-shift report) The physician removed the vaginal pack this morning. Client's vital signs are within normal limits. Her temperature is 37.2° C (99° F). She was able to eat a soft diet for breakfast, including 600 mL of fluids. She was out of bed for two brief periods yesterday. Her pain has been controlled with 75 mg of Demerol used every 4 to 6 hours since surgery, but she took two Vicodin this morning. Skin turgor is brisk.

NANDA Nursing Diagnosis	NOC Expected Outcomes With Indicators	NIC Interventions With Selected Activities	Evaluation Data
RISK FOR URINARY RETENTION **Related Factors:** • Edema, interruption in normal stimulus to void	**URINARY ELIMINATION** • Urinary elimination pattern in expected range of 4-6 voidings in waking hours • Urine passes without hesitancy • Urine passes without urgency • Empties bladder completely	**URINARY RETENTION CARE** • Urinary assessment including voiding pattern, intake, and output per shift • Provide privacy for elimination. • Make use of power of suggestion by running water or flushing toilet. • Insert urinary catheter as appropriate.	• Voided 3 times in 2 hours after Foley removed without burning or hesitancy. • Reported feeling like bladder empty. • After 8 hours, has voided 5 times. • Intake 900 cc; output 800 cc • Urine clear, yellow

CRITICAL THINKING QUESTIONS

1. Mrs. Shireem has resumed a normal pattern of voiding. Would she still be vulnerable to urinary tract infections after discharge? Why?

2. What would you teach about preventing urinary tract infections after discharge?

3. What signs and symptoms of urinary tract infection should she report to her physician?

Nursing outcome and intervention labels from Johnson, M., Bulechek, G., McCloskey Dochterman, J.M., Maas, M., & Moorhead, S. (2001). *Nursing diagnoses, outcomes, and interventions: NANDA, NIC, and NOC linkages.* St Louis, MO: Mosby.

Urinary incontinence in immobile, neurologically impaired older adult clients often cannot be resolved. Evaluation seeks to ensure that the client is clean, dry, and comfortable. Equally important is determining that the skin remains intact. The diet should be free of foods or fluids that irritate the bladder. The client should be well hydrated, and the environment should be free of the odor of stale urine. Measures to prevent and detect urinary tract infection should be in place. If the client develops a urinary tract infection, ask what measures should be added to prevent future occurrences.

Urinary incontinence in many cases can be resolved with exercises or other treatment methods. If the problem is not resolved, evaluation includes asking whether the client has been given all available options and is satisfied with the level of resolution. Management may be considered successful if the number of episodes or the severity of each episode is reduced.

Consider the client's ability to participate in the treatment regimen and the level of participation observed.

Evaluation also includes examining nursing care. Were the methods of teaching appropriate to the client's ability to learn and to the client's value system? Was the immobile client checked for dryness at sufficiently frequent intervals to detect incontinence? How frequently was the client offered a bedpan or assisted to the toilet? What measures were used to control odor? If odor is present, additional measures should be included in the care plan. Was the client offered a sufficient amount of appropriate fluids? Were measures included to ensure the client's privacy and avoid embarrassment over incontinence?

Evaluation of the care of the client with a urinary diversion considers the same parameters for skin care, diet, fluids, odor control, privacy, and embarrassment. However, a major part of the evaluation examines the client's level of self-care and whether the care is managed in a manner that minimally disrupts the client's preferred lifestyle.

Mrs. Shireem is discharged on the third postoperative day. The nurse writes the discharge note below.

SAMPLE DOCUMENTATION NOTE FOR MRS. SHIREEM
Discharged to automobile with husband. Is able to void without difficulty; knows to monitor self for signs and symptoms of UTI and maintain fluid intake of 6-8 glasses of water a day. Has spots of serosanguineous drainage on vaginal pad. Will report increase to physician. Scheduled for physician's office visit in 1 week.

Key Principles

- Understanding problems of urinary dysfunction involves an understanding of the structure and function of the kidneys, ureters, bladder, and urethra.
- Examination of urine provides information relevant to the function of the urinary tract and to the general health and function of the body.
- Substances in the urine are a result of the filtration, reabsorption, and secretion functions of the kidney as an organ of homeostatic balance.
- Dysuria can result from obstruction, infection, neurological injury, or decreased muscle tone.
- Low urine volumes can result from dehydration, hypotension, antidiuretic hormone, renal failure, or urinary retention.
- The diagnosis of *Impaired urinary elimination* requires differentiation between stress, urge, reflex, functional, and total incontinence.
- Urinary tract infection is not a nursing diagnosis because the nurse cannot prescribe definitive therapy, but the nurse can treat the risk for urinary tract infection by instituting measures to prevent the problem and to educate the client about healthy practices.
- A nurse can assist a client in avoiding urinary tract infections by teaching about hygiene, fluid intake, and measures to change the pH of the urine.
- The bladder is a sterile body cavity but is at risk for infection because the entrance to the bladder is in close proximity to the anus. Women have higher risk than men because their urethra is short.
- The concept of cleaning the perineum from clean to dirty, front to back, is key to preventing urinary tract infection, especially in women.
- The bladder feels full when it contains an average of 300 mL, after which it is emptied completely with each voiding.
- An indwelling catheter should be the treatment of last resort for urinary incontinence.
- Urinary tract infections are highly associated with the use of indwelling catheters.
- Incontinence often results from a correctable cause. A medical evaluation may be appropriate before deciding on nursing care to manage incontinence.

Bibliography

Addison, R. (1999). Changing a suprapubic catheter. I. *Nursing Times*, 95(42), Suppl. 1-2.

Agency for Health Care Policy and Research. (1996). *Urinary incontinence in adults: Acute and chronic management—Clinical practice guideline No. 2* (AHCPR Publication No. 96-0682). Rockville, MD: Author. Available at http://text.nhm.nih.gov.

Ball, E. M. (2000). Ostomy guide. I. A teaching guide for continent ileostomy. *RN*, 63(12), 35-40; quiz 42.

Boucher, M. A. (1998). Delegation alert! *American Journal of Nursing*, 98(2), 26-32.

Brandt, D. (2000). Lurking nurses: The perils of post-op. *American Journal of Nursing*, 100(11), 25.

Dorey, G. (2000). Male patients with lower urinary tract symptoms. 1: Assessment. *British Journal of Nursing*, 9(8), 497-501.

Doughty, D. (2000). Show me the data. *Journal of Wound Ostomy and Continence Nursing*, 27(4), 199-200.

Giger, J. N., & Davidhizar, R. E. (1996). *Transcultural nursing: Assessment and intervention.* St Louis, MO: Mosby.

Gray, M. (2000). Urinary retention: Management in the acute care setting, Part 2. *American Journal of Nursing*, 100(8), 36-43; quiz 44.

Guyton, A. C., & Hall, J. E. (2001). *Textbook of Medical Physiology.* Philadelphia: Saunders.

Hardyck, C., & Petrinovich, L. (1998). Reducing urinary tract infections in catheterized patients. *Ostomy/Wound Management*, 44(12), 36-43.

Heavner, K. (1998). Urinary incontinence in extended care facilities: A literature review and proposal for continuous quality improvement. *Ostomy/Wound Management*, 44(12), 46-53.

Jirovec, M. M, & Templin, T. (2001). Predicting success using individualized scheduled toileting for memory-impaired elders at home. *Research in Nursing and Health*, 24(1), 1-8.

Johnson, M., Bulechek, G., McCloskey-Dochterman, J., Maas, M., & Moorhead, S. (2001). *Nursing diagnoses, outcomes, and interventions: NANDA, NOC, and NIC linkages.* St Louis, MO: Mosby.

Johnson, T. M, Ouslander, J. G, Uman, G. C, & Schnelle, J. F. (2001). Urinary incontinence treatment preferences in long-term care. *Journal of the American Geriatric Society*, 49(6), 710-718.

*Jolley, S. (1997). Intermittent catheterization for post-operative urine retention. *Nursing Times*, 93(33), 46-47.

Kirkwood, L. (1999). Continence: Taking charge. *Nursing Times*, 95(6), 63-64.

Lalos, O., Berglund, A. L., & Lalos, A. (2001). Impact of urinary and climacteric symptoms on social and sexual life after surgical treatment of stress urinary incontinence in women: A long-term outcome. *Journal of Advanced Nursing*, 33(3), 316-327.

Lekan-Rutledge, D. (2000). Diffusion of innovation: A model for implementation of prompted voiding in long-term care settings. *Journal of Gerontological Nursing*, 26(4), 25-33.

Lyons, S. S., & Specht, J. K. (2000). Prompted voiding protocol for individuals with urinary incontinence. *Journal of Gerontological Nursing*, 26(6), 5-13.

Newman, D. K. (1998). Managing indwelling urethral catheters. *Ostomy/Wound Management*, 44(12), 26-32.

Nicolle, L. E. (2001). Urinary tract infections in long-term-care facilities. *Infection Control and Hospital Epidemiology*, 22(3), 167-175.

---

*Asterisk indicates a classic or definitive work on this subject.

Nissan, D. (Ed.) (2003). Mosby drug consult. St Louis, MO: Mosby.

Osborne, D. M. (2000). Managing patients with a distended bladder. *Clinical Journal of Oncology Nursing, 4*(2), 103-104.

Ouslander, J. G, Ai-Samarrai, N., Schnelle, J. F. (2001). Prompted voiding for nighttime incontinence in nursing homes: Is it effective? *Journal of the American Geriatric Society, 49*(6), 706-709.

Ouslander, J. G., Greendale, G. A., Uman, G., Lee, C., Paul, W., & Schnelle, J. (2001). Effects of oral estrogen and progestin on the lower urinary tract among female nursing home residents. *Journal of the American Geriatric Society, 49*(6), 803-807.

Pfisterer, M., Kuno, E., Muller, M., Schlierf, G., & Oster, P. (1998). [Urinary incontinence in the elderly. 1: Forms of urinary incontinence—basic diagnosis—additional diagnosis] [Review, in German]. *Fortschritte der Medizin, 116*(17):22-26.

Rhodes, C. (2000). Effective management of daytime wetting. *Paediatric Nurse, 12*(2), 14-17.

Shaw, C., Williams, K. S., Assassa, R. P. (2000). Patients' views of a new nurse-led continence service. *Journal of Clinical Nursing, 9*(4), 574-582.

Steed, C. J. (1999). Common infections acquired in the hospital: the nurse's role in prevention. *Nursing Clinics of North America, 34*(2), 443-461.

Thompson, J. (2000). A practical ostomy guide: Part 1. *RN, 63*(11), 61-66; quiz 68.

Thompson, J. (2000). Urinary incontinence in women: Evaluation and management. *American Family Physician, 62*(11), 2433-2445.

Urinary Incontinence Guideline Panel (1982). *Urinary incontinence in adults.* AHCPR Publication No. 92-0038 and 92-0041. Rockville, MD: Agency for Health Care Policy and Research.

Warner, A. J., Phillips, S., Riske, K., Haubert, M. K., & Lash, N. (2000). Postoperative bladder distention: Measurement with bladder ultrasonography. *Journal of Perianesthesia Nursing, 15*(1), 20-25.

Warren, J. W. (2001). Catheter-associated urinary tract infections. *International Journal of Antimicrobial Agents, 17*(4), 299-303.

Wilson, L., Brown, J. S., Shin, G. P., Luc, K., & Subak, L. L. (2001). Annual direct costs of urinary incontinence. *Obstetrics and Gynecology, 98*(3), 398-406.

30

Managing Self-Care Deficit

Key Terms

alopecia

caries

cerumen

dentures

gingivitis

perineum

plaque

tartar

Learning Objectives

After studying this chapter, you should be able to do the following:

- Describe the structure and function of the skin, hair, nails, and oral cavity
- Discuss problems associated with personal hygiene
- Discuss the life span, physiological, and cultural or lifestyle factors that influence hygiene practices
- Assess the client who is at risk for or has an actual self-care deficit in managing personal hygiene, feeding, toileting, or dressing related to physical, psychological, or cognitive impairment
- Choose appropriate nursing diagnoses related to the client's ability to engage in self-care
- Plan client-centered outcomes to assist the client with meeting self-care deficits
- Describe nursing interventions to promote hygiene of the skin, mouth, and hair, and feeding, toileting, and dressing/grooming
- Evaluate outcomes of nursing care in assisting the client to meet self-care needs

Joy Wilson, age 78, resides with her daughter and son-in-law. Mrs. Wilson is of African-American ancestry. She was admitted to the hospital 2 weeks ago after a sudden onset of weakness, nausea, and left hemiplegia. A stroke (cerebrovascular accident) was diagnosed. Her hospital stay is ending, and she is being prepared for discharge to her daughter's home. Her progress in physical therapy has been only fair. Her left side is dominant, so she is being required to master and adapt motor skills completely foreign to her. She has a great desire to learn to care for herself, but she is weak and able to tolerate only minimal activity before becoming extremely fatigued. Her cognitive status is slightly impaired because of a short-term memory deficit as well as some emotional lability. Her frustration at not being able to care for her hygiene needs is evidenced by tears and anger when she cannot achieve a goal.

Mrs. Wilson's daughter is devoted to her mother and desires to provide home care. Both mother and daughter are opposed to considering nursing home placement at this time. Her daughter is eager to learn to care for her mother and asks pertinent questions that reflect interest in her mother's welfare. Although she plans to be the primary caregiver for Mrs. Wilson, she will use community resources to assist in providing the best possible care. Because Mrs. Wilson has related problems of cognitive impairment, exercise intolerance, and frustration with her altered state of wellness, the nurse assesses that in addition to *Self-care deficit: bathing/hygiene*, there are other nursing diagnoses that must be addressed (see below).

KEY NURSING DIAGNOSES FOR Self-Care Deficit

Bathing/hygiene self-care deficit: Impaired ability to perform or complete bathing/hygiene activities for oneself

Dressing/grooming self-care deficit: Impaired ability to perform or complete dressing or grooming activities for oneself

Feeding self-care deficit: Impaired ability to perform or complete feeding activities

Toileting self-care deficit: Impaired ability to perform or complete own toileting activities

---

CONCEPTS OF SELF-CARE DEFICIT

Self-care is the ability to meet needs related to hygiene, dressing, toileting, and feeding without the assistance of another person. These activities are generally independent functions that an individual maintains daily. For that reason, they are called activities of daily living (ADLs). Usually acquired in early childhood, these skills and abilities become an integral part of adult behavior.

Personal hygiene consists of those activities that an individual undertakes to maintain body cleanliness and freedom from disease—namely, bathing, oral hygiene, and hair care. It is essential to both physical and psychological well-being that hygiene needs be adequately met. If the body is not kept clean, the skin is compromised and the body can be threatened by infection or disease. The individual's self-esteem and body image are also enhanced by cleanliness of the body.

When illness or injury prevents the client from meeting self-care needs, it is the responsibility of the caregiver to assist the client to meet these needs. The act of assisting with self-care also provides you, as the nurse, with an opportunity for other therapeutic activities, such as communicating with the client and developing a therapeutic relationship, performing client assessments, and providing emotional support. The ultimate aim of nursing care is to assist clients in a culturally sensitive manner to be as independent as possible, and to provide clients with information and resources needed to resume self-care abilities to the extent that physical and mental capacities allow.

Skin

The skin is an organ with highly specialized functions that are essential for human survival. Without skin, adaptation to the environment would be impossible because the intricate functions of this vital organ serve to maintain biological integrity and homeostasis. The surface area of the skin makes it one of the larger organs in the body, covering approximately 20 square feet, or 3000 square inches in the average-size adult.

Strata of the Skin. The skin is composed structurally of two layers (Figure 30-1). The outer portion, the epidermis, is composed of stratified squamous epithelium and contains four kinds of cells. Most of these cells are keratinocytes; they produce keratin, a substance that protects skin and underlying tissues and plays a part in immune function. Melanocytes, which are located at the base of the epidermis, produce melanin, a pigment responsible for skin color. Melanin also assumes a protective function by absorbing ultraviolet rays, thereby lessening their harmful effects on the skin. Other epidermal cells, the nonpigmented granular dendrocytes, are made up of two distinct cell types: Langerhans' cells and Granstein cells. These cells interact with T cells to assist in the immune process.

The second layer of skin is the dermis, which is composed of connective tissue containing collagenous and elastic fibers. Numerous blood vessels, nerves, glands, and hair follicles are embedded in this stratum of the skin.

Underneath the dermis lies the subcutaneous tissue, also known as the superficial fascia or the hypodermis. This subcutaneous layer consists of areolar and adipose tissue and provides support and blood supply to the dermis. The strata that make up the skin are connected by fibers that extend from the dermis to the underlying tissues and organs.

Glands of the Skin. Three kinds of glands are associated with the skin. They are the sebaceous glands, sudoriferous glands, and ceruminous glands.

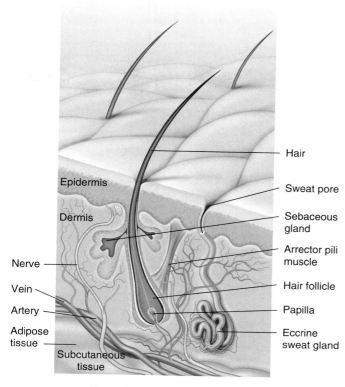

Epidermis

Dermis

Nerve

Vein

Artery

Adipose
tissue

Subcutaneous
tissue

Hair

Sweat pore

Sebaceous
gland

Arrector pili
muscle

Hair follicle

Papilla

Eccrine
sweat gland

Figure 30-1. Anatomy of the skin.

Most sebaceous glands are connected to hair follicles. The secreting portions of these glands lie within the dermis and open into the necks of hair follicles. Those not associated with hair follicles open directly onto the surface of the skin (lips, glans penis, labia minora, and tarsal glands of the eyelids). Their size and shape vary throughout the body, being small in much of the trunk and extremities and larger in the breasts, face, neck, and upper chest. They are absent in the palms and soles.

The sebaceous glands secrete an oily substance called sebum, made up of a mixture of fats, cholesterol, proteins, and inorganic salts. Sebum serves to protect hair from drying and forms a protective film on the skin that prevents excessive evaporation of water. It also helps to keep the skin soft and supple and inhibits the growth of certain bacteria on the skin.

Sudoriferous, or sweat, glands are identified according to their structure and function. Apocrine sweat glands are simple, branched, tubular glands that are distributed primarily in the skin of the axilla, pubic region, and pigmented areas (areolae) of the breasts. The secretory portion of this gland is located in the dermis and the excretory duct opens into hair follicles. Apocrine glands begin to function at puberty and produce a more viscous secretion than eccrine sweat glands.

Eccrine sweat glands are more numerous than apocrine sweat glands and are distributed throughout the skin except for the margins of the lips, nail beds, glans penis, clitoris, labia minora, and eardrums. They are most numerous in the skin of the palms and soles and are easily observed by the wetness of palms when a person is anxious or under stress.

The secretory portion of the gland is located in the subcutaneous layer, and the excretory duct projects upward to terminate at a pore on the surface of the epidermis. Eccrine sweat glands function throughout life and produce a watery secretion known as perspiration, in which small amounts of waste products are excreted.

Ceruminous glands secrete a thick, heavily pigmented, oily substance called cerumen. **Cerumen** is a waxy secretion of the glands of the external ear canal or external acoustic meatus; it is commonly known as earwax.

Functions of the Skin. The skin is the body's first line of defense, and that principle is of paramount importance when considering a client's hygiene needs. Normally, the skin hosts a large contingent of resident bacteria that serve a useful function. On intact skin, these resident organisms prevent excess growth of fungi. Sebum, secreted into the hair follicles by the sebaceous glands, has antibacterial and antifungal properties. Normal skin acidity also inhibits growth of pathogenic organisms.

The skin assists in regulating body temperature through production of perspiration by the sudoriferous glands, which helps to lower body temperature. Perspiration, or sweat, is a mixture of water, salts (mostly sodium chloride), urea, uric acid, amino acids, ammonia, sugar, lactic acid, and ascorbic acid. Its principal function is to help regulate body temperature via evaporation of the water in perspiration; this evaporation carries off large quantities of heat energy from the body surface.

The skin helps screen out harmful ultraviolet (UV) rays from the sun, but it also lets in necessary UV rays that convert 7-dehydrocholesterol (a chemical in the skin) into vitamin D for normal growth of bones and teeth. A lack of UV light and vitamin D impairs absorption of calcium from the intestine into the bloodstream.

The skin is an important sensory organ containing sensory receptors that respond to heat, cold, touch, pressure, and pain. Skin offers protection through its many nerve endings, which warn of environmental sources of harm such as hot coals or sharp blades. The nerve endings also help in sensing the outside world so that physiological adjustments can be made to maintain homeostasis.

Hair

Because it arises from the skin, hair is considered to be an appendage of the skin. In the human, hair covers the entire body with the exception of the palms, soles, lips, tip of penis, inner lips of vulva, and nipples. The hair consists of two major parts: the shaft (the portion protruding from the skin) and the root (embedded in the skin).

About halfway up the length of the hair follicle is an oil gland, which is located between the follicle and the arrector pili muscle. When this muscle contracts, it pulls the follicle and its hair upright, elevating the skin above the follicle and producing what is commonly called gooseflesh.

Rate of hair growth appears to depend on several factors, of which age, seasonal changes, and hair texture are prominent. Rate of hair growth slows with advancing age. Hair grows faster at night than during the day, and faster in warm weather than in cold. Coarse black hairs grow faster than fine blonde hair. Location of the hair is also a determining factor. Scalp hairs may last 3 to 5 years, whereas eyebrow and eyelash hairs may last only 10 weeks. The average scalp contains about 125,000 hairs.

Although humans do not have as much of a need for the protective covering of hair as many other mammals have, hair does serve some protective functions in humans. Scalp hair serves to insulate against cold air and external heat from the sun. Most hair follicles are associated with sebaceous glands, and some sweat gland ducts open into hair follicles. Therefore, the scalp becomes moist and oily in a hot environment.

Hair also serves to protect by providing a cushion for the cranium. Also, the eyebrows are cushions for protecting the eyes. Eyelashes serve to screen the entry of foreign particles or objects. Nostril hairs trap dust particles and foreign matter that are present in inhaled air.

Nails

The nails are composed of hard, keratinized cells of the epidermis that form a clear, solid covering over the dorsal surfaces of the terminal surfaces of the fingers and toes. Each nail consists of three basic parts: the nail body, which is the visible portion; the free edge, which projects beyond the tip of the digit; and the nail root, which is hidden in the proximal nail groove.

Most of the nail body is pink because of the underlying vascular system. The semilunar area at the base (lunula) appears white because the vascular tissue is hidden by the thick stratum there. The eponychium (or cuticle) is a narrow band of epidermis that extends from the margin of the nail bed (lateral border) and is the proximal border of the nail.

The epithelium of the proximal part of the nail bed is known as the nail matrix. Its function is to bring about the growth of nails by transforming superficial cells of the matrix into nail cells. Functionally, nails help with grasping and manipulating small objects in various ways. They also provide protection against trauma to the ends of the digits.

Oral Cavity

The oral cavity is composed of the teeth, the tongue, and the oral mucosa. Eruption of deciduous teeth (baby teeth) begins at approximately 6 months of age. These deciduous teeth are lost in childhood and are replaced by a set of 32 permanent teeth (16 in each jaw) composed of four incisors, two canines, four premolars, and six molars (see Chapter 16). All teeth consist of three parts: a root embedded in a socket (alveolus) in the alveolar process of the jaw bone; a crown projecting upward from the gum; and a neck between the root and the crown, which is surrounded by the gum (Figure 30-2).

Each tooth is composed of dentin, enamel, cementum, and pulp. The dentin is the sensitive portion surrounding the pulp cavity, and it forms the bulk of the tooth. The enamel is the white covering of the tooth. The cementum is the bonelike covering of the neck and root. The pulp is the soft core of

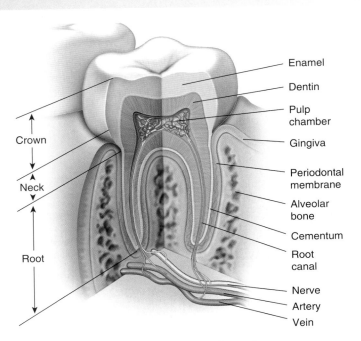

Figure 30-2. Anatomy of a tooth.

connective tissue that contains the nerves and blood vessels of the tooth.

The teeth are held in their sockets by connective tissue called periodontal ligaments. The collagenous fibers of each ligament extend from the alveolar bone into the cement of each tooth, allowing some tooth movement during the process of chewing.

The mouth and teeth play vital roles in mastication (chewing) and digestion, which begins in the mouth as food is mixed with saliva for food breakdown and for further digestion. The muscles in the cheeks aid in chewing. The tongue has taste buds for discerning different tastes of food, and it helps mix saliva with food. The tongue also aids in swallowing by moving the food toward the pharynx. Phonation (the forming of words) is also a function of the tongue.

Problems of Self-Care

Problems of the Skin. Skin types, textures, and conditions are influenced by many factors. Overall health status, age, nutritional status, and activity level may play a big part in determining the client's skin condition. Infants have skin that is delicate and sensitive because it has yet to be exposed to the environmental influences that alter skin texture. Because of this delicacy of skin, infants cannot usually tolerate harsh soaps and extremes of water temperature. Their skin is particularly prone to trauma in the form of abrasions, which are breaks in the skin that may lead to infection.

Adolescents are prone to developing enlarged sebaceous glands of the face because of accumulated sebum, which may take the form of blackheads, pimples, or boils. At puberty, the sebaceous glands, under the influence of androgens (male hormones), grow in size and increase production of sebum. Although testosterone, a male hormone, appears to be the

Table 30-1	Common Problems of the Skin	
Problem	**Description**	**Nursing Implication**
Abrasion	Broken skin that may be weeping or bleeding; may be noted on elbows, heels, sacrum, and other areas that are subject to rubbing motions	Remove source of irritation. Prevent secondary infection; keep wound clean; avoid wearing rings or jewelry when caring for client; lift client when moving rather than pulling across the bed (shearing factor).
Acne	Oversecretion of sebum, which enlarges the gland and plugs the pore with pus; often occurs on face, chest, and back; most common in adolescence.	Prevent secondary infection; instruct client to avoid squeezing and causing additional trauma to tissue; treatment may vary depending on severity of the problem; encourage meticulous skin cleanliness.
Dryness	Flaking and rough skin (generalized or patchy)	Prone to infection if the skin cracks; skin should be kept lubricated; reduce frequency of bathing and hot showers or tub baths; rinse skin thoroughly because soap residue promotes dryness; avoid irritating soaps and alcohol-based lotions; encourage increased fluid intake.
Dermatitis	Inflammation of skin with itching, redness, and blisters; may be allergic reaction to external chemical irritants (fabrics, solutions, plants) or internal (foods or medications)	Identify and remove source of irritation if possible; provide comfort for client with treatment for itching; discourage scratching to prevent breaking of skin and secondary infection.

most potent circulating androgen for sebaceous cell stimulation, adrenal and ovarian androgens can stimulate sebaceous secretions as well.

Acne occurs predominantly in sebaceous follicles that are rapidly colonized by bacteria that thrive in the lipid-rich sebum. When this occurs, the cyst, or sac of connective tissue cells, can destroy and displace epidermal cells, resulting in permanent scarring, a condition called cystic acne. Cystic acne may be treated by a synthetic form of vitamin A called isotretinoin (Accutane). However, it must not be used by females who are pregnant or who intend to become pregnant while undergoing treatment. Major fetal abnormalities have been traced to isotretinoin. This drug may also cause serious side effects in those who take it and should be used only if less toxic forms of therapy have failed.

Dry skin is a problem common to aging. Older adults cannot tolerate harsh soaps because of their delicate skin. Skin of older people is also prone to breakdown. Abrasions may be slow to heal or may become infected.

Skin rashes or dermatitis are common skin problems. They may be due to an allergic or nonallergic contact. It is important to identify the source irritant and to prevent secondary infection from scratching with resultant destruction of the body's first line of defense, the intact skin. Table 30-1 lists some common skin problems and their causes and treatments.

Problems of the Hair. Normal hair loss in an adult scalp is about 70 to 100 hairs per day. The rate of growth and the replacement cycle may be altered by illness, diet, and other factors. High fever, major illness, major surgery, blood loss, or severe emotional stress may increase the rate of shedding and may result in **alopecia,** which is loss of hair and baldness. Rapid weight-loss diets with severe caloric restriction or protein restriction may also increase hair loss. Certain drugs and radiation therapy are also factors in increasing hair loss.

Dandruff is a chronic, diffuse scaling of the epidermis of the scalp. It is characterized by itching and flaking of whitish scales, which are annoying and embarrassing.

Infestation with lice is called pediculosis. Lice may be found on any part of the body that has hair. Lice may be found in the hair of the head, eyebrows, eyelashes, and beard (pediculosis capitis), on the body (pediculosis corporis), and in the pubic hair (pediculosis pubis). Head lice and pubic lice attach their eggs (nits) to the hair shaft with a sticky substance that makes them hard to remove. They may be visible to the naked eye or seen through a magnifying glass as shiny ovals. They may look to the naked eye like dandruff. They live on the skin, and their bites cause itching. Inflamed sores may be visible along the hairline. Body lice suck blood from the skin and live in clothing, making them hard to detect. Scratching and hemorrhagic lesions of the skin are clues that should alert the caregiver to the possibility of infestation. Table 30-2 (p. 730) identifies common problems of the hair.

Problems of the Nails and Feet. Care of the nails is vital to good hygiene. The accumulation of dirt and debris around the cuticle and underneath the fingernail is a potential source of infection, especially if the nail should become torn. Hangnails, ragged cuticles, and long untrimmed nails are hazardous to the client. Confused clients sometimes injure themselves by scratching or otherwise abrading the skin. Dirty fingernails open the avenue to infection.

The nails are affected by aging and disease. Nails become more dry and brittle with age. Fungal infections of the nails are a common problem of the aged, primarily because of dehydrated epidermal cells and decreased sebaceous gland secretion. If nails are thickened and yellow, this may indicate a fungal infection. Increased brittleness and angulation between the nail and the nail bed and changes in the thickness or texture of the nails can indicate illness. Clubbing of the nails or marked curvature and lines in the nails may be indicative of serious health problems.

The toenails are vital for good ambulation. Assessment of the client's gait may point toward sore feet, ingrown toenails, corns, and calluses, which are uncomfortable but not life threatening. However, in a client with circulatory impairment or diabetes, an ingrown toenail may be a source of serious problems.

Table 30-2	Common Problems of the Hair	
Problem	**Description**	**Nursing Implication**
Alopecia	Absence of body hair; may be sudden onset of patchy scalp and beard hair loss without any in-flammation and usually reversible or sudden loss of all scalp hair or total loss of all body hair including scalp and face	Be aware of client's history and treatment to know if condition is likely to be reversible (chemotherapy) or irreversible; recognize significance of hair to client's self-esteem and body image.
Dandruff	A scaly collection of dried sebum and flakes of dried skin on the scalp; characterized by itching of the scalp	Daily brushing and shampooing; medicated shampoos may help; instruct client to avoid scratching scalp.
Pediculosis	Infestation with lice; characterized by itching and scratching	Removal of nits (eggs) from hair shaft; bathing and shampooing with topi-cal medications; careful treatment of clothing and bed linens to prevent reinfestation with lice.

Table 30-3	Common Problems of the Feet and Nails	
Problem	**Description**	**Nursing Implication**
Athlete's foot	Fungal infection of the foot characterized by weeping, itching, excoriated lesions, usually lo-cated between the toes	Medicated antifungal medications may be used; regular washing and drying of feet is important; instruct client to wear white cotton socks during treatment to prevent potential infection from dyes in colored socks and to alternate shoes each day.
Corn/callus	A hardened area on the foot, usually caused by pressure or friction	Instruct client to avoid attempting to remove by cutting; use pumice stone to soften; encourage wearing of well-fitting shoes.
Fungal infection of nails	Nails may be yellow or black and thickened	Observe for signs of side effects of treatment regimen, which consists of oral antifungal medication.

The diabetic client is at high risk for infection from breaks in skin integrity and may have decreased sensation to pain because of peripheral neuropathies. Diabetes is associated with changes in microcirculation in peripheral tissues. Edema may be present because of renal disease or congestive heart failure or other conditions that interfere with blood flow to surrounding tissues. Table 30-3 lists common problems of the nails and feet.

Problems of the Oral Cavity. Table 30-4 lists some common problems of the oral cavity. Halitosis may be an early indica-tor of either poor oral hygiene or a health problem, such as a gastrointestinal (GI) tract disorder. An offensive breath odor caused by inadequate oral hygiene can be alleviated with cleansing of the teeth and oral mucosa. If the origin of the hal-itosis is systemic, oral hygiene will not remove the odor.

Dental **caries** is a destructive process causing decalcifica-tion of the tooth enamel and leading to continued destruction of the enamel and dentin with resulting cavitation of the tooth. When the enamel barrier is breached, cavities develop. Dental caries is a disease of the calcified structure of the tooth. The agent responsible for dental caries is dental plaque. Dental **plaque** is a soft, thin film of food debris, mucin, and dead ep-ithelial cells that is deposited on the teeth and provides a medium for the growth of bacteria. Freshly deposited plaque is transparent unless stained brown by tobacco or coffee or tea. When old dental plaque is present, the teeth appear dull with a dingy, yellowish cast.

Cavity formation results when bacterial enzymes combine with the dental plaque and ferment the dietary carbohydrates

and organic acids. These acids initiate the decalcification of tooth enamel. Once the bacteria have gained access to the tis-sue substance of the tooth, the next step is the development of caries. In infants, dental caries can be caused by allowing the infant to go to bed with a bottle filled with a liquid other than water, sometimes referred to as bottle mouth syndrome.

Plaque and food remaining in the mouth produce an envi-ronment that is conducive to cavity formation. Dental plaque can be removed by brushing and flossing. Food remnants left trapped between the teeth set the stage for the beginning of decay and periodontal disease. When dental plaque remains on teeth, it becomes hardened (calcified) and forms calculus or tartar. **Tartar** is a yellowish film of calcium phosphate, carbonate, food particles, and other organic matter deposited on the teeth by saliva. Calculus must be removed with dental instruments.

Sound nutrition provides some resistance to dental decay. Dietary needs vary with such factors as age and general phys-ical condition. Moderation in diet is important because both deficiencies and excesses can decrease resistance to decay. The use of a nonabrasive dentifrice (toothpaste or toothpow-der) containing fluoride and the consumption of whole-grain foods that contain phosphorus inhibit caries. Dietary fats pro-vide a barrier to acid penetration by forming an oily film on the surface of the tooth.

The gum is also known as the gingiva. It is the firm con-nective tissue covered with mucous membrane that surrounds the alveolar processes of the teeth.

Gingivitis is an inflammation of the gums usually mani-fested by the primary symptom of bleeding of the gums. It is

Table 30-4	Common Problems of the Oral Cavity	
Problem	**Description**	**Nursing Implication**
Halitosis	Offensive odor of breath.	Provide regular oral hygiene or teach client; assess for cause of halitosis.
Caries	Teeth may be dark in carious areas; may be painful.	Advise client to seek dental intervention.
Gingivitis	Gums may be pale and spongy; bleeding may occur with brushing and flossing or may occur spontaneously.	Provide regular oral care or teach client; dental intervention may be necessary.
Periodontal disease	Gums may bleed easily; teeth may be loose.	Advise client to seek dental care.
Stomatitis	Inflammation of oral mucosa; occurs in clients who are in a state of immunosuppression.	Rinse and cleanse mouth at least every 2 hours and after eating; local anesthetic rinses may provide some comfort.
Dryness	Lips and oral mucosa dry and cracked and may bleed; noted in clients who are dehydrated, who are on oxygen therapy, or who are mouth breathers.	Increase fluid intake as appropriate; apply water-based lubricants or petroleum jelly to lips.

an early stage of periodontal disease. Gingivitis may result from waste products and toxins from organisms in the mouth, which may cause initial injury. Then, when plaque and bacteria accumulate, they form calculus, which contains more microorganisms and causes further gingivitis. Those at increased risk for gingivitis include people who breathe through their mouths, diabetics, people who use orthodontic supplies (e.g., braces), and people experiencing hormonal fluctuations (adolescents, pregnant women, and those taking oral contraceptives).

Chronic gingivitis causes the inflammation to spread and destroy the underlying bone, causing periodontitis. In an advanced stage of periodontal disease, the periodontium atrophies so that the gums appear to have receded completely away from the tooth. Without adequate supporting structure, the tooth becomes very loosely attached or falls out.

A large number of young people have dental caries and mouth and gum disease because of excessive dietary sugar and insufficient oral hygiene. During pregnancy, the increased circulating levels of hormones cause gingival hypertrophy, which can increase the incidence of periodontal disease if good oral hygiene is not consistently practiced. Periodontal disease is common among young adults and may be precipitated by emotional stress, which aggravates the inflammatory process.

Tooth loss is not inevitable in older adults; however, half the people over age 65 have no teeth. With age, the gums tend to recede and to develop a brownish pigmentation along the tooth edge. Salivation decreases and many older people complain of a dry mouth. Older adults who have few permanent teeth left will have partial or full dentures. **Dentures** are a complement of teeth, either natural or artificial; the term is ordinarily used to indicate an artificial replacement for the natural teeth.

Alterations in the oral mucosa may have several causes. Healthy mucosa is moist and pink without ulceration, dryness, or bleeding. Dryness of the lips and mucosa may occur in the client who is dehydrated or who is breathing through the mouth. Clients receiving oxygen therapy are prone to this because oxygen tends to dry out the mucosa.

Irritated, reddened, or excoriated mucosa may also result from ill-fitting dentures. Clients who have experienced rapid weight loss or who have sustained significant changes in facial features may have dentures that are loose, which may cause irritation and pain when eating. Stomatitis is a common problem with certain clients. This condition is an inflammation of the oral mucosa and may occur in the following clients:

- Those who receive drugs such as anticholinergics that cause decreased salivation with resultant mouth dryness
- Those who have poor oral hygiene
- Those who are in treatment with chemotherapy or radiotherapy for cancer
- Those who have an immune deficiency.

FACTORS AFFECTING SELF-CARE

Self-care practices vary among individuals, groups, and cultures. It is a mistake to assume that all clients will adhere to similar practices of hygiene or that all have similar beliefs about hygiene and methods of practicing it. Variations in self-care practices also may result from life span factors, physiological factors, or cultural and lifestyle factors.

Risk Factors Across the Life Span

The age of an individual usually provides some expectation of what that person should be able to achieve in self-care. However, the interventions should be in accordance with their identified needs and abilities, whether or not they are congruent with chronological age and stage of development.

A need for independence in self-care is manifested early in childhood as the child takes pride in eating, grooming, dressing, and caring for hygiene needs. The loss of this ability in adulthood can be stressful, even if the loss is temporary.

Self-concept and the feeling of being in control of the body are threatened by the loss of self-care abilities. Being bathed and dressed by a caregiver may be equated with regression to an infantile state. For some individuals, this feeling is not acceptable, particularly if the individual has a strong need for independence. A sense of powerlessness may result from this loss. It is important to be sensitive to the client's emotional needs when providing hygiene and other assistive care.

Newborns and Infants. The infant is totally dependent on the caregiver to meet self-care needs. Crying to signal need for feeding and diapering is the only action the infant can take in the interest of self-care. Bathing, dressing, and grooming are the total responsibility of the caregiver. Frequency of urine and stool elimination may vary, but infants usually urinate about 20 times a day (250 to 500 mL per day). Stools may vary according to amount and consistency; they may be soft or liquid and may occur frequently. Meticulous cleaning is essential because the infant's tender skin is susceptible to breakdown. Keep the skin as dry and clean as possible. Never leave infants in wet or soiled diapers for extended periods. The infant's skin and mucous membranes are easily injured and are susceptible to injury and infection.

> *Action Alert!* Remind parents that they need to take special care to avoid injury and infection to their infant's skin.

Toddlers and Preschoolers. During the toddler/preschool years, the child develops gross and fine motor skills so that some independent grooming and toileting are possible. Bowel and bladder control is usually achieved by the age of 3 years even though some assistance may still be needed with wiping after toileting. Nighttime dryness may not be complete until a few years later. The preschooler is usually eager to help with dressing and derives great satisfaction with learning to master buttons and zippers.

Toddlers and preschoolers may regress in times of illness or stress and resume infantile behaviors related to toileting and self-care. Bed-wetting may occur again during this period of stress. This is a primary infantile means of coping and for securing the comfort needed at this time of crisis. The child will regain the skills previously learned when the child no longer needs to use this coping mechanism.

School-Age Children and Adolescents. The school-age child may be independent in self-care activities but may need occasional adult supervision to see that skin care and oral hygiene are being done completely and correctly. As the child approaches adolescence, assistance with self-care is no longer necessary, but because of the many physical changes that are occurring, a different kind of assistance, supervision, and teaching may be needed. This is a time when hormonal changes bring about the emergence of axillary and pubic hair in both sexes and facial hair in boys. The skin may become more oily because of increased activity of the sebaceous glands. Skin problems such as acne may occur during this period and can be a source of great distress to the adolescent who is becoming increasingly aware of the importance of appearance in being accepted by peers and attractive to the opposite sex. The sweat glands also become functional during adolescence, and the presence of body odor becomes an incentive for daily bathing and shampooing and for wearing clean clothes.

Adults and Older Adults. During early and middle adult life, self-care is usually an independent function unless some temporary or permanent physical or mental impairment prevents the individual from performing self-care. Patterns of hygiene practices are well established by this time, to meet the individual's goals for personal appearance and health.

Developmental considerations related to aging may affect clients' hygiene practices. This is particularly true in older adults because the aging process may limit agility and endurance and therefore the ability to perform safely and capably some aspects of good hygiene. Some older adults who were previously meticulous in their grooming may be noted by family members to be less attentive or even totally negligent in bathing and changing clothing. This could result from mental or physical changes, and it requires attention from a caregiver because the client is no longer able to meet hygiene needs independently.

As physiological changes occur with aging, some hygiene needs and practices must change accordingly. For example, the skin becomes thinner and less elastic, and breaks in the skin tend to occur more readily. Because less oil is being produced, the skin becomes drier. The appearance of the skin also changes with wrinkling and discoloration in the form of age spots, which occur particularly on the face and the dorsal surface of the hands. Skin carcinomas are also prominent in aging skin.

The hair changes with aging, becoming thinner and growing more slowly. Baldness in both men and women may occur. Hair color changes to gray or white as the pigment in the hair is lost. The oral mucosa changes and becomes drier with decreased production of saliva. The teeth may become loose or may even be lost if there is periodontal disease. Many older adults wear dentures.

Care of the nails may be difficult. Nails become thickened and harder to maintain. The older adult may have difficulty with this psychomotor task because of decreased visual acuity and agility. The feet of the older client are of special concern because many older adults cannot see well enough to inspect or care for their feet. Decreased circulation in the extremities due to reduced peripheral blood flow from arteriosclerosis or poor circulation puts them at risk.

> *Action Alert!* Advise older clients and their caregivers to take special care to prevent trauma or infection in the extremities because of decreased circulation.

Many older adults, especially diabetics, use the skills of a podiatrist because of the danger inherent in accidentally traumatizing the feet with manicure tools. Some hospitals and nursing homes prohibit foot care by nurses and require clients to secure the services of a podiatrist because the danger caused by inadvertent foot trauma is so great.

Older adults frequently have to use at least one assistive tool to support sensory function. Hearing aids, glasses, and artificial eyes are common. The care of these devices may be a problem for those older adults who have reduced vision and hearing acuity as well as psychomotor skill. Your role is to assist in the care of these devices, which are useful in enhancing quality of life and safety for the older person.

Physiological Factors

An individual's state of health is a major influence in the practice of self-care. Regardless of the motivation to maintain good hygiene and other ADLs, the client may be so ill or weak that there is insufficient energy to perform self-care activities.

Physical Illness.
Clients may be temporarily weakened by ordinary health problems, such as the flu. Others may have long-term paralysis or weakness and loss of physical mobility from a cerebrovascular accident, a neuromuscular disorder, a spinal cord injury, or other catastrophic event.

The degree of assistance needed varies according to the nature of the neuromuscular involvement and which muscle groups are affected. Muscular movements are classified as either fine motor or gross motor. Fine motor movement involves precise movements, such as applying toothpaste to a toothbrush, whereas gross motor movement involves the coordination of large muscle groups, such as getting in and out of the bathtub or on and off the toilet. These tasks require an intact nervous system for their performance. The pathways from brain to muscle and the muscle fibers themselves must be open and able to give and receive impulses. Neuromuscular diseases may affect any level of this pathway.

Action Alert! Be prepared to assist clients who have neurological changes with activities such as applying toothpaste, getting in and out of the bathtub, or getting on and off the toilet.

Conservation of energy is another factor in self-care. Physicians or nurse practitioners sometimes place clients on bed rest or impose other activity restrictions to help them conserve energy. Examples of pathological conditions that often deplete one's energy level are cardiovascular and respiratory diseases. Fatigue is a prominent symptom of these disorders.

Pain is another physiological factor that limits the ability to perform self-care. Careful pain assessment and management is needed to enable the client to participate as fully as possible in ADLs (see Chapter 36). In some clients, pain is a short-term, acute problem that is easily treated, whereas in others it is so severe that simple movements trigger intense pain and prevent self-care. This is especially true in disorders in which the joints are painful, such as arthritis. It is important to plan for self-care activities while medications or other pain management strategies are exerting their peak effect.

Cognitive dysfunction may vary in degree so that a client may need either simple assistance or total care. It is important to accurately assess the client's potential for self-care. It is important for the client to maintain as much independence as possible. It is also important not to expect too much from clients who are too cognitively impaired to meet their own self-care needs.

Sensoriperceptual problems, such as blindness or deafness, may limit the client's ability to participate in self-care, particularly when placed in an unfamiliar environment such as a hospital. Visually impaired clients may need assistance with eating or getting to the bathroom. Hearing-impaired clients may not be able to follow instructions. Specific strategies, such as verbal cuing for visually impaired clients or using gestures for hearing-impaired clients, can be employed to help counteract these problems (see Chapter 37).

Medical or Surgical Procedures.
Medical or surgical procedures may alter the client's ability to perform self-care. An acutely ill client with a medical or surgical diagnosis usually needs a great deal of help with care. Not only is there impairment caused by the medical or surgical problem but there may be associated weakness or pain from treatments or medications.

Opioid analgesics or sedatives may make the client drowsy or sedated and unable to perform self-care. In addition, a general anesthetic will cause weakness. The client may also have decreased mobility because of problems such as fluid and electrolyte imbalances, hypoxia, or hypovolemia. Equipment that encumbers the client, such as an IV, monitoring equipment, central lines, oxygen, and catheters, may also interfere with self-care and require assistance from the nurse or other health care provider.

Cultural and Lifestyle Factors

Cultural and Religious Factors.
Culture has an important influence on self-care practices (Box 30-1, p. 734). Cultural and social norms as well as the teachings of family create different perspectives on cleanliness and hygiene. There may be wide variation among groups with regard to common bathing rituals and the application of preparations to the skin. In some cultures, bathing is done daily or even more often. In other cultural groups, bathing may not occur daily because it is not deemed necessary, or for reasons such as the reduced availability of an adequate water supply or provisions for bathing. Some groups apply oils and other preparations to the skin and hair. Shaving of leg and axillary hair, which is practiced by most women in the United States, is not necessarily a standard hygiene practice around the world, particularly in some parts of Europe. It is important to understand these individual differences in caring for clients of diverse ethnic and cultural backgrounds. Some personal hygiene practices may be unfamiliar to you, but their significance to the client should be respected.

Religious rituals may also influence the client's hygiene habits. Some religions have prohibitions against the exposure of body parts, the cutting and care of hair, and bathing during menses or immediately after delivery of a child. In some groups, it is forbidden for a male to attend to the hygiene needs of a female. Be aware of and respect these beliefs and practices that vary from those in traditional Western culture.

Psychosocial Factors.
Psychological factors that accompany physical illness may cause the client to need help with self-care, even if it is only in the form of a reminder or

Cross-Cultural Care   CARING FOR AN AFRICAN-AMERICAN CLIENT   Box 30-1

Mrs. Wilson, the client discussed in this chapter, is of African-American ancestry. She grew up in the Deep South as the daughter of sharecroppers who struggled to feed and clothe their 10 children. Mrs. Wilson is the fifth child and the only surviving sibling. She has never lived more than 50 miles from the place of her birth.

Poverty was a reality of her early life, but she says that the difficulties were made bearable by the intensity of love within the family, and she feels that this has been a blessing in her life. She has been a widow for 10 years. Her daughter is her only child, and two granddaughters live nearby.

Several characteristics have been identified in African Americans that demonstrate their values, beliefs, and worldviews. Attributing specific characteristics to groups is not without risks and is not intended to stereotype individuals. African Americans tend to value the following:
- Having a strong will to survive
- Being steeped in a particular culture and tradition

- Showing adaptive behavior
- Showing strong belief in self-reliance
- Avoiding self-blame for failures
- Having major concern for health and ability to maintain activities of daily living
- Tending to overestimate health status
- Seeing trouble as a "cross one must bear"
- Believing that avoidance of worry and tension is the same as problem solving
- Relying on kinship and family networks to cope with health concerns

---

encouragement to take a bath or shampoo. If clients are dealing with the stress of a serious diagnosis for themselves or a loved one, encouraging them to participate in hygiene activities may help them exert control over some facet of their daily life.

Emotional disturbances may cause disruptions in the ability to perform self-care. The client with active psychosis is likely to need assistance because of the break with reality and the resultant inattention to hygiene and other self-care needs. Sometimes a change in grooming is an early indicator of mental illness. Depression can slow a person down because of the lack of psychic energy and therefore physical energy. Poor grooming, lack of interest in appearance, or inappropriate dressing may reflect a need for assistance.

Knowledge Level. Take into account the client's knowledge level in regard to self-care practices. The frequency of bathing, shampooing, and oral care (including flossing and brushing) are usually taught by significant others during childhood. These teachings are not always incorporated into the client's behavior and indicate an opportunity for health teaching about self-care.

Health teaching may be done informally by pointing out to the client ways in which overall health might be improved through specific actions. If family members are present with the client during hospitalization, health teaching is essential if they are to care for the client at home after hospitalization. They need to know principles of aseptic technique as well as specific procedures that will be necessary at home. All of these can be incorporated into teaching and are most easily taught while care is being given.

Territoriality. Caring for the most intimate needs of ill persons requires that you operate within the personal space of each client. Each client has a sense of "space" in which he or she feels comfortable. This space includes not only the physical area surrounding the person but also the emotional possession of the body and personal self-knowledge. Research

has been conducted about clients' needs for physical personal space, and the results have been incorporated into design and allocation of square footage for rooms in hospitals and other health care facilities.

Intrusion into this personal space or territory without permission often causes discomfort. Nursing has implicit permission from society to move into an individual's space as necessary to give care, after obtaining permission whenever possible. This is a rare opportunity not offered to other disciplines and should be considered a privilege. It is important to be aware, however, that some clients may be uncomfortable with this physical and emotional closeness. Assess the client's comfort level so that care can be taken to reduce discomfort and anxiety.

Privacy in an institutional setting is difficult to achieve at times. Respect for the client's privacy is important in preserving dignity and feeling of worth. Carefully drape and screen the client during care, avoid intrusion when the client has visitors or is talking on the telephone, and knock before entering the room to show concern for the right to privacy. Respect the client's personal space also by providing privacy when sensitive matters are to be discussed.

Institutions tend to be very depersonalizing. One of the first events that a hospitalized client encounters is the removal of clothing and personal belongings. Provide an identified space for personal belongings and encourage the inclusion of personal and familiar objects in the client's hospital environment to help make the space psychologically comforting to the client. Pictures, cards, and flowers not only bring a cheerful look to the client's room but also make the space unique for the client. It is a way of defining who that person is as an individual.

Socioeconomic Factors. Socioeconomic factors influence self-care habits and practices in a number of ways. Financial resources to purchase the necessary tools for hygiene may be limited. An environment that is dreary and unclean does not encourage the individual toward meticulous hygiene. Bathing may assume a low priority in an environment with inadequate heat or a lack of privacy for hygiene practices. When a significant amount of physical and emotional energy is required to meet daily subsistence needs for food and shelter, grooming and hygiene may be neglected. This does not imply that the individual no longer values them; it is simply that basic human needs for physical survival become paramount. An example of this may be seen in the homeless person who is hospitalized and finds comfort from being in a warm and comfortable environment where hygiene needs can be met.

ASSESSMENT

General Assessment of Self-Care

Self-care depends on the client's physical and emotional ability to perform feeding, bathing, hair care, oral care, dressing, and toileting. An accurate assessment allows you and the client to mutually determine how much assistance is needed and to what extent the client can participate. If the client has a deficit in self-care ability, it may range from total inability to participate in any self-care activities to a partial deficit, in which case the client may be able to assist a greater or lesser degree in these activities. If you presuppose lack of ability when some ability may be present, it can further reinforce a client's sense of dependence and helplessness. On the other hand, if you expect participation in self-care activities when the client is physically or emotionally exhausted, the result may be increased client frustration or anxiety.

Action Alert! Assess the client's physical and emotional ability to participate in self-care activities as one means of providing a therapeutic environment for recovery or healing.

Health History. The health history is important in that it will give you information on which to base current self-care status. Why was the client admitted for home care services, to an acute care facility, or to a skilled nursing facility? How long has this problem existed? Is it new or long-standing? What was the lifestyle before? What is the history of the illness? What was the previous activity level? What are hygiene habits? The health history provides information about the client's present and past health and illness experiences. The health history interview should include a review of functional health patterns; question the status of and change in patterns. When did the ability to manage ADLs change? Is this a recent change or has it been coming over time? Is the alteration in functional ability of sudden or slow onset?

Note the client's physical status. Observe for the presence of pain or discomfort and whether these are aggravated by movement. Assess the acuity of the client's vision and hearing. Determine the ability to follow your directions. An assessment of cognitive function will provide you

with clues about how to approach the client and how to proceed. Note the presence of neuromuscular weakness or neuromuscular impairment (tics, spasticity, rigidity, palsy, paralysis). If the client's mobility is severely impaired, you may need to involve more than one caregiver. An assessment of the client's energy level is important so that care can be provided while minimizing the client's expenditure of energy.

Assess for factors that place the client at risk for self-care deficit. Risk factors include developmental stage, current health status, mobility, cognitive status, emotional status, and medical plan of care.

Be aware of the client's age. The very young and the very old have special needs for assistance. Infants have no capacity to perform self-care, whereas older adults may have some need for dependency on caregivers when self-care abilities are affected by physical or psychological impairments.

Mobility may be a risk factor if there is any impairment due to neuromuscular weakness or sensory deficits. Some clients may have limited mobility because of the weakness of one or more extremities.

The client's ability to recognize the need for hygiene measures and the ability to implement this knowledge are necessary to prevent a deficit in self-care. A cognitively impaired individual may not be able to focus well enough to plan the essential steps necessary for self-care or to carry them out.

Action Alert! Carefully assess clients' cognitive status; even if they appear to be well oriented and capable of self-care, more careful assessment may reveal short-term memory loss or other deficits.

The client who is very stressed or emotionally unstable may outwardly appear to have self-care skills, but because of the intense focus on the emotional stressor, the client may simply not have enough energy to meet these needs.

The medical plan of care may put the client at risk for self-care deficit. Therapeutic management of illness or trauma, surgical or medical procedures that cause weakness, or pain or nausea may necessitate bed rest and interfere with the client's ability to perform self-care activities.

Action Alert! Anticipate the client's forthcoming therapies and treatment so as to anticipate the risk for self-care deficit.

Gather subjective assessment data by interacting with both the client and family. Functional health pattern assessment provides valuable information about the client's perceived self-care abilities and difficulties and associated feelings about adequacy. The assessment may include the normal routine for feeding, bathing, grooming, and toileting, and the personal satisfaction with this routine. Ask the client what causes problems and what has been done to deal with these problems. What does the client want to happen? Is the client satisfied with the current state of daily self-care activities? What are the client's goals and expectations? Is there hope for improvement in self-care status? What level of dependence on family caregivers is necessary?

Focused Assessment for *Self-Care Deficit*

Defining Characteristics. Assess the client's abilities and deficits in the following areas.

SELF-CARE DEFICIT: BATHING/HYGIENE. Assess the client's ability to wash the body or body parts, to obtain water or regulate the temperature and flow of water, to get bathing supplies, to sit or stand while bathing, and to get to the bathroom [North American Nursing Diagnosis Association (NANDA), 2001]. Total hygiene consists of bathing, skin care, oral care, hair care, perineal care, back massage, shaving, changing the bed linens, and changing gown or pajamas.

SELF-CARE DEFICIT: DRESSING/GROOMING. Assess the ability to choose clothing, put on or take off pieces of clothing including socks and shoes, fasten clothing using zippers and buttons, use assistive devices for dressing, and maintain a satisfactory appearance (NANDA, 2001). Also identify the client's ability to choose or replace clothing.

SELF-CARE DEFICIT: FEEDING. Assess the ability to open containers, prepare food, place food onto utensils, bring food to mouth, chew, and swallow. Also assess the client's ability to take in sufficient food (NANDA, 2001).

SELF-CARE DEFICIT: TOILETING. Assess the ability to get to the toilet or commode, to sit on and rise from it, and to flush. Also assess the client's ability to move clothing to carry out toileting, and to use proper hygiene after toileting (NANDA, 2001).

Related Factors. The related factors for all of these nursing diagnoses are similar, and include fatigue, inadequate or lack of motivation, pain or severe anxiety, perceptual or cognitive impairment, neuromuscular or musculoskeletal impairment, or environmental barriers (NANDA, 2001).

DIAGNOSIS

Use the physical assessment database and your observations to determine the appropriate nursing diagnoses (Table 30-5). When the client presents with a self-care deficit problem, it may be total or partial. If it is total, it includes deficits in feeding, bathing/hygiene, dressing/grooming, and toileting. If it is partial, one or more deficits may be present. The client may have a diagnosis that begins with *Risk for* if there is potential for loss of self-care ability.

Related Nursing Diagnoses

Impaired skin integrity is a problem for the client who cannot manage self-care and hygiene. A good time to assess the skin is during the client's bath. Assess the color and temperature, particularly in the extremities. Note areas that are different from other areas (cooler, warmer, paler, pinker), the texture (dry or oily), any lesions or impaired integrity, any rectal bleeding, and pain or sensitivity in any area as it is bathed or moved. Note the client's sense of touch (temperature of water, pressure with rubbing), limitation of motion or stiffness or pain during range-of-motion (ROM) exercises, emotional state, and ability to communicate.

Impaired oral mucous membranes may apply to a client who is not able to manage oral hygiene for a number of reasons. Persons who have altered states of consciousness are unable to meet self-care needs for oral care. Others have mobility impairment so that it is difficult or impossible to get to the sink or bathroom and to manipulate toothbrush or dental floss (e.g., a client with arthritic hands may have difficulty in picking up and holding small items).

Impaired physical mobility may be caused by acute or chronic illness, trauma, psychological impairment, or the

Table 30-5	*Clustering Data to Make a Nursing Diagnosis*
SELF-CARE DEFICIT	
Data Cluster	**Diagnosis**
A 65-year-old, poorly nourished, fatigued, and listless woman was diagnosed with Alzheimer's disease 5 years ago. She has shown rapid deterioration and now is unable to care for any of her basic hygiene needs.	*Self-care deficit* related to loss of memory and neuromuscular function
A young man, age 30, has metastatic brain tumor secondary to progressive bronchogenic carcinoma. He is totally blind in his right eye. He also has right hemiplegia and is very limited in his self-care abilities.	*Self-care deficit* related to decreased visual and motor ability
A 55-year-old woman has a history of chronic obstructive pulmonary disease and is now in acute congestive heart failure. She has extreme dyspnea and is able to ambulate only to the bathroom and back to recliner.	*Self-care deficit* related to activity intolerance
A 40-year-old woman has had severe rheumatoid arthritis for 20 years. She has severe limitations of the lower and upper extremities. She has difficulty grasping objects because of the malformation of hands and fingers.	*Self-care deficit* related to limited range of motion
A 20-year-old man was hospitalized after a motor vehicle accident; his pelvis, left tibia, and fibula were fractured. He refuses to move because of the intense pain caused by any movement.	*Self-care deficit* related to pain and limited mobility from fractures

need to conserve energy as with bed rest or reduced activity. *Activity intolerance* occurs when the physical or psychological demands of the activity are more than the client can tolerate without manifestations of distress, which may take the form of dyspnea, muscle weakness, fatigue, or tachycardia.

Powerlessness may apply to a client who is dependent on others for activities of daily living. Assess the client's behavior for attempts at establishing control. The client who is demanding and manipulative may be feeling out of control. On the other hand, powerlessness may be expressed as apathy or fastidiousness.

PLANNING

Planning for outcomes should be a collaborative effort between you, the client, and, when appropriate, the client's family. Setting mutually acceptable and attainable goals is essential in assisting the client to attain some degree of independence.

Expected Outcomes for the Client With *Self-Care Deficit*

Planning is essential to help the client meet personal care needs when there is a self-care deficit. For the client who has a total self-care deficit, the goal is to provide measures that will prevent complications. For the client with partial self-care deficit, the goal is to assist the client as needed and to encourage as much independence as possible. The goal is always to encourage independence and to return the client to a state of independent self-care. Take the following factors into account when planning:

- The client's general physical condition and functional status
- Individual specific self-care requirements
- Personal preferences and wishes

Expected Outcomes for Client and Family With *Self-Care Deficit*

Planning with the client and family is important because the desired outcomes may vary with the client's level of illness or with priorities that are different from those you believe to be necessary for the client. Expected outcomes for the client and family with self-care deficit might be the following:

- Client's self-care needs are met.
- Complications are avoided and minimized.
- Client and family members carry out self-care program daily.
- Client and family communicate feelings and concerns.
- Client and family identify resources to help cope with problems after discharge.

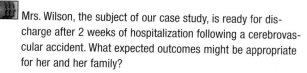
Mrs. Wilson, the subject of our case study, is ready for discharge after 2 weeks of hospitalization following a cerebrovascular accident. What expected outcomes might be appropriate for her and her family?

INTERVENTION

Interventions to Promote Skin Hygiene

Principles of Skin Care. Because the skin is the first line of defense against microbes and other harmful substances, healthy intact skin is important to a client's overall health. Keeping the skin clean and dry helps to protect it from disease and damage. When providing skin care to a client, remember to bathe from cleaner to less-clean areas, working from the head and upper body toward the feet. Keep in mind also that hygiene and grooming are directly related to self-esteem.

BATHING THE CLIENT. Bathing is an important intervention to promote hygiene. Choice of the method of bathing depends on your judgment as well as the medical plan of care in regard to the client's activity level and mental and physical capabilities to perform self-care (Box 30-2). Consider the client's preferences for type of bath and time of day for bathing to allow some degree of control. This may not always be possible because of the client's condition and other factors.

Bathing may be accomplished with a bed bath, a tub or shower, or the client's bathing at a sink or lavatory. Bed baths are less commonly used than in the past as recognition of the need for mobility has assumed precedence over bed rest. Assistive devices such as shower chairs that can be rolled into the shower, and lifting devices that can lift a client in and out of a tub, allow tub and shower bathing for clients who previously would have received bed baths.

Action Alert! The benefits for the client of bathing in a tub or shower are so significant that, if that option is available, you should use it even though it may be more difficult and time consuming. The enhanced physical and emotional state of the client will be worth the effort.

Some of the goals of hygiene care are the following:

- Comfort and relaxation, which help to relax tense muscles and allow the client to feel refreshed
- Stimulation of circulation through friction and massage
- Cleanliness from removal of body waste products and secretions

Bathing a client is a time of close contact that provides you with an opportunity to communicate with the client as well as assess the client's physical and mental status.

Box 30-2	Guidelines for Bathing Clients

- Promote safety and prevent falls.
- Assess psychological and physical needs.
- Determine self-care abilities and limitations.
- Encourage self-help except when contraindicated.
- Allow as much control and involvement as possible; let the client make some choices.
- Provide privacy and warmth at time of bathing; cover and drape sufficiently.
- Use good body mechanics for yourself by keeping a wide base of support, keeping back straight, and using leg and abdominal muscles to move and lift clients.

The client may appreciate your undivided attention for a concentrated period of time and may feel free to express concerns that otherwise would not be expressed. It is a time to provide special skin care and teach the client and family about skin care (Box 30-3).

Several types of baths can be used, depending on the client's need (Table 30-6). Baths may be used for cleansing or for therapeutic measures related to some skin problem.

BATHING THE CLIENT IN BED. Procedure 30-1 provides detailed steps for bathing a client in bed. The bed bath is given for the purpose of providing cleanliness for a client who is unable to be out of bed and who is unable to care for hygiene needs because of physical or mental limitations. It is indicated primarily for clients with restricted mobility (people with casts, traction, or back problems), those who have heart and respiratory problems and thus limited exercise tolerance, or those who are at the first postoperative day and thus may be too weak to get out of bed to bathe.

Methods include the following:

- Complete bed bath: giving the complete bath without any assistance from the client
- Partial bed bath: assisting with key areas such as axilla, back, and perineal care
- Self-help: giving the client help with hard-to-reach areas, such as the back, legs, and feet

A bed bath may be given using a "bag" bath or a towel bath. The client is cleansed with a warm cloth or towel saturated with a quick-drying solution, such as Septi-Soft. An advantage of this type of bath is that it is brief (10 minutes) and can be used for the client who is easily fatigued and who has limited tolerance for any activity. The oil in the solution softens the skin, and clients report a refreshed feeling from this kind of bath.

PROVIDING PERINEAL CARE. Cleaning the genitalia is usually a part of the bath, but it also may be needed after urinary or bowel elimination. If the client is unable to maintain adequate perineal care, this part of the care is your responsibility (Procedure 30-2). Perineal care for women involves washing the labia majora and the labia minora, the inner thighs, the perineum, and the anal area. The **perineum** is the pelvic floor and associated structures occupying the pelvic outlet, bounded anteriorly by the symphysis pubis, laterally by the ischial tuberosities, and posteriorly by the coccyx. For men, perineal care involves cleaning the upper inner thighs, penis, and scrotum. In uncircumcised men, the foreskin must be retracted and the glans penis washed. In both sexes, the perianal area is cleaned last with the client in a side-lying position. Professional behavior helps to reduce anxiety and embarrassment in the client. It is essential to wear gloves for this procedure because of the direct contact with body fluids and exudates and because any open wounds or sores on your hands are avenues for transmission of infections. Clients may receive perineal care while sitting on the bedpan or toilet.

Clients at risk for skin breakdown, and who may have particular needs for meticulous and frequent perineal care, include those with indwelling catheters, postpartum clients, clients with perineal, rectal, or lower urinary tract surgery, and incontinent clients.

ASSISTING THE CLIENT WITH A SHOWER OR TUB BATH. Assess the client to determine the degree of independence to allow in bathing. Safety becomes a priority because injuries caused by

Text continued on p. 744

Teaching for Wellness — Skin Care — Box 30-3

Purpose: To teach client about the care of dry skin, which is susceptible to breaking, and causes itching and roughness.

Expected Outcomes: Client will follow prescribed regimen for skin to alleviate dryness.

Client Instructions

- Sometimes your skin can become dry because you have not taken in enough fluids. Make sure you drink 8 glasses of water a day. Avoid dehydrating fluids, such as sodas and caffeine-containing drinks. These are not substitutes for water.
- Bathing can dry your skin as well. Use a gentle bath lotion or mild soap. No soap is sometimes the best answer.
- Too-frequent bathing may dry the skin. It may be wise to reduce baths from daily to every other day or even twice a week. When bathing, use warm rather than hot water.
- Use bath oils or lubricants immediately after bathing to prevent immediate loss of moisture.
- Pay attention to the way your linens and clothing are being laundered. Harsh detergents and bleaches are irritating to already dry skin. Use mild nondetergent cleaning products rather than harsh detergents. Avoid perfumed fabric softeners.
- Dry skin tends to itch, and you may want to rub or scratch it. Try not to do this because you can hurt your skin. Also avoid rubbing your skin roughly with a towel after bathing. Patting dry is much less harmful to the skin.

Table 30-6	Types of Therapeutic Baths
Type of Bath	**Purpose**
Sitz bath	To decrease pain and inflammation after rectal or perineal surgery or for pain relief from hemorrhoids. Water should be warm to client's comfort level.
Hot-water bath	To relieve muscle spasm and muscle tension. Water should be deep enough for immersion. Warm to client's comfort level.
Warm-water bath	To relax and soothe. Client's comfort will dictate water temperature. Caution client about time limits for soaking (20 minutes) because of vasodilation.
Cool-water bath	To decrease fever and to reduce muscle tension. Avoid chilling. Water should be cool but not cold.
Oatmeal or Aveeno	To soothe irritated skin. Softens and lubricates dry scaly skin. Place 3 cups cooked oatmeal in a cheesecloth bag and place in tub of water.
Corn starch	To soothe skin irritation. Dissolve 1 lb of cornstarch in cold water, then add boiling water until mixture is thick and add to tub water.

| PROCEDURE 30-1 | GIVING THE CLIENT A BATH |

TIME TO ALLOW
Novice: 45 min.
Expert: 20 min.

The bed bath is given to provide cleanliness and comfort to a client who is unable to be out of bed because of physical or mental limitations. The client who is unable to perform any of the bath is given a complete bed bath. Most clients can perform some of the bath and in most circumstances should be encouraged to do so. The bed bath is an opportunity to perform range-of-motion (ROM) exercises and skin assessment.

Standard precautions are followed for all bath procedures. In standard precautions, the nurse wears clean gloves for any contact with blood, body fluids, secretions, excretions, and contaminated items. Put on clean gloves just before touching mucous membranes and nonintact skin. Change gloves between tasks and procedures on the same client after contact with material that may contain a high concentration of microorganisms. Remove gloves promptly after use, before touching noncontaminated items and environmental surfaces, and before going to another client, and perform hand hygiene immediately to avoid transfer of microorganisms to other clients or environments.

DELEGATION GUIDELINES

Once you have assessed your client, you may delegate the performance of a bed bath to a nursing assistant. Remember that although the nursing assistant may be instructed to observe for changes in the client's skin, such as irritation or discoloration, you as the nurse maintain the professional responsibility for assessment and for appropriate action based on assessment. You are responsible for reestablishing any disruption in IV infusions or drainage devices at the completion of the bath.

EQUIPMENT NEEDED

- Washbasin
- Soap or cleansing lotion
- Two towels and two washcloths
- Clean gown or pajamas
- Powder, deodorant, skin lotion
- Oral-care items
- Hair-care items
- Shaving items
- Clean gloves (essential for perineal and oral care; otherwise, as needed)

1. Follow preliminary guidelines for nursing procedures (see inside front cover).

2. Check physician's orders for activity and any special positioning needs or contraindications. Assess for ability to participate in the bath even if on a limited scale. Evaluate client's need for teaching about skin care and plan to incorporate teaching into the procedure. Assess for presence of IV lines, catheters, tubes, casts, and dressings. Assess client's ROM. *Cleansing of skin and teaching about skin care and ROM movements can be smoothly integrated so that time and energy are conserved for you and client. If assessment indicates that the bath can be done more efficiently or safely with two people, it is advisable to secure this help. Allowing the client to participate in the bath provides a source of exercise and ROM movement as well as providing for enhancement of self-worth and feelings of independence.*

3. Prepare the environment.
a. Perform hand hygiene and apply gloves if needed. Change gloves after oral care, perineal care, or washing nonintact skin. *Some agencies adopt a policy of using gloves for the bath without regard to assessing for intact skin. Other agencies leave it to the nurse's judgment.*

b. Gather equipment and take to the bedside. Have all necessary supplies and equipment ready for use. *Having necessary supplies readily at hand enhances organization and efficiency in bathing the client.*

c. Raise bed to a comfortable working height, ensure privacy by closing door or curtains, and regulate temperature of the room for comfort. Keep the side rail up on the side of the bed opposite to where you are working. *Applying principles of body mechanics allows you to work comfortably and efficiently without muscle strain. Privacy, comfort, and safety are prerequisites for making the bed bath a positive experience for the client.*

d. Place articles on over-bed table, within easy reach. *Organization of supplies conserves energy and increases efficiency of movement. Having supplies within reach also promotes client's safety because it eliminates the necessity for your turning away from the client or moving away from the bedside to reach for supplies.*

PROCEDURE 30-1   GIVING THE CLIENT A BATH—CONT'D

4. Prepare the client.

a. Assist client to use bedpan, commode, or urinal. *Bathing, turning, and placement of extremities in warm water may stimulate the need to void.*

b. Place bath blanket over the client, covering the top linen (see illustration). *The bath blanket is warmer and more absorbent than a sheet. If a bath blanket is not available, the top sheet may be used to cover the client.*

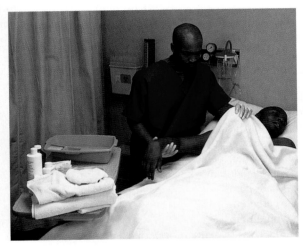

Step 4b. Placing the bath blanket over the client, covering the top linen.

c. Loosen top linen at the foot of the bed and remove from under the bath blanket. To do so, ask the client to grasp the top of the bath blanket. If client is unable to grasp the blanket, grip it with one hand while removing the linen with the other. The client remains covered with the bath blanket while the soiled sheet is pulled out. Refold any linen that is to be reused and place on a chair. Place dirty linen in a laundry hamper or laundry bag.

d. Place bath towel under head. Remove pillow if the client can tolerate it. If removal of pillow causes any discomfort, leave it in place and place the towel over the pillow. *Removal of the pillow allows better access to the back of the neck and skin surfaces. It also prevents the pillow from becoming damp while the face and neck are being washed.*

e. Help client move to the side of the bed nearest you. Be sure that the side rail on the opposite side of the bed is raised. *Having the client close to you lowers your center of gravity and enhances efficiency of movement and energy, and it protects your back muscles from being stretched.*

f. Remove client's gown or pajamas. If an IV is in place, remove the arm without the IV first; then, on the arm with the IV, slide the sleeve down, lower the IV, and slide the IV through the sleeve opening. Rehang the IV and assess the rate of flow.

5. Wash the client's face and neck. *In general, bathe from head to toe (cleanest to dirtiest). Wash, rinse, and dry before moving to the next area.*

a. Fill washbasin ⅓ to ½ full of warm water. Test the temperature of the water with a bath thermometer or with your wrist. It should be comfortably warm, between 109.4° and 114.8° F (43° to 46° C). *If the pan is too full, the basin is difficult to handle and spilling is likely. Too little water cools very quickly and is not sufficient for adequate bathing and rinsing.*

b. Put on clean gloves if there is a possibility of exposure to body fluids during the bath. *Standard precautions should be maintained when any exposure to body fluids is anticipated.*

c. Make a mitt with the washcloth. Use either the triangular or the rectangular method of folding (see illustration). Place your hand in the center of the washcloth. Fold the edges over your hand. Tuck the edges in to make a mitt. *Using the mitt prevents the loose ends of the washcloth from dragging across the client's skin and chilling or irritating the skin.*

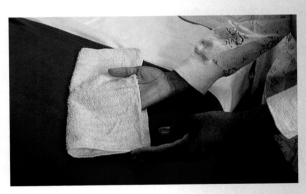

Step 5c. Folding the edges of the washcloth over the hand to make a mitt (rectangular method).

d. Wash and dry the client's face using clear water or a mild soap. *Soap is sometimes drying to the skin, especially in older people. Many people do not want soap on their face. Ask client for preference before using soap.*

e. Wash the client's eyes with clear water. With one corner of the mitt, begin washing the eye at the inner canthus and work toward the outside (see illustration). Change the placement of your hand in the mitt and repeat with the other eye. Dry thoroughly. If crusted secretions are present, place warm washcloth or cotton ball over the eye until secretions are moist enough to be easily removed.

Using different points on the washcloth prevents cross-contamination of the eyes if there is any infection. Infectious secretions are prevented from entering the lacrimal ducts. Moistening dried secretions prevents trauma to the eye on removal of the secretions.

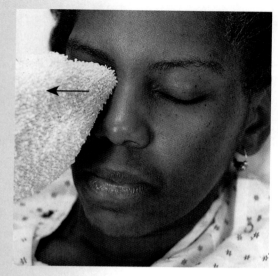

Step 5e. Washing the eye from the inner canthus outward.

f. Wash forehead, cheeks, nose, and perioral areas.
g. Wash the postauricular area. Clean the anterior and posterior ear with the tip of the washcloth.
h. Wash the front and back of the neck.
i. Remove the towel from beneath client's neck.

6. Wash the client's arms. *As you move down the body you can wash larger areas at a time. Wash small to moderate-size sections of the body at a time. The size of the area is determined by the likelihood of the person experiencing the discomfort of chilling.*
a. Place a towel lengthwise under upper arm and axilla. Wash the upper surface of the arm. Use long, firm strokes, proceeding from the distal to the proximal area (see illustration).

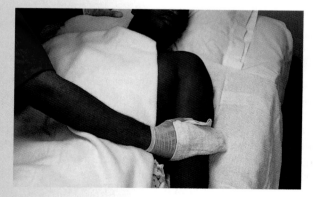

Step 6a. Washing the client's arm.

b. Grasp the client's wrist firmly and elevate the arm to wash its lower surface.
c. Wash the axilla. *Elevating the arm helps with ROM movement, and distal-to-proximal stroking aids venous return. Extremities should be grasped at the joint rather than by the body of the muscle when they are being elevated. Gripping the muscle body may cause great discomfort.*
d. Wash the client's hands. Support the wrist joint and immerse the hand in warm water. Allow it to soak for a few minutes. Do ROM movements with the client's fingers. Dry the hand thoroughly. Nails may be cleaned now or after the bath. Apply lotion if desired. *Moving the joints provides ROM exercise. Soaking the hand is relaxing and pleasant for the client. It also softens the cuticle and makes it easier to clean the nails by loosening any dirt under the nails.*

7. Wash the client's chest.
a. Fold the bath blanket down to the umbilicus.
b. Cover a female client's chest with a towel. Then lift up one side to wash her chest. Dry under the breasts and in any skin folds. Bath powder or cornstarch may be used in small amounts under the breasts if desired. Assess breasts and teach breast self-examination if appropriate. Palpate for axillary node enlargement. *Keeping the client covered protects privacy and prevents unnecessary exposure. Powder or cornstarch serves to absorb perspiration and helps to prevent skin breakdown in body folds, but large quantities of powder under breasts and in skin folds tend to clump.*

8. Wash the client's abdomen.
a. Expose only the areas being washed. Keep remaining areas covered with a towel. Fold the bath blanket down to the symphysis pubis.
b. Use firm strokes to wash the abdomen from side to side, including the umbilicus. *Firm strokes decrease the sensation of tickling, which some people have on light abdominal touching.*
c. Observe for signs of distention or visible peristalsis.
d. Re-cover the client with the bath blanket.

9. Wash the client's legs.
a. Expose one leg at a time. Keep the other leg covered with the bath blanket. Keep the rest of the body covered. Remove bath blanket from the farther leg first.
b. Use firm distal-to-proximal strokes. *Distal-to-proximal stroking stimulates circulation and promotes venous return.*
c. Place the client's foot in the basin for a few minutes to soak. Do ROM movements with the toes. Inspect the feet and nails. When flexing the leg, grasp and support the heel while cradling the calf. *Although it is not essential, soaking the feet can be comforting, especially if the client has been in bed for several days. Soaking aids circulation and*

Continued

PROCEDURE 30-1 | GIVING THE CLIENT A BATH—CONT'D

softens nails and calluses. Supporting the extremity at the joint prevents discomfort that is initiated by grasping the body of a muscle.

d. Dry the feet thoroughly, especially between the toes (see illustration).

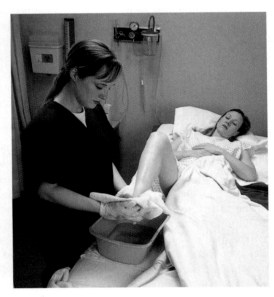

Step 9d. Drying the feet thoroughly.

e. Repeat this process for the other leg. *Pain on flexing of the leg may be suggestive of a positive Homans' sign, which should be reported to the physician immediately.*

10. Provide perineal care.

a. Place the client in a supine position. If the client is able to wash genitalia without assistance, place a basin of warm water, washcloth, and towel within reach and provide privacy. If the client cannot wash the perineal area, drape the area with the bath blanket so that only the genitalia are exposed.

b. Wash the perineal area, as explained in Procedure 30-2.

11. Wash the back, buttocks, and perianal area.

a. Change the bath water.

b. Place the client in a side-lying position.

c. Place a towel lengthwise along the client's back and buttocks.

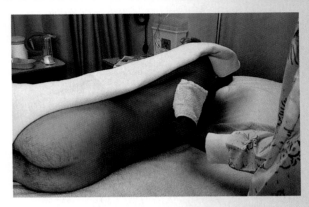

Step 11d. Washing the back and buttocks.

d. Wash, rinse, and dry the client's back and buttocks (see illustration). *The perianal area is considered the dirtiest area of the body and is bathed last to prevent microorganisms from being transferred to cleaner parts of the body.*

e. A back massage with powder or lotion may be done at this time or it may be done at the completion of the bath.

12. Help the client don a clean gown or pajamas.

a. While the client is still on one side, place one arm in the sleeve of the gown.

b. Turn the client to the back and place the other arm in the sleeve.

13. Assist with hair care.

14. Assist with oral care, as explained in Procedure 30-6 (p. 752).

15. Make the bed with clean linens, as explained in Procedures 30-4 (p. 747) and 30-5 (p. 749).

16. Leave the client's environment clean and uncluttered.

17. Document significant observations and assessment findings.

PEDIATRIC CONSIDERATIONS

Regulate the temperature of bath water carefully to avoid burns. Newborn infants do not require tub baths; rather, they should be given sponge baths. Infants should be dried and wrapped immediately after a bath to conserve body heat, because they have an incompletely developed temperature-regulating center. Children should participate in bathing according to their developmental level; for safety, they should never be left unattended in the bath. Adolescents may need assistance in choosing deodorants to reduce odor from perspiration caused by the reaction of bacteria with secretions from newly active sweat glands.

GERIATRIC CONSIDERATIONS

Regulate the temperature of bath water carefully to avoid burns. Avoid excessive use of soap to prevent excessively dry skin. Use moisturizers on the skin immediately after bathing while skin is still slightly damp. Avoid the use of powder, which causes moisture loss and could be hazardous if inhaled. Avoid the use of cornstarch in moist areas because it breaks down into glucose and enhances the growth of microorganisms.

HOME CARE CONSIDERATIONS

In giving a bed bath in the home, follow the same general guidelines for body mechanics, cleaning from clean to dirty, maintaining physical comfort, and working efficiently. However, the typical home environment requires some modification to meet these guidelines. If the client will need bed baths on a long-term basis, obtaining a hospital bed may be a helpful solution. Some modifications to teach the family caregiver include the following:

- Place a worktable at the bedside.
- Sit on the side of the bed instead of bending over.
- Use a minimum amount of soap.
- Use a no-rinse cleansing product.
- Give a complete bath only every 3 days, with axillary and perineal care in between.
- Check and massage the skin daily.

PROCEDURE 30-2   # PROVIDING PERINEAL CARE

TIME TO ALLOW
Novice: 15 min.
Expert: 5 min.

Perineal care is the cleansing of the external genitalia, perineum, and surrounding skin. It is usually part of the bath but is sometimes needed more frequently and is done as a separate procedure. See Procedure 30-1 for standard precautions guidelines.

DELEGATION GUIDELINES

You may delegate the performance of perineal care to a nursing assistant who has received specific training in the performance of this task. You remain responsible and accountable for assessing the client's perineum.

EQUIPMENT NEEDED

- Bedpan
- Two towels
- Two washcloths
- Soap
- Cotton balls
- Warm water or prescribed solution
- Waterproof pad
- Toilet tissue
- Bath blanket
- Clean gloves (required)

FOR A FEMALE CLIENT

1. Follow preliminary guidelines for nursing procedures (see inside front cover).

2. Prepare for the procedure.
a. Organize necessary equipment. Don clean gloves.
b. Place a protective pad or towel underneath the client before placing her on the bedpan if doing perineal care in bed. *Perineal care may be done with the client on a bedpan or sitting on the toilet or in a commode chair.*
c. Place the client in a comfortable position on bedpan, toilet, or commode chair. She may also sit on a bedpan in a semi-Fowler position if the dorsal recumbent position is not possible. *Adapting position to the client's needs ensures a more positive outcome of the procedure.*
d. If care is to be given in bed, ask the client to bend her knees and separate her legs.
e. Drape the client with a bath blanket. Cover her legs and wrap the corners of the bath blanket around her feet so her legs are covered. Leave a flap of drape covering the perineum until you are ready to begin the procedure. *Privacy and respect for the client's dignity are essential; expose as little as possible.*

Conti...d

PROCEDURE 30-2 PROVIDING PERINEAL CARE—CONT'D

3. Clean the perineum.

a. Pour warm water or prescribed solution over the perineum.

b. Separate the labia with one hand to expose the urethral and vaginal openings.

c. With your free hand, wipe from front to back in a downward motion with water and soap, washcloth, or cotton balls. Use a new cloth or cotton ball for each downward stroke. *Wiping in this manner prevents cross-contamination of areas.*

d. Wash the external labia. Turn the client to a side-lying position and wash her anal area.

e. Pat dry with a second towel.

4. Make the client comfortable.

a. Remove equipment and cover the client.

b. Position her for comfort.

FOR A MALE CLIENT

1. Follow preliminary guidelines for nursing procedures (see inside front cover).

2. Prepare for the procedure.

a. Organize necessary equipment. Don clean gloves.

b. Cover the client with a bath blanket. Expose him only as needed to clean the genitalia. *Avoiding unnecessary exposure respects the client's need for privacy.*

3. Clean the perineum.

a. If the client is uncircumcised, retract the foreskin to remove smegma. *Smegma is a cheese-like substance secreted by the sebaceous glands. It collects under the foreskin.*

b. Hold the shaft of the penis firmly but gently with one hand. With the other hand, begin washing at the tip of the penis. Using a circular motion, clean from the center to the outside.

c. Wash down the shaft toward the scrotum. Do not repeat washing an area without changing to a clean area on the washcloth.

d. After washing the penis, replace the foreskin if necessary.

e. Wash around the scrotum.

4. Make the client comfortable.

a. Remove equipment.

b. Cover him and position for comfort.

HOME CARE CONSIDERATIONS

For the client who is unable to provide self-care at home, perineal care should be done daily to prevent unpleasant body odor and for comfort. If the client has a Foley catheter, daily perineal care will help prevent urinary tract infection. Gentle cleansing with soap and water is all that is required. Teach the family how to turn and position the client to work efficiently.

---

falls in a bathtub or shower are common and often have serious consequences. Assess the client for dizziness; weakness in extremities; hypotension; any sensory impairment, particularly visual; mental capacity; degree of judgment; and clarity of thought. You may determine that the client can be left alone for bathing, or you may plan to remain with the client during the bath.

Transport the client to the tub or shower in a wheelchair, on a stretcher, or in a rolling shower chair. If the person is ambulating, use nonskid slippers. If a wheelchair or rolling shower chair is used, take safety precautions such as belt restraints to prevent falling from the chair. Shower chairs are made of metal or plastic so they can be rolled into the shower. Use the hand-held shower nozzle to direct the flow of water. See Procedure 30-3 for details about assisting a client with a tub or shower bath.

Dressings and casts need not always be deterrents to bathing in a tub or shower. Improvised covers and plastic wrap taped over a cast or dressing can afford the person freedom to bathe as desired without damage to cast or dressing.

ASSISTING THE CLIENT WITH A SINK BATH. Sometimes the client is well enough to sit up in a chair and bathe at the sink or can sit on the side of the bed with the bath basin positioned on the over-bed table. Provide privacy by closing the door and using a drape or sheet for cover and warmth. Wash the back, legs, and feet as necessary. If necessary, provide perineal care. Because the client bathes in a seated position, it is wise to stay nearby in case assistance is needed or the client becomes weak or dizzy. If the client is bathing at the sink or in a chair, you may use this opportunity to change the bed linens. If the client is sitting on the side of the bed, you may use this time to prepare for mouth or hair care.

BEDMAKING. In the hospital setting, the changing of bed linens is often included as part of the routine morning care and is done in conjunction with the bath and grooming. At other times, linens are changed as needed when they become wet or soiled. In the home setting, linens may not be changed every day, but care should always be taken to smooth the linens and remove crumbs and foreign objects to ensure comfort and safety for the client.

PROCEDURE 30-3 | HELPING THE CLIENT WITH A TUB BATH OR SHOWER

TIME TO ALLOW
Novice: 30 min.
Expert: 15 min.

Clients are assisted with a tub bath or shower when they are able to bathe themselves and there is no contraindication to bathing in a tub or shower. The client should be carefully monitored because the change in temperature and exertion can precipitate weakness or dizziness. Clients who have had medical or surgical treatments in a hospital setting need orders from a physician. Follow standard precautions.

DELEGATION GUIDELINES

The nursing assistant may help with the performance of a tub bath or shower. In addition to instruction regarding bathing, the nursing assistant should receive safety and mobility training to appropriately assist the client with this task. You remain responsible for the assessment of the client's independence, skin, gait, mobility, and response to this activity.

EQUIPMENT NEEDED

- Bath towel
- Two washcloths
- Soap or bath lotion
- Skin care products (deodorant, talcum powder, lotion)
- Clean gown or pajamas
- Clean gloves (if indicated)

1. Follow preliminary guidelines for nursing procedures (see inside front cover).

2. Assess the client's capacity for self-care. Assess tolerance for activity, cognitive state, and musculoskeletal function. *An assessment of the client's ability prior to initiating the bath procedure is critical to maintaining the client's safety and comfort.*

3. Make sure that the bathroom is prepared and that the tub or shower is clean. Place a disposable bath mat or towel on the floor by the tub or shower. Adjust the room temperature so the client is not chilled during bath. *Cleanliness and safety are primary responsibilities in caring for the client.*

4. Put on clean gloves.

5. Assess the client's ability to access bathroom. Transport the client in a wheelchair or shower chair if ambulation cannot be done safely without assistance. Accompany the client to the bathroom.

6. Keep the client covered with a bath blanket while preparing the water and while transporting (see illustration). *Chilling occurs quickly when skin is uncovered. Keeping the client covered conserves body heat, preventing chilling.*

7. Provide privacy for the client by placing an "occupied" sign on the door. *Bathroom doors are not locked for safety reasons because clients may need unexpected assistance. The need for privacy while bathing is basic to human dignity, and provision for privacy demonstrates respect.*

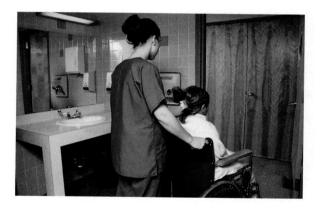

Step 6. Keeping the client covered with a bath blanket during transport to the bathroom.

8. Test the water temperature before the client gets into tub or shower. Adjust the temperature until it is comfortable. Fill the bathtub no more than half full of warm water (105° F). Caution client not to adjust temperature without assistance. *Testing the temperature before the water is entered prevents burns. Attempts to adjust the water temperature without your assistance can result in scalding.*

9. Provide assistance as the client is entering tub or shower. *Falls in the tub or shower are common accidents and must be prevented by safety measures.*

10. Assess whether the client can safely bathe without assistance. If the client can remain unattended, demonstrate the use of the call signal and the safety bars in the tub or shower. The client may wish to sit in a shower chair to conserve energy while bathing. Place all bath supplies within easy reach.

Continued

PROCEDURE 30-3 HELPING THE CLIENT WITH A TUB BATH OR SHOWER—CONT'D

Falls in the tub or shower often occur when client is reaching for an object, such as soap or a towel. Placing everything within easy reach prevents the need to reach.

11. If the client can be safely left to bathe unattended, check every 10 to 15 minutes to determine if help is needed.

12. If independent bathing is not possible, remain with the client at all times. Assist as needed with bathing. Encourage the client to do as much of the bathing as possible. *This encourages independence as well as motor function.*

13. Wash any areas that the client is unable to reach, such as the back and legs. Assist a female client with shaving her legs or axillae if desired.

14. Watch closely for signs of dizziness or weakness while the client is in the tub or shower and immediately on exiting the tub or shower. *Vasodilation and pooling of blood in the extremities occurs with prolonged exposure to warm water. This may manifest as dizziness, weakness, or faintness.*

15. Help the client out of the tub or shower. Assist with drying.

16. Assist with grooming and dressing in clean pajamas or gown.

17. Help the client return to the room.

18. Assess the client's tolerance for the procedure (level of fatigue, musculoskeletal strength, and sensorium).

19. Leave the bathroom clean. Discard soiled linen. Clean the tub or shower according to agency policy.

20. Document the client's response to the activity.

HOME CARE CONSIDERATIONS

The home care client who can get in the tub or shower will have some concerns about mobility and will need modifications for safety. Be sure the bathroom is equipped with grab bars and that a steady stool or shower chair is available. The bathtub should have a nonskid surface. The bath mat should be nonskid and the floor should not be slippery when wet. For showers in a chair, it may be helpful to install a long, hose-type shower head.

In bedmaking, you must incorporate a variety of skills to make the procedure safe, efficient, and coordinated. The use of good body mechanics is important for protection of your back.

> *Action Alert!* Keep your center of gravity close to a wide base of support. Keep the bed at a working height that is comfortable for you so that there is no need to stretch or twist to reach the bed or the client. Use your strong leg and arm muscles to protect weaker back muscles.

The type of bedmaking required depends in large measure on the condition and needs of the client. If the client is able to be out of bed, the bed should be made at this time. Procedure 30-4 outlines the steps in making an occupied bed.

Preparation for bedmaking is important for the sake of efficiency. Stack clean linen on a chair in the order of use so that each item is accessible as needed. Place soiled linens in a hamper as soon as they are removed; *never* place them on the floor. Hold soiled linens away from the uniform at arm's length until they can be placed in the hamper. Do not shake either clean linen or soiled linen because this readily disperses organisms into the air. Do not place soiled linens on the overbed table. This is not only unclean but aesthetically unpleasing because this is the table from which the client eats.

A different type of linen arrangement is needed for the client returning from surgery. Consider the needs of the client and prepare the room accordingly. Make the bed as with any unoccupied bed with a few exceptions. Procedure 30-5 (p. 749) describes the steps in preparing a surgical bed (and an unoccupied bed). The purpose of this linen arrangement is that an easy transfer from stretcher to bed can be made when the client returns from the operating room and the top covers can quickly be put in place. Put the bed in high position, and clear the room of any clutter so that there is no obstruction. Knowing what to anticipate as a result of the surgical procedure is important. If you anticipate that the client will need assistance with turning and moving, place a draw sheet on the bed for use as a lift sheet. Add extra precautions such as incontinent pads if you anticipate drainage, bleeding, or incontinence.

Interventions to Promote Oral Hygiene

The client who is unable to provide for oral hygiene is host to potentially serious problems that are preventable. Assess the client's physical status to determine the degree of assistance needed with oral hygiene. The arthritic client may find it difficult to grasp a small toothbrush handle, so it may be helpful to use an electric toothbrush, which tends to have a bigger handle, or to pad the handle of the toothbrush to make it

Text continued on p. 751

PROCEDURE 30-4   MAKING AN OCCUPIED BED

TIME TO ALLOW
Novice: 20 min.
Expert: 10 min.

If the client cannot be out of bed, the linens are changed at the end of the bed bath. This can be accomplished by turning the client to one side, making half the bed, turning the client to the other side, and making the other half of the bed. In an acute care facility, bed linens are often changed daily for the client's comfort and to eliminate a reservoir of microorganisms. When linens become wet or soiled, they are changed more frequently. In the home setting, linens are not changed daily but should be changed when wet or soiled.

DELEGATION GUIDELINES

Once you have assessed your client's ability to be turned and positioned in a side-lying fashion, you may delegate the performance of an occupied bed change to the nursing assistant. Clients with neurological or orthopedic injuries may have special positioning restrictions that require your direct supervision and assistance with the performance of this task. In the basic training program, the nursing assistant should receive specific instruction in the performance of this task, including safety, client comfort, and infection control.

EQUIPMENT NEEDED

- Top sheet, bottom sheet, draw sheet (optional)
- Bedspread (change if soiled)
- Blanket (if needed; change if soiled)
- Mattress pad (change if soiled)
- Pillowcases
- Waterproof pads

1. Follow preliminary guidelines for nursing procedures (see inside front cover).

2. Organize the environment and position the client to expose half the bed.
a. Perform hand hygiene.
b. Close the door or curtain for privacy.
c. Fold a full-size sheet to be used as a draw sheet.
d. Lower the rail on the near side of the bed. Be sure that the side rail on the opposite side is up and locked. *This ensures safety as the client rolls to the side of the bed. Upright side rails also allow the client something to grasp to help in turning.*
e. Position the bed at a comfortable working height. Move the client toward the near side of the bed. *Having the bed at waist height and the client at the side of the bed allows the use of correct body mechanics by lowering the center of gravity and avoiding stretching of the lower back muscles.*
f. Loosen the top linens.
g. Remove spread, top sheet, and blanket in one movement, at the same time pulling the bath blanket over the client. If top linens are to be reused, fold and place them in a chair. *Linens should always be folded and not fluffed in the air. It is important to prevent the spread of microorganisms.*
h. Place any linen that is not to be reused in a laundry hamper or linen bag. Avoid contact with your uniform. Hold at arm's length while removing from bed to linen hamper. *The spread of microorganisms from soiled linen to uniform to other clients is prevented by avoiding contact with linen.*

i. Loosen bottom sheet on near side of bed. Have the client roll to the opposite side of the bed. Adjust the pillow under the head.
j. Lower the bed position to flat if the client can tolerate it. If the client cannot breathe when lying flat, adjust the bed to as near flat as possible. *The flatter the surface of the bed, the more efficiently the sheets can be tucked under the mattress.*

3. Make half the bed from top to bottom.
a. Fan-fold the dirty bottom sheet and draw sheet, and tuck them under the client's back and buttocks as tightly as possible (see illustration). *This allows space for you to place clean linens, and it moves dirty linen close to the other side of the bed for easy removal.*

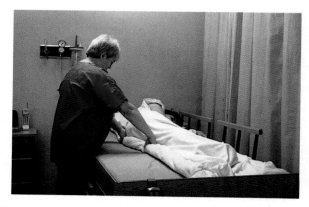

Step 3a. Fan-folding the dirty bottom sheet and draw sheet and tucking them under the client's back and buttocks.

PROCEDURE 30-4   **Making an Occupied Bed**—Cont'd

b. Place the clean bottom sheet on the bed. Start with the bottom edge even with foot end of bed, and with the center fold in the middle of the bed. Unfold to the top and allow the extra length to hang over the top. Tuck the end of the sheet under the mattress.

c. Fan-fold the top layer to the middle of the bed (see illustration). Make the roll of linens as flat as possible. The client will need to roll over the linens gathered in the middle of the bed. Pull the triangular fold over the side of the mattress.

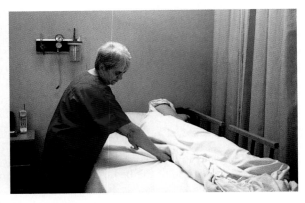

Step 3c. Fan-folding the top layer to the middle of the bed.

d. If contour sheets are to be used, fit the elastic edges under the top and bottom corners of the mattress. If regular sheets are used, make a mitered corner. Tuck the top of the sheet well under the mattress at the head of the bed. To make a mitered corner, lay a triangular fold of sheet on the bed. Tuck the triangular fold under the mattress. Tuck the sheet well under the mattress, working from top to bottom (see illustrations).

4. Place a draw sheet on top of the bottom sheet. The folded edge is placed at the top of the client's shoulders. *The draw sheet should cover the bed from the client's shoulders to below the hips.*

a. Place the center fold along the center of the bed.

b. Fan-fold the top layer toward the client.

c. Tuck the excess under the mattress along with the bottom sheet.

d. Smooth out the wrinkles as much as possible.

e. If an incontinence pad is used, fan-fold and place it on top of the linens near the client's back.

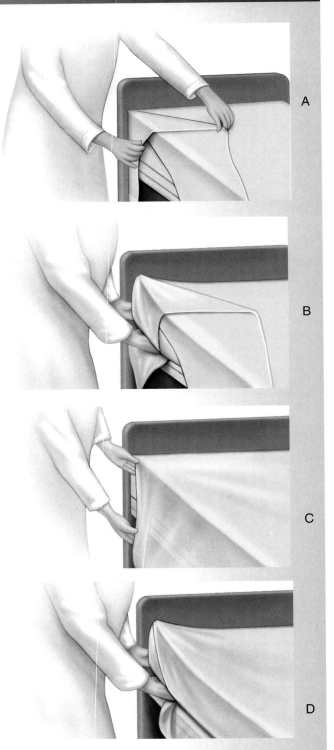

A

B

C

D

Step 3d. A, Beginning a mitered corner by laying a triangular fold of sheet on the bed.**B,** Tucking the end of the sheet under the mattress. **C,** Pulling the triangular fold over the side of the mattress. **D,** Tucking the triangular fold under the mattress.

5. Make the second half of the bed.

a. Help the client turn onto the clean sheets. Raise the side rail and move to opposite side of the bed. Lower the side rail on that side.

b. Remove the dirty linens, folding toward the center or one end of the bed. Holding the linens away from your body, place them in the dirty linen bag or hamper.

c. Pull the clean linens over the exposed half of the bed.

d. Tuck in the bottom sheet. *As you work from top to bottom, pull the linens tight and tuck one section at a time.*

e. Tuck the draw sheet, moving from the middle to the top to the bottom.

6. Put on the top sheet and spread.

a. Help the client move back to the center of the bed.

b. Place the top sheet over the client with the seam side up. The center crease should be at the center of the bed. Unfold the sheet from head to toe.

c. Have the client grasp the top sheet while you pull the soiled sheet or bath blanket from under the clean sheet.

d. Place the blanket and spread evenly over the top sheet. Be sure that they are even on both sides.

e. Make mitered corners at the foot of the bed with the top sheet, blanket, and spread together.

f. Pull the top sheet, blanket, and spread into a tent over the client's toes. *Pleating removes pressure of bed covers on client's toes.*

g. Cuff the spread, blanket, and top sheet at the head of the bed. Be sure that there is adequate sheet at the head of the bed to cover the client's shoulders.

7. Change the pillow case.

a. Grasp the closed end of a clean pillow case at the center point.

b. With the other hand, hold the open end of the case.

c. Invert the case over your hand and forearm (at the closed end) by pulling the open end of case back toward the closed end. Maintain your grasp at the closed end.

8. Return the bed to its low position. Place the call light within the client's reach.

9. Position the client for comfort.

10. Perform hand hygiene and document your care.

HOME CARE CONSIDERATIONS

Help the family make modifications for ease in bedmaking. Both sides of the bed should be accessible. The client may be using a double bed. To move the client from one side to the other, the family caregiver can get on the bed on the knees. A turn sheet can be used to slide the client across the bed without risking damage to the skin. Teach the family about the importance of a wrinkle-free bed. If soiling is a problem, instruct the family about options for protecting the mattress. A heavy-duty lawn and leaf bag can be used to cover the mattress. Any plastic that is used should be covered with a mattress pad to prevent excess perspiration.

PROCEDURE 30-5   MAKING AN UNOCCUPIED BED AND A SURGICAL BED

TIME TO ALLOW
Novice: 10 min.
Expert: 5 min.

In an acute care facility, bed linens are changed daily for the client's comfort and to eliminate a reservoir of microorganisms. When linens become wet or soiled, they are changed more frequently. In the home setting, linens are not changed daily but should be changed when wet or soiled. Bed linens are changed when the client is out of bed. A surgical bed is made for the client who is returning from the operating room on a stretcher. It is an *open bed* as described in this procedure. However, the sheets are fan-folded top to bottom to receive the client from a stretcher.

DELEGATION GUIDELINES
You may delegate the full performance of this task to a nursing assistant.

EQUIPMENT NEEDED
- Top sheet, bottom sheet, draw sheet (optional)
- Bedspread, blanket
- Waterproof pad (if needed)

Continued

PROCEDURE 30-5 | MAKING AN UNOCCUPIED BED AND A SURGICAL BED—CONT'D

MAKING AN UNOCCUPIED BED

1. Follow preliminary guidelines for nursing procedures (see inside front cover).

2. Organize the environment.
a. Raise the bed to a comfortable working height.
b. Lower the side rails.

3. Remove soiled linens. Fold soiled surface inward and place in the hamper.
a. Remove the bedspread and blanket. Fold and put them in a chair if they will be reused. If they are soiled, place them in the laundry hamper or linen bag. Remove the pillow from its pillow case.
b. When handling soiled linens, always hold them away from your body. *This prevents the spread of microorganisms from person to person.*

4. Make one side of the bed, and then move to the other side. *This conserves time, energy, and movement and contributes to the smoothness of the sheets.*
a. If the bottom sheet is a contour sheet, place the elastic bands under the top and bottom corners of the mattress. Tuck along the sides. If the bottom sheet is not a contour sheet, unfold it lengthwise and place the vertical crease at the center of the bed (see illustration). Unfold it toward the opposite side of the mattress. Make the bottom edge even with the bottom edge of the mattress. Smooth any wrinkles out of bottom sheet. Make a mitered corner at the head of the bed as explained in Procedure 30-4.

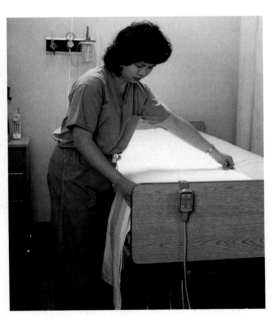

Step 4a. Centering the bottom sheet.

b. Tuck the side in along the mattress.
c. If the client needs a draw sheet, center the draw sheet on the bed and unfold toward the opposite side (see illustration). Tuck under the mattress. If a pull (turn) sheet is needed, fold the draw sheet in halves (a full sheet is folded into four layers), creating a strong sheet to turn and move the client in bed. If an absorbent pad is needed, position at the center of the bed on top of the draw sheet.

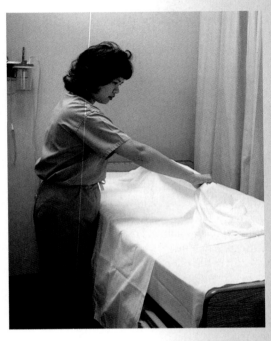

Step 4c. Centering the draw sheet and unfolding toward the opposite side.

d. Move to the other side of the bed. Remove the soiled linen. Fold the soiled side in. Hold the bundle of linen away from your body and place in a linen bag or hamper.
e. Pull the linen to your side. Tuck the top of the sheet at the head of the bed. Make a mitered corner at the head of the bed. If a draw sheet is used, pull and tuck it along with the bottom sheet.

5. Place the top sheet, blanket, and spread over the bed.
a. Leave a cuff at the top of the spread.
b. Miter the corners all together at the foot of the bed.

6. Prepare the bed for the client to return.
a. Make a toe pleat (see illustrations).

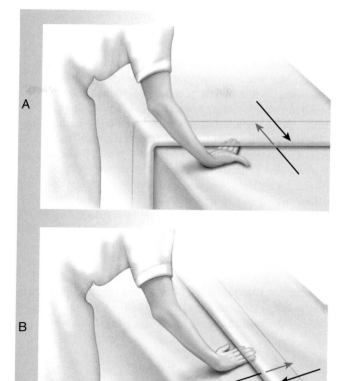

Step 6a. Making a toe pleat. **A,** Vertical toe pleat. **B,** Horizontal toe pleat.

b. Fan-fold the linen to the foot of the bed to create an *open bed.*
c. Change the pillowcase.
d. Return the bed to its low position.
e. Position the call light.
f. Dispose of soiled linens.

7. Perform hand hygiene and document your care.

MAKING A SURGICAL BED

1. Make the bed as in the preceding Steps 1 to 5.

2. Fold the bottom and top corners on the near side to the opposite side, making a triangle (see illustration).

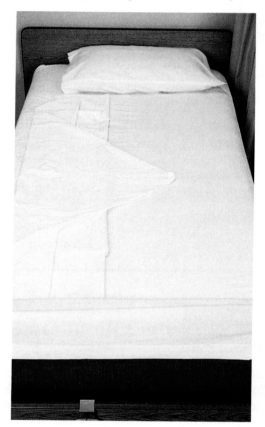

Step 2. Triangle of sheet on surgical bed.

3. Pick up the center point of the triangle and fan-fold the linen to the side of the bed.

4. Leave the bed in high position.

5. Change the pillowcase and leave the pillow at the foot of the bed or on a chair to be accessible for placement under the client's head after the client is transferred to the bed.

6. Move all objects away from bedside area to leave room for the stretcher.

bigger and easier to hold. The blind client may need assistance with knowing where basin, water, and mouthwash are located. The mentally impaired client may need assistance because of a short attention span or an inability to focus on the required components of the task.

The performance of oral hygiene presents an excellent opportunity for teaching (Box 30-4, p. 752). Inadequate oral hygiene may occur because of lack of knowledge of oral hygiene practices, poor nutritional habits, inadequate oral

hygiene practices, or painful oral lesions that are responsible for the neglect. Information about drug interactions, nutrition, and the need for periodic dental assessment can be incorporated into the demonstration of correct oral hygiene measures.

Assisting the Conscious Client. If the client is unable to go to the sink for oral care, it is still possible to provide oral hygiene (Procedure 30-6, p. 752). Clients with dry mouths or lips may need frequent mouth care, sometimes as often as

Teaching for Wellness
Oral Hygiene

Box 30-4

Purpose: To teach the client the importance of good oral hygiene and the need for preventive dentistry to maintain healthy teeth.

Expected Outcomes: The client will perform oral hygiene after each meal, floss daily, and visit the dentist every 6 months for supervision.

Client Instructions

- Brush your teeth thoroughly at least twice a day.
- Floss your teeth once or twice a day.
- Remember that good dental health contributes to your overall well-being.
- Keep in mind that recent studies seem to suggest a relationship between gum disease and heart disease.
- Visit your dentist regularly for preventive care and cleaning. Doing so not only will prevent painful dental problems but also is more cost effective in the long run.
- Certain foods are best for oral health, such as raw fruits and vegetables. Others are not good for oral health, such as sugary drinks and candy. Try to avoid the latter.

every 2 hours, to preserve the integrity of the oral mucosa. Dry lips and mucosa tend to crack and fissure, leading to infection and other problems. Rinsing the mouth with water, saline solution, or mouthwash can be helpful for these clients. Mouthwashes come in several varieties. Use bactericidal mouthwashes with caution because they tend to destroy the normal bacterial flora of the mouth, resulting in overgrowth of fungus. Avoid commercial mouthwashes that contain high concentrations of alcohol that can increase mouth dryness. Saline solution is soothing for some clients. Some clients have stomatitis from radiation or chemotherapy, which leads to mouth ulcerations that are extremely painful. Anesthetic solutions may be soothing for them. Use of hydrogen peroxide solutions is no longer recommended because it can irritate healthy oral mucosa, alter the microflora of the mouth, and cause sponginess of the gums and decalcification of tooth surfaces with excessive use.

Assisting the Unconscious Client. Oral care for the unconscious client is critical for the person's well-being. Clients who have altered sensorium levels often breathe through the

---

PROCEDURE 30-6   PROVIDING ORAL HYGIENE

TIME TO ALLOW
Novice: 10 min.
Expert: 5 min.

Oral hygiene is provided to maintain the integrity of the client's teeth, gums, mucous membranes, and lips. Oral hygiene ideally means brushing the client's teeth or cleaning the dentures according to the client's usual routine. Moistened toothettes can be used for comfort and moisture in between brushing.

DELEGATION GUIDELINES

Generally, you may delegate the performance of providing oral hygiene to a nursing assistant. Knowledge of the client's oral anatomy and any necessary precautions related to the performance of this task are your responsibility. A client having undergone an oropharyngeal procedure or known to have a bleeding disorder should have a careful assessment by you, prior to your considering delegation of this task.

EQUIPMENT NEEDED
- Soft-bristle toothbrush long enough to reach the back teeth
- Toothpaste of client's choice
- Cup of water
- Emesis basin or sink
- Dental floss, regular or fine, waxed or unwaxed
- Tissues
- Towel
- Mouthwash, if desired
- For an unconscious client, petroleum jelly, sponge swab (if desired, instead of a toothbrush), bulb syringe or suction catheter, padded tongue blade

FOR A CONSCIOUS CLIENT

1. Follow preliminary guidelines for nursing procedures (see inside front cover).

2. Prepare for the procedure.
   a. Assess the client's ability to participate in procedure.
   b. Don clean gloves.
   c. Position the client either in high or semi-Fowler's position or in a lateral side-lying position. *These positions decrease the possibility of aspiration and choking.*

3. Place a towel under the client's chin and over the upper chest. *This prevents soiling of the bed linens or the client's gown or pajamas.*

4. Moisten the toothbrush with a small amount of water and apply toothpaste.

5. Either give the toothbrush to the client for brushing or brush the client's teeth if necessary.
a. Ask the client to open the mouth wide and hold an emesis basin under the chin.
b. Position the toothbrush at a 45-degree angle to the gum line (see illustration).

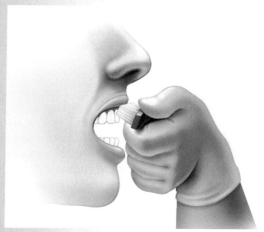

Step 5b. Positioning the toothbrush at a 45-degree angle to the gum line.

c. Directing the bristles of the toothbrush toward the gum line, brush from the gum line to the crown of each tooth, making sure to clean all surfaces (see illustration). *Brushing action removes food particles from the gum line and stimulates the gums.*

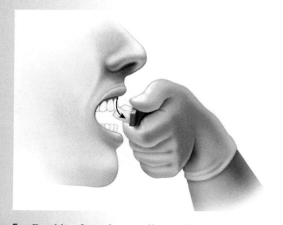

Step 5c. Brushing from the gum line to the crown of the tooth.

d. Using back-and-forth strokes, clean the biting surfaces of the teeth.
e. Gently brush the client's tongue. Do not stimulate the gag reflex by reaching the back surface of tongue. *Bacteria, oral secretions, and food particles accumulate on the tongue and must be removed.*
f. Have the client rinse the mouth with water and expectorate into the emesis basin.

6. Have the client rinse with mouthwash if desired. A solution of half-strength hydrogen peroxide may serve to remove extremely heavy coating on the tongue. Ask the client to hold the solution in the mouth for 10 to 15 seconds before expectorating. This can be repeated at hourly intervals if needed.

7. Remove the tooth-brushing equipment.

8. Floss the client's teeth. *Flossing removes plaque and food particles that collect between teeth and below the gum line and that brushing cannot reach.*
a. Cut a 10-inch piece of floss. Wind the ends of the floss around the middle finger of each of your hands.
b. Holding the floss tightly to provide tension, start with the back lower teeth and floss up and down around the lower teeth from one side of the mouth to the other. Use a gentle sawing motion to get the floss past the point where the teeth meet (see illustration). Avoid a sawing motion at the gum line.

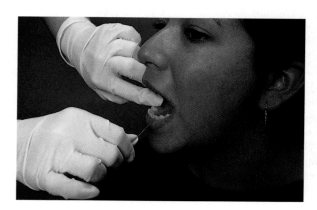

Step 8b. Flossing, using a "sawing" motion.

c. Cut a fresh piece of floss and repeat the process on the upper teeth, moving from one side of the mouth to the other.
d. Ask the client to rinse the mouth and expectorate into the emesis basin.
e. Dry the mouth and help the client to a comfortable position.

9. Remove all equipment and make the client comfortable.

Continued

PROCEDURE 30-6   PROVIDING ORAL HYGIENE—Cont'd

FOR AN UNCONSCIOUS CLIENT

1. Follow preliminary guidelines for nursing procedures (see inside front cover).
a. Don clean gloves.
b. Place the client in a side-lying position. *The lateral position allows for gravity drainage of fluid and decreases the chance of aspiration. A full lateral position may be preferred for the completely unconscious client.*
c. Place the bulb syringe or suctioning equipment nearby for when the client needs to be suctioned.
d. Place a towel or waterproof pad under the client's chin. Place an emesis basin under the chin as well.

2. Clean the client's teeth and mouth.
a. Use a padded tongue blade to open the client's mouth (see illustration). *Never attempt to open an unconscious client's mouth with the fingers. Oral stimulation often causes the biting-down reflex, and serious injuries can occur.*

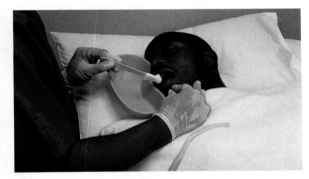

Step 2a. Using a padded tongue blade to open the client's mouth.

b. Swab the inside of the mouth, the tongue, and the teeth with a moist, padded tongue blade.
c. Brush the teeth as directed for a conscious client. A toothbrush or sponge swab may be used (see illustration).

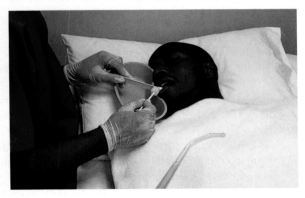

Step 2c. Brushing the client's teeth with a sponge-tipped swab.

d. Rinse the client's mouth using a very small amount of water that can be suctioned readily from the mouth.
e. Lubricate the client's lips with petroleum jelly. *Petroleum jelly may be applied as often as necessary to prevent drying and cracking of the lips.*

3. Remove the equipment and document your care.

4. Leave the client dry and comfortable.

FOR DENTURES

1. Prepare for the procedure as in Step 1 for a conscious client. Don clean gloves.
a. Ask the client to remove the dentures. If this is not possible, place a gauze square on the front of the denture. Grasping the front teeth between your thumb and forefinger, pull down gently until the suction that holds the upper dentures in place is loosened. Loosen lower dentures by lifting up and out. *Use of the gauze square prevents your fingers from slipping. Dentures are slippery. Hold the dentures firmly until they are secured in a basin or denture cup.*

2. Clean the dentures according to client's usual routine or the instructions on your cleaning product. *It is usually acceptable to clean with any gentle toothpaste.*
a. Soak in a denture cleanser. If unavailable, use warm (not hot) water and a gauze square or toothbrush to clean. *Place washcloth in the sink while you are cleaning the dentures, and work close to the bottom of the sink in case you drop them.*
b. Brush the dentures with a soft-bristle brush (see illustration).
c. Rinse under warm water.

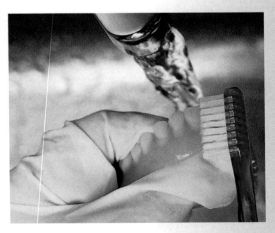

Step 2b. Brushing the dentures with a soft-bristle brush.

3. Help the client replace the dentures. *If you need to put the dentures in, start with the molars and use one edge at a 45-degree angle to open the mouth, then turn to a 90-degree angle and stretch the lips to insert the other side.*

4. Use denture adhesive according to the package directions if the client desires.

5. Clean your work area and make the client comfortable. Document your care.

PEDIATRIC CONSIDERATIONS

Infant dental hygiene should begin when the first tooth erupts. Complete oral hygiene by using a wet washcloth or small gauze moistened with water. Toothbrushing begins at about 18 months of age using water. Toothpaste is generally introduced later, and dentists recommend using one that contains fluoride.

GERIATRIC CONSIDERATIONS

Promoting good oral hygiene can help relieve the dryness of oral mucosa that accompanies the aging process, and can positively affect the older adult's ability to eat.

HOME CARE CONSIDERATIONS

Teach the family the importance of daily oral hygiene. Help them develop methods to prevent choking and aspiration.

mouth, which accentuates the problems related to the mouth and makes frequent oral care essential.

The comatose client can receive adequate oral hygiene with the use of a minimal amount of liquid. Position the client flat in side-lying position to prevent aspiration. Position the back of the head on a pillow so that the face tips forward and fluid will flow out of the mouth, not back into the throat. Swallowing and gag reflexes may not be intact; therefore, it is important to be very careful to prevent aspiration.

Action Alert! Be sure to have oral suction at hand when giving oral care to an unconscious client.

Once the client is safely positioned, brush the teeth in the usual manner to clean them. It will be necessary to find a means to keep the mouth open. An easy way is to tape tongue blades together and cover them with gauze taped in place. Never place your fingers in the mouth of a person with altered level of consciousness. Human bites are very painful and potentially dangerous. After brushing the teeth and cleaning the tongue, apply a water-soluble lubricant, lip balm, or petroleum jelly to the lips.

Assisting With Denture Care. Care of dentures becomes your responsibility when the client is unable to care for them. Dentures are expensive, and it is important that you treat them carefully and with respect.

Clients should be encouraged to wear their dentures at all times. This helps with speech, eating, and appearance. Dentures should be cleaned after each meal. If they are removed at night, they should be placed in a denture cup covered with water. While the dentures are out of the mouth, assess the oral cavity. Improperly fitting dentures can cause irritation and sometimes make the client vulnerable to cancer of the mouth. Rinse dentures and help the client rinse the mouth with water or mouthwash before replacing the dentures. If rinsing and spitting is not possible, clean the mouth with gauze. If dentures will not be returned to the client's

mouth, store them in a water solution. Assess dentures for breaks, cracks, or food debris.

Assisting With Flossing. Flossing as an adjunct to brushing is essential to remove dental plaque and food debris trapped between the teeth that cannot be removed with the toothbrush. Many people do not floss; therefore, instruction may be necessary while demonstrating. Dental floss comes in waxed and unwaxed textures. Unwaxed is easier to use because it is thinner, slides between teeth more easily, and is more absorbent than waxed floss. After flossing, rinse vigorously to remove debris that has come loose in the mouth.

Interventions for Grooming

Caring for Normal Hair. Grooming includes caring for normal hair. The appearance of the hair is important because it influences self-image and makes clients feel better. Clients with a bathing or hygiene self-care deficit are unable to groom or clean their hair. The scalp perspires, oil is secreted, and dirt collects along the hair shaft. Hair care involves daily brushing and combing to remove dead cells and dirt, and periodic shampooing to clean the hair shafts and the scalp. Hair care should be a part of daily care, and shampooing should be done at least once a week.

When brushing the hair, assess for the presence of scalp lesions and abrasions, dandruff, and the overall quality of hair. The hair itself is an excellent measure of general health. Dull, lifeless hair may indicate problems with nutrition as well as self-care deficit. Shiny, healthy hair is usually a valid measure of overall health.

A caregiver may comb and brush the hair if the client is unable to do so. However, if the person is able to handle comb and brush, these activities should be encouraged because they facilitate ROM exercise of upper extremities. If the client is able to sit up in bed or in a chair, styling is facilitated. It is important to learn about caring for hair of various racial and gender groups. Ask the client or family member about grooming preferences, so that the care provided is in keeping with the client's usual routine. Some people prefer oils or other substances to be applied to their hair. Women who are confined to bed for long periods of time may prefer hair to be braided so that tangling does not become a problem, particularly if the hair is long.

Caring for Hair With Special Needs. Very curly hair requires some additional care and handling, such as a wide-toothed comb. African-American clients may prefer to use a large pick comb to prevent damage to their hair (Figure 30-3). An effective way to work with very curly hair is to divide it into small sections and comb and brush to break up tangles. Using a wide-toothed comb or pick, gently lift hair and smooth it out evenly. Work from the tip of the hair, then from the middle to the tip, then from the scalp to the tip. Be very gentle because some people have an extremely sensitive scalp and this can be an uncomfortable procedure if done roughly and with haste. Patience and adequate time are essential. For corn-rowing, make small rows of braids close to the scalp in the client's choice of design. This type of braid is left in the hair for a longer period of time. If hair is tangled, grasp the hair between the head and the tangle to reduce discomfort. Use short, gentle strokes. Work out the tangle from the end of the hair shafts toward the scalp. Work on a small amount of tangle at a time. Working on large tangles results in broken ends and damaged hair shafts. A small amount of vinegar or alcohol may be applied to the hair to make combing of the tangles easier. Style the hair to prevent further tangling.

EXCESSIVELY MATTED OR TANGLED HAIR. If the hair is very matted and tangled, the first impulse is to cut the snarled parts rather than trying to remove the matted hair. This is not acceptable unless the person agrees to have the hair cut. Hair may sometimes be matted with blood in addition to the tangles. First, work with water and alcohol and hydrogen peroxide. Then, divide the hair into sections and clean one section at a time. When combing and brushing, be careful to prevent injury to the scalp. Avoid brushes and combs with sharp bristles and teeth because they are potentially harmful. Clean combs and brushes after each use by soaking them in a solution of ammonia or by washing them with hot water and soap.

BRAIDING THE HAIR. Comb or brush the hair. Before braiding, remove tangles, especially those close to the scalp. Section the hair to equal the number of desired braids. Divide each section into three equal strands. Begin the braid so that the base will not be in a pressure area of the head. If the braid is directly at the base of the scalp, it may be uncomfortable for the client who is bedridden. Weave each of the three strands, alternately placing the right strand over the middle strand, then the left strand over the middle one. Work with smooth motions as you move strands from one hand to the other. Keep the strands in your hands at all times. If the tension is released, the strands become loose and you will need to begin braiding again. Continue until the ends of the strands are reached. Fasten the ends of the braid with a barrette or covered elastic to prevent the braid from coming loose. Avoid use of rubber bands because they damage the hair shaft.

DANDRUFF. Dandruff is usually associated with excessive flaking of the scalp. Brush dry patches loose from the scalp and work them toward the end of the hair. Shampooing every day helps to reduce dandruff in some people; others require a medicated dandruff shampoo. Some conditioners (e.g., petroleum jelly or various oils) may help decrease itching and flaking.

PEDICULOSIS. Pediculosis is infestation with lice. It is associated with poor hygiene, crowded living conditions, and exposure to others with lice. Pediculosis capitis refers to infestation of the head, eyebrows, eyelashes, and beard. Pediculosis corporis refers to infestation of the body. Pediculosis pubis refers to infestation of the perineal area.

Lice live on the skin, attaching their eggs (nits) to hair, and must be removed. Itching and scratching are a response to lice. Lice nits are difficult to remove because the nits are attached to the hair by an adhesive substance. Pediculosis corporis can be treated with complete bathing, application of topical medication, and washing linen and clothing in very hot water. To treat pediculosis capitis, vigorously massage the hair and scalp with gamma benzene hexachloride (Kwell). Pediculosis pubis may be more resistant to treatment because of heavy hair growth. Apply the medication to the involved area and leave it on for 12 to 24 hours. Then bathe the client with soap and water. When lice are discovered, remove and bag clothing and linen to prevent spreading. Assure the person that lice infestation does not necessarily mean that they are unclean. Explain what must be done to treat the problem and prevent reinfestation. The person may need emotional support. If crab lice (pediculosis pubis) are found, emphasize the need for treatment of sexual partners to prevent reinfestation.

Shampooing the Client's Hair. Shampooing may be done in a variety of ways even if the client is confined to bed. Unless there are contraindications related to the medical condition, the client may be shampooed in bed, in a chair at the sink, or at the sink on a stretcher (Procedure 30-7).

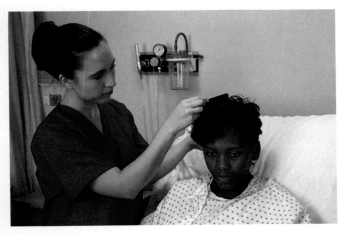

Figure 30-3. Combing the hair of an African-American client.

| PROCEDURE 30-7 | SHAMPOOING THE CLIENT IN BED |

TIME TO ALLOW
Novice: 20 min.
Expert: 10 min.

When a client has undergone a prolonged hospitalization or an emergency admission, the hair may need to be shampooed for cleanliness and comfort. The clients most in need of a hair shampoo are those who have been in a motor vehicle accident and those who lack hygiene facilities, such as the homeless.

DELEGATION GUIDELINES

You may delegate the performance of shampooing to a nursing assistant. The requisite skills should be a component of the nursing assistant's basic training program. Special precautions may be necessary for the client with a scalp laceration or glass fragments in the hair after a traumatic injury. You should supervise the application of medicated shampoo for the removal of parasites from the hair and scalp.

EQUIPMENT NEEDED
- Shampoo/conditioner
- Two bath towels
- Washcloth
- Bath blanket
- Comb and/or brush
- Shampoo board or inflatable basin
- Water pitcher
- Wastebasket or bucket
- Waterproof pads

1. Follow preliminary guidelines for nursing procedures (see inside front cover).

2. Prepare for the procedure.
a. Place waterproof pads under client's head and shoulders. *This helps keep the bed dry.*
b. Remove pins, clips, or barrettes from client's hair. Undo braids and brush the hair thoroughly. *Brushing the hair before wetting it reduces tangling and allows even distribution of shampoo.*
c. Place the bed in its flat position.
d. Place a shampoo board or inflated basin under the client's head. *Pad as needed to absorb water leaks.*
e. Drape one towel over the client's shoulders. If using a board, place a folded washcloth to pad the rim where the client's neck touches the board. *The towel prevents the client from becoming damp and provides neck support for comfort.*
f. Uncover the client's upper body by folding the linens down to waist level. Place a bath blanket over the chest.
g. Place a washcloth over the client's eyes. *The eyes should be protected from irritation from shampoo accidentally getting into them.*
h. Place a receptacle in a position to catch water. *The water receptacle should be at a level lower than the client's head so that water will run away from the head and face. It may need to be emptied several times.*

3. Shampoo the client's hair.
a. Using a water pitcher, pour water over the hair until it is thoroughly wet (see illustration). The water should be comfortably warm (110° F). *Water that is too hot may burn the client, and water that is too cold is uncomfortable and chilling.*

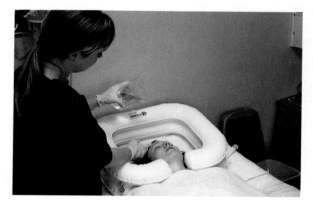

Step 3a. Pouring warm water over the client's hair.

Continued

PROCEDURE 30-7 | SHAMPOOING THE CLIENT IN BED—CONT'D

b. Apply a small amount of shampoo (see illustration). Using your fingertips, gently work it into a lather over the entire scalp. Work from the hairline to the neckline. *Massage is beneficial to scalp circulation, and it aids in the cleansing effect of shampoo throughout the hair.*

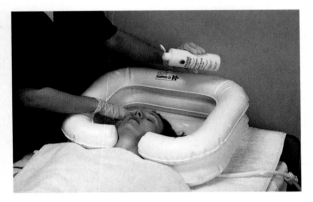

Step 3b. Applying shampoo.

4. Rinse the hair with warm water and reapply shampoo if needed. Repeat until hair is "squeaky clean" when hair shafts are rubbed. *Thorough rinsing is important because shampoo residue is irritating to the scalp and dulls the hair luster.*

5. Apply a small amount of conditioner if desired. *Conditioner serves as a detangler and makes hair easier to comb.*

6. Make a turban by wrapping a towel around the client's head. Pat or towel dry until the hair is free of excess moisture.

7. Change the client's gown and linens if they are wet.

8. Dry and style the client's hair.

9. Help the client assume a comfortable position.

10. Remove all equipment and leave the environment clean.

HINTS

If hair dryer is used to dry hair, avoid the hot setting.

Use electrical equipment only after shampoo trough and water have been removed.

Special care should be taken with an African-American client's hair. It tangles easily, so after shampooing it should be combed while wet. Mineral oil or petroleum jelly can be applied if the hair seems dry. This will make braiding and styling easier.

HOME CARE CONSIDERATIONS

Cleansing sprays are acceptable for short-term use. However, the long-term-care client will need to have the hair shampooed periodically. Obtaining a shampoo board may be the easiest option. However, the same can be accomplished by repositioning the client crosswise on a double bed with the head at the edge of the bed. Use plastic garbage bags to protect the bed and to fashion a drainage system to a pan sitting by the bed. Use a minimum amount of water.

It is helpful to know how to improvise if the client is to be shampooed in bed or at the sink. The one item that is necessary is a "trough." This is an item that may be available in the hospital or at home. If no plastic trough is available, you can easily make one from plastic and newspaper or from a rubber sheet and newspaper. Form a trough with raised edges, place the flat portion on the bed, and make a run-off channel that will drain into a waste receptacle.

Shaving the Client. Shaving is an important grooming measure for men (Procedure 30-8). Most men shave daily and do not feel well groomed when facial stubble is present. If the client is unable to shave himself, determine his preferences for shaving soap, colognes, and aftershave lotions. Determine

also whether the client should use an electric razor instead of a manual razor, such as when taking medications (e.g., anticoagulants) that can cause bleeding as a side effect. In such cases, inquire as to whether the family or a friend can bring an electric razor from home, since health care facilities do not routinely supply these.

Interventions for Nail and Foot Care

Nail care is part of personal hygiene and usually includes trimming nails, cleaning under nails, and thoroughly rinsing and drying skin of the hands and feet, especially between the fingers and toes (Procedure 30-9, p. 760). Filing of nails may be safer than clipping or cutting. Some agencies do not permit you to clip the nails of clients. In this case, families are required

PROCEDURE 30-8	SHAVING THE CLIENT

TIME TO ALLOW
Novice: 15 min.
Expert: 10 min.

Shaving the face is an important grooming measure for men. Most men shave daily and do not feel well groomed when facial stubble is present. Clients who are taking anticoagulants should use electric razors because of the prolonged clotting time.

DELEGATION GUIDELINES

The nursing assistant may be assigned to perform or assist with shaving your client. Special precautions may be necessary if the client has undergone a craniofacial procedure. It is your responsibility to assess the safety of shaving the client in this situation. You may choose to shave this client yourself.

EQUIPMENT NEEDED

- Safety razor or electric razor
- Three towels
- Soap or shaving cream
- Aftershave lotion

1. Follow preliminary guidelines for nursing procedures (see inside front cover).

2. Prepare for the procedure.
a. Place the client in a sitting position, either in bed or in a chair.
b. If using a safety razor, apply a warm, wet towel to the client's face to soften the beard before beginning to shave.
c. Apply a thick layer of soap or shaving cream to the client's face.

3. Shave with even strokes in the direction of hair growth to decrease irritation and prevent ingrown hairs (see illustration). If the skin is not taut, use your opposite hand to hold the skin motionless while you shave.

4. Use a damp washcloth to remove excess shaving cream. Inspect for areas that may have been missed. Apply aftershave lotion if desired.

5. Clean the area, make the client comfortable, and document your care.

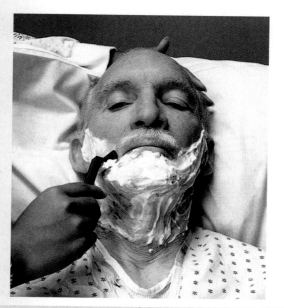

Step 3. Shaving in the direction of hair growth.

PROCEDURE 30-9	PERFORMING FOOT AND NAIL CARE

TIME TO ALLOW
Novice: 20 min.
Expert: 10 min.

Foot and nail care are given to clients to prevent infection and soft tissue trauma from ingrown or jagged nails and to eliminate odors. Older adult and diabetic clients are the most likely to need special attention to their feet.

DELEGATION GUIDELINES

Once you have assessed your client's feet, you may choose to delegate routine foot care. Special consideration may be appropriate for your clients with diabetes or vascular insufficiency. You may deem it more appropriate to perform the nail maintenance part of foot care yourself in such cases because of the risk of injury if improperly performed by a nursing assistant.

EQUIPMENT NEEDED

- Nail clippers, file
- Orange stick and/or cotton-tipped applicator
- Waterproof pad
- Washcloth
- Towels
- Washbasin
- Soap
- Lotion

1. Follow preliminary guidelines for nursing procedures (see inside front cover).

2. Prepare for the procedure.
a. Don gloves if necessary.
b. Help the client to sit in a chair if possible. If the client cannot sit in a chair, elevate the head of the bed.
c. Fill a basin half full of warm water (105° F).
d. Test the temperature with a bath thermometer or by inserting your elbow. *Clients with impaired circulatory status can be burned if water is too hot. Peripheral sensations may be diminished so that pain is not felt.*
e. Place a waterproof pad under the basin.

3. Place the client's foot or hand in the basin. Wash with soap and allow to soak for about 10 minutes. *Warm water serves to soften nails and skin, loosen debris under nails, and comfort the client.*

4. Rinse the foot or hand thoroughly with the washcloth, remove from the basin, and place on a towel.

5. Dry the foot or hand thoroughly but gently, being especially careful to dry between the digits. *Moist skin between the digits tends to encourage maceration of tissue. Harsh rubbing may damage tissues.*

6. Empty the basin, refill it with warm water, and repeat with the other foot or hand.

7. While the second foot or hand is soaking, provide nail care for the first hand or foot.

a. Carefully clean under the nails with a cotton-tipped applicator. Use an orange stick to remove debris. Push the cuticle back with the orange stick. Be careful to avoid injury to the skin under the nail rim.
b. Beginning with the large toe or the thumb, clip the nails straight across. Clip small sections at a time, starting with one edge and working across. File and shape each nail with an emery board or a nail file. *Trimming nails straight across or along the slight curve of the nail prevents splitting and the development of ingrown nails. Filing removes rough edges that might produce trauma and injury.*
c. After completing the manicure or pedicure, apply lotion to the client's feet or hands. Powder may be dusted between the digits.

8. Help the client to a comfortable position, remove all equipment, perform hand hygiene, and document care.

HOME CARE CONSIDERATIONS

Ongoing nail and foot care is especially important for the home care client. For problem feet, a clinical nurse specialist or a podiatrist may be consulted to develop a plan for care.

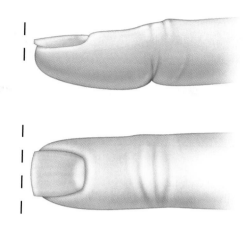

Figure 30-4. Fingernails should be trimmed to a length that is even with the fingertips, and cut straight across to prevent the nails from breaking.

Teaching for Wellness
Nail and Foot Care   Box 30-5

Purpose: To teach the client the importance of good foot care to prevent foot infection and trauma, which can lead to other serious problems.

Expected Outcomes: Client will avoid habits that are dangerous to foot health, such as trimming calluses and wearing poorly fitting shoes. Client will seek professional help from a podiatrist in trimming nails.

Client Instructions

- Inspect your feet daily, or have someone do it for you.
- Wear cotton socks and change them every day.
- Have a podiatrist trim your toenails.
- Wear properly fitted soft shoes.
- Avoid walking barefoot, smoking, and being in extreme cold.
- Avoid garters or stockings that constrict leg circulation.
- Wash your feet with warm, not hot, water.
- Always dry your feet thoroughly, especially between the toes.

---

to provide a podiatrist for the client or one is supplied by the agency (check agency policy). Clients with peripheral vascular disease or diabetes are particularly prone to injury, and nail care must be done with extreme caution since even a minor cut or abrasion on the foot can lead to serious complications, even gangrene, with resultant amputation.

Problems with nail and foot care may occur because of neglect or abuse. Improper trimming of nails and cuticles, frequent exposure to chemicals, trauma, ill-fitting shoes, and inadequate hygiene can cause problems. Be sure to trim fingernails to a length that is even with the fingertips, and cut straight across to prevent the nails from breaking (Figure 30-4).

Some general physical problems, such as diabetes, obesity, and peripheral vascular disease, make a person more prone to nail and foot problems. Poor circulation and altered metabolic function can lead to skin breakdown and infection and alter nail growth and texture. Nails easily grow into soft tissue around them, causing pain, tissue trauma, and infection. Aging also brings about changes in the nails, and older adults often have thick, discolored nails that must be trimmed by a podiatrist. Feet are more susceptible to trauma and prone to infection than other parts of the body. The dark, often moist environment of shoes promotes the growth of bacteria and enhances the chance of infection. Dirty socks or stockings and poorly ventilated shoes also create an environment that encourages bacterial and fungal growth. Box 30-5 provides guidelines for teaching clients about the importance of foot and nail care.

Interventions for Ear Care

Unless the client has an ear infection, the ears require minimal care. The external auricles can be cleaned with a washcloth, and excess cerumen can be removed with the tip of a washcloth. Instruct clients to avoid insertion of objects such as Q-tips and bobby pins to remove cerumen because they may traumatize the ear canal or rupture the tympanic membrane. Assess the ear for signs of inflammation, drainage, or external lesions and for evidence of discomfort.

Interventions for Eye Care

Some clients are unable to maintain their own eye care for a variety of reasons. Those clients who have undergone surgery or who are critically ill or comatose may have lost the blink reflex, which serves to protect the eye from trauma. Assess the eyelids first. Are they encrusted with dried exudate? Are they edematous? Are they inflamed with styes or pustules? Are the lacrimal ducts functioning normally, neither too dry nor tearing excessively? Assess the sclera (the white portion of the eye). It should be white, without redness or jaundice. The conjunctivae should be pink and moist and not reddened. Pupils should be equal, round, and reactive to light and accommodation, not constricted or dilated, and eye movements should be coordinated.

If the eyes are draining or if there is crusted exudate, the eyes must be gently cleaned. Take care to avoid transferring infection from one eye to the other.

Clean a client's eyeglasses at least once daily. Cleaning may be done with warm water and a mild soap. If the lenses are plastic, it is wise to clean them with an appropriate cleaning solution made especially for plastic lenses. Be careful in drying and wiping lenses, especially plastic lenses, because they scratch easily. Dry with a soft nonabrasive cloth or chamois skin. Label eyeglasses with client's name and put them in a safe place.

Contact lenses come in two varieties: hard and soft lenses. Hard lenses are worn during waking hours and must be removed while sleeping. Some soft lenses may be worn for extended periods of time and may be worn while sleeping.

PROCEDURE 30-10 ASSISTING AN ADULT CLIENT WITH EATING

TIME TO ALLOW
Novice: 20 to 30 min.
Expert: 20 to 30 min.

Adequate intake of food is necessary to maintain healthy nutritional status. Clients who are weak or have sensorimotor problems may require partial or total assistance with eating.

DELEGATION GUIDELINES
The task of feeding or assisting a client to eat may be delegated to a nursing assistant. However, as the nurse, you retain the responsibility for assessing the client's ability to eat and any risks to nutritional status, and for evaluating the client's actual intake.

EQUIPMENT NEEDED
- Over-bed table and chair
- Meal tray with correct diet and utensils
- Small towel or extra napkin for protection of clothes
- Straw or any adaptive feeding equipment, such as weighted cup, rimmed plate, or special utensils

1. Follow preliminary guidelines for nursing procedures (see inside front cover).

2. Prepare the client and environment.
a. Explain the procedure.
b. Assist the client with urinary or bowel elimination needs before feeding.
c. Help the client to wash hands and possibly complete oral hygiene. *Oral hygiene can improve the taste in the mouth, positively affecting appetite.*
d. Place meal tray on the over-bed table so that the client can see it. *This allows the client to view foods and participate in food choices.*
e. Check the tray for the client's name, diet, and completeness of dietary items. Check the tray against the diet order and the client's identification bracelet. Remove an incorrect tray from the room immediately.

3. Position the client appropriately.
a. Assist the client to a comfortable position, usually sitting in a supported upright position or in a chair.
b. If the client cannot use a sitting position, place the client in a lateral position. *This position enhances swallowing, and the risk of aspiration is less than in the supine position.*
c. Place yourself in a standing position if setting up the meal tray, or in a sitting position if feeding the client.

4. Assist the client to the degree necessary.
a. Encourage the client to eat as independently as possible. *This promotes client independence and self-esteem.*
b. For a visually impaired client, describe the location of foods on the plate using a clock face analogy.
c. Prepare food items by removing food covers, cutting foods, applying butter, and pouring liquids as needed.
d. Ask client about preferences for the order of eating foods.
e. Monitor the temperature of beverages to be sure they are not too hold or too cold.

f. When assistance is necessary, give small amounts at a time, allowing ample time for chewing and swallowing.
g. Provide liquids at client request, or after every 3 to 4 mouthfuls of food.
h. Do not hurry the mealtime; create a pleasant environment by conversing according to the client's interests and desire to talk.

5. At the completion of the meal, make the client comfortable.
a. Assist the client to clean the mouth and hands.
b. Assist the client to a comfortable semiupright position to prevent regurgitation, if appropriate.
c. Remove the meal tray from the bedside area.

6. Document the client's food and fluid intake, as well as any adverse symptoms experienced (such as nausea or fatigue); report to the nurse if the client does not eat a sufficient diet.

GERIATRIC CONSIDERATIONS
Offer extra seasoning on food to compensate for the age-related decline in ability to taste food. Offer sufficient fluids to prevent dry mouth due to decreased saliva production. Allow sufficient time for mealtime if the client has musculoskeletal problems that hinder joint mobility and speed of movement. Observe for dysphagia if the client has neurological or other problems that could affect swallowing.

HOME CARE CONSIDERATIONS
Ensure that there are adequate facilities for food storage and preparation (working refrigerator and stove). Assess the client for factors that interfere with proper nutrition, such as oral lesions, ill-fitting dentures, or gastrointestinal disturbances. Teach family members about the importance of a nutritious diet in maintaining health, and, when needed, provide written instructions about dietary needs or restrictions. When appropriate, be sure to include guidelines for special feeding techniques.

An unconscious client may require frequent eye care, as often as every 4 hours. Eyes must be kept clean, moist, and protected from the drying effects of the air. If the corneal reflex is lost or decreased, the eye has lost a vital protective mechanism. This reflex is the automatic closing of the eyes in response to a sudden movement of an object toward the eye. In the unconscious client, the eyes may remain open and become dried from the air. Dry eyes can lead to corneal ulceration and possible vision loss. You may need to provide artificial tears or moisture by instilling drops of liquid tear solution or normal saline into the eyes or the conjunctival sac. If the eyes remain completely or partially open, you may need to gently close them and cover them with a protective shield or patch.

Interventions to Promote Feeding

The client who is unable to eat independently needs assistance from others to maintain nutrition necessary for healing and to maintain life (Procedure 30-10). Remove bedside care items and eliminate offensive odors before mealtime. When an adult requires feeding, maintain the client's dignity. Offer food in an unhurried manner, and converse pleasantly. For clients with blindness, describe the food and caution them about hot foods. Allow time for chewing and enjoying the food. Studies show that clients eat more food if you switch from one food to another during feeding.

Interventions to Promote Toileting

A male client who is unable to toilet himself may need to be given a urinal as a receptacle for voiding. A female client who is unable to toilet herself may need to use a bedpan for voiding. Male and female clients may need to use a bedpan for bowel elimination. Examples of clients who have this need include those restricted to bed rest because of fracture, recent surgery, or other illness. A client receiving an enema or one who has diarrhea may need to use a bedpan as well.

Refer to Chapter 28 for additional information about choosing and using bedpans for specific clients. Provide perineal care each time the client uses a bedpan.

EVALUATION

Evaluation of the achievement of self-care outcomes involves determining that the expected outcomes have been met. Safety is an essential outcome. Evaluate both the client and the environment for safety before you leave the room (Figure 30-5).

Typical outcomes that are measured during evaluation are the following:
- Maintains clean and intact skin
- Maintains intact oral mucosa without gingivitis or caries
- Has clean hair without scalp lesions or abrasions
- Actively participates in feeding activities according to ability
- Actively participates in toileting activities according to ability
- States confidence in caregiver's ability to provide safe care at home

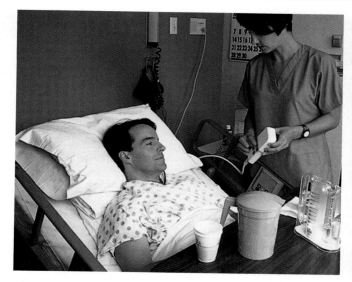

Figure 30-5. A minimum standard of safety is an accessible call light and the knowledge of how to use it.

A sample care plan for the client in this chapter's case study, Mrs. Wilson, is outlined in Box 30-6. The expected outcome for Mrs. Wilson's *Self-care deficit: bathing/hygiene* is that Mrs. Wilson maintains a satisfactory appearance and that hygiene needs are met. Direct observation will allow you to infer a positive outcome. Mrs. Wilson is well groomed and clean. Her skin and hair are clean and odor free. The oral mucosa is intact with no signs of gingivitis or irritation. Subjectively, she indicates a feeling of comfort and well-being and demonstrates a positive feeling about herself as indicated in verbal interaction.

If the outcomes are not achieved or the client is not making sufficient progress toward achievement of the goals within the expected time, reassessment may reveal an explanation for lack of progress. For example, if Mrs. Wilson continues to have halitosis even after adequate brushing and rinsing, assessment for other causes of the odor is necessary.

SAMPLE DOCUMENTATION NOTE FOR MRS. WILSON
"Participated in bath by using right hand to wash face and brush hair, and attempted to brush teeth without assistance. Assisted with washing of upper body. Asked for shampoo and also for a rest period after bathing was complete."

In the example given, you have documented that the client has resolved her difficulty with initiating and implementing oral hygiene, one aspect of the self-care regimen. As goals are met, new ones can be established so that the client can emerge from the experience not only with the resumption of previously acquired skills but with new goals. For Mrs. Wilson, new goals are to pay closer attention to oral hygiene and to pursue regular dental assessments that had not previously been done.

Nursing Care Plan A CLIENT WITH A STROKE

Box 30-6

ADMISSION DATA

Mrs. Wilson was admitted to the unit from the Emergency Department. Her daughter and son-in-law accompanied her. She appeared slightly listless and lethargic and allowed her daughter to answer all the questions. Her daughter stated that when Mrs. Wilson awoke after an afternoon nap, she was slightly disoriented and nauseated and had marked left hemiplegia. Her physician advised immediate hospitalization and she was brought to the hospital by ambulance.

PHYSICIAN'S ORDERS

Admit to Neurology
Dx: Cerebrovascular accident
Regular diet
Skull x-ray stat
MRI in A.M.
Vital signs QID

Up in chair TID with assistance
Physical therapy consult
Tylenol 650 mg q4h × PRN for headache
Milk of magnesia 30 mL QD PRN constipation

NURSING ASSESSMENT

6 Days After Admission: Vital signs: BP 170/86, pulse 76, respiration 14, temperature 98.6° F. Skin moist and warm with good turgor. Appetite good but requires assistance with feeding because she is left-handed. Alert and oriented × 3. Responds appropriately to questions. Has some short-term memory deficit. Affect somewhat flat. Speaks in a monotone. Cries easily, especially when frustrated by inability to use left side. Speech clear; no slurring, hesitancy, or stammering. Bowel and bladder control intact; no incontinence. No difficulty swallowing.

NANDA Nursing Diagnosis	NOC Expected Outcomes With Indicators	NIC Interventions With Selected Activities	Evaluation Data
SELF-CARE DEFICIT: BATHING/HYGIENE **Related Factors:** • Inability to wash body parts because of hemiplegia.	**SELF-CARE: BATHING** • Skin dry and clean. • Hair is clean and free of dandruff. • Oral mucosa is clean; teeth and gums clean; no halitosis.	**SELF-CARE ASSISTANCE** • Bathe daily. Encourage her to use right hand. Prevent fatigue by allowing her to rest at intervals. • Shampoo every week. • Assist with brushing by putting paste on brush and guiding hand.	• Used right hand to wash face. Asked for rest period after bath. Assisted with washing of upper body. • Used right hand to brush hair. Asked for shampoo. • Attempted to brush teeth without assistance.

CRITICAL THINKING QUESTIONS

1. On day 2, Mrs. Wilson says, "Leave me alone. I am just too tired to bathe. I just want to rest." How would you respond?
2. Mrs. Wilson's daughter says that she wants to care for her mother at home, but she is unsure whether she can manage all the care. How would you advise her in regard to the availability of community resources and their accessibility?
3. On day 4, Mrs. Wilson was incontinent of urine for the first time since hospitalization. She says that she just "waited too long" because she knew the nurses were busy and she didn't "want to bother anyone." How would you respond to this comment?

Nursing outcome and intervention labels from Johnson, M., Bulechek, G., McCloskey Dochterman, J. M., Maas, M., & Moorhead, S. (2001). *Nursing diagnoses, outcomes, and interventions: NANDA, NOC, and NIC linkages.* St Louis, MO: Mosby.

Key Principles

• Self-care and hygiene are important to disease prevention and health promotion.
• *Self-care deficit* may be related to physical or mental factors or a combination of both.
• *Self-care deficit* may include a deficit for bathing, dressing/grooming, toileting, and feeding.
• *Self-care deficit* may be partial or total, requiring either total or assisted nursing care. Alterations in functional ability may occur suddenly or over time.

• Inability to bathe oneself, to dress and groom oneself, to feed oneself, or to toilet oneself is validation of *Self-care deficit*.
• Interventions can meet the needs of the client for skin care, hair care, and oral care.
• Interventions can focus on prevention of complications from the inability to maintain adequate self-care.
• Interventions can meet the needs of the client for positive self-image and self-concept.
• Interventions can meet the needs of the client for comfort.
• Evaluation of the achievement of self-care outcomes involves determining that the expected outcomes have been met.

Bibliography

*Adams, R. (1996). Qualified nurses lack adequate knowledge related to oral health, resulting in inadequate oral care of patients in medical wards. *Journal of Advanced Nursing, 24*(3), 552-560.

American Diabetes Association (1999). Position statement on preventive foot care in people with diabetes: Clinical practice recommendations 1999. *Diabetes Care, 22*(Suppl. 1), 22-25.

Anderson, M. A., & Helms, L. B. (1998). Extended care referral after hospital discharge. *Research in Nursing and Health, 21*, 385-394.

Baker, F., & Smith, L. (1999). Giving a blanket bath. *Nursing Times, 95*(3, Suppl.), 1-2.

Baker, F., Smith, L., & Stead, L. (1999). Washing a patient's hair in bed. *Nursing Times, 95*(5, Suppl.), 1-2.

Bennett, J. (1999). Activities of daily living: Old-fashioned or still useful? *Journal of Gerontological Nursing, 25*(5), 22-29.

Carpenito, L. J. (2000). *Nursing diagnosis: Application to clinical practice* (8th ed.). Philadelphia: Lippincott.

Fitch, J. A., Munro, C. L., Glass, C. A., & Pellegrini, J. M. (1999). Oral care in the adult intensive care unit. *American Journal of Critical Care, 82,* 314-316.

Gender, A. (2002). Bowel elimination and regulation. In S. Hoeman (Ed.), *Rehabilitation nursing: Process, application, & outcomes* (3rd ed.). St Louis, MO: Mosby.

Glenn-Molali, N. (2002). Nourishment and swallowing. In S. Hoeman (Ed.), *Rehabilitation nursing: Process, application, & outcomes* (3rd ed.). St Louis, MO: Mosby.

*Hardy, M. A. (1996). What can you do about your patient's dry skin? *Journal of Gerontological Nursing, 22*(5), 10-17.

*Harel, Z., McKinney, E. A., & Williams, M. (Eds.). (1990). *Black aged: Understanding diversity and service needs.* Newbury Park, CA: Sage.

Hoeman, S. (2002). Movement, functional mobility, and activities of daily living. In S. Hoeman *Rehabilitation nursing: Process, application, & outcomes* (3rd ed.). St Louis, MO: Mosby.

Hospital Infection Control Advisory Committee. (1999). *Part II: Recommendations for isolation precautions in hospitals.* Atlanta: Centers for Disease Control and Prevention. Available at http://www.cdc.gov/ncidod/hip/isolat/ispoart2.htm. Accessed June 1, 2002.

Johnson, M., Maas, M., & Moorehead, S. (2000). *Nursing outcomes classification (NOC)* (2nd ed.). St Louis, MO: Mosby.

Johnson, M., Bulechek, G., McCloskey Dochtermann, J., Mass, M., & Moorhead, S. (2001). *Nursing diagnoses, outcomes, & interventions: NANDA, NOC, and NIC linkages.* St Louis, MO: Mosby.

Leuckonette, A. G. (2000). *Gerontological nursing* (2nd ed.). St Louis, MO: Mosby.

McCloskey, J. & Bulecheck, G. (2000). *Nursing interventions classification* (3rd ed.). St Louis, MO: Mosby.

North American Nursing Diagnosis Association. (2001). NANDA *nursing diagnoses: Definitions and classification, 2001-2002.* Philadelphia: Author.

*Pearson, L. S. (1996). A comparison of the ability of foam swabs and toothbrushes to remove dental plaque: Implications for nursing practice. *Journal of Advanced Nursing, 23*(1), 62-69.

Senol, M., & Fireman, P. (1999). Body odor in dermatologic diagnosis. *Cutis, 63*(2), 107-111.

*Skewes, S. M. (1996). Skin care rituals that do more harm than good. *American Journal of Nursing, 96*(10), 33-35.

Smith, S. F., Duell, D. J., & Martin, B. C. (2000). *Clinical nursing skills: Basic to advanced skills* (4th ed.). Stamford, CT: Appleton & Lange.

Stone, C. (1999). Preventing cerumen impaction in nursing facility residents. *Journal of Gerontological Nursing, 24*(10), 35-38.

*Whittle, H., & Goldenberg, D. (1996). Functional health status and instrumental activities of daily living performance in noninstitutionalized elderly people. *Journal of Advanced Nursing, 23*(2), 220-227.

Wong, D., Hockenberry-Eaton, M., Wilson, D., Winkelstein, M., Ahmann, E., & DiVito-Thomas, P. (1999). *Whaley & Wong's nursing care of infants and children* (6th ed.). St Louis, MO: Mosby.

---

*Asterisk indicates a classic or definitive work on this subject.

31

Restoring Physical Mobility

Key Terms

flaccid

hemiparesis

hemiplegia

isometric exercise

isotonic exercise

kyphosis

paraparesis

paraplegia

PQRST model

proprioception

quadriparesis

quadriplegia

range-of-motion exercises

spastic

synovium

Learning Objectives

After studying this chapter, you should be able to do the following:

- Describe the concepts of the structure and function of the musculoskeletal system pertaining to mobility
- Discuss factors affecting mobility
- Describe the assessment of a client with impaired mobility
- Identify appropriate nursing diagnoses for clients with mobility problems
- Identify expected outcomes for permanent and temporary mobility problems
- Intervene to assist a client to restore or improve mobility
- Evaluate nursing care for the nursing diagnoses *Impaired physical mobility* and *Activity intolerance*

Kristina Lasauskas has been in an assisted living facility since her husband died 5 years ago. Last year she had a stroke, which left her weak on the right side. She ambulates independently with a cane. This morning her neighbor found her on the floor, and subsequent examination found that she had fractured her hip. She was admitted to the hospital for emergency surgery to repair the hip.

After the surgery, the nurse assesses her to identify nursing diagnoses and subsequent interventions. Because the client has previous right-sided weakness and has had surgery on her left hip, the nurse considers *Impaired physical mobility* and *Activity intolerance* as potential nursing diagnoses (see below). The nurse also expects the client to have pain.

KEY NURSING DIAGNOSES FOR Mobility

Impaired physical mobility: A limitation in independent, purposeful physical movement of the body or of one of the extremities

Activity intolerance: Insufficient physiological or psychological energy to endure or complete required or desired daily activities

CONCEPTS OF PHYSICAL MOBILITY

No matter which health care setting you choose to practice in, you will care for clients with varying limitations in physical mobility. These limitations commonly result from musculoskeletal or neurological injury, disease, or surgery. However, any severe illness or injury may affect a client's physical mobility. For example, congestive heart failure can cause severe fatigue. Complications of long-term impaired mobility, regardless of cause, can lead to serious or life-threatening conditions, such as pneumonia. You will need to understand the structure and function of the musculoskeletal system to assist the client with problems associated with mobility.

Structure of the Musculoskeletal System

As a body system, the musculoskeletal system is second in size only to the integumentary system. It includes bones, joints, skeletal muscles, and other soft tissues.

Bones. Bone is a highly vascular and dynamic body tissue. Throughout childhood until puberty, many hormones and other substances in the body influence bone tissue growth. Growth hormone, secreted by the anterior lobe of the pituitary gland, determines bone structure formed before puberty. In adults, the parathyroid hormone, estrogens, and glucocorticoids work together to ensure a balance in calcium, phosphorus, and vitamin D. Over 99% of the body's calcium and 90% of the body's phosphorus are stored in a total of 206 bones.

From puberty through young adulthood, the amount of bone formation (osteoblastic activity) is greater than the amount of bone resorption, or destruction (osteoclastic activity). Beginning at about 35 years, osteoclastic activity becomes greater than osteoblastic activity. The resulting decreased bone mass predisposes middle-aged and older adults to bone injury.

Besides forming the skeletal framework for the body and storing vital minerals, bone assists in movement of joints and it produces blood cells in its red marrow. Long bones that bear weight, such as the femur, manufacture more blood cells than short bones, such as the phalanges (fingers and toes). Some of the flat bones, especially the sternum and part of the pelvis, also contain blood-forming cells. These sites are commonly used for bone marrow aspiration and analysis to determine the body's ability to produce blood cells.

Joints. A joint is the point of articulation between two or more bones, and it usually allows voluntary movement. The most common type of joint is the freely movable synovial, or diarthrodial, joint (Figure 31-1). The surface of each bone end of a synovial joint is covered with articular cartilage and attached by ligaments. The **synovium** (synovial membrane) is

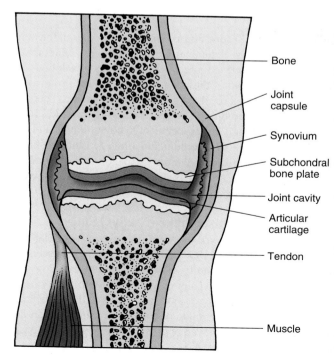

Figure 31-1. Structure of a synovial joint. (From Ignatavicius, D. D., Workman, M. L., & Mishler, M. A. [1999]. *Medical-surgical nursing across the health care continuum* [3rd ed.]. Philadelphia: Saunders.)

Labels: Bone; Joint capsule; Synovium; Subchondral bone plate; Joint cavity; Articular cartilage; Tendon; Muscle the inner layer of the articular capsule surrounding a freely movable joint. It is loosely attached to the external fibrous capsule and it secretes a thick fluid to lubricate the joint and absorb shock.

As adults age, deterioration of cartilage causes pain and possible inflammation. Arthritis, or joint inflammation and degeneration, results from "wear and tear" and can limit mobility.

Some joints are not movable. Joints in the adult skull, for example, are not movable. They are called synarthrodial joints. In the normal newborn infant, however, the cranial bones are separated by fibrous tissue (sutures) in which growth occurs.

Other joints are slightly movable and are called amphiarthrodial joints. Joints within the pelvis must be slightly movable to allow for childbirth. Joints between the ribs and sternum are slightly movable to allow the chest to expand with respiration.

Skeletal Muscles. Unlike the smooth, or nonstriated, muscles in organs and the muscle in the heart, skeletal muscles are voluntarily controlled by the central and peripheral nervous systems. Skeletal muscles are surrounded by dense, fibrous tissue called fascia. Small bundles of muscle tissue, blood vessels, and peripheral nerves make up compartments in the extremities, especially the distal part of each extremity.

During the aging process, muscle fibers decrease in size and number, even when the muscles are regularly exercised. Exercise helps keep the intact fibers from atrophy, which is a decrease in the size of a normally developed tissue or organ as a result of inactivity or diminished function. Muscle atrophy causes weakness that can limit physical mobility.

Soft Tissues. Adjacent fibrous tissues, such as tendons and ligaments, support skeletal muscles and bones. Tendons attach muscles to bone (Figure 31-2); ligaments attach bones to bones at joints. Both of these soft tissue types are prone to injury, especially as a result of contact sports, such as football, or physically demanding activities, such as tennis and skiing.

Cartilage is found on bone ends of synovial joints, and it is also located in the rib–sternum junctions (costal cartilage), nasal septum and trachea (hyaline cartilage), and external ear (yellow cartilage). Cartilage is flexible tissue, but it can withstand enormous tension.

Function of the Musculoskeletal System

Together with the nervous system, the musculoskeletal system enables us to move in a coordinated manner. Muscles are grouped according to the type of movement they allow. For example, *flexors* allow a joint or an extremity to flex or bend; *extensors* allow the joint or extremity to extend or straighten out. The elbow is an example of a synovial joint that can flex and extend. These movements are discussed later under range-of-motion (ROM) exercises.

Regulation of Movement. Movement is regulated by the central and peripheral nervous systems. The primary *motor area* (the motor "strip"), located in the frontal lobe of the

cerebrum, is responsible for voluntary muscle contraction of muscle groups. Adjacent to the motor area is the *premotor area,* which directs new movements or movements that have been changed. Motor neurons and premotor neurons, also referred to as upper motor neurons, synapse with the corticospinal tract nerve fibers and descend into the spinal cord. At the level of the medulla, these fibers cross to the opposite side of the body. Therefore the left motor area in the brain controls the right side of the body, and vice versa.

As the nerve fibers descend into the spinal cord, some synapse with peripheral nerves that supply the head, trunk, and limbs (lower motor neurons). Others synapse with interneurons in the cord. The peripheral nerves contain motor, sensory, and sometimes autonomic fibers. The motor fibers stimulate muscles to contract. Special chemicals called neurotransmitters, such as acetylcholine, facilitate muscle contraction. After muscle contraction, the muscle then relaxes because certain enzymes destroy the neurotransmitters after muscle contraction.

Proprioception. **Proprioception** is sensation pertaining to stimuli originating from within the body regarding spatial position and muscular activity, or to the sensory receptors that they activate. It is our awareness of body position, posture, and movement. Small receptor cells in skeletal muscle, subcutaneous tissue, and the inner ear respond to stimuli within the body, such as pressure or muscle stretch, promoting this awareness. For example, we know if we are standing or sitting, even if our eyes are closed. In a sense, proprioception is a protective function, enabling us to be aware of our bodies without actually seeing them.

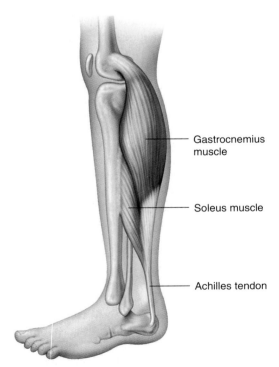

Figure 31-2. Tendons attach to muscles and bone.

Body Mechanics. Body mechanics describes the use of the body in movement and at rest. Improper use can cause fatigue and injury, such as back strain. Back injury among health care workers and others who perform physical activities is a common and costly health problem that commonly results from poor body mechanics. Health care workers must use proper body mechanics to prevent injury, maintain balance, and conserve energy.

COMPONENTS. The *center of gravity,* located within the pelvis, is the point where the body's mass is centered. The body maintains optimal balance and alignment when the *line of gravity* (an imaginary line) passes through the center of gravity. The base of support for the body includes the feet and the distance between the feet.

PRINCIPLES. While sitting, standing, or lying, the body can easily maintain alignment. However, when lifting, pushing, or pulling an object, the center and line of gravity shift, possibly causing poor body alignment and injury from loss of balance or stress on soft tissues.

Large muscle groups in the legs and arms should perform the work required to lift an object. As seen in Figure 31-3, the proper use of these muscles prevents back stress and strain. The back must remain straight during lifting, pulling, or pushing. Moving the feet farther apart broadens the base of support and keeps the body balanced during physical activity. Twisting the body should also be avoided. Pivoting on the ball of one foot keeps the back straight. Table 31-1 summarizes key principles of proper body mechanics.

Body Alignment. When the body is not moving, alignment is also important. When in a standing, sitting, or lying position, the body should be aligned so that the line of gravity passes through the center of gravity and the longer and

Table 31-1 Principles and Benefits of Proper Body Mechanics	
Principle	**Benefit**
• Pull, push, or roll objects rather than lifting them. • Pulling is usually easier than pushing, so pull clients toward you rather than pushing them. • Lower the head of the bed to move a client up in bed.	Reduces the workload Decreases opposition from gravity and decreases friction and shear
• Size up your load to determine whether you need help. • Keep your back straight when moving an object. • Use the longest and strongest muscles of your legs and arms rather than the weaker muscles of your back. • Rock your body to use the weight of your body to enhance the force of your arm muscles. • Move your body as a unit; twisting, stretching, or reaching. • Lower your center of gravity by bending your knees. • Widen your base of support by moving your feet apart. • Maintain your center of gravity (your pelvis) over your base of support. To support a client, stand close; carry an object close to your body.	Prevents muscle strain Maintains stability

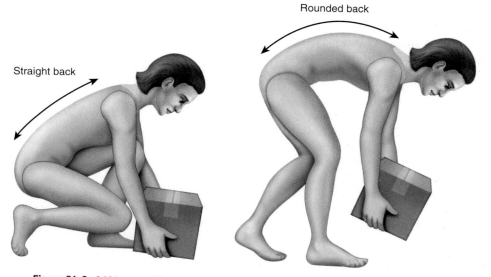

Figure 31-3. Lifting an object using proper *(left)* and improper *(right)* body mechanics.

STANCE PHASE

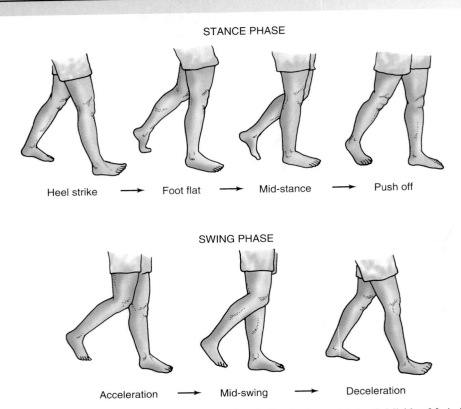

Heel strike $\longrightarrow$ Foot flat $\longrightarrow$ Mid-stance $\longrightarrow$ Push off

SWING PHASE

Acceleration $\longrightarrow$ Mid-swing $\longrightarrow$ Deceleration

Figure 31-4. Normal phases of gait. (From Ignatavicius, D. D., Workman, M. L., & Mishler, M. A. [1999]. *Medical-surgical nursing across the health care continuum* [3rd ed.]. Philadelphia: Saunders.)

stronger muscles do the work. Poor positioning changes the center and line of gravity, causing muscle fatigue and stress. When sitting, standing, or walking, good posture allows the least amount of stress on muscles, joints, and soft tissues because the line of gravity passes perfectly through the center of gravity.

CHILDREN. When an infant sits, the thoracic spine appears curved or convex because of weak chest and truncal muscles. As the muscles strengthen and the child begins to walk, the back straightens. Normal toddlers and preschool children may actually appear to have an increased lumbar concavity because they have protuberant abdomens. Adolescents who grow quickly may slouch forward, producing a round-shouldered appearance.

ADULTS. Good posture for adults means that the head is held erect, the shoulders are back, and the vertebral column is held straight. Poor posture can result in back discomfort from excessive strain. As adults age, especially postmenopausal women, vertebral bone mass decreases and the thoracic spine becomes more convex, or curved.

GAIT. The manner in which we walk is referred to as gait. As a person ages, the long, smooth steps often shorten and become less steady. This change is particularly obvious for older women who have decreased vertebral bone mass. The normal, automatic gait has two phases—the stance phase and the swing phase (Figure 31-4). The *stance phase* includes the heel strike through the push-off action of the first foot. An abnormality in the stance phase is called an antalgic gait. The *swing*

phase includes the action of the second foot from acceleration through deceleration. An abnormality in this phase is called a lurch. Pain, muscle weakness, and limb shortening are common causes of abnormal gait.

FACTORS AFFECTING MOBILITY

Many factors can affect a person's mobility, including lifestyle, the environment, physical development, and pathophysiological conditions.

Lifestyle Factors

Some recreational activities place people at a high risk for injury to the musculoskeletal system. For example, physically demanding sports such as skiing, football, and tennis can result in fractures or soft tissue damage. Failure to adequately train or physically prepare for these activities contributes to injuries. Carelessness and taking unnecessary risks also cause accidents, which in some cases are fatal.

Diet can affect mobility. For example, a diet that is low in calcium, protein, and other vital nutrients prevents bone growth and development in children and contributes to bone loss in older adults. The resulting "brittle" bones are prone to deformity and fracture. Regular exercise helps build strong bones and muscle tissue. Assess the client's cultural beliefs regarding diet and other lifestyle considerations to determine whether any factors might affect your client's mobility. Box 31-1 offers one example.

Environmental Factors

Environmental factors can lead to accidents or injury either in the workplace or at home. You can be instrumental in teaching clients about ways to prevent musculoskeletal injury.

Workplace. In the United States, the Occupational Safety and Health Administration (OSHA) establishes standards for workplace safety. The purpose of OSHA is to protect workers from injuries and accidents. The three major causes of worker injury are repetitive motion, poor body mechanics, and accidents.

When a worker performs the same activity repeatedly over a period of time, repetitive motion injuries can occur. For example, workers who use computers are at risk for carpal tunnel syndrome. The median nerve in the wrist becomes inflamed and entrapped, leading to pain, tingling, and decreased function of the hand. Preventive measures such as a wrist support bar on the keyboard and adjusting the height of the chair and computer station can help minimize the risk of carpal tunnel syndrome.

The use of poor body mechanics in the workplace can also cause musculoskeletal injury. Back supports are commonly required for workers who lift objects as part of their jobs. Classes on proper body mechanics, often provided by occupational health nurses, help workers protect themselves from back and other work-related injuries. Construction workers have the most back injuries of all employees; nurses are second in the number of job-related back injuries.

Accidents in the workplace can cause trauma and possibly lead to death. The workplace building and equipment should be safe and periodically inspected for continued safety. Most accidents can be prevented.

Home. Accidents from environmental hazards also occur in the home. Because OSHA has no jurisdiction in private residences, the homeowner must ensure that the home structure and equipment are safe. For older adults, reducing environmental hazards is especially important for preventing falls (see Chapter 22).

Developmental Factors

Most age groups are at risk for decreased mobility, especially children, young adults, and older adults.

Children. Infants may be born with congenital musculoskeletal deformities that decrease their ability to crawl or walk. Abnormal fixed positions of the feet, such as metatarsus varus (pigeon toe, toes pointing in), metatarsus valgus (duck walk, toes pointing out), and talpes equinovarus (clubfoot or twisted foot), are deformities that can worsen and delay physical development if not corrected.

Congenital dysplasia of the hip is one of the most common musculoskeletal malformations. The femoral head is partially displaced from the pelvic acetabulum. If this condition is not diagnosed until after the child walks, the child will have a limp. If both hips are affected, the child will have a waddling gait.

A small number of infants are born without complete extremities, causing marked problems with learning to sit, crawl, and walk. In other infants, toes or fingers may be webbed, ultimately resulting in decreased function.

Congenital spinal deformities may also occur (Figure 31-5, p. 772). The most common is scoliosis, a lateral deviation of the spine that is typically diagnosed in preadolescent and adolescent children. If not corrected, this deformity can also affect the cardiopulmonary system.

Young Adults. The highest incidence of musculoskeletal injuries is among young men between ages 18 and 25. Young men often take risks, such as reckless driving without a seat belt or operating a motorcycle without a helmet. Alcohol or drug consumption increases the risk of these activities.

Older Adults. Aging typically results in muscle weakness and atrophy, decreased coordination and balance, and loss of bone tissue. These physiological changes decrease mobility but should not prevent the individual from independent function. Staying active and exercising help keep intact muscle fibers strong and promote coordination and balance.

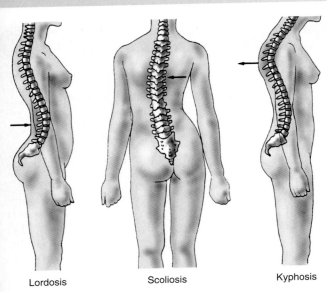

Lordosis   Scoliosis   Kyphosis

Figure 31-5. Common congenital spinal deformities. (From Ignatavicius, D. D., Workman, M. L., & Mishler, M. A. [1999]. *Medical-surgical nursing across the health care continuum* [3rd ed.]. Philadelphia: Saunders.)

As discussed earlier, after the age of 35, bone breakdown exceeds bone formation. After menopause in women, bone mass decreases (osteoporosis), possibly causing painful fractures of the wrist, vertebral column, and hip. Men have large amounts of testosterone, which results in continued formation of bone until about age 80. After age 80, men also have a high risk of hip fractures. Measures to prevent or slow bone loss include calcium supplements, exercise, and precautions to prevent falls.

Physiological Factors

Many acute and chronic health problems can decrease mobility; this discussion is limited to common problems affecting the musculoskeletal and nervous systems.

Musculoskeletal Problems. Musculoskeletal health problems can be divided into inflammatory, degenerative, traumatic, and congenital problems. Rheumatoid arthritis is one of the most common inflammatory problems affecting people at any age and potentially causing joint deformity and chronic pain. This systemic disease also affects major body organs and must be treated aggressively to slow its progress. Degenerative joint disease, sometimes referred to as osteoarthritis, is an example of a degenerative process that is seen most typically in older adults, but it also commonly affects athletes and obese individuals.

Trauma often results in bone fractures or dislocations and soft tissue damage. Fractures occur in any age group, but they heal most readily in infants and young children. A young, healthy adult heals in 4 to 6 weeks; young children heal in 1 to 2 weeks, and older adults may take up to 3 months for bone healing.

Neurological Problems. Damage to the brain or spinal cord is a leading cause of immobility. Depending on the level of injury, the person will be weak (paresis) or paralyzed (plegia). When injured at the cerebral or cervical spine level, the client may experience **quadriplegia**—an abnormal condition characterized by paralysis of the arms, legs, and trunk below the level of an associated injury to the spinal cord. Or the client might experience **quadriparesis,** which is numbness or other abnormal or impaired sensation in all four limbs and the trunk. Lower-level spinal injuries result in **paraplegia**— paralysis characterized by motor or sensory loss in the legs and trunk. Or the client might experience **paraparesis,** which is numbness or other abnormal or impaired sensation in the legs and trunk.

Middle-aged and older adults are at risk for degenerative or thrombotic neurological health problems. Parkinson's disease is a common degenerative, progressive process in which the client eventually becomes completely immobile. Cerebrovascular accidents (strokes) are the most costly disability. Part of the brain becomes damaged (infarcted) as a result of hypoxia due to a thrombus (stationary blood clot), embolus (dislodged blood clot), or hemorrhage. The typical client with a stroke has **hemiplegia** (paralysis of one side of the body) or **hemiparesis** (numbness or other abnormal or impaired sensation experienced on only one side of the body), which may limit mobility and activities of daily living (ADLs).

Recall the case study: Kristina Lasauskas's previous stroke had left her with hemiparesis. What concerns should you have about her postoperative rehabilitation program? Might she be at risk for another stroke?

ASSESSMENT

General Assessment of Physical Mobility
Health problems that impair mobility may affect any body system. To assess physical mobility, collect data related to the musculoskeletal system.

Health History. The health history elicits information about the client's chief complaint, risk of musculoskeletal health problem, previous or current treatment plan, and current condition.

CHIEF COMPLAINT. The most common complaints associated with musculoskeletal health problems are pain, muscle weakness, and inflammation. Pain may be acute or chronic; it may be assessed using the following **PQRST model:**

P— What was the *provoking incident* that caused the pain, if any?

Q— What is the *quality* of the pain? Is it burning, throbbing, stabbing?

R— Where is the *region* of pain? Does it *radiate?* Does anything *relieve* the pain?

S— How *severe* is the pain?

T— What is the *timing* of the pain? When does it occur and how long does it last?

Also assess any history of muscle weakness or inflammation:

- Have you experienced muscle weakness or fatigue? If so, when does it occur?
- Do you find that you drop items or stumble at times when walking?
- Have you noticed any redness or excessive warmth around your joints or over muscles?
- Have you been unable to carry out any usual daily activity? Have you had to restrict some of your usual activities?

RISK FOR MUSCULOSKELETAL HEALTH PROBLEMS. Determine which factors place the client at risk for a musculoskeletal health problem, such as age, environment (both work and home), lifestyle, and personal and family history of musculoskeletal problems. Some health problems tend to recur. A complete history of previous problems and how they were managed could be very important in assisting with the diagnosis and management of the current condition. Box 31-2 (p. 774) provides an example of other therapies that a client may have used.

Ask the client about treatments that have been or are being received that could contribute to the current health problem. You might use the following questions:

- Have you had any surgery? If so, what and when? (Previous surgery could cause nerve or muscle weakness.)
- What medications are you taking, including both prescription and over-the-counter? (Some medications have side effects that cause weakness, lowered blood pressure, or muscle atrophy. Other medications may be given to prevent musculoskeletal problems, such as calcium and alendronate [Fosamax], to prevent or treat osteoporosis.)
- Are you currently under a physician's care? If so, what for and how is it being treated?

Physical Examination. The musculoskeletal physical examination includes assessment of body alignment, gait, joints, and skeletal muscles. For clients who experience musculoskeletal trauma or surgery, you frequently monitor neurovascular function as well.

BODY ALIGNMENT. If possible, observe the client's posture and positioning while sitting, lying, and standing. Assess for scoliosis and kyphosis. In scoliosis, the vertebral column deviates laterally. In children or adolescents, it may result from habit (functional), muscle weakness, contractures, or a tilted pelvis. Have the client bend forward at the waist. If the deviation disappears when the client bends forward, the problem is functional. If it does not disappear, the problem may require treatment.

Kyphosis is an abnormal condition of the vertebral column characterized by increased convexity in the thoracic spine when viewed from the side. It is common in middle-aged and older adult clients. The client's shoulders are slouched and the vertebral bones are very prominent. Check to ensure that this problem is not interfering with breathing.

GAIT. Observe while the client ambulates if the client can walk. Note the stance and swing phases, looking for limps or other abnormalities in gait. If the lower extremities are not the same length, the client will walk with a limp. Ask the client if

there is a congenital abnormality or if surgery was performed on one or both extremities.

JOINTS. The best method for assessing joints is to use a head-to-toe approach, beginning with joints of the head and neck and progressing to the lower extremities. Inspect, palpate, and put through its range of motion every movable joint. Inspect the joints for proper alignment, symmetry, redness, and swelling. Then, palpate each joint for tenderness and masses. Finally, put each joint through its range of motion to determine function and listen for *crepitus,* a continuous grating sound caused by deterioration of the joint.

Assessing the extremities is particularly important because the client needs full use of these joints for performing ADLs. For example, clients with shoulder limitations and pain may not be able to perform hair grooming. Clients with hand deformities due to arthritis may have trouble cutting up food or opening food containers.

Ask the client to move each joint through its range of motion. The normal ROM for each joint is illustrated in Table 31-2 (p. 775). As long as the client can perform ADLs, a slight limitation of ROM is acceptable, especially for older adults.

SKELETAL MUSCLES. Skeletal muscles can be examined at the same time as joints. Observe each major muscle group for symmetry in size, shape, tone, and strength. Palpate the muscle and ask the client to demonstrate its strength—for example, by squeezing your hand or a sphygmomanometer. The latter method provides a numerical score that can be used later for comparison. To check for movement against resistance, ask the client to move an extremity while you are trying to prevent that movement.

Physical and occupational therapists perform more detailed assessments of muscle strength using various scales. Table 31-3 (p. 777) describes Lovett's scale for determining muscle strength. Using this scale, the therapist assesses each muscle and scores it as a rating out of a possible 5. For example, if a muscle is rated as a 3/5, the client has fair strength, can complete ROM, but cannot move against resistance. If it is available, review the client's muscle strength evaluation to help determine how much assistance you might need when getting the client out of bed or ambulating.

NEUROVASCULAR FUNCTION. Your major responsibility is frequent monitoring of neurovascular function, or CMS (circulation, movement, sensation) assessment. Check for skin color, temperature, movement, sensation, pulses, capillary refill, and pain. Always compare the affected limb with the unaffected one. Table 31-4 (p. 778) describes the neurovascular assessment and gives the normally expected findings.

This assessment is especially important when external devices, such as casts and bulky dressings, can compress the compartments created by sheaths of inelastic fascia, causing extensive tissue damage. Excessive tissue fluid from severe burns, insect bites, or infiltration of intravenous fluids can increase compartmental pressure. If this pressure is not relieved, ischemic tissue necrosis can result in 4 to 8 hours. Known as *compartment syndrome,* this phenomenon occurs in the extremities, especially the legs, where a sheath of inelastic

Text continued on p. 777

Box 31-2 *Considering the Alternatives*
Complementary Modalities: Physical Movement and Body Work

Description and History: Exercise and physical movement have recently been linked to general health. In modern times, especially in technologically developed societies, people have led more sedentary lives, which has contributed to a number of chronic diseases and disorders such as cardiovascular disease, diabetes, hypertension, and certain types of cancers. Exercise has been endorsed by a National Institutes of Health consensus committee; children and adults are encouraged to engage in regular physical activity consisting of at least 30 minutes of moderate exercise on most days of the week. Forms of bodywork have been associated with healing and medicine in most cultures. Early healing roles included practitioners of bonesetting and other forms of manual healing. Contemporary awareness of health and fitness has led to the popularity of a number of types of exercise programs and bodywork.

Important Concepts: *Exercise or physical movement:* Exercise programs are aimed at one or more of the following: (1) *Aerobics:* Exercises that increase cardiovascular fitness and include jogging, fast walking, cycling, and swimming. (2) *Strengthening:* Exercises that use weights or machines to build muscles. (3) *Flexibility:* Exercises that enhance range of motion and include stretching and relaxation or perhaps calisthenics or a yoga routine. (4) *Endurance:* Exercises that build stamina and often use a combination of the first three.

Sports activities often employ a combination of types of movement. Other physical movement techniques include the following:

- Alexander technique: This technique was developed by Fredrick Alexander, an actor, as a means of aligning the body with proper posture to allow him to project his voice better. It is popular with actors, dancers, and singers. Classes and individual instruction are available and involve relearning better alignment through repeated practice.
- Feldenkrais method: This method was developed by Joseph Feldenkrais to treat skeletal disorders and has been helpful in a number of neuromuscular disorders. It focuses on awareness of the body while doing simple movement sequences.
- Pilates: This exercise aims to create balance, flexibility, and coordination by focusing on specific muscles and movements. It was developed by Joseph Pilates and is offered in many health clubs.

Other bodywork: Bodywork involves specific physical manipulations that require a trained practitioner. Usually, the client is passive and a therapist performs the bodywork. The most common category is *massage,* which employs a number of techniques such as *effleurage* (a smooth gliding stroke used for relaxation), *sports massage* (specific muscle groups are massaged), *Swedish massage* (particular sets of different strokes are used to work on superficial muscle layers), and Tapotement (percussion-type movements). Some therapists specialize in trigger point massage and neuromuscular massage, which is the application of pressure to particular tender points to release tension in muscle groups. Osteopathic medicine and physical therapists also practice this technique. Other techniques include the following:

- Myofascial release: A technique that originated in osteopathic medicine; the fascia is stretched to correct soft tissue dysfunction.
- Rolfing: Ida Rolf developed this technique. Rolfers use strong pressure on various points to reduce thickness and fusion in the fascia caused by gravity, stress, and inactivity.

- Trager: Developed by Milton Trager; a trained practitioner assists clients in recognizing and relearning movement patterns that are more conducive to good health and function. The therapist gently brings the client into a position of ease and facilitates the relearning of that posture.

Practice of Exercise and Bodywork: Exercise programs are available at many community centers and health clubs and through tapes, books, and so on. Many people can add an exercise regimen to their lifestyle without any formal program. A number of bodywork practitioners may be available through health centers, health clubs, or in private practice in the community.

Practitioners: Many exercise instructors or personal trainers have special training in fitness and physical education. Several universities have advanced programs of study in exercise physiology and/or kinesthesiology. Some may be members of the American Society of Exercise Physiologists. Physical therapists or licensed massage therapists may employ bodywork techniques of massage, myofascial release, and others. Practitioners of the Alexander technique, Feldenkrais method, or Pilates are also certified by their respective organizations. Therapists using Rolfing or Trager may be certified by their respective institutes.

Potential Benefits From Exercise and Bodywork: Exercise has demonstrated benefits in promoting health and is an important lifestyle issue for the prevention of a number of chronic diseases. Bodywork has shown benefits for a number of musculoskeletal disorders. Many consumers find that bodywork makes them feel better and function better, and they use them regularly. Research is being conducted on the efficacy of these techniques for rehabilitative use in neuromuscular disorders.

Concerns Related to the Practice of Exercise and Bodywork: It is important for anyone with a health problem to get their physician's or nurse practitioner's advice prior to starting any exercise program. Bodywork is contraindicated for clients with phlebitis, deep vein thrombosis, burns, skin lesions and wounds, bone fractures, and osteoporosis. Caution should also be used with clients with cancer, arthritic problems, or blood platelet disorders.

Licensed providers generally practice within the scope of their practice and use referrals to treat conditions that warrant more immediate and invasive treatment, such as surgery and pharmaceuticals.

Website Resources
Associated Bodywork and Massage Professionals: http://www.abmp.com.
American Massage Therapy Association: www.amtamassage.org.
Myofascial release online: www.myofascialrelease.com.
The Rolf Institute: www.rolf.org.
The Trager Approach: www.trager.com.
The Pilates Institute: www.pilates.net.
Feldenkrais Guild of North America: www.feldenkrais.com.
The complete guide to the Alexander technique: www.alexandertechnique.com.
National Institutes of Health consensus reports: www.nih.gov.consensus.

Table 31-2 Reviewing Range of Motion

Area of Body/Motion		Area of Body/Motion	
NECK		Circumduction (360 degrees)	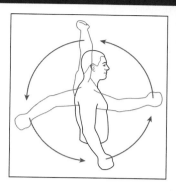
Flexion (45 degrees), extension (45 degrees), hyperextension (50 degrees)	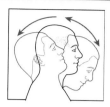		
Lateral flexion (40 degrees)	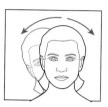	External rotation (90 degrees), internal rotation (90 degrees)	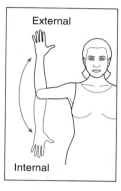
Rotation (70 degrees)	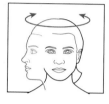	**ELBOW**	
SHOULDER		Flexion (160 degrees), extension (160 degrees)	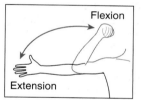
Flexion (180 degrees), extension (180 degrees), hyperextension (50 degrees)	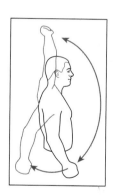	Rotation for supination, rotation for pronation (180 degrees)	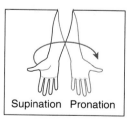
Abduction, adduction	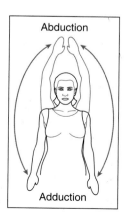	**WRIST**	
		Flexion (90 degrees), extension (90 degrees), hyperextension (70 degrees)	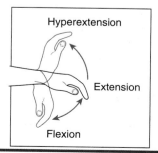

Continued

Table 31-2 Reviewing Range of Motion—cont'd

Area of Body/Motion		Area of Body/Motion		Area of Body/Motion Wrist	

WRIST—CONT'D

Ulnar flexion
  (adduction) (30-50 degrees),
  radial flexion (abduction)
  (30 degrees)

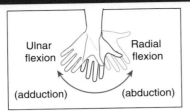

HAND AND FINGERS

Flexion (90 degrees),
  extension (90 degrees),
  hyperextension (150 degrees)

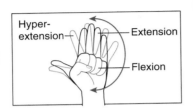

Abduction, adduction
  (spreads to 90 degrees)

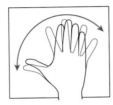

Opposition of thumb (thumb
  touches each finger)

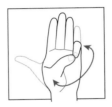

HIP

Flexion (90-120 degrees),
  extension (90-120 degrees),
  hyperextension (30-50 degrees)

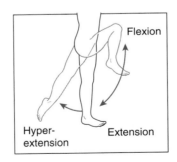

Abduction (30-50 degrees),
  adduction (30-50 degrees)

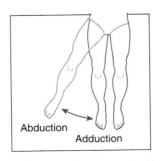

Circumduction
  (foot makes small circle)

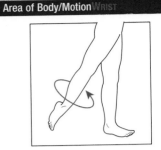

External rotation, internal rotation
  (90 degrees)

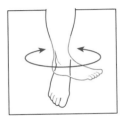

KNEE

Flexion, extension
  (120-130 degrees)

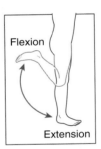

ANKLE

Extension (20-30 degrees),
  flexion (45-50 degrees)

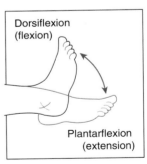

Eversion (10-20 degrees),
  inversion (10-20 degrees)

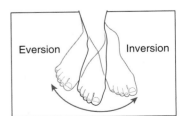

Table 31-2 Reviewing Range of Motion—cont'd

Area of Body/Motion		Area of Body/Motion	
FOOT AND TOES			
Flexion (30-60 degrees), extension (30-60 degrees)	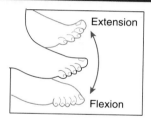	Abduction (15 degrees or less), adduction (15 degrees or less)	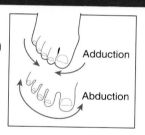

Flexion: bending at a joint in the natural direction of movement
Extension: moving from the flexed position to a neutral or straight position
Hyperextension: moving beyond a straight or neutral position
Rotation: pivoting a body part on its axis
Abduction: movement of a limb in a direction away from the midline of the body
Adduction: movement of a limb in a direction toward the midline of the body
Circumduction: a combination of movements that causes a body part to move in a circle
External rotation: rotation from a joint in the direction away from the midline of the body
Internal rotation: rotation from a joint in the direction toward the midline of the body
Supination: rotation of the palm of the hand upward or in the anterior direction
Pronation: rotation of the palm of the hand downward or in the posterior direction
Opposition: the relationship of the thumb and fingers for the purpose of grasping objects
Eversion: movement of the ankle to turn the sole of the foot laterally (away from the midline)
Inversion: movement of the ankle to turn the sole of the foot medially (toward the midline)
Dorsal flexion: flexion of the ankle in the direction of the dorsal surface
Plantar flexion: flexion of the ankle in the direction of the plantar surface

---

fascia partitions blood vessel, nerve, and muscle tissue, and the pressure in this compartment is normally less than capillary pressure.

Action Alert! Notify the physician immediately of signs of compartment syndrome.

Increased pain on passive motion when compared with active motion, or loss of sensation in the web space between the great and second toes (or between the thumb and second finger on the hand), indicates early compartment syndrome. When the client is in late-stage compartment syndrome and damage is not reversible, the six "Ps" may be present, including the following:
- Pain not relieved
- Paresthesias
- Pallor
- Pulse absent (pulselessness)
- Paralysis
- Palpated tense tissue

Do not wait until these signs and symptoms are present. The earlier compartment syndrome is treated, the better the prognosis is. Compartment syndrome may require amputation of the limb if the neurovascular compromise is not promptly assessed and managed.

Postoperatively, Mrs. Lasauskas has a physician's order to perform "CMS checks" every 4 hours. Why is this client at risk for neurovascular compromise?

Table 31-3 Lovett's Scale of Muscle Strength

Rating	Description
5	Normal: ROM unimpaired against gravity with full resistance
4	Good: Can complete ROM against gravity with some resistance
3	Fair: Can complete ROM against gravity
2	Poor: Can complete ROM with gravity eliminated
1	Trace: No joint motion and slight evidence of muscle contractility
0	Zero: No evidence of muscle contractility

From Ignatavicius, D. D., & Workman, M. L. (Eds.). (2002). *Medical-surgical nursing: Critical thinking for collaborative care* (4th ed.). Philadelphia: Saunders.
ROM, range of motion.

Diagnostic Tests. Diagnostic tests are commonly performed to determine the nature and extent of musculoskeletal health problems that may interfere with mobility.

Radiographs (or x-ray films) are used to detect bone density, swelling, alignment, and continuity. Joint structure can also be visualized, but soft tissues are not always clearly differentiated. Remind the client to remain still during the procedure even though the table may feel cold and hard.

The computed tomography (CT) scan provides a better picture of soft tissues and less-dense bone than standard radiographs, especially in the vertebral column. It is also used

Table 31-4 Assessing Neurovascular Status

Characteristic	Assessment Technique	Normal Findings
Skin color	Inspect the area distal to the injury.	No change in pigmentation compared with other parts of the body
Skin temperature	Palpate the area distal to the injury (the dorsum of the hands is most sensitive to temperature).	The skin is warm.
Movement	Ask the client to move the affected area or the area distal to the injury (active motion).	The client can move without discomfort.
	Move the area distal to the injury (passive motion).	No difference in comfort compared with active movement.
Sensation	Ask the client if numbness or tingling is present (paresthesia).	No numbness or tingling. No difference in sensation in the affected and unaffected extremities.
	Palpate with a safety pin or paper clip, especially the web space between the first and second toes or the web space between the thumb and forefinger.	Loss of sensation in these areas indicates peroneal nerve or median nerve damage.
Pulses	Palpate the pulses distal to the injury.	Pulses are strong and easily palpated; no difference in the affected and unaffected extremities.
Capillary refill	Press the nail beds distal to the injury until blanching occurs (or the skin near the nail blanches if nails are thick and brittle).	Blood returns (return to usual color) within 3 seconds (5 seconds for older adult clients).
Pain	Ask the client about the location, nature, and frequency of pain.	Pain is usually localized and is often described as stabbing or throbbing.

From Ignatavicius, D. D., & Workman, M. L. (Eds.) (2002). *Medical-surgical nursing: Critical thinking for collaborative care* (4th ed.). Philadelphia: Saunders.

to identify problems of the central nervous system, such as strokes and tumors. The test may be performed with or without use of a contrast medium to enhance the views. If a contrast medium is going to be used, check that the client has had nothing by mouth (NPO status) for at least 4 hours and that there is no allergy to iodine or seafood.

Magnetic resonance imaging (MRI) is often more accurate than either the standard radiograph or the CT scan for detecting soft tissue damage. The image is produced by the interaction of radio waves and magnetic fields. As for the CT scan, a contrast medium may be used to enhance the view. Ask the client to remove any metal objects, such as clothing with metal fasteners. Metal joint implants are safe, but pacemakers are not.

An arthrogram is an enhanced radiograph of a joint obtained after injection of contrast medium. The test is performed most commonly for knees and shoulders. Ask the client about allergies to iodine and seafood. Instruct the client that joint swelling caused by the injection fluid will diminish within a day or two. If the joint injury is not severe, usual activities can typically be resumed within 12 to 24 hours.

A myelogram is a radiograph of the vertebral spine obtained after injection of a contrast medium into the lumbar subarachnoid space. The spinal cord, vertebral bones, intervertebral disks, and surrounding soft tissues can be visualized. The client will be asked to take a fetal position or to sit and bend at the waist to open the lumbar intervertebral space before injection.

If a cervical myelogram is done, the client bends the neck forward. The injection site is locally anesthetized. After the contrast medium is injected, the client is moved into various positions while radiographs are taken. After the test, the client must be properly positioned to prevent cerebrospinal fluid leakage and subsequent headaches.

Action Alert! The client must remain flat or in a semi-Fowler's position for at least 4 to 8 hours to prevent spinal headache or meningeal irritation. Check the injection site for cerebrospinal fluid leak. Also, frequently monitor the level of consciousness, ability to move and feel the limbs, and ability to void spontaneously.

An arthrocentesis may be performed for diagnostic or treatment purposes. A sample of synovial fluid from the affected joint is withdrawn and sent to the laboratory for pathological analysis. Clients with rheumatoid arthritis usually have copious synovial fluid that contains antibodies and white blood cells that are characteristic of inflammatory disease. If the joint swells excessively, some of the fluid can be removed to alleviate discomfort. Instruct the client that this test is usually done in the physician's office, in a clinic, or at the bedside. The injection site is locally anesthetized before the larger aspirating needle is inserted. After the aspiration, apply pressure until fluid leakage subsides.

In a healthy person, calcium and phosphorus have an inverse relationship, meaning that when the serum calcium level decreases, phosphorus increases, and vice versa. Bone disease and parathyroid dysfunction can cause alterations in this relationship.

Alkaline phosphatase is an enzyme that tends to increase when bone or the liver is damaged. Increases in serum levels reflect an increase in osteoblastic (bone-building) activity.

When skeletal muscles are damaged or diseased, serum muscle enzymes typically increase, including skeletal muscle creatine kinase, lactate dehydrogenase, aspartate aminotransferase, and aldolase. Muscle trauma, polymyositis, and muscular dystrophy commonly cause increased serum muscle enzymes.

As a medic tending the wounded, I saw the ravages of World War II up close. One day I was treating three or four wounded men in a trench when an enemy mortar shell scored a direct hit. My right leg was gone; my left leg and arm were shredded by shrapnel, which also tore through my spine. If the shrapnel hadn't seared the arteries in my legs, I would have bled to death then and there. My first thought was, "There go my dreams: college, a career in professional basketball, marriage, everything I'd hoped for. I was right about basketball but wrong about everything else."

The first year at home was the hardest, like a dark tunnel, wondering what the future had in store, wanting to be as independent as possible—so much to learn. Fortunately, I had nurses and therapists who took time to get to know me before prescribing just how I should achieve maximum independence. They listened. They understood my disability and the limits it imposed. They tried to get me to do as much as possible for myself but didn't push me too hard or too fast. You need to go at your own speed in learning about assisted living. Each person is different. I'm living proof that with the right care and therapy, the body can rebuild itself marvelously.

The beautiful black-haired girl I was engaged to still wanted to marry me, disabilities and all. We've been together 53 years now. She's the greatest thing that ever happened to me. With her love and support, I

completed a 2-year business college course in accounting and worked as an accountant for a trucking company until 1948, when the poor circulation in my legs and my spinal problems made it impossible to work at a desk job.

From day one, the VA (Veterans Administration) system has done wonders for me, both in the hospital and out. Whatever I needed for assisted living—wheelchairs, prosthetic legs—they've provided. With the support of the VA, I designed my own house with everything on one level and totally accessible. The sidewalks are 48 inches wide so I can go outside, work in the garden, or do projects in my woodworking shop. I've made furniture, cabinets—you name it, I've made it.

Fifty years with a disability have taught me a lot. Probably the most important lesson is that attitude is everything. How you perceive and respond to your situation has a tremendous influence on your life—your physical, emotional, and spiritual well-being.

I've had a wonderful life: marriage to the woman I love, two sons, eight grandchildren, and, just last week, our first great-grandson. Because I've been so blessed, I enjoy giving to others, especially people who are just learning to live with disabilities. Until 2 years ago, I did chaplaincy work in nursing homes and hospitals.

Focused Assessment
for *Impaired Physical Mobility*

Nursing assessment includes interpreting data to help you select meaningful interventions. A client has *Impaired physical mobility* when there is a limited ability to physically move. If the client has a prolonged impairment, complications of immobility may occur (see Chapter 32).

Defining Characteristics. Defining characteristics for the nursing diagnosis *Impaired physical mobility* include the following:

• Postural instability while performing ADLs
• Limited ability to perform gross or fine motor skills, uncoordinated or jerky movements, limited range of motion, or difficulty turning
• Decreased reaction time
• Slowed movement or movement-induced shortness of breath or tremor
• Gait changes (such as decreased walk speed, difficulty initiating gait, small steps, shuffling of feet, exaggerated lateral postural sway)
• Substitutions for movement (such as increased attention to other's activity, controlling behavior, focus on activities that occurred before the illness or disability)

A client's inability to move includes bed mobility, transfers from the bed to chair, and ambulation. Assessing a client's ability to move and perform ADLs is referred to as a *functional assessment.* Several functional assessment tools can be used to determine a client's functional level. A very simple classification system is often used to designate the functional status. This system rates the client's functional ability from a 0 (completely independent) to a 4 (dependent and does not participate in activity). Box

31-3 illustrates the effects of impaired mobility on the life of one person.

Some clients may be able to move but are reluctant to move because of pain or discomfort, fear of falling, or fear that they will dislodge or disrupt equipment that is being used in their care, such as intravenous therapy. Reassure the client that the pain can be controlled and should not be tolerated. If equipment and lines are the concern, secure them so they will not kink, become dislodged, or disconnect.

Diseases such as arthritis and trauma such as fractures limit ROM in synovial joints, which affects the client's ability to move and perform ADLs. ROM is also limited in clients with contractures.

Prolonged immobility can cause muscle atrophy that leads to further impairment in mobility. Neuromuscular diseases, such as Parkinson's disease, muscular dystrophy, and amyotrophic lateral sclerosis, are also characterized by muscle atrophy and subsequent decreased muscle strength. Clients with these disorders often experience respiratory failure because of muscle fatigue.

Spinal cord injuries disrupt nervous system communication between the brain and peripheral muscles. A cervical or high thoracic injury (quadriplegia) spares the lower motor neurons, so reflex activity remains intact. The skeletal muscles below the injury are **spastic**, that is, they contract by reflex activity rather than by central nervous system control.

Injuries that occur in the lower thoracic or lumbosacral spine may result in paraplegia. The lower motor neurons, or reflex arcs, are damaged and the client's muscles are **flaccid**—the state of being weak, soft, and flabby, lacking normal muscle tone, or having no ability to contract. Flaccid muscles tend to atrophy and decrease in mass more quickly than spastic muscles.

Related Factors. Factors related to the diagnosis *Impaired physical mobility* include the following:

- Medications
- Prescribed movement restrictions or lack of knowledge about the value of physical activity
- Discomfort, intolerance to activity, reluctance to initiate movement, limited cardiovascular endurance, or decreased strength and endurance
- Body mass index above the age-appropriate 75th percentile
- Sensoriperceptual, neuromuscular, or musculoskeletal impairments; cognitive impairment; pain
- Depression, anxiety, lack of physical or social environmental supports
- Decreased muscle strength, control, or mass; joint stiffness or contractures
- Sedentary lifestyle, disuse, or deconditioning
- Selective or generalized malnutrition, altered cellular metabolism
- Loss of integrity of bone structures
- Developmental delay
- Cultural beliefs regarding age-appropriate activity

Many chronic diseases, such as coronary artery disease, chronic respiratory disorders, terminal cancer, and neuromuscular diseases, can cause decreased muscle strength and endurance. Assess muscle strength using the Lovett scale or suggest a physical therapy evaluation to assess individual muscle groups.

Acute or chronic pain may prevent a person from moving a part or all of the body. Assess the type, nature, duration, and location of pain as discussed in Chapter 36. Repositioning the client, providing massage, or enhancing imagery may help relieve pain and promote mobility. For more severe pain, administer a prescribed analgesic and evaluate its effectiveness.

Action Alert! For clients who cannot verbalize complaints of pain, especially older adults who have dementia or delirium, use nonverbal cues to assess their pain level, such as moaning, crying, or restlessness. Anticipate the need for pain relief interventions, including medication.

Neuromuscular or musculoskeletal impairments may be acute and reversible or chronic and disabling. In addition to the chronic spinal cord injuries, stroke, and neuromuscular diseases described earlier, clients may experience acute problems that temporarily decrease mobility. Fractures or other soft tissue injuries are common examples of acute musculoskeletal impairments. When these injuries heal, the client usually returns to baseline activity level.

Clients with late-stage dementia, as in Alzheimer's disease, experience *Impaired physical mobility* and usually die as a result of complications of immobility. The client forgets how to perform ADLs and how to ambulate.

 In the case study, Mrs. Lasauskas had been living independently in an assisted living residence. Why might you expect her to be confused immediately after surgery? Did surgery cause her to become demented?

Focused Assessment for *Activity Intolerance*

Activity intolerance results when a client has insufficient physiological or psychological energy to endure or complete a desired activity. It is evidenced when the client reports fatigue or weakness, experiences abnormal vital signs or electrocardiographic (ECG) changes, or has exertional discomfort or dyspnea during or after the activity. If a client has *Activity intolerance,* health care professionals tend to document that the client did not "tolerate" the activity. If the client was able to tolerate the activity without the fatigue or abnormal vital signs and ECG changes, the documentation is usually summarized as "tolerated well."

Action Alert! The term *tolerated well* is a vague judgment. If you are absolutely sure that the client has no fatigue or weakness, and experiences no abnormal vital signs or ECG changes during an activity, then you can use the term.

Defining Characteristics. Before you ask clients to perform any activity, ask if they are tired or weak. Fatigue or weakness can have a number of causes, including pain, hypoxia, fluid and electrolyte imbalances, and decreased muscle tone and strength. If they are willing to perform or participate in the activity, observe them for increased fatigue or weakness and discontinue the activity if necessary.

Monitor the client's vital signs and observe for ECG changes for clients in monitored beds. Clients with coronary artery disease or respiratory disease are particularly likely to experience changes in heart rate or ECG recording while performing ADLs or after a physical therapy plan of care.

Clients experiencing pain may have increased discomfort during activity. Evaluate the change in the client's pain level and discontinue the activity if indicated. Clients with respiratory or coronary artery disease may experience exertional dyspnea during activity. Assess the client before, during, and after the activity for changes in breathing pattern or rate.

Related Factors. Prolonged immobility due to chronic disease or severe injury leads to generalized weakness and subsequent *Activity intolerance*. These clients need to be out of bed and moved as much as possible. Assess changes in muscle tone and joint ROM.

All body tissues require oxygen. When an oxygen deficit occurs or the demand for oxygen exceeds available oxygen, fatigue develops and vital signs change. If the oxygen deficit is severe, ECG changes can occur. For clients with cardiovascular or respiratory problems, use a pulse oximeter to check for oxygen saturation before, during, and after activity. Arterial blood gases provide additional information about the partial pressure of arterial oxygen (see Chapter 33).

DIAGNOSIS

When you care for a client with musculoskeletal, neuromuscular, or neurological problems, analyze the assessment data to identify the common nursing diagnoses that will guide your care. If clients are at risk for any of the diagnoses, add *Risk for* at the beginning of the diagnosis—for example, *Risk for activity intolerance.*

Also identify the related factors for actual nursing diagnoses and the risk factors for potential diagnoses. For example, clients with back injury have *Pain related to muscle spasms.* But they may also be at *Risk for impaired physical mobility* related to pain, depending on how severe the back injury is.

Clients who have had a stroke usually have an actual nursing diagnosis of *Impaired physical mobility* related to hemiparesis or hemiplegia, but they are at *Risk for activity intolerance* related to generalized weakness. The related factors or risk factors help guide nursing interventions.

Adolescents who have suffered a spinal cord injury have *Impaired physical mobility.* However, they may also have *Hopelessness, Self-care deficit, Risk for injury, Risk for impaired skin integrity,* and *Risk for disuse syndrome.*

Clients with *Impaired physical mobility* and *Activity intolerance* often have additional nursing diagnoses. Assess the client comprehensively.

Clients who cannot bathe, dress, groom, toilet, or feed themselves have one or more self-care deficits. The nursing diagnosis *Self-care deficit* may be appropriate for these clients. Clients experiencing neurological, neuromuscular, or musculoskeletal health problems are often unable to move and therefore cannot perform ADLs independently. Perform functional assessments periodically to determine the client's progress in achieving independence, if possible. Do your best to consider each client's situation with an open mind, no matter how difficult the circumstances.

Clients who cannot move are at a high risk for pressure ulcers, especially over bony prominences, and the nursing diagnosis *Risk for impaired skin integrity* may apply. Thin, emaciated, and poorly nourished clients are at the highest risk of any group. Assess the skin for reddened areas. Assess nutritional status, especially laboratory indicators such as serum albumin, prealbumin, and transferrin. When these indicators are decreased, the client has inadequate protein stores to prevent or heal tissue breakdown.

Mrs. Lasauskas is a petite woman, weighing 102 pounds. What preventive measures should you use for Mrs. Lasauskas to help prevent skin breakdown after her surgery?

Exercise, hydration, and fiber are necessary to prevent *Constipation.* Clients who are immobile cannot exercise and often have an inadequate intake of food and water. Assess intake, especially fiber content. Older adult clients are particularly prone to decreased peristalsis and constipation. Monitor bowel habits and the consistency of stools.

The inactive client is at risk for deterioration of all body systems, sometimes referred to as disuse syndrome or complications of immobility. For these clients, the diagnosis *Risk for disuse syndrome* may apply. Assess every body system for possible complications or risk of complications. Chapter 32 discusses disuse syndrome in detail.

The client with *Impaired physical mobility* is at *Risk for injury* from falls and fractures as a result of osteoporosis. Anemia often contributes to the risk. Additionally, the person is at risk for thromboembolic complications.

As described earlier, clients with musculoskeletal trauma or conditions that increase peripheral compartment pressure are at high risk for neurovascular compromise, and the nursing diagnosis *Risk for peripheral neurovascular dysfunction* may apply. Monitor clients frequently for this potentially serious complication.

Musculoskeletal injury, surgery, or disease can be very painful, so you will need to assess acute pain in a client with an injury, such as a fracture, or who has had surgery to repair a fracture. For these clients, the nursing diagnosis *Pain* may apply. Clients with chronic joint diseases such as degenerative or rheumatoid arthritis experience chronic pain, which is often difficult to control. For these clients, the diagnosis *Chronic pain* may apply.

Clients who have chronic musculoskeletal, neuromuscular, or neurological health problems may feel hopeless when they are unable to move or care for themselves. They depend on others for care and often feel that they are a burden to their families and significant others. This sense of hopelessness can result in clinical depression or suicide. Assess the client's response to illness and identify clients at risk for *Hopelessness.*

Table 31-5 shows examples of clustering data to arrive at appropriate nursing diagnoses.

Table 31-5 *Clustering Data to Make a Nursing Diagnosis*	
MOBILITY PROBLEMS	
Data Cluster	**Diagnosis**
An older adult woman who fell, resulting in a fractured hip; history of previous stroke with hemiparesis; cries out when moved; degenerative arthritis in both knees	*Impaired physical mobility* related to muscle weakness, severe pain, and joint degeneration
A 12-year-old girl with rheumatoid arthritis; uses a walker to ambulate short distances but relies on wheelchair most of the time; becomes very fatigued when walking; takes two to three naps each day	*Activity intolerance* related to generalized weakness and fatigue
An older adult woman with acute vertebral compression fractures; complains of severe pain when moved; heart rate 120 and weak, blood pressure 180/90	*Pain* related to muscle spasm and nerve impairment
A 53-year-old woman, first day after total abdominal hysterectomy; requires morphine for pain control; blood pressure low for her	*Activity intolerance* related to pain after surgery and cardiovascular instability

PLANNING

Once the nursing diagnoses have been determined, think about what outcomes can be expected for the client. To the extent possible, outcomes should be individualized, measurable, and realistic. For the client with *Impaired physical mobility,* the overall goal is to improve mobility and prevent complications of immobility. For the client who has *Activity intolerance,* the goal is to improve endurance and tolerance to activities.

Expected Outcomes for the Client
With *Impaired Physical Mobility*

Improvement in mobility depends on several factors. First, try to determine whether the mobility deficit is permanent or temporary. A severed spinal cord results in permanent paralysis below the level of injury. Therefore expecting the client to walk is not likely. However, expecting the client to be able to ambulate in a wheelchair may be very realistic. The client with a total knee replacement is expected to walk with a walker or cane within a few days after surgery. This client's physical mobility impairment is temporary.

Second, look at the causes or related factors that could be managed or resolved. For example, if the client cannot move because of pain and discomfort, then interventions directed at pain relief should improve physical mobility.

Third, assess the client's willingness to participate in the treatment plan. If exercises are expected to increase muscle strength and endurance, the client has to be willing and able to exercise as prescribed.

The outcomes that might be expected for the client with a permanent impairment in mobility may include the following:
- Ambulates independently in a wheelchair
- Transfers independently from the bed to chair and vice versa using a sliding board
- Performs ADLs independently using assistive or adaptive devices
- Maintains intact skin, especially over bony prominences
- Drinks at least 2000 mL of fluid per day to prevent constipation and renal or urinary calculi
- Demonstrates passive and active ROM exercise techniques

Possible expected outcomes for a client with a temporary or less severe impairment in mobility may include the following:
- Ambulates independently in home using a walker, crutches, or cane
- Maintains optimal joint function
- Performs ADLs independently
- States that pain is reduced or relieved

Each of these long-term outcomes can be broken into progressive stages. For example, for the postoperative client with a total knee replacement, a realistic intermediate outcome is that the client is expected to walk in the hospital room using a walker. By discharge from the rehabilitation program several weeks later, the client is expected to walk up and down stairs using the walker or cane.

Expected Outcomes for the Client
With *Activity Intolerance*

The major expected outcome for *Activity intolerance* is that the client tolerates activity without evidence of fatigue or weakness, abnormal vital signs, ECG changes, or exertional discomfort or dyspnea.

INTERVENTION

Interventions to promote mobility and improve activity intolerance are interrelated. Mobility skills cannot improve unless the client can tolerate the interventions that are directed toward building tolerance. Therefore interventions for *Activity intolerance* are discussed first.

You will collaborate with members of the interdisciplinary team, including rehabilitation nurses, physical therapists (PT), occupational therapists (OT), and physicians, when planning and implementing these interventions. The rehabilitation team is discussed in Chapter 43.

Regardless of whether your client is treated by a PT or an OT, you are still responsible for carrying out interventions that help the client achieve the health care team's expected outcomes.

Interventions to Improve Activity Tolerance

Interventions for improving activity tolerance center around building muscle mass and strength while managing other causes of activity intolerance, such as pain and discomfort.

Building Muscle Mass and Strength. A structured, consistent exercise program is started as soon as the client is medically stable. Several types of exercise may be used to build muscle mass and strength, including isometric, isotonic, and isokinetic exercises.

Isometric exercise (Figure 31-6, *A*) is a form of active exercise that increases muscle tension by applying pressure against stable resistance. Isometric contractions can be accomplished by opposing different muscles in the same person. There is no joint movement and the length of the muscle remains unchanged, but the tone and strength are maintained or increased. They are also called static or setting exercises. Ask the client to tighten certain muscle groups without moving the adjacent joints. These exercises are particularly helpful for strengthening leg, hip, and abdominal muscles. Clients who have lower extremity musculoskeletal surgery, such as hip and knee replacements, are taught how to do "quad setting" exercises. Ask the client to tighten the quadriceps muscles and hold for a few seconds. Then repeat this exercise about 10 times in a set at least twice a day.

Isometric exercises also have the advantage of increasing heart rate and cardiac output, but blood flow to other parts of the body is not increased. In addition, these exercises are not helpful in preventing contractures because joints do not move.

Isotonic exercise (Figure 31-6, *B*) is a form of active exercise in which the muscle contracts and moves. There is no significant change in the resistance, so the force of the contraction remains constant. Isotonic exercise has the advantage of increasing cardiopulmonary function and blood flow, preventing contractures, and building muscle mass and strength. These dynamic exercises involve muscle contraction and muscle shortening. Examples of isotonic exercises performed in a hospital are straight leg raises after hip or knee surgery. Swimming, walking, and cycling are also examples of isotonic exercises that can be done by the client independently to continue the physical conditioning of muscles. These exercises are sometimes referred to as *isokinetic* (Figure 31-6, *C*) because they are dynamic exercises performed at a constant velocity.

Mobilizing the Client Progressively. When a client experiences an acute musculoskeletal or neurological health problem, recovery may be gradual. Being confined to bed for more than a day can cause generalized weakness. Anesthesia during surgery also causes weakness and fatigue, sometimes for several weeks after surgery. Infections and other illnesses also deplete the client's energy.

Therefore you will want to slowly build the client's activity tolerance level. For instance, before clients get out of bed for the first time, you will want them to sit on the bed with legs dangling on the side. Clients may be able to tolerate only this simple activity the first time. Once they can tolerate dangling, help them transfer from the bed to the chair. Each time the client gets out of bed, increase the activity, so that eventually the client can walk a few steps.

Action Alert! Monitor the client for vital sign changes, fatigue, and exertional discomfort or dyspnea before, during, and after each activity. If the client's heart is monitored, look for ECG changes. Discontinue the activity immediately if any of these changes occur and notify the physician.

Controlling Pain and Discomfort. If the client experiences pain before, during, or after the activity, there will most likely be reluctance to increase the activity level or even perform the same activity again. Before the client gets out of bed or goes for therapy, administer pain medication or provide other appropriate pain relief measures. Check with your physical therapy department, however, because heavy sedation could prevent client participation in the treatment plan. In some instances, physical therapists do not want clients to have medication because pain is used as an indicator that the client needs to discontinue treatment for that session.

Interventions to Promote Mobility

You and the therapist are responsible for promoting mobility, including ADLs. The goal is that the client will be independent at home or at the facility to which the client will be transferred. Maintaining or improving joint mobility helps with transfer and ambulation skills.

Maintaining Joint Mobility. Range-of-motion exercises include any body action (active or passive) involving the muscles, joints, and natural directional movements, such as abduction, extension, flexion, pronation, and rotation. They are

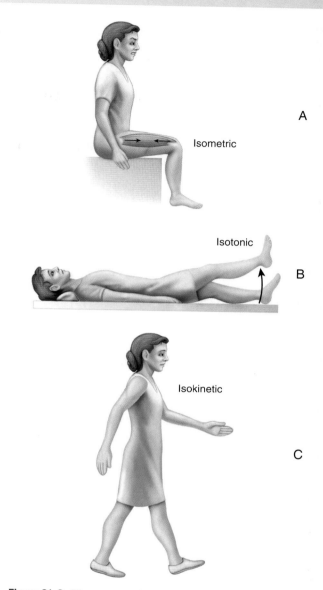

Figure 31-6. Three types of exercise: **A,** Isometric. **B,** Isotonic. **C,** Isokinetic.

the most important interventions to promote and maintain joint mobility. ROM exercises are isotonic exercises in which the client or health care provider moves each synovial joint through its complete range of motion (see Table 31-2). When the client can perform the exercises, they are termed active. When you or the physical therapist performs the exercises on the client's joints, they are termed passive. These exercises also prevent contractures and help build activity tolerance.

If the clients can move, teach them how to perform active ROM exercises. They can move each joint through its range of motion several times a day independently. If they cannot move or exercise their own joints, perform passive ROM exercises for each joint as described in Procedure 31-1 (p. 784). If the clients can assist you, the ROM exercises are called active-assistive.

| PROCEDURE 31-1 | PERFORMING RANGE-OF-MOTION EXERCISES |

TIME TO ALLOW
Novice: 15-30 min.
Expert: 15-30 min.

Range-of-motion (ROM) exercises are performed to maintain joint flexibility and movement in the client who is unable to move or is confined to bed. They have the added benefit of stimulating circulation and relaxing the body. ROM exercises may be full, which includes all the joints, or for selected joints. ROM will not maintain or improve strength. You need to be familiar with the normal range of motion for each joint.

DELEGATION GUIDELINES

Following your assessment of your client's functional status and joint mobility, you may delegate the performance of ROM exercises to a nursing assistant who has received special training in the performance of this skill. Provide special instructions outlining those observations and findings that should be brought to your immediate attention.

EQUIPMENT NEEDED
- Bath blanket to cover the body other than the part being exercised
- Pillows for positioning

1. Follow preliminary guidelines for nursing procedures (see inside front cover).

2. Explain the procedure to the client and assess the client's ability to assist with the exercises. *If the client can assist or can perform the exercises independently, active-assistive or active ROM can be performed rather than passive ROM.*

3. If moving the joints of the entire body through their ROM, use a head-to-toe approach (see Table 31-2, p. 775). *This approach helps to organize the intervention so that all joints are moved through their range of motion.*

4. Support the client's body part by cradling or cupping above and below the joint being moved (see illustration). *Supporting the joint prevents injury and stress on the joint and also promotes client comfort.*

5. Put the joint through its complete ROM, but do not force it beyond where it will move comfortably. *Complete ROM of each joint is beneficial in preventing contractures, maintaining joint flexibility, and building muscle tone.*

6. Throughout the exercises, observe the client for tolerance, including pulse rate and discomfort, if any. Do not exercise to the point of producing pain. *If the client cannot tolerate the exercises, discontinue them immediately.*

HINTS

Use slow, smooth movements. Move joint only to the point where you feel resistance. Stop if you reach the point of pain. Assess for fatigue. Finish with the joint in good alignment. Check physician's instructions about the number of sets and repetitions. A typical protocol is four sets daily, with five repetitions for each joint.

HOME CARE CONSIDERATIONS

ROM exercises should be taught to family caregivers as part of the routine care for a client who has mobility limitations. The family may need help to make ROM part of all activities rather than trying to make room in a crowded schedule for several ROM sessions.

Step 4. Supporting the body part above and below the joint being moved.

Purpose: To promote client independence in transfer skills.

Rationale: Independence in mobility increases self-esteem and maintains muscle tone and endurance.

Expected Outcome: The client will transfer from bed to chair independently.

Client Instructions

- If you have an electric bed, put the bed in its lowest position.
- Raise the head of the bed if needed to decrease the distance to a sitting position.
- Turn onto your side. (If you're stronger on one side than the other, turn toward the stronger side.)

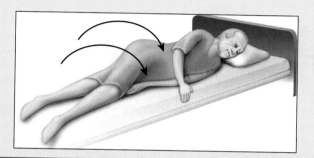

- Push against the mattress with either your elbows or hands to raise your upper body off the bed.

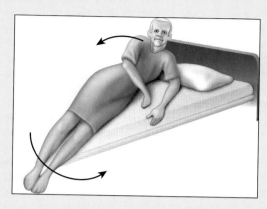

- Once you're in a sitting position, let your legs dangle for a moment over the side of the bed. This will help you get your balance and make sure you aren't dizzy.
- If you aren't dizzy, go ahead and stand up.
- *Hint:* If the client is too weak to push up from the bed, set up an overhead frame and trapeze for the client to pull on. Clients with lower-extremity trauma or surgery, including amputations, especially benefit from this device.

Action Alert! Follow these safety guidelines when putting a joint through its range of motion:

- Position the bed at an appropriate height to maintain good body mechanics.
- Support the limb being moved, above and below the joint.
- Do not force the joint into any position.
- Move the body part smoothly and slowly, observing the client for discomfort and listening for crepitus.

Assisting With Movement. If the clients are strong enough, teach them how to get out of bed independently, as described in Box 31-4. Otherwise you will need to provide assistance.

Transferring the Client. If clients cannot transfer independently, you will need to assist them. Always remember to use good body mechanics (discussed earlier) and size up your load. At least two people are needed to move a client who cannot help with the transfer. Also, if the client is obese or has multiple pieces of equipment, seek extra help with the transfer.

TRANSFERRING FROM BED TO CHAIR. A client may need assistance transferring from the bed to a regular chair, wheelchair, or bedside commode. Transfer belts provide extra security and are the safest way to perform a transfer. Procedure 31-2 (p. 786) describes how to help a client from a bed to a chair with or without a transfer belt. This procedure assumes that the client is strong enough to help you with the transfer.

For clients who are totally immobile and unable to assist with the transfer, two people are needed, as described in Procedure 31-3 (p. 789). One nurse lifts the upper portion of the body while the other lifts the legs and hips. Be sure to lock the brakes on both the bed and the wheelchair before the client is transferred. Also, position the client in the chair in proper alignment using pillows and bath blankets for support. Be sure that the client's feet are supported by the foot rest and that all necessary items are within reach, including the call light.

Another option for transferring an immobile client is using a mechanical, hydraulic lift. Although the lift is designed to be used by one person, you will need an assistant for safety. The lift requires a one- or two-piece sling that is placed under the client. The sling is hooked into the lift device and the client is moved into position over a chair before lowering. As seen in Procedure 31-4 (p. 790), the sling remains under the client at all times.

The physician wants Mrs. Lasauskas out of bed in a chair on the first full postoperative day. Given her weakness, hemiparesis, and pain, what transfer technique would you use? How many people should be used to transfer her?

TRANSFERRING FROM BED TO STRETCHER. Transferring a client from the bed to a stretcher requires at least two people. Transfers are easiest when a turning sheet or

Text continued on p. 788

PROCEDURE 31-2   HELPING A CLIENT GET OUT OF BED

TIME TO ALLOW
Novice: 15 min.
Expert: 10 min.

You can help a client get out of bed with or without a transfer belt. A transfer belt is a woven canvas belt about 2½ to 3 inches wide and 6 feet long. It is fastened around the client's waist and secured with a locking device. The belt is used to maintain control of clients when you help them stand, transfer to a chair, or walk. Transferring with a belt is safer and avoids pulling on the arm and shoulder joints.

DELEGATION GUIDELINES

Once you have assessed the client's ability to stand safely, you may delegate assistance with bed-to-chair transfer to the nursing assistant. The nursing assistant should receive specific instruction in body mechanics and safety concerns related to client mobility. Instruct the nursing assistant to report to you any client complaints of dizziness and any observation of unsteady gait or imbalance.

EQUIPMENT NEEDED

- Transfer belt
- Supportive shoes with rubber soles
- A bathrobe

WITHOUT A TRANSFER BELT

1. Follow preliminary guidelines for nursing procedures (see inside front cover).

2. Place the bed in its lowest position and raise the head of the bed. *Having the bed in the lowest position is safest in case the client falls. The client can sit up more easily if the head of the bed is up.*

3. Place a chair or wheelchair at a 45-degree angle to the bed. Plan for clients to get out of bed on their stronger side. *Having them get out of bed on the strong side helps prevent loss of balance and possible falls.*

4. Using good body mechanics, help clients to a full sitting position while swinging their legs over the edge of the bed in a single, smooth motion (see illustration). Support their upper body as they come to the sitting position. *Moving their legs reduces friction or shearing from the sheets while increasing the force of the movement. Supporting their upper body keeps them from falling backward.*

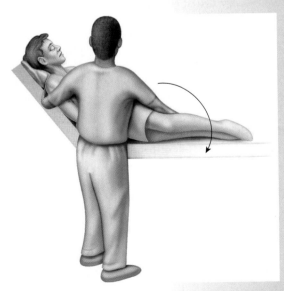

Step 4. Assisting the client to a full sitting position.

5. Support clients in a sitting position on the side of the bed with their feet dangling (see illustration). *Moving from a lying to sitting position can cause postural hypotension, which can lead to dizziness and a subsequent fall unless the client has time to gather equilibrium.*

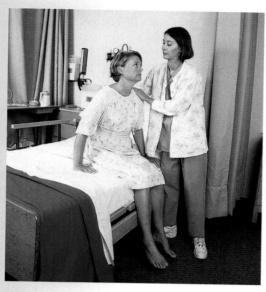

Step 5. Supporting the client in a sitting position.

6. If they are able, have the clients place their hands on your shoulders or on the mattress on either side of their body. *When you help clients stand, they can assist you by balancing against your shoulders while using their leg muscles to stand or by pushing off the mattress with their hands.*

7. Place your hands under their arms. Place your knees in front of their knees and help them rise to a standing position (see illustration). *Keeping your knees against the client's knees prevents them from buckling, thus reducing the risk of a fall. Avoid axillary pressure.*

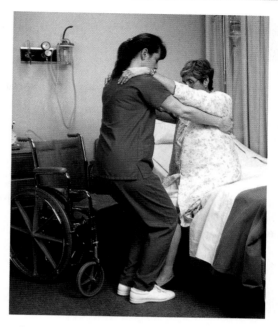

Step 7. Helping the client to a standing position.

8. Pivot with the clients toward the chair or wheelchair, being careful not to dislodge equipment or lines (see illustration). *Pivoting prevents twisting your spine and causing injury.*

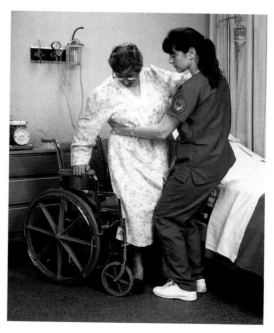

Step 8. Pivoting and turning the client toward the wheelchair.

9. Using good body mechanics, lower the clients into the chair or wheelchair slowly and reposition them in proper body alignment. Make them as comfortable as possible. *Moving slowly helps prevent dizziness or other discomfort.*

Continued

PROCEDURE 31-2   HELPING A CLIENT GET OUT OF BED—CONT'D

WITH A TRANSFER BELT

1. Place a transfer/gait belt around the client's waist. *The transfer belt allows you to guide the client, and it offers support during the transfer.*

2. Standing in front of the clients, grasp the transfer belt on both sides toward their back (see illustration). Assess whether they have the strength to stand. When they are ready, help them to a standing position by rolling your body and arms up-ward, pulling them with the transfer belt. *Favoring the client's weaker side helps prevent falls because most clients drift toward, or lose balance on, their weaker side.*

3. Pivot clients toward the chair and lower them slowly into it. Ideally, they will take two or three small steps to get into position to sit. *Pivoting prevents twisting of your spine.*

4. Have the client reach for the armrests, if available, while lowering into the chair. *Holding on to the armrests provides additional support for the client.*

HOME CARE CONSIDERATIONS

Teach family caregivers how to use good body mechanics to prevent back injuries when transferring the client. Most caregivers can be easily taught how to use a transfer belt. If the family cannot transfer the client to a chair, they can rent a mechanical lift or a geriatric chair. The chair reclines and the feet can be elevated. It also has a tray that fastens on the front for meals and other activities.

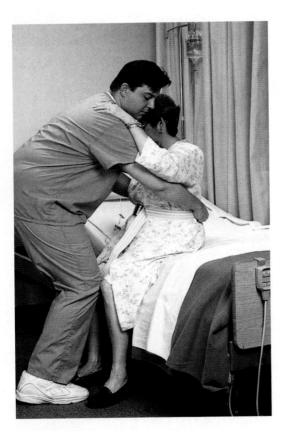

Step 2. Grasping the transfer belt to assist the client to a standing position.

drawsheet is placed under the client. First, adjust the height of the client's bed to be even with the height of the stretcher. Ensure that the wheels on both the bed and the stretcher are locked. Then move the client to the edge of the bed closer to the stretcher. Pull the turning sheet and lift the client onto the stretcher in unison. Place a pillow under the client's head, pull up the stretcher side rails, fasten the strap around the client, and push the stretcher from the head.

Supporting the Ambulating Client. Some clients cannot ambulate independently and require human or mechanical assistance. The transfer belt serves as the gait or walking belt that

PROCEDURE 31-3 | TRANSFERRING AN IMMOBILE CLIENT FROM BED TO WHEELCHAIR

TIME TO ALLOW
Novice: 15 min.
Expert: 10 min.

Immobile clients who cannot bear weight on their feet and legs can be moved to a wheelchair using a two- or three-person lift.

DELEGATION GUIDELINES

The transfer of an immobile client from bed to wheelchair, and back to bed, may be delegated to a nursing assistant who has received training in body mechanics and safety techniques. Two nursing assistants, having received this training, may perform this task without you present.

EQUIPMENT NEEDED

- Wheelchair with locking wheels, removable armrest, and movable leg and feet supports
- Bath blanket to cover the chair and wrap around the client's shoulders

1. Follow preliminary guidelines for nursing procedures (see inside front cover).

2. Obtain an assistant before transferring the client. *At least two people are needed to lift an immobile client to prevent back injury and maintain the client's safety. Assess the client's weight and make sure you can lift that weight safely.*

3. Place the chair parallel to the bed before transferring the client. *A parallel position makes the transfer into the chair easier.*

4. Pull the bed out from the wall, if necessary, so one nurse can get behind the client's shoulders and upper body from the other side of the bed. One nurse lifts the client's hips and legs, and the other nurse simultaneously lifts the torso.

5. In unison and using good body mechanics, you and your colleague should lift the client's shoulders and legs (see illustration). *This technique distributes the weight between two people and thereby prevents injury. A turning sheet will make the lifting easier.*

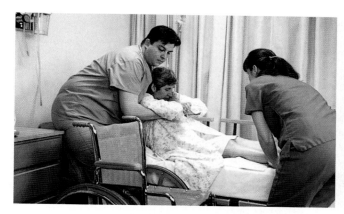

Step 5. Lifting the client from the shoulders and legs.

6. Lower the client into the chair and use pillows and other devices as needed to achieve good body alignment. *Proper body alignment promotes optimal function and prevents discomfort.*

HOME CARE CONSIDERATIONS

Consider the age and physical condition of the caregiver before teaching this transfer technique. If no strong people are present in the home, help the caregiver arrange for assistance with transfers. As an alternative, consider a mechanical lift.

you can hold during ambulation. If the client is weaker on one side than the other, stand on the weaker side. The client can also push a portable intravenous pole and use it as an extra support if needed (Procedure 31-5, p. 791).

If the client starts to fall or faint, support them and ease them to the floor. Make them as comfortable as possible and stay with them until help arrives.

Compensating for Physical Impairments. When human assistance is not available or the client is ready to learn to ambulate independently, assistive devices may be used. If available, a physical therapist will do the initial teaching, but you will need to reinforce the techniques that were taught. Walkers, canes, crutches, and wheelchairs allow independence in ambulation.

PROCEDURE 31-4 | USING A MECHANICAL LIFT

TIME TO ALLOW
Novice: 20 min.
Expert: 15 min.

A mechanical lift uses a hydraulic pump or electric motor to hoist a sling. With the sling around the client, the lift can raise her off the bed and swing her into position above a chair. The lift is then lowered and the client is slowly rolled into the chair. Possible disadvantages of a mechanical lift are the insecurity clients may feel while suspended in the air and the training required to properly use the lift.

DELEGATION GUIDELINES

The use of a mechanical lift for client transfer may be delegated to a nursing assistant who has received training in body mechanics, safety, and the use of this equipment. You should place special emphasis on the client's perception of the experience of being suspended in the air, and on protection of the skin from injury, when reviewing the key aspects of this skill with your assistant.

EQUIPMENT NEEDED
- Mechanical lift
- Bedside chair or wheelchair
- Bath blanket

1. Follow preliminary guidelines for nursing procedures (see inside front cover).

2. Obtain a functioning lift and move it into the client's room (see illustration). *Make sure that the lift works correctly and safely to prevent accidents. Practice before you take it into the client's room.*

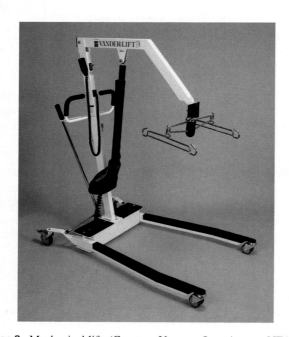

Step 2. Mechanical lift. (Courtesy Vancare, Inc., Aurora, NE.)

3. Place the one- or two-piece sling under the client by turning her onto the side, place the sling along the back, and have her roll onto the sling. Make sure the sling supports the shoulders and buttocks. *Take care not to injure the client's skin with the metal attachments. If the sling is not positioned correctly, the client will not feel secure and may slide out of the sling.*

4. Place the bed in a low position. Securely attach the sling to the lift. Have the client cross the arms across the chest. *Crossing the arms will help prevent injury caused by the client trying to help, thus causing instability of the lift.*

5. Raise the lift to elevate the client enough to clear the bed. *If the client is not completely off the bed, shearing or friction of the skin can result. Promote the client's security by moving slowly and avoiding erratic movements; protect the head if necessary.*

6. Move the lift until the client is aligned with the chair, lock the wheels, release the pressure valve, and lower the client slowly into the chair. *Correct alignment with the chair prevents the client from falling or other injury.*

7. Keep the sling under the client, but position her into comfortable and functional body alignment. *The sling remains under the client until it is used again to return the client to bed. Disconnect the sling from the lift and store the lift in a corner out of the way of traffic.*

HOME CARE CONSIDERATIONS

Teach family caregivers how to use the mechanical lift and help them practice until they are proficient and feel secure before trying to move the client.

PROCEDURE 31-5	SUPPORTING THE AMBULATING CLIENT

TIME TO ALLOW
Novice: 20 min.
Expert: 10 min.

The first time a client gets out of bed after anesthesia, prolonged illness, or bed rest, you will assist with ambulation to ensure the client's safety. It is better to be overly cautious in deciding which clients need assistance than to risk a fall.

DELEGATION GUIDELINES

You may delegate assisting the client with ambulation, after your initial assessment of the client's functional status and the client's risk factors for falling. The nursing assistant should receive training in body mechanics, safety, and assisting with mobility.

EQUIPMENT NEEDED

- Comfortable, supportive shoes with rubber soles
- Bathrobe
- Transfer/gait belt

1. Follow preliminary guidelines for nursing procedures (see inside front cover).

2. Apply a gait belt (also called a transfer or walking belt) around the client's waist and help the client to a standing position as outlined in Procedure 31-2.

3. Stand at the client's side and slightly behind, and walk with the client while holding onto the back of the belt (see illustration). *By holding on to the gait belt while the client is walking, you provide support for the client and you gain some control over ambulation. Grasp the belt from beneath the belt in a manner that will allow you to lift up if the client starts to fall. Your second hand may be used to guide the client's posture to an upright position.*

4. The client with an intravenous pole can push the pole while walking. *The client with an intravenous line will need a portable rolling pole. However, these poles roll freely and should be used to guide, not to support the client's weight.*

5. If the client is weaker on one side than the other, walk on the weak side while grasping the belt and guiding the client's posture. *The client will tend to lean and could fall toward the weaker side. Remind the client to lean toward the strong side.*

6. If the client is especially weak or this is the first time ambulating, ask another person to walk with you to support the client. If necessary, have another assistant follow with a wheelchair in case the client becomes too weak to stand. *An additional person helps by supporting the client from the opposite side or by moving portable equipment that must go with the client.*

7. If the client starts to fall, do not try to prevent the fall by supporting the weight with your own body. Rather, help the client fall safely, without injury to either of you.

8. As the client starts to fall, move your feet so your stronger leg is somewhat behind you. *This action forms a solid base of support for you and allows you to bear most of the weight on your stronger leg.*

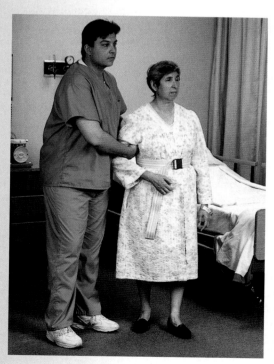

Step 3. Standing at the client's side while holding onto the back of the transfer belt.

Continued

PROCEDURE 31-5	SUPPORTING THE AMBULATING CLIENT—CONT'D

9. At the same time, use the transfer belt to pull the client toward you, allowing her to slide against you, supported, as you ease her onto the floor (see illustration).

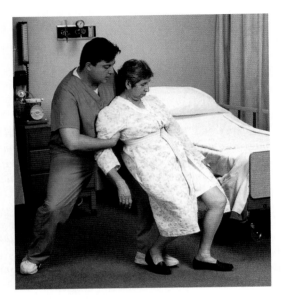

Step 9. Supporting the client and easing her to the floor.

10. Stay with the client until help arrives. Assess her for injury before trying to move her (see illustration). *Even a minor fall can result in a fractured hip for an older adult, especially one who has osteoporosis. You may need to use a three-person lift to a stretcher rather than having the client try to stand. Have the client evaluated by a physician.*

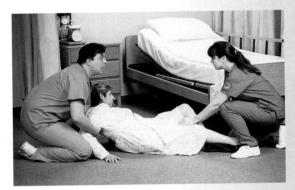

Step 10. Staying with the client until help arrives.

11. Document the events leading up to the fall, your client assessment, notification of the physician, and any action taken.

HOME CARE CONSIDERATIONS

Help the family caregivers assess their home environment for hazards, such as throw rugs, slick floors, or obstructed pathways, before getting the client out of bed to walk. A chair should be available that is sturdy, comfortable, and easily accessible. A high-backed chair is preferable to support the client's neck in anatomic alignment.

USING A WALKER. Walkers provide better support than either a cane or crutches (Figure 31-7). They are used most often for older adults who have decreased muscle strength. The standard walker can be adjusted for the client's height so that the hand bar is just below the client's waist and the client's elbows are slightly flexed. The standard walker is used for clients who can bear partial weight, and it must be picked up to be used correctly. Exercises to strengthen the arms are important. For clients who have insufficient arm strength, roller walkers with two or four wheels can be substituted. Some roller walkers have a seat where the client can sit when fatigued.

When teaching clients how to use a walker, place a gait belt around them and help them to a standing position. Tell them to place both hands on the walker. If a client has severe arthritis in the hands, platforms for resting the arms can be used instead of handgrips. Teach the client to lift the walker and move it about 1 to 2 feet forward, depending on the client's comfort level and strength. While resting on the walker, ask the client to take one or two small steps and check balance. Repeat this procedure while ambulating. You should grasp the gait belt until the client is strong enough to ambulate independently with the walker.

USING A CANE. A variety of canes are available for ambulation, depending on the amount of support the client needs. The quadripod ("quad") and hemicane provide the most support (Figure 31-8). They are used most often for clients who have had strokes. The straight cane provides the least support. All canes should have rubber tips on the end to prevent slipping.

When teaching the client how to use a cane, again use a gait belt and help the client to a standing position. Have the

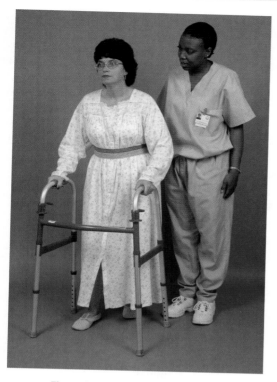

Figure 31-7. Client using a walker.

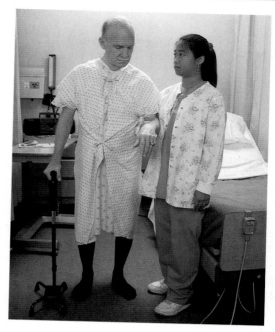

Figure 31-8. Client using a "quad" cane.

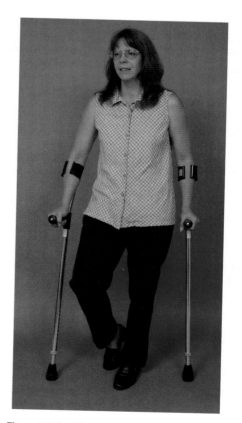

Figure 31-9. Client using Lofstrand crutches.

client place the cane in the hand of the stronger side of the body. The length of the cane should permit the elbow to be slightly flexed. Have the client move the cane forward about a foot and about 6 inches to the side, then move the weaker leg one step forward. Then have the client move the stronger leg forward and check the balance.

Like walkers, canes may be used on a temporary or a permanent basis. Some clients learn to ambulate using a walker and then progress to a series of canes as needed.

USING CRUTCHES. For most clients, crutches are used as a temporary measure until they regain full mobility. However, for clients with permanent disability, they may be needed on a permanent basis. Axillary crutches are used most often when temporary support is needed. Lofstrand crutches are used most often for permanent needs (Figure 31-9). Before use, the client should be measured carefully for adjustments to prevent axillary nerve damage or muscle strain. Each crutch end should have a rubber tip to prevent slipping.

Arm strength needs to be assessed. If needed, the client performs exercises to prepare for the demands of crutch walking. The basic crutch stance is called the *tripod,* or triangle, position. It provides a broad base of support. Several gaits can be used for ambulating, depending on the injury and the client's weight-bearing status. The four-point gait provides the most support, but it requires coordination to maneuver. The three-point gait requires that the client be able to bear full weight on the unaffected leg. The two-point gait is the quickest and requires at least partial weight-bearing ability for both legs. Procedure 31-6 (p. 794) describes these gaits and how to manage stairs and sitting.

Swing-to or swing-through gaits are used for clients who are paralyzed in both legs. Teach the client to move both crutches ahead together by about 2 feet, then lift the body and swing to or past the crutches, whichever is most comfortable and balanced.

Text continued on ■ *798*

PROCEDURE 31-6   WALKING WITH CRUTCHES

TIME TO ALLOW
Novice: 20-30 min.
Expert: 20-30 min.

Crutches are usually used for clients with orthopedic injuries who are unable to bear weight on one or both legs. Using crutches properly requires good upper body strength and balance.

DELEGATION GUIDELINES

The evaluation of the need for crutches and instruction in the use of crutches may not be delegated to a nursing assistant. Assessment and instruction for crutch walking are the domain of a licensed professional, such as you or a physical therapist. Once a client has been instructed and successfully demonstrates crutch walking, you may assign or delegate a nursing assistant to accompany the client, much as you would do with ambulation.

EQUIPMENT NEEDED
- Crutches with rubber tips
- Supportive shoes with rubber soles

1. Follow preliminary guidelines for nursing procedures (see inside front cover).

2. Inspect the prescribed crutch or crutches to make sure that the rubber tips are in place. *Rubber tips prevent slipping and therefore promote safety.*

3. Reinforce the importance of arm exercises, such as flexing and extending the arms, body lifts, and squeezing a rubber ball. *Arm muscles need to be toned to use crutches. Upper body strength is required.*

4. Check that crutches are the correct length (see illustration).
a. First, have the client stand.
b. Next, with the crutch tips and the client in the basic crutch stance (tripod position), check the distance between the axilla and the top of the crutch. It should be at least three finger widths, or 1 to 2 inches (2.5 to 5 cm). If the crutches are not the correct length, the client could sustain axillary nerve damage.

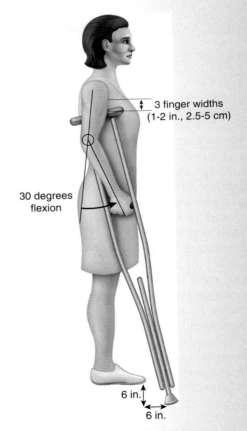

3 finger widths
(1-2 in., 2.5-5 cm)

30 degrees
flexion

6 in.

6 in.

Step 4. Measuring crutch length.

5. Teach the client how to balance using the tripod (triangle) position by placing the crutches 6 inches (15 cm) in front of the feet and out laterally about the same distance. *The tripod position provides a wide base of support and balance to prevent falls.*

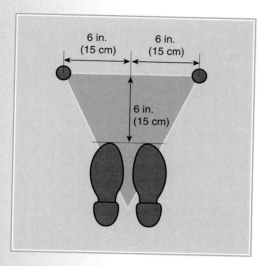

Step 5. Basic crutch stance, tripod position.

6. Check with the physician or physical therapist to determine which gait the client needs: a four-point, three-point, or two-point gait. *The type of injury and the client's balance determine which gait will be recommended.*

a. For a four-point gait, have the client follow this series of steps (see illustration):

(1) Move the right crutch forward about 6 inches (15 cm).

(2) Move the left foot forward.

(3) Move the left crutch forward.

(4) Move the right foot forward.

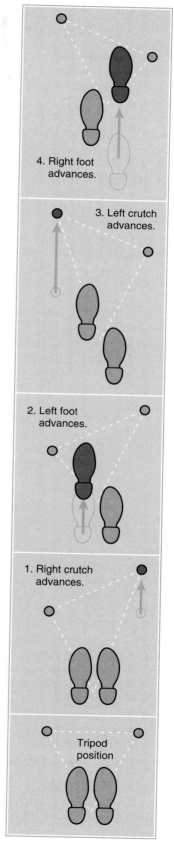

Step 6a. Four-point gait.

Continued

b. For a three-point gait, have the client follow this series of steps (see illustration):
   (1) Move both crutches and the weaker leg forward.
   (2) Move the stronger leg forward.

c. For a two-point gait, have the client follow this series of steps (see illustration):
   (1) Move the left crutch and the right foot forward at the same time.
   (2) Move the right crutch and the left foot forward at the same time.

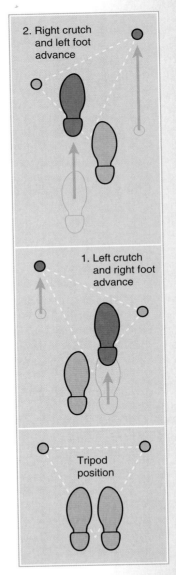

Step 6b. Three-point gait.

Step 6c. Two-point gait.

7. Teach the client how to ascend stairs:

a. Step up first with your stronger leg (see illustration).

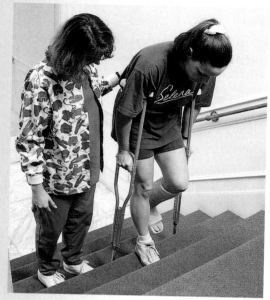

Step 7a. Stepping up first with the stronger leg

b. Shift your weight to the strong leg and move the crutches and the weaker leg onto the same step.

c. Repeat these steps until the stairs are negotiated. The crutches always support the weaker or affected leg.

8. Teach the client how to descend stairs:

a. Shift your weight to the stronger leg and move the crutches and the weaker leg onto the lower step (see illustration).

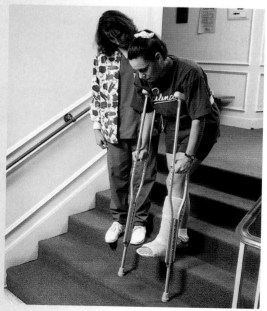

Step 8a. Stepping down first with the weaker leg.

b. Shift your weight to the crutches and move the strong leg onto that step.

c. Repeat these steps until the stairs are negotiated. The crutches always support the weaker or affected leg.

9. Teach the client how to get in and out of a chair. *The following technique supports the weaker leg and provides the best balance for the client:*

a. Stand with the chair behind you, making sure that the back of your stronger leg is against the chair.

b. Transfer your crutches to your weaker side and hold them by the hand bar.

c. Grasp the arm of the chair with the hand on your strong side, then lean forward and flex your hips and knees while lowering yourself into the chair.

d. To get out of the chair, move to the edge of the chair and position the stronger foot to support your weight when arising.

e. Hold both crutches by the hand bar, using the hand on your weaker side. Hold the arm of the chair with the hand on your stronger side.

f. Push down on the crutches and the armrest to push yourself out of the chair.

HOME CARE CONSIDERATIONS

Help the client do a safety check of the home environment for slippery floors, loose throw rugs, or obstructions in walkways. If the client will need to use stairs, it is preferable to have a handrail.

USING A WHEELCHAIR. For some clients, walking is no longer possible. Clients with complete spinal cord injuries, advanced multiple sclerosis, cerebral palsy, or muscular dystrophy are often confined to a wheelchair. These clients ambulate in their wheelchairs using their arms or other part of the body to propel the chair. Some use electric wheelchairs that can be advanced by a hand control or with a slight head movement.

Clients who are confined to wheelchairs are at risk for skin breakdown and other complications of immobility previously described. Teach the client and family or significant others to inspect skin every day and perform wheelchair pushups if possible to decrease pressure on the ischial tuberosities. Pushups also build arm strength, which is essential for propelling a manual wheelchair.

As a result of the federal Americans with Disabilities Act, all public places are wheelchair accessible. Ramps, handicapped toilets, and designated parking spaces have allowed wheelchair-bound people access to places they were previously not able to visit.

EVALUATION

Evaluation involves determining whether expected outcomes have been met. If they have not been met, the plan may need modification.

In our case study, Mrs. Lasauskas required rehabilitation for her fractured hip repair. By the fifth postoperative day, she was discharged to the hospital's transitional care unit (TCU). She was able to transfer from her bed to a chair and walk about 15 feet using a walker. Beyond that distance, she became dyspneic and tired. The plan for her continued rehabilitation in the TCU is to increase her ambulation distance and continue to build her tolerance for activity so that she can return to her assisted living apartment.

In this example, the client has progressed slowly, but is able to ambulate with a walker independently for a short distance. The intermediate expected outcomes were met, but the long-term outcomes still need to be achieved before she can be discharged back into the community. Box 31-5 illustrates Mrs. Lasauskas's care after surgery, when she is ready to get out of bed for the first time.

Nursing Care Plan A CLIENT WITH A FRACTURED HIP — Box 31-5

ADMISSION DATA

Mrs. Kristina Lasauskas is an 80-year-old woman admitted for a fractured left hip. She was taken from the emergency department to the operating room, where she had an open reduction and internal fixation. She was in the recovery room 3 hours and has been admitted to an orthopedic nursing unit.

PHYSICIAN'S ORDERS

$D_5\frac{1}{2}$ NS @ 75 mL per hour
Up in a chair TID as tolerated starting in A.M.
ROM QID
Laxative of choice
Lovenox 30 mg subcutaneous q12h

Regular diet, encourage fluids
Plan for discharge to a rehabilitation unit

NURSING ASSESSMENT

It is now the morning after her surgery. You receive the following report: Mrs. Lasauskas is 1 day post an open reduction and internal fixation of a fractured left hip. Her vital signs are stable. She is awake, alert, and oriented × 3. Lungs clear. Bowel sounds hypoactive. IV site patent and free of inflammation. She has left-sided weakness from a previous cerebrovascular accident but was able to walk with a cane. She is to be up in a chair today and physical therapy will start ROM. She is depressed because she believes she will never walk again.

NANDA Nursing Diagnosis	NOC Expected Outcomes With Indicators	NIC Interventions With Selected Activities	Evaluation Data
IMPAIRED PHYSICAL MOBILITY	**JOINT MOVEMENT**	**EXERCISE PROMOTION**	
Related Factor:			• Data gathered at discharge to rehabilitation setting.
• Right-sided weakness and healing fracture of left hip	• Active • Transfer performance	• Strength training. • Joint mobility.	
	THE CLIENT WILL		
	• Maintain full ROM.	• Full active/passive ROM by physical therapy 0800, 1300. • By nursing 1700, 2100. • Use client's history of self determination to motivate.	• Has full ROM in upper extremities. • Can perform active ROM. • Performs active ROM on right leg. • Straight leg raising to a 30-degree angle. • Can raise left leg by bending knee to 30-degree hip flexion.

Nursing Care Plan A CLIENT WITH A FRACTURED HIP—CONT'D

Box 31-5

NANDA Nursing Diagnosis	NOC Expected Outcomes With Indicators	NIC Interventions With Selected Activities	Evaluation Data
IMPAIRED PHYSICAL MOBILITY	**THE CLIENT WILL** • Increase upper body strength. • Transfer from bed to chair with assistance. • Sit in a chair without fatigue or change in vital signs. • Perform resistance exercises to right leg and ROM to left leg. • Stand at bedside with partial weight bearing to left hip.	**EXERCISE PROMOTION** • Use 3-pound weights to exercise arms during ROM. • Have great-grandchildren bring colored weights and make a game of exercising. • Pivot to chair 1000, 1500, 1900. • Sit in chair as tolerated, increasing to 30 min. • Use light resistance for ROM to right leg.	• Exercises arms with 3-pound weights. • Tolerates flexion at elbow. Raising weight over her head tires right arm. • Can stand and pivot to chair with assistance. • Can raise right leg against light resistance of nurse's hand on knee. • Puts left leg on floor for balance when standing. • Minimal if any weight bearing.

CRITICAL THINKING QUESTIONS

1. Estimate Mrs. Lasauskas's potential for rehabilitation on a scale of 1 to 10, with 10 meaning she will be able to walk as well as she did before she fell.

2. List the criteria you used to make the decision in Question #1.
3. Mrs. Lasauskas refuses to do active ROM exercises with her arms. How would you motivate her?

Nursing outcome and intervention labels from Johnson, M., Bulechek, G., McCloskey Dochterman, J. M., Maas, M., & Moorhead, S. (2001). *Nursing diagnoses, outcomes, and interventions: NANDA, NOC, and NIC linkages.* St Louis, MO: Mosby.

When Mrs. Lasauskas is discharged to the rehabilitation setting, the nurse writes the following note:

SAMPLE DOCUMENTATION FOR MRS. LASAUSKAS
Discharged to Meridian Rehabilitation per stretcher. Transportation provided by a van from Elderly Assistance, Inc. Vital signs stable. Pain controlled with Vicodin given 30 minutes prior to getting out of bed. Can feed self and dress with assistance. Physical therapy reports she is ready to begin walking a few steps with a walker. Report called to Meridian.

Key Principles

• Physical mobility requires functional joints, muscles, and bones.
• Factors affecting mobility include lifestyle, environment, growth and development, and pathophysiological factors, especially musculoskeletal and neurological health problems.
• *Impaired physical mobility* occurs when the client experiences limited ability to move within the physical environment.
• *Activity intolerance* results when a client has insufficient physiological or psychological energy to endure or complete a desired activity.
• Physical examination of a client with impaired physical mobility includes assessment of body alignment, gait, joints, skeletal muscles, and neurovascular function.
• Diagnostic tests help you select appropriate nursing diagnoses for clients with musculoskeletal health problems.

• Functional assessment includes determining a client's ability to move and perform activities of daily living.
• Assessment of the client with *Impaired physical mobility* should be holistic and include assessment of all functional health patterns for emotional as well as physiological responses, including hopelessness and pain or chronic pain.
• Expected outcomes for clients with musculoskeletal problems are that the client will experience improved mobility and tolerance to activities.
• Interventions for improving activity tolerance focus on building muscle mass and strength, progressive mobilization, and controlling pain and discomfort.
• Interventions for improving mobility include maintaining joint mobility, assisting with movement, and compensating for physical impairments.
• Evaluation of outcomes for clients with musculoskeletal problems involves promoting ambulation (including wheelchair ambulation), preventing complications of immobility, and building activity tolerance.

Bibliography

Anonymous. (2000). Lifting devices needed to reduce injury, experts say: OSHA begins hearings with health care panel. *Hospital Employee Health, 19*(5), 51, 60.

Cornman-Levy, D., Gitlin, L. N., Corcoran, M. A., & Schinfeld, S. (2001). Caregiver aches and pains: The role of physical therapy in helping families provide daily care. *Alzheimer's Care Quarterly, 2*(1), 47-55.

*Asterisk indicates a classic or definitive work on this subject or deposited in the muscles and joints. The bones become brittle and porous, and they fracture easily.

Integumentary Effects of Inactivity and Immobility

Damage to the skin from prolonged pressure on bony prominences is the major complication of immobility. Additional damage can result from shear, friction, maceration, and infection.

A **pressure ulcer** is any lesion caused by unrelieved pressure that leads to damage of underlying tissues. When pressure on the skin exceeds capillary pressure, blood flow to the skin is impaired. The supply of oxygen and nutrients is insufficient to maintain the viability of the skin and underlying structures. The cells die and slough, leaving an open crater. Pressure ulcers can range from reddened skin to large, open, deep wounds. Poor nutrition, dehydration, and continued pressure lead to poor wound healing and wound infections. A pressure ulcer can develop in a single day.

The most commonly affected areas are tissues overlying bony prominence (Figure 32-2). The area over the coccyx is probably the most common site of pressure ulcers. However, pressure ulcers also develop over the greater trochanter, shoulder, elbow, back of the skull, heels, ankle, and ear. For a client confined to a wheelchair, the most common sites are the ischial tuberosities and the coccyx. Keep in mind, however, that a pressure ulcer can develop anywhere there is sufficient pressure for a sufficient time.

For a pressure ulcer to occur, the amount of pressure on the capillary bed must exceed the arteriole pressure (the capillary closing pressure is about 35 mm Hg), and the duration of pressure must be long and unrelieved. **Interface pressure** is pressure created in tissues that are compressed between the bones and a support surface by the weight of the body. As the client lies in bed or sits quietly in a chair, interface pressure exerted on tissues by the external surface of the bed or chair interrupts blood flow through the vessels and impairs the delivery of oxygen and nutrients to cells.

Although the development of pressure ulcers has a sole cause (prolonged, unrelieved pressure), additional factors increase the risk for developing a pressure injury. A client who is unable to move independently in bed because of cognitive or musculoskeletal limitations is at high risk. Chronic illnesses, such as renal failure, diabetes, and anemia, further exacerbate the risk. Frail or edematous skin is more likely to sustain damage. Dehydration and poor nutrition (inadequate protein) also decrease the skin's tolerance to injury. Pressure ulcers account for a large proportion of skin injuries that result from bed rest. Because treating these injuries is costly, prevention is always the treatment of choice.

 If Mr. Jackson wears a brace on his knee, how could you help him prevent pressure points?

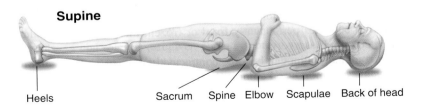

Supine

Heels   Sacrum   Spine   Elbow   Scapulae   Back of head

Figure 32-2. Bony prominences subject to pressure, ischemia, necrosis, and ulceration in the supine, side-lying, and prone positions.

Side-lying

Toes   Medial and lateral condyles   Iliac crest   Ribs   Ear
Malleolus   Greater trochanter   Acromion process

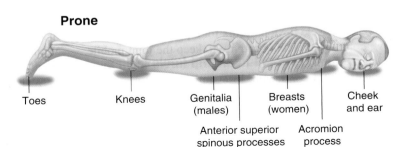

Prone

Toes   Knees   Genitalia (males)   Breasts (women)   Cheek and ear
Anterior superior spinous processes   Acromion process

Nursing Care Plan A CLIENT WITH A FRACTURED HIP—CONT'D

Box 31-5

NANDA Nursing Diagnosis	NOC Expected Outcomes With Indicators	NIC Interventions With Selected Activities	Evaluation Data
IMPAIRED PHYSICAL MOBILITY	THE CLIENT WILL • Increase upper body strength. • Transfer from bed to chair with assistance. • Sit in a chair without fatigue or change in vital signs. • Perform resistance exercises to right leg and ROM to left leg. • Stand at bedside with partial weight bearing to left hip.	EXERCISE PROMOTION • Use 3-pound weights to exercise arms during ROM. • Have great-grandchildren bring colored weights and make a game of exercising. • Pivot to chair 1000, 1500, 1900. • Sit in chair as tolerated, increasing to 30 min. • Use light resistance for ROM to right leg.	• Exercises arms with 3-pound weights. • Tolerates flexion at elbow. Raising weight over her head tires right arm. • Can stand and pivot to chair with assistance. • Can raise right leg against light resistance of nurse's hand on knee. • Puts left leg on floor for balance when standing. • Minimal if any weight bearing.

CRITICAL THINKING QUESTIONS

1. Estimate Mrs. Lasauskas's potential for rehabilitation on a scale of 1 to 10, with 10 meaning she will be able to walk as well as she did before she fell.

2. List the criteria you used to make the decision in Question #1.
3. Mrs. Lasauskas refuses to do active ROM exercises with her arms. How would you motivate her?

Nursing outcome and intervention labels from Johnson, M., Bulechek, G., McCloskey Dochterman, J. M., Maas, M., & Moorhead, S. (2001). *Nursing diagnoses, outcomes, and interventions: NANDA, NOC, and NIC linkages.* St Louis, MO: Mosby.

When Mrs. Lasauskas is discharged to the rehabilitation setting, the nurse writes the following note:

SAMPLE DOCUMENTATION FOR MRS. LASAUSKAS

Discharged to Meridian Rehabilitation per stretcher. Transportation provided by a van from Elderly Assistance, Inc. Vital signs stable. Pain controlled with Vicodin given 30 minutes prior to getting out of bed. Can feed self and dress with assistance. Physical therapy reports she is ready to begin walking a few steps with a walker. Report called to Meridian.

Key Principles

- Physical mobility requires functional joints, muscles, and bones.
- Factors affecting mobility include lifestyle, environment, growth and development, and pathophysiological factors, especially musculoskeletal and neurological health problems.
- *Impaired physical mobility* occurs when the client experiences limited ability to move within the physical environment.
- *Activity intolerance* results when a client has insufficient physiological or psychological energy to endure or complete a desired activity.
- Physical examination of a client with impaired physical mobility includes assessment of body alignment, gait, joints, skeletal muscles, and neurovascular function.
- Diagnostic tests help you select appropriate nursing diagnoses for clients with musculoskeletal health problems.

- Functional assessment includes determining a client's ability to move and perform activities of daily living.
- Assessment of the client with *Impaired physical mobility* should be holistic and include assessment of all functional health patterns for emotional as well as physiological responses, including hopelessness and pain or chronic pain.
- Expected outcomes for clients with musculoskeletal problems are that the client will experience improved mobility and tolerance to activities.
- Interventions for improving activity tolerance focus on building muscle mass and strength, progressive mobilization, and controlling pain and discomfort.
- Interventions for improving mobility include maintaining joint mobility, assisting with movement, and compensating for physical impairments.
- Evaluation of outcomes for clients with musculoskeletal problems involves promoting ambulation (including wheelchair ambulation), preventing complications of immobility, and building activity tolerance.

Bibliography

Anonymous. (2000). Lifting devices needed to reduce injury, experts say: OSHA begins hearings with health care panel. *Hospital Employee Health, 19*(5), 51, 60.

Cornman-Levy, D., Gitlin, L. N., Corcoran, M. A., & Schinfeld, S. (2001). Caregiver aches and pains: The role of physical therapy in helping families provide daily care. *Alzheimer's Care Quarterly, 2*(1), 47-55.

*Asterisk indicates a classic or definitive work on this subject.

Daus, C. (1999). Long-term rehab: Maintaining mobility for the geriatric population. *Rehab Management: The Interdisciplinary Journal of Rehabilitation, 12*(5), 58, 60-61.

Haigh, C., & Peacock, L. (1998). Dilemmas in moving and handling patients. *Community Nurse, 4*(1), 26-28.

Herbert, P., Rochman, D. L., & McAlary, P. W. (1998). Dealing with pain. *Case Review, 4*(6), 16-19.

Ignatavicius, D. D., Workman, M. L., & Mishler, M. A. (1999). *Medical-surgical nursing across the health care continuum* (3rd ed.). Philadelphia: Saunders.

Johnson, M., Bulechek, G., McCloskey Dochterman, J. M., Maas, M., & Moorhead, S. (2001). *Nursing diagnoses, outcomes, and interventions: NANDA, NOC, and NIC linkages.* St Louis, MO: Mosby.

Kachourbos, M. J., & Creasey, G. H. (2000). Health promotion in motion: Improving quality of life for persons with neurogenic bladder and bowel using assistive technology [corrected]. [Published erratum appears in *Scientific Nursing, 17*(4), 221]. *Scientific Nursing, 17*(3), 125-129.

*Leininger, M. M. (1991). *Culture care diversity and universality: A theory of nursing.* New York: National League for Nursing Press.

Love, C. (2001). Using assisted walking devices. *Journal of Orthopaedic Nursing, 5*(1), 45-53.

McCaffery, M., & Ferrell, B. R. (1999). Opioids and pain management. *Nursing99, 29*(3), 48-52.

McCliment, J. K. (2000). Implementing a zero-lift program: This facility invested in learning how electronic lifts affect resident care. *Nursing Homes Long Term Care Management, 49*(11), 20-23, 81-82.

Miller, D., & Sprigle, S. (2001). Long-term rehab. Risk management: Secondary complications, falls, restraints, and transportation are all safety issues for wheelchair users that clinicians must address. *Rehab Management: The Interdisciplinary Journal of Rehabilitation, 14*(5), 58-60.

Nelson, A., Tiesman, H., & Lloyd, J. (2000). Get a handle on safe patient transfer and activity. *Nursing Management, 31*(12), 47.

Neu, M., Browne, J. V., & Vojir, C. (2000). The impact of two transfer techniques used during skin-to-skin care on the physiologic and behavioral responses of preterm infants [corrected]. [Published erratum appears in *Nursing Research, 49*(6), 326]. *Nursing Research, 49*(4), 215-223.

North American Nursing Diagnosis Association. (2001). *NANDA nursing diagnoses: Definitions and classification, 2001-2002.* Philadelphia: Author.

Owen, B. D. (2000). Preventing injuries using an ergonomic approach. *AORN Journal, 72*(6), 1031-1033, 1035-1036.

Raine, E. (2001). Testing a risk assessment tool for manual handling. *Professional Nurse, 16*(9), 1344-1348.

Schiff, L. (2001). Market choices: Lift and transfer devices. *RN, 64*(8), 61-62.

Sloan, H. L., Haslam, K., & Foret, C. M. (2001). Teaching the use of walkers and canes. *Home Healthcare Nurse, 19*(4), 241-246.

Stewart, K. B., & Murray, H. C. (1998). How to use a walker correctly. *Nursing, 28*(9 Hosp Nurs), 32hn22-23.

Tammelleo, A. D. (1999). Hoyer Lift "gives way" on paraplegic: Malpractice limitation not applicable v agency. *Regan Report on Nursing Law, 40*(6), 3.

Thompson, F. (1999). Innovation station: Ceiling track lifting devices. *Scientific Nursing, 16*(3), 103.

Waters, J. (1998). Hidden hazards associated with moving and handling. *Community Nurse, 4*(8), 21.

Wilson, C. B. (2001). Safer handling practice 2: Putting theory into practice. *Nursing & Residential Care, 3*(8), 388-392.

Wood, J., Raudsepp, T., Miller, L., & Dazey, E. (2000). Improving resident transfers. *Nursing Homes Long Term Care Management, 49*(6), 68-72.

Worthington, K. (2000). Health & safety: Watch your back. *American Journal of Nursing, 100*(9), 96.

Preventing Disuse Syndrome

32

Preventing Disuse Syndrome

Key Terms

atrophy
bed rest
contracture
deep vein thrombosis
disuse
excoriation
footdrop
friction injury
hypomotility
hypostatic pneumonia
immobility
inactivity
interface pressure
maceration
orthostatic hypotension
orthostatic intolerance
osteoporosis
pressure ulcer
pulmonary embolus
renal calculi
shear
trochanter roll
wrist drop

Learning Objectives

After studying this chapter, you should be able to do the following:

- Describe the physiological concepts underlying the diagnosis of *Risk for disuse syndrome*
- Discuss the factors that may lead to immobility and disuse
- Assess a client who is at risk for complications from disuse
- Diagnose the client at risk for disuse complications
- Plan goal-directed interventions to prevent complications of disuse
- Describe interventions needed to prevent complications of disuse
- Evaluate outcomes that describe progress toward managing immobility and preventing disuse

Mr. Jackson is a 48-year-old African-American man who has come to the emergency department after being injured on the job. The physician diagnoses a compound fracture of the left tibia and a fractured left clavicle. Mr. Jackson is taken to the operating room where the bone fragments are pinned and a stabilizing device applied. His arm is placed in a sling. After 24 hours, Mr. Jackson is sent home with instructions to keep the left leg elevated at all times, to apply an ice pack to the left knee for 20 minutes every 4 hours, and to bear no weight on the leg. He is to return to the orthopedic clinic in 1 week. It will be at least 3 months before he will be able to return to the heavy construction work he has done since he was 16 years old. He is likely to lose strength and endurance, and the limb is likely to atrophy. Additionally, he is at risk for cardiovascular deconditioning, respiratory infection, urinary tract infection, depression, and skin breakdown. The nurse makes the diagnosis of *Risk for disuse syndrome.*

KEY NURSING DIAGNOSES FOR   Disuse

Risk for disuse syndrome: At risk for deterioration of body systems as the result of prescribed or unavoidable musculoskeletal inactivity

Risk for impaired skin integrity: At risk for skin being adversely altered

Activity and movement develop and maintain the normal functioning of all body systems. In contrast, prolonged inactivity causes physical and mental deterioration. You will care for clients who are inactive from immobility, prescribed bed rest, critical illness, neurological damage, trauma, or pain. Through astute assessment and aggressive interventions, you can prevent many of the complications of disuse.

CONCEPTS OF INACTIVITY AND IMMOBILITY

Disuse is a state (or condition) of decrease or cessation of use of an organ or a body part, restriction of activity, or immobility. Complications of disuse occur in every body system. Disuse can affect a single body part or multiple interrelated body systems. Complications of disuse occur if the client has a prescribed or an unavoidable period of inactivity or immobility. Preventing complications of disuse will decrease both suffering and health care costs.

Immobility is the inability to move the whole body or a body part. It occurs in clients who are paralyzed or unconscious, or who have neuromuscular or orthopedic disorders. Many frail older adults have fewer spontaneous movements because of neurological or musculoskeletal problems. The immobile client is totally dependent on the nurse to maintain safety and body functions.

Bed rest is a prescribed or self-imposed restriction to bed for therapeutic reasons. Complete bed rest is seldom prescribed because of the potential complications of immobility. However, critically ill clients, some orthopedic clients, and clients with severe limitation of movement may be confined to bed. Some clients with prescribed bed rest are able to move about freely in bed, but others require much effort to move or need assistance to move.

Inactivity and immobility have a cyclic relationship with the development of complications. For example, when a client remains inactive, the joints begin to get stiff, and the muscles get weak. The client is less able to participate in activities of daily living (ADLs) and experiences increased risk for immobility. Eventually, the client develops respiratory and cardiovascular deconditioning and is at risk for skin breakdown. The longer the person is immobile, the higher is the risk for complications of disuse. Preventing complications of immobility requires support of all body systems to break the cycle of disuse.

Psychosocial Effects of Inactivity and Immobility

Initially, most people welcome the brief rest and relief from ADLs that accompanies a brief period of inactivity or immobility. However, long-term or permanent inactivity or immobilization can alter that feeling. Often, the client loses motivation or interest in participating in daily living. Losing contact with friends and work can result in loneliness and social isolation. The client who is forced to rely on others for help feels powerless. Loss of self-esteem is associated with the absence of social roles as caregiver, parent, or breadwinner.

A person's behavior changes in response to a prescribed or unavoidable activity restriction. The client may act out negative feelings of dissatisfaction and frustration in the form of irritation, anger, or aggression. Additionally, inactivity can increase mental confusion as a consequence of sensory deprivation. The person is less able to concentrate and focus on learning, memory may be impaired, and problem-solving abilities decline.

Resting in bed 24 hours a day also interferes with the normal circadian rhythm and pattern of sleep. When the client sleeps during the day, the quality of the sleep is not the same as it is during the night. However, having slept during the day, the client may be unable to sleep through the night. The psychological manifestations of sleep deprivation may be present.

Mr. Jackson is the primary financial support for his family. He has good health insurance but does not have sick leave. What psychosocial manifestations would you predict for him?

Musculoskeletal Effects of Inactivity and Immobility

Active use maintains the strength of bones, strength and tone of muscles, and mobility of joints. Much as the trained athlete becomes deconditioned when not in training, the client who is inactive experiences deterioration of bones, muscles, and joints.

Shear is a mechanical force that acts on an area of skin in a direction parallel to the body's surface. Shear injuries are a serious form of pressure injury, as they result in necrosis and ulceration, usually over the coccyx. One cause is improper positioning, which can lead to the client sliding down in bed (Figure 32-3). When that happens, blood vessels in the two sacral tissue layers are stretched and torn, which disrupts the blood supply to these cells and causes skin breakdown. Shearing forces cause deep ulcers. Although they may appear small on the skin surface, considerable necrosis may be present in the underlying tissues.

Injuries can occur to the superficial layers of the skin. In a **friction injury,** the epidermal layer of skin is rubbed off, possibly from a restraint, a dressing, or a tube. Friction injury commonly affects the elbows, which can become irritated as the client moves around in bed. An **excoriation** is an injury to the epidermis caused by abrasion, scratching, a burn, or chemicals, such as sweat, wound drainage, feces, or urine coming in contact with skin. **Maceration** is a softening of the epidermis caused by prolonged contact with moisture, such as from a wet sheet or diaper. Maceration increases the risk for damage by decreasing the skin's ability to resist trauma.

Once the skin's first line of defense is broken, microorganisms can freely invade an ulcer or lesion, causing an infection. Infections slow wound healing and carry the risk for the serious complication of septicemia (infection in the bloodstream). The absence of circulation further decreases the oxygen, immune response, and nutrients necessary for healing.

Cardiovascular Effects of Inactivity and Immobility

When a client is on bed rest, the demands of the cells for oxygen initially decrease. However, the cardiovascular workload may actually increase. Additionally, without exercise, cardiac deconditioning begins. These changes in the cardiovascular system lead to decreased energy and further inactivity.

It is also harder for a client to change positions and perform the ADLs when restricted to bed. Often, during the "work" of moving in bed or using a bedpan, the client will use Valsalva's maneuver, that is, hold the breath (which increases intrathoracic pressure by straining against a closed glottis).

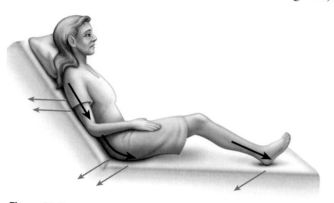

Figure 32-3. Shearing forces pull tissue layers in opposite directions. Tissue near the bone slides downward and forward, whereas the skin tends to be held upward and back by friction from the sheets.

When a breath is taken, the intrathoracic pressure drops, and blood flow suddenly increases to the right heart, causing an increased workload. Reflex bradycardia occurs, which can cause syncope or a heart attack in vulnerable persons.

Unlike arteries, which pump blood forward from the heart, the veins rely on the "squeezing" action of calf muscles to move the venous blood along. In a bedridden client, decreased calf muscle activity and increased external pressure from the bed gradually allow blood to pool in the distal veins. This stasis of blood contributes to three problems: orthostatic intolerance, edema, and thrombus formation.

Orthostatic intolerance is a drop in systolic blood pressure of 20 mm Hg or more and a drop in diastolic blood pressure of 10 mm Hg or more for 1 or 2 minutes after a client stands up. It is also called orthostatic or postural hypotension, and it commonly results from immobility.

In the supine position (lying flat on the back), blood pools in the legs, and venous return and cardiac output decrease. When the client sits or stands up, blood pressure can drop rapidly. Prolonged supine positioning also decreases the sensitivity of baroreceptors in the aortic arch to positional blood pressure changes. These receptors become sluggish and less responsive in stimulating the sympathetic nervous system to maintain normal blood pressure with changes in position. Dehydration can also contribute to this problem by decreasing the blood volume.

Low blood pressure and orthostatic intolerance increase the client's risk for falling. Signs and symptoms of orthostatic intolerance include dizziness, feeling faint, or feeling lightheaded. Orthostatic intolerance is present in about 20% of people over age 65 and in at least 30% of people over age 75.

Stasis of blood in the legs and sacral area increases hydrostatic pressure on vein walls. As the veins dilate in response, the valves open and allow backflow of blood down the veins. Also, this increase in hydrostatic fluid pressure "pushes" more fluid out of the veins into the interstitial spaces, producing edema. Edema constricts blood flow to the tissues and cells, decreasing their oxygen supply.

Stasis of venous blood, viscosity of the blood, and injury to vessel walls predispose the client to thrombus formation in the legs. **Deep vein thrombosis** (DVT) is the condition caused when a blood clot (thrombus) develops in the lumen of a deep leg vein, such as the tibial, popliteal, femoral, or iliac vein. Superficial vein thrombosis is a clot in a superficial vessel.

Deep vein thrombosis can develop when slowed blood flow allows platelets and increased levels of calcium (from the bones) to settle out and come in contact with the intima that lines the vessel. This activates the clotting process, and blood clots form along the vessel wall, particularly if the walls are damaged or if the vessels are tortuous (twisting). Dehydration contributes to thrombus formation by causing the blood to become more viscous.

Signs of deep vein thrombosis are calf tenderness, calf pain with passive dorsiflexion of the foot (Homans' sign), edema that causes one calf to increase in diameter, and slight warmth of the involved leg. The major risk created by DVT is

pulmonary embolism, which results when a piece of the thrombus breaks free, is carried by veins to the right heart and the pulmonary circulation, and lodges in a pulmonary blood vessel. As a result, blood flow and oxygen cannot reach the area of lung tissue served by the blocked vessel.

Signs and symptoms of pulmonary embolism include the sudden onset of dyspnea, a cough, sudden chest pain, hemoptysis, tachycardia over 100 beats per minute, and tachypnea over 20 breaths per minute. A pulmonary embolus can be life-threatening and requires immediate emergency action.

Respiratory Effects of Inactivity and Immobility

The lungs function at their best in the upright position. The recumbent position (lying flat) compromises respiratory function and predisposes the client to respiratory complications, such as hypoventilation, atelectasis, stasis of secretions, and altered gas exchange.

Initially, bed rest decreases the body's metabolic need for oxygen. The respiratory rate slows, and the depth becomes shallow. Eventually, immobility causes the respiratory muscles to weaken, which decreases the bellows effect of the bony structures of the chest. Pressure of the mattress against the thorax decreases the respiratory movement of the chest as well. The abdominal contents also push against the diaphragm, decreasing its effectiveness in contracting and expanding the lungs.

Immobility also compromises the client's ability to cough—the normal mechanism for moving secretions out of the lungs. With a diminished cough effort, secretions accumulate and block the airways. Dehydration causes the secretions to become thick and tenacious, making them even more difficult to mobilize. Gravity contributes to the stagnation of secretions in the dependent areas of the lungs.

Hypostatic pneumonia is an inflammation of the lungs caused by stasis of secretions, which become a medium for bacterial growth. Signs of pneumonia are thickened yellow sputum, crackles, wheezes, fever, and an increased respiratory rate.

Gastrointestinal Effects of Inactivity and Immobility

Immobility or inactivity slows the basal metabolic rate and gastrointestinal (GI) motility, and it decreases nutrient absorption. These effects are manifested as anorexia, constipation, increased storage of fat and carbohydrates, and a negative nitrogen balance.

A client confined to bed may experience a loss of appetite (anorexia) because the metabolic rate slows with rest, thus reducing calorie requirements. With inadequate nutrient intake, the client feels tired and prefers to sit quietly, becoming more and more inactive. If the client does not eat, muscle and subcutaneous tissue are broken down for energy needs. Changes in the client's nutritional status affect endurance and muscle strength. Fatigue and loss of energy lead to further inactivity and immobility.

Anorexia combined with muscle atrophy can produce a negative nitrogen balance when nitrogen excretion exceeds nitrogen intake. The body begins to break down fat for energy,

The client may become malnourished, and the skin may become dry and cracked.

Blood cells cannot be synthesized by bone marrow without sufficient protein; lack of adequate protein occurs with poor intake. Without enough white blood cells (leukocytes), there is increased susceptibility to infections—the immune system is less effective. The red blood cells also decrease, which leads to generalized fatigue, anemia, and poor wound healing. The skin, nails, and hair are also affected and become dull, dry, and brittle. The client loses subcutaneous fat and thereby the ability to effectively conserve heat and protect bony prominences.

Fluid intake may also be affected if the client on bed rest is unable to obtain and drink water. Decreased fluid intake results in dehydration, which causes constipation, decreased blood volume (decreased cardiac output and orthostatic intolerance), decreased tissue perfusion (skin ulceration and poor wound healing), decreased urine output (oliguria and stasis of urine), and stasis of respiratory secretions.

Hypomotility is decreased peristalsis from lack of stimulation of the gastrocolic reflex. Bowel sounds are faint and slowed. With slowed peristalsis, the transient time of food through the GI tract is lengthened, allowing more water to be absorbed. Thus constipation and flatulence often accompany bed rest. This can be compounded by an individual's reluctance to use the bedpan to have a bowel movement, leading to further constipation.

For the first week after his injury, Mr. Jackson is expected to be either in bed or sitting down with his leg elevated. Do you think constipation could be a problem for him?

Genitourinary Effects of Inactivity and Immobility

Immobility diminishes the kidney and bladder function and results in an increased incidence of urinary stasis, retention, renal calculi, and urinary tract infections. Urinary tract infections are the most prevalent hospital-acquired infections in bedridden clients.

The client may also be unable to empty the bladder completely because of an inability to assume a normal voiding position while in bed. The male client with an enlarged prostate gland may be unable to urinate lying flat. Urinary retention results in residual urine remaining stagnant in the bladder for a prolonged time. Residual urine leads to bladder distention, reflux of urine to the kidneys, growth of bacteria, and urinary tract infections.

Placing a client in the supine position can prevent urine from draining from the renal pelvis into the ureters. This allows urine to fill up and accumulate in the kidneys, leading to urinary stasis. Residual urine becomes an excellent medium for bacterial growth.

Alkaline urine and inadequate personal hygiene further predispose the immobile client to urinary tract infections. The end products of metabolism in an inactive client are generally alkaline because of decreased muscle activity. The high pH of the urine promotes bacteria growth. Additionally, personal hygiene and perineal care are difficult for the bedridden client. The accumulation of microorganisms outside the urethra from the anal area encourages bacteria to invade the bladder. Reflux of urine back into the ureters can spread microorganisms from the bladder into the kidneys. Signs of a urinary tract infection are dysuria (pain or burning sensation on voiding), urgency, frequency, fever, and voiding small amounts. Older adults may not exhibit these classic signs but instead develop confusion; this should prompt a more thorough assessment for infection.

Stasis of urine and infection increase the risk for formation of calculi (stones, lithiasis) in the kidneys, renal pelvis, or urinary bladder. **Renal calculi** are stones formed in the kidney when the excretion rate of calcium or other minerals is high, as when osteoclastic activity releases calcium from the bones during immobility. Calculi can occur after only 1 or 2 weeks of inactivity.

FACTORS AFFECTING ACTIVITY AND MOBILITY

An optimal level of activity may be altered by a myriad of factors affecting the client's ability or desire for mobility. These factors place a client at risk for the complications of disuse.

Pain
The immediate response to pain is to keep quiet. The pain of a broken arm causes the person to immobilize the involved limb. For example, postoperative or cancer pain prevents the client from getting up from bed and freely moving around.

Therapeutic or Prescribed Inactivity
Although complete bed rest is seldom prescribed, rest does aid healing for a variety of problems. For example, rest reduces the workload to allow the heart to heal. Immobilization allows a broken bone, skin, or nerve tissue to regenerate and grow together.

Mr. Jackson, the client in our case study, needs to limit his activity, but his cultural values may influence his response to the treatment plan (Box 32-1).

Change in Level of Consciousness
A client who is in a coma or unconscious remains unmoving in bed. An automobile accident that causes a head injury may leave the client immobile. The person who experiences a cerebrovascular accident (stroke) may be unable to move.

Change in Musculoskeletal Functioning
The aging process causes skeletal muscles to atrophy and joints to become more rigid and less flexible during the middle and later adult years. In addition, musculoskeletal disorders often limit mobility. Although paralysis is the most obvious cause of illness-related impaired mobility, other causes include amputation, arthritis, and Parkinson's disease. Muscular dystrophy and multiple sclerosis cause the muscles to lose their ability to function.

Emotional or Psychological Disturbances
A depressed client may lack the emotional energy to participate in ADLs, even to the extent of fixing a meal or getting dressed for the day. Extreme fear may prevent a client from leaving the room or even the house, for days.

Chronic Illnesses
Illnesses that cause physiological changes in the body can affect the person's ability or energy to move. Either from fatigue or physical inability, the client remains inactive for a period. For example, anemia from blood loss or renal failure decreases the oxygen-carrying capacity of the blood, and the person experiences severe fatigue.

ASSESSMENT

General Assessment of Activity and Mobility
There are two purposes in assessing the immobile client. One is to detect the risk for complications of immobility. The other is to determine how much assistance the client will need to manage ADLs and prevent complications. Whether the client is in the hospital or at home, risk for complications of immobility should be identified and treated early.

Health History. Assessment begins with gathering data about the client's ability and motivation to be active. You should do the following:
- Note any medical or surgical conditions that would limit movement before you attempt to move the client or ask the client to move.
- Assess for pain that may be limiting movement.
- Assess the person's ability to understand and follow your instructions for self-care while in bed.
- Assess any risk factors affecting movement.
- Assess for *Risk for disuse syndrome.*
- Determine the client's previous level of functioning to set appropriate goals for care.

The following client questions may be helpful if the client is able to answer them. Alternatively, you may have some ac-

---

Cross-Cultural Care **CARING FOR A SOUTHERN AFRICAN-AMERICAN MAN**

Box 32-1

Mr. Jackson is a 48-year-old African American. He is the head of his household and proud to be its breadwinner. He is active in his job as a construction worker, but he gets no other exercise. He eats a Southern breakfast of eggs, ham, and buttered grits every morning. His wife does all the cooking in the household. Mr. Jackson is slightly overweight but powerfully built.

When Mr. Jackson leaves the hospital, his wife and extended family will take care of him. His wife will "do" everything for him, encouraging him to

rest. Although every client is unique, many African Americans from the South tend to value the following:
- Matriarchal family structure
- Male role as decision maker
- Large, extended families
- Strong tradition of religion

cess to information in the medical records and from a family member.

- Describe your usual activities. Are you limited in your exercise or leisure activities because of fatigue, muscle weakness, joint changes, or breathing problems?
- Describe your usual health practices. Nutrition? Elimination? Exercise?
- Have you noticed any sores on your skin? Do you bruise or injure easily?
- Do you have a history of cardiac, gastrointestinal, respiratory, urinary, or skin problems?

When Mr. Jackson returns for his 1-week clinic visit, you ask him all of these questions. What problems would you anticipate in helping him maintain his ADLs?

Physical Examination. Assess the client's ability to move in bed. Sometimes you can observe the person moving and make a judgment about how much assistance is needed. Other times you may have to ask the client to move his arms and legs, squeeze your hands, hold a glass, or perform another activity. You can observe the speed of movement, strength, and coordination. As you perform a complete physical examination, you are assessing the person's ability to move. This is one of the reasons your daily assessment in the hospital or assessment in the home setting includes a physical examination.

Focus especially on the musculoskeletal system, including the client's muscle strength and tone, and ability to move in bed. Check the range of motion in each joint. Assess the skin carefully; this step is a key element of the physical examination for clients with mobility problems. Examine the skin for lesions and frailty.

Focused Assessment for *Risk for Disuse Syndrome*
Defining Characteristics. *Risk for disuse syndrome* is defined by the presence of its risk factors, and the primary one is immobility. In considering this diagnosis, you will want to assess whether your client is at minimal risk, moderate risk, or high risk for disuse syndrome, as shown in the decision tree (Figure 32-4).

Two important criteria for assessing degree of risk include the client's level of inactivity and the duration of inactivity. The client may experience a combination of these, such as being maximally inactive for a minimal duration. Assessment parameters and interventions should reflect the most aggressive category.

LEVEL OF INACTIVITY. The level of inactivity can be categorized as minimal, moderate, or maximal. A client with minimal inactivity can move about freely within the confines of prescribed rest (in bed or a chair) or in a wheelchair. A client with moderate inactivity can move in the bed or chair but moves slowly, infrequently, or only with assistance. A client with maximal inactivity does not move or is incapable of moving in the bed or chair.

DURATION OF INACTIVITY. Duration can also be categorized as minimal, moderate, or maximal. A minimal duration is short and measured in hours. Moderate duration typically

means inactivity that lasts for days. Maximal duration typically means inactivity that lasts for weeks, months, or years.

Related Factors. The primary related factors for *Risk for disuse syndrome* are the client's level of inactivity and the duration of inactivity. However, other related factors contribute to the risk as well. If the client has one or more of these factors, you will need to increase the frequency of your assessments and the aggressiveness of your interventions to prevent the complications of disuse syndrome. To help remember these risk factors, use the mnemonic ABCDE, which stands for age, body weight, chronic illness, discomfort, and environment.

Using this method of risk assessment, how would you assess Mr. Jackson's risk for disuse problems?

AGE. Age-related changes occur in all systems, making them more prone to deterioration resulting from disuse. For example, an older adult's skin may become dry, fragile, and more easily damaged by shear or pressure. Additionally, the frail older adult may be undernourished from not eating balanced meals because of difficulty obtaining or preparing food.

BODY WEIGHT. The decreased defenses of a malnourished client raise the risk for complications from disuse. A reduced red blood cell count (anemia) decreases the oxygen available to the tissues and causes generalized fatigue. Reduced levels of white blood cells (leukopenia) decrease the immune system's ability to fight off infections. Breakdown may occur because the skin is less resistant to pressure and shearing forces. Ulcers form more easily in older adults because of the loss of subcutaneous fat.

The weight of an obese client places excessive pressure on bony prominences and may raise the risk for pressure ulcers. Joint changes stem from the increased weight as well, making mobility difficult. The overweight client experiences increased efforts to breathe, which may cause respiratory changes.

CHRONIC ILLNESS. Many chronic illnesses can increase the risk for complications from disuse. For example, diseases such as renal failure, cancer, and diabetes (which interfere with metabolic processes) increase the risk for disuse complications. Diseases such as heart disease, respiratory disease, and anemia (which interfere with the transport of oxygen) must also be considered. Neurological problems must be added to the list because they commonly decrease mobility.

DISCOMFORT. A client with discomfort or pain is typically reluctant to move and instead prefers to lie quietly in bed. This compounds the risk for disuse by creating further inactivity. Adequate pain relief can help offset the effects of this risk factor, especially if relief is attained before a scheduled activity.

ENVIRONMENT. Wrinkled sheets or pillows increase the risk for skin breakdown and ulceration by causing uneven pressure on the skin. Excoriation of the skin occurs when the client is exposed to wound drainage, urine, or feces. The enzymes and altered pH of the drainage irritate and chemically burn the skin. Constant contact with a bed made wet by perspiration causes maceration of the skin. Hard surfaces increase the interface pressure, causing the skin to become ischemic and necrotic.

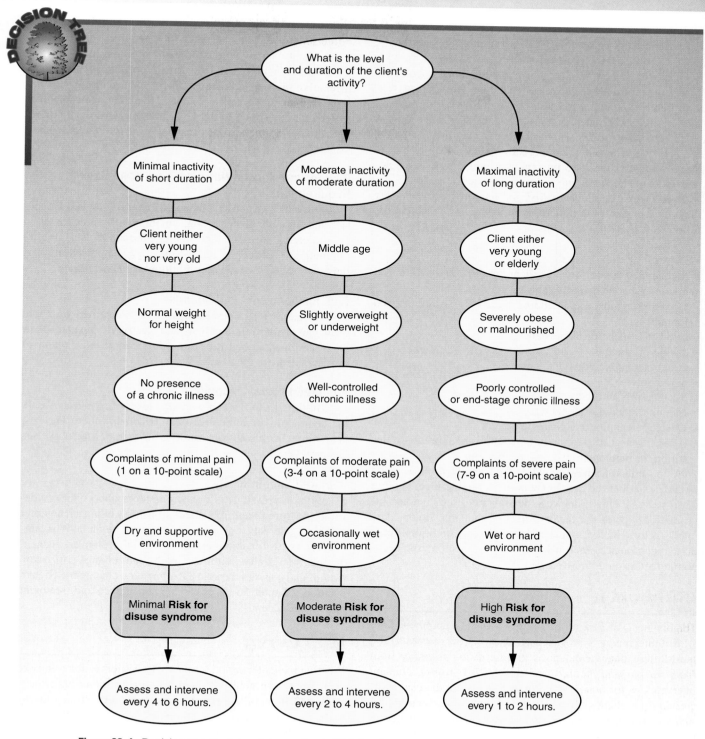

Figure 32-4. Decision tree for determining a client's Risk for disuse syndrome. Diagnoses are shown in rectangles. Within these rectangles, diagnoses shown in **bold** type are NANDA-approved nursing diagnoses; diagnoses shown in regular type are not NANDA-approved nuring diagnoses.

Mr. Jackson is middle-aged, and he has moderate inactivity of moderate duration, normal to slightly increased body weight, no chronic illnesses, minimal discomfort, and low environment risk. These characteristics yield a moderate *Risk for disuse syndrome.* How often should he receive assessment and intervention?

Focused Assessment for
Risk for Impaired Skin Integrity

Assessing your client's risk for developing pressure ulcers is an important nursing role. To help determine your client's risk, use a systematic risk assessment tool. Such tools include the

Norton scale, the Gosnell scale, and the Knoll assessment tool. One of the most commonly used and highly reliable tools is the Braden scale for pressure sore risk (Figure 32-5). It is based on risk factors for clients in a nursing home population.

Using the Braden scale, assess your client in six areas: sensory perception, moisture, activity, mobility, nutrition, and friction and shear. The client's total score may range from 6 to 23. The lower the score, the higher is the client's risk for pressure ulcer development. Agency policy usually dictates that a standard of care to prevent skin breakdown be implemented once the score falls below a predetermined level.

Risk factors common to *Risk for impaired skin integrity* may be internal or external. External factors include the following:

- Radiation
- Physical immobilization
- Mechanical factors, such as shear, pressure, and restraints
- Hypothermia or hyperthermia
- Exposure to moisture, including excretions, secretions, and humidity
- Exposure to chemical substances
- Young or old age

Internal factors include the following:

- Medications
- Skeletal prominence
- Immunological problems
- Developmental or psychogenic factors
- Altered sensation, circulation, metabolism, skin turgor, nutrition, or pigmentation

A conceptual framework called the *web of causation* helps in understanding the development of a pressure ulcer (Figure 32-6, p. 812). This framework demonstrates the complex interrelationships of the factors affecting the skin. It considers many factors, including the client's clinical condition, nutrition, incontinence, mobility, activity, motivation, socioeconomic factors, and knowledge.

DIAGNOSIS

The diagnosis of *Risk for disuse syndrome* is a comprehensive way of intervening to prevent deterioration from inactivity. You must differentiate the diagnosis *Risk for disuse syndrome* from *Impaired physical mobility* and *Activity intolerance.* Nursing interventions for *Impaired physical mobility* are directed at increasing the client's ability to move about. Interventions for *Activity intolerance* are focused on the client's endurance in performing activities. However, because immobility and lack of endurance are risk factors for disuse, these two diagnoses are often written with the *related to* phrase.

With inactivity and immobility, the client's list of problems or potential problems may be long. Instead of writing multiple diagnoses to accommodate this list, the diagnosis *Risk for disuse syndrome* ensures a comprehensive approach.

Mr. Jackson would have the nursing diagnosis *Risk for disuse syndrome* related to prescribed rest secondary to left knee injury and left clavicle break.

Related Nursing Diagnoses
Powerlessness

A client who is confined to bed, paralyzed, or in traction for a broken bone is helpless. A nurse or caregiver needs to meet all of this person's needs. The mere need to use the bathroom or bedpan requires assistance. The client is unable even to get a glass of water to drink. This feeling of loss of control over the basic functions of life can be frustrating and embarrassing.

Risk for Imbalanced Nutrition: Less Than Body Requirements

With a lack of activity, decreased energy, slowed peristalsis, and abdominal distention, an immobilized client often fails to eat an adequate diet. The client complains of not being hungry or of feeling full too quickly. The person may eat only 20% or 30% of the diet. Fluid intake is decreased.

Risk for Deficient Fluid Volume

The inability to obtain fluids or the decreased desire to drink can result in fluid deficits and electrolyte imbalances. A client confined to bed relies on you or another caregiver to provide adequate fluid (see Chapter 25).

Impaired Physical Mobility

Multiple factors affect a client's level of mobility. Assess the degree to which the client can become mobile. The best prevention for disuse syndrome is to maintain activity (see Chapter 31).

Impaired Skin Integrity

With decreased activity, there is more opportunity to develop pressure ulcers if a client's position is not changed at sufficient intervals to prevent excess pressure on bony prominences. Assess for skin breakdown. Do a thorough assessment of the skin daily with the bath and change of linen. Additionally, assess the skin each time you change the client's position. Chapter 26 describes the appearance and treatment of pressure ulcers.

PLANNING

Whether a client's period of inactivity is short or long, the expected outcome goal is to prevent complications from inactivity and immobility. The primary prevention strategy is to maintain activity. Expected outcomes for *Risk for disuse syndrome* are that the client will do the following:

- Participate in decision making about self-care
- Have intact skin and mucous membranes
- Maintain full range of motion of joints
- Maintain optimum cardiac and respiratory function
- Maintain optimal patterns of elimination
- Maintain orientation to person, place, and time
- Consume calories and nutrients to meet energy requirements and promote healing
- Maintain contact with the outer world consistent with physical ability

BRADEN SCALE
For Predicting Pressure Sore Risk

Patient's Name _____ Evaluator's Name _____ Date of Assessment _____

SENSORY PERCEPTION ability to respond meaningfully to pressure-related discomfort	**1. Completely Limited** Unresponsive (does not moan, flinch, or grasp) to painful stimuli, due to diminished level of consciousness or sedation. OR limited ability to feel pain over most of body	**2. Very Limited** Responds only to painful stimuli. Cannot communicate discomfort except by moaning or restlessness OR has a sensory impairment which limits the ability to feel pain or discomfort over ½ of body.	**3. Slightly Limited** Responds to verbal commands, but cannot always communicate discomfort or the need to be turned. OR has some sensory impairment which limits ability to feel pain or discomfort in 1 or 2 extremities.	**4. No Impairment** Responds to verbal commands. Has no sensory deficit which would limit ability to feel or voice pain or discomfort..
MOISTURE degree to which skin is exposed to moisture	**1. Constantly Moist** Skin is kept moist almost constantly by perspiration, urine, etc. Dampness is detected every time patient is moved or turned.	**2. Very Moist** Skin is often, but not always moist. Linen must be changed at least once a shift.	**3. Occasionally Moist:** Skin is occasionally moist, requiring an extra linen change approximately once a day.	**4. Walks Frequently** Walks outside the room at least twice a day and inside room at least once every 2 hours during waking hours.
ACTIVITY degree of physical activity	**1. Bedfast** Confined to bed.	**2. Chairfast** Ability to walk severely limited or non-existent. Cannot bear own weight and/or must be assisted into chair or wheelchair.	**3. Walks Occasionally** Walks occasionally during day, but for very short distances, with or without assistance. Spends majority of each shift in bed or chair	**4. Walks Frequently** Walks outside room at least twice a day and inside room at least once every two hours during waking hours
MOBILITY ability to change and control body position	**1. Completely Immobile** Does not make even slight changes in body or extremity position without assistance	**2. Very Limited** Makes occasional slight changes in body or extremity position but unable to make frequent or significant changes independently.	**3. Slightly Limited** Makes frequent though slight changes in body or extremity position independently.	**4. No Limitation** Makes major and frequent changes in position without assistance.
NUTRITION usual food intake pattern	**1. Very Poor** Never eats a complete meal. Rarely eats more than ⅓ of any food offered. Eats 2 servings or less of protein (meat or dairy products) per day. Takes fluids poorly. Does not take a liquid dietary supplement OR is NPO and/or maintained on clear liquids or IV's for more than 5 days.	**2. Probably Inadequate** Rarely eats a complete meal and generally eats only about ½ of any food offered. Protein intake includes only 3 servings of meat or dairy products per day. Occasionally will take a dietary supplement. OR receives less than optimum amount of liquid diet or tube feeding	**3. Adequate** Eats over half of most meals. Eats a total of 4 servings of protein (meat, dairy products) per day. Occasionally will refuse a meal, but will usually take a supplement when offered OR is on a tube feeding or TPN regimen which probably meets most of nutritional needs	**4. Excellent** Eats most of every meal. Never refuses a meal. Usually eats a total of 4 or more servings of meat and dairy products. Occasionally eats between meals. Does not require supplementation.
FRICTION & SHEAR	**1. Problem** Requires moderate to maximum assistance in moving. Complete lifting without sliding against sheets is impossible. Frequently slides down in bed or chair, requiring frequent repositioning with maximum assistance. Spasticity, contractures or agitation leads to almost constant friction	**2. Potential Problem** Moves feebly or requires minimum assistance. During a move skin probably slides to some extent against sheets, chair, restraints or other devices. Maintains relatively good position in chair or bed most of the time but occasionally slides down.	**3. No Apparent Problem** Moves in bed and in chair independently and has sufficient muscle strength to lift up completely during move. Maintains good position in bed or chair.	

Total Score _____

© Copyright Barbara Braden and Nancy Bergstrom, 1988

Figure 32-5. Braden scale for predicting pressure sore risk. (Courtesy Barbara Braden and Nancy Bergstrom, 1988.)

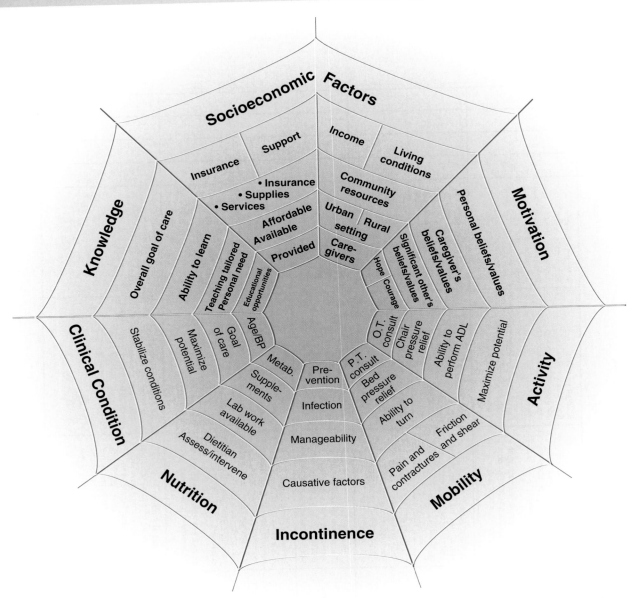

Figure 32-6. The web of causation of pressure ulcer development. (Redrawn with permission from Barbara Oot-Giromini, RN, MS, CETN, Binghamton, NY.)

INTERVENTION

The most important nursing intervention to prevent the complications of disuse syndrome is to keep the client as active and mobile as possible.

Interventions to Prevent Musculoskeletal Disuse

You should position and move the client in bed to maintain maximal function of the joints, stimulate circulation, maximize respiration, and prevent skin breakdown.

Maintain Readiness for Activity. Activity is a priority in preventing the complications of disuse. Make sure that the activity is appropriate to the client's condition and age. Working as a team with the physician, physical therapist, and others,

you will implement a plan of progressive activity that may include some or all of the following interventions. If the client has pain, remember to provide pain relief before engaging in these or any other activities.

- Perform passive, assisted, or active range-of-motion exercises for all joints, in sets of 5 to 10, three times daily. Active range of motion, in which the client moves the limbs rather than having them moved, provides the best level of activity for both muscles and joints.
- A passive range-of-motion machine (Figure 32-7) is prescribed after orthopedic knee or hip surgery to maintain continuous joint motion. Maintain the device at the prescribed speed and degree of joint flexion. Use of continuous passive motion not only maintains range of motion, it actually reduces postsurgical pain.

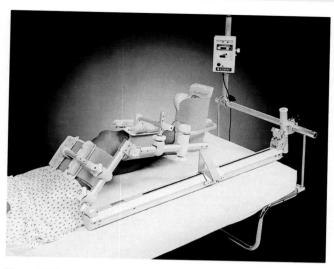

Figure 32-7. A passive range-of-motion, or continuous passive motion, device. (From Phipps, W. J., et al. [2003]. *Medical-surgical nursing: Health and illness perspectives* [7th ed.]. St Louis, MO: Mosby.)

- Perform range-of-motion exercises against resistance. Foot, ankle, and leg exercises can be done every 1 or 2 hours and before changing from a lying position to a sitting position. These exercises include range of motion movements for the ankles and toes, and pushing the feet against a footboard or the end of the bed for about 1 or 2 minutes. A footboard is a board placed at the foot of the bed, perpendicular to the mattress, to prevent the feet from plantar flexion in the supine or Fowler's position.
- Encourage other isometric exercises. Tell the client to tighten his muscles while in bed or in a chair, especially the abdominal muscles used for bowel elimination and the gluteal and quadriceps muscles used for ambulation. Kegel exercises strengthen the perineum muscles. Teach the client to tighten, hold, and release the perineal muscles 10 times, three times daily. This can be done also during voiding. Remember that isometric exercises help maintain muscle strength but not joint integrity.
- Encourage the client to perform ADLs independently, such as the self-care activities of bathing and combing hair. Encourage the client to move independently in bed using the side rails or trapeze.
- With a physician's order, get clients out of bed. While they stand, have them begin to shift their weight back and forth, rocking on both feet. Have them walk to a chair and sit, three times daily. Encourage them to be in the chair as long as they can tolerate sitting. An initial goal would be 30 to 45 minutes. As possible, have clients ambulate with assistance or with an assistive device (such as a walker, cane, or quad cane) four times daily or as much as possible. As the clients progress, encourage them to be up most of the day with ad lib activity.

Action Alert! Prevent the complications of disuse with an aggressive intervention of progressive activity.

Maintain Body Alignment. While in a bed, chair, or wheelchair (or while walking), the client should be positioned in good body alignment. When positioning a client who is unable to move, position the joints in anatomic or functional alignment. Provide support above and below the joints. Alternate the positions frequently, using side-lying, Sims', semisupine, supine, and Fowler's. The prone position is also therapeutic but is rarely used in clinical practice, especially if the client has some type of respiratory impairment (Box 32-2, p. 814).

Action Alert! Perform range-of-motion exercises on each joint to prevent contractures in the client who is immobile. Inactive muscles will contract and become inflexible. The joints will become fixed in a flexed position, making ADLs almost impossible to perform.

Change the client's position every 1 to 2 hours throughout the day and night. Make sure that all joints are positioned in extension (neutral) or in a functional position whenever possible and that you have taken proper precautions (Table 32-1, p. 815). If a joint is in flexion for a period of time, perform active or passive range-of-motion exercises before the next position change. Use positioning devices such as foam boots or high-top tennis shoes, footboards, hand mitts, hand rolls or supports, eggcrate pads, over-bed cradles, **trochanter rolls,** wrist splints, and heel protectors to keep joints in alignment while the client is in bed (Box 32-3, p. 816).

When the client is sitting in a chair, the head should be up, and the shoulders should be back. The arms should be supported to prevent pulling on the shoulders. Make sure that the feet are resting comfortably on the floor or are elevated on a footstool. When it is possible, the client should walk with the head up and facing forward, shoulders back, and feet forward.

Interventions to Reduce the *Risk for Impaired Skin Integrity*

Skin care is influenced by culture, education, socioeconomic status, religion, and individual preference. You should respect the client's desires while trying to prevent skin complications caused by disuse. Several strategies should be used to prevent skin impairments, including activities to monitor the client, cleanse the skin, provide nutrition, reposition the client, and encourage the client to maintain ADLs. Client teaching is also valuable in preventing development of some skin problems.

Monitor the Client. Skin assessment is essential in identifying the client at risk. Perform skin assessment at least once a day, paying special attention to bony prominences.

One of the most important aspects of preventing *Impaired skin integrity* is recognizing which clients are at risk (Box 32-4, p. 818). Also consider environmental factors in the at-risk client. For instance, prolonged supine positioning on a stretcher in the emergency department, skin moisture caused by diaphoresis, and wrinkled bed linens can put a client's skin integrity at risk. When caring for a surgical client, monitor all tubes, catheters, and drains because these may cause skin breakdown or exert excessive pressure on the client's skin.

Box 32-2 Common Client Positions

LATERAL, SEMIPRONE, AND SEMISUPINE POSITIONS

- In the lateral (side-lying) position, the trunk is at a right angle to the bed. To increase the base of support and comfort, one or both legs are bent, and both arms are extended in front of the body. Because the body weight is borne on the shoulders and hips, the semiprone or the semisupine position is preferred.

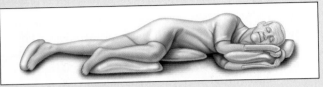

Lateral (side-lying) position.

- In the semiprone position (the Sims' or forward side-lying position), the trunk is rotated 15 to 30 degrees forward from the lateral position, with the superior arm and leg supported in front of the body to form part of the base of support.

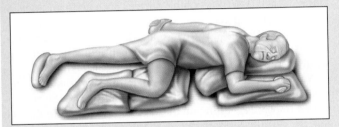

Semiprone (Sims' or forward side-lying) position.

- In the semisupine position (the modified lateral or oblique position), the trunk is rotated 15 to 30 degrees from supine, with the superior arm and leg supported in a comfortable position. The semiprone and semisupine positions minimize pressure on bony prominences of the shoulder and hip.

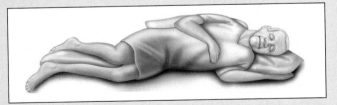

Semisupine (modified lateral or oblique) position, which can be used as a substitute for the side-lying position and results in less pressure on the trochanteric area.

SUPINE AND FOWLER'S POSITIONS

- Both the supine and Fowler's positions are back-lying positions. Supine is a horizontal position, and Fowler's is a sitting position. The supine position prevents lordosis or kyphosis.
- In high Fowler's position, the head of the client's bed is elevated to 90 degrees. In semi-Fowler's position, it is elevated to 45 degrees. In low

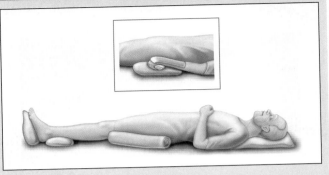

Supine position, including the use of the footboard, trochanter roll, and lumbar support. **Inset:** Correct positioning of the client's arm, which is elevated and has a wrist support.

Fowler's position, it is elevated about 30 degrees. Usually, the client's knees are bent slightly.
- Fowler's position concentrates body weight on the sacrum and creates shearing force. Reducing the angle and the time in the position are preventive measures. Prevent hip and knee contractures by instructing the client to shift positions and perform range-of-motion exercises.

PRONE POSITION

- In the prone position, the client lies front down with his face turned to the side and one or both arms turned up, as shown. This position may be contraindicated in the presence of abdominal distention or wounds

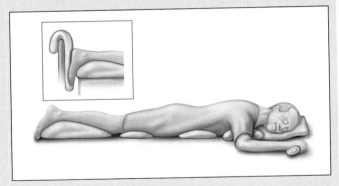

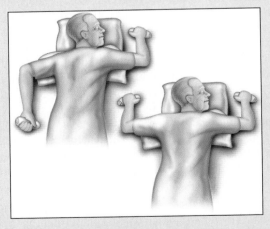

Prone position. The client's arms and shoulders may be positioned in internal or external rotation.

Table 32-1 | Precautions for Proper Positioning

Lateral Position, Semiprone Position, Semisupine Position	Supine Position, Fowler's Position	Prone Position
HEAD AND NECK		
• Prevent forward flexion of head, neck, and cervical spine. • Prevent lateral bending of head, neck, and cervical spine.	• Prevent forward flexion of head, neck, and cervical spine. • Prevent lateral bending of head, neck, and cervical spine. • Avoid pressure on back of head.	• Prevent hyperextension, lateral bending, and pressure on cheek and ear.
SHOULDERS		
• Avoid direct pressure on acromion process. • Prevent adduction of shoulders. • Avoid skin-to-skin contact of axillae.	• Prevent forward flexion. • Avoid pressure on scapulae. • Avoid skin-to-skin contact at axillae by abducting shoulders slightly.	• Prevent forward flexion of neck. • Avoid skin-to-skin contact at axillae.
BREASTS AND MALE GENITALIA		
	• Prevent skin-to-skin contact in presence of moisture.	• Avoid abdominal pressure.
ELBOWS AND WRISTS		
• Prevent flexion or hyperextension. • Avoid pressure on thorax and ribs from upper arms. • Avoid pressure on lateral condyle of humerus. • Prevent edema.	• Prevent flexion. • Prevent edema. • Avoid pressure on elbow.	• Prevent flexion by positioning elbows in extension.
FINGERS AND THUMB		
• Prevent flexion and opposition of fingers and thumb.	• Prevent flexion and opposition of fingers and thumb.	• Prevent flexion and opposition of fingers and thumb.
SPINE		
• Prevent lateral bending. • Prevent rotation.	• Prevent flexion of lumbar spine. • Prevent lateral bending (shoulders and hips in alignment). • Avoid pressure on lumbosacral area.	• Prevent hyperextension of lumbar spine by using a firm mattress or lumbar support.
HIPS AND KNEES		
• Prevent adduction, flexion, and internal rotation of upper leg. • Avoid pressure on iliac crest. • Avoid skin-to-skin contact at perineum.	• Prevent adduction, flexion, and internal rotation of upper legs. • Avoid prolonged flexion. • Avoid skin-to-skin contact at perineum. • Avoid compression of popliteal artery.	• Prevent internal rotation. • Avoid pressure on patella and anterior iliac spine. • Avoid skin-to-skin contact at perineum.
ANKLES AND TOES		
• Prevent inversion and plantar flexion of upper foot. • Avoid pressure on ankle of lower foot.	• Prevent plantar flexion. • Avoid pressure on toes and heels.	• Prevent plantar flexion. • Avoid pressure on toes.

Cleanse the Skin. Keep the client's skin clean. Be sure it is cleansed immediately after soiling and at routine intervals. During cleansing, minimize force and friction to the skin to help prevent skin breakdown. Try to reduce the client's exposure to moisture caused by incontinence, perspiration, and wound drainage. Keep in mind that exposure to moisture may cause skin maceration or breakdown.

If a client is bedridden, a bed bath is indicated. The client can still participate in the bath, however, by performing it as independently as possible. Avoid the use of powder because it may retain moisture and can cause pulmonary damage if inhaled.

INCREASE CIRCULATION. Increase circulation to the skin to enhance transport of nutrients and oxygen to cells in the skin. Increase the temperature in the room to a comfortable level. Use a bath blanket while bathing the client, and keep the bath water between 105° and 110° F to prevent chilling and vasoconstriction.

Action Alert! Do not use hot water and soap to cleanse the client's skin. Tailor the plan for skin cleansing on the basis of the client's preferences and skin care needs.

Box 32-3	**Positioning Devices**

Foam boots or high-top tennis shoes.

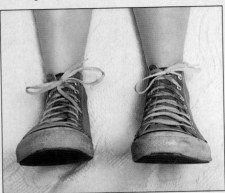

Footboard.

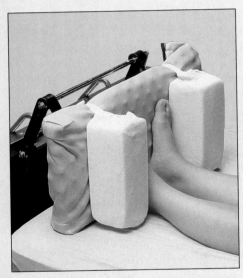

(Courtesy J.T. Posey Co., Arcadia, CA.)

Hand mitt.

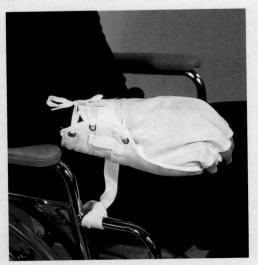

(Courtesy Medline Industries, Mundelein, IL.)

Foam boots or high-top tennis shoes to keep the ankle in dorsiflexion.

Board placed at the end of bed, perpendicular to the mattress, to prevent the feet from assuming plantar flexion in the supine or Fowler's position. May be used for isometric exercises of the foot and leg to prevent deep vein thrombosis.

Mitten that slides over the fingers to keep the fingers from flexion and the thumb from opposition.

Box 32-3   Positioning Devices—cont'd

Hand roll/support.

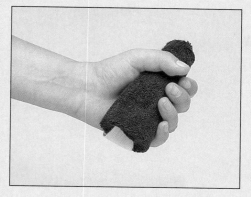

(Courtesy J.T. Posey Co., Arcadia, CA.)

Roll of cloth or manufactured hand grip placed in the palm of the hand used to keep the fingers from flexion and the thumb from opposition.

Over-bed cradle.

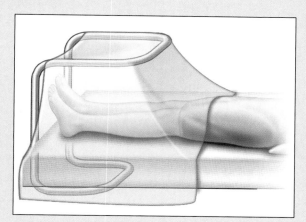

Device placed at the end of the bed to raise the top sheet and thus prevent pressure ulcers on the toes and plantar flexion of the ankles.

Trochanter roll.

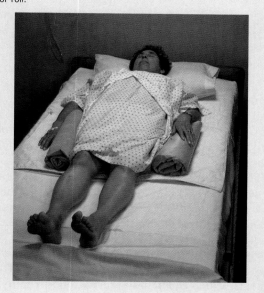

Sheet placed halfway under a client's hip and rolled snugly against the hip to prevent external rotation of the trochanter (hip joint).

| **Box 32-3** | **Positioning Devices—cont'd** |

Wrist splint.

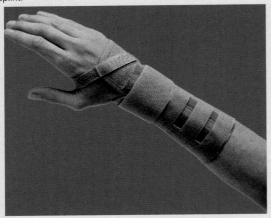

(Courtesy North Coast Medical, San José, CA.)

Support placed on the client's wrist to prevent flexion.

Heel protectors.

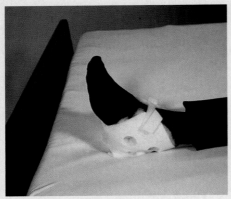

(Courtesy Medline Industries, Mundelein, IL.)

Sheepskin or other padded device to prevent skin breakdown at the heels.

| **Box 32-4** | **Conditions That Increase the Risk for Impaired Skin Integrity** |

- Advanced age
- Altered level of consciousness
- Chronic conditions that limit physical mobility
- Dehydration
- Diabetes
- Fractures
- Short-term or long-term immobility
- Impaired circulation
- Deficient nutrition
- Incontinence
- Multisystem trauma
- Obesity
- Paralysis

Action Alert! Avoid massaging over bony prominences where early signs of pressure ulcers are present. Also, do not massage the legs; this could increase the risk for pulmonary embolism if a deep vein thrombosis is forming.

To minimize dry skin, apply topical moisturizing agents and maintain adequate skin hydration. Keep in mind that although the client may find a gentle massage relaxing and soothing, you must use caution when applying creams and lotions to high-risk or reddened skin areas.

Elevate the client's arms on pillows. If the client cannot brush his own hair, offer to do so twice a day. If the client is cold, offer extra blankets, socks, and other warm clothing. Encourage the client to perform ADLs to increase blood circulation.

DECREASE MICROORGANISMS. Removing dead skin cells decreases the growth and accumulation of microorganisms, which can help to prevent skin irritation and infection and reduce body odor. Most clients need to cleanse the skin in some manner each day and any time

Gently massage the skin but avoid areas that are reddened or are over bony prominences to avoid additional injury. Use long, firm, strokes, and move from distal to proximal areas during the bath. Encourage the client to participate in ADLs to increase blood circulation.

they become soiled. Older adults may need only a partial bath of the back and perineum.

REMOVE EXCESS MOISTURE. To help keep the skin dry, make sure that bed linens are breathable cotton, not plastic. Dry the client's skin well after bathing, particularly in areas where the skin folds over on itself, such as at the axillae, under the breasts, and in the perineal area. Change the client's bed linens immediately if they become wet from diaphoresis (sweating) or incontinence, and bathe the client. Position the client to allow air to circulate to the axillae and perineal areas.

Remember that, although dry skin discourages the growth of microorganisms, overly dry skin can crack open and form lesions. To help the skin from becoming too dry, use a moisturizing lotion after baths. Do not use soap every day for bathing unless it is very mild; clear water may be used instead. Do not use alcohol on the skin because it has a drying effect and can crack the skin.

DECREASE FRICTION AND EXCORIATION. Friction and excoriation can alter the skin's function as a protective barrier. To decrease the risk for friction and excoriation, gently pat the client's skin dry rather than rubbing with a towel after baths. Use a soft washcloth and soft towels during the bath. Linens should be soft and smooth as well. Use a turning sheet (also called a draw sheet) or trapeze when moving the client in bed. Lift clients, rather than dragging them, when moving them in bed. Use extra help to move clients if needed.

Use protective ointment around wounds or on the client's perineum, as needed. According to the physician's order, change the client's wound dressings frequently. Take care when removing the tape. Place a drainage bag on wounds as needed. Check casts, braces, traction, restraints, and splints for irritation.

Provide Nutrition. Promote nutrition and a well-balanced diet. This will help prevent skin breakdown and pressure ulcer development (see Chapters 23 and 24).

Position the Client Properly. Positioning the client at risk for skin breakdown is one of your major roles. You can reduce the risk for skin breakdown with various positioning strategies, including the following:
• Reposition high-risk clients at least every 2 hours.
• Use positioning devices such as pillows to keep bony prominences from touching one another.
• Raise the client's heels completely off the bed.

Action Alert! Do not use doughnut devices to relieve pressure on the client's heels. Instead, suspend the heels off the bed to prevent pressure ulcers there.

• Avoid placing the client's body weight directly on the trochanter when a side-lying position is used. Instead, position the client at a 30-degree angle to reduce pressure on both the trochanter and the sacrum (Figure 32-8).
• Keep the head of the bed as low as the client can tolerate; sacral pressure is reduced when head of bed is 30 degrees or lower.

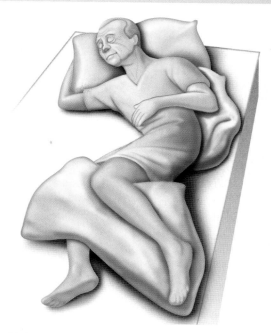

Figure 32-8. Position the client on his or her side at a 30-degree angle to prevent pressure on the trochanter and sacrum. To keep the client in this position, provide support with pillows, as shown.

• When moving the client, use proper positioning, transferring, and turning techniques to minimize friction and shear. For example, use assistive devices such as a trapeze or the bed linens. Consider using lubricants (such as creams and cornstarch), protective films (such as a transparent dressing), and protective devices to help reduce friction.
• Avoid prolonged sitting in a chair or wheelchair by repositioning the client at least every hour.
• Develop a written plan of care for positioning and turning.

PREVENT SHEAR. Placing the head of the bed in a low or flat position reduces the gravitational pull and helps keep the client from sliding down in the bed. As a result, it prevents shearing of the skin on the client's lower back. Lifting the client (rather than dragging) and using a turning sheet helps to prevent shear injuries as well. As needed, ask for help from co-workers when turning or moving a client in bed (Procedure 32-1, p. 822). Limit the time the client spends in Fowler's position to 30 to 60 minutes. During that time, use a footboard, and support the client's arms on pillows.

DECREASE PRESSURE. To relieve pressure, turn the client to a new position every 1 to 2 hours. To ensure pressure relief, follow a 24-hour turning schedule (side to back to other side to supine). Encourage a client who can sit in a chair to shift position every 15 minutes or to do pushups on the arms of the chair.

Action Alert! Reposition the client on bed rest every 1 to 2 hours, keep the bed dry and wrinkle free, and keep the client dry to help prevent pressure ulcers.

THE STATE OF NURSING RESEARCH: Protecting the Body's Largest Organ
Box 32-5

What Are the Issues?

The skin is the largest organ in the body. It protects the person from infection and acts as a major sense organ. Prolonged pressure on the skin can reduce blood flow and cause ischemic damage. Breaks in the skin then allow microorganisms to enter, putting the person at risk for local and systemic infection. Institutionalized older adults are at risk for impaired skin integrity, as are people who have impaired mobility. Nurses are constantly on the lookout for ways to prevent skin breakdown in such clients. One method of reducing the risk for pressure ulcers is to position the client on an alternative surface. Equipment to accomplish this comes in many forms and is marketed as a way to reduce pressure ulcers. Research is needed to demonstrate which types of equipment are most effective in reducing pressure ulcer development.

What Research Has Been Conducted?

Russell (2001) reviewed the literature on pressure-reducing surfaces, including (1) studies that used healthy volunteers and measured interface pressure changes on points of contact, (2) case studies that described changes in clients after using the new products, and (3) randomized clinical trials (RCTs) that attempted to control for extraneous influences. An RCT is considered the strongest research design for intervention studies. One RCT was a pilot study of the effects of different types of pressure-reducing seat cushions used by older adults in wheelchairs (Geyer, Brienza, Karg, Trefler, & Kelsey, 2001). The researchers studied at-risk older adult residents at a nursing home who were able to sit in a wheelchair at least 6 hours a day. Participants were randomly assigned to the control (foam cushion) or treatment (variety of commercial types) group. The staff that collected pressure ulcer measurements did not know which type of cushion each resident used. This "blind" study is a way to reduce bias and ensure more accurate results.

What Has the Research Concluded?

Most of the studies reviewed by Russell (2001) had flaws and the results cannot be relied on for clinical guidance. There seems to be some effect on the incidence of pressure ulcers, but sample sizes were too small to show statistical significance. The pilot study by Geyer et al. (2001) demonstrated a decrease in ischial pressure ulcers and helped the researchers decide how many subjects to use in a subsequent larger study. They also found that interface pressures were helpful in identifying people at risk for pressure ulcer development.

What Is the Future of Research in This Area?

There is a critical need to explore the use of pressure-reducing products used by clients while seated in chairs. A large-scale study of such devices is planned to fill this need (Geyer et al., 2001). Cost factors need to be included in such studies to help institutions make informed decisions. The cost analysis should include savings seen when pressure ulcers are prevented, as well as quality-of-life measures from the point of view of the client.

References

Geyer, M. J., Brienza, D. M., Karg, P., Trefler, E., & Kelsey, S. (2001). A randomized control trial to evaluate pressure-reducing seat cushions for elderly wheelchair users. *Advances in Skin & Wound Care, 14*(3), 120.

Russell, L. (2001). Overview of research to investigate pressure-relieving surfaces. *British Journal of Nursing, 10*(21), 1421.

If needed, have the client set a timer to remember to shift weight. Remember that standard mattresses exert considerable pressure against the skin. As needed, use a special mattress to reduce the pressure, such as an eggcrate, foam, sheepskin, gel, flotation, or waterbed. Keep the bed linens and pillows free of wrinkles.

Use Support Surfaces When Indicated. Support surfaces are therapeutic devices used to control pressure and protect bony prominences. These devices serve many functions, including reducing pressure, friction, and shear, controlling moisture, and inhibiting bacterial growth (Box 32-5). Many support surfaces are available in various sizes and shapes for use on beds and in chairs (Figure 32-9). Use them in conjunction with meticulous turning and repositioning to prevent development of pressure ulcers and, if indicated, to enhance healing of existing pressure ulcers. Be aware that a hand mitt is also considered a form of restraint, so follow agency policy with regard to its use.

Be aware that no single support surface eliminates the effects of pressure on the skin. Assess your client carefully to determine the most appropriate support surface. Keep in mind that *pressure-relieving devices* reduce the interface pressure

between the body and the support surface below 32 mm Hg (thus capillary closing pressure). *Pressure-reducing devices* also reduce the interface pressure—but not below the capillary closing pressure. Support surface therapy must be tailored to the client's individual needs. Foam overlays that are 3 to 4 inches thick may also help reduce pressure. Support surface characteristics and cost are important factors to consider. Static air overlays—mattresses that are blown up—also serve to reduce pressure. Low-air-loss beds can benefit a client who needs moisture control and prevention of maceration and friction.

Interventions to Maintain Circulatory Function

Interventions are needed to maintain the circulatory status and prevent complications.

Decrease Edema Formation. Unless contraindicated, elevate the clients' legs to counteract gravity and assist with venous return. This position can prevent dependent edema formation and can reduce edema if present. Keep clients' legs at heart level while they are in bed. Place their feet on a footstool while they sit in a chair. Elevate their arms to prevent edema formation or decrease edema in their hands.

Text continued on p. 826

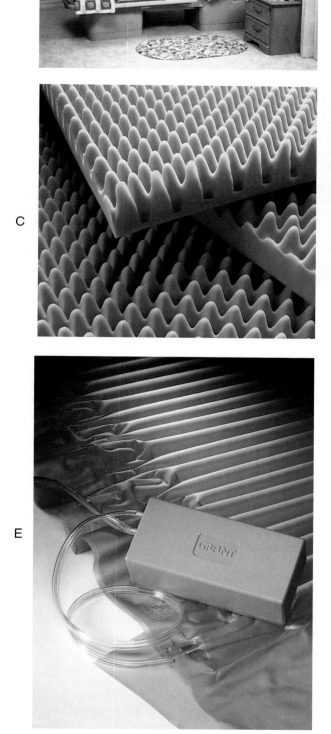

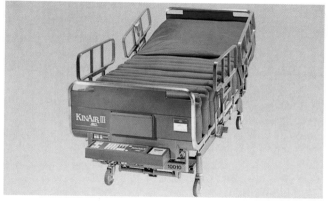

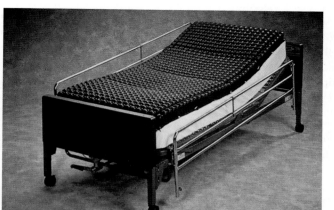

Figure 32-9. Specialty support surfaces. **A,** Air-fluidized bed (Clinitron At-Home Therapeutic Bed). **B,** Low-air-loss (The KinAirIII Bed). **C,** Eggcrate mattress. **D,** Static air mattress (Roho Dry Flotation Mattress System). **E,** Alternating air mattress (Grant Dyna-CARE). (**A** courtesy Hill-Rom Home Care, Charleston, SC; **B** courtesy Kinetic Concepts, San Antonio, TX; **C** courtesy Medline Industries, Mundelein, IL; **D** courtesy Roho Incorporated, Belleville, IL; **E** courtesy Grant Airmass Corporation, Stamford, CT.)

PROCEDURE 32-1   # TURNING AND MOVING A CLIENT IN BED

TIME TO ALLOW
Novice: 10 min.
Expert: 5 min.

Especially for a client with a *Risk for disuse syndrome,* you will need to pay special attention to proper turning and positioning. Often, you will perform these activities on a schedule tailored to the client's condition and needs. Each time, you must follow appropriate steps to avoid injuring the client or yourself. This procedure describes proper methods for turning a client in bed (alone and with another nurse), moving a client up in bed (alone and with another nurse), and transferring a client from bed to stretcher.

DELEGATION GUIDELINES

The routine positioning and repositioning of a client in bed may be delegated to a nursing assistant. For clients with mobility or positioning restrictions, however, you must first assess the client and then determine the appropriateness of delegation on the basis of risk to the client. For a client requiring multiple personnel for turning and moving, you may perform the procedure together with multiple nursing assistants.

EQUIPMENT NEEDED
- Turning sheet
- Pillows or wedges for positioning
- Trapeze
- Transfer board

1. Follow preliminary guidelines for nursing procedures (see inside front cover).

2. Before turning or moving a client in bed or transferring him to a stretcher, lock the bed's wheels and assess the client's condition.
a. Can the client assist with turning, moving, or transferring?
b. Do any joints have contractures or need special handling?
c. Can the client tolerate having the head of the bed lowered briefly?
d. Can you turn or move the client alone, or will you need help from colleagues? *Turning or moving a client alone requires that you be sure you can manage the client's weight. If the procedure requires two or three nurses, one nurse should take charge of the procedure.*

TURNING A CLIENT ALONE

1. Lower the head of the bed and the bed's knee-raising (gatch) device until the bed is flat. Raise the bed to a comfortable working height. *You will be better able to handle the client's weight on a flat surface. Also, the flat position allows you to avoid moving uphill against gravity. Raising the bed height reduces strain on the nurse's back.*

2. Move the client to one side of the bed. *This allows room to turn the client to the opposite side.*
a. First, slide your arms under the client's shoulders and back, and move the client's upper body to one side of the bed (see illustration).

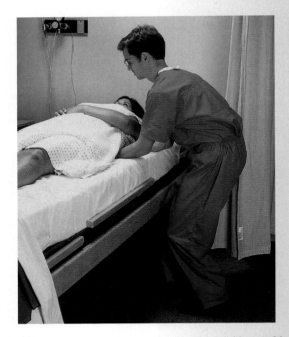

Step 2a. Sliding the arms under the client's shoulders and back.

b. Then, slide your arms under the client's hips, and slide the hips to the side.
c. Finally, move the client's feet and legs to the side of the bed.

3. Cross the client's arms across the chest, and cross the legs at the ankle (see illustration). Position a pillow or wedge at the head or foot of the bed to be used behind the client's back after turning. *Crossing the client's arms and legs helps the body turn as a unit.*

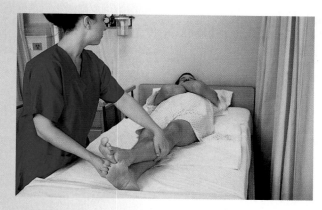

Step 3. Crossing the client's arms and legs.

4. Place one hand on the client's shoulder and the other hand on the client's hip, and roll the client toward you. *Pulling is easier than pushing.*

5. Turn the client far enough forward so that you can release one hand and position a pillow or wedge behind the client's back.

6. You may need to go to the opposite side of the bed and pull the client's hips toward the center of the bed to make the position more stable. Check the position according to Table 32-1 (p. 815).

TURNING A CLIENT WITH ANOTHER NURSE

1. Bring the bed to a comfortable working height. With the bed in a flat position, move the client to one side of the bed. *This allows room to turn the client to the opposite side.*

a. If the client is on a turning sheet (a sheet that extends from the shoulders to below the hips), stand on opposite sides of the bed so that each nurse can grasp the top and bottom of the sheet (see illustration).

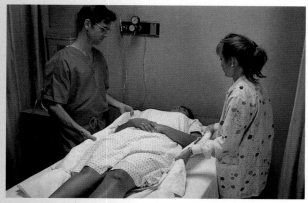

Step 1a. Two nurses grasping the top and bottom of a turning sheet.

b. If the client is not on a turning sheet, both nurses should stand on the same side of the bed. One nurse should slide her arms under the client's shoulders while the other slides her arms under the client's hips. On the count of three, both nurses should slide the client to one side of the bed. *When turning a client, make sure you stand with your knees somewhat bent and your feet spread so that you have a wide base of support.*

2. Bend the client's knee on the side opposite the one to which you will be turning. Fold the client's arms over the chest. One nurse is positioned on each side of the bed.

3. Turn the client.

a. If you do not have a turning sheet, the nurse positioned on the side of the bed toward which the client will turn should place one hand on the client's shoulder and one hand on the client's hip. He then pulls the shoulder and hip toward himself. At the same time, the nurse on the opposite side of the bed slides her hands under the client's bottom hip, pulls the hip toward her, and places a pillow at the client's back (see illustration).

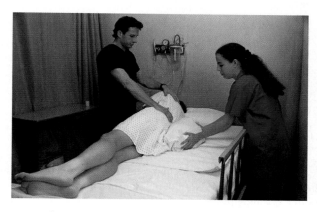

Step 3a. Placing a pillow at the client's back.

b. If you have a turning sheet, use it to pull the client's hips and shoulders in the direction of the turn.

4. Place a pillow between the client's legs (see illustration). *The pillow at the back supports the client in the side-lying*

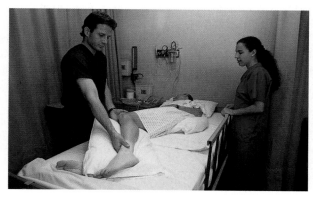

Step 4. Placing a pillow between the client's legs.

PROCEDURE 32-1   TURNING AND MOVING A CLIENT IN BED—CONT'D

position. The pillow between the legs maintains alignment of the spine and hips and prevents skin-to-skin contact.

5. Check the client's position against Table 32-1 (p. 815) to make sure that the client is properly positioned.

6. If the client's condition demands that you maintain anatomic alignment of the spine during turns, you may need three nurses working together to turn the body and head as a unit. The spine is kept straight as the client is turned (see illustration).

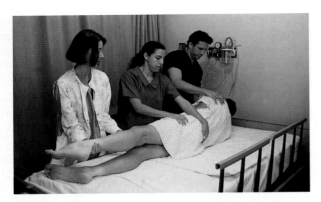

Step 6. Keeping the spine straight as the client is turned.

7. After turning a client, make sure to document that the client was turned. Also document the position assumed. *Proper documentation helps to maintain continuity of care. The next nurses to work with the client will know what positions have been used and the amount of time in the position.*

MOVING A CLIENT UP IN BED

1. Before moving a client up in bed, determine whether you can do it alone or whether you need help from another nurse. If you can do it alone, determine whether to stand at the side of the bed or at the head of the bed. Lower the head of the bed as far as the client can tolerate.

a. For one nurse to assist a client move up in bed from the side of the bed, have the client bend her knees and place her feet flat on the bed so she can push. Place one hand under the client's back and one under the thighs, close to the hips. Tell the client to push with her legs on a count of three. When she does, slide her up toward the head of the bed. (See illustration.)

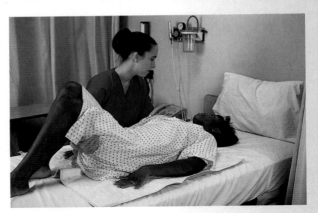

Step 1a. One nurse assisting a client to move up in bed from the side of the bed.

b. For one nurse standing at the head of the bed to move a lightweight client, start by removing the headboard from the bed. Place the bed in a slight Trendelenburg position (head lower than the feet). When possible, use a turning sheet to move the client; otherwise, slide your hands under the client's shoulders, and pull the client toward you. (See illustration.)

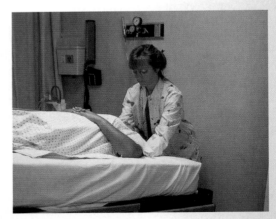

Step 1b. One nurse assisting a client to move up in bed from the head of the bed, using the force of gravity created by a slight Trendelenburg position.

2. If the client has good upper body strength, use a trapeze to move her up in bed.

a. Place a trapeze over the bed.

b. Have the client bend her knees and place her feet flat on the bed so she can push.

c. Have the client hold onto the trapeze and pull with her arms to lift her hips slightly off the bed (see illustration).

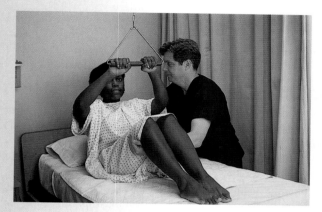

Step 2c. One nurse assisting a client to move up in bed using a trapeze.

d. With hips lifted, have the client push with her legs to move up in bed.
e. You may assist by placing your hands under the client's thighs, close to the hips.

3. If the client is too heavy to move by yourself, get help from a colleague.
a. Stand on opposite sides of the client's bed.
b. With the client's knees bent and feet flat on the bed, each nurse grasps the turn sheet with one hand at the level of the shoulders and the other hand at the level of the hips.
c. On the count of three, the client pushes with the legs as the two nurses slide the torso up in bed (see illustration).

4. After moving the client up, raise the head of the bed, and check the position against Table 32-1 (p. 815).

5. Document that the client was repositioned and the position assumed.

MOVING A CLIENT FROM A BED TO A STRETCHER

1. If a client is unable to move from the bed to a stretcher on his own, you will need to move him.
a. Two caregivers should be positioned on each side of the stretcher.
b. One person should be designated to ensure that the client's head is protected during movement, while another should ensure the feet are protected. *Make sure the wheels are locked on both the bed and the stretcher. Position the bed and stretcher next to each other without any gaps in between.*

2. Use a sheet to make the transfer easier.
a. Untuck the sheet from the client's bed.
b. Have one nurse grasp the sheet under the client's shoulders while another on the same side grasps it at the client's hips and legs. The nurses on the opposite side of the bed should do the same.
c. On a count of three, the nurses on the stretcher side should lift and pull the client onto the stretcher. The nurses on the opposite side of the bed provide minimal assistance because it is more difficult to push than pull.

3. As an alternative, use a transfer board.
a. Two nurses standing on the same side of the bed turn the client away from the stretcher.
b. Place the transfer board where the client was lying, and turn the client back onto the board (see illustration).

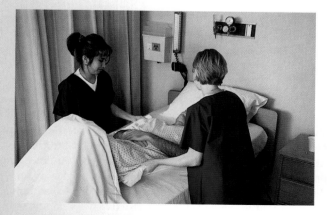

Step 3c. Two nurses assisting a client to move up in bed.

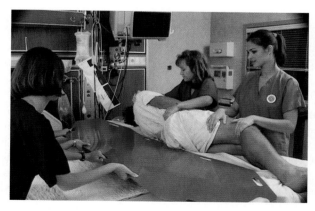

Step 3b. Placing the transfer board where the client was lying.

Continued

PROCEDURE 32-1   TURNING AND MOVING A CLIENT IN BED—CONT'D

c. Pull the board onto the stretcher with the client on it.

d. Turn the client again to remove the board.

4. Raise the side rails on the outside of the stretcher, then move between the bed and stretcher and raise the remaining side rails.

5. If the stretcher cannot be positioned adjacent to the bed but can be positioned at a right angle to the bed, use a three-person lift to transfer the client.

a. Position three nurses on the same side of the bed.

b. One nurse slides her hands and arms under the client's head and shoulders. The second slides his hands under the client's back and buttocks, and the third one slides her hands under the legs and thighs. On the count of three, the nurses simultaneously lift the client. *In this procedure, each nurse bears only a third of the client's weight.*

c. The three nurses then move as a unit to rotate and transfer the client to the stretcher (see illustration).

6. Cover the client with a sheet. Supply a pillow, and raise the head of the stretcher if needed for the client's comfort. Fasten a safety strap over the client. It can be fastened loosely if the client is fully alert. Put side rails up.

HOME CARE CONSIDERATIONS

Work closely with family caregivers to teach methods of turning and methods of preventing back strain in the caregiver. The family must understand the importance of a regular schedule of turning, even through the night. A single caregiver is not sufficient to provide care around the clock to a family member who is unable to turn and move in bed. All family members must understand the importance of skin integrity and agree to participate in maintaining it. Families must also understand that pressure ulcers can form in a chair or wheelchair; the client must periodically shift weight to relieve pressure.

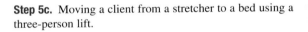

Step 5c. Moving a client from a stretcher to a bed using a three-person lift.

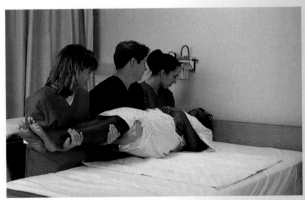

Decrease Blood Stasis. Elastic antiembolism stockings and sequential compression devices can be used to apply external pressure on the client's legs to prevent blood from pooling in the veins. These devices, with the assistance of the calf muscles, "milk" venous blood back up to the heart. They decrease blood stasis and prevent the formation of thrombi and edema.

Antiembolism stockings are elasticized stockings that provide varying degrees of pressures at different areas of the leg. To provide the optimal amount of pressure, the stockings should fit properly and be free of wrinkles. Periodically inspect the feet for evidence of poor circulation, and remove the stockings two to three times daily to inspect the skin (Procedure 32-2).

Leg exercises can supplement the effect of antiembolism stockings in preventing venous stasis. One exercise that can be done by most clients is to flex and extend the foot five times per hour. A second exercise is to bend the knee and draw the foot up to the thigh, then extend the leg again. A third exercise is to raise the leg off the bed, one leg at a time. These exercises can be active or passive.

Sequential compression devices are plastic sleeves that are wrapped around the client's legs. The sleeves have air tubes that are inflated in sequence from the bottom of the leg to the top, helping to move venous blood out of the leg veins and toward the heart (Procedure 32-3, p. 829). Once the client can ambulate, the device is discontinued.

PROCEDURE 32-2 | APPLYING ANTIEMBOLISM STOCKINGS

TIME TO ALLOW
Novice: 20 min.
Expert: 10 min.

Antiembolism stockings increase venous return, decrease venous stasis, and decrease dependent edema by applying external pressure to the lower legs. They are used to prevent deep vein thrombosis.

DELEGATION GUIDELINES

The application and maintenance of antiembolism stockings may be delegated to a nursing assistant who has been properly trained in this skill. Periodic removal of the stockings and inspection of the skin may be delegated to the nursing assistant, with specific attention to findings that necessitate immediate RN notification.

EQUIPMENT NEEDED

- Measuring tape
- Calf-length or thigh-length antiembolism stockings of correct size

1. Follow preliminary guidelines for nursing procedures (see inside front cover).

2. Check physician's orders.

3. Place client supine in bed with the legs horizontal for 15 minutes. After first use, they should be applied daily before getting out of bed. *This prevents blood from pooling in the legs.*

4. Measure the client's legs to determine the correct stocking size.

a. If the client needs calf-length stockings, measure calf circumference and the distance from the foot to the knee (see illustration).

b. If the client needs thigh-length stockings, measure calf and thigh circumference and the distance from the foot to the thigh (see illustration). *Determining the correct size ensures that the client will receive firm support but no restriction of the circulation.*

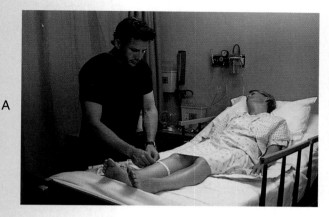
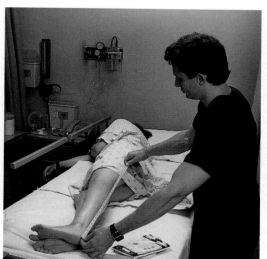

Step 4b. A, Measuring calf circumference. **B,** Measuring foot-to-thigh distance.

Continued

PROCEDURE 32-2 **APPLYING ANTIEMBOLISM STOCKINGS—CONT'D**

5. Place a stocking on the client's foot.

a. Insert one hand into the top of the stocking and slide it down as far as the heel pocket.

b. Grasp the center of the heel pocket and turn the stocking inside-out down to the heel area (see illustration).

6. Pull the body of the stocking up the client's ankle and calf, making sure as you work that there are no wrinkles that could restrict the circulation (see illustration).

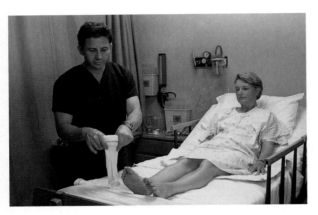

Step 5b. Grasping the center of the heel pocket.

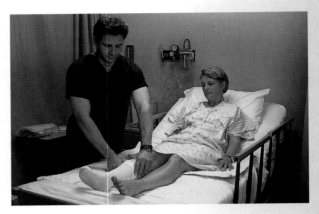

Step 6. Pulling the stocking firmly up the leg.

c. Carefully slide the stocking onto the foot and ankle, making sure that the client's heel is centered in the heel pocket (see illustration).

7. Check the client's toes for pressure. *Pull the stocking away from the toes to release pressure on them.*

8. Repeat with the other leg.

9. Assess the client to make sure the stockings are functioning properly.

a. Make sure the stockings have no wrinkles. *Wrinkles can cause uneven pressure and ulcerations.*

b. Prevent the stockings from rolling down. *Rolls create a tourniquet effect that decreases arterial blood flow and impedes venous return.*

c. Remove the stockings at bath times and before bed to provide skin care and a more complete assessment. Assess the skin for temperature, color, capillary refill, pulses, redness, irritation, and lesions. Ask whether the client feels any tingling or numbness.

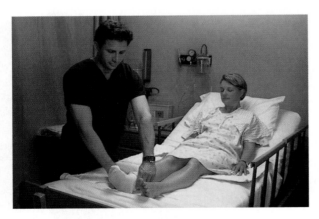

Step 5c. Sliding the stocking onto the foot and ankle.

10. Document the size and length of the stockings, the time they were applied, the condition of the client's skin, any client complaints, and times the stockings were removed and reapplied.

HOME CARE CONSIDERATIONS

For clients at risk for thrombophlebitis, antiembolism stockings should be worn at home. Suggest that the client keep two pairs on hand so one pair can be washed (in mild soap, by hand) while the other pair is being worn.

PROCEDURE 32-3	USING A SEQUENTIAL COMPRESSION DEVICE

TIME TO ALLOW
Novice: 15 min.
Expert: 7.5 min.

A sequential compression device creates waves of external pressure that move from distal to proximal areas of the legs. By doing so, the device enhances venous return, decreases venous stasis, and prevents deep vein thrombosis. Typically, you will use a sequential compression device with a bedridden client who is at high risk for thrombosis.

DELEGATION GUIDELINES

The application and maintenance of a sequential compression device may be delegated to a nursing assistant who has been properly trained in this skill. Periodic removal of the device to promote mobility or inspection of the skin may be delegated to the nursing assistant, with specific attention to findings that necessitate immediate RN notification.

EQUIPMENT NEEDED

- Antiembolism stockings of the correct size
- Tape measure
- Sequential compression sleeves
- Compression controller

1. Follow preliminary guidelines for nursing procedures (see inside front cover).

2. Check physician's order.

3. Place the client in a supine position with her legs horizontal. *This keeps blood from pooling in the legs.*

4. Apply antiembolism stockings. *Antiembolism stockings protect the legs from overheating and sustaining skin damage. Cotton also absorbs excess moisture from the skin, helping to prevent maceration.*

5. Measure the circumference of the client's upper thigh. *This ensures that the device is the correct size.*

6. Open the inflatable sleeve on the flat bed, cotton-side up, and place the client's leg on the sleeve (see illustration). Avoid positioning the sleeve so that it places direct pressure on the popliteal artery. Also, avoid positioning it in a manner that could cause skin breakdown on the client's ankle.

Step 6. Placing the client's leg on the sleeve.

7. Wrap the sleeve snugly around the client's leg, beginning with the side that does not contain tubes (see illustration). Fasten the sleeve closed with the Velcro fasteners. *Make sure you can fit two fingers between the sleeve and the client's skin. If the sleeve is too loose, it will function less effectively. If it is too tight, it could cause skin breakdown, compression of the arteries, and neurological changes.*

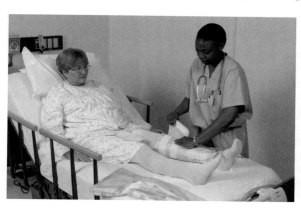

Step 7. Wrapping the sleeve snugly around the client's leg.

8. Connect the tubing on the sleeve to the compression controller.

9. Follow the physician's orders in setting the controller to the correct amount and time of compression. After turning it on, observe to make sure the unit is working properly.

10. Remove the client's antiembolism stockings three times daily, and perform skin care during this time. Assess for skin breakdown and pressure ulcers. Examine the toes for arterial changes, such as coolness, pallor, and decreased capillary refill. Ask whether the client feels tingling or numbness.

11. Document the date and time the sleeves were applied or removed. Also, document your assessment findings.

Maintain Venous Return. Avoiding compression of leg veins maintains blood flow and prevents venous stasis. To avoid compressing the leg vessels, teach the client not to cross the legs at the knee, either while in bed or sitting in a chair. Also teach the client to avoid tight knee socks or garters.

Also, do not routinely use the Gatch bed's knee-raising device, or pillows behind the client's knees, because they could put pressure on the popliteal artery at the back of the knee. If you use pillows under the client's legs, use them to support the entire length of the leg, not just under the knee. Assess the client's antiembolism stockings frequently to make sure they have not rolled down.

Encourage Correct Breathing. The change in pressure in the thorax during inspiration pulls blood into the inferior vena cava, thus promoting venous return. If the client holds his breath and bears down, blood is unable to return to the heart and can cause decreased blood pressure and cardiac disturbances. When the client moves in bed, instruct him to breathe out through his mouth rather than holding his breath. He can also use an over-bed frame, a trapeze, or the bed's side rails when changing positions or moving in bed.

Prevent Orthostatic Intolerance. Provide clients with a planned program of gradual adjustment to vertical positioning in order to recondition the baroreceptors and help stabilize blood pressure. Have clients perform foot and leg exercises for 1 to 2 minutes before beginning any position change. If they have been lying flat for a long time, elevate the head of the bed for 15 minutes three times daily for a few days before sitting them up or getting them out of bed. When you do sit them up, let their feet dangle over the edge of the bed for a few minutes until they are not dizzy or lightheaded before standing.

Action Alert! If a client is experiencing orthostatic intolerance, return him to the sitting position and take his blood pressure. Do not leave the client, because he may fall. The dizziness, lightheadedness, and feeling of fainting experienced on standing usually resolve within a few minutes.

If the client experiences severe hypotension after a prolonged time in the supine position, a physical therapist may need to use a tilt table for position changes.

Interventions to Maintain Respiratory Function

Without enough oxygen, the client does not have the endurance to be active. Interventions aim to maximize respiratory function by encouraging lung expansion and mobilizing secretions.

Encourage Lung Expansion. To help maximize your client's lung expansion, elevate the head of the bed to 45 or 90 degrees (Fowler's or high Fowler's position) for short intervals. Remember that although this position supports lung expansion, it also increases pressure on the skin over the coccyx. Support the client's arms on pillows. Remind the client to per-

form deep breathing 10 times every 2 hours while awake. If necessary, have the client use an incentive spirometer 10 times every 1 to 2 hours while awake (see Chapter 33). Reposition the bedridden client every 2 hours. With a physician's order, begin progressive activity and ambulation as soon as possible.

Mobilize Secretions. Thin, watery secretions are easier to expectorate than thick, sticky sputum. Teach the client to drink 2000 to 3000 mL of fluid daily help keep secretions more liquid, unless this is contraindicated by a fluid restriction order to treat a coexisting cardiac or renal disorder. A forceful cough is the most effective method for removing sputum. For a more effective cough, teach the client cascade coughing or huff coughing (see Chapter 33). Coughing should be done five times every 2 hours.

Regular position changes can also help to mobilize secretions by using the pull of gravity. Turn the client every 1 to 2 hours. Also, perform chest physiotherapy and postural drainage two or more times daily (see Chapter 33). Humidify the client's inspired air. As needed, obtain an order for aerosol therapy and a liquefying inhaler medication.

EVALUATION

Risk for disuse syndrome is the nursing diagnosis used to keep the body systems healthy if the client's activity status is suddenly altered. Interventions are implemented to prevent the complications of disuse from occurring, as suggested in Box 32-6. For a more specific and complete list of interventions for each of the nursing diagnoses and correlative problems, consult the appropriate chapter in this book.

Evaluation of outcomes should be done on a daily basis. Because this a *Risk* diagnosis, achievement of the health outcomes occurs if no problems develop. If the outcome is not met because a problem does occur, add the appropriate nursing diagnosis. For example, if the client experiences deterioration of the psychosocial system, the appropriate additional nursing diagnoses might be *Anxiety, Ineffective role performance, Self-care deficit, Powerlessness, Low self-esteem, Disturbed sensory perception,* or *Deficient diversional activity.*

If the client experiences deterioration of nutrition and metabolism, you might add *Imbalanced nutrition: less than body requirements, Risk for infection,* or *Risk for fluid volume deficit.* If the client experiences deterioration of the skin, you might add *Impaired skin integrity, Risk for infection,* or *Impaired tissue integrity.* If the client experiences deterioration of the musculoskeletal system, you might add *Impaired physical mobility, Activity intolerance, Self-care deficit,* or *Risk for injury.* If the client experiences deterioration of the cardiovascular system, you might add *Ineffective tissue perfusion, Activity intolerance,* or the collaborative problems orthostatic intolerance, deep vein thrombosis, pulmonary embolism, or decreased cardiac output.

If the client experiences deterioration of the respiratory system, you might add *Ineffective breathing pattern, Ineffective airway clearance, Impaired gas exchange,* or the

Nursing Care Plan A CLIENT WITH WORK-RELATED INJURIES

Box 32-6

ADMISSION DATA

Mr. Jackson is a 48-year-old African-American man who presents to the emergency department following an injury on the job. The emergency department physician diagnoses a compound fracture of the left tibia and a fractured left clavicle. Mr. Jackson is taken to the operating room where the bone fragments are pinned and a stabilizing device applied. Mr. Jackson is sent home to rest, elevate the left leg, and apply an ice pack to his knee. He has a sling to prevent him from moving his left arm. He is to return to the orthopedic clinic in 1 week.

PHYSICIAN'S ORDERS

Apply ice pack to left knee for 20 minutes every 4 hours.
No weight bearing on left leg.

Return to clinic in 1 week.
Fill prescription for pain medication.
Do not use left arm and keep in sling at all times (including sleeping) except for bathing.
Elevate left leg 90% of the time.

NURSING ASSESSMENT

Vital signs were temperature 98.4° F, pulse 88, respiration 16, BP 136/86. All WNL for him. He appears in minimal distress. C/o pain in his left knee (4 out of 10-point pain scale) and in his left shoulder (8 of 10). Toes pink, capillary refill <3 seconds, and normal movement. Unable to perform ROM on his left shoulder.

NANDA Nursing Diagnosis	NOC Expected Outcomes With Indicators	NIC Interventions With Selected Activities	Evaluation Data
RISK FOR DISUSE SYNDROME **Related Factor:** • Prescribed rest secondary to left knee injury and left clavicle break	**MOBILITY LEVEL** • Muscles will remain strong, without contractures. • Unaffected joints will have full ROM.	**EXERCISE THERAPY: JOINT MOBILITY** • Encourage right arm and leg exercises against resistance three times daily. • Encourage full ROM for right arm and leg at least three times daily. Keep left shoulder immobilized.	**AT HOME AFTER 24 HOURS OF CARE** • No evidence of muscle changes in upper or lower extremities. • Mr. Jackson has full ROM in right arm and leg. Left shoulder is immobilized with sling. Pain is 3 on a scale of 10. Left knee is still slightly swollen but not red. Movement is painful (2 of 10) on flexion and limited.
RISK FOR IMPAIRED SKIN INTEGRITY	**SKIN INTEGRITY** • Skin will be free of irritation, redness, ulceration, or edema.	**PRESSURE ULCER PREVENTION** • Inspect skin under sling, around pins, back, and sacrum twice daily. Teach client to shift weight every 15 minutes while sitting in the chair. Support arm on a pillow while sitting in chair.	• No evidence of skin irritation. No edema present in hands or ankles. States that he does shift his weight every 15 minutes or so while in a chair.

CRITICAL THINKING QUESTIONS

1. What other discharge instructions should have been given to Mr. and Mrs. Jackson? Does he need a home health referral?
2. Mrs. Jackson calls the clinic stating that Mr. Jackson has a fever, feels warm, and is not feeling well. What do you tell her? Should he come to the clinic or be sent to the hospital? Can Mrs. Jackson drive him safely?
3. What other nursing interventions should be done for Mr. Jackson to prevent the complications of immobility?

Nursing outcome and intervention labels from Johnson, M., Bulechek, G., McCloskey Dochterman, J., Maas, M., & Moorhead, S. (2001). *Nursing diagnoses, outcomes, and interventions: NANDA, NOC, and NIC linkages.* St Louis, MO: Mosby.

---

collaborative problems atelectasis or pneumonia. If the client experiences deterioration of the gastrointestinal system, you might add *Constipation* or *Incontinence.* Finally, if the client experiences deterioration of the genitourinary system, you might add *Impaired urinary elimination, Bowel incontinence,* or *Risk for infection.*

Documenting the outcomes of care is essential. A sample note for Mr. Jackson, the case study client, reads as shown.

> **SAMPLE DOCUMENTATION NOTE FOR MR. JACKSON**
> Full ROM present in right arm and leg. Left shoulder is immobilized in sling. Left leg has painful movement (2 on a scale of 0-10) and flexion is limited. Left knee is still slightly swollen but no redness is present. No evidence of skin irritation or edema. Patient states he shifts weight in chair approximately every 15 minutes.

Key Principles

- Disuse syndrome refers to clients at risk for deterioration of body systems from inactivity and immobility.
- Short periods of rest are beneficial.
- Prolonged inactivity causes behavioral changes of anger, hostility, loneliness, and social isolation.
- Independence in performing activities of daily living is lost during immobility.
- Muscle is broken down for energy in states of decreased protein intake.
- Malnutrition causes a decrease in red blood cells, causing anemia, and a decrease in white blood cells, causing infection.
- Lack of activity leads rapidly to muscle weakness and atrophy.
- Bone decalcification causes weak bones and increased serum levels of calcium.
- Immobilization of joints leads to stiffness and limited movement.
- Skin breakdown occurs with increased pressure, shear, friction, excoriation, and maceration.
- Loss of skin integrity allows microorganisms to invade and produce infection.
- Stasis of blood in dependent limbs leads to edema and thrombus formation.
- The development of deep vein thrombosis and subsequent pulmonary embolism can lead to client's death.
- Sudden changes in a client's position can cause blood pressure to drop sharply, a condition known as orthostatic intolerance.
- Hypoventilation and stasis of respiratory secretions can lead to atelectasis and hypostatic pneumonia.
- Hypomotility of the gastrointestinal tract causes abdominal distention, discomfort, constipation, and flatulence.
- Difficulty in voiding leads to urinary retention, residual urine, and urinary tract infections.
- The best treatment for complications from disuse is prevention.
- Increased activity and exercise can prevent most of the complications of disuse.
- When positioning a client who is unable to move, position joints in anatomic alignment or functional alignment. Provide support above and below the joints.

Bibliography

Ayello, E., & Braden, B. (2001). Why is pressure ulcer risk assessment so important? *Nursing 2001, 31*(11), 74-79.

*Bright, L. D., & Georgi, S. (1994). Protect your patient from DVT. *American Journal of Nursing, 94*(12), 28-32.

Burke, S. (2001). Boning up on osteoporosis. *Nursing 2001, 31*(10), 36-42.

---

*Asterisk indicates a classic or definitive work on this subject.

Christie, F. (1998). Clinical snapshot: Pulmonary embolism. *American Journal of Nursing, 98*(11), 36.

Church, V. (2000). Staying on guard for DVT and PE. *Nursing 2000, 30*(2), 35-42.

Collier, M., & Brevet, T. (1999). Antiembolism stockings for prevention and treatment of deep vein thrombosis. *British Journal of Nursing, 8*(1), 44.

Ebersole, P., & Hess, P. (1998). *Toward healthy aging: Human needs and nursing response* (5th ed.). St Louis, MO: Mosby.

Geyer, M. J., Brienza, D. M., Karg, P., Trefler, E., & Kelsey, S. (2001). A randomized control trial to evaluate pressure reducing seat cushions for elderly wheelchair users. *Advances in Skin and Wound Care, 14*(3), 120.

*Hangartner, T. N. (1995). Osteoporosis due to disuse. *Physical Medicine and Rehabilitation Clinics of North America, 6*(3), 579-594.

*Hunter, S. M., Langemo, D. K., Olson, B., Hanson, D., Cathcart-Silberberg, T., Burd, C., et al. (1995). The effectiveness of skin care protocols for pressure ulcers. *Rehabilitation Nursing, 20*(5), 250-255.

Johnson, M., Bulechek, G., McCloskey-Dochtermann, J., Mass, M., & Moorehead, S. (2001). *Nursing diagnoses, outcomes, & interventions: NANDA, NOC, and NIC linkages.* St Louis, MO: Mosby.

Johnson, M., Maas, M., & Moorehead, S. (2000). *Nursing outcomes classification* (NOC) (2nd ed.). St Louis, MO: Mosby.

Leuckonette, A. G. (2000). *Gerontological nursing* (2nd ed.). St Louis, MO: Mosby.

Marion, B. S. (2001). A turn for the better: "Prone positioning" of patients with ARDS. *American Journal of Nursing, 101*(5), 26-33.

McCloskey, J., & Bulechek, G. (2000). *Nursing interventions classification* (3rd ed.). St Louis, MO: Mosby.

McConnell, E. A. (2002). Clinical do's & don'ts. Applying antiembolism stockings: Proper measurements and application help protect your patient against deep vein thrombosis. *Nursing, 32*(4), 17.

O'Hanlon-Nichols, T. (1998). A review of the adult musculoskeletal system. *American Journal of Nursing, 98*(6), 48-52.

*Olson, E. V. (1967). The hazards of immobility. *American Journal of Nursing, 67*(4), 779-796.

Rawsky, E. (1998). Review of the literature on falls among the elderly. *Image, the Journal of Nursing Scholarship, 30*(1), 47-54.

*Rondorf-Klym, L. M., & Langemo, D. (1993). Relationship between body weight, body position, support surface, and tissue interface pressure at the sacrum. *Decubitus, 6*(1), 22-25.

Russel, L. (2001). Overview of research to investigate pressure-reducing surfaces. *British Journal of Nursing, 10*(1), 1421.

*Skewes, S. M. (1996a). Skin care rituals that do more harm than good. *American Journal of Nursing, 96*(10), 33-35.

*Skewes, S. M. (1996b). Spotting pressure ulcers in patients with dark skin. *Nursing96, 26*(6), 24q-24r.

*Topp, R., Mikesky, A., & Bawel, K. (1994). Developing a strength training program for older adults: Planning, programming, and potential outcomes. *Rehabilitation Nursing, 19*(5), 266-273.

*Winslow, E. H. (1994). Mattresses that spell pressure R-E-L-I-E-F. *American Journal of Nursing, 94*(9), 48.

33

Supporting Respiratory Function

Key Terms

bronchospasm
chest percussion
chest physiotherapy
cough
cyanosis
diaphragmatic (abdominal) breathing
dyspnea
endotracheal tube
hemoptysis
hypercapnia
hyperventilation
hypoventilation
hypoxemia
hypoxia
incentive spirometer
postural drainage
pulse oximetry
pursed-lip breathing
respiration
sputum
ventilation
vibration

Learning Objectives

After studying this chapter, you should be able to do the following:

- Describe the physiological concepts underlying the respiratory nursing diagnoses
- Discuss the most common lifestyle, environmental, developmental, and physiological factors affecting respiration, as well as contributing pathologies
- Assess the client who has risk for experiencing a respiratory problem and the client's responses to the respiratory problem
- Diagnose the client's respiratory needs that are amenable to nursing care
- Plan goal-directed interventions to prevent or correct the respiratory diagnoses
- Describe and practice key interventions for respiratory care, including positioning, suctioning, providing supplemental oxygen, and maintaining a patent (open) airway
- Evaluate the outcomes that describe progress toward the goals of respiratory nursing care

Anna Wilheim is 88 years old and lives alone since her sister died last year. She called her daughter this morning to say that she did not feel well. Because Mrs. Wilheim had assured her daughter that there was no cause for concern, it was noon before the daughter arrived. Mrs. Wilheim had a temperature of 38.9° C (102° F), and she was pale, cold, and weak. She complained of pain with breathing. Her daughter called the doctor and drove her to the emergency department. She was admitted to the hospital with a diagnosis of pneumonia. Both the daughter and Mrs. Wilheim were frightened.

The nurse makes plans to assist Mrs. Wilheim to manage the effects of her illness and support her recovery. Because Mrs. Wilheim is having difficulty breathing, the nurse considers the diagnosis of *Ineffective breathing pattern* from the list of nursing diagnoses for respiratory function (see below). Because pneumonia is likely to increase the secretions in her lungs and could interfere with the oxygenation of her blood, the nurse also assesses for *Ineffective airway clearance* and *Impaired gas exchange*.

KEY NURSING DIAGNOSES FOR Respiratory Function

Ineffective breathing pattern: A state in which the rate, depth, timing, rhythm, or chest/abdominal wall excursion during inspiration, expiration, or both, does not maintain optimum ventilation for the individual

Ineffective airway clearance: A state in which an individual is unable to clear secretions or obstructions from the respiratory tract

Impaired gas exchange: A state in which the individual experiences an excess or deficit in oxygenation and/or carbon dioxide elimination at the alveolar–capillary membrane (specify: hypercapnia or hypoxemia)

CONCEPTS OF RESPIRATION

Nurses encounter clients with respiratory problems in virtually every area of practice and virtually every practice setting. Nursing care of clients with respiratory problems may range from prevention of the spread of the common cold in a school setting to sustaining the life of a client in respiratory failure in the intensive care unit. Respiratory problems are potential or actual problems in the majority of clients admitted to hospitals and nursing homes. Public health and community health nurses screen for respiratory problems and plan community programs for the prevention of respiratory disease. A respiratory diagnosis may be related to a medical diagnosis of respiratory disease or it may be present as a complication of a medical or surgical condition. Regardless of the area of practice or the practice setting, many of these client situations can be described using one, two, or three of the respiratory nursing diagnoses.

Physiology of Breathing

As we begin to consider the physiology of breathing, it is important to differentiate between two important concepts: respiration and breathing. The term **respiration** refers to two processes. The first is the exchange of oxygen and carbon dioxide between the atmosphere and the cells of the body. The second process is actually a series of metabolic activities by which living cells break down carbohydrates, amino acids, and fats to produce energy in the form of adenosine triphosphate. The term *breathing* refers strictly to *ventilation*—the process of exchanging air between the ambient air and the lungs. The term *pulmonary ventilation* refers to the total exchange of air, whereas the term *alveolar ventilation* refers to the effective ventilation of the alveoli.

Air enters the body through the nose or the mouth. The nose is designed to warm and moisten the air as well as to filter debris from the air. The air then passes through the

pharynx and trachea before entering the bronchi. The right and left bronchi divide into smaller bronchioles, which in turn branch into millions of tiny air sacs called alveoli. Each alveolus is surrounded by a capillary bed. Gas exchange occurs where the capillary meets the alveolus.

Figure 33-1 illustrates gas exchange in the alveoli. The alveolar wall and the capillary membrane are only a single cell thick. Exchange of oxygen and carbon dioxide between the alveolus and the capillary bed depends on contact between oxygen-laden air in the alveoli and hemoglobin-rich blood in the capillary. The thickness of the capillary membrane is therefore critical to the rate of gas exchange.

Ventilation. Ventilation refers to the cycle of inspiration and expiration of air into and out of the lungs. Air moves into the lungs when the atmospheric pressure is greater than the pressure in the air passages. Two things happen simultaneously to create this pressure gradient:

- Elevation of the ribs and movement of the diaphragm enlarge (expand) the chest cavity. The diaphragm moves downward when it contracts, thus creating more intrathoracic space.
- As the chest wall expands, it pulls away from the lungs, creating negative pressure, which draws the lungs open. As the lungs are pulled open, negative pressure is created in the airways inside the lungs, and the air is drawn into the lungs.

Figure 33-2 (p. 836) illustrates chest wall expansion during inspiration. The chest wall and the lungs must remain intact (no air allowed in the pleural space) for the negative pressure to be created.

Inspiration is a more active process than expiration, because in inspiration the diaphragm contracts, moving downward, and the intercostal muscles contract to elevate the ribs. When the intercostal muscles and the diaphragm relax, the chest cavity becomes smaller and air passively leaves the lungs.

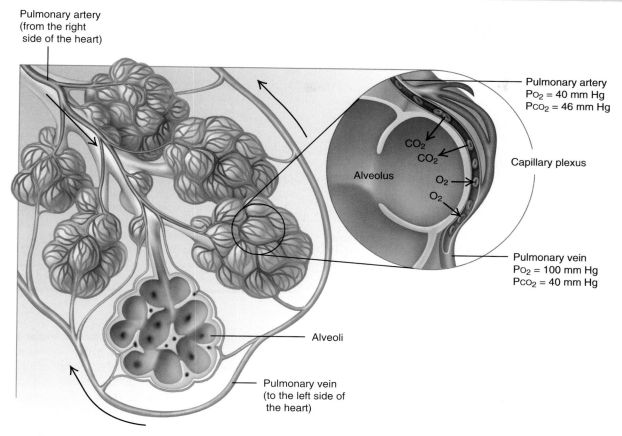

Figure 33-1. Millions of alveoli interface with the capillary bed, providing a tremendous surface for gas exchange. Rapid diffusion of oxygen and carbon dioxide saturates the blood with oxygen and removes excess carbon dioxide.

Muscles of Respiration. The primary muscle of respiration is the *diaphragm.* When the diaphragm is relaxed, it assumes a dome shape that ascends into the thorax. As we have seen, when the diaphragm contracts, it flattens along the lower border of the ribs. Again, relaxation of the diaphragm is associated with exhalation, and contraction of the diaphragm is associated with inhalation.

The additional muscles that assist the diaphragm are called the *accessory muscles of respiration.* Three important sets of accessory muscles are the sternocleidomastoid, the scaleni, and the intercostals. During inspiration, the *sternocleidomastoid* muscle raises the sternum, the *scaleni* muscles elevate the first two ribs, and the external *intercostal* muscles elevate the remaining ribs. During quiet respiration, these inspiratory muscles exert little observable activity. The muscles that assist expiration are the internal intercostal muscles and the abdominal muscles. The expiratory muscles become more active during forceful expiration.

Compliance and Elasticity. Normal ventilation depends on compliance and elastic recoil of the lung tissue. *Compliance* is a measure of the distensibility of the lungs—the degree to which the lungs can stretch. *Elastic recoil* is the tendency of the lungs to return to a nonstretched state. This rebound effect contributes to expiration.

Surface Tension. In the lungs, elastic recoil is produced by elastic fibers in lung tissue and by the surface tension of the fluid that lines the alveoli. This surface tension causes a continuous tendency of the alveoli to collapse. Surface tension is the attraction between the molecules on the surface of a fluid. If you observe various fluids in a glass, you will notice that some have a convex surface (upward curve) created by surface tension. Fluids with less surface tension have a concave surface (downward curve). *Surfactant,* a lipoprotein mixture secreted by the alveolar epithelium, acts likes a detergent to reduce the surface tension and hold the alveoli open. Stretching of the alveoli through periodic deep breaths, known as sighing, stimulates the production of surfactant. For this reason, periodical sighing is an essential physiological mechanism to maintain open alveoli. Surfactant is absent or diminished in premature newborns.

Airway Resistance. The work of breathing is directly related to the amount of *airway resistance,* which is the amount of opposition to airflow within the air passages. The diameter and the length of the airways determine airway resistance. It is normally low; however, any obstruction in the respiratory passages, whether a foreign body, a mass, or mucus, narrows the diameter and increases airway resistance. Contraction of the smooth muscles of the bronchi also decreases the diameter.

Inspiration

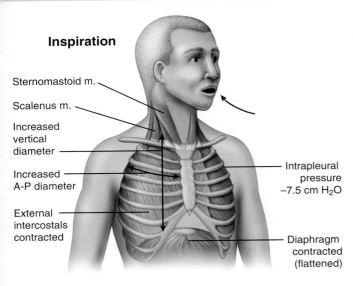

Sternomastoid m.

Scalenus m.

Increased vertical diameter

Increased A-P diameter

External intercostals contracted

Intrapleural pressure −7.5 cm H_2O

Diaphragm contracted (flattened)

Expiration

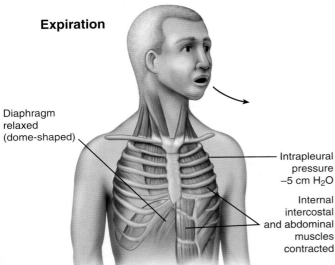

Diaphragm relaxed (dome-shaped)

Intrapleural pressure −5 cm H_2O

Internal intercostal and abdominal muscles contracted

Figure 33-2. During inspiration, the diaphragm and the external intercostal muscles contract to increase the intrathoracic space, decreasing the intrapleural pressure to about −7.5 cm H_2O, which expands the lungs. During expiration, the diaphragm relaxes, and the internal intercostal and abdominal muscles contract to reduce the size of the thoracic cavity. A negative intrapleural pressure of about −5 cm H_2O holds the lungs in a somewhat inflated position.

Dead Space. *Dead space* is any surface of the airways that contains air but does not participate in gas exchange. On inspiration, a tidal volume of 500 mL of air (in the adult) fills the nose, pharynx, trachea, bronchi, bronchioles, and alveoli. However, only the air that reaches the alveoli is available for gas exchange. The remaining air is said to occupy dead space. Therefore the volume of air that enters the alveoli with each breath is equal to the inhaled air minus the dead space volume. Normal dead space volume in the average adult is approximately 150 mL.

Control of Respiration. Ventilation is controlled by a combination of neurological and chemical mechanisms. Neuro-

Table 33-1	Common Symbols Used in Respiratory Care
Symbol	**Interpretation**
A	Alveolar
a	Arterial
CO_2	Carbon dioxide
O_2	Oxygen
V	Ventilation
V_T	Tidal volume
$\dot{V}/\dot{Q}$	Ventilation/perfusion ratio
VC	Vital capacity
FEV_1	Forced expiratory volume/time
Sao_2	Percentage hemoglobin oxygen saturation
PA_{O_2}	Partial pressure of alveolar oxygen
Pa_{O_2}	Partial pressure of arterial oxygen
Pa_{CO_2}	Partial pressure of arterial carbon dioxide
pH	Hydrogen ion concentration, acidity or alkalinity
FI_{O_2}	Fraction of inspired oxygen, expressed in decimal form (0.40 = 40% oxygen)

logical control is in the respiratory centers in the pons and medulla of the brain stem. Several groups of neurons exert different influences on respiration. The medullary rhythmicity area controls the rhythmicity of inspiration and expiration. The apneustic and pneumotaxic areas of the medulla smooth the pattern of respiration into a short inspiration and a longer expiration. These respiratory control centers respond to changes in carbon dioxide (CO_2) and oxygen (O_2) in the blood but are more sensitive to carbon dioxide. Increased carbon dioxide can increase ventilation sevenfold. Additionally, chemoreceptors, present primarily in the aortic arch and the carotid artery, respond to changes in CO_2 and O_2 but are more sensitive to oxygen deficit. Together these neurological and chemical mechanisms control ventilation almost exactly to the demands of the body.

Pulmonary Symbols. Symbols are used in respiratory care as a shorthand method of representing the parameters of ventilatory function. Table 33-1 lists common symbols used in respiratory care.

Physiology of Airway Clearance

The ability to maintain clean, clear airways is an important defense mechanism of the body. Because the lungs are open to polluted atmospheric air, foreign matter and microorganisms are a constant threat. The design of the respiratory tract protects the body from invasion.

Respiratory Defense Mechanisms

UPPER AIRWAYS. The upper airways are designed to maintain an internal environment essentially free of microorganisms and foreign matter. As air enters the nose, the upper airways begin the defensive function of the respiratory system. The hairs of the anterior nostrils and the mucus remove large foreign particles from the air. The irregular surfaces of the turbinates, septum, and pharynx create obstruction to the

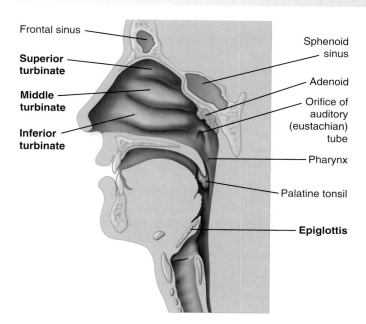

Figure 33-3. Upper airway defense mechanisms. The irregular turbinates trap debris that would otherwise fall into the pharynx. The epiglottis protects foreign matter from entering the lower respiratory tract.

Frontal sinus

Superior turbinate

Middle turbinate

Inferior turbinate

Sphenoid sinus

Adenoid

Orifice of auditory (eustachian) tube

Pharynx

Palatine tonsil

Epiglottis

Box 33-1   Threats to Normal Airway Clearance

CHRONIC PERSISTENT IRRITATION

- Air pollution
- Cigarette smoking

ACUTE TRAUMATIC INJURY

- Endotracheal suction
- Aspiration of vomitus or other foreign body
- Endoscopic examination
- Endotracheal or tracheostomy tubes

OTHER

- Dehydration
- Extreme heat or cold
- Medications that depress the cough reflex
- Pathology that causes increased mucus, irritation, edema

---

passage of smaller particles that escaped the hairs and remained suspended in the air. Figure 33-3 illustrates the structural upper airway defenses.

The upper airways are lined with a mucous membrane that protects the lungs by cleaning, moisturizing, and warming the air. The upper airways are lined with a mucous membrane that secretes mucopolysaccharides that trap the foreign particles. Its ciliated epithelium, extending from the nose to the bronchioles, propels the mucus into the pharynx, where it can be expelled from the body or swallowed. The mucus also humidifies the air. Finally, the high vascularity of the mucous membrane contributes to warming of the inspired air.

The sneeze reflex provides added protection against larger particles and more irritating substances. A *sneeze* is stimulated by irritation to the nasal passageway caused by foreign bodies, chemicals, or temperature extremes. During a sneeze, the uvula is depressed, allowing a large volume of air to be forced through the nose and mouth, thus clearing the offending substance. Increased pressure is created in the lungs by taking a deep breath and holding the breath immediately before the sneeze.

LOWER AIRWAYS. The *glottis* is the opening at the top of the larynx between the resting vocal folds. It divides the upper from the lower respiratory tract. The glottis is open with inspiration, but when we speak, the vocal folds come together, temporarily eliminating the glottis. When we swallow, the epiglottis tips downward to seal off the glottis. This reflex sometimes fails when we try to talk and swallow food or fluids at the same time. However, if foreign particles do pass the glottis, additional protection exists: cilia propel the particles upward, phagocytes engulf the particles, and the cough reflex produces a forceful exhalation to expel the irritating matter.

The cleaning and moisturizing activity of the upper airways continues in the lower respiratory tract. A ciliated epithelium interspersed with mucus-secreting cells lines the lungs down to the level of the bronchioles. Thus the air reaches the alveoli essentially clean, 100% humidified, and at body temperature (Guyton & Hall, 1996).

The cough reflex is the last line of defense. A **cough** (a sudden, audible, forceful expulsion of air from the lungs, usually an involuntary, reflexive action in response to an irritant) is stimulated when foreign particles or infection irritates the airways. Further down, a cough control center exists in the carina where the bronchus bifurcates into the right and left primary bronchi. If the irritating substance passes the bronchi, the bronchioles and alveoli, which are particularly sensitive to chemical stimulation, will trigger a cough.

The automatic sequence of events in a cough is triggered in the medulla. The person simultaneously takes a deep breath, closes the vocal cords to trap the large volume of air in the lungs, and contracts the abdominal muscles and other accessory muscles of respiration to increase the pressure in the lungs. When the pressure in the lungs rises to an uncomfortable level, the vocal cords and epiglottis are forced open, and the air, with a velocity equivalent to a speeding car, expels foreign particles. The cough reflex is weak or absent in a person with central nervous system depression, such as occurs in comatose clients or in clients on high doses of narcotics for pain management.

Threats to Airway Defenses. The natural defense mechanisms of the airways are vulnerable to damage or destruction from a variety of causes. Box 33-1 lists threats to normal airway clearance. Physical damage that destroys or inflames respiratory cilia or mucus-secreting cells renders these defense mechanisms ineffective. A sudden overwhelming assault or persistent irritants can cause such damage. Although respiratory defense depends on a moist mucous membrane, an overproduction of mucus threatens the ability of the respiratory tract to clear the airways.

Physiology of Gas Exchange

The exchange of carbon dioxide and oxygen depends on adequate ventilation, which requires not only the movement of air, but a clear air passage. Inefficient patterns of breathing or obstruction of airways can be severe enough to impair gas exchange. *Impaired gas exchange* results in **hypoxemia** (deficient oxygenation of the blood) or **hypercapnia** (high carbon dioxide level in the blood, usually resulting from failure of the lungs to remove carbon dioxide), or both.

Diffusion. Gas exchange depends on efficient transport of oxygen and carbon dioxide across the alveolocapillary membrane by the process of diffusion. Diffusion is a passive process by which molecules move through a cell membrane from an area of higher concentration to an area of lower concentration without the expenditure of energy. For oxygen and carbon dioxide to diffuse across the semipermeable alveolocapillary membrane, there must be both adequate ventilation and adequate blood flow. Oxygen-rich air must reach the alveoli as unoxygenated blood flows into the capillary bed.

The relative concentration of the gases, the thickness of the membrane, and the surface area of the alveoli also affect diffusion. Carbon dioxide is highly concentrated in the blood entering the capillary bed. It crosses the alveolocapillary membrane into the alveoli where the carbon dioxide concentration is lower. Similarly, since the partial pressure of oxygen is greater in the alveoli than in the pulmonary capillaries, oxygen readily diffuses across the membrane from the air sacs into the blood. The thin alveolocapillary membrane and the extremely large surface area across the capillary bed allows rapid, efficient diffusion.

Ventilation/Perfusion Ratio. As we have seen, for optimal transport of oxygen and carbon dioxide, the amount of blood flow *(perfusion)* must be matched to the amount of airflow *(ventilation)*. The upright position is the anatomic position of the body that is optimal for ventilation and perfusion matching. In fact, the overall ventilation/perfusion ratio in the normal upright lung is 0.9, or slightly less than 1:1. This ratio occurs because ventilation is at the maximum in the apices of the lungs and perfusion is at the maximum in the bases of the lung. This phenomenon reflects the relative weights of air and blood in response to gravity. Any condition that upsets this balance may result in a mismatch of ventilation to perfusion and in a less than optimal exchange of oxygen and carbon dioxide.

Oxygen-Carrying Capacity of the Blood. Additionally, gas exchange depends on the presence of hemoglobin. Hemoglobin in the red blood cells carries 97% of the oxygen; the remaining 3% is dissolved in plasma. The hemoglobin combines with the oxygen to form oxyhemoglobin. Oxygenation of tissues depends on the perfusion of oxygen-rich blood to those tissues (see Chapter 34).

FACTORS AFFECTING RESPIRATION

A number of factors affect a person's respiratory function. They include lifestyle factors, environmental factors, developmental factors, and physiological factors.

Lifestyle Factors

Lifestyle factors that affect respiratory function include smoking and the person's general state of health.

Smoking. The primary lifestyle factor affecting respiration is smoking. Inhaling tobacco or marijuana smoke from cigarettes, pipes, or cigars is a chronic irritant to the lungs. Irritation causes increased mucus production. Smokers have varying degrees of reduced ciliary function, bronchoconstriction,

---

THE STATE OF NURSING RESEARCH: Do you smoke? Do you want to quit?   Box 33-2

What Are the Issues?

Tobacco use is one health risk that can be modified. Clinical practice guidelines for health care providers encourage them to assess the smoking status of all of their clients. For all smokers, a follow-up question about intent to quit is next (Fiore, Bailey, & Cohen, et al., 2000). Knowledge of the health effects of tobacco use alone is not enough to help people quit unless they are ready to quit. Studies that examine the stage of readiness indicate that only 20% are in the preparation stage that is the focus of most cessation programs. New strategies are needed that help motivate people to stop using tobacco.

What Research Has Been Conducted?

A recent review of studies that used the transtheoretical model (TTM) to design their interventions located 16 studies. The TTM includes five stages of readiness to change: "precontemplation, contemplation, preparation, action, and maintenance" (Andersen, Keller, & McGowan, 1999). (The model has also been used in studies of weight loss.) The reviewers evaluated the strength and quality of the interventions. Quality was determined by how closely the intervention matched the TTM.

What Has the Research Concluded?

The reviewers concluded that the model is useful to clinicians in assessing which stage clients are in but that few studies clearly tested interventions for each of the stages. Current efforts (e.g., giving social support) are geared toward people in the preparation stage.

What Is the Future of Research in This Area?

The reviewers recommend more studies on the differences between the stages and a person's movement between stages. Additional research on culturally sensitive interventions for various populations is also needed.

References

Andersen, S., Keller, C., & McGowan, N. (1999). Smoking cessation: The state of the science—The utility of the transtheoretical model in guiding interventions in smoking cessation. *On-line Journal of Knowledge Synthesis in Nursing, 6*(9) [internet www.nursingsociety.org].

Fiore, M. C., Bailey, W. C., Cohen, S. J., et al. (2000). *Treating tobacco use and dependence: Quick reference guide for clinicians.* Rockville, MD: U.S. Department of Health and Human Services, Public Health Service.

and decreased compliance and elasticity. Smoking increases the heart and respiratory rates, constricts blood vessels, and increases blood pressure. Smoking is highly associated with emphysema and lung cancer as well as other respiratory diseases. Seventy-eight to 90% of lung cancers occur in people who smoke (National Cancer Institute, 1999) (Box 33-2).

Smoking is a potential hazard to nonsmokers. Passive smoke in the home has been linked to the incidence of respiratory symptoms, episodes in asthmatics, and acute lower respiratory tract infections in schoolchildren. Breathing in children can be affected through frequent exposure in the homes of friends, in restaurants, and in crowded housing situations that are common among those in low socioeconomic groups.

Nicotine is a highly addictive substance. Once a person starts smoking, quitting is not easy (Box 33-3). In addition to the addiction to nicotine, other barriers to quitting include the following:

- Strong link to habits
- Other smokers in personal environment
- Facing stressful situations without a cigarette

The best defense against the effects of inhaled smoke from tobacco products is to never start smoking in the first place. Adolescents are the highest risk group for starting to smoke. Most people who smoke started as adolescents, often around the age of 12. Box 33-4 (p. 840) provides some guidelines for helping a client stop smoking.

General Health. Exercise and proper nutrition are important to respiratory function. Aerobic exercise increases maximal exercise ventilation (the most that the person can *actually* breathe). It also increases the ratio of maximal exercise ventilation to maximal *voluntary* ventilation (the most that the person *typically* breathes during exercise). As the ratio of possible ventilation to voluntary respiration increases, the person experiences less dyspnea with exercise. Endurance training improves the efficiency of breathing even in older adults. Besides general health benefits from nutrition, nutrition is directly related to obesity, which decreases the ventilatory capacity and increases the work of breathing.

Environmental Factors

Risk for respiratory disease is highly associated with the quality of the air that we breathe. Air pollution increases the incidence of respiratory disease and the exacerbation of respiratory diseases. Additional hazards can occur in the workplace or home.

Workplace Exposure. The risk for respiratory disease from environmental exposure can be associated with a specific occupation or avocational activities. Acute respiratory injury can occur from exposure to sulfuric acid, ammonia, or hydrochloric acid. Fungal diseases may be associated with a particular occupation, such as "farmer's lung disease" in Midwestern farmers. Often the damage done by environmental exposure does not manifest itself in signs and symptoms for years after the exposure has occurred. The person who has been exposed to asbestos, dust from grinding heavy metals, or caustic chemicals may have no evidence of the disease for years, but the stress of anesthesia or serious illness may precipitate symptoms. Thus a history of exposure

---

A PATIENT'S PERSPECTIVE
"I Get Out of Breath Just Walking to the Front Door."

Box 33-3

When I moved from the Midwest to Las Vegas, I thought I had found the perfect retirement spot, complete with longtime friends, a couple I had known for years. Before long, however, things began to go sour. Our friends separated and went their separate ways, leaving me a stranger in a strange land. Then, in September 1996, I was diagnosed with lung cancer, and my world turned upside down. Cancer shouldn't have surprised me; I was a smoker, so I have no one to blame but myself. But you always think cancer only happens to other people.

Doctors said the cancer was too close to my heart for surgery. So I had months of chemotherapy, then weeks of radiation. Both left me feeling down and out; I just let myself go. In February 1998, my son came to Las Vegas, took one look at me, and realized I was in trouble. After being hospitalized and treated for dehydration, malnutrition, and anemia, I went back to live with my son and his family. They have a big house, and it's nice to have young people around, especially my three granddaughters and my grandson.

I'm having more radiation treatment now, and the cancer seems to be contained in one lung, but my breathing is severely impaired. I used to be real active. I biked and walked a lot; I walked at least two miles several times a week. Now I get out of breath just walking to the front door, and it's worse in humid weather. I'm not totally incapacitated, and I try to help around the house, like loading the dishwasher. It may take me 2 hours, but at least it makes me feel a little bit useful.

In June, I developed another smoking-related problem: blood clots in my legs. Because of the cancer, I couldn't take blood thinners, so I had to have surgery.

My legs are better, but I still have trouble with them. Wearing those heavy elastic stockings helps a lot, and I have a hospital bed that can be elevated at the foot if my legs start to swell.

Since I came to live with my son, I've had wonderful care from visiting nurses. After my surgery, one of the visiting nurses noticed that I was kind of "out of it." When she checked my prescriptions, she saw that the doctor had prescribed a heavy dose of morphine, even though I wasn't in much pain, so she talked to him and got the prescription changed.

Twice a week, a home health aide comes to help me with my bath. I can still use the shower and the bathtub, but I need someone to help me in and out. Sometimes I wonder if I really need a tub bath, but when it's over, I feel so much better I know it was worth the effort.

Physical therapy has helped me, too. Right after the surgery, my legs felt really wobbly, and I had to use a walker. But the physical therapist had me do exercises with weights, and now I don't have to use the walker.

It was nurses who put us in touch with all of the resources available in the community. If I had known there was so much help available when I was first diagnosed, I wouldn't have ended up in such bad shape.

It's hard being housebound when you've always been independent, especially when you're only 63 years old. But both my sons are here, and we have a lot of other family in the area so there's always someone to take me where I need to go. I'm just glad to be alive and surrounded by people I love. I've already lived longer than the doctors thought I would, and I plan on enjoying life just as long as I can.

Teaching for Wellness
Helping a Client Stop Smoking

Box 33-4

Purpose: To support the client's motivation to stop smoking.

Expected Outcome: The client will develop a plan to stop smoking.

Client Instructions

Nicotine is a highly addictive substance. While addiction is the primary reason people smoke, smoking is also associated with relaxation, pleasurable activities, relief of boredom, and coping with stress.

Nicotine Replacement: While nothing delivers nicotine as effectively as a cigarette, about 30% of people receiving nicotine replacement along with support and counseling are able to quit smoking. Nicotine replacement is available as gums, patches, and nasal sprays. Gums and nasal sprays may work better for people who have trouble controlling the immediate urge to smoke, because these forms get nicotine into the bloodstream faster than patches. Nasal sprays have the fastest absorption. However, some people will be more successful with the constant nicotine levels provided by the patches, which keep the craving for nicotine under control. People with gum disease or dentures also may prefer the patches.

Some side effects are associated with the use of nicotine gums, sprays, and patches. Some of these side effects are unique to each form of nicotine replacement; other side effects are related to the nicotine itself. The most common problem with nicotine gum is using the product incorrectly. The user should chew the gum by biting it one or two times and then "parking" it between the cheek and gums. If it is rapidly chewed and the nicotine is swallowed, it causes nausea. The nasal spray can irritate the nose, causing a hot, peppery feeling and sneezing. The patch can irritate the skin. Patches that provide 24 hours of nicotine coverage have been associated with sleep disturbances and strange dreams.

Tips for Helping People Quit Smoking: Most people know that smoking is harmful to health, that it is sometimes offensive to others, and that it is costly. However, because some smokers will use any excuse for not quitting ("My doctor has never told me I should quit"), health professionals should use every opportunity to reinforce the wisdom of quitting.

Consider the following gentle reinforcers as part of discharge instructions for a respiratory client:

- "And of course you know you need to quit smoking."
- "I would like to see you quit smoking."
- "Have you thought about quitting?"
- "How can I help you quit smoking?"
- "What methods have you tried to quit smoking?"

The common theme in these statements is that each one places the control with the client and does not make a negative value judgment of the person.

When a client indicates the need for suggestions about how to stop smoking, assess the client's smoking behavior and offer specific suggestions:

- If smoking is strongly associated with specific activities, it may help to change the person's routine. For example, if the strongest urge to smoke comes with morning coffee when the person has just gotten out of bed, suggest a change in routine. On arising, the client might take a bath, brush the teeth, and eat a light breakfast in a different location (on the patio, or in the dining room, rather than in front of the morning news on the couch).
- If smoking is associated with social activities, especially seeking company in a bar or tavern, joining a support group may be a good suggestion. The support group provides an avenue for social interaction that reinforces the client's desire to quit smoking. Eventually, however, the person has to learn to control the urge to smoke in a variety of social situations where others are smoking.
- Increased exercise is an important suggestion. An exercise program may confirm the negative effects of cigarettes, it will give the client something to do rather than smoking, and it will help reverse the cardiovascular and respiratory effects of smoking, thus shortening the time before the client begins to feel a tangible benefit from quitting.
- If the person reports smoking as a response to stress, learning relaxation techniques and coping skills may help.
- Help the smoker find rewards for quitting: reduction of lines in the face, clearer skin, improved taste and smell, reduced stains on the hands and teeth, easier housecleaning, reduced cough, and reduced incidence of respiratory illness. Sometimes living to see grandchildren grown is a motivating force.

---

is an essential component of assessment of risk for respiratory complications.

Home Exposure. Besides the presence of tobacco smoke, other hazards exist in the home. For people who have allergies, allergens in the home can precipitate asthma attacks. The use of strong chemicals for cleaning, paint fumes, insecticides, and sources of carbon monoxide should be monitored.

Developmental Factors

Risk for respiratory disease is present throughout the life span, with the very young and the very old being the most vulnerable. Exposure to specific respiratory risk factors is related to the age of the person, however.

Infants and Children. Respiratory risk factors in infants and children are generally confined to exposure to common upper respiratory infections. Preschool children who attend day-

care centers are more likely to be exposed to respiratory infections than children raised at home. School-aged children are likely to pick up colds and flu viruses from classmates. Fortunately, respiratory infections in infants and young children are usually not serious, and most children are able to recover quickly without complications.

Certain respiratory conditions are potentially more serious in infants and children. Pneumonia is always a serious infection, but it is especially dangerous in babies under the age of 1 year. It can be fatal for premature infants, especially when surfactant production has not sufficiently developed (hyaline membrane disease).

Other than infections, reactive airway disease (asthma) is the most common respiratory condition in infants and children. It appears as early as 6 months of age, ranges from mild to severe, and can be fatal. The incidence of asthma is on the rise from multiple allergens. For example, dead roaches have been investigated as an allergen in low-income housing.

Adolescents and Middle Adults. The most prominent risk factor in adolescents and adults is smoking. Most people who smoke start smoking in adolescence, and the age of starting to smoke is younger than in previous generations. Inhaling substances, such as glue or paint, to get "high" can cause damage to the lungs. For adults, respiratory risks include smoking and occupational exposure as described earlier.

Older Adults. As a person ages, a decreasing amount of surfactant is produced in the lungs and there is a decrease in compliance, elasticity, and total lung capacity. In addition, the rib cage is less mobile. These physiological changes increase the risk for respiratory dysfunction by reducing the reserve capacity to compensate for increased need for oxygen. Among older adults, exercise tolerance may be compromised by inactivity. The older adult client who is immobilized has a high risk for developing the respiratory complications associated with any illness that requires bed rest. Thus age alone does not produce respiratory dysfunction but does increase the risk.

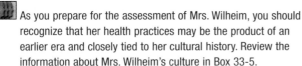 As you prepare for the assessment of Mrs. Wilheim, you should recognize that her health practices may be the product of an earlier era and closely tied to her cultural history. Review the information about Mrs. Wilheim's culture in Box 33-5.

Physiological Factors
Normal Physiological Variations.
Respiration varies to meet the demands of the body for oxygen and elimination of carbon dioxide at different levels of activity. An increased rate and depth of breathing is especially noticed with exercise because exercise increases the demand for oxygen and generates carbon dioxide as a byproduct of metabolism. At rest, breathing becomes slower and quieter.

Body position also affects respiration. As a person assumes different positions throughout the day, ventilation and perfusion shift to maintain the optimal ratio. When a person sits slumped in a comfortable chair, the lungs cannot fully expand, but the oxygen demand is low. When the carbon dioxide level reaches a certain point, the person will sigh or shift position to establish a better balance of ventilation and perfusion. Turning and moving during sleep accomplishes the same physiological purpose.

Respiration changes to compensate for changes in body size and shape. When a person gains weight or is pregnant,

the metabolic demand for oxygen increases. In the 9th month of pregnancy, the uterus may displace the diaphragm enough that the woman becomes short of breath with usual activities or lying down in some positions in bed. Severe obesity is associated with shortness of breath with moderate activity and a preference for sleeping with the upper torso elevated. The severely obese person has an increased risk for respiratory infection.

Respiratory Disorders. Physiological factors affecting ventilation generally fall in one of two categories. The problem is either restrictive to lung expansion or obstructive to the movement of air into and out of the lungs. Restriction to chest wall expansion can be from muscle dysfunction, nerve dysfunction, skeletal abnormalities, decreased intrathoracic space, or changes in lung compliance. Obstructive disorders produce difficult breathing because reduction in the size of the airway increases airway resistance.

Restrictive airway disease is any pathology that decreases the ability to expand the lungs. Paralysis, muscle weakness, and fatigue limit changes in the size of the thoracic cavity. Chest wall abnormalities can restrict expansion, particularly when the problem produces pain. Examples of chest wall abnormalities include fractured ribs and thoracic surgery. Expansion can also be impaired by hemothorax (blood in the pleural space) or pneumothorax (air in the pleural space). The lungs cannot expand because the space in the thorax is diminished and the lungs are atelectatic (collapsed). Fibrotic changes in the lungs decrease expansion because compliance is decreased. Pulmonary fibrosis is the formation of scar tissue (fibers) as a sequel to any inflammation or irritation.

Restriction to expansion can be from factors other than respiratory disease. Bed rest restricts lung expansion, as does a cast, brace, or rib binder used to treat orthopedic injuries. Abdominal distention, whether from pregnancy, abdominal surgery, or ascites (fluid in the abdominal cavity), inhibits movement of the diaphragm, thus restricting expansion of the lungs. Some examples of restrictive disorders are shown in Box 33-6 (p. 842).

Airway obstruction can be from mucus, inflammation or infection, a tumor, a foreign body, or constriction of the bronchi. Infection or inflammation causes swelling and increased production of **sputum,** the mucus secreted from the lungs, bronchi, and trachea. A tumor or foreign body can partially or totally occlude an airway. Bronchoconstriction is

Box 33-6   **Common Respiratory Disorders**

RESTRICTIVE DISORDERS

Atelectasis: A collapsed or airless state of the lung or a portion of a lung, caused by obstruction, hypoventilation, restriction to expansion, or absence of surfactant. May be a whole lung, a lobe, or a lobule, or it may be diffuse microatelectasis (scattered microscopic areas of collapse that cumulatively represent significant nonfunctional lung tissue).

Pleural effusion: Accumulation of fluid in the space between the visceral pleura and porietal pleura of the thorax, usually from an inflammatory process secondary to pneumonia, malignancy, or trauma.

Hemothorax: Bleeding into the pleural space secondary to trauma to the chest. May occur in a motor vehicle accident or fall, or it may follow thoracic surgery.

Pneumothorax: Air from the lung leaking into the pleural space, or atmospheric air entering the pleural space through a traumatic opening in the chest wall. Spontaneous pneumothorax can occur at high altitudes in depressurized airplane cabins.

Pneumoconiosis: A group of fibrotic lung diseases caused by prolonged inhalation of dust particles, usually from industrial dust (silica, asbestos); eventually develops a chronic obstructive component.

OBSTRUCTIVE DISORDERS

Pneumonia: Inflammation of the lung with consolidation and exudation. May be infectious (viral, bacterial, fungal) or inflammatory (aspiration of vomitus, chemicals, gases, oily substances, foreign bodies). The airways are reduced by consolidation and fill with edema, exudate, and sputum.

Asthma: An inflammatory response that constricts the bronchi and causes edema and increased production of sputum. Asthma can be caused by an allergic response to allergens, such as pollen, dust, smoke, and animal dander, or secondary to chronic infections or heart disease. Marked by recurrent attacks of dyspnea, with wheezing due to spasmodic constriction of the bronchi and increased production of sputum.

Emphysema: Pathological accumulation of air in tissues or organs, usually refers to pulmonary emphysema where air (carbon dioxide) accumulates in the alveoli because of loss of elasticity. Fatigue and dyspnea are the most prominent symptoms.

Tuberculosis: An infectious, inflammatory, reportable disease that is chronic in nature and commonly affects the lungs, although it may occur in almost any part of the body. The causative agent is *Mycobacterium tuberculosis*.

Lung cancer: Malignant growths of the lung tissue. Early symptoms are vague or may not appear at all. The earliest and most common symptom is a dry, hacking cough.

caused by contraction of the smooth muscles of the bronchi or bronchioles in response to an irritant or allergen. Box 33-6 also gives some examples of obstructive disorders.

ASSESSMENT

General Assessment of Respiration

As a nurse, you will perform a respiratory assessment as part of a general health screening, as a baseline review of a client just admitted to a hospital or clinic, or in response to cues to possible respiratory problems. The general health screening focuses on risk factors for respiratory disease and evidence of any current problems. For the client being admitted to the hospital, you will be looking for evidence that the client has a risk for the development of a respiratory complication or for the manifestations of respiratory disease. When a cue, such as a cough or shortness of breath, prompts the assessment, you will conduct a focused assessment to determine the nature and extent of the problem.

Regardless of the circumstances, the assessment begins with reviewing available data. Because nurses encounter clients at various stages of wellness and illness, the type and amount of data will vary. Pertinent cues to the risk for respiratory problems in the database would include history of cardiovascular or respiratory disorder, advanced age, anticipated use of anesthetics or narcotics, obesity, inability to cooperate with instructions, and immobility.

When assessing respiratory status, you need to be able to determine whether immediate, definitive action is needed. Cues to significant respiratory problems may suggest the need for emergency response to prevent or treat respiratory arrest. You can reduce the need to treat respiratory complications or

even respiratory failure by taking preventive action early in the client's illness.

Health History

CHIEF COMPLAINT. The assessment begins with the chief complaint. Respiratory complaints are difficulty breathing, cough, and pain. Identify the subjective findings by asking the questions necessary to analyze the symptom, such as the following:

- Are you having any difficulty breathing?
- When did it start? How long have you had the problem?
- Is it worse with activity? How much or what kind of activity?
- Is there anything that seems to relieve your difficult breathing?
- Have you tried anything to manage the problem? Medications? Breathing moist air?
- Any pain associated with breathing? Describe the pain. Where is the pain?
- Do you have a cough? Is it productive? Describe the sputum. Color? Amount? Is the cough nonproductive? Hacking? Does it occur at a particular time of day? Does it disturb sleep?

RISK FOR RESPIRATORY DISEASE. When the client's problems have not been identified, begin a screening history by assessing for factors that place the client at risk for specific respiratory disorders. Risk factors include age, environment, lifestyle, family history, and a history of respiratory problems.

AGE. Note the client's age. The very young and the very old have the highest risk for respiratory complications. Ask about recent exposure to respiratory infections.

ENVIRONMENT. Ask about the client's home and work environments. Take an occupational history and a history of travel, particularly to foreign countries, where exposure to uncommon diseases may have occurred.

LIFESTYLE. Assess for lifestyle factors that contribute to respiratory disorders. Respiratory assessment should include a complete history of smoking behaviors. Not only is smoking associated with lung cancer and emphysema, but it also increases the risk for a person having anesthesia. The smoking history is calculated by multiplying the number of packs per day by the number of years the person has smoked and is expressed as pack-years. For example, someone who has smoked 1½ packs a day for 20 years has smoked 30 pack-years. If you ask about the use of tobacco products rather than smoking, the client may be prompted to give information about cigars and smokeless tobacco. Additionally, any history of smoking should include marijuana use, because marijuana is even more harmful to the lungs than tobacco.

FAMILY HISTORY. Taking a family history is important because of the possibility of genetically or environmentally transmitted disease. Asthma is an example of a respiratory disease that tends to run in families and may have a genetic component. Additionally, family history may suggest the need to screen for infectious diseases like tuberculosis that can be contacted by exposure within the family. Family history may also suggest the need to screen for cystic fibrosis or ciliary defects.

HISTORY OF RESPIRATORY PROBLEMS. Ask if the client has a history of respiratory problems, especially asthma and emphysema. Particularly, ask about a history of tuberculosis.

PHYSICIAN'S TREATMENT PLAN. Knowledge of the physician's diagnostic and treatment plan will guide the assessment. Interventions that have a risk for respiratory complications include the use of sedatives and narcotics, diagnostic procedures in which an instrument is passed into the gastrointestinal tract or airways, bed rest, and intravenous fluids. Any surgical procedure requiring general or spinal anesthesia has a risk of respiratory complications.

CURRENT CONDITION. Observe the client's general condition. The person may be described as in excellent or good health, debilitated, or having a high stress level. The general nutritional status may have an impact. It may be sufficient to note that the person appears well developed and well nourished, obese, or undernourished. A history of chronic illness may reveal risk factors. Fatigue and the severity of the current illness can add to the risk. Assess the level of consciousness.

Physical Examination
The physical examination focuses on assessing for abnormal respiratory findings, the effects on vital signs, and signs of oxygen deficit in all body systems. The following help identify objective findings.

ORIENTATION, LEVEL OF CONSCIOUSNESS, AND BEHAVIOR. A sudden or gradual change in the person's level of consciousness or behavior can indicate that the person is not getting enough oxygen.

VITAL SIGNS. An increase or decrease in pulse, respiration, and blood pressure indicates that the client is compensating for an oxygen deficit or can no longer compensate for the deficit.

SKIN AND MUCOUS MEMBRANES. Check for color, warmth, turgor, and moisture. Cold, pale, clammy (moist) skin is a compensatory mechanism for oxygen deficit. Decreased skin turgor indicates dehydration.

BREATHING PATTERN. Check breathing for unusually quiet, labored, noisy, or shallow breathing; shortness of breath; and dyspnea.

LUNG AUSCULTATION. Listen for crackles, diminished sounds, rhonchi, and wheezes. Adventitious sounds help identify the cause of the change in breathing pattern.

ABDOMINAL ASSESSMENT. Listen to bowel sounds. Assess for abdominal distention. Diminished bowel sounds and distention may be associated with oxygen deficit.

URINE OUTPUT. Check the amount and concentration. If the client has a Foley catheter, observe the urine directly. Otherwise, ask when the person last urinated and ask for a description of the amount and color. Diminished urinary output is associated with insufficient oxygenated blood flow to the kidneys.

Recall the case of Mrs. Wilheim, introduced at the beginning of the chapter. The nursing assessment for Mrs. Wilheim on admission to the emergency room was as follows: "88-year-old white female in acute respiratory distress. Temperature 38.9° C (102° F), P 100, R 36, BP 106/70. Diminished breath sounds left lower base. Wheezes and rhonchi left lower lobe. Fremitus present. Oxygen saturation 87%. Oxygen started per face mask at 6 L. Oxygen saturation 91%. Skin pale, diaphoretic. Skin turgor sluggish. Complaining of feeling cold. Denies pain. Oriented to person, place, and time. Extremely weak and frightened. Abdomen soft, flat. Hypoactive bowel sounds. Foley catheter inserted. Returned 200 mL concentrated urine. Daughter at bedside. Blood drawn for electrolytes, CBC, chest film, and blood cultures."

Diagnostic Tests
Review the client's chart and correlate your clinical findings with any available diagnostic data. The physician uses the tests to make a medical diagnosis, whereas you will use the tests to assist in making nursing diagnoses and decisions about nursing interventions.

COMPLETE BLOOD COUNT. A *complete blood count* provides information about the oxygen-carrying capacity of the blood expressed as a red blood cell (RBC) count, a hematocrit index (the volume percentage of RBCs in the total plasma), and a hemoglobin concentration. The white blood cell count provides clues to the presence of an infection, which may be the primary cause of the respiratory problem or secondary to the problem.

CHEST RADIOGRAPH. Chest radiography provides basic diagnostic information about chest disorders and is used for health screening. Pneumonia, pneumothorax, atelectasis, fractured ribs, foreign bodies, and tumors can be distinguished on radiograph. A follow-up chest film may be used to monitor the progress of the disease. Chest radiography is used to screen for tuberculosis when the client has a positive tuberculin skin test.

To prepare the client for a chest film, have the client remove clothing and jewelry from the waist up and don a hospital gown. Advise the client that the quality of the radiograph will depend on the client's ability to take a deep breath and hold it. A portable chest radiograph can be taken with the client in a high Fowler's position. You may need to assist with placing the x-ray film behind the client, but then you will need to leave the room to avoid exposure to radiation.

Mrs. Wilheim's chest film shows pneumonia in the left lower lobe. Notice that she had pain with breathing when her daughter found her. Can you correlate the location of her pain with her chest film? How do you think an 88-year-old woman would feel about having pneumonia?

PULMONARY FUNCTION TESTS. *Pulmonary function tests* measure lung volumes associated with the mechanics of breathing when the client performs a series of respiratory maneuvers. The volumes are recorded using a spirometer (an instrument for measuring air taken into and expelled from the lungs). Pulmonary function tests may be simple measurements performed at the bedside, in the home, or in a clinic. The full scope of pulmonary function tests requires more sophisticated equipment available only in a pulmonary function laboratory.

The expected lung capacity and volumes are calculated for each client using a formula that includes height, weight, sex, and age. Results are reported as a percentage of the expected value. Table 33-2 describes basic measurements of pulmonary function and illustrates the relationships of lung volumes and

Table 33-2	Basic Measurements of Pulmonary Function	
Measurement	**Description**
MEASUREMENT OF LUNG VOLUME	
Tidal volume (V_T)	Volume of air inhaled and exhaled with each quiet respiration
Residual volume (RV)	Volume of air remaining in the lungs after a maximum exhalation
MEASUREMENT OF LUNG CAPACITY	
Total lung capacity (TLC)	Volume of air in lungs after maximal inhalation
Vital capacity (VC)	Volume of air that can be exhaled after a maximal inhalation
Functional residual volume (FRV)	Volume of air remaining in the lungs at the end of normal expiration
Inspiratory capacity (IC)	Largest volume of air that can be inspired in one breath from the resting expiratory
MEASUREMENTS RELATED TO THE MECHANICS OF BREATHING	
Forced vital capacity (FVC)	Volume of air forcefully (with maximum effort) exhaled after a maximum inhalation
Forced expiratory volume in 1 second (FEV_1)	Amount of air expelled from the lungs during the 1st second of the FVC

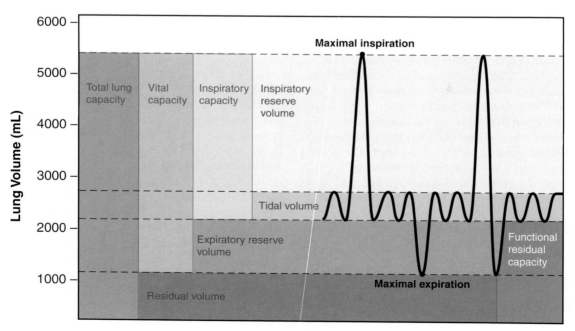

Spirographic representation of the relationship of lung volumes and capacities. Notice that the lungs always have a residual volume of approximately 1000 mL and a vital capacity far in excess of the tidal volume.

capacities. The tests used for bedside monitoring are tidal volume and vital capacity.

ARTERIAL BLOOD GASES. *Arterial blood gases* are measured to determine the partial pressures of oxygen and carbon dioxide as an indicator of respiratory function. Full interpretation of arterial blood gases is an advanced skill, but it is possible to quickly learn a beginning level of interpretation.

Drawing arterial blood is an invasive procedure usually performed by respiratory therapists and specially trained nurses. Arteries are deep under the surface of the skin and are located adjacent to nerves; therefore insertion of the needle is highly painful. Use of a heparinized syringe prevents the blood from clotting before the test can be run. A glass syringe may be selected because the plunger will move easily, allowing the pressure of the arterial blood to fill the syringe. The needle must be occluded after drawing the blood to prevent the escape of the blood gases; the blood is chilled, especially if the laboratory is a distance from the bedside.

Subcutaneous bleeding is a likely complication even after the needle has been withdrawn. Uninterrupted pressure is applied to the artery for a minimum of 5 minutes to prevent a hematoma from forming.

Blood gas results provide information about oxygenation. The normal value of the arterial partial pressure of oxygen (Pa_{O_2}) is based on room air; therefore it can be interpreted only with knowledge of the amount of oxygen the person is breathing. The percentage saturation is the percentage of hemoglobin saturated with oxygen. If the client is on oxygen therapy, the liter flow and delivery device are written on the report. The physician may order the blood gases to be drawn on room air if the client can tolerate having the oxygen removed. It takes about 30 minutes for the arterial oxygen level to become stable on room air.

Blood gas results also provide information about acid–base balance. The arterial partial pressure of carbon dioxide (Pa_{CO_2}) is directly correlated with the pH, or acidity, of the blood. The respiratory system helps maintain the acid–base balance of the body by controlling the carbon dioxide level in the blood. If the carbon dioxide level is high, indicating acidosis, and the pH is normal, the kidneys have compensated for the acidosis by retaining the bicarbonate ion as a buffer. Renal compensation is observed by an elevation of the bicarbonate level (H_2CO_3) in the reported blood gases. Acidosis or alkalosis can result from metabolic problems, so it is important to distinguish pH changes as having a metabolic or respiratory cause.

PULSE OXIMETRY. Pulse oximetry (Sp_{O_2}) is a method of measuring the oxygen saturation of hemoglobin in the blood. It can be used at the hospital bedside, in the home, or in a clinic. A sensing device is clipped to a finger or an earlobe. Within this device, a photoelectric detector records the amount of light transmitted or reflected by deoxygenated versus oxygenated hemoglobin. Figure 33-4 shows placement of a finger sensor.

Pulse oximetry is a useful clinical tool for monitoring oxygen level. Arterial saturation measured with the pulse oximeter is reliable because it has a close correlation with the saturations obtained from the blood gases when the saturation is above 70%. A saturation of 90% is the critical value for oxygenation to support life. Arterial blood does not develop any significant degree of desaturation until the Pa_{O_2} falls below 60; therefore, when the percentage of saturation falls below 90, the Pa_{O_2} may be below 60.

Pulse oximetry is a helpful tool but should be used only in conjunction with other assessment data. Hypotension, vasoconstriction, hypothermia, reduced blood flow, thick acrylic nails, some dark nail polishes, bright florescent lights, and movement of the finger can interfere with the measurement. Because pulse oximetry does not provide as much information as arterial blood gases, arterial blood is still drawn for analysis in some situations.

SPUTUM CULTURE. Sputum culture means growing microorganisms from sputum. When the client has a productive cough, sputum may be collected for a culture and sensitivity test. It takes 24 to 72 hours to grow a culture of the organisms in laboratory conditions. The organism is then identified and tested for sensitivity to a list of antibiotics. In the meantime, the physician makes a judgment of the most likely causative organism on the basis of the presenting signs and symptoms and starts an antibiotic regimen. A Gram stain may be done to narrow the choice of antibiotic within a few hours. Often an appropriate antibiotic has been chosen and the infection is resolving by the time the culture and sensitivity report is available. If the antibiotic needs to be changed, then no further time is lost identifying an appropriate antibiotic.

Any sputum specimen is best collected early in the morning when the sputum has collected in the lungs during the night. For the client who cannot cough deeply enough to obtain sputum rather than pharyngeal mucus, endotracheal suctioning is sometimes requested. Use of a sterile container will prevent cross-contamination. The specimen is sent to the laboratory within 30 minutes of collection.

THROAT CULTURES. Throat cultures are grown from material swabbed from the throat. The most common use of a throat culture is to evaluate a possible streptococcal infection.

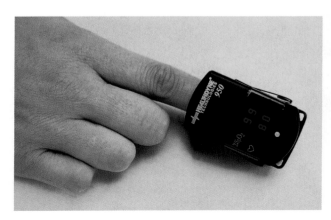

Figure 33-4. A pulse oximeter. Before you attach the sensor, clean the client's finger with an alcohol wipe, and remove any nail polish or artificial nails. (Courtesy Respironics, Pittsburgh, PA.)

Because infections with β-hemolytic streptococci can result in rheumatic fever or acute glomerulonephritis, permanent damage to the heart or kidneys can occur. A Gram stain may be used to aid in promptly beginning appropriate therapy. Throat cultures can screen for asymptomatic carriers of organisms.

To obtain a specimen for culture, tilt the head to expose the tonsillar surfaces, and with a sterile cotton-tipped applicator swab the area from side to side, including any inflamed or purulent sites (Figure 33-5). Return the swab to the culture tube. To ensure that the swab is not cross-contaminated by your hands, touch only the cap and the outside of the culture tube, not the swab. Break the ampule of fluid in the bottom of the tube and send it directly to the laboratory.

BRONCHOSCOPY. *Bronchoscopy* is the direct visualization of the larynx, trachea, and large bronchi using a flexible, fiberoptical scope passed into the lungs. It is used to visually guide the physician in obtaining specimens of secretions or tissue for biopsy, removing foreign bodies and mucus plugs, or implanting medications for treating tumors.

After bronchoscopy, the client is positioned for maximum respiratory function (usually in a semi-Fowler's position) and monitored for complications. Vital signs and breath sounds are helpful in detecting problems. Complications are usually minor but may include bleeding, edema, **bronchospasm,** aspiration, and temporary hoarseness. Less often, bronchoscopy can result in pneumothorax. Box 33-7 provides guidelines for assisting the client experiencing a bronchoscopy.

THORACENTESIS. In a *thoracentesis,* the physician punctures the chest wall and enters the pleural space. When pleural effusion or blood in the pleural space has been demonstrated on a chest film, thoracentesis drains the fluid and relieves the respiratory distress. Thoracentesis may also be used to obtain a specimen for diagnostic studies. The fluid is examined for abnormal cells, white blood cells, red blood cells, glucose,

and microorganisms. Box 33-7 describes the steps for assisting the client undergoing a thoracentesis and shows the most common position for a thoracentesis.

Focused Assessment
for *Ineffective Breathing Pattern*

Because oxygenation is a high-priority problem, you will need to recognize problems and intervene before the person has an oxygen deficit or before the deficit becomes critical. Keep in mind that the diagnoses are closely interrelated.

Breathing patterns can vary in rate, depth, timing, rhythm, and chest wall and abdominal excursion during inspiration, expiration, or both. Abnormal breathing patterns are those that produce less than optimal ventilation for the individual. *Ineffective airway clearance* describes a client who has difficulty maintaining a clear airway. The airway may be obstructed with secretions, edema, a foreign body, or a tumor or because it has collapsed. *Impaired gas exchange* is a defect in the ability to oxygenate the blood or eliminate carbon dioxide from the blood, or both.

Defining Characteristics

HYPOVENTILATION. When a client is not breathing well, assess for hypoventilation. **Hypoventilation** is a decrease in the rate and depth of breathing, clinically defined as $PaCO_2$ greater than 45 mm Hg. Assessment of the breathing pattern includes rate of breathing, depth of breathing, breath sounds, and sometimes the relationship of inspiration to expiration.

Assess the rate, rhythm, and depth of respiration. The normal pattern of breathing includes inspiration lasting about 2 seconds and expiration lasting about 3 seconds at a rate of 11 to 24 cycles per minute. Normal tidal volume, the amount of air inhaled and exhaled with each breath, is 500 mL. The rhythm should be regular with periodic sighing. The rate that is considered normal varies across the life span. Normal tidal volume is based on age, sex, and body size.

The presence of hypoventilation is inferred at a respiratory rate less than 10 per minute, a depth of respiration that diminishes breath sound, or as a combination of both. Although a rate of less than 10 is generally considered a critical level, the client's baseline rate and associated symptoms should be considered. Rapid, shallow breathing reflects hypoventilation at the alveolar level because the person is not inflating as much as the lower two thirds of the lung. Auscultation for breath sounds reveals absent or diminished sounds in the bases.

To be clinically significant, hypoventilation must produce a change in minute ventilation. Minute ventilation is the total amount of air that enters the respiratory passages in 1 minute, and it is calculated as a product of tidal volume and respiratory rate. At a respiratory rate of 12, the minute ventilation would be 500 mL multiplied by 12, or 6 L.

However, even if you could measure the total volume of air moving into and out of the lungs, it would not be sufficient information to decide whether adequate ventilation is occurring throughout the lung fields. Diminished breath sounds are most frequently detected in the bases of the lungs when the

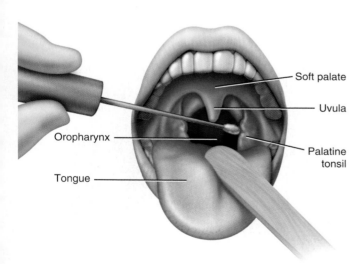

Figure 33-5. To collect a specimen for a throat culture, depress the tongue with an applicator, and swab the tonsillar area. Work quickly to prevent gagging.

Soft palate

Uvula

Oropharynx

Palatine tonsil

Tongue

person is not taking deep enough breaths to fill the alveoli. Breath sounds could also be diminished in a specific area because of a mucus plug, edema, bronchial constriction, or other obstruction to airflow. Table 33-3 describes the interpretation and management of abnormal breath sounds.

Oxygen deficit and carbon dioxide retention are closely associated with hypoventilation. From a physiological perspective, hypoventilation is defined as a pattern of breathing producing a $PaCO_2$ of more than 45 mm Hg. It is sometimes referred to as alveolar hypoventilation. The carbon dioxide level, rather than the oxygen level, is used because the respiratory control center is more sensitive to carbon dioxide.

Action Alert! For the client with rapid, shallow breathing, institute measures to increase ventilation, and assess for oxygen deficit.

HYPERVENTILATION. Hyperventilation is an increase in the rate and depth of breathing, clinically defined as $PaCO_2$ less than 35 mm Hg. Under normal conditions, the physiological respiratory control mechanisms return rapid respiration to normal. In some circumstances, however, rapid deep breathing continues to a point that causes a change in the blood gases. Alveolar hyperventilation is defined as deep, rapid respirations sufficient to lower the $PaCO_2$ and produce respiratory alkalosis. From a physiological perspective,

hyperventilation is defined as a pattern of breathing producing a $PaCO_2$ less than 35 mm Hg. The signs and symptoms of alkalosis are feeling lightheaded, muscle twitching, numbness, tetany, and, in severe cases, convulsions.

Action Alert! The hyperventilating client who has rapid, deep respirations and complains of numbness and tingling in the fingers is in a state of alkalosis. Assist the client to slow the respiration.

Respirations are increased by metabolic need, exercise, fever, acidosis, hypoxemia, or hypercapnia. Hyperventilation can result from any metabolic disease that causes acidosis (increased blood acidity). The body attempts to reduce the acid by elimination of carbon dioxide.

DYSPNEA. Rather than being a specific pattern of breathing, **dyspnea** is the subjective sensation of difficulty in breathing and is usually associated with increased rate of breathing. The client reports dyspnea when the work of breathing necessary to meet metabolic demands reaches conscious awareness. Dyspnea is important to consider in a discussion of breathing patterns because it is more closely related to the ventilatory component of pulmonary function than to the gas exchange component. Dyspnea may be acute or chronic. The abnormal breath sounds described in Table 33-3 (p. 848) may be associated with dyspnea.

Box 33-7   Assisting With Bronchoscopy and Thoracentesis

BRONCHOSCOPY

Bronchoscopy is an invasive procedure requiring informed consent and performed by a physician.

1. Keep the client NPO for 4-6 hours before the procedure. Have the client remove any dentures.
2. Administer an analgesic or sedative, if ordered, 30 minutes before the procedure.
3. The physician will apply a local anesthetic to the throat. Keep in mind that the gag and swallowing reflexes will be impaired while the effects of the anesthetic are present.
4. Withhold fluids and food until the swallowing reflex has returned.
5. After the procedure, provide warm saline gargles to relieve a sore throat.
6. Observe for complications of bronchoscopy: hemoptysis, atelectasis, and bronchitis.

THORACENTESIS

Thoracentesis is an invasive procedure requiring informed consent and performed by a physician under sterile conditions.

1. Take baseline vital signs before the procedure. The client may have a drop in blood pressure, especially when a large volume of fluid is withdrawn.
2. Advise the client that a local anesthetic will be injected subcutaneously, but that the client will feel pressure from insertion of a large-bore needle.
3. Position the client on the side of the bed, with the arms folded and supported by an over-bed table at nipple height.
4. Assist the client to remain still during the puncture to help prevent damage to lung tissue. Coughing or taking a deep breath during the procedure increases the risk of puncturing the lung.

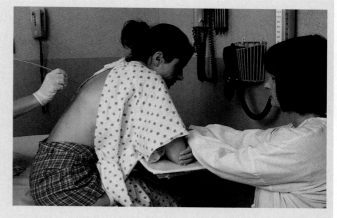

The most common position for a thoracentesis. Gravity allows the fluid to accumulate in the lower thoracic cavity. The spine is slightly curved. The needle must enter the fluid to avoid puncturing the lungs.

5. If a large amount of fluid is removed from the lungs, observe the client for hemodynamic changes. Take the client's vital signs.
6. Assess the client for atelectasis and pneumothorax.
7. Keep the specimen-filled test tubes upright. Label them and send them to the laboratory.

Table 33-3	Interpreting and Managing Abnormal Breath Sounds	
Abnormal Sound	**Etiology**	**Management**
Diminished or absent	Hypoventilation, atelectasis, consolidation of lung tissue	Bronchial hygiene, coughing, deep breathing, position changes, ambulation
Abnormal location of bronchial or bronchovesicular sounds	Consolidation or compressed lung tissue	Provide rest to decrease oxygen need. Assist to cough and deep-breathe until definitive medical therapy reestablishes ventilation.
Crackles (fine): a discontinuous fine crackling sound at the middle or end of inspiration; the sound of alveoli popping open	Atelectasis, mucus in small airways, fluid overload, left ventricular heart failure, or interstitial fibrosis	Diuretics, fluid restriction, a low-sodium diet, or treatment for heart failure
Crackles (coarse): a discontinuous, bubbling sound (sometimes called coarse rales or bubbling rhonchi)	Mucus in the bronchioles	Bronchial hygiene; hydration to loosen mucus; may clear with coughing
Rhonchi: a continuous sonorous or sibilant sound, like air through a hollow tube	A sound in the larger airways (bronchi), produced by vibration of narrowed airways; narrowing could result from edema, bronchospasm, or mucus	Measures to open the airways such as administration of bronchodilators, coughing, or humidification
Wheezes: continuous, high-pitched musical sounds	Bronchoconstriction or bronchospasm, or other obstruction	Bronchodilators; diuretics if the airways are narrowed by edema
Pleural friction rub: the grating, rubbing sound of two inflamed surfaces rubbing together	Inflammation of the pleura	Treatment for the underlying inflammatory process, possibly antibiotics; disappearance may indicate the development of pleural effusion

With normal pulmonary function, the increased work of breathing with exercise will produce dyspnea. Dyspnea becomes a symptom when the level of activity necessary to produce dyspnea is a level of activity that would not usually produce it in a given individual. Dyspnea is an important diagnostic cue for the respiratory nursing diagnoses and for the nursing diagnoses *Activity intolerance* (see Chapter 31) and *Decreased cardiac output* (see Chapter 34).

Dyspnea is difficulty in breathing and it can be acute or chronic. Signs of acute dyspnea are increased rate and depth of breathing, struggling to breathe, use of accessory muscles of respiration, flared nostrils in infants, and, in severe distress, paradoxical respirations. The person may need to sit up to breathe. Assess for pain and gather information about the pain if present. Chronic dyspnea is evidenced by hypertrophy of accessory muscles, sitting in a forward position with the hands supported on the knees (three-point position), and pursed-lip breathing.

Although dyspnea can occur with or without hypoxemia, the assessment of dyspnea should include assessing for signs and symptoms of diminished tissue oxygenation. Hypoxemia occurs when the compensatory mechanisms that produce dyspnea fail to provide enough oxygen.

Related Factors

FACTORS RELATED TO HYPOVENTILATION

IMMOBILITY. Bed rest or immobility compromises the ventilation/perfusion ratio, decreases the tidal volume, and decreases the total lung capacity. The part of the lung resting against the bed cannot fully expand. Ventilation is best in the upper portion of the lungs. Secretions become stagnant in the lower airways where the alveoli may not be filled by the diminished volume of inspired air.

PAIN. Pain or discomfort will prevent the client from taking a deep breath. Pain in the abdomen or thorax causes the client to splint the chest and decrease expansion of the lungs. The presence of abdominal distention, whether from surgery or disease, should prompt assessment of respiratory status. High or lengthy abdominal incisions may compromise respiratory function. Obesity, pregnancy, and severe *ascites* (lymphatic fluid accumulation in the abdomen secondary to cirrhosis of the liver) can compromise respiratory function by exerting pressure on the diaphragm.

MEDICATIONS. Furthermore, the measures to *treat* pain carry a risk of respiratory depression. Narcotics and anesthetic agents are the most prominent among the central nervous system depressants causing hypoventilation. The first dose or a high dose of central nervous system depressants demands close monitoring of the client during the administration. Elderly patients, patietns with liver disease, and patients with respiratory disease also require close monitoring. *Obtundation* describes the client rendered insensitive to painful stimuli because the level of consciousness has been reduced by a narcotic or anesthetic.

MUSCLE OR NERVE DYSFUNCTION. Muscle or nerve damage may compromise respiratory function. High spinal cord injuries result in paralysis of accessory muscles of respiration or may even affect the medulla to depress respiration. Muscle-weakening diseases such as multiple sclerosis, Guillain-Barré syndrome, and myasthenia gravis result in hypoventilation.

RESTRICTIONS TO EXPANSION. Trauma to the chest or abdomen should be a cue for assessment. Chest wall damage, hemothorax, pneumothorax, kyphoscoliosis, or fractured ribs can be the cause of hypoventilation. The client is not able to fully expand the lungs or may have a significant portion of the lungs that is collapsed (atelectatic).

FATIGUE. The client may be so physically overwhelmed by an illness that decreased energy and fatigue contribute to hypoventilation. This phenomenon is seen in the critically ill, especially when the person has had a prolonged episode of difficulty in breathing.

FACTORS RELATED TO HYPERVENTILATION. Hyperventilation may be in response to severe anxiety, fear, or metabolic disease, but other causes should be ruled out before deciding that anxiety is the cause. Acidosis resulting from metabolic disease such as renal failure or diabetes can be the underlying cause of hyperventilation. Metabolic acidosis means that excess acids have been produced through a metabolic process. The respiratory system attempts to compensate for the excess acid by eliminating carbonic acid in the form of carbon dioxide. Lactic acid produced by the skeletal muscles during exercise contributes to the increase in respiration with exercise. Head injury, salicylate overdose, and hypoxemia result in increased respiration.

FACTORS RELATED TO DYSPNEA. The underlying causes of dyspnea are a variety of neurological, respiratory, metabolic, and cardiac conditions. Obstructed or restricted breathing can cause dyspnea. Obstructed breathing is discussed next, under *Ineffective airway clearance.*

Focused Assessment for *Ineffective Airway Clearance*

Defining Characteristics. You may be prompted to assess for clear airways when the person complains of dyspnea, has a change in rate or depth of respiration, complains of feeling "congested," has a cough, or complains of pain. Because the client is not taking deep breaths, fluid may accumulate in the airways. When the fluid remains stagnant, infection may develop, resulting in hypostatic pneumonia. A fever may be present before infection occurs and is a cue that should prompt respiratory assessment. Therefore risk factors for hypoventilation also apply to *Ineffective airway clearance.* Additionally, any respiratory disease that results in increased production of sputum carries the risk for *Ineffective airway clearance.*

The most obvious signs of failure to clear the airways are the audible signs of obstructive breathing. *Stridor* is a shrill, harsh sound, especially the respiratory sound heard during inspiration in laryngeal obstruction. Stridor indicates a narrowing of the larynx or trachea, and secretions are probably retained below the obstruction. *Wet respirations* refer to an audible, bubbling sound with inspiration and expiration. *Audible wheezing* also indicates obstructive breathing that is resulting in the retention of secretions.

When the respirations are quiet, you can detect *Ineffective airway clearance* using a stethoscope to auscultate the lung fields.

Action Alert! Rhonchi indicate the retention of secretions that can be coughed out. Have the client cough and take deep breaths to reduce rhonchi and an associated fever.

A cough is an attempt to clear the airway; therefore it is a cardinal sign of *Ineffective airway clearance.* A wet- or loose-sounding cough suggests mucus retention. A dry, hacking cough generally indicates airway irritation, but it may result from an obstructive disorder. Sometimes a cough is the only sign of asthma (constricted airways) observable without a stethoscope. A harsh, barky cough suggests upper airway obstruction secondary to subglottic inflammation, especially edema, as in bronchitis. A cough that results in the expectoration of sputum is described as *productive.* A productive cough that does not clear rhonchi, or that clears the rhonchi for only a short period of time, is appropriately described as *Ineffective airway clearance.* Absence of a cough reflex is highly associated with *Ineffective airway clearance.*

Related Factors

SPUTUM ABNORMALITIES. Pathology of the lungs carries the risk for *Ineffective airway clearance,* especially when excess sputum is produced. As defined earlier, sputum is the mucus secreted from the lungs, bronchi, and trachea. Interventions are directed at reducing the amount of sputum or helping the client manage expectoration of sputum.

The characteristics of the sputum should be monitored. As sputum is removed from the lungs by ciliary action, the lung is cleared of dead cells and debris. When an infection is present, sputum also contains microorganisms and white blood cells. The volume of the sputum and the tenacity of the sputum are directly related to the ability to clear the airway. The normal daily production of approximately 100 mL of sputum cannot be coughed out. Foreign matter that irritates the respiratory passage increases the production of sputum and stimulates a cough. Detailed observations of sputum help you assess the problem and monitor the course of illness.

ABNORMAL QUANTITY. The *quantity of sputum* can be measured as the frequency of the productive cough or directly measured as milliliters produced in a 24-hour period. Clients are more likely to describe the volume of sputum using the more familiar terms of teaspoons, tablespoons, or cups. Intensive care nurses may describe the quantity on the basis of the frequency of the need for suctioning. A reduction in the quantity of sputum indicates progress or, in the case of chronic respiratory disease when excess sputum is always present, may be the desired outcome.

ABNORMAL COLOR. The *color of sputum* should be clear or somewhat white. Purulent (yellow or green) mucus indicates infection (e.g., lung abscess or pneumonia). Mucopurulent sputum contains both the increased mucus from an airway disease (e.g., bronchitis, bronchiectasis) and the pus from infection. Blood-streaked sputum indicates airway irritation that can result from excessive coughing with rupture of pulmonary capillaries from high intravascular pressures. Pink, watery, frothy sputum is typical of an acute episode of pulmonary edema. Rusty sputum is from blood that has been in the airways for a period of time. Pneumococcal pneumonia characteristically produces rusty sputum.

HEMOPTYSIS. Hemoptysis is defined as coughing and spitting up of blood as a result of bleeding from any part of the lower respiratory tract. It may indicate a potentially life-threatening bleeding problem, cardiopulmonary disease, or irritation of the mucous membrane as occurs with frequent endotracheal suctioning. On the other hand, an overdose of an anticoagulant can result in hemoptysis. A small amount (5 to 10 mL) of frankly bloody sputum may be present in tuberculosis, lung cancer, or pulmonary embolism. Large amounts (60 mL or more) are more likely to be chest trauma with rupture of a larger blood vessel.

Abnormal Consistency. The *consistency of sputum* may help diagnose the client's problem. Thick, tenacious sputum is difficult to cough out. Lack of moisture causes it to stick to the alveoli and the surfaces of airways and predisposes the person to mucus retention. Thick, tenacious sputum is often associated with chronic obstructive pulmonary disease (COPD) or may be caused by dehydration. Thin, watery sputum is associated with allergic responses.

Abnormal Odor. The *odor of the sputum* is an important observation. Normal sputum is odorless. Sputum may have a sweet, foul, or decomposed stench. The odor of sputum may be detected as *halitosis*. Other causes for halitosis (bad breath) are poor oral hygiene, infection in the mouth, or dental caries. A sweet odor to the breath is a reason to suspect diabetic ketoacidosis.

Fatigue or Decreased Energy. When the client's energy level is a related factor, nursing interventions are directed at conserving energy. The prescription for bed rest in the client who is weak or fatigued is sufficient reason to assess for *Ineffective airway clearance*. The client's energy need is a factor in the decision to treat a cough. Recovery is compromised in the client who lacks the energy to cough out sputum or even to take deep breaths. On the other hand, coughing is tiring and may need to be treated to conserve the client's energy. Energy needed for other activities of getting well must be balanced against the need to cough.

Altered Level of Consciousness. When *Ineffective airway clearance* is related to a decreased level of consciousness, more aggressive nursing intervention may be necessary to maintain a clear airway. Both the respiratory control center and the bronchial cough reflex can be suppressed from a neurological cause. A client in a coma, or unconscious from anesthesia or narcotics, does not have a cough reflex. At a higher level of consciousness, the client may be unable to consciously produce a cough but retains the cough reflex and will cough when the epiglottis is stimulated with a suction catheter. A decreased level of consciousness is also associated with the inability to spontaneously change position in bed. Stagnation of secretions is further exacerbated by a reduction in the sighing mechanism.

Pain. Pain can contribute to *Ineffective airway clearance;* therefore pain management may be helpful in maintaining respiratory function. Chest wall or abdominal pain is aggravated by coughing or even by deep breathing. The client attempts to control the pain by splinting the chest and fails to take the deep breaths necessary to clear the airways and prevent atelectasis. Additionally, pain is exhausting, depleting the client's energy store and psychological reserves needed for recovery.

Focused Assessment for *Impaired Gas Exchange*

Defining Characteristics. Any factor that predisposes a client to altered respiratory function can be a risk factor for *Impaired gas exchange*. High-risk clients include those who have undergone surgery, have sustained severe trauma, are seriously ill, or have severe respiratory disease. Hypoventilation and *Ineffective airway clearance* are primary risk factors both for the retention of carbon dioxide and for inadequate oxygenation.

Hypoxemia. As indicated, hypoxemia refers to low oxygen levels in the blood. **Hypoxia** refers to inadequate oxygenation at the level of body tissues. Hypoxemia is the usual cause of hypoxia. Hypoxemia is definitively diagnosed with arterial blood gases or pulse oximetry, or it is inferred from signs and symptoms of hypoxia. Holistic assessment is well illustrated in the examination for hypoxemia, because every body system is affected.

Recognize any sign or symptom of hypoxia as a cue to thoroughly assess respiratory status, particularly when the client has multiple predisposing factors. It is easy to think of hypoxemia when the client has multiple signs of oxygen deficiency, but if you are aware of the client's risk, you will consider subtle cues.

Action Alert! If your at-risk client is restless, call the respiratory therapy department for a pulse oximeter if your nursing unit does not have one. Restlessness in a semiconscious or unconscious client suggests the need for a thorough assessment for an oxygen deficit.

Changes in Mental Status. The mental status of the client may be the first cue to diagnosis. Restlessness is the earliest and most often missed sign of hypoxia. A diminishing level of consciousness may progress from difficulty concentrating to confusion, lethargy, and finally coma. The older adult client who becomes restless and confused after surgery should be assessed for hypoxemia.

Changes in Vital Signs. Vital signs change to compensate for hypoxemia. The respiratory rate is initially elevated as a compensatory response to hypoxemia and then may drop as the level of oxygen becomes insufficient to support life. The blood pressure and heart rate will initially increase and then drop. A narrow pulse pressure (i.e., a small difference between the diastolic and systolic pressures) is a warning sign that may be quickly followed by shock. If the client is on a heart monitor, heart block or bradycardia (slow rate) may be seen.

Changes in the Skin. Cyanosis is a blue color to the skin that results from the concentration of deoxygenated hemoglobin close to the surface of the skin. It is usually a late sign of hypoxemia. Cyanosis may be absent when the skin is vasoconstricted or if the hemoglobin level is low. Cyanosis may be present without hypoxemia if there is an abnormal elevation of red blood cells (polycythemia vera). Cyanosis is most frequently seen as central cyanosis—that is, in the earlobes, in the mucous membranes of the mouth, or circumorally (around the mouth). A pale skin color is associated with the compensatory mechanism of peripheral vasoconstriction that occurs in the physiological stress response, which shunts blood away from the skin to the vital organs.

CHANGES IN GASTROINTESTINAL FUNCTION. Gastrointestinal symptoms are not of immediate concern in identifying hypoxemia but may be considered as secondary symptoms or complications. The gastrointestinal tract slows either from the physiological stress response or from the lack of oxygen. Constipation, abdominal distention, and even paralytic ileus may occur.

CHANGES IN RENAL FUNCTION. Lack of oxygen to the kidney may be from hypoxemia or from decreased renal blood flow secondary to shock or congestive heart failure. Renal function is assessed by the volume of urinary output. A Foley catheter may be ordered to assist in assessing renal function. Less than 30 mL per hour of urine output suggests renal failure. Blood urea nitrogen (BUN) and blood creatinine levels may be ordered by the physician to determine the effect on the kidneys.

HYPERCAPNIA. Hypercapnia, the retention of carbon dioxide, is synonymous with acidosis from a respiratory cause. In the body fluids, carbon dioxide combines with water to become carbonic acid; therefore the pH immediately drops (respiratory acidosis) when the client hypoventilates or stops breathing. Diminished breath sounds and confusion are cues that alert you to consider the diagnosis.

Hypercapnia is defined as a $PaCO_2$ greater than 45 mm Hg. Clinical signs and symptoms occur in the cardiac, respiratory, and neurological systems. However, the signs and symptoms are not definitive for hypercapnia; therefore the signs and symptoms must be accompanied by a reason to believe carbon dioxide retention has occurred. The cardiovascular signs are increased pulse rate, increased blood pressure, bounding pulse, and palpitations. Cardiac arrhythmias can result from potassium depletion. The respiratory response to hypercapnia is an increased respiratory rate often resulting in a complaint of dyspnea. With persistently elevated levels of carbon dioxide, cerebral edema can cause headache, dizziness, and a feeling of pressure in the head. The client may have lethargy, disorientation, and confusion and may be uncooperative. The result can be convulsions and coma.

Related Factors

FACTORS RELATED TO HYPOXEMIA. The factors related to hypoxemia are risk factors that, if left untreated, will result in hypoxemia. Refer to the sections on *Ineffective breathing pattern* and *Ineffective airway clearance.* The client's care is managed as a collaborative problem because the physician must order the definitive treatment to restore oxygenation and to remove the underlying cause. Table 33-4 describes the causes of hypoxemia.

FACTORS RELATED TO HYPERCAPNIA. Hypercapnia is associated with hypoxemia caused by hypoventilation, apnea, and trapping of air in the alveoli. It is not associated with hypoxemia from other causes. The client with chronic airflow limitation (CAL) is prone to retention of carbon dioxide and may live with chronic hypercapnia.

Table 33-4	**Causes of Hypoxemia**
Cause	**Example**
Inadequate inspiration of oxygen	Airway obstruction with secretions, foreign objects, or tumors; high altitude
Hypoventilation	Impaired ventilation due to disease, injury, medications, or anesthesia
Impaired diffusion	Interstitial lung disease, pulmonary edema, destruction of lung tissue
Impaired perfusion and transport	Anemia, decreased cardiac output, hemorrhage, pulmonary emboli
Altered uptake of oxygen by the tissues	Fever, carbon monoxide poisoning, cyanide poisoning, blood transfusion

Focused Assessment for *Respiratory Failure*

Recognizing the client who should be closely observed to prevent respiratory arrest or respiratory failure requires synthesis of information about the client. Seldom does one factor suggest the need for close monitoring. The severity of the pathology, and the client's general condition, medical or surgical treatment (especially medications), and age must be considered together. However, even in an otherwise healthy person, a single factor may be sufficient. For example, a history of allergies may suggest the need to monitor for an anaphylactic reaction that could result in obstructive edema of the airway.

It is crucial that a nurse recognize impending respiratory failure and sudden respiratory arrest. Respiratory failure is a term used to indicate that the respiratory system is unable to exchange enough oxygen and carbon dioxide to sustain life. More technically speaking, *respiratory failure* is a PaO_2 of less than 60 mm Hg or a $PaCO_2$ of greater than 55 mm Hg. *Respiratory arrest* means the absence of spontaneous ventilation. It will result from mechanical obstruction of the airway or from respiratory failure. See Table 33-5 (p. 852) for guidelines for recognizing and managing airway obstruction. Prevention of respiratory failure is a priority in any client with hypoxemia, especially when the person's condition is deteriorating.

The client who cannot exchange air may have no respiratory movement or may have exaggerated chest wall movement with no discernible air movement felt at the nose or mouth. Establishing a patent airway can often start respiration. Lack of a patent airway from upper airway obstruction is a life-threatening emergency. Airway obstruction is defined as any significant interruption in airflow through the nose, mouth, pharynx, or larynx. A partial obstruction may be obvious, or the client may have vague symptoms. Unexplained or persistent symptoms warrant evaluation even if the symptoms are vague.

Respiratory failure is also an emergency, but it is more difficult to identify. Observe for signs of progressive deterioration in the client's condition to anticipate and prevent respiratory failure. Because signs of hypoxia are often subtle, an emergency can exist before they are detected. To prevent death, respiratory failure must be identified before it is complete.

Table 33-5 Recognition and Management of Airway Obstruction

Etiology	Recognition	Management
Loss of control of the tongue and cricopharyngeal muscles	Noisy, snoring inspiratory sound (partial obstruction) Marked inspiratory effort without ventilation; forceful contraction of the thorax and neck muscles (complete obstruction)	Place the client in a side-lying position with the neck extended. Insert an oral airway. If respiration is not established, initiate the emergency response system.
Retention of mucus	A wet, gurgling noise with respiration or with cough	Assist the client to cough, or suction the client.
Paralysis, edema, or other obstruction of the vocal cords, larynx, or epiglottis; foreign object	Stridor, inability to produce sound, hoarseness, restlessness, dyspnea, anxiety, respiratory effort without moving air	Call the physician for stat orders: high Fowler's position, oxygen, and vasoconstrictive or antiinflammatory drugs. Prepare for emergency endotracheal intubation or tracheostomy. The Heimlich maneuver may remove a large foreign object from the upper airway.
Aspiration of stomach contents	Evidence of vomitus in or around the mouth, odor of vomitus, dyspnea, cyanosis, respiratory distress, diminished breath sounds, coarse rales or bubbling rhonchi, crackles	Suction stat; call the physician by stat orders as above. Monitor closely.

The related factors are the same as the respiratory problems previously discussed. The *severity of the condition* and *fatigue* are predictive factors. The client who is severely ill and has been struggling to breathe for a prolonged time finally becomes exhausted with the work of breathing and is at risk for respiratory failure. Additionally, decreased ventilatory drive, edema, and laryngospasm are especially important.

In particular, consider a decreased ventilatory drive from narcotics, sedatives, anesthetics, and tranquilizers in the client who has multiple risk factors. The client with CAL is vulnerable to decreased ventilatory drive when oxygen is administered. The client who is heavily sedated (*obtunded*) may have relaxation of the muscles of the throat and neck that allow the tongue to drop into the back of the throat and obstruct the airway.

Edema is part of the inflammatory response and therefore can be caused by any condition that produces inflammation. *Laryngeal edema* can result from a burn, smoke inhalation, or an anaphylactic reaction to allergens. Even the client with tracheobronchitis should be observed for severe laryngeal edema. Additionally, any irritation to the larynx can cause *laryngospasm,* which tightens the throat and obstructs the airway.

DIAGNOSIS

The choice of diagnosis is based on a philosophy of early detection and prevention of health problems. For example, a postoperative client is at risk for hypostatic pneumonia. The diagnosis could be written as *Risk for ineffective breathing pattern: Hypoventilation* related to recovery from anesthesia, narcotic side effects, and immobility. If the client develops hypoventilation with no signs of retention of secretions, the diagnosis would be *Ineffective breathing pattern: Hypoventilation.* If secretions are present, the diagnosis is *Ineffective airway clearance,* and if signs of hypoxemia are present, the diagnosis is *Impaired gas exchange.* See the decision tree in Figure 33-6 for making a nursing diagnosis.

The nursing diagnosis is made with thought to the focus of care and interventions that are appropriate to the stage of the client's illness. For example, the client with COPD lives with a low oxygen level and a high carbon dioxide level. Oxygen therapy is used only in selected cases, particularly those in which oxygen can be expected to increase activity tolerance. In such cases, a diagnosis of *Impaired gas exchange* would be appropriate. However, the goals of treatment are more likely to be aimed at improving ventilation by altering the breathing pattern and clearing the airway.

Sometimes other nursing diagnoses may depict the goals of care more accurately than any of the three respiratory diagnoses. For the client with COPD living at home, the focus may be *Activity intolerance,* even though the underlying cause is chronic hypoxemia. For the nonemergent care of the asthmatic child, a diagnosis of *Risk for ineffective health maintenance* may be appropriate because the child is likely to ignore health activities. *Powerlessness* is appropriate for the child who feels helpless to control the asthma. Table 33-6 provides examples of how to cluster data to formulate an appropriate nursing diagnosis.

Related Diagnoses

Anxiety. Anxiety is an expected response to *Ineffective breathing pattern,* whether that pattern is hypoventilation, hyperventilation, or dyspnea. It is also commonly seen in clients with *Ineffective airway clearance,* especially when caused by asthma, anaphylactic shock, and other conditions of rapid onset. If the client's dyspnea, wheeze, or cough is severe, the level of anxiety can reach panic. Because anxiety can further increase the difficulty in breathing, you must assist the client to constructively manage both the respiratory symptoms and the anxiety.

Anxiety may be the underlying cause of hyperventilation rather than a response. This response is outside the parameters of a normal anxiety response and requires prompt intervention directed toward controlling anxiety (see Chapter 41).

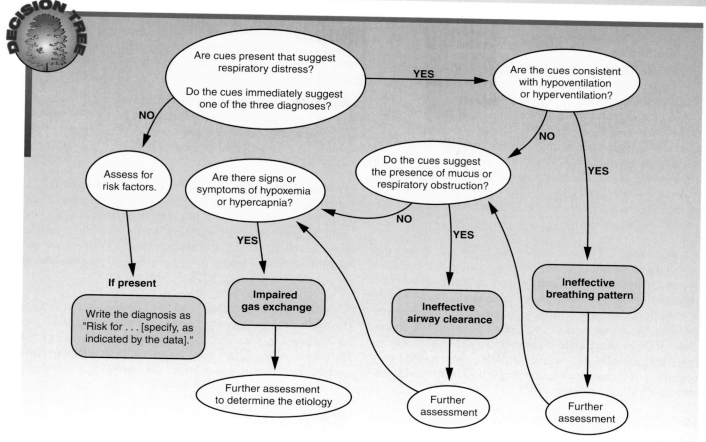

Figure 33-6. Decision tree for respiratory nursing diagnoses. Diagnoses are shown in rectangles. Within these rectangles, diagnoses shown in **bold** type are NANDA-approved nursing diagnoses; diagnoses shown in regular type are not NANDA-approved nursing diagnoses.

Table 33-6	*Clustering Data to Make a Nursing Diagnosis*

RESPIRATORY PROBLEMS

Data Cluster	Diagnosis
First postoperative day, respiratory rate 30, shallow, lungs clear, elevated BP and pulse, no spontaneous cough, taking narcotics q4h for pain	*Ineffective breathing pattern: hypoventilation* related to fatigue, use of narcotics, and residual effects of anesthesia
A 10-year-old asthmatic boy needs cromolyn sodium for exercise tolerance to play soccer, refuses medication, does not want to be different from peers. Has dropped out of the team after getting "benched" because of an asthma attack	*Ineffective health maintenance* related to self-esteem interfering with health care regimen
History of COPD, tachypnea, barrel chest, hypertrophy of accessory muscles; unable to prepare own meals because of dyspnea; refuses Meals on Wheels or residential care facility	*Activity intolerance* related to increased work of breathing
Admitted to hospital following a motor vehicle accident with three fractured ribs and multiple contusions; vomited and aspirated; oxygen saturation 85%	*Impaired gas exchange* related to inflammation in the lungs, decreased lung expansion
First postoperative day, midline abdominal incision, splinting chest, refuses to turn, coarse crackles throughout lung fields; temperature 38.8° C (102° F)	*Ineffective airway clearance* related to pain, inability to cough

Hopelessness. The client with chronic respiratory disease has no hope for recovery. The best that can be expected is to adapt and to live well with the disease. The ability to live with hope in the face of an incurable illness may be further diminished each time the client is admitted to the hospital for treatment of yet another exacerbation, complication, or episode (see Chapter 48).

Additionally, for the client with severe chronic respiratory disease, situational depression is not an unexpected response, and you must be alert to the possibility of depression in these clients. Living with chronic breathlessness and fatigue severe enough to interfere with activities of daily living prohibits the client from gainful employment, an active social life, and even the small pleasures of daily living. Complex, time-consuming daily routines for self-care use up the client's small amount of energy.

Disturbed Thought Processes. Chronic hypoxemia reduces the ability to concentrate and may even produce delusions and hallucinations. Although it has not been objectively demonstrated, the hallucinations and confusion that occur after open-heart surgery or other major surgery, particularly in older adults, may result from an undetected episode of hypoxemia. At the least, hypoxemia may be a contributing factor. These symptoms may be obvious to you and the client's family or may go undetected because the client is reluctant to describe abnormal thoughts and feelings (see Chapter 39).

Powerlessness. The sensation of not being able to breathe, especially if the client is too weak to describe the sensation, is the ultimate feeling of helplessness, of having no control over the body. Although an acute episode of *Ineffective breathing pattern* temporarily produces a situation of powerlessness, this feeling is not expected to last beyond the immediate situation. But for the client with chronic respiratory disease, the powerlessness evoked by the acute episode may continue and be compounded by the feelings generated by recurrent episodes (see Chapter 42).

Ineffective Health Maintenance. As a client recovers from any episode of illness, give extra attention to the need for health maintenance. The client with a single, isolated episode of respiratory disease that resolves without complications or residual effects does not necessarily need interventions to maintain health beyond the period of convalescence. For example, a healthy 30-year-old man who develops a postoperative fever from hypoventilation, is treated with antibiotics and respiratory therapy, and spends one extra day in the hospital probably has minimal need for interventions for *Ineffective health maintenance* on discharge. However, if the same man has frequent episodes of asthma, requiring constant adjustment of his lifestyle and medication regimen, he will need assistance to manage the problem of *Ineffective health maintenance* (see Chapter 19).

Imbalanced Nutrition. The client with a respiratory problem may need assistance with maintaining nutrition for a number of reasons. First, the physiological stress response to illness suppresses the appetite at a time when energy reserves are already depleted and proper nutrition is especially important. Second, the client with a respiratory problem may find it difficult to breathe while trying to eat. Finally, if the gastrointestinal tract has slowed, the resulting abdominal distention often produces a sensation of fullness that further suppresses the desire to eat.

Deficient Fluid Volume. The client with respiratory problems is at risk for dehydration (a deficit in body water) resulting from an increased insensible water loss from hyperventilation or the diaphoresis associated with an infection. Oxygen

therapy compounds the problem because oxygen is drying to the mucous membrane. Also, with an oxygen mask, taking fluids is as difficult as eating. Just when clients need more fluids, they are less likely to remember or to have the energy to obtain them (see Chapter 25).

 Mrs. Wilheim is started on an intravenous solution of D$_5$/1/4 NS at 100 mL per hour. Does this therapy meet her needs for fluid? How much fluid should she have in addition to the IV fluids? Would you anticipate having difficulty meeting her fluid needs?

Fatigue. Because the work of breathing is increased, fatigue often accompanies prolonged ineffective breathing patterns. The fatigue may also result from the illness that underlies the ineffective breathing pattern. Overwhelming, debilitating fatigue is a major finding in chronic respiratory disease. For the client with COPD fatigue is one of the major contributors to *Activity intolerance* (see Chapter 31).

Constipation. If gastrointestinal function has slowed and dehydration is present, constipation is a likely problem. The risk is increased in the client who does not have the energy for defecation. The exertion required can cause the client to postpone having a bowel movement, thus increasing the likelihood of *Constipation* (see Chapter 28).

PLANNING

The nursing diagnosis selected is an integral part of planning. For the client who has difficult or ineffective breathing, the goal is to improve the breathing. For the client who is unable to maintain clear airways, the goal is to establish clear airways. For the client who has hypoxemia or hypercapnia, the goal is to establish acceptable levels of oxygen and carbon dioxide in the blood.

Careful planning can improve the client's progress, thus reducing the cost of care. Box 33-8 will help you make this connection.

Expected Outcomes for the Client With *Ineffective Breathing Pattern*

The overall expected outcome for *Ineffective breathing pattern* is that the client resume normal respiratory rate, rhythm, and depth. Usually, a positive outcome can be inferred from an adequate rate and depth of respiration, an absence of diminished breath sounds, and a subjective experience of comfortable breathing. This outcome is easily achieved when the problem is related to an acute situation and the cause is eliminated in the natural course of recovery. For example, if the cause is anesthesia, then as the client recovers, the breathing patterns return to normal. The nursing care involves monitoring and supporting the client's physiological processes. If the cause is bed rest, ambulation will reestablish a normal breathing pattern.

When the problem has a longer duration, intermediate outcomes are used to show progress toward the goal. In some cases, an improved tidal volume or vital capacity measured with bedside spirometry is an intermediate outcome.

In 1994 the cost of treating community-acquired pneumonia was estimated at 10 billion dollars (Anonymous, 1999). Most of this cost is directly related to length of hospital stay. McCormick, Fine, and Coley (1999) attempted to answer the question, "Are shorter lengths of stay associated with worse medical outcomes?" In 1188 adults with community-acquired pneumonia, they found the length of stay varied from 7.8 to 9.8 days, but they found no appreciable difference in medical outcomes.

Nurses play a role in the strategies for decreasing the cost of treating community-acquired pneumonia. Three strategies are identifying low-risk clients who can safely be treated as outpatients, decreasing hospital length of stay, and reducing the use of the emergency department as the entry into the health care system.

Hospital nurses affect the length of stay in the following ways:
- Assessing physical, psychological, and environmental risk factors
- Providing the most effective administration of antibiotics
- Early planning and discharge teaching
- Early detection and prevention of complications
- Moving the client toward self-care through promoting physiological and psychological readiness
- Treating the whole person to promote health behaviors (e.g., nutrition, activity and rest, fluid balance)

For the goal of increasing ventilation by stimulation or by opening airways, the outcome is an observation of increased depth of respiration and auscultation of increased breath sounds. Measuring depth is a subjective judgment, and it depends on your having observed the respiration or auscultated the lungs before the intervention.

Improving the efficiency of respiration and managing energy requirements are long-term goals that may result in an improved quality of life for the client with chronic disease. The measures are usually a subjective report from the client that dyspnea has decreased and activity tolerance has improved. Quality of life is measurable only through the subjective report of the client.

If the problem is a direct result of an acute illness, such as hypoventilation in the postoperative client during the first 24 hours after surgery, the outcome of normal respiration by discharge from the hospital is usually sufficient. However, if the problem can be expected to return—that is, if the client is at continued risk or the problem is the result of a chronic illness—the outcomes need to include evidence that the person is prepared to manage the risk.

The client with a respiratory infection should be evaluated for risk for recurrence. The outcomes may include the following:
- Demonstrates understanding of benefits of flu and pneumonia vaccines
- States that she will contact an appropriate agency for assistance in weatherproofing home
- Has made an appointment with Meals on Wheels
- States daughter will provide transportation to doctor's appointment next Thursday

Expected Outcomes for the Client With *Ineffective Airway Clearance*

The expected outcome for *Ineffective airway clearance* is that the client demonstrate no evidence of airway obstruction or secretion retention as indicated by normal breath sounds. Wheezing, crackles, or rhonchi have disappeared.

A short-term outcome is that the client coughs out sputum without fatigue and vital signs return to normal in 10 minutes. A long-term plan would include the outcome that the client demonstrates regular use of a regimen for maintaining airway clearance.

Expected Outcomes for the Client With *Impaired Gas Exchange*

The expected outcome for *Impaired gas exchange* is that the client have normal arterial blood gases or show no evidence of hypoxia or hypercapnia on room air, or both. An intermediate outcome would be that while on oxygen therapy, the client has an oxygen saturation of greater than 95% by pulse oximetry.

Expected Outcomes for the Client With Respiratory Failure

The expected nursing outcome for respiratory failure is that the client be able to breathe unassisted by an artificial airway or ventilatory support. The short-term outcomes include that the client has a patent airway and breath sounds throughout the lung fields. Normal blood gases would be included in the criteria for adequate ventilatory support.

INTERVENTION

The choice of interventions for the respiratory client is derived through a team approach that includes the physician, respiratory therapist, nurse, and dietitian. Many of the interventions that provide definitive therapy are within the medical treatment plan. Respiratory therapy includes a broad range of respiratory interventions, and in many institutions the respiratory therapist provides many of these interventions. Today's respiratory care practitioners graduate from American Medical Association–accredited programs. They are either certified respiratory therapy technicians or registered respiratory therapists. A person with the registered respiratory therapist credential has passed an advanced national registry test and is the most qualified individual to practice respiratory therapy. Respiratory therapists also provide home care for persons with chronic illness. The active role of the respiratory therapist in the hospital or home setting, however, does not relieve you of responsibility for the client's respiratory needs.

Interventions to Change the Breathing Pattern
Intervention when the client has an ineffective breathing pattern is based on the related or etiological factor. There are also general goals that can be applied to the care of any person with an ineffective breathing pattern.

Positioning for Maximum Respiratory Function. Positioning implies both the position and the frequency of position changes. Maximal chest expansion is possible and the ventilation/perfusion ratio is optimal in the upright unsupported position. Lying down limits lung expansion in the dependent portion (subordinate part) of the lung, but, at the same time, it helps increase ventilation in the nondependent portion of the lung. Perfusion is greatest in the dependent lung. Turning and repositioning redistributes pulmonary blood and airflow, thus compensating for the recumbent position to maintain function throughout the lungs.

The client should be positioned for maximum ventilatory function. Because it is natural to shift positions on the basis of respiratory need, a client who is having difficulty breathing should be allowed to assume the most comfortable position. On the other hand, a weak or debilitated client may not be able to self-reposition. When the client is having difficulty breathing, the first thing to do is raise the head of the bed. Positioning is particularly important in clients with obesity, abdominal distention, or ascites. Elevating the head of the bed for these clients will allow gravity to eliminate the impediment of the abdominal organs on the lungs (Burns, Egolff, Ryan, Carpenter, & Burns, 1994).

A second factor to consider in positioning the client is stagnation of secretions. Drainage of secretions is improved by positioning to allow drainage of all the lobes of the lung over time. For most clients, this is accomplished by turning every 2 hours. Others may need postural drainage (discussed under Chest Physiotherapy, later). Box 33-9 lists possible benefits to be gained from positioning.

In positioning the client, the client's ability to tolerate changing position and different positions should be considered. The best positioning regimen for respiratory function should be determined for each client individually and evaluated on the basis of data indicating respiratory function. The person who is positioned to increase drainage and expectoration may tire from the coughing induced by the drainage of mucus and may need to be repositioned. The person who seeks the position of maximal comfort for pain relief may need to be encouraged to periodically change positions to increase drainage and improve ventilation. For the critically ill

client, vital signs may help assess the person's ability to tolerate the repositioning (Yeaw, 1992).

 Again consider the case of Mrs. Wilheim. As soon as she arrives on the unit, the nurse elevates Mrs. Wilheim's head 30 degrees. Mrs. Wilheim thanks the nurse, saying that she is more comfortable with her head elevated and is grateful for the nurse's help. You notice that her skin is thin and fragile. How will you plan for preventing skin breakdown?

Stimulating Respiration. Stimulating respiration means increasing the client's rate and depth of breathing to meet the needs of respiratory function. It opens alveoli and distributes the airflow throughout the lungs.

AMBULATION. Ambulation is an effective, noninvasive, and inexpensive method of stimulating respiration. While walking, the client is in the optimal physiological position to breathe. Additionally, respiration is stimulated by the client's increased metabolic need (Guyton & Hall, 1996). Be careful to confine ambulation to the limits of the client's tolerance (see Chapter 31).

INCENTIVE SPIROMETRY. An **incentive spirometer** is a device that provides a visual goal for and measurement of inspiration, thus encouraging the client to execute and sustain maximal inspiration. Achieving and sustaining a maximal inspiration opens airways, reduces atelectasis, and stimulates coughing. The client benefits from active participation in recovery by developing a feeling of control over the recovery process.

For any of the available incentive spirometers, the goal is to achieve and maintain a maximal inspiration. Correct use requires a slow, voluntary, deep breath. When full or maximal inhalation is reached, the breath is held for at least 3 seconds. This sequence is repeated up to 20 times per hour; the client is usually started with five repetitions per session. Incentive exercises are most effective when used every hour while the person is awake. Each device has a means of setting an inspiratory goal derived from a formula based on height, weight, and sex. Lights, balls rising in a column, or other indicators of success provide visual reinforcement. While the client will initially need instruction and supervision, most people learn the skill quickly. However, occasionally watch the client performing incentive spirometry to ensure continued correct use.

Incentive spirometer therapy is often used postoperatively or when physical mobility is limited. It is most effectively used when people are alert, cooperative, coordinated, and motivated, and when they have sufficient strength to generate an inspiratory flow rate that will produce a deep breath and activate the indicator on the incentive device. Repetitions of the deep breaths must be slow to avoid overbreathing, which will lead to dizziness and tremors as a result of sudden hypocapnia. Box 33-10 provides guidelines for teaching the client to use an incentive spirometer.

MEDICATIONS. Naloxone (Narcan) is used to stimulate respirations in the client whose respirations have been severely depressed by narcotics. The physician's guideline for administering naloxone is usually to administer as necessary

---

Box 33-9	Possible Respiratory Benefits To Be Gained From Positioning

- The cough reflex may be activated by positioning the client on the right side to encourage sputum to come in contact with the cough control center in the right bronchi at the carina.
- Positioning on a painful affected side may help reduce the pain.
- Positioning with the good lung up may increase ventilatory compensation for pathology.
- Positioning on the unaffected side allows drainage of the area of pathology.
- The Sims' position, with the jaw falling forward, is useful for maintaining a patent airway.
- Frequent repositioning will help accomplish multiple purposes.